Critical Care Compendium

Critical Care Compendium

1001 Topics in Intensive Care & Acute Medicine

J. F. Cade

Emeritus Consultant in Intensive Care, Royal Melbourne Hospital; Professorial Fellow,
Department of Medicine, University of Melbourne

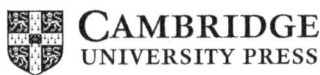

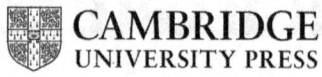

Shaftesbury Road, Cambridge CB2 8EA, United Kingdom

One Liberty Plaza, 20th Floor, New York, NY 10006, USA

477 Williamstown Road, Port Melbourne, VIC 3207, Australia

314–321, 3rd Floor, Plot 3, Splendor Forum, Jasola District Centre, New Delhi – 110025, India

103 Penang Road, #05–06/07, Visioncrest Commercial, Singapore 238467

Cambridge University Press is part of Cambridge University Press & Assessment, a department of the University of Cambridge.

We share the University's mission to contribute to society through the pursuit of education, learning and research at the highest international levels of excellence.

www.cambridge.org
Information on this title: www.cambridge.org/9781009237420

DOI: 10.1017/9781009237451

© J. F. Cade 2023

This publication is in copyright. Subject to statutory exception and to the provisions of relevant collective licensing agreements, no reproduction of any part may take place without the written permission of Cambridge University Press & Assessment.

previously published 9780521189415 - *Acute Medicine - Uncommon Problems and Challenges 2011*
This edition published 2023

A catalogue record for this publication is available from the British Library.

Library of Congress Cataloging-in-Publication Data

ISBN 978-1-009-23742-0 Paperback

....

Cambridge University Press & Assessment has no responsibility for the persistence or accuracy of URLs for external or third-party internet websites referred to in this publication and does not guarantee that any content on such websites is, or will remain, accurate or appropriate.

Every effort has been made in preparing this book to provide accurate and up-to-date information that is in accord with accepted standards and practice at the time of publication. Although case histories are drawn from actual cases, every effort has been made to disguise the identities of the individuals involved. Nevertheless, the authors, editors, and publishers can make no warranties that the information contained herein is totally free from error, not least because clinical standards are constantly changing through research and regulation. The authors, editors, and publishers therefore disclaim all liability for direct or consequential damages resulting from the use of material contained in this book. Readers are strongly advised to pay careful attention to information provided by the manufacturer of any drugs or equipment that they plan to use.

To my family

Contents

Preface page xix

A Abciximab 1
Abdominal compartment syndrome 1
Abortion 1
Abruptio placentae (placental abruption) 1
Acanthosis nigricans 1
ACE 1
Acetazolamide 1
Acetylsalicylic acid 1
Achlorhydria 1
Acidosis, lactic 1
Acidosis, renal tubular 1
Acquired immunodeficiency syndrome 1
Acromegaly 3
ACTH 4
Actinomycete infections 4
Actinomycosis 4
Acute brain syndrome 5
Acute fatty liver of pregnancy 5
Acute flaccid myelitis 5
Acute lung irritation 5
Acute pulmonary oedema 6
Acute respiratory distress syndrome 7
Acyclovir 7
Addison's disease 8
Adenosine 8
Adrenal insufficiency 9
Adrenocorticotropic hormone 12
Adult respiratory distress syndrome 12
Agammaglobulinaemia 12
Agranulocytosis 13
AIDS 13
Air embolism 13
Alcohol, methyl 13
Aldosterone 13
Alkaloids 13
Allergic bronchopulmonary aspergillosis 13
Allergic granulomatosis and angiitis 13
Alopecia 14
Alpha-fetoprotein 14
Alpha$_1$-antitrypsin deficiency 15
Altitude 16
Aluminium 16

Alveolar hypoventilation 17
Alzheimer's disease 17
Amanita 17
Amenorrhoea 17
Aminoaciduria 17
Aminocaproic acid 17
Ammonia 17
Amnesia 17
Amniotic fluid embolism 18
Amoebiasis 19
Amphetamines 19
Amyloid 21
Amyotrophic lateral sclerosis 21
Anaemia 21
Anaphylaxis 25
ANCA 25
Aneurysms, mycotic 25
Angiodysplasia 25
Angioedema 25
Angiotensin 27
Angiotensin-converting enzyme 27
Animal bites 28
Anion gap 28
Ankylosing spondylitis 28
Anorectal infections 29
Anorectic agents 29
Anorexia nervosa 29
Anthrax 30
Antibiotic-associated colitis 31
Anticardiolipin antibody 31
Anticholinergic agents 31
Anticholinesterases 32
Anticoagulants 33
Antidiuretic hormone 36
Antinuclear antibodies 36
Antiphospholipid syndrome 36
Antiplatelet agents 39
Antiprotease 40
Antithrombin 40
Aortic coarctation 41
Aortic dissection 42
Aortitis 43

vii

Contents

Aplastic anaemia 43
Arachnids 43
ARDS 43
Argatroban 43
Arnold–Chiari malformation 43
Arsenic 43
Arteriovenous malformations 45
Arteritis 46
Arthritis 47
Arthropathies 48
Arthropods 48
Arthus reaction 48
Asbestos 48
Aspergillosis 50
Aspiration 51
Aspirin 52
Asplenia 53
Asthma 53
Asthmatic pulmonary eosinophilia 55
Atrial natriuretic factor 55
Autacoids 56
Auto-erythrocyte purpura 56
Autoimmune disorders 56
Autoinflammatory disease 58
Autonomic dysreflexia 58
Avian influenza 58

B Bacillary angiomatosis 58
Bacillary peliosis hepatis 58
Bacitracin 58
Baclofen 59
BAL 59
Barotrauma 59
Basophilia 60
Bat bites 60
Bathing 60
Bed rest 60
Bee stings 61
Behcet's syndrome 61
Bell's palsy 61
Bence Jones protein 62
Benign intracranial hypertension 62
Beriberi 62
Beryllium 63
Beta$_2$-microglobulin 63
Bicarbonate therapy 64
Biliary cirrhosis 64
Biomarkers 64
Bioterrorism 65
Bird fancier's lung 65
Bird flu 65
Bismuth 65

Bites and stings 66
Bivalirudin 71
Black cohosh 71
Bleeding 71
Bleomycin 71
'Blind as a bat …' 72
Blisters 72
Boerhaave's syndrome 72
Bone failure 72
Bornholm disease 72
Botulism 72
Bovine spongiform encephalopathy 73
Bradykinin 73
Brodifacoum 73
Bromhidrosis 73
Bromocriptine 73
Bronchiectasis 73
Bronchiolitis obliterans 74
Bronchocentric granulomatosis 75
Broncholithiasis 75
Bronchopleural fistula 75
Brucellosis 75
Brugada syndrome 75
Budd–Chiari syndrome 76
Bullae 77
Burns, respiratory complications 77
Buruli ulcer 77
Byssinosis 77

C **Cadmium** 77
Caeruloplasmin 77
Calciphylaxis 77
Calcitonin 78
Calcium 79
Calcium disodium edetate 79
Cancer 79
Cancer complications 80
Carbon monoxide 81
Carbon tetrachloride 83
Carbonic anhydrase inhibitors 83
Carboxyhaemoglobin 84
Carcinoembryonic antigen 84
Carcinoid syndrome 84
Cardiac tumours 86
Cardiomyopathies 87
Cardiopulmonary bypass 89
Cardiorenal syndrome(s) 89
Cardiovascular disorders 90
CAR T-cell therapy 91
Cat bites 92
Cat-scratch disease 92
Cathinones 93

Contents

Cavitation 93
Cellulitis 94
Central pontine myelinolysis 94
Cerebellar degeneration 95
Cerebral arterial gas embolism 95
Cerebral arteritis 95
Cerebral salt wasting 95
Charcot–Marie–Tooth disease 96
Chelating agents 96
Chemical exposures 98
Chemical poisoning 98
Chest wall disorders 99
Chest X-ray 99
Cheyne–Stokes respiration 100
Chikungunya 100
Chlorine 100
Cholangitis 100
Cholera 101
Cholestasis 102
Cholinergic agonists 102
Cholinergic crisis 103
Cholinolytic agents 103
Christmas disease 103
Chromium 103
Chronic fatigue syndrome 103
Churg–Strauss syndrome 104
Chylothorax 104
Ciguatera 104
CINMA 105
Circadian rhythm 105
Climate change 105
Clopidogrel 106
Clostridial infections 106
Clostridium difficile 107
Coagulation disorders 108
Coagulation factors 110
Cobalt 110
Cocaine 111
Coeliac disease 112
Colchicine 113
Cold 114
Cold agglutinin disease 114
Colitis 114
Collagen-vascular diseases 115
Complement deficiency 115
Conjunctivitis 116
Connective tissue diseases 117
Conn's syndrome 117
Constipation 118
Copper 118
Coronavirus 119
Costochondritis 119
Coturnism 119
Cough 119
COVID-19 120
C-reactive protein 120
CREST syndrome 121
Creutzfeldt–Jakob disease 121
Cricoarytenoid arthritis 122
Critical illness myopathy 122
Critical illness neuromuscular abnormality 123
Critical illness polyneuropathy 123
Crohn's disease 123
Crustaceans 123
Cryoglobulinaemia 123
Cryptococcosis 123
Cushing's syndrome 124
Cyanide 125
Cystic fibrosis 126
Cytomegalovirus 128

D   Dantrolene 129
Decompression sickness 129
Defibrotide 129
Delirium 129
Dementia 131
Demyelinating diseases 132
Dengue 134
Dermatitis 135
Dermatology 135
Dermatomyositis 137
Desferrioxamine 137
Desmopressin 137
Dextrocardia 137
Diabetes insipidus 137
Diaphragm 138
Diarrhoea 138
DIC 140
Differentiation syndrome 140
Diffuse alveolar haemorrhage 140
Diffuse fibrosing alveolitis 141
Diffuse parenchymal lung diseases 141
Digoxin-specific antibody 141
Dimercaprol 142
Dioxins 142
Diphtheria 142
Dipyridamole 143
Dissecting aneurysm 143
Disseminated intravascular coagulation 143
Disulfiram 144
Diving 144
Dog bites 145
Drowning 145
Drug allergy 147

Contents

Drug–drug interactions 148
Drug fever 149
Drugs 149
Drugs and the kidney 151
Drugs and the lung 152
Dysentery 154
Dysphagia 154
Dysproteinaemias 154

E Eating disorders 154
Eaton Lambert syndrome 154
Ebola haemorrhagic fever 154
Echinacea 155
Echinococcosis 155
Ecstasy 156
Ecthyma 156
Ectopic hormone production 156
Eculizumab 157
EDTA 157
Eisenmenger syndrome 157
Embolism, air 157
Emphysema 157
Empyema 157
Encephalitis 157
Encephalomyelitis 158
Encephalopathy 158
Endarteritis 159
Endocarditis 159
Endocrinology 162
Energy expenditure 164
Enterocolitis 164
Enteropathogenic E. coli 164
Enteropathy 165
Envenomation 165
Environment 165
Eosinopenia 165
Eosinophilia 165
Eosinophilia and lung infiltration 166
Eosinophilic fasciitis 167
Eosinophilic granuloma 167
Eosinophilic pneumonia 167
Epidermolysis bullosa 168
Epididymitis 168
Epidural abscess 168
Epstein–Barr virus 169
Eptifibatide 169
Equine morbilliform virus 169
Ergot 169
Ergotamine 170
Erysipelas 170
Erythema marginatum 170
Erythema migrans 170

Erythema multiforme 170
Erythema nodosum 171
Erythrocytosis 171
Erythromelalgia 171
Erythropoietin 171
Ethylene glycol 172
Euthyroid sick syndrome 173
Exfoliative dermatitis 174
Exophthalmos 175
Exotic pneumonia 175
Extrinsic allergic alveolitis 175

F Fabry's disease 175
Factitious disorders 176
Factor V 176
Factor VIII 176
Faecal calprotectin 176
Faecal lactoferrin 177
Faecal transplantation 177
Familial hypocalciuric hypercalcaemia 177
Familial Mediterranean fever 177
Fanconi's syndrome 178
Farmer's lung 178
Fasciitis 178
Favism 178
Feeding intolerance 178
Felty's syndrome 178
Ferritin 179
Fetal haemoglobin 179
Fetomaternal haemorrhage 179
Fever 179
Fever of unknown origin 179
Fibrinolysis 179
Fish envenomation 181
Fleas 181
Flushing 181
FODMAPs 181
Folic acid deficiency 182
Folliculitis 182
Food poisoning 182
Formaldehyde 183
Fournier's gangrene 183
Frailty 183
Friedreich's ataxia 183
Frostbite 183
Furunculosis 184

G Gamma-hydroxybutyric acid 184
Ganciclovir 184
Gangrene 184
Gas gangrene 186
Gas in soft tissues 186

Contents

Gastric emptying 187
Gastrinoma 187
Gastroenteritis 187
Gastroenterology 187
Gastrointestinal tumours 189
Gastroparesis 189
Gaucher's disease 189
Genomics 189
Germ warfare 189
Ghrelin 189
Giant cell arteritis 190
Gingivitis 190
Glomerular diseases 190
Glossitis 191
Glucagonoma 191
Glucose-6-phosphate dehydrogenase deficiency 191
Glycocalyx 192
Glycogen storage diseases 192
Goodpasture's syndrome 193
Gout 193
Graft-versus-host disease 196
Granulomatosis with polyangiitis 196
Graves' disease 196
Growth hormone 196
Guillain–Barré syndrome 196

H   **Haemangioma** 198
Haematology 198
Haematuria 200
Haemochromatosis 201
Haemodilution 203
Haemoglobin disorders 203
Haemoglobinopathy 205
Haemoglobinuria 205
Haemolacria 205
Haemolysis 205
Haemolytic–uraemic syndromes 205
Haemophagocytic lymphohistiocytosis (HLH) 207
Haemophagocytic syndrome 207
Haemophilia 208
Haemoptysis 209
Haemostasis 210
Hamman–Rich syndrome 211
Hand–Schuller–Christian disease 211
Hantavirus 211
Heat 211
Heat cramps 212
Heat exhaustion/stress 212
Heat rash 212
Heat shock proteins 212
Heat stroke 213

Heavy chains 214
Heavy metal poisoning 214
HELLP syndrome 214
Helminths 215
Hemianopia 215
Hendra virus 215
Henoch–Schonlein purpura 216
Heparin(s) 216
Heparin-induced thrombocytopenia 217
Hepatic diseases 219
Hepatic necrosis 221
Hepatic vein thrombosis 221
Hepatitis 221
Hepatocellular carcinoma 226
Hepatoma 227
Hepatopulmonary syndrome 227
Hepatorenal syndrome 228
Hepcidin 228
Herbicides 228
Hereditary haemorrhagic telangiectasia 228
Herpesviruses 228
High altitude 228
Hirsutism 230
Hirudin(s) 231
Histiocytosis 231
Histocompatibility complex 232
Histoplasmosis 233
HIV 233
Horner's syndrome 233
Hot flushes 233
Hot tubs 233
Human bites 233
Human immunodeficiency virus 233
Hydatid disease 233
Hydrocephalus 234
Hydrogen sulphide 234
Hyperammonaemia 234
Hyperbaric oxygen 235
Hypercalcaemia 235
Hyperdynamic state 237
Hypereosinophilic syndrome 237
Hyperhidrosis 237
Hyperhomocystinaemia 237
Hyperparathyroidism 237
Hyperphosphataemia 239
Hypersensitivity pneumonitis 239
Hypersplenism 241
Hyperthermia 241
Hyperthyroidism 241
Hypertrichosis 243
Hyperuricaemia 243
Hyperviscosity 243

xi

Contents

Hypocalcaemia 243
Hypoglycaemia 244
Hypokalaemia 245
Hyponatraemia 245
Hypoparathyroidism 246
Hypophosphataemia 246
Hyposplenism 247
Hypothalamic–pituitary–adrenal axis 247
Hypothermia 247
Hypothyroidism 250

I **ICU-acquired weakness** 251
Idiopathic inflammatory myopathy (IIM) 252
Idiopathic interstitial pneumonias 252
Idiopathic pulmonary fibrosis 252
Idiopathic pulmonary haemosiderosis 254
Idiopathic thrombocytopenic purpura 254
Immotile cilia syndrome 254
Immune complex disease 254
Immune thrombocytopenic purpura 255
Immunodeficiency 257
Immunology 257
Immunomodulation 259
Immunothrombosis 259
Inborn errors of metabolism 259
Infections 260
Inflammatory bowel disease 263
Inflammatory myeloid neoplasia 266
Influenza 266
Inhalation injury 268
Insect bites and stings 269
Insecticides 270
Insects 270
Insulinoma 270
Intensive Care Unit–acquired weakness 270
Interstitial lung diseases 270
Interstitial nephritis 271
Interstitial pneumonia 271
Intra-abdominal hypertension 272
Iron 273
Iron deficiency 273
Iron overload disease 274
Irritable bowel syndrome 274
Irukandji syndrome 274
Islet cell tumour 274
Isolation 275
ITP 275

J Japanese encephalitis 275
Jarisch–Herxheimer reaction 275
Jellyfish envenomation 275

K Kaposi's sarcoma 275
Kartagener's syndrome 275
Katayama fever 276
Kawasaki disease 276
Kennedy's disease 276
Khat 276
Korsakoff syndrome 276
Kyphoscoliosis 276

L **Lactase deficiency** 277
Lactic acidosis 277
Langerhans cell histiocytosis 279
Lassa fever 279
Lateral medullary syndrome 280
Latex allergy 280
Lead 280
Leflunomide 281
Lemierre's syndrome 281
Leprosy 281
Leptin 282
Leptospirosis 282
Leukocytoclastic vasculitis 282
Leukoencephalopathy 282
Lewisite 283
Lice 283
Lichenoid skin reaction 283
Light chains 283
Lightning 283
Lipoid pneumonia 283
Liquorice 284
Listeriosis 284
Lithium 285
Livedo reticularis 286
Liver abscess 287
Loeffler's syndrome 287
Ludwig's angina 287
Lung tumours 287
Lupus anticoagulant 288
Lyme disease 288
Lymphadenopathy 289
Lymphangioleiomyomatosis 289
Lymphocytosis 290
Lymphomatoid granulomatosis 290
Lymphopenia 291
Lyssavirus 291

M Macrophage activation syndrome (MAS) 291
'Mad Hatter' syndrome 291
Magnesium 291
Malabsorption 293
Malaria 294
Malignant hyperthermia 296

Contents

Mallory–Weiss syndrome 297
Manganese 297
Marfan's syndrome 297
Marine vertebrate and invertebrate stings 298
Mast cells 298
Mastocytosis 298
May–Thurner syndrome 298
Mediastinal diseases 298
Mediastinitis 299
Mediterranean fever 300
Medullary sponge kidney 300
Medullary thyroid cancer 300
Megaloblastic anaemia 300
Melatonin 300
Meleney's progressive synergistic gangrene 302
Melioidosis 302
Mendelson's syndrome 302
Meningococcaemia 302
Meningoencephalitis 302
Mercury 302
MERS 303
Mesothelioma 303
Metabolic acidosis 303
Metabolism and nutrition 303
Metastatic calcification 305
Methaemoglobinaemia 305
Methanol 306
Methylene blue 307
Methysergide 308
Microangiopathic haemolysis 308
Microbiome 308
Microcirculation 310
Microscopic polyangiitis 310
Microvascular dysfunction 310
Middle East respiratory syndrome 310
Mifepristone 310
Miller Fisher syndrome 311
Mites 311
Mitochondrial diseases 311
Mixed connective tissue disease 312
Monkey bites 312
Monosodium glutamate 312
Mosquitoes 312
Motor neuron disease 313
Mouth diseases 314
Multidisciplinary topics 315
Multifocal motor neuropathy 316
Multiorgan failure 316
Multiple endocrine neoplasia 317
Multiple myeloma 318
Multiple organ dysfunction/failure 321
Multiple sclerosis 321
Multiple system atrophy 323
Multisystem inflammatory syndrome in children 323
Munchausen syndrome 323
Murray Valley encephalitis 323
Muscular dystrophies 323
Mushroom poisoning 324
Mustards 325
Myalgic encephalomyelitis 325
Myasthenia gravis 325
Mycetism 327
Mycetoma 327
Mycobacterium ulcerans 327
Mycoplasma hominis 327
Mycoplasma pneumoniae 327
Mycotic aneurysms 327
Myelitis 328
Myelopathy 328
Myoglobinuria 328
Myopathy 328
Myositis 329
Myotonia 330
Myxoedema 330
Myxoma 330

N **Nails** 330
Necrolytic migratory erythema 331
Necrotizing cutaneous mucormycosis 331
Necrotizing fasciitis 331
Necrotizing granulomatous vasculitis 331
Necrotizing pneumonia 331
Necrotizing soft-tissue infection 331
Nephrogenic fibrosing dermopathy 331
Nephrogenic systemic fibrosis 331
Nephrolithiasis 331
Nephrology 332
Nephrotic syndrome 333
Neural tube defects 333
Neurofibromatosis 334
Neuroleptic malignant syndrome 334
Neurology 335
Neuromyelitis optica 337
Neuropathy 337
Neutropenia 340
Neutrophilia 342
Newcastle disease 342
Nitric oxide 342
Nitrous oxide 342
Nocardiosis 342
Non-alcoholic fatty liver disease 343
Non-alcoholic steatohepatitis 343
Non-respiratory thoracic disorders 344

Contents

Norovirus 344
Norwalk virus 344
Nutrition 344

O **Obstetrics and gynaecology** 344
Occupational lung diseases 345
Octreotide 347
Olmesartan 348
Oncofetal antigen 348
Ophthalmoplegia 348
Optic neuritis 348
Oral contraceptives 348
Orchitis 348
Organophosphates 348
Orthodeoxia 348
Osler–Weber–Rendu disease 349
Osmotic demyelination syndrome 349
Osteomalacia 349
Ovarian hyperstimulation syndrome 349
Oxytocin 349

P **PADIS** 349
Paget's disease 350
Palmar erythema 351
Pancreatic stone protein 351
Pancreatitis 351
Pancytopenia 352
Pandemics 352
Papilloedema 353
Paraganglioma 353
Paragonimiasis 353
Parahaemophilia 353
Paralytic shellfish poisoning 353
Paraneoplastic syndromes 354
Paraquat 355
Parasitic infections 356
Parathyromatosis 356
Parotitis 356
Paroxysmal nocturnal haemoglobinuria 357
Pectus excavatum 357
Pediculosis 357
Pelvic inflammatory disease 357
Pemphigus 358
Penicillamine 358
Pericarditis 358
Periodic breathing 359
Periodic fever 359
Periodic paralysis 359
Pernicious anaemia 359
Peroneal muscular atrophy 359
Persistent critical illness 359
Pesticides 360

Petechiae 360
Peutz–Jeghers syndrome 360
Phaeochromocytoma 360
Phosgene 361
Phrenic nerve 361
Phthiriasis 361
Physical exposures 361
Pigmentation disorders 361
Pink urine 362
Pituitary 362
Pituitary apoplexy 364
Placental abruption (abruptio placentae) 364
Plague 364
PLAID syndrome 365
Plasmacytoma 365
Plasmapheresis 365
Plasminogen 365
Platelet function disorders 366
Platelets 367
Platypnoea–orthodeoxia syndrome 368
Pleiotropic effects 368
Pleural disorders 368
Pleural effusion 369
Pleurisy 371
Plumbism 371
Plummer–Vinson syndrome 371
Pneumatosis coli 371
Pneumoconiosis 371
Pneumomediastinum 371
Pneumonia, exotic 371
Pneumonia in pregnancy 371
Pneumothorax 372
Poisoning 373
Poliomyelitis 374
Polyarteritis nodosa 375
Polycystic kidney disease 376
Polycystic ovary syndrome 376
Polycythaemia 376
Polymyalgia rheumatica 377
Polymyositis/dermatomyositis 378
Polyneuritis 379
Polyneuropathy 379
Porphyria 379
Portopulmonary hypertension 381
Posterior reversible encephalopathy 381
Post–Intensive Care syndrome 381
Post-transfusion purpura 382
Pre-eclampsia 382
Pregnancy 384
PRES 388
Priapism 388
Primary alveolar hypoventilation 388

Contents

Primary ciliary dyskinesia 388
Probiotics 389
Procalcitonin 389
Proctitis 389
Progressive multifocal leukoencephalopathy 389
Propofol 389
Prostacyclin 390
Protein C 390
Protein S 392
Protein Z 392
Proteinuria 393
Prothrombin G20210A abnormality 394
Prothrombin complex concentrate 394
Protozoa 394
Pruritus 394
Prussian blue 395
Prussic acid 395
Pseudogout 395
Pseudohyperkalaemia 395
Pseudohyponatraemia 395
Pseudohypoparathyroidism 396
Pseudolymphoma 396
Pseudomembranous colitis 396
Pseudomyxoma peritonei 396
Pseudo-obstruction of the colon 396
Pseudoporphyria 396
Pseudo primary aldosteronism 396
Psittacosis 396
Psoriasis 397
Psychiatric issues 398
Ptosis 398
Pulmonary alveolar proteinosis 399
Pulmonary hypertension 399
Pulmonary infiltrates 404
Pulmonary infiltration with eosinophilia (PIE) 404
Pulmonary Langerhans cell histiocytosis 404
Pulmonary nodules 404
Pulmonary oedema 405
Pulmonary veno-occlusive disease 405
Purpura 406
Pyoderma gangrenosum 406
Pyrexia 407
Pyroglutamic acid 412

Q Q fever 412
Quarantine 412

R **Rabies** 412
Radiation injury 413
Ramsay Hunt syndrome 414
Rat bites 414
Raynaud's phenomenon/disease 414

Reactive arthritis 414
Refeeding syndrome 414
Reiter's syndrome 415
Relapsing fever 415
Renal artery occlusion 416
Renal calculous disease 417
Renal cortical necrosis 417
Renal cystic disease 417
Renal tubular acidosis 418
Renal vein thrombosis 419
Renin–angiotensin–aldosterone 419
Respiratory burns 421
Respiratory diseases 421
Restless legs syndrome 423
Reticulocytes 423
Retinal haemorrhage 424
Retrobulbar neuritis 424
Retroperitoneal fibrosis 424
Reversible posterior leukoencephalopathy 424
Reye's syndrome 424
Rhabdomyolysis 425
Rheumatology 426
Rickettsial diseases 427
Rituximab 428
Ross River virus disease 429

S Salicylism 429
Salpingitis 429
Sarcoidosis 430
SARS 433
Scalded skin syndrome 433
Scarlet fever 433
Schistosomiasis 433
Schonlein–Henoch purpura 434
Scleredema 434
Scleroderma 434
Scombroid 436
Scorpion stings 436
Scrotal fire 436
Scurvy 436
Selenium 436
Serositis 437
Serotonin syndrome 437
Serpins 438
Serum sickness 438
Severe acute respiratory syndrome 439
Sheehan's syndrome 439
Short bowel syndrome 439
Shy–Drager disease 440
Sicca syndrome 440
Sickle cell anaemia 440
Sideroblastic anaemia 440

Contents

Silicosis 440
Situs inversus 440
Sjogren's syndrome 440
Skin necrosis 441
Skin signs of internal malignant disease 442
SLE 442
Sleep 442
Sleep disorders of breathing 442
Smallpox 446
Smoke inhalation 446
Snake bites 446
Sodium nitroprusside 446
Somatomedin C 446
Somatostatin 446
Spider bites 446
Splenomegaly 446
Spondyloarthritis 447
Spotted fevers 447
Sprue-like enteropathy 447
Staphylococcal scalded skin syndrome 447
Star fruit poisoning 447
Statins 448
Stevens–Johnson syndrome 448
Still's disease 448
Stings 448
Stomatitis 448
Storage disorders 448
Stridor 448
Strontium 449
Strychnine 449
Sturge–Weber syndrome 449
Subacute sclerosing panencephalitis 450
Sucralfate 450
Sweating 450
Sweet's syndrome 451
Swimming 451
Swine flu 451
Syndrome of inappropriate antidiuretic hormone 451
Syphilis 452
Syringomyelia 453
Systemic diseases and the lung 453
Systemic lupus erythematosus 454
Systemic sclerosis 456

T Takayasu's disease 456
Takotsubo cardiomyopathy 456
Tardive dyskinesia 457
Telangiectasia 457
Temporal arteritis 457
Tetanus 457

Tetrachlorethylene 459
Tetrachlormethane 459
Tetrahydroaminoacridine (THA) 459
Tetralogy of Fallot 459
Tetrodotoxin 459
Thalassaemia 459
Thallium 459
Thermoregulation 459
Thesaurosis 460
Thiamine deficiency 460
Thrombasthenia 460
Thrombocythaemia 460
Thrombocytopenia 460
Thrombocytosis/thrombocythaemia 463
Thromboembolism 463
Thrombohaemorrhagic disorders 464
Thromboinflammation 464
Thrombolysis 464
Thrombomodulin 464
Thrombophilia 465
Thrombopoietin 466
Thrombotic microangiopathy 466
Thrombotic thrombocytopenic purpura 466
Thymoma 468
Thyroid function 468
Thyroid storm 468
Ticks 468
Tinnitus 469
Tirofiban 469
Tisagenlecleucel 469
Tocilizumab 469
Tongue 469
Torulosis 469
Toxic epidermal necrolysis 469
Toxic erythemas 469
Toxic gases and fumes 469
Toxic shock syndrome 469
Toxoplasmosis 471
Trace elements 471
Tranexamic acid 472
Transverse myelitis 472
Trauma 472
Trauma-induced coagulopathy 473
Trauma in pregnancy 473
Trench fever 474
Trichlorethylene 474
Tropical pulmonary eosinophilia 474
Tuberculosis 474
Tuberous sclerosis 475
Tubulointerstitial diseases 475
Tumour-lysis syndrome 477

Tumour markers/biomarkers 477
Tumour necrosis factor 478
Typhoid fever 479
Typhus 479

U Ulcerative colitis 479
Ulcers 479
Urea cycle disorders 480
Urticaria 480
Uveitis 482
Uveoparotid fever 482

V Valerian 482
Valproate 482
Vaping 482
Vaptans 483
Varicella-zoster 483
Vasculitis 484
Vasopressin 487
Vertigo 487
Vesiculobullous diseases 487
Vincent's angina 488
VIPoma 488
Viral haemorrhagic fever 488
Vitamin deficiency 488
Vitamin B_{12} deficiency 489
Vitamin C deficiency 489
Vitamin D deficiency 490
Vitamin K deficiency 491
Vitiligo 492

Von Recklinghausen's disease 492
Von Willebrand's disease 492

W Waldenstrom's macroglobulinaemia 493
Warfare agents 493
Warfarin 495
Wasp stings 495
Water-related accidents 495
Waterhouse–Friderichsen syndrome 495
WDHA syndrome 496
Wegener's granulomatosis 496
Weil's disease 497
Wernicke–Korsakoff syndrome 497
West Nile virus encephalitis 498
Whipple's disease 498
Whipple's triad 499
Wilson's disease 499
Women's health 499
Woolsorter's disease 499

X **X-linked disorders** 499

Y **Yellow fever** 499
Yellow nail syndrome 500

Z **Zika virus infection** 500
Zinc 500
Zollinger–Ellison syndrome 501
Zoonoses 501
Zoster 502

Main entries are in bold text; cross-references are in plain text.

Preface

Uncommon clinical problems can present serious challenges in any medical specialty, particularly in those areas providing acute care. These problems tend to be overlooked even in major textbooks, they can be difficult to identify fully elsewhere and even an experienced clinician cannot be expected to remember all their relevant details. Yet these problems in total can be numerous and varied, and they may have a direct impact on patient care.

This book offers a solution. Uncommon problems relevant to intensive care and acute medicine have been gathered into a single volume, in which they have been described in sufficient detail to obviate much of the need to refer to specialized sources. The individual topics have been arranged alphabetically, as in an encyclopaedia and with ample cross-referencing to facilitate rapid access. The book is thus intended to provide an easy and practical reference for the clinician at any level faced with an uncommon acute medical problem at the bedside.

On the other hand, there are many things that this book is not intended to do. It does not replace major specialized texts, for it is not designed to cover the frontline disorders and emergencies which underpin the care of the acutely ill patient. Nor does it replace published in-depth specialist reviews or more importantly consultant opinion of specialist colleagues – rather it is hoped to be a partner with these in the large and important boundary between intensive care and the many other medical and surgical specialties which contribute to the care of the acutely ill patient.

Recent years have seen an emphasis on intensive care without walls and on medical emergency or rapid response teams based in intensive care units but operating hospital-wide. Thus, the traditional role of intensive care medicine has become increasingly merged with acute medicine in general, and the topics in this book reflect that overlap.

The author was fortunate to be able to persuade Mr Ron Tandberg, one of Australia's leading political cartoonists, to illustrate the previous editions of this book, and his cartoons have carried over as they are more timeless than any text. His incisive wit has enlivened an otherwise perhaps tedious text to the extent that his cartoons have been referred to by some as the book's main attraction!

Finally, the author again thanks the editorial staff at Cambridge University Press for their continued support and expertise.

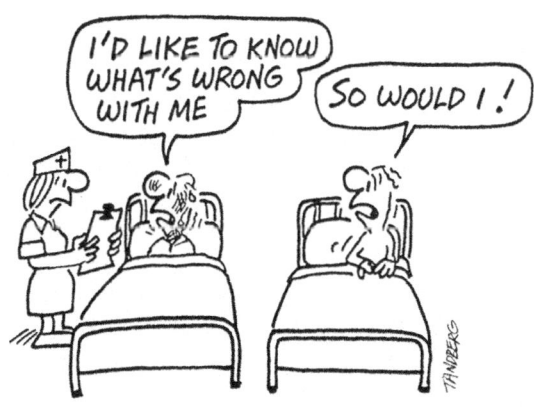

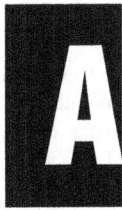

A

Abciximab See
- Antiplatelet agents.

Abdominal compartment syndrome See
- Intra-abdominal hypertension.

Abortion See
- Pregnancy.
  See also
- Amniotic fluid embolism,
- Antiphospholipid syndrome,
- Immune thrombocytopenic purpura,
- Salpingitis,
- Systemic lupus erythematosus,
- Tetanus.

Bibliography
Levens ED, DeCherney AH. Ectopic pregnancy and spontaneous abortion. In: *Scientific American Medicine. Women's Health*. Hamilton: Dekker Medicine. 2020.

Abruptio placentae (placental abruption) See
- Trauma in pregnancy – Placental abruption.
  See also
- Amniotic fluid embolism,
- Haemolytic–uraemic syndromes,
- HELLP syndrome,
- Pre eclampsia.

Acanthosis nigricans See
- Pigmentation disorders.
  See also
- Lung tumours,
- Paraneoplastic syndromes.

ACE See
- Angiotensin-converting enzyme.

Acetazolamide See
- Carbonic anhydrase inhibitors.
  See also
- Benign intracranial hypertension,
- High altitude,
- Periodic paralysis.

Acetylsalicylic acid See
- Aspirin.

Achlorhydria

Achlorhydria refers to the lack of secretion of gastric acid. The diagnosis of achlorhydria may be less than rigorous if it is based on the pH of spot samples of gastric contents rather than on formal testing of basal or stimulated gastric secretion.

The absence of gastric acid even after stimulation (i.e. absolute achlorhydria) has a number of associations, including
- gastric carcinoma,
- gastric polyps,
- pernicious anaemia (q.v.),
- iron deficiency (q.v.),
- hypogammaglobulinaemia (see Agammaglobulinaemia),
- increased susceptibility to gastrointestinal infection.

Achlorhydria is of course also seen after
- extensive gastric surgery or irradiation (permanently),
- potent proton pump (H^+/K^+ ATPase) inhibitors (PPIs) (temporarily).

Gastric acid is a prerequisite for peptic ulceration, and **increased acid secretion** is a feature of refractory or recurrent peptic ulceration (see Zollinger–Ellison syndrome).
See also
- Anaemia.

Bibliography
Wolfe MM, Jensen RT. Zollinger–Ellison syndrome: current concepts in diagnosis and management. *N Engl J Med* 1987; 317: 1200.

Acidosis, lactic See
- Lactic acidosis.

Acidosis, renal tubular See
- Renal tubular acidosis.

Acquired immunodeficiency syndrome

Acquired immunodeficiency syndrome (AIDS) has become a well-recognized entity throughout all of clinical medicine and beyond. The cumulative worldwide mortality from AIDS pandemic has far exceeded 30 million, with 800,000 deaths still occurring annually, as the overall mortality has been about 40%. Nearly 40 million people currently live with HIV infection, to which are added about 1.7 million new cases each year.

Sophisticated computer modelling of viral phylogenetics has suggested that the causative virus, the **human immunodeficiency virus** (HIV-1), originated in Africa perhaps in 1931, presumably via interspecies transfer from chimpanzees, though the first positive serology can be dated only from 1959 in Africa and the first cases did not reach the developed world until nearly 10 years later.

HIV infection is now regarded as a chronic condition, and patients in the developed world at least can have a relatively normal lifespan following viral suppression with combined antiretroviral therapy (ART or cART). These ART regimens must be continued indefinitely to prevent viral re-emergence. Current antiviral therapy is so successful that HIV-AIDS control has been effectively achieved even without the development of an effective vaccine. Moreover, treated patients with an undetectable viral load (i.e. <200 copies/mL in blood) do not pose a risk of transmission to others.

Pre-exposure prophylaxis (PrEP) is also available for those at risk, e.g. in serodiscordant sexual partnerships, on either a daily or an episodic basis. PrEP using a combination of tenofovir and emtricitabine has an effectiveness of over 90%, as also is post-exposure prophylaxis with an effectiveness of over 80%. The widespread availability of targeted PrEP has led to a marked fall in new HIV diagnoses, at least in developed countries.

> Given the large number of otherwise well patients in the population nowadays with HIV stabilized on ART in developed countries, it is now estimated that most such patients will be cared for in ICUs following surgery, trauma, infection or any of the other conditions that prompt admission to ICU generally. In addition, in patients being treated long term with combined highly active antiretroviral agents, there is an increased occurrence of a range of serious chronic conditions, including accelerated cardiovascular disease, COPD and non-AIDS-defining cancers. For all these patients, special considerations apply in the use of ART if they become critically ill, and there are now published guidelines for this.

The traditionally most common presentation to Intensive Care, namely, **opportunistic infection**, has now been relegated to second place. Patients presenting with these, even if their HIV status is unknown and provided they have no other known immunodeficiency, are generally not difficult to recognize as likely to have AIDS.

These infections are often unusually chronic, recurrent, invasive or multiple. In many such patients presenting with fever and a presumptive diagnosis of infection, a specific microbiological cause is never identified. Although the patient may be a risk to others, particularly if tuberculosis is not promptly recognized, the patient is clearly also at risk of acquiring other, nosocomial infections while in hospital and especially while in Intensive Care.

Respiratory infections are the most common infections suffered by AIDS patients admitted for Intensive Care, but the clinical presentation is dependent on the patient's immune status, most simply assessed by the CD4 count.

- If the CD4 count is normal or nearly so, the infection is most likely to be bacterial or perhaps tuberculosis (TB).
- If the CD4 count is <200/µL, the infection is most likely to be caused by, in order,
    - *Pneumocystis jirovecii (P. carinii)*,
    - bacteria (especially pneumococci, but also legionella, listeria, nocardia, salmonella),
    - mycobacteria (either TB or *Mycobacterium avium* complex (MAC)),
    - fungi (candida, aspergillus),
    - protozoa (toxoplasma),
    - viruses (herpesviruses).

Bacillary angiomatosis and bacillary peliosis hepatis are serious infective complications of cat-scratch disease (q.v.), seen in immunocompromised patients such as those with AIDS.

AIDS-defining **neoplastic conditions** remain a major clinical problem. These cancers include

- Kaposi's sarcoma, due to HSV8 (see Herpesviruses),
- non-Hodgkin's lymphoma and primary cerebral lymphoma.

In disadvantaged communities, presenting features may still occasionally represent the **direct effects** of HIV infection. A very broad collection of such features may be seen, including

- an acute infectious mononucleosis-like illness
    - which commonly persists for several months,
- thrombocytopenia (q.v.),
- wasting,
- neurological disease
    - subacute encephalitis (q.v.),
    - encephalopathy (q.v.),
    - myelopathy (q.v.),
    - peripheral neuropathy (q.v.),
    - aseptic meningitis,
- abnormalities of
    - myocardium,
    - kidneys,
    - gut,
    - thyroid,
    - joints.

Bibliography

Barbier F, Mer M, Szychowiak P, et al. Management of HIV-infected patients in the intensive care unit. *Intens Care Med* 2020; 46: 329.

Brookmeyer R. Reconstruction and future trends of the AIDS epidemic in the United States. *Science* 1991; 253: 37.

Cheruvu S, Holloway CJ. Cardiovascular disease in human immunodeficiency virus. *Intern Med J* 2014; 44: 315.

Dickson D. Tests fail to support claims for origin of AIDS in polio vaccine. *Nature* 2000; 407: 117.

Karpatkin S, Nardi M, Green D. Platelet and coagulation defects associated with HIV-1 infection. *Thromb Haemost* 2002; 88: 389.

Korber B, Muldoon M, Theiler J, et al. Timing the ancestor of the HIV-1 pandemic strains. *Science* 2000; 288: 1789.

Levine SJ, White DA. Pneumocystis carinii. *Clin Chest Med* 1988; 9: 395.

Mann JM. AIDS – the second decade: a global perspective. *J Infect Dis* 1992; 165: 245.

Miller R. HIV-associated respiratory diseases. *Lancet* 1996; 348: 307.

Panlilo AL, Cardo DM, Grohskopf LA, et al. Updated U.S. public health service guidelines for the management of occupational exposures to HIV and recommendations for postexposure prophylaxis. *MMWR* 2005; 54: 1.

Pitman MC, Lewin SR. Towards a cure for human immunodeficiency virus. *Intern Med J* 2018; 48: 12.

Rosen MJ. Pulmonary complications of HIV infection: a review. *Respirology* 2008; 13: 181.

Suffredini DA, George JM, Masur H. Management of antiretrovirals in critically ill patients: great progress but potential pitfalls. *Crit Care Med* 2018; 46: 663.

Thompson MA, Aberg JA, Cahn P, et al. Antiretroviral treatment of adult HIV infection: 2010 recommendations of the International AIDS Society-USA panel. *JAMA* 2010; 304: 321.

Yarwood T, Russell DB. HIV: almost gone, but still forgotten. *Intern Med J* 2020; 50: 269.

Acromegaly

Acromegaly is a rare condition, produced in adults by excessive growth hormone which is usually derived from a pituitary adenoma. Its incidence is about 4 per million of the population per year, and its prevalence is about 50 per million of the population.

The pituitary adenoma usually arises from somatic mutation of the gene coding for part of a regulatory G protein, thus causing the production of growth hormone to become continuous instead of varying greatly during the day as it normally does in response to many stimuli, including exercise, stress, hypoglycaemia and adrenergic influences. Excessive growth hormone in children may produce **gigantism** as an occasional phenomenon.

Growth hormone (GH, somatotropin, somatropin) is a 191 amino acid peptide, which is secreted by the anterior pituitary and which acts by stimulating the hepatic production of **somatomedin C** (or insulin-like growth factor 1, IGF-1), one of the body's many growth factors which circulate and bind to target cell receptors. IGF, which as an ultimate anabolic agent was called the wonder drug of the late twentieth century, is now described as a system and is the subject of an extensive literature.

The pituitary secretion of growth hormone is regulated by two neuropeptides secreted by the hypothalamus into the pituitary portal circulation, namely, **growth hormone-releasing hormone** (GHRH) which is stimulatory and **somatostatin** (q.v.) which is inhibitory. Acromegaly may thus also occur from excessive pituitary stimulation by GHRH either from the hypothalamus or ectopically from tumours, particularly benign foregut tumours such as bronchial carcinoid (q.v.) or pancreatic adenoma.

> The clinical features of acromegaly include both local (mechanical or parasellar) and distal (hormonal) changes, as for all pituitary tumours.
> - **Local** (mechanical or parasellar) features include headache and visual impairment (both of fields and of acuity).
> - **Distal** (hormonal) features include acral and soft tissue overgrowth (affecting especially the face, hands and feet), increased bodily hair (see Hirsutism), sweating (q.v.) and odour, sleep apnoea (q.v.), husky voice, diabetes and skin tags (fibroma molluscum). Concomitant vascular disease may occur, with both atherosclerosis and microvascular dysfunction (q.v.).
>
> Most patients have sleep apnoea (q.v.), and both the obstructive and central forms of this condition may occur.
>
> Since the hormonal changes of acromegaly which lead to clinical recognition tend to develop slowly, the adenoma is generally a macro-adenoma (i.e. >10 mm) and parasellar features are usual when the diagnosis is made.

Investigations show an elevated plasma growth hormone level which is not suppressed after a glucose load (i.e. >3 μg/L, despite glucose 75 g 1–2 hr previously in a standard oral glucose tolerance test). The plasma somatomedin C level which reflects average growth hormone activity is increased. The sella itself is best imaged by CT or MRI. If pituitary hyperplasia rather than a discrete adenoma is present, the source of GHRH should be sought either in the hypothalamus or an ectopic site.

Treatment of a pituitary adenoma is usually by trans-phenoidal **resection**.
- Postoperative **radiotherapy** is required if the GH and IGF-1 remain elevated, as is often the case.
- If GH levels still remain elevated, symptoms may be improved by medical treatment, using agents such as **bromocriptine** (a dopamine agonist, given in a dose of 2.5–10 mg bd) or **octreotide** (a synthetic analog of somatostatin, given in a dose of 200 mcg SC bd or tds). Bromocriptine is particularly useful in patients with prolactin-secreting tumours (but see Ergot).
- Second-generation **dopamine agonists** (e.g. cabergoline), **somatostatin analogs** (e.g. pasireotide) and **growth hormone receptor antagonists** (e.g. pegvisomant) provide newer pharmacological options for biochemical control when surgery is not feasible or is incomplete. More recently, a long-acting analog of **somatostatin-release-inhibitor factor** (SRIF) has been found to be effective in resistant cases.

> **Pituitary apoplexy** is an emergency condition which can complicate any pituitary tumour.
> It presents with headache, coma, shock and abnormal eye signs.
> It requires urgent treatment with **corticosteroids** and **surgery**.

See also
- Pituitary.

Bibliography
Bach LA. The insulin-like growth factor system: basic and clinical aspects. *Aust NZ J Med* 1999; 29: 355.
Burt MG, Ho KKY. Newer options in the management of acromegaly. *Intern Med J* 2006; 36: 437.
Bills DC, Meyer FB, Laws ER, et al. A retrospective analysis of pituitary apoplexy. *Neurosurgery* 1993; 33: 602.
Colao A, Ferone D, Marzullo P, et al. Systemic complications of acromegaly: epidemiology, pathogenesis, and management. *Endocr Rev* 2004; 25: 102.
Cheung NW, Taylor L, Boyages SC. An audit of long-term octreotide therapy for acromegaly. *Aust NZ J Med* 1997; 27: 12.
Lamberts S, van der Lely AJ, de Herder WW, et al. Octreotide. *N Engl J Med* 1996; 334: 246.
Melmed S. Medical progress: acromegaly. *N Engl J Med* 2006; 355: 2558.
Randeva H, Schoebel J, Byrne J, et al. Classical pituitary apoplexy: clinical features, management and outcome. *Clin Endo* 1999; 51: 181.

ACTH *See*
- Adrenocorticotropic hormone.
See also
- Adrenal insufficiency.
- Aldosterone,
- Conn's syndrome,
- Cushing's syndrome,
- Ectopic hormone production,
- Hirsutism,
- Paraneoplastic syndromes.

Actinomycete infections *See*
- Actinomycosis,
- Nocardiosis,
- Whipple's disease.

Actinomycosis

Actinomycosis is due to infection with a Gram-positive bacterium, *Actinomyces israelii*, previously thought to be a fungus because of its filamentous hyphae-like appearance. It is an obligate anaerobe, related to *Nocardia* (q.v.) and often part of the normal oral flora.

Infection arises when there is injury to the mucosal barrier, especially in association with necrotic tissue or a foreign body. Most infections are facio-cervical, but occasionally the infection may involve the lungs or become disseminated. It is also an uncommon cause of pelvic inflammatory disease in women.

It is a chronic deep granulomatous infection with sinus formation. Inspection of exuded material may show the characteristic 'sulphur granules', tiny pale particles which on microscopy are masses of filaments.

Laboratory identification can sometimes be difficult, as the organisms on smear may fragment to give cocco-bacilli appearing like diphtheroids and on culture they are slowly growing under anaerobic conditions.

Treatment is with **penicillin** 7.2–14.4 g (12–24 million U) IV per day in divided doses for 2–4 weeks, then orally in reduced dose for 3–6 months. In penicillin-sensitive patients, **tetracycline** may be used.
- **Surgical clearance** may be required, and **hyperbaric oxygen** should be considered in severe infections.

The prognosis is generally good.

Bibliography
Weese WC, Smith IM. A study of 57 cases of actinomycosis over a 36-year period. *Arch Intern Med* 1975; 135: 1562.

Acute brain syndrome *See*
- Delirium.

Acute fatty liver of pregnancy

Acute fatty liver of pregnancy (AFLP) is a rare and potentially fatal condition of the third trimester and is usually associated with pre-eclampsia. It presents with nausea, vomiting, abdominal pain and jaundice.

Liver function tests are abnormal, and there is usually a coagulopathy. Hypoglycaemia can be severe and sustained. The liver biopsy shows diffuse panlobular fatty change (i.e. steatosis).

Treatment is with emergency **delivery** *and Intensive Care support.*

See also
- HELLP syndrome,
- Pre-eclampsia.

Bibliography
Chang MS, Rutherford AE. Liver disease in pregnancy. In: *Scientific American Medicine. Hepatology.* Hamilton: Dekker Medicine. 2020.

Acute flaccid myelitis *See*
- Poliomyelitis.

Acute lung irritation

Acute lung irritation can be produced by a large number of chemical pollutants in the form of noxious gases and fumes (see Occupational lung diseases). Irritation generally occurs in the upper respiratory tract (and often elsewhere, such as the skin), as well as in the lung. Water-soluble gases (e.g. ammonia, sulphur dioxide) particularly affect the upper airway and produce immediate symptoms, whereas less soluble gases (e.g. oxides of nitrogen, ozone) primarily affect the peripheral airways and may produce delayed symptoms (i.e. about 12 hr later). Heavy exposure to any agent causes effects throughout the entire respiratory system.

Clinical features of acute lung irritation thus include
- sneezing, rhinorrhoea, lacrimation,
- stridor (q.v.),
- cough,
- wheeze,
- dyspnoea.

Systemic effects may also be seen on occasion, including
- fever,
- chills,
- leukocytosis.

Bronchiolitis (q.v.), pulmonary oedema (q.v.) and subsequent bronchopneumonia are possible consequences of acute lung irritation.

Toxic gases and fumes include
- ammonia,
- chlorine (q.v.),
- sulphur dioxide,
- oxides of nitrogen,
- ozone,
- hydrogen sulphide (q.v.),
- isocyanates
  - which may also cause occupational asthma (q.v.),
- osmium tetroxide,
- metal fumes
  - especially oxides of copper (q.v.), magnesium (q.v.) and zinc (q.v.),
  - also oxides of antimony, beryllium (q.v.), cadmium (q.v.), cobalt (q.v.), iron (q.v.), manganese (q.v.), nickel, selenium (q.v.), tin, tungsten and vanadium,
- mercury (q.v.),
- platinum salts,
- polymer fumes (Teflon degradation products),
- warfare agents (q.v.).

The treatment of toxic gas exposure is focussed on airway protection, intubation and lung protective modes of mechanical ventilation. Corticosteroids have not been of value acutely, though benefit has been reported during the later reparative phase. Interestingly, simple drugs such as aminophylline, ibuprofen, N-acetylcysteine, nebulized heparin and salbutamol have been recommended, but formal documentation of their efficacy is lacking.

Systemic abnormalities are also produced following the inhalation of
- carbon monoxide (q.v.),
- cyanide (q.v.).

Asphyxia may be caused by excess
- carbon dioxide,
- nitrogen,
- methane.

Bibliography

Dennekamp M, Abramson MJ. The effects of bushfire smoke on respiratory health. *Respirology* 2011; 16: 198.

Kales SN, Christiani DC. Acute chemical emergencies. *New Engl J Med* 2004; 350: 800.

Schwartz DA. Acute inhalational injury. *Occup Med* 1987; 2: 297.

Acute pulmonary oedema

Pulmonary oedema is defined as an increased amount of extravascular fluid (water and solute) in the lung, where it may be interstitial or alveolar or both.

Pulmonary oedema is one of the commonest respiratory disorders and may follow a wide variety of local and systemic insults. Although pulmonary oedema due to left heart failure is the classical clinical picture, pulmonary oedema also occurs in a number of other common settings. In these, the left atrial pressure may be normal or even low.

These non-cardiac settings include
- serious medical or surgical illness in the form of the **acute respiratory distress syndrome** (ARDS) (q.v.),
- an important component in
  - viral pneumonia,
  - aspiration pneumonitis (q.v.),
  - respiratory burns (q.v.),
  - uraemia,
  - endotoxaemia (a systemic inflammatory response syndrome),
  - drowning (q.v.),
  - head injury,
  - severe upper airway obstruction (see Asthma),
  - altitude-related illness (see High altitude).

Pulmonary oedema may therefore present in diverse settings with different pathogenetic mechanisms and thus with different therapeutic implications.

The causes of pulmonary oedema are
1. **Increased capillary hydrostatic pressure**
   - cardiogenic (left heart failure),
   - blood volume overload,
   - pulmonary veno-occlusive disease (q.v.).
2. **Increased capillary permeability**
   - acute respiratory distress syndrome (ARDS)(q.v.),
   - viral and other pneumonia,
   - inhaled toxic substances (including oxygen),
   - circulating toxic agents (including sepsis),
   - disseminated intravascular coagulation (q.v.),
   - uraemia, radiation (q.v.), burns (q.v.), non-fatal drowning (q.v.),
   - vaping-associated respiratory disease after using e-cigarettes (see Vaping).
3. **Decreased plasma oncotic pressure**
   - hypoalbuminaemia.
4. **Decreased tissue hydrostatic pressure (i.e. negative-pressure pulmonary oedema)**
   - rapid lung re-expansion, after
     - drainage of a pneumothorax or large pleural effusion,
     - pneumonectomy,
   - laryngospasm (and other causes of acute upper airway obstruction, when associated with strong inspiratory effort).
5. **Decreased lymphatic drainage**
   - lymphangitis carcinomatosa,
   - lymphangioleiomyomatosis (q.v.),
   - lung transplantation.
6. **Uncertain mechanisms**
   - high altitude (q.v.),
   - neurogenic (raised intracranial pressure),
   - drug overdose (especially IV heroin),
   - pulmonary embolism,
   - maximal exercise (occasionally),
   - scuba diving, usually in cold water (occasionally).

In practice,
- the first two groups of causes are by far the most commonly encountered,
- the third group is probably not a cause in its own right, but lowers the threshold for pulmonary oedema from other causes,
- groups four, five and six are less common.

Bibliography

Adir Y, Shupak A, Gil A, et al. Swimming-induced pulmonary edema: clinical presentation and serial lung function. *Chest* 2004; 126: 394.

Albertson TE, Walby WF, Derlet RW. Stimulant-induced pulmonary toxicity. *Chest* 1995; 108: 1140.

Bhattacharya M, Kallet RH, Ware LB, et al. Negative-pressure pulmonary edema. *Chest* 2016; 150: 927.

Busl KM, Bleck TP. Neurogenic pulmonary edema. *Crit Care Med* 2015; 43: 1710.

Colice GL. Neurogenic pulmonary edema. *Clin Chest Med* 1985; 6: 473.

Esper A, Martin GS, Staton GW. Pulmonary edema. In: *Scientific American Medicine. Pulmonary & Critical Care Medicine – Pulmonary*. Hamilton: Dekker Medicine. 2020.

Gehlbach BK, Geppert E. The pulmonary manifestations of left heart failure. *Chest* 2004; 125: 669.

Harms BA, Kramer GC, Bodai BI, et al. Effect of hypoproteinemia on pulmonary and soft tissue edema formation. *Crit Care Med* 1981; 9: 503.

Kollef MH, Pluss J. Noncardiogenic pulmonary edema following upper airway obstruction. *Medicine* 1991; 70: 91.

McConkey PP. Postobstructive pulmonary oedema. *Anaesth Intens Care* 2000; 28: 72.

Richalet JP. High altitude pulmonary oedema: still a place for controversy? *Thorax* 1995; 50: 923.

Scherrer U, Vollenweider L, Delabays A, et al. Inhaled nitric oxide for high-altitude pulmonary edema. *N Engl J Med* 1996; 334: 624.

Schoene RB. Pulmonary edema at high altitude: review, pathophysiology, and update. *Clin Chest Med* 1985; 6: 491.

Schwarz MI, Albert RK. 'Imitators' of the ARDS: implications for diagnosis and treatment. *Chest* 2004; 125: 1530.

Sibbald WJ, Cunningham DR, Chin DN. Non-cardiac or cardiac pulmonary edema? *Chest* 1983; 84: 452.

Simon RP. Neurogenic pulmonary edema. *Neurol Clin* 1993; 11: 309.

Sporer KA, Dorn E. Heroin-related noncardiogenic pulmonary edema. *Chest* 2001; 120: 1628.

Steinberg KP, Hudson LD. Acute lung injury and acute respiratory distress syndrome: the clinical syndrome. *Clin Chest Med* 2000; 21: 401.

Taylor JR, Ryu J, Colby TV, et al. Lymphangioleiomyomatosis. *N Engl J Med* 1990; 323: 1254.

Timby J, Reed C, Zeilender S, et al. Mechanical causes of pulmonary edema. *Chest* 1990; 98: 973.

Acute respiratory distress syndrome

Acute respiratory distress syndrome (adult respiratory distress syndrome, ARDS) has been recognized as the hallmark respiratory complication of critical illness since its first description in 1967. Its pathogenesis, clinical features, diagnosis and management have been extensively described, studied and reviewed in the literature over the past four decades.

It has become apparent that there has been a major decline (about 4-fold) in the incidence and mortality of ARDS over the past 20 years. This decline has been attributed to improved resuscitation and early treatment of sepsis, trauma and other precursor conditions, to more restrictive fluid and blood product practices, and to improved ventilator protocols focussed on lung protection. This improvement has occurred despite the failure of any specific pharmacological measure to alter its outcome.

It should be remembered that even later definitions of ARDS (e.g. Berlin 2012) have limited accuracy and that its differential diagnosis includes a number of other conditions associated with diffuse alveolar changes (see Pulmonary infiltrates). The syndrome thus incorporates considerable heterogeneity.

See
- Acute pulmonary oedema.

Bibliography

Beitler JR, Schoenfeld DA, Thompson BT. Preventing ARDS: progress, promise, and pitfalls. *Chest* 2014; 146: 1102.

Esper A, Martin GS, Staton GW. Pulmonary edema. In: *Scientific American Medicine. Pulmonary & Critical Care Medicine*. Hamilton: Dekker Medicine. 2020.

Guerin C, Thompson T, Brower R. The ten diseases that look like ARDS. *Intens Care Med* 2015; 41: 1099.

Jaber S, Slutsky AS, eds. Mechanical ventilation in intensive care. *Intens Care Med* 2020; 46: Special Issue.

Rittayamai N, Brochard L. What's new in ADRS (clinical studies). *Intens Care Med* 2014; 40: 1731.

Thompson BT, Chambers RC, Liu KD. Acute respiratory distress syndrome. *N Engl J Med* 2017; 377: 562.

Various. ARDS birthday issue. *Intens Care Med* 2016; 42: 637.

Acyclovir

Acyclovir (aciclovir) is one of the most important antiviral drugs. It replaced vidarabine (ara-A), the first available antiviral agent for systemic use in serious infections. It is a synthetic purine nucleoside analog, structurally related to guanosine. Its unique mechanism of action inhibits DNA synthesis and thus viral replication, so that it does not affect the latent virus. There is a low incidence of development of resistance, but unwarranted use is unwise.

The antiviral effects of acyclovir are particularly relevant for herpesviruses (q.v.), as follows. It is
- especially effective against **herpes simplex virus** (HSV) types 1 and 2,
- less effective but still very useful for **varicella-zoster virus** (VZV) (q.v.),
- of intermediate efficacy against **Epstein–Barr virus** (EBV) (q.v.),
- ineffective against **cytomegalovirus** (CMV) (q.v.), but the related agent, **ganciclovir**, is however effective against CMV – see below.

The greatest value of acyclovir is in **HSV encephalitis**, in which trial results have shown a survival rate of about 80% and complete neurological recovery in about 50%.

> It is also of value in oral-labial, genital, rectal and neonatal HSV infections.

In **VZV infections**, it is helpful in
- the elderly, especially those with widespread lesions or trigeminal involvement,
- herpes zoster encephalitis,
- varicella pneumonia,
- immunocompromised patients (in whom interferon alpha and/or VZV immune globulin are also useful).

Acyclovir
- is not indicated in **infectious mononucleosis**, except perhaps in severe cases,
- is not indicated in **cytomegalovirus infections**, except for prophylaxis after bone marrow transplantation in seropositive patients, in whom it is effective when given in high dosage, i.e. 500 mg/m^2 tds IV for the first month),
- is not effective in the **chronic fatigue syndrome** (q.v.).

Acyclovir is not protein-bound but is distributed evenly throughout the total body water, except in the CSF in which the level is 25–50% of that in plasma. The urinary concentration is about 10 times the plasma concentration. It has a half-life of about 3 hr, which rises 6-fold in severe renal failure, since it is primarily excreted in the urine. It is 60% removed by dialysis. It is probably not mutagenic or carcinogenic. Although fetal risk has not been shown, it crosses the placenta and should be used in pregnancy only if there is a strong maternal indication. It is excreted into breast milk.

It is available as a powder for IV administration, as capsules for oral use and as an ointment for mucocutaneous lesions or keratitis. Intravenously, it is given as 5–10 mg/kg 8 hrly for 5–10 days. Typically, 500 mg are reconstituted in 20 mL, diluted to 100 mL and administered over 1 hr, giving a mean steady-state peak plasma concentration of 20 mcg/mL.

Although the solution is widely compatible, it undergoes irreversible crystallization if refrigerated. Intravenous acyclovir is normally well tolerated, but it is potentially phlebitic because of its alkaline nature unless given diluted and slowly, and it can sometimes give rise to nausea or a rash. Rarely, reversible encephalopathy or renal dysfunction may occur from very high concentrations.

Later nucleoside analogs include
- **valacyclovir** (a prodrug of acyclovir) and **famciclovir**, which are useful alternative agents,
- **foscarnet**, which may be used in chronic acyclovir-resistant HSV type 2 infections.

Ganciclovir is structurally similar to acyclovir and is given in similar dosage. Its chief difference is that it is active against cytomegalovirus (q.v.). It is therefore used, often with immune globulin, in CMV retinitis or pneumonia, for example after bone marrow transplantation. Unlike acyclovir, it can produce bone marrow depression. It is teratogenic and mutagenic in animals. The usual dosage is 5 mg/kg IV 12 hrly.

Valganciclovir is a prodrug of ganciclovir with much higher bioavailability.

See also
- Bell's palsy,
- Encephalitis.

Bibliography

Dwyer DE, Cunningham AL. Herpes simplex and varicella-zoster virus infections. *Med J Aust* 2002; 177: 267.

Ernest ME, Franey RJ. Acyclovir and ganciclovir-induced neurotoxicity. *Ann Pharmacother* 1998; 32: 111.

Hirsch MS. Herpesvirus infections. In: *Scientific American Medicine. Infectious Diseases.* Hamilton: Dekker Medicine. 2020.

Jackson JL, Gibbons R, Meyer G, et al. The effect of treating herpes zoster with oral acyclovir in preventing postherpetic neuralgia: a meta-analysis. *Arch Intern Med* 1997; 157: 909.

Jacobson M. Treatment of cytomegalovirus retinitis in patients with the acquired immunodeficiency syndrome. *N Engl J Med* 1997; 337: 105.

Laskin OL. Acyclovir: pharmacology and clinical experience. *Arch Intern Med* 1984; 144: 1241.

Prentice HG, Gluckman E, Powles RL, et al. Impact of long-term acyclovir on cytomegalovirus infection and survival after allogenic bone marrow transplantation: European Acyclovir for CMV Prophylaxis Study Group. *Lancet* 1994; 343: 749.

Addison's disease See
- Adrenal insufficiency.

Adenosine

Adenosine is an autacoid (q.v.). It is an endogenous purine nucleoside of molecular weight 267 Da, and it has receptors (A1 or A2) on most cell membranes. It is released when ATP is used and may thus help maintain the balance between oxygen availability and utilization. It is involved in many local regulatory processes, and in particular it is a vasodilator and an inhibitor of neuronal discharge. Adenoreceptors are present on phagocytes as well as in cardiac myocytes, and there is evidence that their modulation may prevent tissue injury in ischaemia and sepsis.

Its cardiac effects were first recognized in 1929 and are extensive. They especially involve decreased conduction and ventricular automaticity, coronary vasodilatation and the blunting of the effects of catecholamines. On balance, it is thus 'cardioprotective'. Both A1 and A2 receptors are present in the heart – A1 in the cardiomyocytes and A2 in the endothelial cells and vascular smooth muscle cells.

> Clinically, its particular use is in the diagnosis and treatment of **tachyarrhythmias**.
> - It is of most value in the treatment of supraventricular tachycardia, especially that associated with the WPW syndrome, with an average time to termination of arrhythmia of 30 sec.
> - It has no effect in atrial fibrillation or atrial flutter.
> - It is not of value in ventricular tachycardia unless catecholamine induced.

Its effects are antagonized by theophylline and potentiated by dipyridamole, but it may be administered without altered efficacy in the presence of other cardiac drugs or in liver or renal disease.

It is of potential clinical use in electrophysiological studies, in cardiac stress testing and in the assessment of coronary blood flow reserve. It has no useful effect on coronary ischaemia.

Since its half-life is only 10 sec, it is given as a rapid IV bolus of 3–6 mg. A further bolus of up to 12 mg may be given 1–3 min later if necessary.

It can produce unpleasant and marked though transient side-effects, including flushing (q.v.), sweating (q.v.), tingling, headache, light-headedness, nausea and apprehension. Bronchospasm may be precipitated in asthmatics. It can also produce cardiac pain, which is angina-like but not in fact ischaemic.

Bibliography
Belardinelli L, Linden J, Berne RM. The cardiac effects of adenosine. *Prog Cardiovasc Dis* 1989; 167: 1186.
Cronstein BN. Adenosine, an endogenous anti-inflammatory agent. *J Appl Physiol* 1994; 76: 5.
McCallion K, Harkin DW, Gardiner KR. Role of adenosine in immunomodulation: review of the literature. *Crit Care Med* 2004; 32: 273.

Adrenal insufficiency

Acute adrenal insufficiency is an uncommon condition and is usually due to haemorrhage (especially from heparin – q.v.), hypotension or shock (as in the Waterhouse–Friderichsen syndrome – q.v.).

> It thus occurs mostly in seriously ill patients, in whom it should remembered as an uncommon cause of the **hyperdynamic state** (q.v.).

The clinical features include nausea, weakness and abdominal pain, as well as circulatory failure. Typically, there is hyponatraemia (q.v.) with hyperkalaemia, and the plasma urea may be elevated.

Relevant investigations include failure of the plasma cortisol level to increase after the injection of synthetic ACTH (see below) and direct imaging with CT.

Treatment is with physiological doses of **hydrocortisone** *IV.*

Relative adrenal insufficiency (RAI) refers to a clinical scenario that has been increasingly recognized in seriously ill patients since the 1990s, though there remains controversy about its definition, its relevance and even its existence. Unlike (absolute) acute adrenal insufficiency (see above), it is probably frequent, but it has no particular set of clinical features. Instead, it represents an exacerbation of the responses to severe illness or injury and is chiefly manifest in retrospect as circulatory improvement in catecholamine-dependence after physiological doses of hydrocortisone, particularly in sepsis. Presumably, like other organs and pathways, the hypothalamic–pituitary–adrenal (HPA) axis (q.v.) has been impaired in this setting, although paradoxically the basal cortisol levels in critically ill patients are generally high and independent of the usually low ACTH level at this time (probably because some cytokines have ACTH-like activity).

A task force developing consensus guidelines in 2008 (and updated in 2017) coined the term **critical illness-related corticosteroid insufficiency** (CIRCI) to reflect the additional concept of an inadequate cellular or tissue response to endogenous corticosteroid contributing to the severity of the patient's illness. However, since the diagnosis of tissue corticosteroid resistance remains difficult, practical diagnosis relies on the principles described below.

The identification of relative adrenal insufficiency requires a high level of suspicion and the demonstration of an abnormal synthetic ACTH test (see below). However, like most laboratory tests which have been developed in well subjects or stable patients, the interpretation of this test can be controversial, especially in seriously ill patients, i.e. the very ones in whom the test is most important. This difficulty is compounded by

- hypoalbuminaemia, because most circulating total cortisol is protein-bound and it is the free cortisol

which is active (but which is not currently measurable in most laboratories), and
- a commonly blunted ACTH response, presumably because of existing maximal stimulation.

Nevertheless, the practical implication is that physiological doses of glucocorticoid appear to be of therapeutic benefit, especially in improving inotrope responsiveness in circulatory failure. This is an area of ongoing clinical research. A common practice has been that if the synthetic ACTH is not clearly normal (see below), a therapeutic trial of hydrocortisone (e.g. 100 mg IV 8 hrly or 200 mg per day by IV infusion) can be warranted. However, given the controversy about the ACTH test in this situation (see above), those who prescribe hydrocortisone in such cases most commonly do so empirically and without a prior ACTH test. Such cases include septic shock, ARDS, trauma, community-acquired pneumonia, bacterial meningitis, cardiopulmonary bypass and after cardiac arrest. However, given the heterogeneity of steroid-responsiveness among patients with these conditions, it is likely that genomic studies will be needed to clarify optimal treatment regimens.

An additional point of interest in this area is that the greatly increased risk of relative adrenal insufficiency in patients who have been given the sedative agent, **etomidate**, now provides a contraindication to the use of that drug in Intensive Care practice.

Chronic adrenal insufficiency (Addison's disease) is due to
- autoimmune disease (sometimes polyglandular),
- a space-occupying lesion, typically a metastasis or granuloma (e.g. TB),
- pituitary deficiency, due to
  - global hypopituitarism (when hypothyroidism (q.v.) is also typically present), or
  - previous administration of corticosteroids in pharmacological doses (when diabetes is commonly associated),
- HIV infection (q.v.), with associated CMV adrenal infection,
- drugs, such as ketoconazole, rifampicin.

Clinical features comprise
- weakness,
- weight loss,
- pigmentation (q.v.), especially in body creases,
- hypotension,
- hypovolaemia (except that blood volume remains normal in pituitary deficiency (q.v.), since aldosterone secretion is primarily controlled by the renin–angiotensin system (q.v.)).

Investigations show mild hyperkalaemia and proneness to hyponatraemia (q.v.) from water overload. In patients who are sufficiently hypovolaemic to have pre-renal renal failure, there is more marked hyperkalaemia with hypovolaemia, raised plasma urea and raised haematocrit.

Specific testing shows a low plasma cortisol, which fails to rise after **synthetic ACTH** 250 mcg IV (normal >150 nmol/L and a rise at 30 min by at least 300 nmol/L to a peak of >550 nmol/L). This short synthetic ACTH stimulation test is simple and safe. In septic patients, the cortisol rise rather than the basal level has correlated best with outcome (but see above).

If adrenal insufficiency is clinically overt and corticosteroids have been commenced, confirmatory testing is very difficult, unless dexamethasone can be temporarily substituted and then ceased pending a long (i.e. 3-day) synthetic ACTH stimulation test.

The plasma ACTH level is >20 pmol/L in primary adrenal failure, but in hypopituitarism it is low (as are the other pituitary hormones – q.v.). A rise in plasma cortisol still occurs in hypopituitarism following ACTH, though this may be subnormal due to chronic ACTH deficiency.

*Treatment of adrenal insufficiency is urgent if there is circulatory failure (i.e. adrenal crisis), with **hydrocortisone** 100 mg IV then 10–15 mg/hr, together with fluids, electrolytes and glucose. Chronic treatment requires maintenance therapy with cortisone (approximately 35 mg per day given about 2/3 in the morning and 1/3 in the evening), together with fludrocortisone 100 mcg per day.*

Patients with adrenal insufficiency exposed to stress require increased doses of corticosteroids.

Typically, double the usual dose is used for minor stress and hydrocortisone 100 mg IV 8 hrly for severe stress, though recently it has become recognized that these doses are excessive. In fact, doses of 25–150 mg of hydrocortisone per day for a maximum of 3 days are adequate.

Hypothalamic–pituitary–adrenal (HPA) (q.v.) function is suppressed by previously administered corticosteroids in pharmacological doses (even in the inhaled form in children).
- This may not recover for a year or more after such steroids are ceased.
- There is no simple and accurate prediction of hormonal reserve function, based on the previous dose or duration of steroid treatment.
- Prophylactic hydrocortisone (as above) is also routinely recommended in such patients exposed to

stress. This cover is continued for 2 days, and then if the clinical situation is satisfactory it is tapered over the next few days.

If time permits, the cortisol response to ACTH may be assessed prior to anticipated stress, such as elective major surgery, but a normal value after ACTH does not necessarily imply a normal response to other stress. A more relevant adrenal assessment used to be provided by the cortisol response to insulin-induced hypoglycaemia, but this test is nowadays considered to be unsafe.

Bibliography

Al-Kurd A, Mazeh H. The endocrine system: adrenal glands. In: *Scientific American Medicine. Organ Systems: Anatomy & Physiology*. Hamilton: Dekker Medicine. 2020.

Amrein K, Martucci G, Hahner S. Understanding adrenal crisis. *Intens Care Med* 2018; 44: 652.

Annane D, Pastores SM, Rochwerg B, et al. Guidelines for the diagnosis and management of critical illness-related corticosteroid insufficiency (CIRCI) in critically ill patients (Part 1): Society of Critical Care Medicine (SCCM) and European Society of Intensive Care Medicine (ESICM) 2017. *Crit Care Med* 2017; 45: 2078 and *Intens Care Med* 2017; 43: 1751.

Annane D, Pastores SM, Arlt W, et al. Critical illness-related corticosteroid insufficiency (CIRCI): a narrative review from a Multispecialty Task Force of the Society of Critical Care Medicine (SCCM) and the European Society of Intensive Care Medicine (ESICM). *Crit Care Med* 2017; 45: 2089 and *Intens Care Med* 2017; 43: 1781.

Annane D, Sebille V, Charpentier C, et al. Effect of treatment with low doses of hydrocortisone and fludrocortisone on mortality in patients with septic shock. *JAMA* 2002; 288: 862.

Claussen MS, Landercasper J, Cogbill TH. Acute adrenal insufficiency presenting as shock after trauma and surgery: three cases and review of the literature. *J Trauma* 1992; 32: 94.

Cohen J, Venkatesh B. Relative adrenal insufficiency in the intensive care population; background and critical appraisal of the evidence. *Anaesth Intens Care* 2010; 38: 425.

Editorial. Corticosteroids and hypothalamic-pituitary-adrenocortical function. *BMJ* 1980; 280: 813.

Hamrahian AH, Oseni TS, Arafah BM. Measurement of serum free cortisol in critically ill patients. *N Engl J Med* 2004; 350: 1629.

Jung C, Inder WJ. Management of adrenal insufficiency during the stress of medical illness and surgery. *Med J Aust* 2008; 188: 409.

Keller-Wood M. Hypothalamic-piuitary-adrenal axis-feedback control. *Compr Physiol* 2015; 5: 1161.

Ligtenberg JJM, Zilstra JG. The relative adrenal insufficiency syndrome revisited: which patients will benefit from low-dose steroids? *Curr Opin Crit Care* 2004; 10: 456.

Lipiner-Friedman D, Sprung CL, Laterre PF, et al. Adrenal function in sepsis: the retrospective Corticus cohort study. *Crit Care Med* 2007; 35: 1012.

Loriaux DL. The polyendocrine deficiency syndromes. *N Engl J Med* 1985; 312: 1568.

Loriaux DL. Adrenal insufficiency. In: *Scientific American Medicine. Endocrinology & Metabolism*. Hamilton: Dekker Medicine. 2020.

Malerba G, Romano-Girard F, Cravoisý A, et al. Risk factors of relative adrenocortical deficiency in intensive care patients needing mechanical ventilation. *Intens Care Med* 2005; 31: 388.

Marik PE. Unravelling the mystery of adrenal failure in the critically ill. *Crit Care Med* 2004; 32: 569.

Marik PE, Pastores SM, Annane D, et al. Recommendations for the diagnosis and management of corticosteroid insufficiency in critically ill adult patients: consensus statements from an international task force by the American College of Critical Care Medicine. *Crit Care Med* 2008; 36: 1937.

Marik PE, Zaloga GP. Adrenal insufficiency in the critically ill: a new look at an old problem. *Chest* 2002; 122: 1784.

Marik PE, Zaloga GP. Adrenal insufficiency during septic shock. *Crit Care Med* 2003; 31: 141.

Pastores SM, Annane D, Rochwerg B, et al. Guidelines for the diagnosis and management of critical illness-related corticosteroid insufficiency (CIRCI) in critically ill patients (Part 2): Society of Critical Care Medicine (SCCM) and European Society of Intensive Care Medicine (ESICM) 2017. *Crit Care Med* 2018; 46: 146 and *Intens Care Med* 2017; 43: 1751.

Peeters B, Meersseman P, Perre SV, et al. Adrenocortical function during prolonged critical illness and beyond: a prospective observational study. *Intens Care Med* 2018; 44: 1720.

Puar TH, Stikkelbroeck NM, Smans LC, et al. Adrenal crisis: still a deadly event in the 21st century. *Am J Med* 2016; 129: 339.

Rai R, Cohen J, Venkateash B. Assessment of adrenocortical function in the critically ill. *Crit Care Resusc* 2004; 6: 123.

Rygard SL, Butler E, Granholm A, et al. Low-dose corticosteroids for adult patients with septic shock: a systematic review with meta-analysis and trial sequential review. *Intens Care Med* 2018; 44: 1003.

Salem M, Tainsh RE, Bromberg J, et al. Perioperative glucocorticoid coverage: a reassessment 42 years after emergence of a problem. *Ann Surg* 1994; 219: 416.

Szalados JE, Vukmir RB. Acute adrenal insufficiency resulting from adrenal hemorrhage as indicated by post-operative hypotension. *Intens Care Med* 1994; 20: 216.

Vance ML. Hypopituitarism. *N Engl J Med* 1994; 330: 1651.

Vella A, Nippoldt TB, Morris JC. Adrenal hemorrhage: a 25-year experience at the Mayo Clinic. *Mayo Clin Proc* 2001; 76: 161.

Venkatesh B, Finfer S, Cohen J, et al. Adjunctive glucocorticoid therapy in patients with septic shock. *N Engl J Med* 2018; 378: 797.

Venkatesh B, Prins J, Torpy D, et al. Relative adrenal insufficiency: match point or deuce? *Crit Care Resusc* 2006; 8: 376.

Vita JA, Silverberg SJ, Goland RS, et al. Clinical clues to the cause of Addison's disease. *Am J Med* 1985; 78: 461.

Volbeda M, Wetterslev J, Gluud C, et al. Glucocorticoids for sepsis: systematic review with meta-analysis and trial sequential analysis. *Intens Care Med* 2015; 41: 1220.

Webb SAR. Relative adrenal insufficiency exists and should be treated. *Crit Care Resusc* 2006; 8: 371.

Zaloga GP, Marik P. Hypothalamic-pituitary-adrenal insufficiency. *Crit Care Clin* 2001; 17: 25.

Adrenocorticotropic hormone

Adrenocorticotropic hormone (corticotropin, ACTH) is the main controlling factor for the adrenal production of cortisol and androgens. It is produced in the anterior pituitary by cleavage of a large and complex polypeptide (241 amino acids) called **propiomelanocortin** (POMC), which also includes melanocyte-stimulating hormone (MSH), beta-endorphin, met-enkephalin, beta-lipotropin and a number of other peptides of currently unknown function.

The secretion of ACTH is controlled primarily by the hypothalamus-derived **corticotropin-releasing hormone** (CRH) and secondarily by catecholamines and vasopressin. ACTH release is also stimulated by stress and by hypoglycaemia. CRH production and ACTH release are inhibited by both natural and synthetic corticosteroids, which suppress mRNA for POMC synthesis. ACTH is released in pulses, especially in the mornings, thus explaining the diurnal rhythm of cortisol secretion.

The normal level of ACTH is 1.3–16.7 pmol/L.

See
- Adrenal insufficiency,
- Aldosterone,
- Conn's syndrome,
- Cushing's syndrome,
- Ectopic hormone production,
- Hirsutism,
- Paraneoplastic syndromes.

Bibliography

Editorial. Corticosteroids and hypothalamic-pituitary-adrenocortical function. *BMJ* 1980; 280: 813.

Imura H. Control of biosynthesis and secretion of ACTH: a review. *Horm Metab Res* 1987; 16 (suppl.): 1.

Orth DN. Corticotropin-releasing hormone in humans. *Endocr Rev* 1992; 13: 164.

Adult respiratory distress syndrome *See*
- Acute respiratory distress syndrome.

See also
- Acute pulmonary oedema.

Agammaglobulinaemia

Agammaglobulinaemia (Bruton's agammaglobulinaemia) was the first described immunodeficiency disorder (q.v.). It is a congenital X-linked condition, caused by mutations in the *BTK* gene on the long arm of the X chromosome which encodes for a tyrosine kinase expressed in pre–B cells.

- There is a lifelong **susceptibility to infection**
  - particularly with encapsulated pyogenic microorganisms,
  - less so with viruses, fungi and even most Gram-negative bacteria (except for *Haemophilus influenzae*).
- Infections, particularly of the respiratory tract, show a(n)
  - increased frequency,
  - increased severity,
  - increased recurrence rate,
  - decreased responsiveness to treatment.

Chronic meningoencephalitis, due to an echovirus, can be a particularly troublesome complication (see Encephalitis).

In about 30% of patients, agammaglobulinaemia is associated with a rheumatoid arthritis-like disease and sometimes with dermatomyositis (q.v.), probably due to an enterovirus.

On investigation, all the immunoglobulins are decreased (with IgA, IgM and IgD often undetectable and IgG < 1 g/L) and there are no B cells. There is no antibody response (e.g. to diphtheria–pertussis–tetanus immunization), but there is normal cell-mediated immunity.

Treatment with intravenous **immunoglobulin** *(30 mg/kg/month IV)* significantly improves the prognosis.

Screening of at-risk family members is recommended.

Bibliography
Buckley RH, Schiff RI. The use of intravenous immune globulin in immunodeficiency diseases. *N Engl J Med* 1991; 325: 110.
Van der Meer JWM, Kullberg BJ. Defects in host-defense mechanisms. In: Rubin RH, Young LS, eds. *Clinical Approach to Infection in the Compromised Host*. 4th edition. New York: Plenum. 2002; p 5.

Agranulocytosis

Agranulocytosis for practical purposes is synonymous with neutropenia (q.v.). Theoretically, the term also includes deficiency of the other granulocytes, namely, eosinophils (q.v.) and basophils (q.v.).

Bibliography
Vincent PC. Drug-induced aplastic anemia and agranulocytosis. *Drugs* 1986; 31: 52.

AIDS *See*
- Acquired immunodeficiency syndrome.

Air embolism *See*
- Diving – Gas embolism.

Alcohol, methyl *See*
- Methanol.

Aldosterone

Aldosterone is produced in the zona glomerulosa of the adrenal gland from cholesterol and acetate precursors. It is the chief mineralocorticoid and promotes the renal tubular reabsorption of sodium and water.
- It is stimulated chiefly by angiotensin (q.v.) but also by ACTH (q.v.), hyperkalaemia, hyponatraemia (q.v.) and hypovolaemia.
- It is inhibited by dopamine in low doses which thus causes a natriuresis, an important phenomenon in Intensive Care patients, in whom secondary aldosteronism is common.

Aldosterone circulates in the free form and is metabolized in the liver, so that its level is increased in many liver disorders. Aldosterone causes an increased blood volume and cardiac output via sodium and water retention, and there may be associated increased blood pressure from the vasoconstrictor effects of angiotensin II. These volume and blood pressure signals cause the juxtaglomerular apparatus in the kidney to reduce renin release, a negative feedback effect.

See
- Conn's syndrome,
- Renal tubular acidosis,
- Renin–angiotensin–aldosterone.

Bibliography
Melby JC. Diagnosis of hyperaldosteronism. *Endocrinol Metab Clin North Am* 1991; 20: 247.
Quinn SJ, Williams GH. Regulation of aldosterone secretion. *Ann Rev Physiol* 1988; 50: 409.
White PC. Disorders of aldosterone biosynthesis and action. *N Engl J Med* 1994; 331: 250.

Alkaloids

Alkaloids are a class of organic compounds containing carbon, hydrogen and nitrogen and often possessing powerful physiological effects. They are usually derived from flowering plants and are complex structures generally containing some type of ring. They are chemically basic (i.e. alkaline), hence their name. Their role in nature is unknown.

Alkaloids of clinical interest include substances such as
- ephedrine,
- ergot (q.v.),
- morphine,
- nicotine,
- quinine,
- strychnine (q.v.).

Some plant alkaloids are common cancer chemotherapy agents (e.g. vincristine, vinblastine). They bind to structural proteins in the cytoplasm and thus prevent the formation of microtubules and the spindle apparatus in mitosis.

Alkaloids of the pyrrolizidine class are found in many plants and are sometimes ingested in herbal or bush teas, following which they may produce hepatic veno-occlusive disease (q.v.).

Allergic bronchopulmonary aspergillosis *See*
- Aspergillosis.
  See also
- Asthma,
- Eosinophilia and lung infiltration.

Allergic granulomatosis and angiitis *See*
- Churg–Strauss syndrome.

Alopecia

Alopecia refers to loss of bodily hair. It can have many causes and may vary in extent from the loss of an area of hair on the scalp to the loss of all bodily hair, even including eyebrows and eyelashes.

1. **Alopecia areata**

This is a localized condition of unknown cause, occurring in young people and with one or more areas of complete hair loss, usually on the scalp. There is minimal inflammation clinically (although histological examination shows lymphoid cells around the hair bulbs), and the process is usually reversible within 3 years.

As it can be associated with several autoimmune diseases (q.v.), especially Addison's disease (q.v.), thyroiditis and pernicious anaemia (q.v.), it is probably an autoimmune phenomenon itself.

*It is treated with **local steroids**.*
- Local irritants assist, and phototherapy and/or minoxidil may help in some patients.

2. **Androgenetic alopecia**

This is male baldness and it has well-known features, though an underlying endocrine disorder should be sought if it occurs in young women. Iron deficiency (q.v.) should be excluded, as iron is an important cofactor for the development of hair matrix cells.

*If the result is cosmetically unacceptable, it may be treated with **oestrogens** in women and **antiandrogens** (e.g. finasteride 1 mg per day) in men, or with **minoxidil** topically (1 mL of 2% or 5% bd) in either sex. **Spironolactone** may produce some useful degree of androgen blockade.*

3. **Stress alopecia**

This is referred to as telogen effluvium. It is a diffuse thinning of the hair following a severe physiological insult which has altered the growth cycle of hairs so as to convert the majority in the active phase to the resting phase.

- It is well known to follow severe clinical disease, such as fever, haemorrhage, surgery, trauma, starvation, childbirth or psychiatric illness.
- It may also accompany specific diseases, such as iron deficiency (q.v.), thyroid disease and secondary syphilis (q.v.).
- It may follow the use of a number of drugs, most notably cytotoxic agents (which interfere with mitosis in the hair follicles, rather than converting them to the resting phase) but also allopurinol, heparin (q.v.), indometacin, lithium (q.v.), nitrofurantoin, propranolol and valproate (q.v.). Oral contraceptives (q.v.) on the other hand can give an androgenetic alopecia.

Treatment with zinc-containing multivitamin preparations can improve this condition by strengthening the hair shaft.

4. **Cicatricial alopecia**

This is permanent loss of hair due to destruction of the hair follicles from severe viral, bacterial or fungal infection.

It is also associated with trauma, neoplasia, scleroderma (q.v.), discoid lupus, atrophic lichen planus or occasionally severe acne.

5. **Traction alopecia**

This refers to local hair loss from mechanical trauma, sometimes from fingers (i.e. trichotillomania).

Bibliography

Del Rosso JQ. Disorders of hair. In: *Scientific American Medicine. Dermatology.* Hamilton: Dekker Medicine. 2020.

Kaufman KD. Long-term (5-year) multinational experience with finasteride 1 mg in the treatment of men with androgenetic alopecia. *Eur J Dermatol* 2002; 12: 38.

Paus R, Cotsarelis G. The biology of hair follicles. *N Engl J Med* 1999; 341: 491.

Rusting RL. Hair: why it grows, why it stops. In: *The Frontiers of Biotechnology.* New York: Scientific American. 2002; p 66.

Shapiro J, Price VH. Hair regrowth: therapeutic options. *Dermatol Clin* 1998; 16: 341.

Tosti A, Piraccini BM. Androgenetic alopecia. *Int J Dermatol* 1999; 38 (suppl. 1): 1.

Wolff K, Goldsmith L, Katz S, et al., eds. *Fitzpatrick's Dermatology in General Medicine.* 7th edition. New York: McGraw-Hill. 2007.

Alpha-fetoprotein

Alpha-fetoprotein (AFP, tumour-associated antigen) is an oncofetal antigen, present in fetal tissue but not in the corresponding normal adult tissue. It is, however, elaborated in a number of adult malignant cells, because most of the antigen is carbohydrate-determined and post-translational modification is readily achieved by differential glycosylation (which becomes similar to that in fetal tissue). It is thus an important **tumour marker** (q.v.).

The normal level is <7.75 µg/L. Its half-life is 6 days.

Increased levels of alpha-fetoprotein may be found in
- hepatocellular carcinoma (q.v.),
- liver metastases from gastrointestinal cancer,
- acute and chronic hepatitis (q.v.),
- non-seminoma testicular cancer,

- extragonadal germ cell tumour (e.g. in the anterior mediastinum),
- fetal neural tube defects (q.v.), when it may be demonstrated in both the maternal blood and in the embryonic fluid.

Bibliography

Locker GY, Hamilton S, Harrus J, et al. ASCO 2006 update of recommendations for the use of tumor markers in gastrointestinal cancer. *J Clin Oncol* 2006; 24: 5313.

McIntire KR, Waldmann TA, Moertel CG, et al. Serum alpha-fetoprotein in patients with neoplasms of the gastrointestinal tract. *Cancer Res* 1975; 35: 991.

Alpha$_1$-antitrypsin deficiency

Alpha$_1$-antitrypsin deficiency (AATD, α_1-ATD) was first described as a serum electrophoretic abnormality by Laurell and Eriksson in Scandinavia in 1963 and was soon recognized to be associated with chronic airway obstruction.

Alpha$_1$-antitrypsin (α_1AT) is one of the major plasma antiproteases. It is thus a member of the superfamily of **serpins** (q.v.), which include inhibitors controlling coagulation, fibrinolysis and complement activation. It is also an acute phase reactant. It has a 394 amino acid sequence, and its molecular weight is 52 kDa. It is synthesized mainly in the liver and has a plasma concentration of about 1–2 g/L. In the alveolar wall, it is presumed to function to inactivate proteases, especially neutrophil elastase, and thus to prevent interstitial injury from the recurrent release of this enzyme from phagocytes.

Alpha$_1$-antitrypsin has a complex inheritance with over 30 autosomal codominant alleles at a single locus called Pi ('protease inhibitor') on chromosome 14 producing gene products which are separately identifiable by their different electrophoretic mobility, though most are associated with a normal concentration of the protein in plasma. The most frequent protein is Pi^M, i.e. of medium mobility, and is found in 90% or more of the population. However, homozygous Pi^{ZZ} occurs in 1:1000 or less of the population and is associated with only 10–15% of the normal plasma concentration. The Z variant has only a single amino acid difference from the normal M protein, but this difference impairs hepatic excretion of the molecule, so that there are granular cytoplasmic inclusion bodies in the liver associated with the plasma deficiency in affected subjects.

The clinical importance of alpha$_1$-antitrypsin deficiency (α_1-ATD) is its association with **emphysema** in most patients (80%). The prevalence is 100% in those who also smoke. The emphysema occurs early, i.e. by 35–40 yr in smokers and by 45–55 yr in non-smokers. It is usually panacinar and especially affects the lower lobes. It is responsible for about 2% of cases of emphysema.

Hepatic cirrhosis also occurs in 10–20% of patients, mainly in those over 50 yr.

In severe α_1-ATD, there may be an increased incidence of asthma.

The heterozygotes Pi^{MZ} have about 50% of the normal plasma concentration, which is now considered not to be associated with clinical disease, the threshold for which is probably about 40% of normal.

*Treatment consists of **replacement (augmentation) therapy**, which is purified plasma enriched for AAT, preparations of which have been commercially available since the 1980s. It is given as 60 mg/kg IV weekly or 250 mg/kg IV monthly, based on original confirmation of biochemical efficacy and later demonstration of improved lung function. However, even in the absence of trial evidence of mortality reduction, replacement therapy although expensive has been calculated to be probably cost-effective when given to patients with abnormal lung function.*

- *Clearly smoking should be avoided.*
- *Successful **lung transplantation** has been reported.*

Screening has been recommended in younger adults with emphysema, but also with chronic obstructive lung disease in general, including poorly reversible asthma.

Bibliography

Alkins SA, O'Malley P. Should health-care systems pay for replacement therapy in patients with α1-antitrypsin deficiency? *Chest* 2000; 117: 875.

Burdon JGW, Knight KR, Brenton S, et al. Antiproteinase deficiency, emphysema and replacement therapy. *Aust NZ J Med* 1996; 26: 769.

Carrell RW, Whisstock J, Lomas DA. Conformational changes in serpins and the mechanism of alpha1-antitrypsin deficiency. *Am J Respir Crit Care Med* 1994; 150: S171.

Eden E, Mitchell D, Mehlman B, et al. Atopy, asthma, and emphysema in patients with severe α-1-antitrypsin deficiency. *Am J Repir Crit Care Med* 1997; 156: 68.

Gadek JE, ed. Alpha1-antitrypsin: A world view. *Chest* 1997; 110 (suppl.).

Hogarth DK, Rachelefsky G. Screening and familial testing of patients for α1-antitrypsin deficiency. *Chest* 2008; 133: 981.

Hutchison DCS, Hughes MD. Alpha-1-antitrypsin replacement therapy: will its efficacy ever be proved? *Eur Respir J* 1997; 10: 2191.

Larsson C. Natural history and life expectancy in severe α1-antitrypsin PiZ. *Acta Med Scand* 1978; 204: 345.

Laurell C-B, Erikson S. The electrophoretic α1-globin pattern of serum in α1-antitrypsin deficiency. *Scand J Clin Lab Invest* 1963; 15: 132.

Stoller JK. Clinical features and natural history of severe α1-antitrypsin deficiency. *Chest* 1997; 111: 123S.

Altitude See

- High altitude.

Aluminium

Aluminium (Al, atomic number 13, atomic weight 27, first called **aluminum**) is a light metal of the boron group, first isolated in 1825. Although it is the most abundant metal in the Earth's outer crust, comprising 8% by weight (and exceeded in abundance only by the elements oxygen and silicon), it is never found pure in nature because of its great reactivity, and it is usually obtained as hydrated oxides (bauxite). Following modern production in 1886, it progressively became the most used non-ferrous metal, and from 1960 it was exceeded only by iron in world metal production.

> Aluminium is important in clinical medicine because of
> - its use in gastric medications, and
> - its toxicity.

Aluminium-containing antacids are commonly prescribed but should be used with care, particularly in renal failure, because they are very constipating and because of the possibility of aluminium absorption.

Aluminium is also contained within multiple negatively charged sulphated groups in **sucralfate**, which is a basic aluminium salt of sulphated sucrose used for the treatment of peptic ulceration. Although aluminium can be released from sucralfate with the production of detectable levels in serum, clinical harm from this phenomenon is unlikely, except perhaps in patients with renal failure in whom toxic levels (i.e. >3.7 μM, 100 mcg/L) have been reported.

Aluminium toxicity is seen primarily in patients with renal failure, since it is normally excreted via the kidney. It has occurred either because of intake from aluminium-contaminated dialysis solution or from oral aluminium-containing phosphate binders. The normal serum aluminium is usually <10 mcg/L and toxicity is seen at levels >50–100 mcg/L. However, serum levels are an indirect indication of body load and can be normal even if tissues such as bone and brain are loaded.

Toxicity is manifest by
- encephalopathy (q.v.),
- osteomalacia,
- anaemia (q.v.).

The **encephalopathy** (q.v.) has been termed dialysis dementia (see Dementia) and may be a progressive and eventually fatal process. Increased neurological difficulty occurs with confusion, aphasia, myoclonus and focal signs, which typically are worse after each dialysis. However, it should be remembered that an encephalopathy of non-specific nature is also seen in uraemia and following dialysis. This latter encephalopathy does not correlate with identifiable biochemical changes but is probably related to rapid dialysis-induced biochemical dysequilibrium, when the serum osmolality becomes less than the cerebral osmolality with resultant cerebral oedema causing stupor, fits and raised intracranial pressure.

The **osteomalacia** is vitamin D-resistant, typically with a slightly increased plasma calcium level, a low PTH level, weakness and proximal myopathy (q.v.), and severe bone pain with pathological fractures. This arises because aluminium blocks the mineralization of osteoid. Since the process is vitamin D-resistant, the administration of vitamin D may result in marked hypercalcaemia. Osteomalacia of a similar nature has been reported with long-term total parenteral nutrition, also from aluminium deposition.

The **anaemia** (q.v.) is usually normochromic and normocytic and occurs because aluminium inhibits iron utilization and thus the erythroid precursors. The iron stores and serum ferritin levels are normal.

The diagnosis of aluminium toxicity is made by challenge with desferrioxamine (DFO) (q.v.) and is confirmed by bone biopsy. The DFO challenge consists of the administration of 40 mg/kg IV over 30 min and the demonstration of an increase in serum aluminium level of >200 mcg/L at 48 hr. Bone biopsy shows the typical changes of aluminium-induced osteomalacia, with decreased bone formation and aluminium deposits on the calcifying front on trabecular surfaces.

*The treatment of aluminium toxicity is also with **desferrioxamine** (DFO), in a dose 2 g IV over 30 min after dialysis. The DFO-aluminium complex is removed by the next dialysis, though aluminium itself is not normally removed by dialysis because it is protein-bound. Improvement can take 6 months or more, and in the meantime DFO treatment can cause hypotension, retinal and auditory toxicity, proneness to opportunistic infections (especially with Yersinia) and increased dialysis encephalopathy (see Chelating agents).*

Bibliography
Alfrey AC. Aluminum intoxication. *N Engl J Med* 1984; 310: 1113.
Ciba Foundation. *Aluminium in Biology and Medicine*. London. 1992.
Cooke K, Gould MH. The health effects of aluminium – a review. *J R Soc Health* 1991; 111: 163.
Kaiser L, Schwartz KA. Aluminum-induced anemia. *Am J Kidney Dis* 1985; 6: 348.
McCarthy DM. Drug therapy (sucralfate). *N Engl J Med* 1991; 325: 1017.
Mulla H, Peek G, Upton D, et al. Plasma aluminum levels during sucralfate prophylaxis for stress ulceration in critically ill patients on continuous venovenous hemofiltration: a randomized controlled trial. *Crit Care Med* 2001; 29: 267.
Wills MR, Savory J. Aluminium poisoning: dialysis encephalopathy, osteomalacia, and anaemia. *Lancet* 1983; 2: 29.

Alveolar hypoventilation See
- Sleep disorders of breathing.

Alzheimer's disease See
- Anticholinesterases,
- Dementia.

Amanita See
- Mushroom poisoning.

Amenorrhoea

Primary amenorrhoea (i.e. failure of periods to commence) is relatively rare.

Secondary amenorrhoea (i.e. the cessation of periods) is of much greater clinical importance. The commonest causes are pregnancy or the menopause, but otherwise the condition is probably due to anovulation.

Failure of ovulation can be due to a variety of disorders and can occur at several levels, namely,
- **hypothalamus**
  - this probably includes both athlete's amenorrhoea, which appears to be a reversible neuroendocrine disturbance, and amenorrhoea due to significant weight loss,
- **pituitary**
  - especially due to a microadenoma, which is associated with hyperprolactinaemia,
  - increased prolactin levels prevent release of gonadotrophin-releasing hormone (GnRH) and thus the follicle-stimulating hormone (FSH) and luteinizing hormone (LH) required for follicular development and ovulation,
- **ovary**
  - associated with the polycystic ovary syndrome (q.v.) or with systemic problems, such as autoimmune disease (q.v.), or cytotoxic therapy.

See
- Anorexia nervosa,
- Cushing's syndrome.

Bibliography
Hall JE. Normal and abnormal menstruation. In: *Scientific American Medicine. Women's Health*. Hamilton: Dekker Medicine. 2020.
Nattiv A, Agostini R, Drinkwater B, et al. The female athlete triad: the inter-relatedness of disordered eating, amenorrhea, and osteoporosis. *Clin Sports Med* 1994; 13: 405.
Ng E, Sztal-Mazer S, Davis SR. Functional hypothalamic amenorrhoea: a diagnosis of exclusion. *Med J Aust* 2022; 216: 73.
Tan SL, Jacobs HS. Recent advances in the management of patients with amenorrhoea. *Clin Obstet Gynaecol* 1985; 12: 725.

Aminoaciduria

Aminoaciduria occurs in many forms of renal disease. These include some types of
- glomerulonephritis (q.v.), e.g. focal GN,
- tubulointerstitial disease (q.v.), e.g. Fanconi syndrome.

It is often associated with normoglycaemic glycosuria.

Aminocaproic acid

Epsilon **aminocaproic acid** (EACA) has been used since the 1960s as a fibrinolytic inhibitor in a number of conditions, but it has now been superseded by the related but 10-fold more potent analog **tranexamic acid** (q.v.).

See
- Angioedema,
- Fibrinolysis,
- Von Willebrand's disease.

Ammonia See
- Hyperammonaemia.

See also
- Acute lung irritation,
- Inhalation injury.

Amnesia

Amnesia (memory impairment) may be due to a variety of disorders, which may grouped as follows,
- drugs

- such as classically with alcohol or sedatives (particularly benzodiazepines),
- but also unexpectedly sometimes with ranitidine, simvastatin, selective serotonin reuptake inhibitors (SSRIs),
- metabolic disorders
  - such as hypoglycaemia or multiorgan failure (q.v.),
- structural problems
  - such as cerebrovascular disease, dementia (q.v.), head injury, organic psychosis,
- transient global amnesia
  - a brief and benign state with a good prognosis,
- miscellaneous conditions
  - such as narcolepsy (uncommonly).

Amniotic fluid embolism

Amniotic fluid embolism (AFE) is an uncommon but serious complication of labour, delivery or the early postpartum state. Although it may accompany any obstetric procedure, it is most frequently seen following Caesarean section. It may also occur in prolonged labour, following fetal death in utero or with elective evacuation of a missed second trimester abortion. Its overall prevalence is 1 in 8000–80,000 live births. The development of registries in the USA and in the UK has assisted understanding of this dramatic condition.

It presents acutely, and its severity may range from subclinical to fulminating.

Typically, the clinical features are of the sudden onset of
- respiratory failure, with an ARDS-like picture,
- disseminated intravascular coagulation (q.v.).
There may be shock, coma or fits.

Haemodynamic findings include pulmonary hypertension, elevated pulmonary artery wedge pressure and impaired left ventricular function (e.g. decreased left ventricular stroke work index (LVSWI). As with any venous embolic phenomenon, systemic features may be prominent if there is a potential right-to-left shunt, e.g. patent foramen ovale.

Diagnosis is clinical, as laboratory evidence of circulating fetal material in the mother is non-specific. More importantly, the relevant fetal material is not necessarily particulate in the traditional sense of squames or hair but is more demonstrably humoral in its effect (i.e. procoagulant, immunological and vasoactive). Thus, the more recent term 'anaphylactoid reaction of pregnancy' has some merit. In addition to the laboratory finding of a generalized coagulopathy, a number of blood tests have been reported to be highly sensitive diagnostically for AFE, such as the serological identification in maternal serum of sialyl TN (STN) antigen.

The differential diagnosis includes
- placental abruption (abruptio placentae) (q.v.),
- septic shock,
- pulmonary embolism,
- tension pneumothorax,
- myocardial ischaemia,
- anaphylaxis,
- aspiration.

Treatment is prompt **resuscitation**, *and cardiorespiratory and haematological support, since the condition is self-limited.*

The mortality in severe cases used to be about 80%, with up to half dying in the first hour. It is doubtful if the prognosis is nowadays as poor as this, but the condition is still the cause of about 10% of all maternal deaths.

Bibliography
Choi DMA, Duffy BL. Amniotic fluid embolism. *Anaesth Intens Care* 1995; 23: 741.
Clark SL. Amniotic fluid embolism. *Obstet Gynecol* 2014; 123: 337.
Clark SL, Hankins GDV, Dudley DA, et al. Amniotic fluid embolism: analysis of the national registry. *Am J Obstet Gynecol* 1995; 172; 1158.
Clark SL, Romero R, Dildy GA, et al. Proposed diagnostic criteria for the case definition of amniotic fluid embolism in research studies. *Am J Obstet Gynecol* 2016; 215: 408.
Gist RS, Stafford IP, Leibowitz AB, et al. Amniotic fluid embolism. *Anesth Analg* 2009; 108: 1599.
Locksmith GJ. Amniotic fluid embolism. *Obstet Gynecol Clin North Am* 1999; 26: 435.
McDougall RJ, Duke GJ. Amniotic fluid embolism syndrome: case report and review. *Anaesth Intens Care* 1995; 23: 735.
Monga M. Amniotic fluid embolism: a diagnostic dilemma. *Crit Care Med* 2012; 40: 2236.
Moore J, Baldisseri MR. Amniotic fluid embolism. *Crit Care Med* 2005; 33 (suppl.): S279.
Morgan M. Amniotic fluid embolism. *Anaesthesia* 1979; 34: 20.
Oi H, Kobayashi H, Hirashima Y, et al. Serological and immunohistochemical diagnosis of amniotic fluid embolism. *Semin Thromb Hemost* 1998; 24: 479.
Tuffnell DJ. Amniotic fluid embolism. *Curr Opinion Obstet Gynecol* 2003; 15: 119.

Amoebiasis

Amoebiasis is due to infection with the protozoan *Entamoeba histolytica*, the main human pathogen in this class. Infection occurs following the ingestion of cysts from infected human faeces and is thus via water-borne or food-borne routes. There is a worldwide prevalence of up to 10% of the population, and only malaria and schistosomiasis are more important parasitic causes of death worldwide. In developed countries, it is seen predominantly in travellers to or immigrants from an endemic area (such as South-East Asia or India) or in homosexual men.

Clinical infection usually involves either the colon or the liver.

- Although most cases of colitis are asymptomatic, abdominal discomfort and diarrhoea, even to the extent of dysentery, may be seen. In these cases, there is extensive colonic invasion with necrosis and ulceration. Occasionally, an abdominal mass (amoeboma) may be felt.
- The liver is involved via haematogenous spread. The right lobe is particularly affected, and there is often a solitary abscess which may be up to 20 cm in diameter. In most such cases, the colitis has been asymptomatic and instead there is abdominal pain and hepatomegaly. There are marked systemic symptoms if the abscess ruptures into the chest, when in addition there may be expectoration of the characteristic chocolate sputum with the consistency of anchovy paste.

Investigations typically show anaemia, leukocytosis and raised alkaline phosphatase. The faeces are positive for occult blood and may show Charcot–Leyden crystals (produced when eosinophils coalesce and fragment). Imaging confirms a liver mass. However, definitive diagnosis requires microscopic examination of faeces or biopsy material for cysts or trophozoites. Serology is sensitive and specific for invasive disease, though not for colitis alone. Culture, antigen detection and molecular techniques are available in specialized laboratories.

> The differential diagnosis of amoebic colitis includes
> - diverticulitis,
> - ulcerative colitis (q.v.),
> - Crohn's disease (q.v.),
> - infection with campylobacter, salmonella or shigella,
> - irritable bowel syndrome (see Colitis).
>
> The differential diagnosis of an amoebic liver mass includes
> - pyogenic or hydatid abscess (see Hydatid disease).

Treatment is with **metronidazole** *750 mg orally tds for 5–10 days*. This is so effective even for liver abscess that drainage is not usually necessary. However, metronidazole may be associated with unpleasant side-effects, including nausea, headache, dizziness, a metallic taste, dark urine and a disulfiram-like effect following ingestion of alcohol. **Tinidazole** *2 g per day is an effective alternative to metronidazole.*

Asymptomatic patients are carriers for up to 12 months and should be treated with a luminal agent, e.g. **paromomycin** *500 mg orally tds for 7 days.*

Bibliography

Adams EB, Macleod IN. Invasive amebiasis. *Medicine* 1977; 56: 315 & 325.

Van Hal SJ, Stark DJ, Fotedar R, et al. Amoebiaisis: current status in Australia. *Med J Aust* 2007; 186: 412.

Amphetamines

Amphetamine (alpha-methylphenethylamine) has few medical indications approved nowadays (e.g. narcolepsy, childhood hyperactivity). Its main use is non-medical, as a CNS-stimulant. It has thus been popular with long-distance truck drivers and with students prior to examinations. It was used effectively to prevent military fatigue during WWII, when dexamphetamine (Benzedrine) was used by US soldiers and methamphetamine (Pervitin) was used by German soldiers. Nowadays, amphetamines are one of the commonest illicit drugs of abuse, either for recreational purposes or because of addiction.

The amphetamines are racemic β-phenolisopropylamine, although the d-isomer (**dexamphetamine**) is the main therapeutic agent. It is a sympathomimetic amine, structurally related to the more familiar catecholamines.

Related drugs are

- 3.4-methylenedioxyamphetamine (**MDMA** or 'ecstasy'), a derivative synthesized in 1912 as an appetite suppressant but never commercially marketed, until it appeared as a psychedelic agent in the 1970s and recreational drug in the 1980s,
- parametoxyamphetamine (PMA), synthesized as a substitute for MDMA,
- **methamphetamine** (its crystalline form is popularly referred to as 'ice' or 'crystal meth'), which has an increased central to peripheral effect ratio compared with dexamphetamine.

CNS stimulation gives psychic effects of alertness, euphoria, increased concentration, increased mental performance (but only for simple tasks), increased physical performance (but not aerobic power), but also anorexia, headache and confusion. MDMA (ecstasy) prompts abnormal behaviour, such as marathon dancing, especially when taken by a group (aggregation toxicology) as at 'rave' parties. PMA has been sold either as a substitute or as a flow-on agent for MDMA, but it is even more toxic.

> The toxic effects of amphetamines are numerous and can be life-threatening. They include the following.
> - **central effects**
>   - Those described above are accompanied by an acute psychosis.
>   - This consists of aggression, hallucinations, paranoia and enhanced libido, followed later by depression and fatigue.
>   - Fatal coma, seizures or cerebral haemorrhage may occur.
>   - Hyponatraemia may result from vasopressin stimulation.
> - **cardiovascular features**
>   - These are usually prominent because of the drug's sympathomimetic effects.
>   - Hypertension, arrhythmias, angina and vasculitis are seen.
> - **hyperthermia and rhabdomyolysis**
>   - These are followed by coagulopathy and acute renal failure.
>   - These features are seen especially with MDMA and PMA and resemble the 'serotonin syndrome' (q.v.).
> - **dry mouth, metallic taste and abdominal pain**
> - **acute liver failure, with damage resembling hepatitis**

The toxic effects of amphetamine are not simply related to excess dosage, as they can be either
- severe following a dose as low as 30 mg (which is only a maximum daily therapeutic dose), or
- not fatal at doses as high as 300 mg.

Acute treatment consists of **urinary acidification** *(e.g. with ammonium chloride, which increases excretion), sedation and blood pressure control.*

Dantrolene and serotonin antagonists may be useful in the management of MDMA-induced hyperthermia.

Dialysis and haemoperfusion are not effective.

Chronic use can result in considerable tolerance. Thus, despite increasingly high doses, euphoria disappears, and fatigue, depression, irritability and even paranoia appear. Headache, nausea, tremor, dilated pupils and hypertension are common.

Abrupt withdrawal leads to profound psychological though not physical consequences, in particular with depression which may be severe and prolonged.

Recently, a many-fold increase in the risk of idiopathic pulmonary arterial hypertension (q.v.) has also been found among patients who have used amphetamine, methamphetamine and cocaine (q.v.). Similarly, the related anorectic drugs, **fenfluramine**, **dexfenfluramine** and **phentermine**, were withdrawn from the market worldwide in 1997, because of the discovery of an increased incidence of pulmonary hypertension (20-fold risk above baseline) and a potentially important association with acquired heart valve abnormalities. The valvulopathy typically caused mitral and/or aortic regurgitation and sometimes required valve replacement. The pathogenesis of this latter unexpected effect is unknown, but it has been postulated to be similar to the cardiac impact of the carcinoid syndrome or ergot derivatives. Neither its progression nor its reversibility is currently known. These serious adverse effects are not thought to apply to the newer anorectic amine, **sibutramine**, a selective serotonin and noradrenaline (norepinephrine) reuptake inhibitor (SNRI).

Synthetic **cathinones** are related structurally to amphetamine and have recently become novel drugs of abuse. A number of chemical variants have become street drugs, known by such subterfuge names as 'bath salts'. They produce amphetamine-like effects and have similar toxicity, as described above.

On the other hand, although **MDMA** is a psychedelic recreational drug with no approved therapeutic indications, it has undergone extensive research for its potential as an adjunct to psychotherapy in the treatment of PTSD and perhaps other neuropsychiatric disorders.

Bibliography

Byard RW, Rodgers NG, James RA, et al. Death and paramethoxyamphetamine – an evolving problem. *Med J Aust* 2002; 176: 496.

Chin KM, Channick RN, Rubin LJ. Is methamphetamine use associated with idiopathic pulmonary arterial hypertension? *Chest* 2006; 130: 1657.

Connolly HM, Crary JL, McGoon MD, et al. Valvular heart disease associated with fenfluramine-phentermine. *N Engl J Med* 1997; 337: 581.

Fishman AP. Aminorex to fen/phen: an epidemic foretold. *Circulation* 1999; 99: 156.

Henry JA, Jeffreys KJ, Dawling S. Toxicity and deaths from 3, 4-methylenedioxy methamphetamine ('ecstasy'). *Lancet* 1992; 340: 384.

Milroy CM. Ten years of 'ecstasy'. *J R Soc Med* 1999; 92: 68.

Mokhlesi B, Garinella, PS, Joffe A, et al. Street drug abuse leading to critical illness. *Intens Care Med* 2004; 30: 1526.

Mokhlesi B, Leikin JB, Murray P, et al. Adult toxicology in critical care: part II: specific poisonings. *Chest* 2003; 123: 897.

Parrott AC, ed. *MDMA (Methylenedioxy-methamphetamine)*. Basel: Karger. 2000.

Screaton GR, Cairns HS, Sarner M, et al. Hyperpyrexia and rhabdomyolysis after MDMA ('ecstasy') abuse. *Lancet* 1992; 339: 677.

Amyloid *See*

- Multiple myeloma.
  See also
- Ankylosing spondylitis,
- Asthma – Stridor,
- Beta$_2$-microglobulin,
- Cardiomyopathy,
- Familial Mediterranean fever,
- Fibrinolysis,
- Glomerular diseases,
- Glycogen storage diseases,
- Interstitial lung diseases,
- Malabsorption,
- Mouth diseases – Glossitis,
- Nails,
- Pseudo-obstruction of the colon,
- Pulmonary hypertension,
- Pulmonary nodules,
- Purpura,
- Sarcoidosis,
- Splenomegaly.

Amyotrophic lateral sclerosis *See*

- Motor neuron disease.

Anaemia

Anaemia refers to decreased circulating haemoglobin, but as for many biological parameters any definition is of limited value if based on a single number. Thus, acute blood loss is not initially associated with a decreased haemoglobin concentration, while haemodilution (e.g. in pregnancy) can cause a decreased haemoglobin concentration while being associated with an increased red blood cell mass.

Nevertheless, anaemia is defined as a haemoglobin level below the lower limit of normal for the sex and age of the patient, which in turn depends on the range determined in a specific clinical laboratory (the typical normal range being 130–170 g/L for men and 115–150 g/L for women). For practical purposes, anaemia is commonly considered to be relevant if the Hb is <100 g/L in men and <90 g/L in women.

The normal lifespan of red blood cells (RBCs) in the circulation is about 115 days, with thus about 1% or the equivalent of 50 mL of blood being destroyed and replaced daily. The bone marrow reserve is normally less than 2-fold, but it can rise up to 8-fold in chronic, severe haemolysis (see below). The lifespan of transfused RBCs is about 50% of normal, with an initial clearance of up to 25% in the spleen due to storage lesions. The principles of blood transfusion have been progressively revised in recent years, and current recommendations support a restrictive policy in most circumstances. However, research is ongoing to clarify a number of still unanswered questions in the area of blood management.

The cardinal features of anaemia are weakness, fatigue and pallor. However, while typical of anaemia, especially of recent onset, these features are clearly non-specific.

> Anaemia is very common, indeed almost universal, in critically ill patients, in whom its cause is usually multifactorial, including
> - prior illness,
> - prior and current nutritional state,
> - acute blood loss (gastrointestinal tract, surgery, trauma),
> - iatrogenic blood loss (repeated venesection),
> - haemodilution (from IV fluids),
> - haemolysis (including neocytolysis), and
> - impaired bone marrow function (related chiefly to decreased levels of erythropoietin – q.v.).

In this setting, despite the apparent clinical advantage of increased oxygen delivery in critical illness, blood transfusion in non-bleeding patients is generally recommended to be restrictive, with a commonly accepted haemoglobin threshold of 70 g/L.

> Anaemia is traditionally classified on the basis of red blood cell kinetics and morphology into three main aetiological groups, namely, those due to
> 1. blood loss,
> 2. haemolysis,
> 3. impaired production.

1. Anaemia due to blood loss

Although blood loss is usually readily apparent, sometimes it may be occult, especially from the gastrointestinal tract. Blood loss whether overt or occult is most commonly from the gastrointestinal tract or in women from obstetric or gynaecological causes.

In Intensive Care patients, blood loss may be iatrogenic from repeated venepuncture for laboratory testing.

Rarer causes of a similar anaemia include
- long-distance athletic performance,
- paroxysmal nocturnal haemoglobinuria (q.v.).

> In acute blood loss, the haemoglobin concentration may take up to 3 days to reach its new (lower) plateau.

After acute blood loss, the bone marrow reserve is less than 2-fold (unlike in chronic haemolysis when it is up to 8-fold), because iron is mobilized less easily from the tissues than from the destroyed red blood cells. Moreover, the maximum amount of iron that can be mobilized from stores is insufficient to replace even normally senescent red blood cells, so that continued iron intake is required to maintain normal haemoglobin levels.

The clinical features of blood loss or iron deficiency anaemia are those of any form of hypoxia. In addition, there may be non-haematological manifestations of **iron deficiency** (q.v.).

> The differential diagnosis of anaemia due to blood loss includes
> - the anaemia of chronic disease (see below),
> - haemoglobinopathy (especially thalassaemia) (q.v.),
> - sideroblastic anaemia (q.v.).

Unless the condition is mild, when diagnosis may be difficult, there is
- hypochromia and microcytosis on the peripheral blood film,
- low serum iron,
- low iron-binding saturation (the ratio of serum iron to serum transferrin, or iron-binding capacity, is <20%) – a more important finding,
- low serum ferritin (which reflects iron stores) – also a more important finding.

See Iron, see Ferritin.

However, the serum iron, transferrin and iron-binding (transferrin) saturation are also low in anaemia of chronic disease, and the serum ferritin may be elevated as an acute phase reactant in concomitant disease, such as infection or malignancy.

*Treatment with **iron** supplementation is straightforward, but failure of response suggests*
- *persistent bleeding,*
- *concurrent inflammation,*
- *associated folic acid deficiency,*
- *failure of iron absorption (malabsorption or iron-binding foods),*
- *an alternative diagnosis.*

Symptomatic improvement commences within a few days, but the haemoglobin may not start to rise for a week and may take up to 6 weeks to normalize.

2. **Anaemia due to haemolysis**

Haemolytic anaemia occurs when the rate of red blood cell destruction exceeds the bone marrow's productive capacity. Thus, although the normal lifespan of red blood cells in the circulation is about 115 days, the marrow reserve is such that it can compensate for a red blood cell lifespan of only 30 days or even less. The marrow reserve is thus considerable, being normally up to 5-fold and rising to perhaps 8-fold with severe and prolonged stimulation, provided there is an adequate haematinic supply.

> The hallmarks of haemolysis are
> - anaemia,
> - jaundice (with increased LDH and decreased haptoglobin),
> - a marked reticulocytosis on peripheral blood film,
> - renal damage, thrombosis and tissue hypoxia in severe cases,
> - pigment gallstones in long-standing cases.

Haemolysis is due to either **intracorpuscular** or **extracorpuscular** red cell defects. The sites of destruction are usually **extravascular** (i.e. the reticuloendothelial system), except in severe cases when it can be **intravascular** (with resultant haemoglobinaemia, haemoglobinuria and disseminated intravascular coagulation).

Intracorpuscular defects indicate an abnormal red blood cell. All such conditions are hereditary, except for paroxysmal nocturnal haemoglobinuria (q.v.).

Intracorpuscular defects may be of haemoglobin, cell membrane or cell metabolism.
- **Haemoglobin defects**

These are numerous (see Haemoglobin disorders) and particularly include thalassaemia and sickle cell anaemia.
- **Red blood cell membrane defects**
- These include
   - hereditary spherocytosis,
   - **paroxysmal nocturnal haemoglobinuria** (PNH) (q.v.),
- **Red blood cell metabolic defects**

These particularly include glucose 6-phosphate dehydrogenase (G6PD) deficiency (q.v.).

Extracorpuscular defects include the following.
- **Autoimmune haemolytic anaemia** (AHA)

This may be either idiopathic or secondary to conditions such as lymphoma, multiple myeloma (q.v.), systemic lupus erythematosus (q.v.), ulcerative colitis (q.v.).

The direct Coombs test is positive, and there may be jaundice, hepatosplenomegaly and lymphadenopathy (q.v.) in severe cases. In addition to spherocytosis, there is macrocytosis and sometimes leukopenia or thrombocytopenia (q.v.). Blood cross-matching is difficult.

*The condition usually responds to **corticosteroids**, but sometimes splenectomy or immunosuppressive therapy may be needed. **Rituximab** (q.v.) has been shown to be helpful in refractory cases.*

- **Microangiopathic haemolysis** (q.v.)
- **Cold agglutinin disease** (q.v.)
- **Drug-induced haemolysis**

Methyldopa in particular, but also laevodopa and procainamide, can cause an acquired haemolytic anaemia.

Aspirin, beta-lactam antibiotics, isoniazid, quinidine, rifampicin and sulphonamides can contribute to immune haemolysis.

Nitroglycerin, 'recreational' nitrites and dapsone can occupy the oxygen-binding cleft of haemoglobin and generate free radicals with the consequent production of methaemoglobin (q.v.) and possibly haemolysis due to membrane damage. A similar picture has been reported after paraquat ingestion (q.v.).

Haemolysis similar to that induced by drugs may also be found with
- exposure to toxins (e.g. snake venom),
- physical agents (e.g. cardiopulmonary bypass, fresh water drowning, burns, intravenous water),
- liver disease,
- renal disease,
- lead poisoning (q.v.),
- infections, including clostridial infections (q.v.), infectious mononucleosis, *H. influenzae* type b infection, malaria (q.v.),
- hypophosphataemia (<0.3 mmol/L) (q.v.).

A similar picture has also been reported following lipid emulsion overdose.

- **Incompatible blood transfusion**
- **March haemoglobinuria**

This is similar to microangiopathic haemolysis (q.v.), except that it occurs after prolonged running, especially on a hard surface. It is presumed to be due to destruction of red blood cells in the vessels in the soles of the feet.

There is haemoglobinaemia and haemoglobinuria, which may be clinically apparent for up to 24 hr.

- **Hypersplenism** (q.v.)

3. **Anaemia due to impaired production**

Anaemia due to impaired production may be associated with a bone marrow which is

- hypoplastic,
- normal,
- hyperplastic.

Marrow hypoplasia usually results in concomitant neutropenia and/or thrombocytopenia (and thus infection and/or haemorrhage) as well as anaemia. Compensatory extramedullary haemopoiesis is evident from the leukoerythroblastic peripheral blood film. There is typically immunological damage to pluripotential haematopoietic stem cells in the bone marrow, regardless of the causative trigger. Molecular testing is now used to dissect out these complex issues.

The chief form of this condition is referred to as **aplastic anaemia**, which is a rare but serious form of acquired bone marrow failure.

Aplastic anaemia may have a variety of causative associations, including
- drugs
  - cytotoxics, sometimes chloramphenicol, gold, and previously phenylbutazone,
- toxic inhalants
  - e.g. organic solvents, such as benzene,
- irradiation,
- infections
  - especially hepatitis C (q.v.),
- immune diseases
  - systemic lupus erythematosus (q.v.), graft-versus-host disease,
- pre-leukaemia or paroxysmal nocturnal haemoglobinuria (q.v.),
- thymoma
  - which is typically associated with a pure red cell aplasia (see Myasthenia gravis).

*The treatment of aplastic anaemia may require **bone marrow transplantation**, which has a cure rate of over 90% if the donor is matched. This is the only curative treatment modality.*

Alternatively, immunosuppression with ciclosporin or anti-thymocyte globulin (ATG) can lead to a useful remission, though relapse is common.

Pure red cell aplasia (PRCA) is a separate condition on cytogenetic testing and appears to be a prodrome to acute myeloid leukaemia or a myelodysplastic disorder. It is an occasional complication of erythropoietin treatment for the anaemia of chronic renal failure and is due to antierythropoietin antibody formation.

Normal-appearing bone marrow may be associated with defective red cell production and thus anaemia in systemic disease and in renal disease.

Systemic diseases, such as inflammation, neoplasia and trauma, cause **anaemia of chronic disease**. This is normochromic and normocytic, with both the serum iron and iron-binding capacity low and ferritin normal. The serum erythropoietin level is often low. The anaemia is generally mild and may be multifactorial, with interleukin 1 (IL-1) causing the trapping in macrophages of the iron from senescent red blood cells.

In chronic renal disease, especially during haemodialysis programs, the anaemia is generally moderate (50–80 g/L) and is erythropoietin-responsive. However, the use of erythropoietin to achieve normal haemoglobin levels in chronic renal disease has been associated with an increased incidence of adverse cardiovascular events, so that a modest level of residual anaemia is the preferred goal of such therapy.

Marrow hyperplasia may paradoxically be associated with anaemia if there is ineffective erythropoiesis. An erythroid defect causes premature cell death in the bone marrow and thus some of the features of haemolysis.

This condition is seen in some cases of
- megaloblastic anaemia (q.v.),
- sideroblastic anaemia (q.v.),
- thalassaemia (q.v.),
- myelofibrosis (agnogenic myeloid metaplasia).

Bibliography
Anderson KC, Weinstein HJ. Transfusion-associated graft-versus-host disease. *N Engl J Med* 1990; 323: 315.
Barrett-Connor E. Anemia and infection. *Am J Med* 1972; 52: 242.
Berliner N, Gasner JM. Anemia: production defects. In: *Scientific American Medicine. Hematology.* Hamilton: Dekker Medicine. 2020.
Boutboul D, Touzot F, Szalat R. Understanding therapeutic emergencies in acute hemolysis. *Intens Care Med* 2018; 44: 482.
Clucas DB, Fox LC, Wood EM, et al. Revisiting acquired aplastic anaemia: current concepts in diagnosis and management. *Intern Med J* 2019; 49: 152.
Corwin HL, Gettinger A, Pearl RG, et al. The CRIT study: anemia and blood transfusion in the critically ill – current clinical practice in the United States. *Crit Care Med* 2004; 32: 39.
Editorial. Paroxysmal nocturnal haemoglobinuria. *Lancet* 1992; 339: 395.
Eichner ER. Fatigue of anemia. *Nutr Rev* 2001; 59: S17.
Engelfriet CP, Overbeeke MAM, von dem Borne AEGK. Autoimmune hemolytic anemia. *Semin Hematol* 1992; 29: 3.
Fazio D, Gropper MA. Anemia and transfusion in critical care. *Pulmonary Perspect* 2003; 20: 4.
Finch CA. Erythropoiesis, erythropoietin, and iron. *Blood* 1982; 60: 1241.
Henry DH, Spivak JL. Clinical use of erythropoietin. *Curr Opinion Hematol* 1995; 2: 118.
Hillmen P, Lewis SM, Bessler M, et al. Natural history of paroxysmal nocturnal hemoglobinuria. *N Engl J Med* 1995; 333: 1253.
Krantz SB. Erythropoietin. *Blood* 1991; 77: 419.
Lopez A, Cacoub P, Macdougall IC, et al. Iron deficiency anaemia. *Lancet* 2016; 387: 907.
Low MSY, Grigoriadis G. Iron deficiency and new insights into therapy. *Med J Aust* 2017; 207: 81.
Marmont AM. Therapy of pure red cell aplasia. *Semin Hematol* 1991; 28: 285.
Marsh JCW, Socie G, Schrezenmeier H, et al. Haemopoietic growth factors in aplastic anaemia: a cautionary note. *Lancet* 1994; 344: 172.
Means RT. Advances in the anemia of chronic disease. *Int J Hematol* 1999; 70: 7.
Means RT. Red blood cell function and disorders of iron metabolism. In: *Scientific American Medicine. Hematology.* Hamilton: Dekker Medicine. 2020.
Means RT, Krantz SB. Progress in understanding the pathogenesis of the anemia of chronic disease. *Blood* 1992; 80: 1639.
Mueller MM, Van Remoortel H, Meybohm P, et al. Patient blood management: recommendations from the 2018 Frankfurt consensus conference. *JAMA* 2019; 321: 983.
Nacui FE, Della Torre V, Bhowmick K. Anaemia in the critically ill. *ICU Management & Practice* 2021; 21: 262.
Otis S, Price EA. Hemoglobinopathies and hemolytic anemias. In: *Scientific American Medicine. Hematology.* Hamilton: Dekker Medicine. 2020.
Pasricha SR, Flecknoe-Brown SC, Allen KJ, et al. Diagnosis and management of iron deficiency anaemia: a clinical update. *Med J Aust* 2010; 193: 525.
Pearl RG, Sibbald WJ, eds. Anaemia and blood management in critical care. *Crit Care Med* 2003; 31: S649.
Pieracci FM, Barie PS. Diagnosis and management of iron-related anemias in critical illness. *Crit Care Med* 2006; 34: 1898.
Vincent PC. Drug-induced aplastic anemia and agranulocytosis. *Drugs* 1986; 31: 52.
Vlaar AP, Oczkowski S, de Bruin S, et al. Transfusion strategies in non-bleeding critically ill patients: a clinical practice guideline from the European Society of Intensive Care Medicine. *Intens Care Med* 2020; 46: 673.

Young NS. The problem of clonality in aplastic anaemia: Dr. Damashek's riddle, restated. *Blood* 1992; 79: 1385.

Young NS, Meyers G, Schrezenmeier H, et al. The management of paroxysmal nocturnal hemoglobinuria: recent advances in diagnosis and treatment and new hope for patients. *Semin Hematol* 2009; 46: S1.

Anaphylaxis *See*

- Drug allergy.
  See also
- Angioedema,
- Asthma – Stridor,
- Bites and stings – Bees and wasps, Marine invertebrates, Snakes, Spiders,
- Chelating agents – Penicillamine,
- Digoxin-specific antibody,
- Echinococcosis,
- Flushing,
- Urticaria.

ANCA *See*

- Wegener's granulomatosis.
  See also
- Churg–Strauss syndrome,
- Vasculitis – Microscopic polyangiitis.

Aneurysms, mycotic *See*

- Mycotic aneurysms.

Angiodysplasia

Angiodysplasia refers to the condition of multiple acquired vascular lesions within the bowel wall. They are similar to but separate from arteriovenous malformations (q.v.), which are congenital in origin. They can occur anywhere in the gastrointestinal tract, though they are most frequently found in the caecum and ascending colon. The lesions are usually small and comprise a cluster of dilated mucosal capillaries. Angiodysplasia is an uncommon but important cause of acute or chronic gastrointestinal blood loss, especially in older patients.

Diagnosis is by colonoscopy, angiography, nuclear scan or video capsule endoscopy (for small bowel lesions). Patients should be screened for acquired von Willebrand's disease (q.v.), especially if they also have aortic stenosis (i.e. Heyde syndrome) or lymphoproliferative disease. The lack of von Willebrand factor, either inherited or acquired, can cause increased endothelial cell proliferation with consequent angiogenesis and the development of vascular malformations.

*Acute bleeding generally stops spontaneously, but **surgical resection** or **colonoscopic electrocoagulation** is required for continued haemorrhage, although rebleeding is common after local treatment techniques. The presence of associated von Willebrand's disease provides an opportunity for specific haemostatic therapy (see Von Willebrand's disease). **Anti-angiogenic agents**, such as thalidomide or the related lenalidomide, have been reported to be of benefit in refractory cases.*

See also
- Arteriovenous malformations – Osler–Weber–Rendu disease (hereditary haemorrhagic telangiectasia).

Bibliography

Boey JP, Hahn U, Sagheer S, et al. Thalidomide in angiodysplasia-related bleeding. *Intern Med J* 2016; 45: 972.

Franchini M, Mannucci PM. Gastrointestinal angiodysplasia and bleeding in von Willebrand disease. *J Thromb Haemost* 2014: 112: 427.

Heyde EC. Gastrointestinal bleeding in aortic stenosis. *N Engl J Med* 1958; 259: 196.

Hochter W, Weingart J, Kuhner W, et al. Angiodysplasia in the colon and rectum: endoscopic morphology, localisation and frequency. *Endoscopy* 1985; 17: 182.

Hodgson H. Hormonal therapy for gastrointestinal angiodysplasia. *Lancet* 2002; 359: 1630.

Jackson CS, Gerson LB. Management of gastrointestinal angiodysplastic lesions (GIADs): a systematic review and meta-analysis. *Am J Gastroenterol* 2014; 109: 474.

Randi AM, Smith KE, Castaman C. Von Willebrand factor regulation of blood vessel formation. *Blood* 2018; 132: 132.

Warkentin TE, Moore JC, Morgan DG. Aortic stenosis and bleeding gastrointestinal angiodysplasia: is acquired von Willebrand's disease the link? *Lancet* 1992; 340: 35.

Angioedema

Angioedema arises from increased vascular permeability, which produces a local oedema of a non-dependent and non-pitting nature. It is acute and self-limited, though it may be life-threatening if there is airway compromise. There are many conditions which may cause angioedema itself or which may mimic angioedema, but the two most important are the hereditary and the drug-induced varieties.

Hereditary angioedema (HAE) is due to a deficiency or dysfunction of C1 inhibitor (C1-INH, C1INH), a serine protease like many activated coagulation factors (q.v.). HAE is a rare autosomal dominant condition, with affected heterozygotes having 5–30% of the normal concentration of C1-INH. It was described by Osler in 1888, and the underlying enzyme defect was reported in

1963. A similar condition may occasionally be acquired, generally in association with a lymphoproliferative malignancy. Absence of this enzyme is thought to cause increased vascular permeability due to unregulated activation of **bradykinin** (BK), a vasoactive peptide. This process occurs when the contact system is triggered, with factor XII then activating prekallikrein (PK) to cleave high-molecular-weight kininogen (HK) and thus release BK (see Coagulation disorders).

- Clinically, there are recurrent attacks of non-pitting oedema, lasting 48–72 hr and affecting the skin (especially the face), respiratory tract (typically the upper respiratory tract) and gut (visceral angioedema).
- The most dramatic feature is laryngeal oedema, causing potentially fatal upper airway obstruction (see Asthma – stridor).
- The oedema is not associated with erythema, pruritus or local discomfort (except sometimes for intestinal colic, due to associated visceral angioedema).
- There is typically no associated urticaria.
- The attacks are classically initiated by trauma, though more commonly no obvious precipitant is identified.

Drug-induced angioedema is of course well known as one of the major features of anaphylaxis, the most dramatic manifestation of **drug allergy** (q.v.). Unlike HAE, it is generally associated with urticaria. Cases of angioedema have been reported to have been caused by **ACE inhibitors** (see Angiotensin-converting enzyme), by the anti-smoking drug bupropion, and occasionally by the complementary medicine echinacea, as well as by some foods and by latex in susceptible subjects. This adverse event to ACE inhibitors can represent a major therapeutic problem. It occurs in 0.1–0.2% of patients, though it is more common and more severe in patients with HAE. Its onset is usually within 2 weeks of starting the drug, though it may be delayed for several months or more. Like the much more common side-effects of cough and rhinitis (which interestingly tend to occur in different patients), it is thought to be due to accumulated BK. Although it has been considered a class effect, it has also occurred (though less severely) with angiotensin II inhibitors (ARBs) and with the gliptin class of oral hypoglycaemic agents.

Investigations show elevated C1 and decreased C4 and C2 during the attack. Since C1-INH also inhibits factor XIIa and kallikrein (PKa), the coagulation, fibrinolytic and kinin systems are also activated. The formation of the vasoactive peptide BK appears to be the main pathogenetic mechanism for the increased vascular permeability.

*Prophylactic treatment is not generally used, but the antifibrinolytic agent **tranexamic acid** (q.v.) (or formerly **epsilon aminocaproic acid**) may be helpful. Its mechanism of action in this setting is unknown, though it is a well-recognized inhibitor of fibrinolysis. **Anabolic steroids** (e.g. danazol) may also be used for prophylaxis.*

There is no specific treatment for acute episodes (apart from enzyme replacement – see below), but fresh frozen plasma has been reported to be helpful. Adrenaline (epinephrine), corticosteroids and antihistamines have no effect in hereditary or drug-induced angioedema (unlike in anaphylaxis).

Purified C1 inhibitor *(Berinert) is available, but it is very expensive. Hypersensitivity reactions, thrombosis and paradoxical exacerbation of angioedema have been sometimes reported following its use. Interestingly, there are also case reports of this inhibitor helping ameliorate both graft failure after lung transplantation and streptococcal toxic shock syndrome.*

Icatibant*, a competitive bradykinin antagonist, is also effective in bradykinin-related angioedema, but it too is very expensive.*

Lanadelumab*, a recently introduced monoclonal antibody to kallikrein, reduces bradykinin production and has been shown to be of prophylactic value in reducing attacks in HAE when given every 2 weeks.*

See also
- Complement deficiency,
- Urticaria.

Bibliography

Agah R, Bandi V, Guntupalli KK. Angioedema: the role of ACE inhibitors and factors associated with poor clinical outcome. *Intens Care Med* 1997; 23: 793.

Banerji A, Busse P, Shennak M, et al. Inhibiting plasma kallikrein for hereditary angioedema prophylaxis. *N Engl J Med* 2017; 376: 717.

Bas M, Greve J, Stelter K, et al. A randomized trial of icatibant in ACE-inhibitor-induced angioedema. *N Engl J Med* 2015; 372: 418.

Chen JR, Khan DA. Urticaria and angioedema. In: *Scientific American Medicine. Allergy & Immunology.* Hamilton: Dekker Medicine. 2020.

Colten HR. Hereditary angioneurotic edema, 1887 to 1987. *N Engl J Med* 1987; 317: 43.

Craig TJ, Levy RJ, Wasserman RL, et al. Efficacy of human C1 esterase inhibitor concentrate compared with placebo in acute hereditary angioedema attacks. *J Allergy Clin Immunol* 2009; 124: 801.

De Maat S, Hofman ZLM, Maas C. Hereditary angioedema: the plasma contact system out of control. *J Thromb Haemost* 2018; 16: 1674.

Donaldson VH, Evans RR. A biochemical abnormality in hereditary angioneurotic edema: absence of serum inhibitor of C1-esterase. *Am J Med* 1963; 35: 37.

Frigas E. Angioedema with acquired deficiency of the C1 inhibitor: a constellation of syndromes. *Mayo Clin Proc* 1989; 64: 1269.

Fronhoffs S, Luyken J, Steuer K, et al. The effect of C1-esterase inhibitor in definite and suspected streptococcal toxic shock syndrome. *Intens Care Med* 2000; 26: 1566.

Gabb GM, Ryan P, Wing LMH, et al. Epidemiological study of angioedema and ACE inhibitors. *Aust NZ J Med* 1996; 26: 777.

Javaud N, Floccard B, Gontier F, et al. Bradykinin-mediated angioedema: factors associated with admission to an intensive care unit, a multicenter study. *Eur J Emerg Med* 2016; 23: 219.

LoVerde D, Files DC, Krishnaswamy G. Angioedema. *Crit Care Med* 2017; 45: 725.

Nzeako UC, Frigas E, Tremaine WJ. Hereditary angioedema. *Arch Intern Med* 2001; 161: 2417.

Osler W. Hereditary angioedema. *Am J Med Sci* 1888; 95: 362.

Schmaier AH. The contact system and kallikrein/kinin systems: pathophysiologic and physiologic activities. *J Thromb Haemost* 2016; 14: 28.

Waytes AT, Rosen FS, Frank MM. Treatment of hereditary angioedema with a vapor-heated C1 inhibitor concentrate. *N Engl J Med* 1996; 334: 1630.

Angiotensin *See*
- Renin–angiotensin–aldosterone.
  See also
- Aldosterone,
- Angiotensin-converting enzyme,
- Atrial natriuretic factor,
- Conn's syndrome.

Angiotensin-converting enzyme

Angiotensin-converting enzyme (ACE) is a membrane-bound enzyme in the pulmonary vessels which converts angiotensin I to angiotensin II in a single passage through the lungs (see Renin–angiotensin–aldosterone). Interestingly, an identical enzyme degrades bradykinin (BK), the vasodilator peptide of the kallikrein-kinin system.

> The plasma ACE level is characteristically increased in active sarcoidosis, and also sometimes in biliary cirrhosis, leprosy, pneumoconiosis and tuberculosis.

The **ACE inhibitors** (captopril, enalapril, and the later agents, fosinopril, lisinopril, perindopril, quinapril, ramipril, trandalopril) have become major therapeutic agents in cardiovascular disease, especially for hypertension and cardiac failure. In hypertension, they have become the most commonly prescribed drugs. In cardiac failure, deterioration and mortality are reduced by ACE inhibitors, not just because of vasodilatation but perhaps also because of remodelling and normalized cell growth. This could occur because angiotensin II is a growth factor, contributing to the maladaptation and thus changed molecular composition rather than just the hypertrophy seen in cardiomyopathic processes (see Renin–angiotensin–aldosterone). Cough and angioedema (q.v.) are two interesting side-effects of ACE inhibition, perhaps caused by decreased kinin catabolism. Severe hyperkalaemia may occur if other potassium-sparing agents are used concomitantly, particularly in patients with renal dysfunction. Renal failure may occur when ACE inhibitors (or angiotensin II receptor antagonists, ARBs) are combined with a diuretic in patients then given an NSAID, particularly if they are dehydrated or acutely unwell.

In addition, there is evidence that ACE inhibitors reduce proteinuria in diabetic patients, independent of their effect of blood pressure, and slow the progression of renal failure in nondiabetics.

See also
- Renin–angiotensin–aldosterone – Angiotensin II receptor antagonists, ARBs.

Bibliography

Curry SC, Arnold-Capell P. Nitroprusside, nitroglycerin, and angiotensin-converting enzyme inhibitors. *Crit Care Clin* 1991; 7: 555.

Editorial. Are ACE inhibitors safe in pregnancy? *Lancet* 1989; 2: 482.

Franzosi MG, Santoro E, Zuanetti G, et al. Indications for ACE inhibitors in the early treatment of acute myocardial infarction: systematic overview of individual data from 100,000 patients in randomized trials. *Circulation* 1998; 97: 2202.

ISIS-4 (Fourth International Study of Infarct Survival) Collaborative Group. ISIS-4: A randomised factorial trial assessing early oral captopril, oral mononitrate, and intravenous magnesium sulphate in 58 050 patients with suspected acute myocardial infarction. *Lancet* 1995; 345: 669.

Lewis EJ, Hunsicker LG, Bain RP, et al. The effect of angiotensin-converting-enzyme inhibition on diabetic nephropathy. *N Engl J Med* 1993; 329: 1456.

Luiz W, Wiemer G, Gohlke P, et al. Contributions of kinins to the cardiovascular actions of angiotensin-converting enzyme inhibitors. *Pharmacol Rev* 1995; 47: 25.

Palmer B. Managing hyperkalemia caused by inhibitors of the renin-angiotensin-aldosterone system. *New Engl J Med* 2004; 351: 585.

Pfeffer MA, Lamas GA, Vaughan DE, et al. Effect of captopril on progressive ventricular dilatation after anterior myocardial infarction. *N Engl J Med* 1988; 319: 80.

Pitt B, Segal R, Martinez FA, et al. Randomised trial of losartan versus captopril in patients over 65 with heart failure (Evaluation of Losartan in the Elderly Study, ELITE). *Lancet* 1997; 349: 747.

Quinn SJ, Williams GH. Regulation of aldosterone secretion. *Ann Rev Physiol* 1988; 50: 409.

Sharpe N, Smith H, Murphy J, et al. Early prevention of left ventricular dysfunction after myocardial infarction with angiotensin-converting-enzyme inhibition. *Lancet* 1991; 337: 872.

Vaughn DE, Pfeffer MA. Angiotensin converting enzyme inhibitors and cardiovascular remodelling. *Cardiovasc Res* 1994; 28: 159.

Animal bites See
- Bites and stings.

Anion gap See
- Lactic acidosis.

Ankylosing spondylitis

Ankylosing spondylitis is a subgroup of the **spondyloarthropathies** (q.v.), conditions characterized by the combination of chronic progressive sacroiliitis and seronegative peripheral arthropathy (q.v.).

Although the aetiology is unknown, it may possibly be precipitated by a number of bacterial antigens. There is also a presumed immunogenetic susceptibility, as evidenced by clustering in families and some ethnic groups. There is a strong correlation with the HLA antigen B27 (see Histocompatibility complex). Thus, 95% of patients with ankylosing spondylitis are B27-positive and ankylosing spondylitis occurs in 10–20% of B27-positive individuals. B27-positive adults comprise about 10% of Caucasian populations and from <1% to about 50% of different ethnic groups around the world. On the other hand, the HLA-B27 genotype has been strongly associated with long-term non-progression of HIV infection (see also Acquired immunodeficiency syndrome). Ankylosing spondylitis has also been strongly associated with genetic variants in the interleukin 23 (IL-23) receptor pathway, a finding which has led to new therapeutic options. The overall population prevalence of ankylosing spondylitis is 0.1–0.4% of the population.

There is a predominance in men (70%), especially younger men. The clinical presentation usually is of chronic back discomfort. Typically, there is night pain, morning stiffness and improvement after exercise. Early in its course, the condition is often misdiagnosed as mechanical back disease. If it progresses, there is obvious limitation of lumbar spinal mobility and chest expansion. Peripheral arthropathy occurs in 20–30% of cases, usually in large, lower limb joints. There may be associated inflammation at sites of ligamentous insertion into bone, namely enthesitis. Amyloidosis (q.v.) or IgA nephropathy (see Glomerular diseases) may occur late in the disease.

> More severe disease may be associated with both systemic symptoms and multiorgan changes.
> **Systemic symptoms** include
> - mild fever,
> - fatigue,
> - weight loss.
>
> **Multiorgan changes** especially involve the
> - eye
>   - uveitis,
> - cardiovascular system
>   - aortic valve incompetence,
>   - conduction defects,
> - lung
>   - cystic changes, sometimes with aspergillus superinfection,
>   - pulmonary fibrosis.

The X-ray shows sacroiliitis and sometimes involvement higher in the spine. Laboratory results may be normal, though usually there is a raised ESR or increased IgA. Synovial biopsy shows non-specific changes similar to those of rheumatoid arthritis, with inflammatory cell infiltrate, lymphoid follicles and intimal cell hyperplasia.

The diagnosis can sometimes be difficult. Radiological evidence of sacroiliitis remains the strongest evidence, when combined with the clinical features of back pain and stiffness, decreased spinal flexion and decreased chest expansion. However, typical radiological changes lag many years behind the onset of clinical symptoms and are therefore not helpful in the diagnosis of early disease. MRI scanning provides the opportunity for earliest diagnosis and may guide the assessment of prognosis. The chief value of HLA-B27 gene testing is not in individual diagnosis but in epidemiological studies.

Treatment is primarily with physical measures and **NSAIDs***.*

- Sometimes, sulphasalazine, methotrexate and/or corticosteroids are indicated.
- **Radiotherapy** was used successfully in the past, but this led to an increased incidence of leukaemia.
- Inhibition of tumour necrosis factor with the anti-TNF antibodies **infliximab** and **etanercept**, originally introduced for other conditions (Crohn's disease and rheumatoid arthritis, respectively), has also been found to be effective in refractory cases of ankylosing spondylitis (and in psoriatic arthritis – q.v.). Clinical improvement with these expensive new agents has been rapid and has been associated with reduced radiological and biochemical evidence of inflammation, though long-term benefit and safety remain to be fully established.
- The new agent, **secukinumab**, which is an IL-17 inhibitor (IL-17 being related to IL-23, see above), has been found to be at least as effective as TNF inhibitor treatment. On the other hand, neutralization of IL-17 has been reported to exacerbate inflammatory bowel disease.
- Chronic sacroiliac joint pain may be relieved by **radiofrequency denervation** of the joint.

The prognosis is generally favourable, as the course of the disease is usually very long, and only mild involvement of the sacroiliac joints is seen for periods of up to 30 yr. However, the natural history is variable, and in some patients the condition progresses to involve the entire spine and there are extra-articular manifestations. If permanent spinal stiffness occurs, the spine is more 'brittle' and fractures can occur with relatively minor trauma. Unfortunately, none of the current treatment options can lead to cure or even complete remission.

See
- Chest wall disorders,
- Inflammatory bowel disease – Ulcerative colitis,
- Systemic diseases and the lung,
- Vasculitis.

Bibliography

Brown M, Bradbury LA. New approaches in ankylosing spondylitis. *Med J Aust* 2017; 206: 192.

Callin A, Ellswood J, Riggs S, et al. Ankylosing spondylitis – an analytical review of 1500 patients: the changing pattern of disease. *J Rheumatol* 1988; 15: 1234.

Davies D. Ankylosing spondylitis and lung fibrosis. *Q J Med* 1972; 41: 395.

Kapasi K, Chui B, Inman RD. HLA-B27/microbial mimicry: an in vivo analysis. *Immunology* 1992; 77: 456.

Khan MA. Update on spondyloarthropathies. *Ann Intern Med* 2002; 136: 896.

McEwen C, DiTata D, Lingg C, et al. Ankylosing spondylitis and spondylitis accompanying ulcerative colitis, regional enteritis, psoriasis and Reiter's disease. *Arthritis Rheum* 1971; 14: 291.

Robinson PC, Benham H. Advances in classification, basic mechanisms and clinical science in ankylosing spondylitis and axial spondyloarthritis. *Intern Med J* 2015; 45: 127.

Schachna L. Dispelling the myths about ankylosing spondylitis. *Intern Med J* 2004; 34: 591.

Sheehan NJ. The ramifications of HLA-B27. *J R Soc Med* 2004; 97: 10.

van der Linden S, van der Heijde D. Ankylosing spondylitis: clinical features. *Rheum Dis Clin North Am* 1998; 24: 663.

Anorectal infections

Anorectal infections are most commonly seen in homosexual men. Thus, such infections are often sexually transmitted diseases.

They include
- chancroid,
- chlamydial infection,
- condylomata acuminata,
- gonorrhoea,
- granuloma inguinale,
- herpes (HSV)(q.v.),
- HIV infection (see Acquired immunodeficiency syndrome),
- syphilis (q.v.).

Rectal inflammation, **proctitis**, may be associated with
- the anorectal infections described above,
- campylobacter-like organisms,
- meningococci,
- more proximal inflammatory bowel disease (q.v.),
- radiation.

Anorectic agents *See*

- Amphetamines,
- Pulmonary hypertension.

Anorexia nervosa

Anorexia nervosa is an uncommon but potentially severe eating disorder, associated with a major decrease in food intake due to self-starvation and with resultant weight loss, perhaps up to 30% or more of the ideal body weight. There may be associated vomiting or laxative use, and compulsive exercise. Its greatest incidence is in adolescent women.

Its aetiology is unknown, but it is thought that it could be related to a distortion of the modern perception of an ideal body image. This view would be consistent with its increased incidence in recent decades, especially in the more affluent. Some familial clustering suggests the possibility of a genetic predisposition, which may involve either anorexia nervosa or bulimia nervosa.

Bulimia nervosa involves binge eating with induced vomiting or purgation but without weight loss.

Eating disorders have complex psychopathologies and are associated with increased rates of psychosocial difficulty and psychiatric comorbidity. As well as the better known conditions of anorexia nervosa and bulimia nervosa, the classification of eating disorders has recently been extended to include irregular **binge eating disorder** (BED) and **avoidance/restrictive food intake disorder** (ARFID), neither of which is necessarily associated with distorted body image perceptions. ARFID is important as a cause of nutritional deficiency.

The clinical features of anorexia nervosa are those of starvation, with associated secondary changes, such as endocrine disturbances (including hypothalamic dysfunction, and amenorrhoea – q.v.), lanugo and depression. Clinical features also include coldness, bradycardia, hypotension and cognitive impairment.

Investigations typically show anaemia (q.v.), leukopenia, hypokalaemia, possibly cardiomyopathy (q.v.) with failure and/or arrhythmias, and occasionally fatty liver, pancreatitis (q.v.), seizures and parotitis (see Mouth diseases). Steroid sex hormones are suppressed. Recently, the associated malnutrition of prolonged anorexia nervosa has been shown to lead to respiratory muscle weakness and impaired gas transfer related to enlargement of the peripheral lung units (changes not typical of emphysema but similar to those seen in the elderly). Osteopenia also occurs with prolonged weight loss and may be irreversible.

Treatment derived from clinical trials is not available, but the usual therapeutic principles include motivation, decreased physical activity and restoration of nutrition. If the process is severe, the daily intake may need to be high (e.g. over 3000 kCal or 12,500 kJ) to ensure progress. Care should be taken to avoid the refeeding syndrome (q.v.), which comprises complications such as fluid and electrolyte abnormalities. Nasogastric tube feeding is rarely required, but drugs such as cyproheptadine or currently the newer antipsychotics, fluoxetine or olanzapine, may assist.

The prognosis is often disappointing, with only about two thirds of the patients being normal after 5 yr and about 25% having a continuing poor outlook.

The mortality is up to 10%, with half the deaths from suicide.

Interestingly, in about 2% of the patients, the outcome is obesity.

Bibliography
Gardenghi GG, Boni E, Todisco P, et al. Respiratory function in patients with stable anorexia nervosa. *Chest* 2009; 136: 1356.
Gilchrist PN, Ben-Tovim DI, Hay PJ, et al. Eating disorders revisited. 1: anorexia nervosa. *Med J Aust* 1998; 169: 438.
Hay P. Current approach to eating disorders: a clinical update. *Intern Med J* 2020; 50: 24.
Herzog DB, Greenwood DN, Dorer DJ, et al. Mortality in eating disorders. *Int J Eat Disord* 2000; 28: 20.
Hilbert A, Hoeck HW, Schmidt R. Evidence-based clinical guidelines for eating disorders: international comparison. *Curr Opin Psychiatry* 2017; 30: 423.
Powers PS, Santana C. Available pharmacologic treatment for anorexia nervosa. *Expert Opin Pharmacother* 2004; 5: 2287.
Striegel-Moore RH, Leslie D, Petrill SA, et al. One-year use and cost of inpatient and outpatient services among female and male patients with an eating disorder. *Int J Eat Disord* 2000; 27: 381.
Strober M, Freeman R, Lampert C, et al. Controlled family study of anorexia nervosa and bulimia nervosa: evidence of shared liability and transmission of partial syndromes. *Am J Psychiatry* 2000; 157: 393.

Anthrax

Anthrax is chiefly a disease of animals which is sometimes transmitted to humans from contact with animal products, particularly hides and wool. It is thus one of the zoonoses (q.v.). It is caused by the large, aerobic and highly pathogenic Gram-positive rod, *Bacillus anthracis*, first identified by Koch in 1877. The organism also produces long-lived and resistant spores in the external environment though not in its host. Anthrax is a disease of documented antiquity and may have been the cause of some of the plagues of Egypt recorded in the Bible 3500 years ago. Currently, about 100,000 cases occur worldwide annually.

The particular current interest in anthrax relates to its potential role in germ warfare and especially in bioterrorist attack. For example, about 100,000 people could be killed by a single strategically dispersed bomb containing only 50 kg of spores. The largest recent outbreak of anthrax, in Russia in 1979 with 96 cases and 64 deaths, may have been due an accident in a germ-warfare factory, since subsequent polymerase chain reaction (PCR) analysis of tissue samples from some of the victims showed multiple strains of the organism, suggestive of a manufactured origin of the spores. Subsequently, the bioterrorist attack in the USA in 2001 caused infection in 22 patients with five deaths. More recently, there was an outbreak of anthrax among IV heroin users in Europe in 2010, with a 33% mortality rate and recognition of a new form of soft tissue infection, referred to as **injectional anthrax**.

The classic clinical manifestations can be several.

1. **Cutaneous**

The classical presentation is with a necrotic and oedematous but painless ulcer at the site of an infected abrasion.

2. **Pulmonary**

More rarely, inhalational anthrax causes a serious flu-like pulmonary infection, but with characteristic haemorrhagic mediastinitis, respiratory distress, pleural effusions, meningitis and shock. This form of anthrax was previously called 'woolsorter's disease' and is the form which would be seen in modern germ warfare. It can be produced by the inhalation of as few as 10,000 spores and results in intense bacteraemia.

3. **Intestinal**

Occasionally, intestinal anthrax may occur due to the ingestion of infected meat.

The diagnosis may be late because its clinical features are initially non-specific and it may be unsuspected. The organism is readily identified from blood cultures, and serology is positive.

Treatment is with **antibiotics** (high dose penicillin) and ICU with isolation. The organism is also sensitive to tetracycline, amoxicillin, erythromycin and ciprofloxacin but not third-generation cephalosporins.

Vaccination is available for people at risk. Animal vaccination was introduced by Pasteur in 1881. Without prompt antibiotic therapy, inhalational anthrax is generally fatal and cutaneous anthrax has a mortality of 20% if untreated.

See also
- Bioterrorism,
- Germ warfare.

Bibliography

Dixon TC, Meselson M, Guillemin J, et al. Anthrax. *New Engl J Med* 1999; 341: 815.

Guarner J, Jernigan JA, Sheih W, et al. Pathology and pathogenesis of bioterrorism-related inhalational anthrax. *Am J Pathol* 2003; 163: 701.

Hicks CW, Sweeney DA, Cui X, et al. An overview of anthrax infection including the recently identified form of disease in injection drug users. *Intens Care Med* 2012; 38: 1092.

Inglesby TV, O'Toole T, Henderson DA, et al. Anthrax as a biological weapon, 2002: updated recommendations for management. *JAMA* 2002; 287: 2236.

Keim PS, Walker DH, Zilinskas RA. Time to worry about anthrax again. *Sci Am* 2017; 316: 61.

LaForce FM. Anthrax. *Clin Infect Dis* 1994; 19: 1009.

Penn CC, Klotz SA. Anthrax pneumonia. *Semin Respir Infect* 1997; 12: 28.

Pile JC, Malone JD, Eitzen EM, et al. Anthrax as a potential biological warfare agent. *Arch Intern Med* 1998; 158: 429.

Shafazand S, Doyle R, Ruoss S, et al. Inhalational anthrax: epidemiology, diagnosis, and management. *Chest* 1999; 116: 1369.

Swartz MN. Recognition and management of anthrax – an update. *N Engl J Med* 2001; 345: 1621.

Whitby M, Ruff TA, Street AC, et al. Biological agents as weapons 2: anthrax and plague. *Med J Aust* 2002; 176: 605.

Antibiotic-associated colitis *See*

- Colitis.

Anticardiolipin antibody *See*

- Antiphospholipid syndrome.

See also
- Behcet's syndrome.

Anticholinergic agents

Anticholinergic (cholinolytic) effects are produced by the following agents

- atropine and related compounds, including
  - the belladonna alkaloids, such as scopolamine,
  - the synthetic quaternary ammonium compounds with antimuscarinic action, such as homatropine, ipratropium and propantheline,
- antidepressants (tricyclics),
- antipsychotics (phenothiazines),
- antiparkinsonian drugs (especially benztropine),
- disopyramide,
- mushroom poisons (q.v.),
- plant products taken nutritionally (e.g. untreated lupins or pulses, usually as flour),
- plant products taken recreationally for their psychoactive effects, e.g. deadly nightshade (*Atropa*

belladonna), angel's trumpet (*Datura stramonium*), diviner's sage (*Salvia divinorum*), black henbane (*Hyoscyamus niger*) and mandrake (*Mandragora officinarum*),
- nerve agent antidotes,
- oxybutynin (an antimuscarinic agent for urinary frequency due to an overactive bladder).

Anticholinergic effects comprise three actions, namely,
- **antimuscarinic**,
- **ganglion-blocking**,
- **neuromuscular blocking**.

Clinically, anticholinergic effects are manifest as
- dry mouth,
- tachycardia,
- constipation,
- urinary retention,
- delirium (q.v.), particularly in the elderly,
- predisposition to heat stroke (q.v.).

They are picturesquely described by the mnemonic:

'blind as a bat, dry as a bone, hot as a hare, mad as a hatter and red as a beet'.

These effects are particularly likely to occur in the presence of polypharmacy, including antispasmodics, antidiarrhoeals, antihistamines and some sedatives.

Overdoses of anticholinergic drugs are treated with the anticholinesterases (q.v.), **physostigmine** (a tertiary amine which penetrates the blood brain barrier) and **pyridostigmine** (a quaternary amine which has poor cerebral penetration). Both reversibly inhibit acetylcholinesterase and thus protect it.

Physostigmine reverses the CNS effects of anticholinergic drugs, though other effects of such poisoning (e.g. cardiac) are not reversed. It is given in a dose of 1–2 mg IV over 5 min and repeated if necessary each 20 min. Since pyridostigmine does not penetrate the blood brain barrier, it does not impair CNS performance like physostigmine and is therefore useful as prophylaxis.

Since the entire cholinergic spectrum is particularly seen with **nerve agents** (see Warfare agents), they are antagonized by the anticholinergic agents. Typically, atropine is given (in doses up to 6 mg), though newer antagonists with greater CNS effects have been developed. These newer antagonists particularly include the oximes, e.g. **pralidoxime**, organic compounds which complex with anticholinesterase agents and thus free the enzyme, acetylcholinesterase, so that cholinergic function is restored.

Bibliography
Eddleston M, Szinicz L, Eyer P, et al. Oximes in acute organophosphorus pesticide poisoning: a systematic review of clinical trials. *Quart J Med* 2002; 95: 275.
Goldfrank L, Flomenbaum N, Levin N, et al. Anticholinergic poisoning. *J Toxicol Clin Toxicol* 1982; 19: 17.

Anticholinesterases

Anticholinesterases comprise

- neostigmine and pyridostigmine,
- edrophonium,
- tetrahydroaminoacridine (THA, tacrine),
- nerve agents (e.g. insecticides, chemical warfare agents – q.v.).

Acetylcholinesterase (AChE) terminates the action of acetylcholine at cholinergic nerve endings. Therefore, anticholinesterases allow acetylcholine to accumulate at its extensive central and peripheral sites.

Neostigmine and **pyridostigmine** are the main therapeutic anticholinesterases. They permit the accumulation of acetylcholine at neuromuscular junctions and autonomic synapses. They also give rise to muscarinic effects of salivation, lacrimation, urination, diarrhoea, GI cramps, emesis (summarized by the mnemonic 'SLUDGE'), as well as sweating, bronchospasm, blurred vision and bradycardia (even to the point of asystole).

Their use and that of **edrophonium** is discussed in the section on myasthenia gravis (q.v.).

THA (tetrahydroaminoacridine, tacrine) acts at the neuromuscular junction without a muscarinic effect. THA is also a mild analeptic, prolongs the paralysis induced by suxamethonium and can be used with neostigmine to reverse curarization. It has been withdrawn from the market because of hepatotoxicity.

Because of its central actions, it was considered to provide modest therapeutic benefit in **Alzheimer's disease** (see Dementia), but this benefit was not confirmed in subsequent studies. The newer anticholinesterases, **donepezil**, **rivastigmine** and **galantamine**, have however been confirmed in large studies to provide symptomatic benefit, though these benefits are only modest, improvement may require doses which produce adverse effects, there has been no evidence of decreased disease progression, and long-term efficacy is unknown.

Rivastigmine has also been used for delirium management in ICU patients, but this indication has become controversial.

Bibliography

Cladwell JE. Reversal of residual neuromuscular block with neostigmine at one to four hours after a single intubating dose of vecuronium. *Anesth Analg* 1995; 80: 1168.

Davis KL, Powchik P. Tacrine. *Lancet* 1995; 345: 625.

Mayeux R, Sano M. Drug therapy: treatment of Alzheimer's disease. *N Engl J Med* 1999; 341: 1670.

Peter JV, Cherian AM. Organic insecticides. *Anaesth Intens Care* 2000; 28: 11.

Anticoagulants

Anticoagulants have traditionally comprised **heparin** (q.v.) and **warfarin** (q.v., and see Skin necrosis, see Vitamin K). Both agents have a narrow therapeutic window and a variable dose–response relationship, so that laboratory monitoring is required. Even so, therapeutic failure from under-anticoagulation and bleeding from over-anticoagulation are common.

Newer anticoagulants without these limitations have therefore been sought, a number have been recently introduced, and many more are undergoing investigation. This has been a burgeoning field, because the complex coagulation cascade provides a rich source of targets for potential therapeutic attack. The most promising agents in the future may target the furthest upstream coagulation steps involving factor XII and factor XI, since the contact system is more important in thrombosis than in haemostasis (see Coagulation disorders).

> The newer anticoagulant agents currently include
> 1. new heparins and heparin-like agents,
> 2. hirudin and derivatives,
> 3. direct-acting oral anticoagulants,
> 4. other agents (argatroban, defibrotide),
> 5. natural anticoagulants.

1. New heparins and heparin-like agents

As heparin is a large polydisperse molecule (a glycosaminoglycan) with much of its structure inactive therapeutically, fractionation into smaller and more active components has led to the development of the **low molecular weight heparins** (LMWHs, e.g. enoxaparin, dalteparin and several others). These agents are about one third of the molecular weight of unfractionated heparin (i.e. average 4–5000 Da compared with 15,000 Da), but they retain the pentasaccharide sequence responsible for most of heparin's anticoagulant activity.

The LMWHs have a greater Xa to IIa effect than unfractionated heparin (which has a 1:1 effect), though they still act via antithrombin III (AT-III)(q.v.) like all heparins. However, they have greater bioavailability when given subcutaneously, more predictable dose-response effects, improved efficacy/bleeding ratio and no requirement for laboratory monitoring. The usual heparin antagonist, protamine, provides partial antagonism for the LMWHs.

LMWHs have become the standard anticoagulant for thromboembolism prophylaxis and treatment in most circumstances. Their cost is about double that of unfractionated or standard heparin.

Fondaparinux is a synthetic pentasaccharide of molecular weight 1728 Da, which replicates the binding site of heparin for AT-III. It is a pure Xa inhibitor. It is at least as effective and safe as the low molecular weight heparins in the prophylaxis and treatment of thromboembolism. It is also effective in heparin-induced thrombocytopenia (q.v.). As for all heparins, clearance is renal. It is given in a dose of 2.5 mg SC per day for prophylaxis and average 7.5 mg SC per day (range 5–10 mg) for treatment of thromboembolism. Laboratory monitoring is not required. Its cost is about double that of the LMWHs.

Idraparinux, a long-acting derivative of fondaparinux which may be given once weekly, has undergone successful clinical trials. A biotinylated form, **idrabiotaparinux**, was later introduced, because it can be reversed if necessary with the egg protein, avidin.

Danaparoid is a heparinoid, i.e. a mixture of heparin-related glycosaminoglycans (namely, heparan sulphate, dermatan sulphate and chondroitin sulphate). It acts via both AT-III and heparin cofactor II, and it has even more selective Xa to IIa activity than the low molecular weight heparins. It is effective and safe both for the prophylaxis and treatment of thromboembolism. Because of its very low cross-reactivity with heparin (<5% in vivo), it has been recommended for the treatment of heparin-induced thrombocytopenia (q.v.). However, it is expensive and in persistently short supply.

2. Hirudin and derivatives

Hirudin is a protein of 65 amino acids derived from the saliva of the medical leech, *Hirudo medicinalis*. It binds directly to thrombin (i.e. without the requirement for AT-III) and it inactivates clot-bound as well as circulating thrombin (whereas the heparins inactivate only the latter). Although an effective anticoagulant, it was found to be no more effective clinically than heparin, its therapeutic margin was even narrower, and it is antigenic.

Hirudin is at present available in two recombinant forms.

- **Desirudin** has been shown to be effective in preventing thromboembolism after hip replacement surgery. It is given in a dosage of 15 mg SC bd. It is not widely available.
- **Lepirudin** has been recommended for heparin-induced thrombocytopenia (q.v.) and has been used successfully with thrombolysis in acute myocardial infarction. Clearance is renal, and the dose should be reduced in patients with renal impairment. The usual dosage is 0.4 mg/kg IV bolus, followed by 0.15 mg/kg/hr, with the maintenance dose controlled to give an APTT of about 2 × control. However, its manufacture recently ceased and its residual stock is limited.

Bivalirudin (hirulog) is a synthetic analog of hirudin and consists of 20 amino acids (molecular weight 1980 Da). It is not immunogenic, but it can react with any prior antibodies to hirudin. It has been shown to be an effective anticoagulant in acute cardiology (myocardial infarction, percutaneous coronary intervention) and in cardiopulmonary bypass. It has also been used successfully in heparin-induced thrombocytopenia (q.v.). Clearance is renal, and the dose should be reduced in patients with renal impairment. The recommended dosage varies from 0.5 to 1 mg/kg IV bolus, followed by 1.75–2.5 mg/kg/hr, with the maintenance dose controlled to give an ACT about 2.5 × control or an APTT of about 2 × control. It is expensive.

3. **Direct-acting oral anticoagulants**

Direct-acting oral anticoagulants (DOACs), formerly called **non-vitamin K** (or **novel**) **oral anticoagulants** (NOACs), are those in the group which currently includes **dabigatran**, **rivaroxaban**, **apixaban**, **edoxaban** and **betrixaban**. They were designed to be able to replace warfarin due to their novel properties of
- wider therapeutic window, and thus fixed oral dosage without laboratory monitoring,
- rapid onset (about 2 hr to Cmax) and offset of action (T1/2 8–12 hr), thus avoiding the need for either initial bridging or later antidotes in emergencies, and
- much fewer drug interactions, being limited to strong CYP3A4 (cytochrome P450) or P-glycoprotein inhibitors or inducers (e.g. ketoconazole, ciclosporin, HIV protease inhibitors, rifampicin, carbamazepine).

Their commonest role is now in the prevention of stroke in patients with non-valvular atrial fibrillation, in which they have been found to be about 20% more effective than warfarin and to be associated with about 50% less intracranial bleeding. They are also commonly used in both the prevention and the treatment of venous thromboembolism. Their use in critically ill patients can be challenging, because none of the published studies directly involved patients in ICU and because dosages need to be adjusted or the drug avoided in the presence of either renal or liver impairment. They are less effective than warfarin in patients with artificial heart valves or acute coronary syndrome.

Dabigatran is an oral IIa inhibitor (i.e. DTI), first introduced in 2010. It is effective in the prevention of venous thromboembolism after joint replacement surgery, in the prevention of systemic embolism in atrial fibrillation and in the treatment of venous thromboembolism. For prophylaxis after joint replacement surgery, it is given in a dose of 220 mg per day. In atrial fibrillation, doses of 150 mg bd have been shown to be more effective (but similarly safe) and doses of 110 mg bd more safe (but similarly effective) when compared with conventional warfarin therapy. In the treatment of venous thromboembolism, a dose of 150 mg bd for 6 months after the completion of usual treatment with heparin and warfarin for 6–18 months has been shown to prevent further late recurrence. Caution is required in elderly patients and in those with impaired renal function. It is dialyzable. The manufacturer of dabigatran has recently introduced a specific antidote, **idarucizumab** (see below). Although routine laboratory monitoring is not required, its anticoagulant effect can be shown in vitro using the APTT or dilute thrombin time.

Rivaroxaban is an oral Xa inhibitor, first introduced in 2011 and now the most widely used of the DOACs. It is effective in the prevention of venous thromboembolism after joint replacement surgery, in the prevention of systemic embolism in atrial fibrillation and in the treatment of venous thromboembolism. For prophylaxis, it is given in a dose of 10 mg per day. In atrial fibrillation, it is given in a dose of 20 mg per day. In the treatment of venous thromboembolism, the dosage is 15 mg bd for up to 3 weeks (instead of heparin), followed by 20 mg per day for 3–12 months (instead of warfarin). It is the DOAC least affected by extreme variations in patient weight, especially obesity. Caution is required in patients with greater than mildly impaired renal or hepatic function. It is not usefully dialyzable. Bleeding is less than with traditional anticoagulants, and there is now a validated antidote, **andexanet alfa** (see below), which may be given to reverse any Xa inhibitor. Although routine laboratory monitoring is not required, its anticoagulant effect can be shown in vitro using the INR.

Apixaban is another oral Xa inhibitor, first introduced in 2015. For prophylaxis in the prevention of thromboembolism after joint replacement surgery, it is given in a dose of 2.5 mg bd. In atrial fibrillation, it is given in a dose of 5 mg bd.

Edoxaban is an oral Xa inhibitor, also first introduced in 2015. In atrial fibrillation, it is given in a dose of 60 mg per day.

Betrixaban is the most recently introduced oral Xa inhibitor, launched in 2017. For prophylaxis in the prevention of thromboembolism in high-risk patients, it is given in a dose of 80 mg per day after a loading dose of 160 mg.

Specific **antidotes** are now available for the DOACs following the introduction of **idarucizumab** (a specific monoclonal antibody) for dabigatran and of **andexanet alfa** (an inactivated or decoy factor Xa) for rivaroxaban and apixaban. These expensive new agents provide about 80% effective haemostasis but with a 5–10% thrombotic risk. Although potential reversal is not generally an issue with prophylactic regimens, untoward bleeding can occur when therapeutic doses are given or when patients present with other emergencies (e.g. trauma). Under such circumstances, prothrombin complex concentrate (q.v.), activated factor VIIa (see Haemophilia), tranexamic acid (q.v.) and desmopressin (q.v.) have also been reported to be helpful while awaiting elimination of the culprit drug. International guidelines have been published to assist clinicians in these circumstances. However, it should be remembered that the mortality from serious anticoagulant-relating bleeding (especially intracranial haemorrhage) remains high despite the availability of reversal agents, since these agents can prevent ongoing bleeding only, and they cannot treat any pre-existing haemorrhagic damage.

4. **Other agents**

Argatroban is a direct thrombin inhibitor (DTI) which is able to neutralize both soluble and clot-bound thrombin. It has been shown to be effective in heparin-induced thrombocytopenia (q.v.). It has also been used successfully with thrombolysis in acute myocardial infarction, in percutaneous coronary intervention and for renal replacement therapy. Clearance is hepatic, and the dose must be reduced (by up to 90%) in critically ill patients with multiorgan failure. The usual dosage is 2 mcg/kg/min IV, with the maintenance dose controlled to give an APTT of about 2 × control. It is not widely available.

Defibrotide is a mammalian polydeoxyribonucleotide with fibrinolytic and angiogenic as well as anticoagulant effects (though it causes little systemic anticoagulant activity). It is an adenosine agonist and affects multiple endothelial, platelet and prostaglandin pathways. It is thus a broadly based antithrombotic agent. It has been used successfully in the prevention and treatment of hepatic veno-occlusive disease (hepatic sinusoidal obstruction syndrome), particularly after autologous bone marrow transplantation (see Budd–Chiari syndrome). However, it is very expensive, and its cost-effectiveness has been challenged.

5. **Natural anticoagulants**

The **natural anticoagulants** could also be potentially useful therapeutic anticoagulants, but because of the cross-talk between the body's processes of thrombosis and inflammation (and other responses, see Coagulation disorders), they have been studied mainly for their possible utility in sepsis. The agents studied have included

- **antithrombin III** (AT-III),
- **tissue factor pathway inhibitor** (TFPI, tifacogin),
- **activated protein C** (drotrecogin alpha), and
- **recombinant thrombomodulin** (rhTM, ART-123).

However, although the natural anticoagulants have exacerbated bleeding, they have not been found in controlled trials to have therapeutically useful antithrombotic properties, significant anti-inflammatory effects or mortality benefit. Interestingly, **heparin** itself has not been formally studied in this context, though indirect evidence points to its potential anti-inflammatory effect.

Bibliography

Allingstrup M, Wetterslev J, Ravn FB, et al. Antithrombin III for critically ill patients: a systematic review with meta-analysis and trial sequential analysis. *Intens Care Med* 2016; 42: 505.

Fredenburgh JC, Weitz JI. New anticoagulants: moving beyond the direct oral anticoagulants. *J Thromb Haemost* 2021; 19: 20.

Frontera JA, Lewin JL, Rabinstein AA, et al. Guideline for reversal of antithrombotics in intracranial hemorrhage: Executive summary. A statement for health care professionals from the Neurocritical Care Society and the Society of Critical Care Medicine. *Crit Care Med* 2016; 44: 2251.

Guyatt G, Akl EA, Crowther M, et al., eds. Antithrombotic therapy and prevention of thrombosis, 9th ed: ACCP evidence-based clinical practice guidelines. *Chest* 2012; 141: no. 2 (suppl.).

Hirsh J, Bauer KA, Donati MB, et al. Parenteral anticoagulants. *Chest* 2008; 133 (suppl.): 141S.

Marder VJ, Aird WC, Bennett JS, et al., eds. *Hemostasis and Thrombosis: Basic Principles and Clinical Practice*. 6th edition. Philadelphia: Lippincott Williams & Wilkins. 2012.

McKenzie J-L, Douglas G, Bazargan A. Perioperative management of anticoagulation in elective surgery. *ANZ J Surg* 2013; 83: 814.

Oakley CM. Anticoagulants in pregnancy. *Br Heart J* 1995; 74: 107.

Rali P, Gangemi A, Moores A, et al. Direct-acting oral anticoagulants in critically ill patients. *Chest* 2019; 156: 604.

Schaden E, Kozek-Langenecker SA. Direct thrombin inhibitors: pharmacology and application in intensive care medicine. *Intens Care Med* 2010; 36: 1127.

Schulman S, Beyth RJ, Kearon C, et al. Hemorrhagic complications of anticoagulant and thrombolytic treatment. *Chest* 2008; 133 (suppl.): S257.

Tran H, Joseph J, Young, L, et al. New oral anticoagulants: a practical guide on prescription, laboratory testing and peri-procedural/bleeding management. *Intern Med J* 2014; 44: 525.

Weitz JI, Hirsh J, Samama MM. New antithrombotic drugs. *Chest* 2008; 133 (suppl.): 234S.

Willcox A, Ho L, Jones D. Implications of direct oral anticoagulation and antiplatelet therapy in intensive care. *Crit Care Resusc* 2020; 22: 181.

Zarychanski R, Abou-Setta AM, Kanji S, et al. The efficacy and safety of heparin in patients with sepsis: a systematic review and metaanalysis. *Crit Care Med* 2015; 43: 511.

Antidiuretic hormone

Antidiuretic hormone (ADH, vasopressin – q.v.) is secreted by the posterior pituitary (q.v.). It is important in controlling water conservation in terrestrial species. However, it also acts at sites other than the kidney, and it is thus additionally a vasopressor (hence the name, vasopressin), a neurotransmitter and an oxytocic, and it can release clotting factors from endothelial cells.

Natural **vasopressin** is a nonapeptide, i.e. 8-arginine vasopressin in humans, hence its name arginine vasopressin (AVP). Vasopressin is also referred to as **oxytocin**.

AVP has a precursor peptide, the C-terminal portion of which is called **copeptin**. Unlike AVP which cannot be usefully measured in clinical practice because of its short half-life, copeptin can be readily measured by immunoassay, thus providing a surrogate marker of the AVP level.

See
- Desmopressin,
- Diabetes insipidus,
- Vasopressin.

See also
- High altitude – Pulmonary oedema,
- Pituitary,
- Syndrome of inappropriate antidiuretic hormone.

Antinuclear antibodies

Antinuclear antibodies (ANA) are most characteristically associated with systemic lupus erythematosus (SLE) (q.v.), but in fact they are also diagnostically useful in other autoimmune diseases, including Sjogren's syndrome (q.v.), scleroderma (q.v.) and mixed connective tissue disease (q.v.).

Several nuclear antigens are recognized by autoantibodies in SLE, with the resultant circulating immune complexes able to injure a number of organs and structures, especially renal glomeruli. Antibodies to native double-strand DNA and soluble (extractable) nuclear antigen called Sm are specific for SLE. Other antibodies include those to denatured single-strand DNA, RNA, nucleoprotein, histones and nucleoli.

While the presence of antinuclear antibodies is diagnostically useful, their pathogenetic role is doubtful, except as described above and in congenital heart block which is strongly associated with placental passage of maternal autoantibodies to Ro(SS-A) and La(SS-B).

Antiphospholipid syndrome

The **antiphospholipid syndrome** (APS) is a hypercoagulable state associated with the presence of anticardiolipin antibody, lupus anticoagulant and possibly other autoantibodies. It is a complex autoimmune condition. Its prevalence is about 1 in 2000 of the population.

In the 1950s, some patients with SLE (q.v.) were observed to have a long clotting time but a paradoxical thrombotic tendency. In the 1970s, the responsible substance became referred to as the lupus anticoagulant (LA) and was found to be present in up to one third of cases of SLE. Subsequently, LA was observed in other (especially autoimmune) diseases and even in some healthy people (1–5%), so that it was then referred to as the 'lupus-like anticoagulant' (LLA). This 'anticoagulant' was later found to be closely related to antibodies to negatively charged phospholipids, such as cardiolipin (the antibody responsible for the positive VDRL test in syphilis – q.v.), so that the syndrome was then referred to as the anticardiolipin syndrome. In 1983, the broader name antiphospholipid syndrome (APS) was given to describe the clinical propensity to arterial and venous thrombosis in association with such antibodies. Subsequently, the name 'Hughes' syndrome' has been proposed. Clinical consequences of APS occur eventually in up to 70% of patients with SLE and antibodies.

Although the anticardiolipin antibody and the lupus anticoagulant antibody are both antiphospholipids, the immune response appears to be directed to modified proteins rather than to lipids, since a cofactor (most commonly, beta-2 glycoprotein I, β2-GPI, an activator of lipoprotein lipase) is required for anionic phospholipid binding prior to antibody formation. The lipid-binding peptide of β2-GPI is similar to those found in some bacteria and viruses, implying the potential for an infection to have stimulated anticardiolipin antibody formation. β2-GPI is a 50 kDa glycoprotein which is synthesized in the liver and which has a plasma concentration of 50–500 mg/L. Although originally described in 1961 and since found to be conserved in evolution back to reptiles and fish, no biological function had been identified for it in humans until recently, when it was reported to play a role as a scavenger of circulating particulates. It thus participates in innate immunity and host defence against microorganisms.

The antibodies themselves are heterogeneous and usually polyclonal IgG or IgM. Although many different mechanisms have been postulated to explain their in vitro anticoagulant but in vivo thrombotic effects, it is likely that the antibodies themselves are directly responsible for the clinical effects and that the clotting test results are artefacts of non-flowing blood.

Clinical features of APS comprise
- thromboses
  - including recurrent DVT and other forms of venous thrombosis,
  - APS is thus one of the causes of thrombophilia (q.v.),
- pulmonary hypertension (q.v.),
- cerebral artery occlusion
  - with TIA, stroke, ischaemic dementia, ocular ischaemia,
- livedo reticularis (q.v.)
  - i.e. necrotizing purpura,
- heart valve disease
  - including valvular degeneration and verrucous endocarditis,
  - resembling culture-negative bacterial endocarditis (q.v.),
- spontaneous abortion (q.v.) and fetal death,
- miscellaneous problems
  - such as labile hypertension, epilepsy, migraine, transverse myelopathy (q.v.), thrombocytopenia (q.v.), haemolytic anaemia (see Anaemia), and depression.

The condition may also be
- drug-related, especially to chlorpromazine or hydralazine,
- associated with opportunistic infections, as in AIDS (q.v.),
- an associated phenomenon in septic or shocked patients in ICU.

There is an increased incidence of anticardiolipin antibodies in Behcet's disease (q.v.).

In Intensive Care patients, a form of APS referred to as 'catastrophic APS' (CAPS) may sometimes be seen. It is associated with
- ARDS (q.v.),
- multiorgan failure (q.v.),
- thrombocytopenia (q.v.),
- Budd–Chiari syndrome (q.v.).

These are all considered to be related to a widespread thrombotic tendency (specifically, a thrombotic microangiopathy – q.v.), with an associated systemic inflammatory response related to complement activation. It has a fulminant course with a reported mortality of about 40% despite maximal therapy.

Investigations typically show a prolonged APTT, although this is an in vitro phenomenon only and due to the antibody effect on cephalin which is the phospholipid source in the APTT test. Although not associated with a bleeding tendency, the prolonged APTT is of clinical significance in patients requiring heparin therapy, since it makes control difficult. Perhaps of interest, another cause of an isolated prolonged APTT without clinical consequence is inherited prekallikrein deficiency (see Angioedema).

By current international consensus, the diagnosis of APS requires the presence of one or more of the three common antiphospholipid antibodies, namely lupus anticoagulant (LAC), anticardiolipin antibodies (aCL) and anti beta-2 glycoprotein I antibodies (aβ2-GPI). The presence of a LAC is confirmed by mixing studies, because the APTT becomes normal in this way if its prolongation is due to a circulating inhibitor. The aCL and aβ2-GPI antibodies may be directly assayed, usually by ELISA.

Treatment issues have as much uncertainty as do those related to pathogenesis and investigation. Moreover, the laboratory monitoring of effective anticoagulation can present a variety of technical challenges.
- ***Anticoagulation** with even full doses of heparin is often insufficient and long-term **warfarin** is probably best (except in pregnancy when heparin is the only generally acceptable anticoagulant). The optimal dose of warfarin appears to be high, with a required INR of at least 3 in complex or severe cases. The new*

- *anticoagulant, rivaroxaban, failed to show efficacy in this condition, and the DOACs (see Anticoagulants) are not recommended for anticoagulation in APS.*
- *Low-dose **aspirin** may be ineffective, and **corticosteroids** are contraindicated in some settings (e.g. in pregnancy they are associated with an increased incidence of pre-eclampsia).*
- *In cases with associated SLE, **hydroxychloroquine** is recommended for both primary and secondary thrombotic prophylaxis.*
- *Immune globulin and **plasmapheresis** (q.v.) have been reported to be helpful, especially in catastrophic APS. Immunotherapy with **rituximab** (q.v.) in severe cases and with **eculizumab** (q.v.) in catastrophic APS has been reported to be of benefit.*
- *Recently, **statins** (q.v.) have been shown to offer novel benefit in APS. This is because they prevent the antiphospholipid antibody-induced tissue factor upregulation of endothelial cells and monocytes, thereby decreasing the release of adhesion molecules (and interestingly also pro-inflammatory cytokines). This interrupts a main pathway to thrombosis (and also to pathogen response). This prevention of endothelial cell activation to various stimuli is independent of the lipid-lowering effects of statins.*

Bibliography

Arnout J, Vermylen J. Current status and implications of autoimmune antiphospholipid antibodies in relation to thrombotic disease. *J Thromb Haemost* 2003; 1: 931.

Asherson RA, Cervera R, Piette J-C, et al. Catastrophic antiphospholipid syndrome: clinical and laboratory features of 50 patients. *Medicine* 1998; 77: 195.

Asherson RA, Cervera R, Piette J-C, et al., eds. *The Antiphospholipid Syndrome II: Autoimmune Thrombosis*. Amsterdam: Elsevier. 2002.

Bick RL. Antiphospholipid thrombosis syndromes. *Clin Appl Thromb Hemost* 2001; 7: 241.

Brey RL. New treatment options for the antiphospholipid antibody syndrome? More pleiotropic effects of the statin drugs. *J Thromb Haemost* 2004; 2: 1556.

Brighton TA, Chesterman CN. The clinical significance of antiphospholipid antibodies in patients without autoimmune disease. *Aust NZ J Med* 2000; 30: 693.

Briley DP, Coull BM, Goodnight SH. Neurological disease associated with antiphospholipid antibodies. *Ann Neurol* 1989; 25: 221.

Cohen H, Efthymiou M, Devreese KMJ. Monitoring of anticoagulation in thrombotic antiphospholipid syndrome. *J Thromb Haemost* 2021; 19: 892.

Cowchock FS, Reece EA, Balaban D, et al. Repeated fetal losses associated with antiphospholipid antibodies: a collaborative randomised trial comparing prednisolone with low dose heparin treatment. *Am J Obstet Gynecol* 1992; 166: 1318.

de Groot PG, Derksen RHWM. Specificity and clinical relevance of lupus anticoagulant. *Vessels* 1995; 1: 22.

de Groot PG, Meijers JCM. β2-Glycoprotein 1: evolution, structure and function. *J Thromb Haemost* 2011; 9: 1275.

Galli M. The antiphospholipid triangle. *J Thromb Haemost* 2009; 8: 234.

Galve E, Ordi J, Barquinero J, et al. Valvular heart disease in the primary antiphospholipid syndrome. *Ann Intern Med* 1992; 116: 293.

Giannakopoulos B, Krilis SA. The pathogenesis of the antiphospholipid syndrome. *N Engl J Med* 2013; 368: 1033.

Ginsberg JS, Brill-Edwards P, Johnston M, et al. Relationship of antiphospholipid antibodies to pregnancy loss in patients with systemic lupus erythematosus. *Blood* 1992; 80: 975.

Hoi AY, Ross L, Day J, et al. Immunotherapeutic strategies in antiphospholipid syndrome. *Intern Med J* 2017; 47: 250.

Hughes GR. The antiphospholipid syndrome: ten years on. *Lancet* 1993; 342: 341.

Khamashta MA, Cuadrado MJ, Mujic F, et al. The management of thrombosis in the antiphospholipid-antibody syndrome. *N Engl J Med* 1995; 332: 993.

Laskin CA, Bombardier C, Hannah ME. Prednisolone and aspirin in women with autoantibodies and unexplained recurrent fetal loss. *N Engl J Med* 1997; 337: 148.

Levine JS, Branch W, Rauch J. The antiphospholipid syndrome. *N Engl J Med* 2002; 346: 752.

Mezhov V, Segan JD, Tran H, et al. Antiphospholipid syndrome: a clinical review. *Med J Aust* 2019; 211: 184.

Miyakis S, Lockshin MD, Atsumi T, et al. International consensus statement on an update of the classification criteria for definite antiphospholipid syndrome (APS). *J Thromb Haemost* 2006; 4: 295.

Rand JH, Wu X-X, Andree HAM, et al. Pregnancy loss in the antiphospholipid-antibody-syndrome – a possible thrombogenic mechanism. *N Engl J Med* 1997; 337: 154.

Roubey RAS. Autoantibodies to phospholipid-binding plasma proteins: a new view of lupus anticoagulants and other 'antiphospholipid' autoantibodies. *Blood* 1994; 84: 2864.

Ryan P, Street A. Thrombosis and antiphospholipid antibodies – an evolving story. *Aust NZ J Med* 1993; 23: 148.

Wenzel C, Stoiser B, Locker GJ. Frequent development of lupus anticoagulants in critically ill patients treated under intensive care conditions. *Crit Care Med* 2002; 30: 763.

Antiplatelet agents

Antiplatelet agents provide a major component of antithrombotic therapy, with a particular efficacy in arterial thromboembolism.

Many drugs impair platelet function (see Platelet function disorders), but few have an effect sufficient to cause clinical bleeding and even fewer can provide a useful antithrombotic effect. Clinical bleeding associated with antiplatelet agents may be treated with **desmopressin** (q.v.).

> Antiplatelet agents are usually classified according to their mechanism of action, so that the main groups of therapeutically useful agents are
> 1. glycoprotein IIb/IIIa inhibitors,
> 2. ADP receptor inhibitors,
> 3. cyclo-oxygenase (COX) inhibitors,
> 4. prostaglandin analogs,
> 5. phosphodiesterase inhibitors.

1. **Glycoprotein IIb/IIIa inhibitors**

GP IIb/IIIa is the receptor (an integrin) which, following platelet activation, binds fibrinogen and other adhesive molecules, so that platelet aggregation can proceed. This is the final common pathway of platelet aggregation regardless of the particular initiating stimulus. Inhibition of this receptor causes a temporary thrombasthenia-type platelet function defect (q.v.).

The available inhibitors of this receptor include
- **abciximab**, a monoclonal antibody to the GPIIb/IIIa receptor,
- **tirofiban**, a non-peptide receptor inhibitor derived from tyrosine,
- **eptifibatide**, a small peptide receptor inhibitor derived from rattlesnake venom.

These expensive IV agents have been effective in acute coronary syndromes, particularly with associated percutaneous transluminal coronary angioplasty (PTCA) as an adjunct to heparin and aspirin (and also with thrombolytic therapy in myocardial infarction). They have been to some extent overtaken by the availability of the new rapid-onset and much cheaper oral agents prasugrel and ticagrelor (see below). Their chief adverse effects are bleeding and sometimes thrombocytopenia (q.v.).

A GP IIb/IIIa inhibitor is best avoided in patients with a higher risk of bleeding, when the use of the direct thrombin inhibitor **bivalirudin** (see Anticoagulants) is preferable.

2. **ADP receptor inhibitors**

P2Y12 is the relevant platelet receptor for ADP in the pathogenesis of arterial thrombi, and it is the target for this group of drugs.

The available inhibitors of this receptor include
- **ticlopidine**, now superseded,
- **clopidogrel**, but about 30% of patients have a suboptimal response to this drug,
- **prasugrel**, like clopidogrel a thienopyridine and prodrug,
- **ticagrelor**, from a new class of cyclopentyl-triazolo-pyrimidines (CPTP).

These oral agents are used in association with aspirin for long-term prevention of arterial thromboembolism, particularly after percutaneous coronary intervention (PCI).

3. **Cyclo-oxygenase (COX) inhibitors**

The archetypal agent in this class is **aspirin** (q.v.), which is by far the most widely used of all the antiplatelet agents.

It is a non-selective COX-1 and COX-2 inhibitor, a mechanism which causes decreased production of thromboxane A2 (TXA2). The clinical use of aspirin can be associated with variable individual responses and with occasional resistance.

It should be noted that the selective COX-2 inhibitors increase the risk of vascular events.

4. **Prostaglandin analogs**

The chief agent in this class is **prostacyclin**, but it is used clinically more for its associated vasodilator properties (e.g. see Pulmonary hypertension) than for its antiplatelet activity.

5. **Phosphodiesterase inhibitors**

The only current agent in this class is **dipyridamole**, but nowadays it is used only in combination with aspirin for cerebral ischaemia.

Bibliography

Adgey AA. An overview of the results of clinical trials with glycoprotein IIb/IIIa inhibitors. *Am Heart J* 1998; 135: S43.

Capodanno D, Ferreiro JL, Angiolillo DJ. Antiplatelet therapy: new pharmacological agents and changing paradigms. *J Thromb Haemost* 2013; 11 (suppl. 1): 316.

Cattaneo M. Response variability to clopidogrel: is tailored treatment, based on laboratory testing, the right solution? *J Thromb Haemost* 2012; 10: 327.

Chew DP, Bhatt DL. Optimizing glycoprotein IIb/IIIa inhibition: lessons from recent randomized controlled trials. *Intern Med J* 2002; 32: 338.

Coller BS. Anti-GPIIb/IIIa drugs: current strategies and future directions. *Thromb Haemost* 2001; 86: 427.

Coller BS, Anderson KM, Weisman HE. The anti-GPIIb/IIIa agents: fundamental and clinical aspects. *Haemostasis* 1996; 26: 285.

Davi G, Patrono C. Platelet activation and atherothrombosis. *N Engl J Med* 2007; 357: 2482.

Gachet C. Antiplatelet drugs: which targets for which treatments? *J Thromb Haemost* 2015; 13: S313.

Guyatt G, Akl EA, Crowther M, et al., eds. Antithrombotic therapy and prevention of thrombosis, 9th ed: ACCP evidence-based clinical practice guidelines. *Chest* 2012; 141: no. 2 (suppl.).

Huxtable LM, Tafreshi MJ, Rakkar AN. Frequency and management of thrombocytopenia with the glycoprotein IIb/IIIa receptor antagonists. *Am J Cardiol* 2006; 97: 426.

Marder VJ, Aird WC, Bennett JS, et al., eds. *Hemostasis and Thrombosis: Basic Principles and Clinical Practice.* 6th edition. Philadelphia: Lippincott Williams & Wilkins. 2012.

McKenzie J-L, Douglas G, Bazargan A. Perioperative management of anticoagulation in elective surgery. *ANZ J Surg* 2013; 83: 814.

Patrono C. Aspirin resistance: definition, mechanisms and clinical read-outs. *J Thromb Haemost* 2003; 1: 1710.

Patrono C, Baigent C, Hirsh J, et al. Antiplatelet drugs. *Chest* 2008; 133 (suppl.): 199S.

The EPIC investigation. Use of a monoclonal antibody directed against the platelet glycoprotein IIb/IIIa receptor in high-risk coronary angioplasty. *N Engl J Med* 1994, 330. 956.

Weitz JI, Hirsh J, Samama MM. New antithrombotic drugs. *Chest* 2008; 133 (suppl.): 234S.

Willcox A, Ho L, Jones D. Implications of direct oral anticoagulation and antiplatelet therapy in intensive care. *Crit Care Resusc* 2020; 22: 181.

Antiproteases *See*

- Serpins.
  See also
- Alpha$_1$-antitrypsin deficiency,
- Antithrombin III.

Antithrombin

Antithrombin is a circulating plasma protein of molecular weight 58 kDa. A number of forms of antithrombin were originally described nearly 70 yr ago, but only antithrombin III is of clinical relevance, so that the terms antithrombin and antithrombin III are currently used interchangeably.

Antithrombin III (AT-III) is the most important natural inhibitor of several serine proteases, including activated coagulation factors II, X, IX, XI and XII, as well as plasmin, trypsin and kallikrein. It is thus one of the natural anticoagulants (see Anticoagulants). However, its antiprotease activity is slow, except in the presence of heparin, which binds to a lys residue and produces an allosteric effect, which in turn results in greater accessibility of the active site for stoichiometric protease binding. Anti-protease activity is thereby enhanced 1000-fold by heparin, and this is the main mechanism by which heparin exerts its anticoagulant effect.

Antithrombin also has important anti-inflammatory as well as anticoagulant effects, and this property is a reflection of the extensive cross-talk between the pathways of coagulation and inflammation (see Coagulation disorders). The potential clinical relevance of the anti-inflammatory effects of antithrombin has been supported by the observation that the levels of plasma AT-III are low in sepsis and correlate with outcome. However, study of the use of **antithrombin III concentrates** in the treatment of sepsis yielded variable results initially, and the results of subsequent larger trials were disappointing, possibly related to subgroup heterogeneity. Antithrombin III concentrates have perhaps more usefully been used by some clinicians in the treatment of disseminated intravascular coagulation (q.v.).

Antithrombin III is normally present in a plasma concentration of about 150 mcg/mL (2.5 µM), corresponding to 100% activity, and is sufficient to neutralize all the thrombin that can be generated from the same volume of blood. Its half-life is about 60 hr.

Antithrombin III deficiency may be hereditary or acquired.

Hereditary AT III deficiency is an autosomal dominant condition with over 250 reported gene mutations causing either a quantitative (type I) or a qualitative (type II) deficiency. There is a positive family history and the onset of a thrombotic tendency from early adult life, especially following stimuli such as surgery or pregnancy. Although heterozygotes are generally asymptomatic carriers, the disease is manifest even at levels of circulating AT-III up to 60% of normal. By middle age, there is a 90% prevalence of thrombosis. It is the most severe of the inherited thrombophilias (q.v.).

Acquired AT III deficiency occurs
- in disseminated intravascular coagulation (q.v.) (or other major consumptive disorders, such as extensive thromboembolism or trauma),
- in the postoperative state,
- in liver disease,
- in the nephrotic syndrome (see Glomerular diseases),

- in vasculitis (q.v.),
- after asparaginase (which is better known for causing hypofibrinogenaemia).

*Treatment of an acute thrombosis in AT-III deficiency requires **heparin**, plus **AT-III replacement** if there is heparin resistance (i.e. the APTT does not increase as expected with the usual doses of heparin). AT-III may be given as specific concentrate (20–50 U/kg is required to raise the level to 100%) or fresh frozen plasma. Recombinant human AT has recently been produced from transgenic animals.*

For prevention of thrombosis, lifelong warfarin is required. Since warfarin is contraindicated in pregnancy, heparin and AT-III concentrate are given at labour. Asymptomatic patients are usually not given prophylaxis, though oral anabolic steroids may be helpful in some.

Bibliography

Eisele B, Lamy M, Thijs LG, et al. Antithrombin III in patients with severe sepsis. *Intens Care Med* 1998; 24: 663.

Levi M, ten Cate H. Disseminated intravascular coagulation. *N Engl J Med* 1999; 341: 586.

Levy JH, Weisinger A, Ziomek CA, et al. Recombinant antithrombin: production and role in cardiovascular disorder. *Semin Thromb Hemost* 2001; 27: 405.

Rezale AR, Giri H. Antithrombin: an anticoagulant, anti-inflammatory and antibacterial serpin. *J Thromb Haemost* 2020; 18: 528.

Vinazzer H. Antithrombin concentrates: clinical indications. *Clin Appl Thromb Hemost* 1998; 4: 7.

Wheeler AP, Bernard GR. Treating patients with severe sepsis. *N Engl J Med* 1999; 340: 207.

Aortic coarctation

Aortic coarctation refers to narrowing of the aorta, usually distal to the origin of the left subclavian artery in the vicinity of the ligamentum arteriosum. It is usually congenital, but rarely it can follow aortitis or blunt trauma.

- Congenital aortic coarctation may be associated with a bicuspid aortic valve, ventricular septal defect or Turner's syndrome.
- Coarctation due to aortitis (q.v.) occurs most commonly in young women with idiopathic Takayasu's disease (q.v.), though occasionally it may be associated with a collagen-vascular disease (q.v.) and involve the abdominal and lower thoracic aorta.
- Coarctation following trauma is usually mild and is referred to as pseudocoarctation.

Clinical consequences arise because of the high-pressure zone proximal to the coarctation and the low-pressure zone distal to it. Thus, clinical features comprise hypertension, sometimes associated with headache, and coldness and fatigue of the lower extremities. The femoral pulses are reduced and delayed compared with the radial pulses. A bruit may be heard over the back.

The hypertension is detectable only in the arms, in which the systolic pressure is at least 20 mmHg higher than in the legs. The blood pressure rises markedly on exertion, much more so than for essential hypertension of similar degree. The hypertension may be irreversible, if surgical correction is late or if there is residual or recurrent coarctation. Clearly, examination for aortic coarctation should be included in the assessment of patients with hypertension.

The complications of aortic coarctation include
- cardiac failure,
- intracranial haemorrhage,
- aortic dissection (q.v.),
- bacterial endocarditis (q.v.).

Chest X-ray shows
- cardiomegaly,
- rib notching from dilated collateral intercostal vessels,
- an abnormal silhouette of the aortic knob (the so-called figure-of-three).

Diagnosis is confirmed by angiography and/or CT scanning.

The obstruction is usually moderate, though it can occasionally be complete. Sometimes it is mild, as in pseudocoarctation.

*Significant obstruction has traditionally been treated by surgical **resection**, which is usually very successful, though aneurysm formation, recurrent coarctation and persistent hypertension may occur postoperatively.*

***Angioplasty** with or without stenting is nowadays the preferred treatment. It is especially appropriate for narrowing after aortitis or for recurrence after surgery.*

Bibliography

Arend WP, Michel BA, Bloch DA, et al. The American College of Rheumatology 1990 criteria for the classification of Takayasu arteritis. *Arthritis Rheum* 1990; 33: 1129.

Booher AM, Eagle KA. Diseases of the aorta. In: *Scientific American Medicine. Cardiovascular Medicine.* Hamilton: Dekker Medicine. 2020.

Calhoun DA, Oparil S. Treatment of hypertensive crisis. *N Engl J Med* 1990; 323: 1177.

Harrison DA, McLaughlin PR, Lazzam C, et al. Endovascular stents in the management of coarctation of the aorta in the adolescent and adult: one year follow up. *Heart* 2001; 85: 561.

Hijazi ZM, Geggel R. Balloon angioplasty for postoperative recurrent coarctation of the aorta. *J Interv Cardiol* 1995; 8: 509.

Kerr GS, Hallahan CW, Giordano J, et al. Takayasu arteritis. *Ann Intern Med* 1994; 120: 919.

Rothman A. Coarctation of the aorta: an update. *Curr Probl Pediatr* 1998; 28: 33.

Aortic dissection

Aortic dissection, sometimes erroneously referred to as a dissecting aneurysm, is a spontaneous tear in the aortic intima, giving rise to a false channel within the aortic wall. The blood in this channel dissects along the aorta, including its branches, and eventually ruptures either back into the lumen or out through the adventitia.

The most common sites of the initial tear are in the ascending aorta (type A dissection) and in the descending aorta immediately distal to the origin of the left subclavian artery (type B dissection).

Type A dissection
- is caused by medial degeneration, or cystic medionecrosis, of the aortic wall,
- usually occurs in middle age,
- is not associated with hypertension,
- may be associated with Marfan's syndrome (q.v.),
- may dissect retrograde to the sinuses of Valsalva, then possibly either causing aortic regurgitation or rupturing into the pericardium causing tamponade,
- may dissect antegrade to any of the major aortic branches, including spinal, mesenteric and other arteries, with consequent distal ischaemia.

Type B dissection
- occurs primarily in elderly hypertensive and/or atherosclerotic patients,
- typically presents with chest pain radiating to the back,
- usually dissects antegrade and extends as far as the abdomen.

The clinical features of aortic dissection include
- sudden chest pain mimicking acute myocardial infarction but without ECG changes,
- unequal pulses,
- aortic regurgitation,
- neurological signs,
- a widened mediastinum on chest X-ray.

The diagnosis is confirmed by transoesophageal echocardiography, CT scanning (especially CT angiography), angiography or MRI.

Treatment is either medical or surgical.
- **Medical treatment** may be in preparation for surgery or may be the primary therapy, especially for type B dissection. Treatment emphasis is to decrease the physical stress on the aortic wall by potent antihypertensive agents and beta blockers.
- **Surgery** is indicated for type A dissection as an emergency and for chronic dissection electively. Surgery for type B dissection generally carries a higher mortality than nonoperative treatment. Operative mortality for type A dissection is reported to be 10–35%, depending on comorbidities and the frequent requirement for associated aortic valve replacement and reimplantation of the coronary arteries.
- **Endovascular stenting** can be successfully employed in many cases of dissection of the descending aorta.

Mortality is said to be 1% per hour for the first 24 hr, especially in type A dissections involving the ascending aorta. Peripheral ischaemia is a poor prognostic sign. In patients who survive, the prevalence of recurrence of dissection is considerable, ranging from 15% to 40%. Aneurysmal dilatation may become a late problem.

Bibliography

Armstrong WE, Bach DS, Carey LM, et al. Clinical and echocardiographic findings in patients with suspected acute aortic dissection. *Am Heart J* 1998; 136: 1051.

Booher AM, Eagle KA. Diseases of the aorta. In: *Scientific American Medicine. Cardiovascular Medicine*. Hamilton: Dekker Medicine. 2020.

Crawford ES. The diagnosis and management of aortic dissection. *JAMA* 1990; 264: 2537.

DeSanctis RW, Doroghazi RM, Austen WG, et al. Aortic dissection. *N Engl J Med* 1987; 317: 1060.

Hagan PG, Nienaber CA, Isselbacher EM, et al. The international registry of aortic dissection (IRAD): new insights into an old disease. *JAMA* 2000; 283: 897.

Hayter RG, Rhea JT, Small A, et al. Suspected aortic dissection and other aortic disorders: multidetector row CT in 373 cases in the emergency setting. *Radiology* 2006; 238: 841.

Khan IA, Nair CK. Clinical, diagnostic and management perspectives of aortic dissection. *Chest* 2002; 122: 311.

Mehta RH, Suzuki T, Hagan PG, et al. Predicting death in patients with acute type A aortic dissection. *Circulation* 2002; 105: 200.

Treasure T, Raphael MJ. Investigation of suspected dissection of the thoracic aorta. *Lancet* 1991; 338: 490.

Trimarchi S, Nienaber CA, Rampoldi V, et al. Contemporary results of surgery in acute type A aortic dissection: the international registry of aortic dissection experience. *J Thorac Cardiovasc Surg* 2005; 129: 112.

Aortitis *See*

- Aortic coarctation,
- Arteritis,
- Vasculitis.

Bibliography
Booher AM, Eagle KA. Diseases of the aorta. In: *Scientific American Medicine. Cardiovascular Medicine.* Hamilton: Dekker Medicine. 2020.

Aplastic anaemia *See*

- Anaemia.
  See also
- Reticulocytes,
- Thrombocytopenia.

Arachnids

Arachnids are one of the main groups of arthropods (q.v.). They have four pairs of legs. Those arachnids which are important in human disease, because they are either vectors or directly venomous, include

- mites (q.v.),
- scorpions (see Bites and stings – Scorpions),
- spiders (see Bites and stings – Spiders),
- ticks (q.v.).

ARDS *See*

- Acute respiratory distress syndrome.
  See also
- Acute pulmonary oedema.

Argatroban *See*

- Anticoagulants,
- Heparin-induced thrombocytopenia.

Arnold–Chiari malformation

The **Arnold–Chiari malformation** is one of the congenital **neural tube defects** (q.v.). These also include meningomyelocoele, syringomyelia and stenosis of the aqueduct of Sylvius. The most severe form is anencephaly.

There is an increased incidence of neural tube defects in babies of mothers who are folic acid deficient (q.v.) or who fail to take folic acid supplementation during pregnancy.

The Arnold–Chiari malformation comprises downward displacement of the lower medulla and cerebellar tonsils through the foramen magnum. Half of the cases are associated with syringomyelia (q.v.).

Although developmental, it commonly presents initially in adults, with pain in the back of the head, extending down over the shoulders and arms and exacerbated by coughing.
There may be associated
- bulbar symptoms,
- blurred vision,
- nystagmus,
- vertigo (q.v.),
- ataxia,
- respiratory failure (occasionally),
- sleep apnoea (occasionally).

*Treatment is with surgical **decompression**.*

Bibliography
Lemire RJ. Neural tube defects. *JAMA* 1988; 259: 558.
Milunsky A, Ulcickas M, Rothman K, et al. Maternal heat exposure and neural tube defects. *JAMA* 1992; 268: 882.
Paul KS, Lye RH, Strang FA, et al. Arnold-Chiari malformation. *J Neurosurg* 1983; 58: 183.
Wald NJ, Bower C. Folic acid, pernicious anaemia, and prevention of neural tube defects. *Lancet* 1994; 343: 307.

Arsenic

Arsenic (As, atomic number 33, atomic weight 75) is a non-metallic element in the nitrogen family. Although arsenic-containing compounds have been known since antiquity and arsenic is widely distributed in nature in various forms, the element was not identified until 1649. Arsenicals are used in herbicides, pesticides and various manufacturing processes.

Arsenic poisoning may be occupational, accidental or deliberate (the latter in a suicide attempt, as a classical criminal agent or as a military poison).

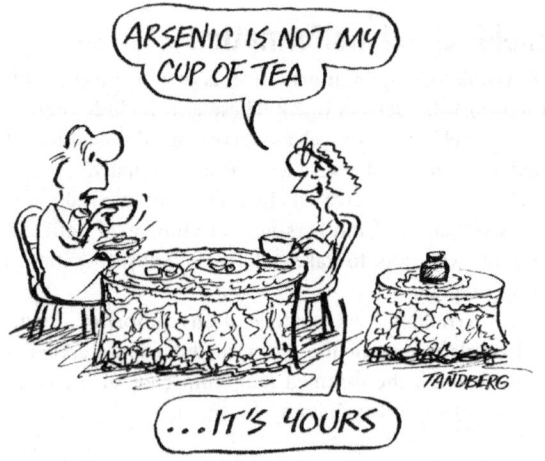

Toxicity from arsenic arises from inactivation of cellular enzymes, though there is great individual variation in susceptibility and many famous cases of tolerance. Most such preparations are arsenates.

- Arsenious oxide (As_4O_6) is a colourless, odourless and tasteless compound, much beloved in detective fiction and presumably as commonly in reality.
- Arsine (arsenic hydride, AsH_3) is a colourless gas, used as a doping agent for semi-conductors and also as a military poison.
- Potassium arsenate was known pharmaceutically as Fowler's solution, a tonic promoted for a variety of ailments, though such arsenicals are not nowadays used clinically.
- Arsenic may also be contained in tobacco, from which it is oxidized like other heavy metals as the tobacco is burned.
- **Arsenic trioxide** (originally found in a traditional Chinese medicine for leukaemia) has been introduced for the treatment of relapsed acute promyelocytic leukaemia. Numerous side-effects are common, but the most serious have been prolonged QT interval and **differentiation syndrome** (q.v.), the latter with pulmonary infiltration, pleural effusions and fever.

Arsenate is isostructural with orthophosphate and thus can become misincorporated into DNA. Various international standards recommend the limitation of exposure to inorganic arsenic to not >10 mcg/m^3/8 hr or 2 mcg/m^3/15 min, beyond which dermatitis and cancer of the lung and of the lymphoid tissues may occur. A urinary concentration of >0.67 μmol/L (>50 mcg/L) confirms a diagnosis of acute arsenic poisoning.

Arsenic poisoning may be either acute or chronic.

Acute poisoning is manifest by
- nausea,
- burning of the mouth,
- abdominal pain,
- acute haemolytic anaemia (q.v.),
- shock and death within an hour.

Chronic poisoning is manifest by
- weakness,
- paralysis,
- confusion,
- toxic neuropathy (q.v.),
- skin pigmentation (q.v.), keratoses and cancer,
- streaking of the nails (q.v.).
- anaemia (q.v.),
- hepatic cirrhosis,
- renal failure.

The **neuropathy** is similar to that produced by many toxic agents and indeed drugs.

The **skin pigmentation** is bronze in colour and is the characteristic skin lesion, with 'rain drop' areas of hypopigmentation due to hypomelanotic macules.

In addition to keratoses, there may be **skin cancer**, either basal cell carcinoma or squamous cell carcinoma. Although Bowen's disease, which resembles superficial basal cell carcinoma, usually arises from solar exposure, when it follows arsenic ingestion it can occur in covered areas of the skin.

The **anaemia** of chronic poisoning is due to decreased red blood cell production.

The **hepatic cirrhosis** is similar to that produced by excess vitamin A and methotrexate.

The **renal failure** is due initially to tubular damage and later to residual tubulointerstitial scarring giving rise to a chronic nephropathy, similar to that produced by mercury (q.v.).

The treatment of arsenic poisoning is with **gastric lavage** if recently ingested.

Both acute and chronic poisoning are treated with **dimercaprol** (BAL)(q.v.).

See also
- Occupational lung diseases,
- Paraneoplastic syndromes,
- Warfare agents.

Bibliography

Duenas-Laita A, Perez-Miranda M, Gozalez-Lopez M, et al. Acute arsenic poisoning. *Lancet* 2005; 365: 1982.

Kyle RA, Pease GL. Hematologic aspects of arsenic intoxication. *N Engl J Med* 1965; 273: 18.

Arteriovenous malformations

Arteriovenous malformations (AVMs) may occur either as a widespread phenomenon (the Osler–Weber–Rendu disease) or as isolated lesions (usually affecting either the cerebral or pulmonary circulation).

- **Osler–Weber–Rendu disease (hereditary haemorrhagic telangiectasia**, HHT) is an autosomal dominant condition causing ectasia of small blood vessels. There is multisystem vascular dysplasia and recurrent haemorrhage. Its prevalence is 1 in 5–10,000 of the population.

Genetically, the condition is heterogeneous with a variety of responsible mutations reported. Genetic testing is available. The end-result appears to be impairment of the function of endoglin, a membrane glycoprotein which assists the binding to various cells, particularly endothelial cells, of transforming growth factor β (TGF-β).

The condition becomes manifest after puberty, with a penetrance of almost 100% by the age of 40 yr. It presents particularly as spider naevi on the skin of the face and fingers and on the mucous membranes of the mouth and nose. Ectatic vessels may also develop in the gut, urinary tract, liver, brain and spinal cord. The lung is involved in about 20% of cases (see below). There may be associated platelet dysfunction, but coagulation is normal.

Patients commonly present with bleeding, either acute and local or chronic with anaemia. Recurrent epistaxis is typical. Surveillance of suspected or confirmed cases is recommended.

Recent reports suggest that **bevacizumab**, *a recombinant monoclonal antibody to vascular endothelial growth factor (VEGF), may offer effective treatment.* **Thalidomide** *and subsequently* **propranolol** *(propanolol) have also been reported to be of benefit.* **Tranexamic acid** *(TXA) (q.v.) is effective in reducing the duration but not the frequency of epistaxes.*

- **Cerebral AVMs** are congenital but usually do not present until early adult life (average age 35 years).

Most become manifest as intracerebral and/or intraventricular or subarachnoid haemorrhage. The annual rate of recurrent bleeding from such lesions is about 4%.

The AVM should be obliterated by **surgery** *or* **embolization** *or, if these are not successful or feasible, by stereotactic* **irradiation**.

- **Pulmonary AVMs** or arteriovenous fistulae are one of the causes of single pulmonary nodules either small or large (q.v.). However, in about one third of the cases, the lesions are multiple and often bilateral. As with cerebral AVMs, the condition is often congenital but becomes apparent only in adult life. About half the cases with multiple lesions in fact have Osler–Weber–Rendu disease (see above) with multiple AVMs elsewhere throughout the body. Other cases may be due to trauma, infection or hepatopulmonary syndrome (q.v.).

Clinical features include hypoxaemia (from right-to-left shunting), haemoptysis, paradoxical systemic embolization and exertional dyspnoea if the condition is severe and especially if there is associated anaemia. Cyanosis and clubbing may be seen and also polycythaemia if there is no systemic bleeding. Pulmonary hypertension, cardiac failure and AVM rupture with haemoptysis or haemothorax are uncommon.

The condition should be suspected if the lesion on chest X-ray is seen to have a leash (containing the feeding artery and draining vein). Pulmonary angiography has been replaced by CT scanning for definitive diagnosis. Transthoracic contrast echocardiography has very good negative predictive value for the identification of right-to-left shunting.

Surgical **resection** *may be considered if the lesion is single and large, but resection is usually unsatisfactory because other small lesions may subsequently enlarge.*

Radiological **embolization** *provides a more satisfactory solution. It is currently the recommended treatment, as soon as an AVM is identified with a feeding artery >3 mm in diameter and even before a complication has occurred. Since recanalization or enlargement of collaterals can occur, long-term follow-up is recommended.*

Antibiotic prophylaxis *is advised for procedures (as for endocarditis – q.v.) to reduce the risk of subsequent cerebral abscess.*

See also
- Hepatopulmonary syndrome.

Bibliography

Begbie ME, Wallace GM, Shovlin CL. Hereditary hemorrhagic telangiectasia (Osler–Weber–Rendu syndrome): a view from the 21st century. *Postgrad Med J* 2003; 79: 18.

Bose P, Holter JL, Selby GB. Bevacizumab in hereditary hemorrhagic telangiectasia. *N Engl J Med* 2009; 360: 2143.

Brier G. Propanolol and angiogenesis inhibition in hereditary haemorrhagic telangiectasia. *Thromb Haemost* 2012; 108: 1.

Cartin-Ceba R, Swanson KL, Krowka MJ. Pulmonary arteriovenous malformations. *Chest* 2013; 144: 1033.

Dines DE, Arms RA, Bernatz PE, et al. Pulmonary arteriovenous fistulas. *Mayo Clin Proc* 1974; 48: 460.

Dupuis-Girod S, Bailly S, Plauchu H. Hereditary hemorrhagic telangiectasia: from molecular biology to patient care. *J Thromb Haemost* 2010; 8: 1447.

Gossage JR, Kanj G. Pulmonary arteriovenous malformations. *Am J Respir Crit Care Med* 1998; 158: 643.

Gupta S, Faughnan ME, Bayoumi AM. Embolization for pulmonary arteriovenous malformation in hereditary hemorrhagic telangiectasia. *Chest* 2009; 136: 849.

Guttmacher AE, Marchuk DA, White RI. Hereditary hemorrhagic telangiectasia. *N Engl J Med* 1995; 333: 918.

Lacombe P, Lagrange C, Beauchet A, et al. Diffuse pulmonary arteriovenous malformations in hereditary hemorrhagic telangiectasia: long-term results of embolization according to the extent of lung involvement. *Chest* 2009; 135: 1031.

Ondra SL, Troupp H, George ED, et al. The natural history of symptomatic arteriovenous malformations of the brain. *J Neurosurg* 1990; 73: 387.

Sabba C. A rare and misdiagnosed bleeding disorder: hereditary hemorrhagic telangiectasia. *J Thromb Haemost* 2005; 3: 2201.

Salaria M, Taylor J, Bogwitz M, et al. Hereditary haemorrhagic telangiectasia, an Australian cohort: clinical and investigative features. *Intern Med J* 2014; 44: 639.

Shovlin CL. Hereditary haemorrhagic telangiectasia: pathophysiology, diagnosis and treatment. *Blood Rev* 2010; 24: 203.

Shovlin CL, Condliffe R, Donaldson JW, et al. British Thoracic Society clinical statement on pulmonary arteriovenous malformations. *Thorax* 2017; 72: 1154.

Terry PB, Barth KH, Kaufman SL, et al. Balloon embolization for the treatment of pulmonary arteriovenous fistulas. *N Engl J Med* 1980; 302: 1189.

White RJ, Lynch-Nyhan A, Terry P, et al. Pulmonary arteriovenous malformation: techniques and long-term outcome of embolotherapy. *Radiology* 1988; 169: 663.

Arteritis

Most types of **arteritis** are more appropriately discussed in the general section on **vasculitis** (q.v.).

> However, three conditions may be considered as specifically arteritic, namely,
> - cerebral arteritis,
> - giant cell arteritis,
> - endarteritis.

Cerebral arteritis is a diffuse inflammation of the intracranial arteries which may be either primary or secondary.

- **Primary arteritis** is an isolated condition causing a fluctuating encephalopathy (q.v.) over weeks or months, with headache, confusion and focal neurological signs. The diagnosis is made angiographically. *Treatment is with* **corticosteroids** *and* **immunosuppression**.
- **Secondary arteritis** occurs in giant cell arteritis (see below), AIDS (q.v.), HZV infection (see Herpesviruses), TB (see Tuberculosis), sarcoidosis (q.v.), collagen-vascular diseases (q.v.) and Hodgkin's disease.

Giant cell arteritis (temporal arteritis) is the most common and important form of arteritis because it may have serious complications if untreated.

It usually presents in patients older than 50 years and is associated with both

- systemic features of fever, anorexia and weight loss,
- local features of headache and scalp tenderness with palpable nodules.

There may be associated **polymyalgia rheumatica** (q.v.).

Clinical features may be present for many weeks, and blindness, neuropathy (q.v.), cerebral ischaemia, vertigo (q.v.) or depression may occur before the diagnosis is made. In particular, the blindness which is due to ischaemic neuritis is sudden and irreversible and may sometimes be bilateral.

Diagnosis is assisted by the finding of mild anaemia and raised ESR and is confirmed by temporal artery biopsy. New imaging modalities and novel therapies are being studied.

Treatment with **corticosteroids** *is the mainstay of therapy and provides a rapid response.* **Tocilizumab** *(q.v.), a monoclonal antibody to interleukin 6 (IL-6) receptors, may be used for steroid-sparing.*

Endarteritis is an infective lesion of the endothelium, analogous with endocarditis (q.v.).

It usually affects the abdominal aorta (i.e. aortitis) or iliofemoral arteries and may involve atherosclerotic plaques and aneurysms, as well as the normal vessel wall.

- Endarteritis is usually bacterial (especially from salmonella), but it can be due to fungi, rickettsiae or chlamydiae.
- Endarteritis may also be produced by irradiation, which causes inflammation and eventually fibrosis of the vasa vasorum, though initially the condition may be steroid-responsive.

Bibliography

Bahlas S, Ramos-Remus C, Davis P. Clinical outcome of 149 patients with polymyalgia rheumatica and giant cell arteritis. *J Rheumatol* 1998; 25: 99.

Booher AM, Eagle KA. Diseases of the aorta. In: *Scientific American Medicine. Cardiovascular Medicine.* Hamilton: Dekker Medicine. 2020.

Calabrese L, Dune G, Lie J. Vasculitis in the central nervous system. *Arthritis Rheum* 1997; 40: 1189.

Denny KJ, Kumar A, Timsit J-F, et al. Extra-cardiac endovascular infections in the critically ill. *Intens Care Med* 2020; 46: 173.

Deipolyi AR, Czaplicki CD, Oklu R. Inflammatory and infectious aortic diseases. *Cardiovasc Diagn Ther* 2018; 8: 561.

Hamilton CR, Shelley WM, Tumulty PA. Giant cell arteritis: including temporal arteritis and polymyalgia rheumatica. *Medicine* 1971; 50: 1.

Hunder GG, Bloch DA, Michel BA, et al. The American College of Rheumatology 1990 criteria for the classification of giant cell arteritis. *Arthritis Rheum* 1990; 33: 1122.

Moore PM. Diagnosis and management of isolated angiitis of the central nervous system. *Neurology* 1989; 39: 167.

Ninan JV, Lester S, Hill CL. Giant cell arteritis: beyond temporal artery biopsy and steroids. *Intern Med J* 2017; 47: 1228.

Oz MC, Brener BJ, Buda JA, et al. A ten-year experience with bacterial aortitis. *J Vasc Surg* 1989; 10: 439.

Zilko PJ. Polymyalgia rheumatica and giant cell arteritis. *Med J Aust* 1996; 165: 438.

Arthritis

Arthritis (and arthropathies – q.v.) describe conditions affecting joints, though strictly arthritis refers to conditions which are inflammatory in nature. Such conditions are traditionally classified as

- **degenerative**
  - primary or secondary,
- **infective** (or septic)
  - usually direct viral, bacterial, fungal or parasitic infection in joints,
  - polymicrobial in about 10% of cases,
  - arthroscopic drainage is usually recommended, as well as antibiotics and initial immobilization,
  - sometimes indirect (i.e. **'reactive'** arthritis), with an infection at some other site precipitating arthritis by a presumed immunological mechanism (see Reiter's syndrome).
- **metabolic disorders**
  - including crystal-induced arthritis (e.g. gout and pseudogout – q.v.),
- **connective tissue diseases** (q.v.)
  - including rheumatoid arthritis, systemic lupus erythematosus (SLE), scleroderma, polyarteritis nodosa, Sjogren's syndrome, Behcet's syndrome, overlap syndromes,
  - see these separate conditions,
- **neuropathic**
- **spondyloarthritis**
  - q.v.,
- **miscellaneous** conditions
  - such as drug-induced joint manifestations, as in SLE (q.v.) or serum sickness (q.v.).

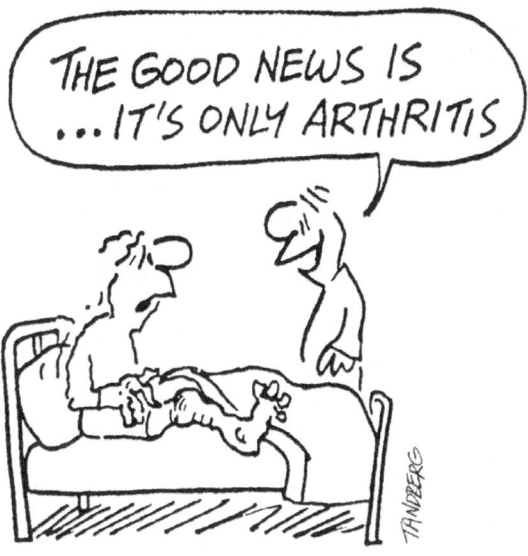

Acute **monoarthritis** is typically infective, though it may often be associated with systemic disease, especially if there are other concomitant clinical features.

Thus, the additional presence of
- erythema nodosum (q.v.) suggests inflammatory bowel disease (q.v.), sarcoidosis (q.v.), SLE (q.v.),
- mouth ulcers (see Ulcers) suggest Behcet's syndrome (q.v.), Reiter's syndrome (q.v.), SLE (q.v.),
- splinter haemorrhages suggest bacterial endocarditis (q.v.).

Fever is absent in 40% of cases of septic arthritis, whereas it may occur in crystal-induced arthritis. Thus, synovial fluid examination is diagnostically important in all cases of acute, painful joint swelling.

It is generally recommended that NSAIDs are avoided in the early stages of suspected septic arthritis, as they can blunt an inflammatory response and therefore mimic a response to concomitantly administered antibiotics (which might not therefore have been effective in their own right).

Infection in a prosthetic joint is a particularly difficult problem.

Bibliography

Ashbaugh C. Septic arthritis, septic bursitis, and osteomyelitis. In: *Scientific American Medicine. Infectious Diseases or Rheumatology*. Hamilton: Dekker Medicine. 2020.

Editorial. Reactive arthritis. *BMJ* 1980; 281: 311.

Gibofsky A, Zabriskie JB. Rheumatic fever and poststreptococcal reactive arthritis. *Curr Opin Rheumatol* 1995; 7: 299.

Gupta MN, Sturrock RD, Field M. Prospective comparative study of patients with culture proven and high suspicion of adult onset septic arthritis. *Ann Rheum Dis* 2003; 62: 327.

Hamerman D. The biology of osteoarthritis. *N Engl J Med* 1989; 320: 1322.

Lidgren L, Knutson K, Stefansdottir A. Infection and arthritis: infection of prosthetic joints. *Best Practice Res Clin Rheumatol* 2003; 17: 209.

Smith JW. Infectious arthritis. *Infect Dis Clin North Am* 1990; 4: 523.

Weston VC, Jones AC, Bradbury N, et al. Clinical features and outcome of septic arthritis in a single UK health district 1982–1991. *Ann Rheum Dis* 1999; 58: 214.

Winblad S. Arthritis associated with Yersinia enterocolitica infections. *Scand J Infect Dis* 1975; 7: 191.

Arthropathies

Arthropathy refers to any joint disease, whereas **arthritis** refers to inflammatory joint disease. Since most joint diseases are in fact inflammatory, at least to some degree, the two terms are for practical purposes interchangeable, and most such diseases have therefore been considered under arthritis (q.v.).

See also
- Haemochromatosis,
- Lung tumours,
- Selenium deficiency,
- Vasculitis,
- Whipple's disease.

Arthropods

Arthropods are invertebrates with an exoskeleton, segmented body and jointed legs. The phylum of arthropods includes several subphyla which in turn contain several of importance in a number of human diseases, including
- insects, which have three pairs of legs,
- arachnids, which have four pairs of legs,
- crustaceans, which have five pairs of legs.

Insects (q.v.) of importance include ants (see Bites and stings – insects), fleas (q.v.), lice (q.v.) and mosquitoes (q.v.). These are either vectors of disease or venom-carrying.

Arachnids (q.v.) of importance include mites (q.v.), scorpions (see Bites and stings – scorpions), spiders (see Bites and stings – spiders) and ticks (q.v.). Like insects, these can be either vectors of disease or venom-carrying.

Crustaceans may harbour organisms causing human disease, e.g. hepatitis (q.v.), norovirus (q.v.), paragonimiasis (q.v.), paralytic shellfish poisoning (q.v.).

See also
- Platelets – haemocytes.

Arthus reaction *See*

- Immune complex disease.

See also
- Drug allergy.

Asbestos

Asbestos is a natural mineral fibre freed from crushed rock, usually chrysotile, and composed of magnesium silicate. It is resistant to fire, acid and alkali. Because it is virtually indestructible, its smooth brittle fibres have been widely used commercially since the nineteenth century both for building and for thermal insulation.

After the association of asbestos exposure with mesothelioma was first described in 1960, its use declined markedly from the 1980s onwards due to workplace safety regulations. In the body, the silicate groups gradually dissociate and then substitute for phosphates, thus deranging DNA. Safe exposure limits of $<100–200,000$ fibres of $>5 \, \mu/m^3/8$ hr have been set.

Calculations of the worldwide health burden from occupational and environmental exposure to asbestos suggest a projected 5–10 million cancers, with 30,000 in Australia alone (two thirds lung cancer, one third mesothelioma). Because of this and because there are now safe and economic alternatives, an international ban on all mining and use of asbestos has been recommended. However, the continuing widespread use of asbestos in developing countries is expected to result in a rising burden of asbestos-related diseases for many decades into the future. Moreover, the popularity of amateur home renovations is considered an ongoing risk in developed countries, since a variety of asbestos-containing materials were commonly used in many older buildings.

> The risks from asbestos exposure include
> - lung cancer (see Lung tumours),
> - mesothelioma (though some cases may be due to radiation),
> - pneumoconiosis (asbestosis) (see Occupational lung diseases),
> - pleural plaques (see Pleural disorders).

Lung cancer follows heavy exposure, and the risk is enhanced 8-fold by concomitant cigarette smoking.

Mesothelioma (malignant mesothelioma, MM) is usually pleural but sometimes it may be peritoneal. Unlike lung cancer, it can occur even after a single exposure and may have a latent period of up to 30 or more years. About 80% of cases of mesothelioma are caused by asbestos. Since the average time from exposure to diagnosis is so long and since exposure to asbestos did not decline until relatively recently, the incidence of mesothelioma is still rising and is not expected to peak until the 2020s. A sensitive diagnostic blood test for soluble mesothelin-related protein (SMRP) has been developed, and a number of other biomarkers (q.v.) are also being assessed. However, diagnosis can be difficult, with differentiation either from other primary or metastatic malignancies or from reactive mesothelial hyperplasia often challenging. Moreover, treatment options are limited, though novel immunotherapeutic strategies are currently being explored. At present, the median survival is still only 9–12 months.

Pneumoconiosis (asbestosis) consists of a diffuse pulmonary infiltrate. The risk is dose-related, with a long latent period of 20 years or more, followed by a slowly progressive fibrosis, with cough and dyspnoea. The characteristic findings include particularly decreased gas transfer, also decreased lung volumes and impaired gas exchange, but normal lung mechanics. The lung function abnormalities precede both symptoms and radiographic changes. Asbestos bodies can be recovered in bronchoalveolar lavage fluid.

Pleural plaques are discrete connective tissue collections on the parietal pleura and follow heavy exposure to asbestos or sometimes other inorganic fibres. Histologically, they contain collagen but not asbestos. They are usually seen on the lateral posterior or basal pleural surfaces and not in the costophrenic angle nor in the upper third of the thorax. They vary greatly in diameter and have an average thickness of 5 mm. Most are bilateral and calcified. If not calcified, they may be seen only in tangential views. They develop slowly with a latent period of 20 years or more. They are a marker only of asbestos exposure and do not predispose to symptoms, functional changes or malignancy. If non-calcified, they should be distinguished from other causes of local pleural thickening, such as inflammation, trauma or malignancy. Sometimes there may be more diffuse pleural fibrosis rather than discrete lesions. Since the chest X-ray has relatively low sensitivity for the detection of pleural plaques, they are best identified by CT scanning.

See
- Occupational lung diseases.

Bibliography

Banks DE, Shi R, McLarty J, et al. American College of Chest Physicians consensus statement on the respiratory health effects of asbestos. *Chest* 2009; 135: 1619.

Berry G. Environmental mesothelioma incidence, time since exposure to asbestos and level of exposure. *Environmetrics* 1995; 6: 221.

Bowman R, Relan V, Hughes B. Medical management of mesothelioma. *Aust Prescriber* 2011; 34: 144.

Cagle PT, Allen TC. Pathology of the pleura: what the pulmonologists need to know. *Respirology* 2011; 16: 430.

Creaney J, Robinson BWS. Malignant mesothelioma biomarkers: from discovery to use in clinical practice for diagnosis, monitoring, screening, and treatment. *Chest* 2017; 152; 143.

Cugell DW, Kamp DW. Asbestos and the pleura. *Chest* 2004; 125: 1103.

Jamrozik E, de Klerk N, Musk AW. Asbestos-related disease. *Intern Med J* 2011; 41: 372.

Kao SC-H, Reid G, Lee K, et al. Malignant mesothelioma. *Intern Med J* 2010; 40: 742.

Mossman BT, Bignon J, Corn M, et al. Asbestos: scientific developments and implications for public policy. *Science* 1990; 247: 294.

Musk AW, de Klerk N, Brims FJ. Mesothelioma in Australia: a review. *Med J Aust* 2017; 207: 449.

Ohar J, Sterling DA, Bleecker E, et al. Changing patterns in asbestos-induced lung disease. *Chest* 2004; 125: 744.

Olsen NJ, Franklin PJ, Reid A, et al. Increasing incidence of malignant mesothelioma after exposure to asbestos during home maintenance and renovation. *Med J Aust* 2011; 195: 271.

Peto J, Decarli A, La Vecchia C, et al. The European mesothelioma epidemic. *Br J Cancer* 1999; 79: 566.

Park EK, Sandrini A, Yates DH, et al. Soluble mesothelin-related protein in an asbestos-exposed population: the dust diseases board cohort study. *Am J Respir Crit Care Med* 2008; 178: 832.

Pistolesi M, Rusthoven J. Malignant pleural mesothelioma: update, current management, and newer treatment strategies. *Chest* 2004; 126: 1318.

Ray M, Kindler HL. Malignant pleural mesothelioma: an update on biomarkers and treatment. *Chest* 2009; 136: 888.

Robinson BW, Creaney J, Lake R, et al. Soluble mesothelin-related protein – a blood test for mesothelioma. *Lung Cancer* 2005; 49 (suppl. 1): S109.

Robinson BW, Musk AW, Lake RA. Malignant mesothelioma. *Lancet* 2005; 366: 397.

Singhal S, Kaiser LR. Malignant mesothelioma: options for management. *Surg Clin North Am* 2002; 82: 797.

Sterman DH, Kaiser LR, Albelda SM. Advances in the treatment of malignant pleural mesothelioma. *Chest* 1999; 116: 504.

Teirstein AS. Diagnosing malignant pleural mesothelioma. *Chest* 1998; 114: 666.

van Ruth S, Baas P, Zoetmulder FA. Surgical treatment of malignant pleural mesothelioma: a review. *Chest* 2003; 123: 551.

Zellos LS, Sugarbaker DJ. Multimodality treatment of diffuse malignant pleural mesothelioma. *Semin Oncol* 2002; 29: 41.

Aspergillosis

Aspergillosis is caused by the fungus aspergillus, most commonly *A. fumigatus* but occasionally others, e.g. *A. flavus*. Aspergillus is a ubiquitous saprophyte in nature, and infection arises only when it is aerosolized into a normally sterile site, so that it is usually a pulmonary infection. Moreover, its isolation from normal subjects may not be significant, whereas its presence in an immunocompromised patient should be taken seriously.

> Aspergillosis may produce one of three pulmonary conditions, namely,
> - mycetoma,
> - allergic disease,
> - invasive disease.

Mycetoma is a fungus ball which occupies an existing cavity. Aspergillus is the most common cause of a fungus ball (then often called an **aspergilloma**), though sometimes other fungi may produce a similar condition. Haemorrhage occurs in more than half the patients and can be fatal. There is an overall mortality of 5–10%. The sputum is usually negative for the organism.

Treatment is with **surgery**.

Allergic bronchopulmonary aspergillosis (ABPA) is associated with wheeze, eosinophilia and brown plugs of sputum. Typically, the patient presents with chronic asthma.

The sputum is usually positive for the organism, and skin tests and serum precipitins are also usually positive. There are recurrent pulmonary infiltrates on chest X-ray.

Treatment is with **corticosteroids**. The oral antifungal agent **itraconazole** (200 mg bd) has been shown to add further improvement without toxicity in patients with this condition who were steroid-dependent.

See
- Asthma,
- Eosinophilia and lung infiltration – asthmatic pulmonary eosinophilia.

Invasive aspergillosis (IA) usually occurs only in immunocompromised hosts, particularly the neutropenic. There is a necrotizing pneumonia with haemorrhagic infarction and cavitation, and sometimes systemic metastases. Sputum cultures are positive for the organism in only about 30% of cases, and blood cultures are always negative, but culture of BAL (q.v.) fluid is generally positive. Serology is unhelpful, but β-D-glucan testing in serum is a useful screening test for fungal infection in general. If positive, the specific diagnosis may be confirmed by an ELISA test for Aspergillus galactomannan antigen in serum or BAL fluid, though the accuracy and particularly the sensitivity of this test have been questioned. PCR testing for specific fungal nucleic acids is available in some centres.

Treatment is with **voriconazole** as the first-line agent or with **amphotericin** B or **itraconazole** as alternative agents. Other antifungal drugs, such as **caspofungin** and **anidulafungin**, may be considered for salvage therapy.

See also
- Acquired immunodeficiency syndrome,
- Exotic pneumonia,
- Sweating – Night sweats,
- Wegener's granulomatosis – Bronchocentric granulomatosis.

Bibliography

Agarwal R. Allergic bronchopulmonary aspergillosis. *Chest* 2009; 135: 805.

Chatzimichalis A, Massard G, Kessler R, et al. Bronchopulmonary aspergilloma: a reappraisal. *Ann Thorac Surg* 1998; 65: 927.

Douglas AP, Smibert OC, Bajel A, et al. Consensus guidelines for the diagnosis and management of invasive aspergillosis, 2021. *Intern Med J* 2021; 51: 143.

Janssen JJWM, Strack van Schijndel RJM, van der Poest Clement EH, et al. Outcome of ICU treatment in invasive aspergillosis. *Intens Care Med* 1996; 22: 1315.

Koulenti D, Vogelaers D, Blot S. What's new in invasive pulmonary aspergillosis in the critically ill. *Intens Care Med* 2014; 40: 723.

Levitz SM. Aspergillosis. *Infect Dis Clin North Am* 1989; 3: 1.

Oakley EJ, Petrou M, Goldstraw P. Indications and outcome of surgery for pulmonary aspergilloma. *Thorax* 1997; 52: 813.

Patterson KC, Strek ME. Diagnosis and treatment of pulmonary aspergillosis syndromes. *Chest* 2014; 146: 1358.

Ricketti AJ, Greenberger PA, Mintzer RA, et al. Allergic bronchopulmonary aspergillosis. *Arch Intern Med* 1983; 143: 1553.

Schuyler MR. Allergic bronchopulmonary aspergillosis. *Clin Chest Med* 1983; 4: 15.

Soubani AO, Chandrasekar PH. The clinical spectrum of pulmonary aspergillosis. *Chest* 2002; 121: 1988.

Stevens DA, Schwartz HJ, Lee JY, et al. A randomized trial of itraconazole in allergic bronchopulmonary aspergillosis. *N Engl J Med* 2000; 342: 756.

Aspiration

Aspiration pneumonitis (chemical pneumonia, Mendelson's syndrome) refers to the inhalation of gastric contents. The original description of this condition was in obstetric patients in 1946, in whom it is still a significant problem. Aspiration remains the second most common cause of death directly related to anaesthesia, with an incidence nearly as high as for anaphylaxis (the commonest cause of anaesthetic-related death).

Aspiration pneumonitis describes the initial chemical injury of the lung, whereas **aspiration pneumonia** refers to any subsequent complicating bacterial infection of the lung. Other aspiration-related problems are also recognized, since aspiration refers broadly to the entry of any foreign material into the respiratory tract.

Aspiration of gastric contents is a serious complication in the patient whose airway is unprotected because of impaired consciousness or other causes of impaired airway defence and/or disturbance of gastro-oesophageal function. Many of the procedures in caring for the unconscious patient, particularly in Anaesthesia and in Intensive Care, relate to airway protection and thus prevention of aspiration. The risk of aspiration particularly applies during emergency intubation, when a rapid sequence procedure should be used or cricoid pressure (Sellick's manoeuvre) may be considered.

The pathogenesis of aspiration is related to the acidity of the gastric contents and is especially significant when the pH is less than 2.5. Acid inhalation causes immediate chemical damage to the bronchial mucosal cells or alveolar epithelial cells, with resulting inflammatory exudate and cellular infiltrate (i.e. pneumonitis).

The clinical features start with the aspiration event itself, which may be witnessed.

- Immediate asphyxia may occasionally result, especially if the aspiration is large and particulate.
- More typically, cough, frothy sputum, dyspnoea and wheeze occur, usually within an hour or so.
- Hypoxaemia occurs and is sometimes severe.
- There may be circulatory failure due to hypovolaemia or reflex responses.
- The features of bronchopneumonia become apparent within 24–48 hr. Secondary aerobic or anaerobic infection may occur in the next few days.
- Subsequently, more chronic inflammatory consequences may occasionally be seen, including bronchiectasis (q.v.) or even bronchiolitis obliterans (q.v.).
- Specific problems occur if the aspiration is infected or if large food particles are retained.
- If the aspirate includes mineral oil, formerly a popular night-time laxative, chronic **lipoid pneumonia** (q.v.) can be produced by repeated aspiration, particularly in the elderly.

> Diagnosis of aspiration is often straightforward. However, it may be difficult if
> - the aspiration has not been witnessed,
> - the patient is already ill for other reasons,
> - no food particles and only patchy inflammation are found in the tracheobronchial tree at fibreoptic bronchoscopy.
>
> Conversely, if food particles are found in the oropharynx, a mistaken diagnosis of aspiration may be made.

The treatment of aspiration is supportive.
- *Since the chemical reaction is immediate, measures such as instillation of bicarbonate or saline lavage are not helpful.*
- *Corticosteroids have been shown to be ineffective.*
- *Prophylactic antibiotics are not generally helpful, unless the aspirate is already or later becomes bacterially contaminated.*
- *Treatment thus consists of oxygenation, cardiovascular resuscitation if necessary, intubation and mechanical*

ventilation in seriously affected patients, and bronchodilators when bronchospasm is prominent.
See also
- Acute pulmonary oedema,
- Asthma,
- Cavitation – Necrotizing pneumonia,
- Pneumonia in pregnancy,
- Polymyositis,
- Pulmonary infiltrates,
- Tetanus.

Bibliography
Baron SE, Haramati LB, Rivera VT. Radiological and clinical findings in acute and chronic exogenous lipoid pneumonia. *J Thorac Imaging* 2003; 18: 217.
DiBardino DM, Wunderink RG. Aspiration pneumonia: a review of modern trends. *J Crit Care* 2015; 30: 40.
Hu X, Lee JS, Pianosi PT, et al. Aspiration-related pulmonary syndromes. *Chest* 2015; 147: 815.
Lee A, Festic E, Park PK, et al. Characteristics and outcomes of patients hospitalized following pulmonary aspiration. *Chest* 2014; 146: 899.
Marik PE. Aspiration pneumonitis and aspiration pneumonia. *N Engl J Med* 2001; 344: 665.
Rimawi RH. Distinguishing pneumonia from pneumonitis to safely discontinue antibiotics. *Crit Care Med* 2017; 45: 1408.
Samhouri BF, Tandon YK, Hartman TE, et al. Presenting clinicoradiologic features, causes, and clinical course of exogenous lipoid pneumonia in adults. *Chest* 2021; 160: 624.
Wright BA, Jeffrey PH. Lipoid pneumonia. *Semin Respir Infect* 1990; 5: 314.

Aspirin

Aspirin (acetylsalicylic acid, ASA) was first prepared by Hoffman at Bayer and introduced into clinical medicine in 1899 as an anti-inflammatory agent. It had been preceded by sodium salicylate, which had been used since 1875 for its antipyretic and uricosuric as well as anti-inflammatory properties. This in turn had been preceded in previous centuries by the use of willowbark (salicylate-containing) as an antipyretic for ague, i.e. fever. Aspirin consists of benzoic acid with an acetyl group at the ortho position, i.e. it is the salicylate ester of acetic acid.

Its use as an analgesic (for integumental but not visceral pain), anti-inflammatory drug, antipyretic and antiplatelet agent (q.v.) are well known.

Review of previous evidence has supported the tantalizing suggestion that aspirin (and probably to a lesser extent NSAIDs) may be beneficial in both preventing and treating sepsis and perhaps other organ dysfunction (e.g. ARDS), as these conditions may have a platelet-mediated component of pathogenesis.

In the ICU, common but important issues include
- drug interactions (q.v.),
- toxic effects,
- side-effects,
- Reye's syndrome (q.v.).

Drug interactions (q.v.) are common, because the acetyl group of aspirin acetylates proteins and thus displaces protein-bound drugs.

Toxic effects of aspirin in high doses are widespread, since the drug is distributed in most tissues and fluids. Toxicity commences at serum levels which are only about twice the therapeutic level. Toxic effects occur earlier after chronic administration or in the elderly. The lethal dose is only about 150 mg/kg or 35 tablets in the average adult.

The constellation of toxic effects of aspirin is referred to as **salicylism** (i.e. salicylate toxicity), and if not promptly recognized these features can be misinterpreted as due to other serious illnesses, including sepsis.

These toxic effects may include
- circulatory depression and peripheral vasodilatation,
- respiratory stimulation initially but depression with very high doses, the initial hyperventilation comprising some increase in tidal volume but a much greater increase in respiratory rate,
- tinnitus (q.v.), vertigo (q.v.) and confusion, with coma after very high dose,
- nausea, vomiting and diarrhoea (q.v.),
- impaired haemostasis (q.v.), often with gastrointestinal bleeding,
- noncardiogenic pulmonary oedema (q.v.),
- hypoglycaemia, including low CSF glucose,
- increased renal loss of sodium, potassium and water,
- increased metabolic rate and metabolic acidosis, due to uncoupling of phosphorylation and the accumulation of metabolic products.

Treatment of salicylate toxicity includes
- *gastric lavage,*
- *correction of fluid, electrolyte, acid–base, haemostasis and temperature disturbances,*
- *forced alkaline diuresis, as urine pH >6 decreases salicylate half-life 3-fold,*
- *dialysis or charcoal haemoperfusion in severe cases.*

Side-effects of aspirin are associated with therapeutic rather than excessive doses and may include
- gastric irritability,
- salicylism, with nausea and tinnitus (q.v.),
- exacerbation of asthma (q.v.) and also of rhinitis, even possibly leading to angioedema (q.v.) or anaphylaxis (q.v.),
- exacerbation of the rare systemic mastocytosis (see Urticaria),
- an enhanced bleeding tendency (see Platelet function disorders),
- more rarely, hepatotoxicity, with a reversible and asymptomatic 'transaminitis', especially in the presence of collagen-vascular diseases (q.v.), though it has also occasionally been implicated in chronic drug-induced hepatitis (q.v.),
- contribution to analgesic nephropathy, i.e. chronic interstitial nephritis (see Tubulointerstitial diseases),
- decreased mucociliary clearance, though the clinical significance of this phenomenon is unknown.

The respiratory side-effects described above are thought to be due to deranged arachidonic acid metabolism, with decreased cyclo-oxygenase-1 (COX-1) and thus increased leukotriene production. This effect is dose-dependent and is shared by other structurally related NSAIDs, but not by paracetamol (acetaminophen) or selective COX-2 inhibitors.

Bibliography

Casey JD, Semler MW, Bastarache JA. Aspirin for sepsis prevention: an ounce of prevention? *Crit Care Med* 2017; 45: 1959.

Chen W, Janz DR, Bastarache JA, et al. Prehospital aspirin use is associated with reduced risk of acute respiratory distress syndrome in critically ill patients: a propensity-adjusted analysis. *Crit Care Med* 2015; 43: 801.

Eisen DP. Manifold beneficial effects of acetyl salicylic acid and nonsteroidal anti-inflammatory drugs on sepsis. *Intens Care Med* 2012; 38: 1249.

Gabow P, Anderson RJ, Potts DE, et al. Acid-base disturbances in the salicylate-intoxicated adult. *Arch Intern Med* 1978; 138: 1481.

Heffner JE, Sahn SA. Salicylate-induced pulmonary edema. *Ann Intern Med* 1981; 95: 405.

Heptinstall S. How important is it to keep taking the aspirin? *Thromb Haemost* 2013; 110: 1298.

Hill JB. Salicylate intoxication. *N Engl J Med* 1973; 288: 1110.

Leatherman JW, Schmitz PG. Fever, hyperdynamic shock, and multiple-system organ failure: a pseudo-sepsis syndrome associated with chronic salicylate intoxication. *Chest* 1991; 100: 1391.

Mokhlesi B, Leikin JB, Murray P, et al. Adult toxicology in critical care: part II: specific poisonings. *Chest* 2003; 123: 897.

Namazy JA, Simon RA. Sensitivity to nonsteroidal anti-inflammatory drugs. *Ann Allergy Asthma Immunol* 2002; 89: 542.

Prescott LF, Balali-Mood M, Critchley JA, et al. Diuresis or urinary alkalinisation for salicylate poisoning? *BMJ* 1982; 285: 1383.

Temple AR. Acute and chronic effects of aspirin toxicity and their treatment. *Arch Intern Med* 1981; 141: 364.

Zimmerman JL. Poisonings and overdoses in the intensive care unit: general and specific management issues. *Crit Care Med* 2003; 31: 2794.

Asplenia *See*
- Hyposplenism.

Asthma

Asthma-like symptoms can develop in any subject given a severe enough stimulus, such as a toxic gas. The presence of a viral infection heightens the susceptibility of normal subjects as well as of asthmatics to such stimuli.

Since anyone can develop asthma-like symptoms given a sufficient stimulus, it is clearly important that the definition of clinical asthma includes the concept of abnormally increased bronchial reactivity. This concept is relevant to the recent recognition of occasional epidemics of severe '**thunderstorm asthma**' which may affect a variety of patients, including many with no prior history of overt asthma.

Clearly, asthma is not a single disease but a syndrome of considerable heterogeneity, with consequent implications for different phenotype presentations and for treatment options. Updated management guidelines for asthma are regularly published by several professional bodies, including most recently the Global Initiative for Asthma. These initiatives have been particularly important, since it has been calculated that about 358 million people worldwide have asthma and about 10% of the population in developed countries will suffer from asthma at some time in their lives.

First-line therapy includes
- ***inhaled short-acting bronchodilators** ('relievers')*
  - *short-acting β2-agonists (SABAs) or ipratropium (short-acting antimuscarinic agent, SAMA),*
- ***inhaled corticosteroids** (ICSs) ('preventers')*
  - *or cromoglycate or nedocromil (mast cell stabilizers),*

- **long-acting inhaled bronchodilators** ('controllers')
    - long-acting β2-agonists (LABAs),
- **combinations** (typically LABA and ICS).
    Additional modalities, particularly for severe or uncontrolled asthma, include
- **long-acting antimuscarinic antagonists** (LAMAs)
    - e.g. tiotropium,
- **leukotriene antagonist**
    - montelukast, for aspirin sensitivity asthma,
- **anti-IgE antibody**
    - omalizumab, for atopic asthma,
- **anti-interleukin 5 (IL-5) antibody**
    - mepolizumab or reslizumab, for eosinophilic asthma, and
- **other biologics**
    - including benralizumab, dupilumab.

The differential diagnosis of asthma includes other conditions producing dyspnoea with wheeze, i.e. airways obstruction, namely,
- chronic bronchitis and emphysema,
- acute pulmonary oedema (q.v.)
    - 'cardiac asthma',
- pulmonary embolism,
- aspiration (q.v.),
- drugs (see Drugs and the lung)
    - hypersensitivity,
    - irritation,
    - smooth muscle cell contraction,
    - prostaglandin inhibition,
- acute lung irritation (q.v.),
- cystic fibrosis (q.v.),
- pulmonary infiltration with eosinophilia (q.v.)
    - specifically, allergic bronchopulmonary aspergillosis (q.v.),
- some restrictive lung diseases
    - with bronchial involvement, e.g. sarcoidosis (q.v.), rheumatoid lung,
- polyarteritis nodosa (q.v.)
    - including Churg–Strauss syndrome (q.v.),
- bronchocentric granulomatosis
    - see Wegener's granulomatosis,
- carcinoid tumour (q.v.)
    - especially with liver metastases,
- local obstruction
    - giving local wheeze.

Stridor (i.e. upper airway obstruction) needs to be excluded. Upper airway obstruction can sometimes be variable and may even be exacerbated by exercise and improved with corticosteroids, thus mimicking asthma.

The most common causes of stridor are
- extrinsic compression
    - e.g. goitre,
- foreign body,
- infection
    - croup, epiglottitis, diphtheria (q.v.),
- inflammation
    - tonsils, granulations, cricoarytenoid arthritis (q.v.), tracheomalacia, stenosis, relapsing polychondritis, sarcoidosis (q.v.), amyloid (q.v.),
- laryngeal oedema
    - e.g. anaphylaxis (q.v.), angioedema (q.v.),
- laryngospasm,
- mediastinal diseases (q.v.),
- neoplasia,
- neurological disease
    - laryngospasm, vocal cord paralysis,
- toxic gases and fumes (see Acute lung irritation),
- vocal cord dysfunction.

The clinical features of upper airway obstruction include a history of local disease and findings of hoarse voice and abnormal cough as well as stridor. Gas exchange is normal, but there is an abnormal flow-volume loop. Specific investigations include inspection by bronchoscopy and CT imaging. Of course, in patients with symptoms severe enough to warrant endotracheal intubation, there is immediate relief of the features of airway obstruction following this procedure. Moreover, the patient is able to be ventilated at normal pressures and flows and with normal gas exchange.

See also
- Churg–Strauss syndrome,
- Eosinophilia,
- Myopathy – Acute necrotizing myopathy,
- Occupational lung diseases – Occupational asthma.

Bibliography
Asthma Management Handbook. Melbourne: National Asthma Council Australia. 2006.
Barrett GE, Koopman CF, Coulthard SW. Retropharyngeal abscess. *Laryngoscope* 1984; 94: 455.
Bush A, Pavord JD. The Lancet Asthma Commission: towards the abolition of asthma? *Eur Med J* 2018; 3: 10.
Clayton-Chubb D. Hidden risk population for thunderstorm asthma. *Med J Aust* 2017; 206: 280.
Draikiwicz S, Oppenheimer J. Use of biological agents in asthma: pharmacoeconomic lessons learned from omalizumab. *Chest* 2017; 151: 249.

Editorial. Cardiac asthma. *Lancet* 1990; 335: 693.

Ernst A, Rafeq S, Boiselle P, et al. Relapsing polychondritis and airway involvement. *Chest* 2009; 135: 1024.

Gibson PG, McDonald VM. Management of severe asthma: targeting the airways, comorbidities and risk factors. *Intern Med J* 2017; 47: 623.

Hew M, Sutherland M, Thien F, et al. The Melbourne thunderstorm asthma event: can we avert another strike? *Intern Med J* 2017; 47: 485.

Kryger M, Bode F, Antic R, et al. Diagnosis of obstruction of the upper and central airways. *Am J Med* 1976; 61: 85.

Lindstrom SJ, Silver JD, Sutherland MF, et al. Thunderstorm asthma outbreak of November 2016: a natural disaster requiring planning. *Med J Aust* 2017; 207: 235.

Maciag MC, Phipatanakul W. Prevention of asthma: targets for intervention. *Chest* 2020; 158: 913.

Martin RJ, Kraft M, eds. Asthma in the new millennium. *Chest* 2002; 123 (suppl.): 339S.

Mayo-Smith M, Hirsch PJ, Wodzinski SF, et al. Acute epiglottitis in adults. *N Engl J Med* 1986; 314: 1133.

McCaughan BC, Martini N, Bains MS. Bronchial carcinoids. *J Thorac Cardiovasc Surg* 1985; 89: 8.

Murray DM, Lawler PG. All that wheezes is not asthma: paradoxical vocal cord movement presenting as severe acute asthma requiring ventilatory support. *Anaesthesia* 1998; 53: 1006.

Papi A, Brightling C, Pedersen SE, et al. Asthma. *Lancet* 2018; 391: 783.

Pavord JD, Beasley R, Agusti A, et al. After asthma: redefining airways disease. *Lancet* 2018; 391: 350.

Randall KW, Spiering BA. Inspiratory stridor in elite athletes. *Chest* 2003; 123: 468.

Reddel HK. Common conditions that mimic asthma. *Med J Aust* 2022; 216: 337.

Shapiro J, Eavey RD, Baker AS. Adult supraglottitis: a prospective analysis. *JAMA* 1988; 259: 563.

Schoettler N, Strek ME. Recent advances in severe asthma: from phenotypes to personalized medicine. *Chest* 2020; 157: 516.

Upham J, Gibson P, Silverstone Z, eds. Severe asthma in Australia. *Med J Aust* 2018; 209: Suppl.

Wenzel SE. Asthma phenotypes: the evolution from clinical to molecular approaches. *Nat Med* 2012; 18: 716.

Asthmatic pulmonary eosinophilia *See*

- Eosinophilia and lung infiltration.

Atrial natriuretic factor

Atrial natriuretic factor (ANF, ANP) is a peptide which is stored in the atrial myocardial cells and released during atrial dilatation. It is one of a family of five structurally related natriuretic peptides of 22–53 amino acids, each peptide being secreted by different tissues. ANP is a natural antagonist to the renin–angiotensin–aldosterone system (q.v.) and thus promotes renal excretion of sodium and water. It is also a potent vasodilator and may thus play a homeostatic role in vascular control.

Excess release of ANF may contribute to hypotension in right ventricular infarction and like inappropriate ADH (q.v.) this may contribute to hyponatraemia. Experimentally, ANP helps to prevent and may even reverse post-ischaemic acute kidney injury (AKI, acute tubular necrosis), and there is some evidence that recombinant human ANP may provide renal benefit after complicated cardiac surgery. Theoretically, circulating natriuretic peptides and their degradation products may be useful biological markers of tissue injury, though such a role has yet to be confirmed by major clinical trial.

A purified preparation of recombinant human **brain natriuretic peptide** (BNP, nesiritide) has been shown to be a potent vasodilator in patients with congestive cardiac failure.

A high circulating level of natural BNP has been proposed as useful in distinguishing cardiac from pulmonary causes of dyspnoea. Thus, cardiac failure is likely if the plasma level is >500 pg/mL (>145 pmol/L) and unlikely if it is <100 pg/mL. However, both BNP and N-terminal pro-BNP (NT-proBNP) are elevated in critical illness generally, and in this situation they should be considered markers of severity rather than diagnostic indices.

Bibliography

Cavallazzi R, Nair A, Vasu T, et al. Natriuretic peptides in acute pulmonary embolism: a systematic review. *Intens Care Med* 2008; 34: 2147.

Davidson NC, Naas AA, Hanson JK, et al. Comparison of atrial natriuretic peptide, B-type natriuretic peptide, and N-terminal proatrial natriuretic peptide as indicators of left ventricular dysfunction. *Am J Cardiol* 1996; 77: 828.

de Denus S, Pharand C, Williamson DR. Brain natriuretic peptide in the management of heart failure: the versatile neurohormone. *Chest* 2004; 125: 652.

Diringer M, Ladenson PW, Stern BJ, et al. Plasma atrial natriuretic factor and subarachnoid hemorrhage. *Stroke* 1988; 19: 1119.

Jason P, Keang LT, Hoe LK. B-type natriuretic peptide: issues for the intensivist and pulmonologist. *Crit Care Med* 2005; 33: 2094.

Levin ER, Gardner DG, Samson WK. Natriuretic peptides. *N Engl J Med* 1998; 339: 321.

Moores LK. CHF or COPD: can BNP decide? *Pulmonary Perspect* 2004; 21: 1: 4.

Mueller C, Scholer A, Laule-Kilian K, et al. Use of B-type natriuretic peptide in the evaluation and management of acute dyspnoea. *N Engl J Med* 2004; 350: 647.

Needleman P, Greenwald JE. Atriopeptin: a cardiac hormone intimately involved in fluid, electrolyte, and blood-pressure homeostasis. *N Engl J Med* 1986; 314: 828.

Phua J, Jason P, Lim TK, et al. B-type natriuretic peptide: issues for the intensivist and pulmonologist. *Crit Care Med* 2005; 33: 2094.

Stein BC, Levin RI. Natriuretic peptides: physiology, therapeutic potential, and risk stratification in ischemic heart disease. *Am Heart J* 1998; 135: 914.

Sudoh T, Kangawa K, Minamino N, et al. A new natriuretic peptide in porcine brain. *Nature* 1988; 332: 78.

Suttner SW, Boldt J. Natriuretic peptide system: physiology and clinical utility. *Curr Opin Crit Care* 2004; 10: 336.

Sward K, Valsson F, Odencrants P, et al. Recombinant human atrial natriuretic peptide in ischaemic acute renal failure. *Crit Care Med* 2004; 32: 1310.

Wei C-M, Heublein DM, Perrella MA, et al. Natriuretic peptide system in human heart failure. *Circulation* 1993; 88: 1004.

Yap LB, Mukerjee D, Timms PM, et al. Natriuretic peptides, respiratory disease, and the right heart. *Chest* 2004; 126: 1330.

Autacoids

Autacoids are a broad range of substances normally present in the body and functioning in humoral regulation at a local level (and thus separate from hormones, neurotransmitters and cytokines).

Autacoids have short half-lives, since they act near to their site of synthesis and are not blood-borne. Examples of autacoids include
- adenosine (q.v.),
- bradykinin (q.v.),
- eicosanoids,
- histamine,
- platelet-activating factor (PAF),
- serotonin.

Auto-erythrocyte purpura See
- Purpura.

Autoimmune disorders

Autoimmune disorders comprise a large group of about 80 diseases caused by an immune reaction to a self (or auto) antigen. Self-reactive lymphocytes, both T cells and B cells, are largely eliminated during development, but some appear to persist in a mature state in peripheral lymphoid tissue, where they can be activated to cause autoimmunity.

Mechanisms of activation of autoimmunity include
- exposure of a normally sequestered self-antigen,
- structural alteration of a self-antigen (e.g. by drugs or viruses),
- molecular mimicry in which an appropriate immune response occurs to bacterial or viral proteins which are closely related to host antigens,
- reduced activation threshold, particularly for B cells (conversely, an increased activation may be responsible for the lymphoproliferative complications sometimes seen in patients with autoimmune disease).

Genetic predisposition to autoimmunity is important, and the MHC (HLA) locus is the best-defined risk factor for most such diseases (see Histocompatibility complex). Hormonal factors are also involved, as autoimmune disorders are much more common in women, perhaps related to factors required for fetal tolerance during pregnancy.

In general, the mechanism of antibody production requires both a genetic predisposition and then a trigger, presumably of environmental origin, since concordance for autoimmune disease is only about 30–50% in identical twins.

Pathology may be caused by
- cell damage from the binding of antibodies to cell surface antigens,
- agonist or antagonist actions of autoantibodies binding to cell surface receptors,
- immune complex disease (especially with nuclear antigens),
- cell-mediated immunity.

The prevalence of autoimmune disorders ranges from
- more than 1 in 100 of the population for psoriasis (q.v.), to
- about 1 in 100 for coeliac disease (q.v.), Graves' disease (q.v.), Hashimoto's thyroiditis (see Hypothyroidism) and rheumatoid arthritis, to
- 1 in 1000 for alopecia areata (q.v.), idiopathic thrombocytopenic purpura (q.v.), multiple sclerosis (q.v.), pernicious anaemia (q.v.), rheumatic fever, type 1 diabetes mellitus and vitiligo (q.v.), to
- 1 in 10,000 to 1 in 1 million or less for the many least common autoimmune disorders.

Autoimmune disorders may be either
- organ-specific, or
- systemic.

The antigens recognized are usually correspondingly organ-specific or widespread.

Organ-specific disorders are commonly multiple, with overlapping syndromes seen in many patients.

The most frequent organ-specific conditions include
- **insulin-dependent diabetes mellitus** (IDDM), in which antibodies recognize islet cells (ICA), and the specific proteins recognized include insulin (IAA), glutamic acid decarboxylase (anti-GAD) or the later described tyrosine phosphatase, IA-2,
- **Graves' disease** (see Hyperthyroidism), in which the antibody is to TSH receptors (TRAb),
- **Hashimoto's thyroiditis,** in which the main antibody specificity is to thyroid peroxidase (anti-TPO, formerly called microsomal antibody),
- **pernicious anaemia** (q.v.), in which there are antibodies to intrinsic factor due to autoimmune gastritis,
- **vitiligo** (see Pigmentation disorders), in which there are antibodies to melanocyte surface antigens.

Other organ-specific conditions include
- Addison's disease (q.v.),
- autoimmune haemolytic anaemia (see Anaemia),
- chronic active hepatitis (q.v.),
- coeliac disease (q.v.),
- hypoparathyroidism (q.v.),
- idiopathic thrombocytopenic purpura (q.v.),
- lymphocytic hypophysitis,
- multiple sclerosis (q.v.),
- myasthenia gravis (q.v.),
- pemphigus (q.v.),
- primary biliary cirrhosis (q.v.).

Many organ-specific disorders are thus endocrine, with autoantigens often being enzymes or receptors. Polyglandular syndromes may occur in some families.

Non-organ-specific disorders, i.e. multisystem or systemic disorders, include
- systemic lupus erythematosus (q.v.),
- Sjogren's disease (q.v.),
- scleroderma (q.v.),
- rheumatoid arthritis,
- rheumatic fever,
- polymyositis (q.v.),
- Goodpasture's syndrome (q.v.).

*Therapeutic opportunities for useful **immunomodulation** in autoimmune disorders include*
- *non-specific immune suppression*
  - *corticosteroids,*
  - *immune globulin (IVIG),*
  - *plasmapheresis (plasma exchange, PEX) (q.v.),*
  - *interferons,*
  - *drugs such as azathioprine, ciclosporin, cyclophosphamide, leflunomide, mycophenolate, tacrolimus, thalidomide,*
- *semi-specific therapy*
  - *e.g. TNF inhibition using anti-TNF antibodies, such as infliximab, etanercept and adalimumab (see Tumour necrosis factor),*
- *specific manipulation using targeted biological therapy*
  - *monoclonal antibodies to CD20 (rituximab) and CD52 (alemtuzumab),*
  - *monoclonal antibodies to interleukin 6 (IL-6) receptors (tocilizumab), IL-17 (ixekizumab, secukinumab), IL-23 (guselkumab, tildrakizumab, ustekinumab),*
  - *monoclonal antibodies to integrins (natalizumab).*

The more specific agents are very attractive because of their greater efficacy and safety compared to previously available non-specific modalities. There is thus a large number of new immunosuppressive agents with specific molecular targets either available for or being trialled in virtually all autoimmune disorders, many of which overlap in various molecular mechanisms of pathogenesis.

However, the newer immunomodulatory agents are generally very expensive, and moreover they carry the risk of increased opportunistic infections and of the development of malignancies.

Bibliography
Abbas AK, Lichtman AHH, Pillai S. *Cellular and Molecular Immunology.* 9th edition. Amsterdam: Elsevier. 2017.
Austen KF, Burakoff SJ, Rosen FS, et al., eds. *Therapeutic Immunology.* 2nd edition. Cambridge: Blackwell. 2001.
Davies PJ, Martin SJ, Burton DR, et al. *Roitt's Essential Immunology.* 13th edition. Hoboken: Wiley 2018.
Dwyer JM. Manipulating the immune system with immune globulin. *N Engl J Med* 1992; 326: 107.
Loriaux DL. The polyendocrine deficiency syndromes. *N Engl J Med* 1985; 312: 1568.
Lundy SK, Gizinski A, Fox DA. Introduction to clinical immunology: overview of immune response, autoimmune conditions, and immunosuppressive therapeutics for rheumatic diseases. In: *Scientific American Medicine. Allergy & Immunology.* Hamilton: Dekker Medicine. 2020.
Naparstek Y, Plotz PH. The role of autoantibodies in autoimmune disease. *Annu Rev Immunol* 1993; 11: 79.

Nossal GJV. Immunologic tolerance: collaboration between antigen and lymphokines. *Science* 1989; 245: 147.

Reimann PM, Mason PD. Plasmapheresis: technique and complications. *Intens Care Med* 1990; 16: 3.

Shoenfeld Y, Meroni PI, Gershwin M, eds. *Autoantibodies*. 3rd edition. Amsterdam: Elsevier. 2013.

Tan EM. Autoantibodies in pathology and cell biology. *Cell* 1991; 67: 841.

Various. The body against itself. *Sci Am* 2021; 325: 22.

Yu Z, Lennon VA. Mechanism of intravenous immune globulin therapy in antibody-mediated autoimmune diseases. *N Engl J Med* 1999; 340: 227.

Autoinflammatory disease *See*
- Familial Mediterranean fever.

Autonomic dysreflexia

Autonomic dysreflexia is syndrome of sympathetic hyperactivity which commonly occurs in patients with a spinal cord injury at or above the level of T6. The specific cord injury is usually traumatic, though it may be surgical, neoplastic or demyelinating.

It is considered to be due to an exaggerated response to afferent sympathetic stimulation below the lesion, as the pre-ganglionic neurones have become separated from their normal hypothalamic control. The most common stimuli are bladder or rectal distension, but irritation of any pelvic or distal structure can precipitate the syndrome.

Paroxysmal and potentially malignant hypertension is the most prominent clinical consequence. If unrecognized and untreated, it can lead to an uncontrolled rise in blood pressure with consequent fatal cerebral haemorrhage or acute myocardial infarction. It is thus a medical emergency due to its life-threatening potential.

Other clinical manifestations include headache, anxiety, impaired consciousness, flushing, sweating, nasal congestion, piloerection and cardiac arrhythmias (especially bradycardia, sometimes tachycardia and occasionally atrial fibrillation). In pregnancy, uteroplacental constriction may occur with consequent fetal hypoxia.

Treatment includes
- sitting upright to promote an orthostatic decrease in blood pressure,
- urgent search for a reversible precipitant, and
- antihypertensive medication (e.g. nifedipine, labetalol, sodium nitroprusside).

Magnesium has been reported to be helpful. ACE inhibitors should be used with care as the patient may be very sensitive to these.

Pregnancy and delivery present particular challenges, and epidural anaesthesia is recommended even if the patient is unable to experience labour pain.

Bibliography

Naftchi NE, Richardson JS. Autonomic dysreflexia: pharmacological management of hypertensive crises in spinal cord injured patients. *J Spinal Cord Med* 1997; 20: 355.

Showkathali R, Antionios TFT. Autonomic dysreflexia: a medical emergency. *J R Soc Med* 2007; 100: 382.

Avian influenza *See*
- Influenza.

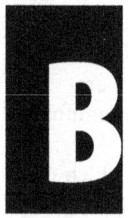

Bacillary angiomatosis *See*
- Cat-scratch disease.
See also
- Acquired immunodeficiency syndrome,
- Rickettsial diseases.

Bacillary peliosis hepatis *See*
- Cat-scratch disease.
See also
- Acquired immunodeficiency syndrome.

Bacitracin

Bacitracin is a polypeptide antibiotic produced from the microorganism *Bacillus subtilis*. It is active against Gram-positive bacteria, but it is nephrotoxic, so that it is not nowadays used parenterally.

Its local administration remains useful, either
- orally for *Clostridium difficile* diarrhoea (q.v.), or
- as an ointment for a variety of infected dermatological conditions, when it is usually combined with other antibacterial agents, such as neomycin and/or polymyxin and often also with corticosteroids.

Baclofen

Baclofen is an analog of the inhibitory neurotransmitter, gamma aminobutyric acid (GABA). It specifically activates GABA-B receptors. Since these receptors reside in presynaptic muscle spindle afferents, it acts as a skeletal muscle relaxant in cases of spasticity due to upper motor neurone damage (i.e. following cerebral or spinal injury). It has thus been used chiefly in multiple sclerosis and spinal cord injury, though it has also been effective in a variety of spastic conditions (e.g. spinal tumour, cerebral palsy, bladder spasticity, Huntington's chorea). Interestingly, it has also been found to be useful in alcohol dependence, particularly in suppressing withdrawal symptoms and relapse.

It may be given either orally (5–25 mg tds) or by intrathecal infusion (100–200 mcg per 24 hr), the latter route because of poor penetration of the blood–brain barrier.

Baclofen is relevant to Intensive Care practice in two settings.

1. **Overdose** produces a serious and complex problem, especially with doses >200 mg. The dominant features are neurological, with coma, seizures, hypotonia, absent reflexes, vomiting, salivation, respiratory depression.

    *Treatment is with **atropine** and/or **physostigmine** (see Anticholinergic agents) and with general support, often including the need for prolonged mechanical ventilation.*

    Reversibility may be eventually expected.

2. **Withdrawal** may lead to a life-threatening state of rebound excitability. GABA-B receptors are rapidly down-regulated within a week after baclofen therapy commences. Withdrawal symptoms may appear as soon as 12 hr or as late as several days after dose cessation or even reduction, and they recede 1–3 days after dosage resumption. The features of withdrawal include fever (q.v.), delirium (q.v.), spasticity, rhabdomyolysis (q.v.), autonomic instability and organ failure.

    This complication can mimic the neuroleptic malignant syndrome (q.v.) or the serotonin syndrome (q.v.).

    *Treatment with either **dantrolene** or **cyproheptadine** has been reported to be helpful while the appropriate baclofen dosage is being re-established.*

Bibliography

Cooper DJ, Bergman J. Massive baclofen overdose. *Crit Care Resusc* 2000; 2: 195.

Cunningham JA, Jelic S. Baclofen withdrawal: a cause of prolonged fever in the intensive care unit. *Anaesth Intens Care* 2005; 33: 534.

Leo RJ, Baer D. Delirium associated with baclofen withdrawal: a review of common presentations and management strategies. *Psychosomatics* 2005; 46: 503.

Leung NY, Whyte IM, Isbister GK. Baclofen overdose: defining the spectrum of severity. *Emerg Med Australasia* 2006; 18: 77.

BAL

BAL refers to dimercaprol, a chelating agent (q.v.), which can be used in some cases of heavy metal poisoning.

BAL is also an acronym for bronchoalveolar lavage, which is an important diagnostic procedure in respiratory diseases (e.g. see Hypersensitivity pneumonitis).

See also
- Warfare agents.

Barotrauma

Barotrauma refers to air forced outside the normal air spaces.

It thus comprises
- pneumothorax (q.v.), i.e. as in bronchopleural fistula,
- interstitial emphysema,
- pneumomediastinum,
- pneumopericardium,
- pneumoperitoneum,
- subcutaneous emphysema,
- gas embolism (via pulmonary veins)(see also Diving).

More subtle abnormalities may be seen histologically or on CT scan and include
- alveolar rupture,
- emphysema,
- pseudocysts (pneumatocoeles).

Barotrauma is a potential complication of mechanical ventilation, especially if inspired pressures or volumes are high or excessive positive end-expiratory pressure (PEEP) is used. An alveolar distending pressure of 30–35 mmHg is the injury threshold in most animal studies, so that the end-inspiratory plateau pressure in ventilated patients should be kept below this level if possible.

However, there is no direct correlation of clinical injury with the level of pressure used, and indeed it preferable to use the term **volutrauma** rather than barotrauma when discussing pneumothorax, etc. in ventilated patients to indicate that the problem is considered to be an overdistended volume rather than an over-distending pressure. Thus, prevention of this complication is one of the goals of the low tidal volume strategies which are a key element of modern ventilator management.

Bibliography
Abolnik I, Lossos IS, Breuer R. Spontaneous pneumomediastinum. *Chest* 1991; 100: 93.
Grotberg JC, Hyzy RC, De Cardenas J, et al. Bronchopleural fistula in the mechanically ventilated patient: a concise review. *Crit Care Med* 2021; 49: 292.
Maunder RJ, Pierson DJ, Hudson LD. Subcutaneous and mediastinal emphysema: pathophysiology, diagnosis, and management. *Arch Intern Med* 1984; 144: 1447.

Basophilia

Basophilia refers to an increased number of circulating basophils ($>0.1 \times 10^9$/L). These cells originate from the pluripotent stem cell via the myeloblast. They have prominent granules containing heparin, histamine and leukotrienes. Like the closely related tissue mast cells, they mediate hypersensitivity reactions.

Basophilia is seen in
- myeloproliferative disorders (most commonly),
- iron deficiency (q.v.),
- lung cancer (see Lung tumours),
- varicella infection (q.v.).
  See also
- Immune complex disease.

Bibliography
Denburg JA. Basophil and mast cell lineage in vitro and in vivo. *Blood* 1992; 79: 846.
Echtenacher B, Mannel DN, Hultner L. Critical protective role of mast cells in a model of acute septic peritonitis. *Nature* 1996; 381: 75.

Bat bites *See*

- Bites and stings.
  See also
- Coronavirus,
- Hendra virus,
- Lyssavirus,
- Rabies,
- Severe acute respiratory syndrome,
- Zoonoses.

Bathing

Bathing or swimming may be associated with folliculitis from contaminated water or with swimmer's ear.

Exposure to hot tubs or saunas may give hyperthermia (q.v.). This is particularly important in patients with cardiac disease, who may suffer failure or arrhythmias, and in pregnancy, when a raised core temperature during the first trimester may give rise to neural tube defect (q.v.) in the fetus.

Bibliography
Allison TG, Miller TD, Squires RW, et al. Cardiovascular responses to immersion in a hot tub in comparison with exercise in male subjects with coronary artery disease. *Mayo Clin Proc* 1993; 68: 19.
Castle SP. Public health implications regarding the epidemiology and microbiology of public whirlpools. *Infect Control* 1985; 6: 418.
Kosatsky T, Kleeman J. Superficial and systemic illness related to a hot tub. *Am J Med* 1985; 79: 10.
Lemire RJ. Neural tube defects. *JAMA* 1988; 259: 558.
Milunsky A, Ulcickas M, Rothman K, et al. Maternal heat exposure and neural tube defects. *JAMA* 1992; 268: 882.
Ridge BR, Budd GM. How long is too long in a spa pool. *N Engl J Med* 1990; 323: 835.

Bed rest

Bed rest is an important therapeutic measure for a number of disorders (particularly cardiac failure and pre-eclampsia – q.v.), but it is more often nowadays a consequence of illness rather than a prescribed therapy.

Bed rest may be regarded as the opposite of exercise training and may thus result in a number of physiological derangements. These may be seen in the elderly within 48 hr and in other patients by 1–3 weeks.

The adverse changes of bed rest include the following effects.
- **Circulatory**, with
  - decreased cardiac output,
  - decreased blood volume (by an average of 750 mL),
  - orthostatic hypotension,
  - decreased red blood cell mass,
  - increased blood viscosity,
  - increased venous stasis with thromboembolism.
- **Respiratory**, with
  - decreased lung volumes, especially vital capacity and functional residual capacity,
  - decreased arterial saturation.
- **Muscular**, with
  - decrease in muscle mass and contractility.
- **Metabolic**, with
  - loss of bone mineralization,
  - impaired glucose tolerance,
  - increased blood cholesterol.

- **Neurological**, with
  - blunted sensation and motor activity, due to sensory deprivation and seen especially in Intensive Care,
  - emotional lability.

Clearly, these changes are undesirable but equally clearly they are inevitable, particularly in Intensive Care patients, when the changes are often compounded by a septic or catabolic state.

Bee stings *See*
- Bites and stings.

Behcet's syndrome

Behcet's syndrome (Behcet's disease) is a chronic, inflammatory, multisystem disease of unknown cause, affecting primarily young adults of Eastern Mediterranean or Japanese origin. It was first described in Turkey in 1937.

Clinical features comprise most commonly
- painful mouth ulcers (similar to aphthous stomatitis) and genital ulcers (see Ulcers),
- eye signs (uveitis – q.v., including iritis and episcleritis; retinal vasculitis; optic neuritis – q.v.).

Less commonly, there may be
- seronegative, non-destructive arthritis (q.v.),
- colitis (q.v.),
- vasculitis (q.v.) and/or thrombophlebitis, sometimes associated with anticardiolipin antibodies (q.v.) and arterial or venous thrombosis (and possibly infarction),
- neurological involvement, with cranial nerve palsy, brainstem dysfunction or meningoencephalitis (q.v.).

The diagnosis is based on the clinical features.

In Intensive Care practice, it should be considered in the differential diagnosis of multisystem dysfunction, if the cause is not otherwise apparent and the clinical setting is appropriate.

Treatment consists of **corticosteroids**, with added cytotoxic therapy in cases of recurrence or relapse.
- *Colchicine, thalidomide, ciclosporin and subsequently interferon alpha have been reported to be of benefit in some patients.*
- *The inhibition of tumour necrosis factor with the anti-TNF antibodies, **infliximab** or **etanercept**, may rapidly and effectively suppress all the clinical manifestations of this disease.*

The prognosis is mostly favourable over several years, apart from the risk of visual loss in those with relapsing ocular involvement and of severe bleeding in those anticoagulated when pulmonary vasculitis has been mistakenly diagnosed as pulmonary thromboembolism.

Bibliography
International Study Group for Behcet's Disease. Criteria for diagnosis of Behcet's disease. *Lancet* 1990; 35: 1078.
James DG. Behcet's syndrome. *N Engl J Med* 1979; 301: 431.
Kaklamani VG, Vaiopoulos G, Kaklamanis PG. Behcet's disease. *Semin Arthritis Rheum* 1998; 27: 197.
Lee S, Bang D, Lee E, et al. *Behcet's Disease*. Berlin: Springer-Verlag. 2000.
Rosenbaum M, Rosner I, Portnoy E. Remission of Behcet's syndrome with TNFa blocking treatment. *Ann Rheum Dis* 2002; 61: 283.
Shimizu T, Ehrlich GE, Inaba G, et al. Behcet's disease (Behcet's syndrome). *Semin Arthritis Rheum* 1979; 8: 223.
Uzun O, Akpolat T, Erkan L. Pulmonary vasculitis in Behcet's disease. *Chest* 2005; 127: 2243.
Yazici H. Behcet's syndrome: where do we stand? *Am J Med* 2002; 112: 75.

Bell's palsy

Bell's palsy refers to paralysis of the facial (cranial VII) nerve. It is produced by inflammation in the facial canal within the temporal bone, but the cause of this process is uncertain. Herpes simplex virus type 1 (q.v.) has been implicated. Several cases of Bell's palsy were reported following the intranasal administration of an inactivated influenza vaccine, which was later withdrawn from the market.

There is the rapid onset of paralysis, which is sometimes complete. There is no sensory change, though there may be impaired lacrimation, salivation and taste.

The differential diagnosis includes
- 7th nerve herpes zoster (Ramsay Hunt syndrome) (see Varicella-zoster),
- diabetic 7th nerve palsy,
- neoplastic or vascular lesions of the pons or cerebellopontine angle,
- Guillain–Barré syndrome (q.v.),
- Lyme disease (q.v.),
- sarcoidosis (q.v.),
- carcinomatous meningitis.

*Treatment with **corticosteroids** is commonly given, but significant benefit has been difficult to confirm in controlled trials. Generally, a short tapered course is given over 2 weeks.* ***Cytotoxic agents*** *(azathioprine, methotrexate, mycophenolate, rituximab (q.v.), in that order) may be of benefit in refractory cases.*

- ***Acyclovir*** *(q.v.) has been shown to be helpful.*
- *The eye should be covered if the cornea is exposed.*

Most cases recover, at least sufficiently to give a good cosmetic result, though 5–10% have some permanent weakness.

Bibliography

Adour KK. Diagnosis and management of facial paralysis. *N Engl J Med* 1982; 307: 348.

Devriese PP, Schumacher T, Scheide A, et al. Incidence, prognosis and recovery of Bell's palsy. *Clin Otolaryngol* 1990; 15: 15.

Halperin J, Luft BJ, Volkman DJ, et al. Lyme neuroborreliosis: peripheral nervous system manifestations. *Brain* 1990; 113: 1207.

Murakami S, Mizobuchi M, Nakashiro Y, et al. Bell palsy and herpes simplex virus identification of viral DNA in endoneurial fluid and muscle. *Ann Intern Med* 1996; 124: 27.

Mutsch M, Zhou W, Rhodes P, et al. Use of the inactivated intranasal influenza vaccine and the risk of Bell's palsy in Switzerland. *N Engl J Med* 2004; 350: 896.

Bence Jones protein

Bence Jones protein is a low molecular weight protein originally described in the urine of patients with multiple myeloma. It was noted to coagulate on gentle heating of the urine but to redissolve on boiling, only to precipitate again on cooling below 60°C.

Its presence is virtually pathognomonic of **multiple myeloma**, though it is present in only 50% of such cases. The urine shows a positive dipstick test for protein, and there is a single band on urine electrophoresis. The protein is also present in serum but in low concentration.

The protein is the kappa or lambda light chain of IgG. Its presence is regarded as mild if the daily urinary excretion is <4 g and severe if it is >12 g.

Bence Jones protein can cause renal tubular damage either directly or associated with cast production. Casts occur from the aggregation of the Bence Jones protein with the locally produced 14 kd glycoprotein, nephrocalcin. Distal tubular obstruction and inflammation may result.

See
- Multiple myeloma.

Benign intracranial hypertension

Benign intracranial hypertension (idiopathic intracranial hypertension, pseudotumour cerebri) refers to chronically increased intracranial pressure without hydrocephalus (q.v.).

It usually occurs in obese young women and without known cause.
  It can also be related to
- some drugs
  - including indometacin, isotretinoin, nitrofurantoin, oral contraceptives – q.v., tetracycline (especially minocycline, the most lipid-soluble member of the group),
- cerebral venous thrombosis,
- endocrine disorders (sometimes).

Clinical features include
- headache,
- visual impairment, with
  - visual loss (sometimes permanent),
  - peripheral field defects,
  - diplopia,
  - papilloedema (q.v.).

Treatment is with **CSF drainage, diuretics** *or, if refractory,* **corticosteroids** *(in moderate doses for about 3 months).*

- *CSF drainage may be by repeated lumbar puncture (e.g. 20–40 mL taken several times weekly) or a shunt (e.g. lumboperitoneal).*
- *Suitable diuretics include furosemide or acetazolamide (q.v.). Glycerol orally can be effective.*
- *Weight reduction is recommended.*
- ***Surgical decompression*** *is sometimes required, e.g. optic nerve sheath decompression if vision is threatened.*

Bibliography

Giuseffi V, Wall M, Siegel PZ, et al. Symptoms and disease associations in idiopathic intracranial hypertension (pseudotumor cerebri). *Neurology* 1991; 41: 239.

Lyons MK, Meyer FB. Cerebrospinal fluid physiology and the management of increased intracranial pressure. *Mayo Clin Proc* 1990; 65: 684.

Wall M, George D. Idiopathic intracranial hypertension. *Brain* 1991; 114: 155.

Beriberi

Beriberi is vitamin B_1 (thiamine) deficiency, and the name is derived from the Sinhalese meaning extreme weakness. In developed countries, it is sometimes seen as part of the nutritional deficiency associated with alcoholism. It is thus usually accompanied by other stigmata of alcoholism, especially Wernicke's encephalopathy (q.v.).

So-called dry beriberi causes neurological disease (especially polyneuropathy – q.v.), and wet beriberi is manifested by a dilated cardiomyopathy (q.v.) with hyperdynamic circulatory failure.

> In Intensive Care, beriberi should thus be remembered as one of the uncommon causes of the hyperdynamic state (q.v.).
>
> Its importance lies in its rapid response to thiamine (100 mg IV), but severe disease should be treated with higher doses for the first week (e.g. 300 mg IV tds).

See also
- Vitamin deficiency.

Bibliography
Blankenhorn MA. The diagnosis of beriberi heart disease. *Ann Intern Med* 1945; 23: 398.

Beryllium

Beryllium (Be, atomic number 4, atomic weight 9) is a light, brittle, alkaline–earth metal and was discovered in 1798. It is not free in nature and there are no large deposits, so that beryllium most frequently appears in compounds, such as beryllium aluminium silicate in gem stones (including emeralds). It has a very high melting point (1278°C) and is a good conductor of both heat and electricity. It has unusual physical properties, in that it is a very light but mechanically strong metal. Its particular use has been as a hardening agent in metallurgy, hence its widespread application in the aerospace, electronics and defence industries. It has no known biological role.

Exposure levels of not >0.5–2 mcg/m^3/8 hr were traditionally recommended, as soluble beryllium compounds are toxic. Recently, the recommended limitation on exposure levels has been reduced 10-fold, based on revised epidemiological data.

Acute toxicity occurs in mining or metallurgy and consists of a burning rash, nose and eye irritation, cough and chest tightness, with an acute pneumonitis. Fatal respiratory failure within 72 hr may occasionally occur, but more commonly there is recovery over a few months.

Chronic toxicity (chronic beryllium disease, CBD) is seen in scientific or industrial workers and follows a variable latent period of up to 15 yr. Permanent, though often mild, respiratory disability occurs with cough and dyspnoea, though about 25% of patients develop progressive disease which is eventually fatal. The development of diffuse pulmonary changes is referred to as **berylliosis**, in which granulomas histologically identical to sarcoidosis (q.v.) are seen and even bilateral hilar lymphadenopathy. This diagnosis can be difficult to make and is easily overlooked, but a beryllium-lymphocyte proliferation test (LPT) can assist diagnostic accuracy in centres where it is available. The LPT may become positive early in the course of chronic disease and suggests beryllium sensitization as a mechanism of CBD. The chest X-ray may be normal during early disease, and lung function tests show variable abnormalities. *Treatment with corticosteroids is of benefit.*

Chronic beryllium exposure can also predispose to lung cancer (see Lung tumours).

See
- Occupational lung diseases.

Bibliography
Alberts WM. Lung disease and the lightest of metals. *Chest* 2004; 126: 1730.

Balmes JR, Abraham JL, Dweik RA, et al. An official American Thoracic Society statement: diagnosis and management of beryllium sensitivity and chronic beryllium disease. *Am J Respir Crit Care Med* 2014; 190: e34.

Infante PF, Newman LS. Beryllium exposure and chronic beryllium disease. *Lancet* 2004; 363: 415.

Kriebel D, Brain JD, Sprince NL, et al. The pulmonary toxicity of beryllium. *Am Rev Respir Dis* 1988; 137: 464.

Lundgren RA, Maier LA, Rose CS, et al. Indirect and direct gas exchange at maximum exercise in beryllium sensitization and disease. *Chest* 2001; 120: 1702.

MacMurdo MG, Mroz MM, Culver DA, et al. Chronic beryllium disease: update on a moving target. *Chest* 2020; 158: 2458.

Rossman MD, Kern JA, Elias JA, et al. Proliferative responses of bronchoalveolar lymphocytes to beryllium: a test for chronic beryllium disease. *Ann Intern Med* 1988; 108: 687.

Sood A, Beckett WS, Cullen MR. Variable response to long-term corticosteroid therapy in chronic beryllium disease. *Chest* 2004; 126: 2000.

Beta$_2$-microglobulin

Beta$_2$-microglobulin is the beta or light-chain of the HLA Class I molecule required for cell–cell recognition. It is a small protein of 11.5 kDa and is present on most cell membranes though not on mature red blood cells. There is considerable amino acid sequence homology between beta$_2$-microglobulin, the heavy chain of the

MHC Class I antigen and the constant region of the heavy chain of IgG.

Beta$_2$-microglobulin is released during cell breakdown and is then metabolized and cleared by the kidney. Its plasma level is thus increased with renal impairment. It is also increased following complement activation and IL-1 generation, due to increased synthesis.

> The proteinuria in tubulointerstitial disease (q.v.) is predominantly low molecular weight material, such as beta$_2$-microglobulin, rather than albumin as in glomerular diseases.

Beta$_2$-microglobulin provides the protein subunit for dialysis-related amyloid (q.v.). As a middle molecule, its effective plasma removal thus requires a high-flux dialysis membrane. However, its slow transfer rate from the extracellular fluid compartment where it is chiefly located to the intravascular compartment from where it can be removed limits its total removal by any individual dialysis session.

The serum level of beta$_2$-microglobulin also guides the staging classification in multiple myeloma (q.v.).

See
- Histocompatibility complex,
- Proteinuria.

Bicarbonate therapy See
- Lactic acidosis.

Biliary cirrhosis

Biliary cirrhosis may be either primary or secondary.

Primary biliary cirrhosis is an autoimmune disease. It is thus also associated with other autoimmune diseases (q.v.), particularly scleroderma (q.v.), CREST syndrome (q.v.), Sjogren's syndrome (q.v.) and renal tubular acidosis (q.v.). There is a genetic predisposition because of the association with the HLA-DR8 haplotype.

> Clinical features of primary biliary cirrhosis typically occur in women aged 30–50 yr, with the gradual onset of pruritus, fatigue and increased skin pigmentation (q.v.).
>
> Late features include jaundice, hepatosplenomegaly, multiple xanthomas and osteoporosis (with bone pain and pathological fractures). Eventually, ascites and oedema occur.

Investigations show liver function disturbance with chiefly an increased alkaline phosphatase. Antimitochondrial antibody is typically present, and the serum cholesterol is raised, as is the serum ACE level (q.v.). Liver biopsy shows a specific histological picture in only a few patients, as in most the findings are similar to those seen in chronic active hepatitis (q.v.).

The differential diagnosis includes
- secondary biliary cirrhosis (see below),
- cholangitis (q.v.),
- chronic biliary obstruction,
- drug-induced cholestasis.

Treatment modalities, including corticosteroids, cytotoxic agents, colchicine, penicillamine (q.v.) and ciclosporin, are all at best poorly effective and are associated with significant side-effects.
- ***Colestyramine*** *(cholestyramine) may alleviate pruritus, for which antihistamines are usually ineffective.*
- *The bile acid,* ***ursodeoxycholic acid*** *(ursodiol) 12–15 mg/kg per day orally, diminishes the potentially toxic endogenous bile acid pool and is moderately effective as well as safe, though it is expensive.*
- *Vitamin supplementation is required.*

The course of the disease is slow, with a median survival of 10 years.

Secondary biliary cirrhosis arises from chronic biliary tract disease due to obstruction or prolonged inflammation. This leads to the irreversible histological changes of cirrhosis.

See
- Cholangitis,
- Cholestasis.

Bibliography

Heathcote EJ. Management of primary biliary cirrhosis: the American Association for the Study of Liver Diseases practice guidelines. *Hepatology* 2000; 31: 1005.

James SP, Hoofnagle JH, Strober W, et al. Primary biliary cirrhosis: a model autoimmune disease. *Ann Intern Med* 1983; 99: 500.

Poupon RE, Poupon R, Balkau B. Ursodiol for the long-term treatment of primary biliary cirrhosis. *N Engl J Med* 1994; 330: 1342.

Biomarkers

A **biomarker** is a substance whose presence in the blood (or biological tissues or fluids) can be used to identify the presence of a particular disease or to predict its outcome. The development of effective biomarkers is a key requirement for the eventual establishment of personalized medicine.

Biomarkers that are well recognized and in common use include
- specific autoimmune antibodies (see Autoimmune disorders),
- sepsis biomarkers (such as C-reactive protein – q.v., procalcitonin – q.v.),
- cardiovascular biomarkers (such as BNP or NT-proBNP, see Atrial natriuretic factor).

Some less common biomarkers may be used in critical care research studies, such as those for
- haemostasis (e.g. von Willebrand factor, vWF (q.v.) and thrombomodulin, TM (q.v.)),
- renal injury (e.g. neutrophil gelatinase–associated lipocalcin, NGAL), or
- endothelial permeability (e.g. vascular endothelial growth factor, VGEF),
- idiopathic pulmonary fibrosis (q.v.) (e.g. CA 125, chitinase-3-like protein-1 (YKL-40), C-X-C motif chemokine 13 (CXCL13), matrix metalloproteinase 7 (MMP7), osteopontin (OPN), surfactant protein D (SP-D) and vascular cell adhesion molecule-1 (VCAM-1)).

Studies of panels of biomarkers and of serial measurement of a single biomarker have been reported. There are continued developments in biomarkers, and the new techniques of functional genomics and proteomics are expected to expand these future horizons greatly. Meanwhile, the general utility of biomarkers in ICU is subject to ongoing pro–con debate.

Tumour markers/biomarkers (q.v.) are considered separately.

Bibliography
Bellomo R, See EJ. Novel renal biomarkers of acute kidney injury and their implications. *Intern Med J* 2021; 51: 316.
Legrand M, Januzzi JL, Mebazaa A. *Critical research on biomarkers: what's new? Intens Care Med* 2013; 39: 1824.
Moran JL, Solomon PJ. The search for biomarkers in the critically ill: a cautionary tale. *Crit Care Resusc* 2018; 20: 85.
Seymour CW, Yende S, Scott MJ, et al. Metabolomics in pneumonia and sepsis: an analysis of the GenIMS cohort study. *Intens Care Med* 2013; 39: 1423.
Sweeney TE, Khatri P. Generalizable biomarkers in critical care: towards precision medicine. *Crit Care Med* 2017; 45: 934.
Various. Biomarkers in ICU: less is more? Yes, no, not sure. *Intens Care Med* 2021; 47: 94.

Bioterrorism

Bioterrorism is a potential consequence of the widespread knowledge of the technology involved in the now banned field of germ warfare (q.v.). Terrorist groups or rogue nations with relatively limited resources could manufacture and distribute a range of virulent organisms with catastrophic results.

It has been considered that the optimal approach to bioterrorism has much in common with that required to deal with large and unexpected natural epidemics, such as the outbreak of SARS in 2002–3 (q.v.).

See
- Anthrax,
- Botulism,
- Germ warfare,
- Plague,
- Warfare agents.

Bibliography
Antosia R, Cahill J, eds. *Handbook of Bioterrorism and Disaster Medicine.* Berlin: Springer. 2006.
Duchin J, Malone JD. Bioterrorism. In: *Scientific American Medicine. Interdisciplinary Medicine.* Hamilton: Dekker Medicine. 2020.
Karwa M, Bronzert P, Kvetan V. Bioterrorism and critical care. *Crit Care Clin* 2003; 19: 279.
Kvetan V, Farmer JC, et al., eds. Critical care medicine for disasters, terrorism, and military conflict. *Crit Care Med* 2005; 33 (1, suppl.).
Rotz LD, Khan AS, Lillibridge SR, et al. Public health assessment of potential bioterrorism agents. *Emerg Infect Dis* 2002; 8: 225.
Ursano RJ, Norwood AE, Fullerton CS, eds. *Bioterrorism: Psychological and Public Health Interventions.* Cambridge: Cambridge University Press. 2004.
Waterer GW, Robertson H. Bioterrorism for the respiratory physician. *Respirology* 2009; 14: 5.
Wenzel RP, Edmond MB. Managing SARS amidst uncertainty. *N Engl J Med* 2003; 348: 1947.
Whitby M, Ruff TA, Street AC, et al. Biological agents as weapons 2: anthrax and plague. *Med J Aust* 2002; 176: 605.

Bird fancier's lung *See*

- Hypersensitivity pneumonitis.

Bird flu *See*

- Influenza.

Bismuth

Bismuth (Bi, atomic number 83, atomic weight 209, melting point 271°C) is the most metallic of the elements in the nitrogen family. It was first described in 1450 and is a hard, brittle, greyish substance, which does not tarnish in air and which is difficult to magnetize. In addition to its widespread use in manufacturing, its salts in a variety of colloidal forms have long been in common use in medicine as a gastrointestinal soothing agent, in ointments and as a radio-opaque medium. It is also commonly used as an antibacterial in the prevention or treatment of diarrhoea, e.g. in travellers.

It has been used for peptic ulceration, despite its lack of antacid effect. In this setting, it inhibits pepsin, increases mucus and most importantly detaches *Helicobacter pylori* from the gastric epithelium thus permitting its lysis.

Non-absorbable preparations are used, because systemic levels can cause encephalopathy (q.v.) and osteodystrophy. It should not be used in renal failure, as any small amounts that may be absorbed are normally excreted in the urine. The oral administration of bismuth compounds can produce a dark mouth, a phenomenon which is reversible.

The most common therapeutic compound is **bismuth subcitrate** (tripotassium dicitratobismuthate), but subnitrate, subgallate and subsalicylate compounds are also prepared.

Bites and stings

Bites and stings may be inflicted by many creatures. Their clinical effects depend on
- the site and severity of the bite or sting itself,
- the injection of toxin (venom),
- the injection of potentially pathogenic organisms.
  Infecting organisms may come from the biting mouth or stinging part of the attacking creature or from the recipient's skin.

Venom refers to a poisonous secretion from specialized glands, often associated with the teeth, spines, stingers or other piercing parts of the attacking creature. Venoms are a mixture of toxic enzymes and other proteins. In nature, venoms are used for attacking prey or for defence. When injected into humans, they produce the syndrome of **envenomation**.

Venomous creatures may be found worldwide and are represented in most major animal phyla, although they are especially found in the rural tropics. The best-known such creatures are snakes, spiders, scorpions, insects and marine vertebrates and invertebrates. The most venomous creatures reside in Australia, which has some 2000 such species.

Nevertheless, death from envenomation is rare in a developed country (e.g. about two deaths per year in Australia, all without appropriate first-aid), though it has been estimated that over 100,000 people die worldwide each year from envenomation, particularly from snakes. In developed countries, anaphylaxis from bee or wasp venom is a more common cause of death.

Snake bites alone have been calculated to afflict 5 million people worldwide per year, particularly in Asia and Africa. Although about 50% of bites are thought to be 'dry', the number of deaths from snake bite is similar to that from many of the major infectious diseases (e.g. dengue), but with permanent disability including limb loss occurring in an additional four times as many people. This large health care burden arises mainly because of the limited availability and quality of antivenoms in the rural areas where most envenomation occurs, even though a comprehensive range of snake, spider and other antivenoms have been increasingly made and have become widely available in developed countries since the 1930s.

Bites and stings are seen most frequently in children and are much less common in adults over 25 years of age. They are most commonly caused by insects and next most commonly by dogs and spiders. Bites and stings leading to hospitalization are most commonly from spiders (38%), bees and wasps (28%), and snakes (16%). Numerically, they cause less than 1 hospital admission per day per 1 million population in a developed country.

> The clinical features of envenomation may be
> - neurotoxic,
> - haemotoxic,
> - allergic.
>
> These features may vary greatly in severity from asymptomatic to serious or even fatal.

The general principles of treatment of bites and stings relate to local trauma (if any) and to the risks of infection or of envenomation.
- ***Potentially infected bites**, especially on the hand, should be treated with prophylactic oral antibiotics (e.g. amoxicillin/clavulanic acid), though these may safely be omitted if the bite is minor. Prophylactic antibiotics should always be given if the patient has diabetes, peripheral vascular disease or immunocompromise. If infection actually occurs or if the patient presents late, intravenous antibiotics are preferable. Since the Gram stain from the wound usually provides inadequate information, microbiological culture is important. Appropriate tetanus prophylaxis is required, as is basic wound care.*

- *Potentially venomous bites* should be treated with bodily rest and immobilization of the affected part by the bandage and splint technique (except after fish, red-back spider or Crotalid envenomation, because local pressure increases pain and possibly local tissue damage). Transport should be arranged to a hospital, and unless the injury is minor, the patient should be admitted to Intensive Care for circulatory, respiratory, renal and coagulation support. Treatment of circulatory failure (due especially to hypovolaemia), respiratory failure (due primarily to paralysis), coagulopathy, haemolysis and rhabdomyolysis (q.v.) are the chief priorities.

> If there are clinical or investigational features of systemic envenomation, specific antivenom (antivenene) should be urgently given, following species identification (if necessary using a venom detection kit). If the responsible species cannot be identified with confidence, polyvalent antivenom should be given. The antivenom is given diluted and IV, and the dose is based on the amount of venom injected and not on the patient's body size. The dose in one container is designed to neutralize the amount of venom in a standard or milked bite; this dose needs to be increased or repeated if there have been multiple bites, delay in treatment or relapse.
>
> *Adrenaline* (epinephrine) is required either for anaphylaxis or prior to antivenom in patients with a previous reaction.
>
> **Corticosteroids** and **antihistamine** should be given IV if the patient is hypersensitive to horse serum or has had a previous exposure.
>
> *Tetanus prophylaxis* is required, but antibiotics are not indicated.

The bites and/or stings from a number of creatures may present specific problems.
- **Bats** from all continents except Australia have been recorded to harbour **rabies** (q.v.). However, some fruit bats in Australia have been found to carry a related organism, **lyssavirus** (q.v.). This can cause encephalitis in humans, which should be managed as for rabies.

Bats also harbour a number of other viruses which can cause disease in humans, including the **Hendra virus** (q.v.) and the coronaviruses responsible for **severe acute respiratory syndrome** (SARS) (q.v.) and for **COVID-19** (q.v.).
- **Bees and wasps** may give acute allergic reactions and even anaphylaxis (q.v.) in some patients. This is because Hymenoptera venom contains enzymes (proteins), as well as vasoactive amines and small peptides. Even a large local reaction is generally allergic, as infectious cellulitis is rare after insect stings. If very numerous, such stings may produce severe systemic toxicity with hypotension.

Insect-venom allergy may be formally diagnosed by either skin tests or RASTs (radioallergosorbent tests) using Hymenoptera venom, but both tests can sometimes be difficult to interpret. Serum IgE antibody levels may best predict the risk of anaphylaxis (q.v.).

*Acute treatment of a clinically significant reaction is with an anti-H1 **antihistamine** and if severe with **corticosteroids**, as well as with symptomatic measures such as ice and analgesia.*

*Either **desensitization** (venom immunotherapy) or self-administered adrenaline (epinephrine) should be offered to those who have had a previous severe reaction.*
- **Cats** can give an infective bite, the risk being higher than for a dog bite because of the cat's sharper teeth (and thus the bite and anaerobic inoculum are generally deeper). Cats are responsible for about 7% of all mammalian bite injuries presenting to hospital. The usual pathogen in domestic cats is *Pasteurella multocida*, though organisms similar to those in the human mouth (see below) may also be present, as may be Capnocytophaga *canimorsus* found in dogs (see below).

Similar flora ('fang flora') exist in the mouths of large cats, though clearly the bites from these animals are also associated with much more severe injuries, including particularly spinal damage from a crushing bite to the neck.

A cat bite can also lead to cat-scratch disease (q.v.).
- **Dog** bites are usually from a known animal and are on an extremity, except in children when the face is commonly bitten. Dogs are responsible for about 80% of all mammalian bite injuries presenting to hospital. Although the dog mouth contains many aerobic and anaerobic bacteria, the main pathogens are *P. multocida* and *C. canimorsus* (formerly called DF-2), a slowly growing Gram-negative rod. The latter can cause death even in normal hosts and is especially prone to cause sepsis in alcoholics or in patients with significant underlying disease. The sepsis is indistinguishable clinically from other forms of severe sepsis, except for the presence of a wound usually with painful cellulitis. Systemic symptoms occur 1–8 days after the bite, and the reported mortality is about 30%.

Despite this potential, most dog bites are in fact not infectious and prophylaxis is often unnecessary.
- **Wild animal** bites should be considered a risk for rabies, unless in a rabies-free country (see Rabies).

- **Human** bites may occur anywhere on the body but most commonly on the fingers. Similar lesions may also occur on the knuckles of a clenched fist or may be self-inflicted on the hands or lips. Humans are responsible for about 9% of all mammalian bite injuries presenting to hospital. The organism most commonly involved is *Streptococcus viridans*. Other organisms are also commonly involved, including *Staphylococcus aureus, Haemophilus influenzae, Eikenella corrodens*, and a variety of anaerobes, including bacteroides, fusobacteria and peptostreptococci.

  Human bites have had a reputation for serious and frequent complications due to infection, but apart from bites to the hand, they may be no more prone to infection than lacerations in general.

  *Prophylaxis with **amoxicillin/clavulanic acid** (or flucloxacillin, penicillin or a cefalosporin) is recommended for serious bites, including to the hand.*

- **Insects** and **arachnids** (see Arthropods), including mosquitoes, ticks, lice and mites, are the vectors for the transmission to humans of a wide variety of infectious diseases (q.v.). The bites of **jack jumper ants** and of **red fire ants** are painful and may cause anaphylaxis.

  In particular, **ticks** may inject a neurotoxin, which can produce diplopia, weakness and ataxia, similar to Guillain–Barré syndrome (q.v.), sometimes with associated rhabdomyolysis, myocarditis or lymphadenopathy (see also Lyme disease).

  Antitoxin treatment is available for tick bites.

- **Marine invertebrates** which can cause envenomation in humans particularly include members of the Coelenterata phylum, such as **jellyfish** (the best known being the Portuguese Man of War and the most toxic being the Box Jellyfish, *Chironex fleckeri*). Their sting can cause local pain (which may be extreme) and cutaneous eruption (which may be followed by skin necrosis), as well as systemic features of vomiting, sweating, dyspnoea, hypotension and even anaphylaxis. Following contact with Box Jellyfish tentacles, hypotension, paralysis and cardiorespiratory failure may develop within minutes.

  Recently, deaths due to the Irukandji syndrome have been reported from the stings of a number of small box jellyfish species, particularly *Carukia barnesi*. In this condition, while the sting itself may appear trivial, severe systemic symptoms occur within 30 minutes, with sweating, anxiety, nausea, headache, palpitations and painful generalized muscle cramps. There is marked hypertension, probably due to noradrenaline (norepinephrine) release, with the consequent risk of intracranial haemorrhage and acute cardiac failure.

  Emergency treatment of jellyfish stings is with local vinegar and immobilization. Ice-packs are recommended if available. Analgesia, volume expanders, inotropes and ventilatory support may be required in hospital until antivenom becomes available. The hypertension of the Irukandji syndrome requires urgent treatment.

  The blue-ringed **octopus** may inject tetrodotoxin (a neuromuscular blocking neurotoxin). The bite itself may be painless, but paralysis may result.

  Treatment of an octopus bite is supportive, as no antivenom is currently available, though anticholinesterase therapy (q.v.) has been reported to be possibly helpful.

- **Marine vertebrates** can also produce venom, particularly in fish spines.

  The **puffer fish** contains tetrodotoxin (see blue-ringed octopus above), though most cases of human injury are poisonings from ingestion of the fish rather than from a sting. Such poisonings have generally occurred in Asia and particularly in Japan, where the fish is considered a delicacy but can be prepared safely only by a specialist chef.

  Stone fish spines are typically a risk to humans from being trodden on. There is severe local pain (and possibly skin necrosis subsequently) and sometimes major systemic symptoms, such as paralysis and circulatory collapse.

  Antivenom should be given, except in mild cases, and local anaesthesia is symptomatically effective.

- **Monkey** bites can potentially cause infection with herpesvirus simiae (monkey B virus), which is a fatal neurotropic viral infection.

- **Rat** saliva may contain the organisms, *Spirillum minus* (mainly in Asia) or *Streptobacillus moniliformis* (mainly in the West). These anaerobic Gram-negative bacilli may cause rat-bite fever, often with rash and arthralgia and sometimes with endocarditis (q.v.). They are sensitive to penicillin or tetracycline.

- **Scorpion** stings are common in tropical and subtropical countries. There are over 1000 species of scorpions worldwide, with variable potential to harm humans. The venom is a complex mixture of mucopolysaccharides and mediators with potent neurotoxicity. The sting causes considerable local pain and often general intoxication, but the mortality is generally less than 1%. The general intoxication comprises neurological, respiratory and especially cardiovascular responses. The latter is due to intense adrenergic stimulation, which causes arrhythmias, cardiac failure and even shock.

*Treatment is supportive, with ICU management (if available) in severe cases. **Antivenom** treatment has been shown to reduce the serum venom concentration, but its effect on outcome has been less convincing. Importantly, antivenom is expensive, and it is thus not widely available in developing countries.*

Interestingly, scorpion venom and more lately some of its synthesized constituents have been shown to have potentially valuable antimicrobial qualities.

- **Snake** bite is a potential emergency, although the mortality is in fact low in developed countries (see envenomation above). In untreated cases, up to 10% of deaths occur within 3 hr, though over 80% occur after 7 hr (and thus usually well after medical assistance can be obtained) and nearly half occur after 24 hr.

The fang marks themselves may be difficult to identify, but there is usually local pain and inflammation. Local tissue damage is most evident following cobra or rattlesnake bites. Following a suspected snake bite, the patient should be observed for at least 12 hr for signs of envenomation.

Snake venoms are complex products, generally with neurotoxins, but also commonly with haemotoxins (either procoagulant or anticoagulant), myotoxins, nephrotoxins, cardiotoxins and proteolytic enzymes which cause local tissue damage.

Systemic symptoms generally appear within 4 hours and sometimes by 30 minutes.
   They include
- neurological features
   - including headache, paraesthesiae, weakness, paralysis, strange taste, drowsiness, bulbar signs, ptosis, fits,
- nausea,
- bleeding
   - including intracranial haemorrhage,
- dyspnoea
   - related to respiratory paralysis, pulmonary oedema or pulmonary haemorrhage,
- shock.

Anaphylaxis may occur in patients who have been similarly envenomated on a previous occasion (e.g. snake handlers).

Investigations include full blood examination (especially for haematocrit and platelet count), coagulation screen, electrolytes, muscle enzymes, renal function and urinalysis. These should be carried out initially and then 8 hrly until any major acute changes have resolved. Persistently negative results at 12 hr exclude severe envenomation. A **snake venom detection kit** should be used to identify the snake type responsible and thus to target specific antivenom.

*Treatment principles are outlined above, with particular emphasis on the prompt administration of appropriate **antivenom**.*

***Heparin** is ineffective in treating the procoagulant effects of snake venoms, because these can cause clotting directly and not via thrombin (and the classic coagulation sequence).*

***Factor replacement** in venom-induced coagulopathy has been controversial because of fears of 'feeding the fire' until the venom has disappeared either spontaneously or following antivenom neutralization.*

***DMPS**, a chelating agent (q.v.), may be able to neutralize viper venom, since these snakes have zinc-containing toxic metalloproteinases. The zinc may be captured and the toxin neutralized by this particular drug, offering the potential for simple oral treatment in the field.*

- **Spider** bites mostly are harmless, though there are some major exceptions.

The **Sydney funnel-web spider** is the world's most deadly spider. The best-known species is *Atrax robustus*, and specific antivenom was first produced for it in 1981. Its bite may cause potentially lethal envenomation, with a dramatic clinical picture of tachycardia, hypertension, salivation, muscle spasm, pulmonary oedema, raised intracranial pressure and acidosis. This is sometimes referred to as an autonomic storm.

*Treatment of a funnel-web spider bite consists of immobilization, support of respiratory and circulatory failure, and the administration of **antivenom**, the beneficial effects of which are rapid.*

Red-back spider bites cause severe and prompt local pain (which is sometimes prolonged beyond 24 hr), followed by sweating, nausea, vomiting, headache, and sometimes tachycardia, hypertension and paralysis. This spider is a member of the *Lactrodectus* genus, which includes the American black widow spider, and envenomation from such species is referred to as '**latrodectism**'.

*Treatment of a red-back spider bite is with local ice packs, diazepam and specific **antivenom**.*

Extensive local tissue damage (**necrotic arachnidism**) may sometimes be produced by the bites of some spiders (e.g. recluse), but two former putative culprits (white-tailed and wolf spiders) have recently been exonerated from blame for this complication.

Treatment of this injury is primarily on its local merits, but associated vasculitis may be helped with heparin and/or corticosteroids. Useful measures for necrosis probably include hyperbaric oxygen but not debridement, grafting or antibiotics.

Brown recluse and **black widow** spiders are important causes of envenomation in the USA.

Tarantulas have become common household 'pets', and the bites of these large hairy creatures are correspondingly frequent. Local pain, erythema and swelling are accompanied by systemic features of anaphylaxis in those allergic to the venom. Eye injuries from released barbs can occur.

- **Toad bites** may occasionally cause envenomation.

*Successful treatment of toad envenomation with **digoxin-specific antibody** (q.v.) has been reported.*

Bibliography

Abroug F, Ouanes-Besbes L, Tilouche N, et al. Scorpion envenomation: state of the art. *Intens Care Med* 2020; 46: 401.

Auerbach PS. Marine envenomation. *N Engl J Med* 1991; 325: 486.

Bailey PM, Little M, Jetliner GA, et al. Jellyfish envenoming syndromes: unknown toxic mechanisms and unproven therapies. *Med J Aust* 2003; 178: 34.

Barnes JH. Cause and effect in Irukandji singings. *Med J Aust* 1964; 1: 897.

Berling I, Isbister GK. Hematologic effects and complications of snake envenoming. *Transfus Med Rev* 2015; 29: 82.

Bonefish F, Jute M, Belo BM, et al. Prevention and treatment of Hymenoptera venom allergy: guidelines for clinical practice. *Allergy* 2005; 60: 1459.

Broacher JR, Ravikumar PR, Bania T, et al. Treatment of toad venom poisoning with digoxin-specific Fab fragments. *Chest* 1996; 110: 1282.

Brooder J, Jerald D, Locker J, et al. Low risk of infection in selected human bites treated without antibiotics. *Am J Emerg Med* 2004; 22: 10.

Burnett JW, Calton GJ. Jellyfish envenomation syndromes updated. *Ann Emerg Med* 1987; 16: 1000.

Callahan M. Dog bite wounds. *JAMA* 1980; 244: 2327.

CSL Ltd. *Treatment of Snake Bite in Australia and Papua New Guinea Using Antivenom.* Melbourne: Commonwealth Serum Laboratories. 1992.

Cummings P. Antibiotics to prevent infection in patients with dog bite wounds: a meta-analysis of randomized trials. *Ann Emerg Med* 1994; 23: 535.

Cuthbertson BH, Fisher M. Envenomation. *Int J Intens Care* 1998; 5: 64.

Dire DJ. Cat bite wounds: risk factors for infection. *Ann Emerg Med* 1991; 20: 973.

Fanner PJ, Haddock JC. Fatal envenomation by jellyfish causing the Irukandji syndrome. *Med J Aust* 2002; 177: 362–363.

Fanner PJ, Williamson JA. Worldwide deaths and severe envenomation from jellyfish stings. *Med J Aust* 1996; 165: 658.

Fisher MM, Bowery CJ. Urban envenomation. *Med J Aust* 1989; 150: 695.

Fisher MM, Carr GA, McGuinness R, et al. *Atrax robustus* envenomation. *Anaesth Intens Care* 1980; 8: 410.

Flicker H. Irukandji sting to North Queensland bathers without production of weals but with severe general symptoms. *Med J Aust* 1952; 2; 89.

Ghanaian RV, Conte JE. Mammalian bite wounds. *Ann Emerg Med* 1980; 9: 79.

Goldstein EJC. Bite wounds and infection. *Clin Infect Dis* 1992; 14: 633.

Griego RD, Rosen T, Orengo IF, et al. Dog, cat, and human bites. *J Am Acad Dermatol* 1995; 33: 1019.

Hamilton RG. Diagnostic methods for insect sting allergy. *Cur Open Allergy Clin Immune* 2004; 4: 297.

Having S, Tulleken JE, Moller LVM, et al. Dog-bite induced sepsis: a report of four cases. *Intens Care Med* 1997; 23: 1179.

Healy J, Winkel KD, eds. *Venom: Fear, Fascination and Discovery.* Melbourne: Medical History Museum, University of Melbourne. 2013.

Hunt GR. Bites and stings of uncommon arthropods. *Postgrad Med* 1981; 70: 91 & 107.

Huynh TT, Seymour J, Pereira P, et al. Severity of Irukandji syndrome and nematocyst identification from skin scrapings. *Med J Aust* 2003; 178: 38.

Isbister GK, Bawaskar HS. Scorpion envenomation. *N Engl J Med* 2014; 371: 457.

Isbister GK, Brown SGA, Page CB, et al. Snakebite in Australia: a practical approach to diagnosis and treatment. *Med J Aust* 2013; 199: 763.

Isbister GK, Gray MR. A prospective study of 750 definite spider bites with expert spider identification. *QJM* 2002; 95: 723.

Isbister GK, Gray MR. Latrodectism: a prospective cohort study of bites by formally identified red back spiders. *Med J Aust* 2003; 179: 88.

Isbister GK, Gray MR, Bali CR, et al. Funnel-web spider bite: a systematic review of recorded clinical cases. *Med J Aust* 2005; 182: 407.

Isbister GK, Volschenk ES, Seymour JE. Scorpion stings in Australia. *Intern Med J* 2004; 34: 427.

Isbister GK, Whyte IM. Suspected white-tail spider bite and necrotic ulcers. *Intern Med J* 2004; 34: 38.

Ismail M. The scorpion envenoming syndrome. *Toxicon* 1995; 33: 825.

Janda DH, Ringler DH, Hilliard JK, et al. Nonhuman primate bites. *J Orthop Res* 1990; 8: 146.

Javaid M, Feldberg L, Gipson M. Primary repair of dog bites to the face. *J R Soc Med* 1998; 91: 414.

Johnston CI, Ryan NM, Page CB, et al. The Australian snakebite project, 2005–2015 (ASP-20). *Med J Aust* 2017; 207: 119.

Klein M. Nondomestic mammalian bites. *Am Fam Physician* 1985; 32: 137.

MacBean C, Taylor DM, Ashby K. Animal and human bite injuries in Victoria, 1998–2004. *Med J Aust* 2007; 186: 38.

McHugh TP, Bartlett RL, Raymond JI. Rat bite fever. *Ann Emerg Med* 1985; 14: 1116.

McKinney PE. Out-of-hospital and interhospital management of crotaline snakebite. *Ann Emerg Med* 2001; 37: 168.

Moffitt JE, Golden DB, Reiaman RE, et al. Stinging insect hypersensitivity: a practice parameter update. *J Allergy Clin Immunol* 2004; 114: 869.

O'Hehir RE, Douglass JA. Stinging insect allergy. *Med J Aust* 1999; 171: 649.

Pennell TC, Babu S-S, Meredith JW. The management of snake and spider bites in the southeastern United States. *Ann Surg* 1987; 53: 198.

Pers C, Gahrm-Hansen B, Frederiksen W. Capnocytophaga canimorsus septicaemia in Denmark, 1982–1995: review of 39 cases. *Clin Infect Dis* 1996; 23: 71.

Possani LD. Antivenom for scorpion sting. *Lancet* 2000; 355: 67.

Reisman RE. Insect stings. *N Engl J Med* 1994; 331: 523.

Rodrigo C, Gnanathasan A. Management of scorpion envenomation: a systematic review and meta-analysis of controlled clinical trials. *Syst Rev* 2017; 6: 74.

Sofer S. Scorpion envenomation. *Intens Care Med* 1995; 21: 626.

Sutherland SK, Coulter AR, Harris RD. Rationalisation of first-aid measures for elapid snakebite. *Lancet* 1979; 1: 183.

Sutherland SK, Leonard RL. Snakebite deaths in Australia 1992–1994 and a management update. *Med J Aust* 1995; 163: 616.

Sutherland S, Nolch G. *Dangerous Australian Animals.* Sydney: Hyland House. 2000.

Sutherland SK, Sutherland J. *Venomous Creatures of Australia.* 5th edition. Melbourne: Oxford University Press. 2006.

Sutherland SK, Tibbals J. *Australian Animal Toxins: The Creatures, Their Toxins and the Care of the Poisoned Patient.* 2nd edition. Melbourne: Oxford University Press. 2001.

Sutherland SK, Trinca JC. Survey of 2144 cases of red-back spider bites: Australia and New Zealand, 1963–1976. *Med J Aust* 1978; 2: 620.

Tibballs J. Severe tetrodotoxic fish poisoning. *Anaesth Intens Care* 1988; 16: 215.

Tibballs J. Diagnosis and treatment of confirmed and suspected snake bite. *Med J Aust* 1992; 156: 270.

Underhill D. *Australia's Dangerous Creatures.* Sydney: Reader's Digest. 1990.

Walker JP. Venomous bites and stings. In: *Scientific American Medicine. Interdisciplinary Medicine.* Hamilton: Dekker Medicine. 2020.

Warrell DA, Fenner PJ. Venomous bites and stings. *Br Med Bull* 1993; 49: 423.

Weiner S. Redback spider bites in Australia. *Med J Aust* 1961; 2: 44.

White J. *CSL Antivenom Handbook.* 2nd edition. Melbourne: CSL. 2001.

White J. Necrotising arachnidism. *Med J Aust* 1999; 171: 98.

White J. Debunking spider bite myths. *Med J Aust* 2003; 179: 180.

White J, Edmonds C, Zborowski P. *Australia's Most Dangerous Spiders, Snakes and Marine Creatures.* Sydney: Australian Geographic. 2001.

Williamson JA, Le Ray LE, Wohlfahrt M, et al. Acute management of serious envenomation by box-jellyfish (*Chironex fleckeri*). *Med J Aust* 1984; 141: 851.

Bivalirudin See

- Anticoagulants.

Black cohosh See

- Hepatitis.

Bleeding See

- Haemostasis.

Bleomycin

Bleomycin is a mixture of related glycopeptides used in cancer chemotherapy, especially for squamous cell carcinomas, as well as for lymphoma and testicular cancer. It produces little bone marrow or immune suppression. Its unique action is to fragment DNA, and it is commonly used in multidrug combinations.

Its side-effects include fever, stomatitis (q.v.), alopecia (q.v.), and rash with pruritus and vesiculation. When the rash is associated with linear scratch marks, it is referred to as flagellate dermatitis (see Dermatitis).

> In the ICU, two uncommon but important side-effects can be relevant.
> 1. A **fulminant reaction** may be seen in about 1% of patients overall and in 5% of patients with lymphomas.
> This reaction occurs within a few hours of the first or second dose and is characterized by confusion, fever, wheeze and hypotension.
> It does not appear to be anaphylactic and may be related to the release of endogenous pyrogens.
> 2. **Pulmonary toxicity** which can be severe and even fatal may be a late complication.
> It occurs 4–10 weeks after the start of treatment in 5–10% of patients. The risk is increased with higher doses, in the elderly, with oxygen and with irradiation. It is characterized by cough, crackles on auscultation and a diffuse basal infiltrate on chest X-ray.
> The value of corticosteroids is unknown, but they are probably helpful. Recent experimental studies have suggested that recombinant human erythropoietin may ameliorate the development of this form of pneumonitis. If recovery occurs, pulmonary function returns to normal.
> Nevertheless, the risk of post-anaesthetic ARDS persists for 6–12 months after treatment, and it is important in such patients to avoid excessive fluid administration and to keep the inspired oxygen concentration below 30% (though the added pulmonary risk from 'hyperoxia' is controversial).

Bibliography
Mathes DD. Bleomycin and hyperoxia exposure in the operating room. *Anesth Analg* 1995; 81: 624.
Sleijfer S. Bleomycin-induced pneumonitis. *Chest* 2001; 120: 617.

'Blind as a bat, dry as a bone, hot as a hare, mad as a hatter and red as a beet'

This colourful mnemonic is used to describe **anticolinergic** excess.
See
- Anticholinergic agents.

Blisters See
- Vesiculobullous diseases.

Boerhaave's syndrome See
- Mallory–Weiss syndrome.

Bone failure

Bone failure, as shown by increased bone resorption, has been reported to be common in critically ill patients, though its routine assessment is problematic. It may be considered another component of **multiorgan failure** (q.v.), especially in patients with sepsis. There may be a consequently increased risk of fractures in survivors.

Bibliography
Lee P, Nair P, Eisman JA, et al. Bone failure in critical illness. *Crit Care Med* 2016; 44: 2270.

Bornholm disease See
- Pleurisy.

Botulism

Botulism is produced by the neurotoxin from the anaerobic Gram-positive bacillus, *Clostridium botulinum*, which blocks acetylcholine release at peripheral nerve endings.

The use of **botulinum toxin** in hemifacial spasm and other disorders of dystonia (i.e. involuntary and sustained muscle contraction, or spasticity) is an interesting and valuable clinical application of this otherwise undesirable toxin. Not unexpectedly, this therapeutic application has become extensively adopted for facial and other cosmesis since it became available for this purpose in 1989. The dose used in such therapeutic or cosmetic applications is far too small to cause systemic symptoms, though occasional toxicity (rarely serious) has been reported due to dosage or administration errors.

Although the toxin is labile, the spores are heat-stable and may thus produce new toxin if cooked food is left at room temperature for more than 16 hr. Most commonly, botulism arises from the ingestion of poorly processed home foods (historically sometimes called ptomaine poisoning), though it occasionally occurs as a wound infection. Cases have been reported following the ingestion of fish gut. The incubation period ranges from 6 hr to 8 days, though it usually 18–36 hr.

The patient experiences diplopia, ptosis, dysphagia, dysarthria and descending paralysis. The mouth is dry and there are usually gastrointestinal symptoms. There is no fever.

The diagnosis is clinical, and the differential diagnosis includes
- Guillain–Barré syndrome (q.v.),
- myasthenia gravis (q.v.),
- brainstem stroke,

- poisoning,
- diphtheria (q.v.).

*Treatment is with **antitoxin** (if available), administered as soon as the diagnosis is established, and with mechanical ventilation. An experimental vaccine has been prepared for military use.*

The mortality is still about 20%.

Like anthrax (q.v.) (and perhaps plague and smallpox), botulism offers potential for germ warfare (q.v.) and thus bioterrorism (q.v.). In such a scenario, the toxin would be distributed in aerosolized form for inhalation, but the clinical consequences would be similar to the more typical food-borne condition described above except for the absence of gastrointestinal symptoms.

See also
- Clostridial infections,
- Food poisoning,
- Germ warfare.

Bibliography

Arnon SS, Schechter R, Inglesby TV, et al. Botulinum toxin as a biological weapon: medical and public health management. *JAMA* 2001; 285: 1059.

Hatheway CL. Botulism: the present status of the disease. *Curr Top Microbiol Immunol* 1995; 195: 55.

Jankovic J, Brin MF. Therapeutic uses of botulinum toxin. *N Engl J Med* 1991; 324: 1186.

Lecour H, Ramos H, Almeida B, et al. Food-borne botulism: a review of 13 outbreaks. *Arch Intern Med* 1988; 148: 578.

Merson MH, Dowell VR. Epidemiologic, clinical and laboratory aspects of wound botulism. *N Engl J Med* 1973; 289: 1005.

Scheinberg A. Clinical use of botulinum toxin. *Aust Prescriber* 2009; 32: 39.

Whitby M, Street AC, Ruff TA, et al. Biological agents as weapons 1: smallpox and botulism. *Med J Aust* 2002; 176: 431.

Bovine spongiform encephalopathy See
- Creutzfeldt–Jakob disease.

Bradykinin See
- Adenosine,
- Angioedema,
- Angiotensin-converting enzyme,
- Carcinoid syndrome,
- Renin–angiotensin–aldosterone.

Brodifacoum

Brodifacoum is a vitamin K antagonist, introduced as a second-generation anticoagulant pesticide for use in warfarin-resistant rodents. It has been referred to as 'super-warfarin' because of its potency and long duration of action. Its LD_{50} in rodents is several hundred-fold greater than warfarin, and its half-life can be up to several months.

Human poisoning has occurred from both occupational exposure and deliberate overdose. It has also been reported from contaminated cannabis. Animal poisoning of pets and wildlife has occurred after the consumption of dead rodents.

The chief clinical manifestation is bleeding, but occasionally it may cause a serotonin syndrome (q.v.) or a DIC-like picture (see Disseminated intravascular coagulation). Laboratory investigation shows a prolonged prothrombin time (PT) or INR. A specific assay for brodifacoum is available in some specialized laboratories.

*Treatment is with **vitamin K**, which may need to be given daily (e.g. 10 mg bd) for up to 6 months, as brodifacoum may persist for weeks in the blood and for months in the liver.*

See
- Vitamin K deficiency.

Bromhidrosis

Bromhidrosis refers to the foul body odour which is typically associated with increased axillary sweating, particularly **hyperhidrosis** (q.v.).

Bromocriptine See
- Acromegaly,
- Ergot,
- Neuroleptic malignant syndrome.

Bronchiectasis

Bronchiectasis is defined on anatomical grounds as chronic abnormal dilatation of larger bronchi. It may be focal or diffuse.

It has sometimes been described as an 'orphan disease', and a large US database (the Bronchiectasis Research Registry) was established in 2007 to collate cases which were non-CF (i.e. without cystic fibrosis). A non-tuberculous mycobacteria (NTM) component was later added in 2011.

The bronchiectatic process comprises airway obstruction and damage following chronic inflammation, because the pooling of bronchial secretions rich in inflammatory products and in released intracellular proteases weakens the bronchial wall. In addition to severe, necrotizing lung infections, the aetiology probably also includes congenital factors, although most cases remain idiopathic.

The association of bronchiectasis with congenital dextrocardia and sinusitis is referred to as **Kartagener's syndrome** (q.v.).

Bronchiectasis may also complicate
- cystic fibrosis (q.v.),
- hypogammaglobulinaemia,
- rheumatoid lung,
- asthmatic pulmonary eosinophilia (q.v.),
- non-tuberculous mycobacterial infection.

The clinical features are cough, purulent sputum and proneness to recurrent or persistent lower respiratory tract infection. The sputum can be copious and particularly offensive. Haemoptysis, dyspnoea and wheeze may occur, and there are crackles on auscultation and clubbing of the fingers.

The diagnosis was confirmed formerly by bronchography (or autopsy) but is made nowadays by CT scanning, in which bronchi can be seen to be larger than the associated artery. The former bronchographic distinction of cylindrical, varicose (fusiform) and cystic (saccular) changes probably has little clinical significance.

Treatment is primarily with **physiotherapy** and **antibiotics**.
- **Physiotherapy** using manual techniques such as chest percussion and postural drainage is commonly supplemented by a variety of instrumental airway clearance techniques (ACTs) using devices providing chest oscillations or positive expiratory pressure.
- **Antibiotics** in most patients should preferably be used only for exacerbations.

Mucolytic therapy (e.g. with dornase alfa or hypertonic saline) may be helpful in patients with particularly viscid tracheobronchial secretions. Airway inflammation may be reduced with **inhaled corticosteroids** (but not bronchodilators or anticholinergic agents) or **oral macrolides** (but these should be avoided in cases of NTM). Recent studies have shown that **statins** (q.v.) may be helpful in some patients.

Surgical resection is only occasionally indicated nowadays.

Prevention is of major importance and includes particularly the prompt and effective treatment of respiratory infections and of airway obstruction by foreign bodies.

Bibliography

Afzelius BA. A human syndrome caused by immotile cilia. *Science* 1976; 193: 317.

Agasthian T, Deschamps C, Trastek VF, et al. Surgical management of bronchiectasis. *Ann Thorac Surg* 1996; 62: 976.

Angrill J, Agusti C, Torres A. Bronchiectasis. *Curr Opin Infect Dis* 2001; 14: 193.

McShane PJ. Bronchiectasis: an orphan finds a home. *Chest* 2017; 151: 953.

McShane PJ, Tino G. Bronchiectasis. *Chest* 2019; 155: 825.

Mygind N, Nielsen MH, Pedersen M. Kartagener's syndrome and abnormal cilia. *Eur J Respir Dis* 1983; 64 (suppl. 127): 1.

O'Donnell AE. Bronchiectasis. *Chest* 2008; 134: 815.

Polverino E, Goeminne PC, McDonnell MJ, et al. European Registry Society guidelines for the management of adult bronchiectasis. *Eur Respir J* 2017; 50: 1700629.

Visser SK, Bye P, Morgan L. Management of bronchiectasis in adults. *Med J Aust* 2018; 209: 177.

Bronchiolitis obliterans

Bronchiolitis obliterans (BO) (obliterative bronchiolitis, bronchiolitis fibrosa obliterans) is a rare condition and probably a very severe form of chronic obstructive bronchitis with pathological changes implied by its name, namely chronic organizing inflammation of small airways. Its pathogenesis is presumably bronchiolar epithelial injury followed by an excessively proliferative repair process.

It is most usually due to the inhalation a few weeks previously of a toxic gas, for example an industrial chemical (such as nitrogen dioxide, as in silo-filler's disease) or a military poison. In such circumstances, treatment is generally ineffective, and the prognosis is poor.

It has occasionally followed severe infections, usually viral pneumonia, when it may sometimes take the additional form of what was formerly called **bronchiolitis obliterans organizing pneumonia** (BOOP). More recently, this condition has been renamed **cryptogenic organizing pneumonia** (one of the forms of **interstitial pneumonia** – q.v.).

See also
- Acute lung irritation – Toxic gases and fumes,
- Warfare agents.

Bibliography

Boehler A, Kesten S, Weder W, et al. Bronchiolitis obliterans after lung transplantation: a review. *Chest* 1998; 114: 1411.

Epler GR, Colby TV, McLoud TC, et al. Bronchiolitis obliterans organizing pneumonia. *N Engl J Med* 1985; 312: 152.

Ramirez J, Dowell AR. Silo-filler's disease: nitrogen dioxide-induced lung injury: long-term follow-up and review of the literature. *Ann Intern Med* 1971; 74: 569.

Schwartz DA. Acute inhalational injury. *Occup Med* 1987; 2: 297.

Theodore J, Starnes VA, Lewiston NJ. Obliterative bronchiolitis. *Clin Chest Med* 1990; 11: 309.

Wohl MEB, Chernick V. Bronchiolitis. *Am Rev Respir Dis* 1978; 118: 759.

Bronchocentric granulomatosis *See*
- Wegener's granulomatosis.

Broncholithiasis

Broncholithiasis refers to the presence of calcified or stone-like material in the tracheobronchial tree. It is a rare phenomenon of unknown aetiology, though its pathogenesis is likely to involve the erosion into a major airway of an adjacent chronic inflammatory process (e.g. paratracheal or peribronchial lymph node granuloma). The stones in this setting are composed of calcium phosphate.

Occasional cases are related to **primary ciliary dyskinesia** (q.v.), but not to other chronic inflammatory airways diseases, such as COPD or cystic fibrosis (q.v.). The stones in this setting are composed of calcium carbonate.

Broncholithiasis is unrelated to the rare infiltrative condition of **pulmonary alveolar microlithiasis** (see Interstitial lung diseases).

Clinical features include cough, wheeze, sometimes haemoptysis and rarely lithoptysis. The diagnosis is suspected on chest X-ray and confirmed on bronchoscopy.

Bronchoscopic removal is generally recommended.

Bibliography
Alshabani K, Ghosh S, Arrossi AV, et al. Broncholithiasis: a review. *Chest* 2019; 156: 445.
Kennedy MP, Noone PG, Cardon J, et al. Calcium stone lithoptysis in primary ciliary dyskinesia. *Respir Med* 2007; 101: 76.

Bronchopleural fistula *See*
- Barotrauma,
- Pneumothorax.

Brucellosis

Brucellosis is due to infection with a small slowly growing Gram-negative aerobic bacillus, discovered by Bruce in 1887. It is chiefly found in domesticated animals – *Brucella abortus* in cattle, *B. suis* in pigs, *B. melitensis* in goats and *B. canis* in dogs, as well as other strains later identified strains in different animals, including marine mammals. Brucellosis is thus a bacterial zoonosis (q.v.), and infection usually arises following exposure to animals and so particularly affects meat workers. Dairy products are not nowadays a source of infection in most countries, except for goat milk in poorer societies. Laboratory staff can also be at risk.

Following a variable incubation period of days to months, there is an insidious onset of fever and variable local findings, e.g. endocarditis (q.v.), meningitis, osteomyelitis.

Investigations may show a normal white cell count and ESR. The microbiological diagnosis is made from blood cultures or from an increased titre of serum agglutinins. Specimens must be handled with special care in the laboratory, so as to avoid accidental infection of the staff.

Treatment is with **tetracycline** *(e.g. doxycycline 100 mg bd) and/or* **rifampicin** *(600–900 mg per day) for 3–6 weeks. Monotherapy is less effective than dual or probably even triple antibiotic therapy. If there is severe local disease, such as endocarditis or meningitis, combination therapy of tetracycline with added cotrimoxazole and/or rifampicin and/or an aminoglycoside is used for several months.*

The prognosis is nowadays good, with a mortality of <1%. There is no currently available vaccine.

Bibliography
Corbell MJ. Brucellosis: an overview. *Emerg Infect Dis* 1997; 3: 2.
Fiori PL, Mastrandrea S, Rappelli P, et al. *Brucella abortus* infection acquired in microbiology laboratories. *J Clin Microbiol* 2000; 38: 2005.
Liles WC. Infections due to brucella, francisella, yersinia pestis, and bartonella. In: *Scientific American Medicine. Infectious Diseases.* Hamilton: Dekker Medicine. 2020.
Pappas G, Akritidis N, Bosilkovski M, et al. Brucellosis. *N Engl J Med* 2005; 352: 2325.
Radolf J. Brucellosis: don't let it get your goat! *Am J Med Sci* 1994; 307: 64.

Brugada syndrome

The **Brugada syndrome** is a serious cardiac condition with potentially fatal electrical instability despite structural normality. It was first described in 1992 by the Spanish cardiology family, Brugada, and it is characterized by a distinctive ECG, with ST elevation in the right precordial leads. It is a genetic disorder and is inherited as an autosomal dominant. Its prevalence of about 1 in 2000 of the population, and it is most common in South East Asian countries, where it is a recognized cause of death in young adults, particularly men.

Although there is some phenotypic variation, there is always an alteration in the transmembrane ion channels, with consequently increased propensity for supraventricular and particularly ventricular arrhythmias. This propensity is readily exacerbated by classic antiarrhythmic agents, beta blockers, nitrates, many psychotropic drugs, alcohol excess, electrolyte disturbance and fever.

The chief clinical features are syncope, palpitations or sudden death, typically occurring in a young otherwise well adult.

The only effective treatment is an **implantable cardioverter-defibrillator** *(AICD). This procedure is indicated in patients who have suffered an arrhythmia.*

Quinidine may help suppress ventricular tachyarrhythmias in some patients. In shocked patients, an isoprenaline infusion is recommended, despite the tachycardia, as it increases cyclic AMP and thus reduces the ion channel abnormality.

In asymptomatic patients, lifestyle changes are recommended, including avoidance of alcohol and prompt treatment of fever.

Bibliography
Antzelevitch C, Brugada P, Borgreffe M, et al. Brugada syndrome: report of the second consensus conference. *Circulation* 2005; 111: 659.
Brugada P, Brugada J. Right bundle branch block, persistent ST elevation and sudden cardiac death: a distinct clinical and electrocardiographic syndrome. *J Am Coll Cardiol* 1992; 20: 1391.
Carey SM, Hocking G. Brugada syndrome – a review of the implications for the anaesthetist. *Anaesth Intens Care* 2011; 39: 571.

Budd–Chiari syndrome

The **Budd–Chiari syndrome** arises from hepatic vein thrombosis. This leads to **hepatic veno-occlusive disease** (hepatic sinusoidal obstruction syndrome). It is the least common form of **splanchnic vein thrombosis**, which also includes portal, splenic and mesenteric vein thromboses.

> The Budd–Chiari syndrome is seen
> - in thrombophilias (q.v.)
>   - such as antiphospholipid syndrome or antithrombin III deficiency,
> - in myelodysplastic disorders
>   - such as polycythaemia vera (q.v.),
> - in veno-occlusive disease
>   - such as in poisoning from plant alkaloids (q.v.), as are found in herbal or bush teas,
> - following high-dose chemotherapy
>   - in association with bone marrow transplantation.

Secondary Budd–Chiari syndrome may be caused by extrinsic compression, e.g. from the local effect of an intra-abdominal malignancy.

The clinical features comprise acute tender hepatomegaly, with jaundice, ascites and peripheral oedema.

Treatment is traditionally with **anticoagulation** (heparin followed by warfarin), but there have been case reports of successful **thrombolytic therapy** given either locally or systemically. Useful mechanical decompression of the congested liver sinusoids can be achieved radiologically with **transjugular intrahepatic portosystemic shunting** (TIPS).

The new antithrombotic agent, **defibrotide** (an adenosine receptor agonist), has shown therapeutic promise both for prevention and treatment of this difficult condition (see Anticoagulants). The synthetic bile acid, **ursodeoxycholic acid**, has also been used prophylactically with success.

Gene therapy (with the agent Difitelio) has been approved for use in cases which occur following bone marrow transplantation.

Liver transplantation may be indicated as a final rescue therapy in advanced cases.

Even if acute recovery occurs, cardiac cirrhosis may result and may then become a longer-term problem.

Bibliography
Ageno W, Dentali F, Pomero F, et al. Incidence rates and case fatality rates of portal vein thrombosis and Budd–Chiari Syndrome. *Thromb Haemost* 2017; 117: 794.
Bach N, Thung SN, Schaffner F. Comfrey herb tea-induced hepatic veno-occlusive disease. *Am J Med* 1989; 87: 97.
Bearman SI. The syndrome of hepatic veno-occlusive disease after marrow transplantation. *Blood* 1995; 85: 3005.
Broughton BJ. Hepatic and portal vein thrombosis closely associated with myeloproliferative disorders. *BMJ* 1991; 302: 192.
Di Nisio M, Valeriani E, Riva N, et al. Anticoagulant therapy for splanchnic vein thrombosis: ISTH SSC Subcommittee Control of Anticoagulation. *J Thromb Haemost* 2020; 18: 1562.
Klein AS, Sitzmann JV, Coleman J, et al. Current management of the Budd–Chiari syndrome. *Ann Surg* 1990; 212: 144.
Kumar S, DeLeve LD, Kamath PS, et al. Hepatic veno-occlusive disease (sinusoidal obstruction syndrome) after hematopoietic stem cell transplantation. *Mayo Clin Proc* 2003; 78: 589.
Mitchell MC, Boitnott JK, Kaufman S, et al. Budd–Chiari syndrome: etiology, diagnosis and management. *Medicine* 1982; 61: 199.
Shulman HM, Hinterberger W. Hepatic veno-occlusive disease – liver toxicity syndrome after bone marrow transplantation. *Bone Marrow Transpl* 1992; 10: 197.
Valla D, Casadevall N, Lacombe C, et al. Primary myeloproliferative disorder and hepatic vein thrombosis. *Ann Intern Med* 1985; 103: 329.
Vassal G, Hartmann O, Benhamou E. Busulfan and veno-occlusive disease of the liver. *Ann Intern Med* 1990; 112: 881.
Wadleigh M, Ho V, Momtaz P, et al. Hepatic veno-occlusive disease: pathogenesis, diagnosis and treatment. *Curr Opin Hematol* 2003; 10: 451.

Bullae See
- Vesiculobullous diseases.
  See also
- Cavitation,
- Pneumothorax.

Burns, respiratory complications See
- Inhalation injury.

Buruli ulcer See
- Mycobacterium ulcerans.

Byssinosis See
- Occupational lung diseases.

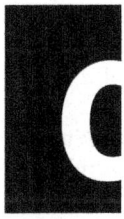

Cadmium

Cadmium (Cd, atomic number 48, atomic weight 112) is a soft, highly polishable metal of the zinc group with a low melting point (321°C). It was discovered in 1817 and is associated in nature with zinc. It is widely used in metallurgy, the most common compounds being cadmium oxide and cadmium sulphide (artist's yellow). It is also present in air pollution and in cigarette smoke.

Its vapour and dust are toxic, with recommended levels not >0.1 mg/m^3/8 hr for fumes and 0.2 mg/m^3/8 hr for dust. A urinary excretion of >10 mcg per day or probably a blood level of >0.09 mcmol/L (10 mcg/L) confirms toxicity. The biological half-life of cadmium in humans can be as long as 10–30 years.

The clinical features of toxicity depend upon the route and duration of exposure.
- **Acute toxicity** from ingestion produces prompt but transient nausea, diarrhoea and prostration (onset within 15 min and offset by 24 hr).
- **Acute toxicity** from inhalation can produce a potentially fatal pneumonitis.
- **Chronic inhalation** at a lower level gives rise to anosmia, cough, dyspnoea, weight loss, renal damage (tubulointerstitial damage like that from other heavy metals, especially lead), liver damage and increased risk of cancer of the lung, kidney and prostate.

Treatment of cadmium toxicity is with **calcium edetate** *(q.v.).*
  See also
- Heavy metal poisoning,
- Tubulointerstitial diseases.

Bibliography
Ellis KJ, Yuen N, Yasumura S, et al. Dose-response analysis of cadmium in man: body-burden vs. kidney dysfunction. *Environ Res* 1984; 33: 216.
Lin J-L, Lin-Tan D-T, Chu P-H, et al. Cadmium excretion predicting hospital mortality and illness severity of critically ill medical patients. *Crit Care Med* 2009; 37: 957.
Pinot F, Kreps SE, Bachelet M, et al. Cadmium in the environment: sources, mechanisms of biotoxicity, and biomarkers. *Rev Environ Health* 2000; 15: 299.

Caeruloplasmin See
- Copper.

Calciphylaxis

Calciphylaxis (calcific uraemic arteriopathy) refers to localized areas of skin necrosis due to vascular calcification in patients with chronic renal failure. Initially, the lesions are painful purple patches, sometimes resembling livedo reticularis (q.v.). Later, they may ulcerate and even lead to amputation. It may be exacerbated in patients taking warfarin (see Vitamin K).

Metastatic calcification is the broad term which includes both calciphylaxis, which comprises non-visceral calcification, and visceral calcification, which affects the lungs, kidneys, muscles, gastrointestinal tract. In chronic renal failure, it is due to the interplay of abnormalities of calcium, phosphate and vitamin D.

Treatment with **parathyroidectomy** *may promote healing. Chelation with* **sodium thiosulphate** *has been found to be effective in younger patients. Vitamin K deficiency should be avoided.*

Bibliography
Floege J, Ketteler M. Vascular calcification in patients with end-stage renal disease. *Nephrol Dial Transplant* 2004; 19 (suppl. 5): V59.
Guldbakke KK, Khachemoune A. Calciphylaxis. *Int J Dermatol* 2007; 46: 231.

Calcitonin

Calcitonin is a polypeptide hormone secreted by the parafollicular cells of the thyroid gland and is one of the three regulators of calcium balance, together with parathyroid hormone and vitamin D. Calcitonin blocks the release of calcium and phosphorus from bone by inhibiting osteoclastic bone reabsorption, so that it opposes the effects of parathyroid hormone and vitamin D.

However, neither abnormally increased plasma levels of calcitonin (e.g. with tumours) nor abnormally decreased levels (e.g. following thyroidectomy) result in detectable changes in serum calcium level or in any apparent clinical effect, so that the physiological role of calcitonin and of its controls remain unknown. In fact, its synthesis is closely related to that of several other peptides with probable neurotransmitter rather than hormonal roles, including calcitonin gene-related peptide, the most potent natural vasodilator.

> Nevertheless, the clinical significance of calcitonin is 2-fold.
> 1. Its level is increased in medullary thyroid carcinoma, for which it is a marker.
>   It is also produced ectopically from a number of other tumours, particularly phaeochromocytoma (q.v.) and thus especially in patients with MEN type II (q.v.).
> 2. It has considerable pharmacological value in **Paget's disease** (q.v.), in which it produces an immediate response of falling serum and urine hydroxyproline levels.
>   Side-effects include local discomfort, as well as flushing, nausea and abnormal taste. The synthetic salmon polypeptide preparation, unlike the synthetic human form, may induce antibodies.

Procalcitonin (PCT, ProCT), the precursor of calcitonin, has been found to be a new and unexpected marker of severe infection. Procalcitonin is a 116 amino acid glycoprotein with a molecular weight of 13 kDa, derived from the larger preprocalcitonin (141 AA). Cleavage by a specific protease produces calcitonin (32 AA from the mid region) and other fragments of unknown function. The half-life of procalcitonin is 25–30 hr (compared with 10 min for calcitonin), but plasma levels are undetectable in normal subjects (i.e. <0.1 ng/mL). However, PCT may rise to 100 ng/mL or more in severe sepsis and septic shock, in which its rise is similar to that of the cytokines, except for a slower onset and greater duration. In these circumstances, it is probably produced by extra-thyroid cells, perhaps leukocytes or neuroendocrine cells of the lung or intestine, and is not degraded to calcitonin.

Despite numerous clinical trials and meta-analyses, the clinical utility of tests for PCT has been difficult to assess because of multiple research problems, especially with trial design, bias, confounders and industry sponsorship. However, PCT levels (in conjunction with clinical and other laboratory data) may be useful in providing individual patient guidance in the diagnosis of infection, in the need for ICU management of these patients and in deciding the optimal duration of antibiotic therapy in existing infection.

Bibliography
Assicot M, Gendrel D, Carsin H, et al. High serum procalcitonin concentrations in patients with sepsis and infection. *Lancet* 1993; 341: 515.
Becker KL, Snider R, Nylen ES. Procalcitonin assay in systemic inflammation, infection, and sepsis: clinical utility and limitations. *Crit Care Med* 2008; 36: 941.
De Jong E, van Oers JA, Beishuizen A, et al. Efficacy and safety of procalcitonin guidance in reducing the duration of antibiotic treatment in critically ill patients: a randomised, controlled, open-label trial. *Lancet Infect Dis* 2016; 16: 819.
de Werra I, Jaccard C, Corradin SB, et al. Cytokines, nitrite/nitrate, soluble tumor necrosis factor receptors, and procalcitonin concentrations: comparison in patients with septic shock, cardiogenic shock, and bacterial pneumonia. *Crit Care Med* 1997; 25: 607.
Kalil AC, Lisboa T. To procalcitonin or not to procalcitonin. *Chest* 2019; 155: 1085.
Kalil AC, Van Schooneveld TC. Is procalcitonin-guided therapy associated with beneficial outcomes in critically ill patients with sepsis? *Crit Care Med* 2018; 46: 811.
Maves RC. Procalcitonin is not an adequate tool for antimicrobial de-escalation in sepsis. *Crit Care Med* 2020; 48: 1848.
McDermott MT. Calcitonin and its clinical applications. *Endocrinologist* 1992; 2: 366.
Povoa P, Kalil AC. Any role for biomarker-guided algorithms in antibiotic stewardship programs? *Crit Care Med* 2020; 48: 775.
Scheutz P, Wirz Y, Sager R, et al. Effect of procalcitonin-guided antibiotic treatment on mortality in acute respiratory infections: a patient level meta-analysis. *Lancet Infect Dis* 2018; 18: 95.
Stevenson JC, Hillyard CJ, MacIntyre I, et al. A physiological role for calcitonin: protection of the maternal skeleton. *Lancet* 1979; 2: 769.
Torres A, Artigas A, Ferrer R. Biomarkers in the ICU: less is more? No. *Intens Care Med* 2021; 47: 97.

Uzzan B, Cohen R, Nicolas P, et al. Procalcitonin as a diagnostic test for sepsis in critically ill adults and after surgery or trauma: a systematic review and meta-analysis. *Crit Care Med* 2006; 34: 1996.

Calcium *See*

- Hypercalcaemia,
- Hypocalcaemia.
  See also
- Aluminium,
- Calcitonin,
- Hyperparathyroidism,
- Hyperphosphataemia,
- Hypoparathyroidism,
- Magnesium,
- Nephrolithiasis,
- Rhabdomyolysis.

Bibliography
Becker C. Diseases of calcium metabolism and metabolic bone disease. In: *Scientific American Medicine. Endocrinology & Metabolism.* Hamilton: Dekker Medicine. 2020.

Calcium disodium edetate *See*

- Chelating agents.

Cancer

Patients with the common **cancers** are frequently seen in Intensive Care, either because of concomitant disease or because of specific cancer complications, procedures or treatments.

Less common tumours or complications are considered in this book, including

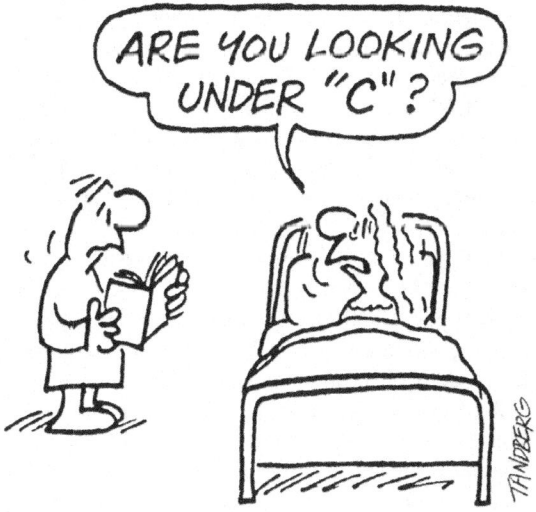

- Alpha-fetoprotein,
- Amyloid,
- Bence Jones protein,
- Cancer complications,
- Carcinoembryonic antigen,
- Carcinoid syndrome,
- CAR T-cell therapy,
- Cryoglobulinaemia,
- Differentiation syndrome,
- Dysproteinaemias,
- Ectopic hormone production,
- Gastrinoma,
- Gastrointestinal tumours,
- Glucagonoma,
- Graft-versus-host disease,
- Haemangioma,
- Heavy chains,
- Hepatocellular carcinoma,
- Hepatoma,
- Insulinoma,
- Islet cell tumour,
- Kaposi's sarcoma,
- Light chains,
- Lung tumours,
- Medullary thyroid cancer,
- Mesothelioma,
- Multiple myeloma,
- Myxoma,
- Paraganglioma,
- Paraneoplastic syndromes,
- Phaeochromocytoma,
- Plasmacytoma,
- Pseudomyxoma peritonei,
- Skin signs of internal malignant disease,
- Tisagenlecleucel,
- Tumour-lysis syndrome,
- Tumour markers/biomarkers,
- Waldenstrom's macroglobulinaemia.

Bibliography
Aaronson SA. Growth factors and cancer. *Science* 1991; 254: 1146.
Adjei AA, ed. Oncology. In: *Scientific American Medicine.* Hamilton: Dekker Medicine. 2020.
Angell M. The quality of mercy. *N Engl J Med* 1982; 306: 98.
Holzman D. New cancer genes crowd the horizon, create possibilities. *J Natl Cancer Inst* 1995; 87: 1108.
Kerr JFR, Winterford CM, Harmon BV. Apoptosis: its significance to cancer and cancer therapy. *Cancer* 1994; 73: 2013.
Krontiris TG. Oncogenes. *N Engl J Med* 1995; 333: 303.

Lowe S, Bodis S, McClatchey A, et al. Status and efficacy of cancer therapy in vivo. *Science* 1994; 266: 807.

Pardoll DM. Tumour antigens: a new look for the 1990s. *Nature* 1994; 369: 357.

Rosenberg SA. The immunotherapy and gene therapy of cancer. *J Clin Oncol* 1992; 10: 180.

Seleznick MJ. Tumor markers. *Prim Care* 1992; 19: 715.

Smith RA, Cokkinides V, Brooks D, et al. Cancer screening in the United States, 2010: a review of current American Cancer Society guidelines and issues in cancer screening. *CA: A Cancer Journal for Clinicians* 2010; 60: 99.

Solomon E, Borrow J, Goddard AD. Chromosome aberrations and cancer. *Science* 1991; 254: 1153.

Sturgeon CM, Lai LC, Duffy MJ. Serum tumour markers: how to order and interpret them. *BMJ* 2010; 339: 852.

Weinberg RA. Tumor suppressor genes. *Science* 1991; 254: 1138.

zur Hausen H. Viruses in human cancers. *Science* 1991; 254: 1167.

Cancer complications

By far the majority of patients with cancer seen in an ICU present with concomitant or incidental problems. The most frequently encountered concomitant problems are opportunistic infections and postoperative complications.

Uncommonly, more specific problems of Intensive Care relevance are encountered. These may be classified as follows.

- **cardiac**
  - non-bacterial endocarditis (q.v.), pericardial tamponade,
- **cutaneous**
  - various dermatoses (see Paraneoplastic syndromes),
- **endocrine/metabolic**
  - adrenal insufficiency, diabetes insipidus, ectopic hormone production, hypercalcaemia, hyperuricaemia (see these separate conditions),
- **general**
  - fever (q.v.), metastases, weight loss,
- **haematological**
  - anaemia, disseminated intravascular coagulation, neutropenia, thrombocytopenia, thromboembolism (see these separate conditions),
- **neurological**
  - myopathy (q.v.), neuropathy (q.v.),
- **renal**
  - tumour-lysis syndrome (q.v.).

In addition, **toxicities due to cancer treatment** are both frequent and varied, and some of these complications can present difficulties for Intensive Care clinicians. Of particular concern are some of complications related to new immunotherapeutic and targeted agents.

- **Monoclonal antibodies** (mABs) may cause cardiac, neurological, pulmonary and renal toxicity, as well as cytokine release syndrome and infusion reactions. This group includes rituximab (q.v.) as well as seven other newer anti-cancer agents.
- **Immune checkpoint inhibitors** (ICIs) include four particular mABs which additionally can cause hepatotoxicity and endocrine dysfunction.
- **Chimeric antigen receptor T-cell therapy** (CAR T-cell therapy – q.v.) may cause a dramatic cytokine release syndrome and neurotoxicity. CAR T-cell therapy is one of the forms of immune effector cell (IEC) therapy, whereby autologous T cells are modified to recognize a tumour antigen (either a specific receptor or a major histocompatibility complex).
- **Tyrosine kinase inhibitors** (TKIs) have expanded from the original imatinib to 14 related agents, which can cause cardiac, neurological, pulmonary and renal toxicity.

Bibliography

Adelstein DJ, Hines SG, Carter SF, et al. Thromboembolic events in patients with malignant superior vena cava syndrome and the role of anticoagulation. *Cancer* 1988; 62: 2258.

Arrambide K, Toto RD. Tumor lysis syndrome. *Semin Nephrol* 1993; 13: 273.

Barton JC. Tumor lysis syndrome in nonhematopoietic neoplasms. *Cancer* 1989; 64: 738.

Bell DR, Woods, RL, Levi JA. Superior vena cava obstruction. *Med J Aust* 1986; 145: 566.

Bick RL. Coagulation abnormalities in malignancy: a review. *Semin Thromb Hemost* 1992; 18: 353.

Carrier M, Khorana AA, Zwicker JI, et al. Management of challenging cases of patients with cancer-associated thrombosis including recurrent thrombosis and bleeding: guidance from the SSC of the ISTH. *J Thromb Haemost* 2013; 11: 1760.

Cascino TL. Neurologic complications of systemic cancer. *Med Clin North Am* 1993; 77: 265.

Chan A, Woodruff RK. Complications and failure of anticoagulation therapy in the treatment of venous thromboembolism in patients with disseminated malignancy. *Aust NZ J Med* 1992; 22: 119.

Coiffier B, Mounier N, Bologna S, et al. Efficacy and safety of rasburicase (recombinant urate oxidase) for the prevention and treatment of hyperuricemia during

induction chemotherapy of aggressive non-Hodgkin's lymphoma. *J Clin Oncol* 2003; 21: 4402.
Colman RW, Rubin RN. Disseminated intravascular coagulation due to malignancy. *Semin Oncol* 1990; 17: 172.
Gutierrez C, McEvoy C, Munshi L, et al. Critical care management of toxicities associated with targeted agents and immunotherapies for cancer. *Crit Care Med* 2020; 48: 10.
Howard SC, Jones DP, Pui C-H. The tumor lysis syndrome. *N Engl J Med* 2011; 364: 1844.
Langstein HN, Norton JA. Mechanisms of cancer cachexia. *Hematol Oncol Clin North Am* 1991; 5: 103.
Lazarus HM, Creger RJ, Gerson SL. Infectious emergencies in oncology patients. *Semin Oncol* 1989; 16: 543.
McCurdy MT, Shanholtz CB. Oncologic emergencies. *Crit Care Med* 2012; 40: 2212.
Pizzo PA. Management of fever in patients with cancer and treatment-induced neutropenia. *N Engl J Med* 1993; 328: 1323.
Rosen PJ. Bleeding problems in the cancer patient. *Hematol Oncol Clin North Am* 1992; 6: 1315.
Silverman P, Distelhorst CW. Metabolic emergencies in clinical oncology. *Semin Oncol* 1989; 16: 504.
Silverstein RL, Nachman RL. Cancer and clotting – Trousseau's warning. *N Engl J Med* 1992; 327: 1163.
Weiss HW, Walker MD, Wiernik PH. Neurotoxicity of commonly used antineoplastic agents. *N Engl J Med* 1974; 291: 75 & 127.
Zacharski LR, Wojtukiewicz MZ, Costantini V, et al. Pathways of coagulation/fibrinolysis activation in malignancy. *Semin Thromb Hemost* 1992; 18: 104.
Zafrani L, Canet E, Darmon M. Understanding tumor lysis syndrome. *Intens Care Med* 2019; 45: 1608.

Carbon monoxide

Carbon monoxide is a colourless, odourless, non-irritant and flammable gas with physical properties similar to nitrogen. It is produced from the incomplete combustion of carbon-containing fuels and is thus a common product in motor vehicle exhausts, faulty domestic heating and cooking devices, and in industry. In most countries, its predominant source is motor vehicle exhaust fumes, from which death can occur within 15 min if inside a confined space.

> Carbon monoxide is the most common lethal poison in all societies.
> - Poisoning has an estimated incidence of about 1 in 25,000 of the population per year.
> - Nearly one third of cases are fatal.
> - Most cases nowadays are suicidal, though some can be accidental (e.g. from faulty gas heaters).

Although carbon monoxide poisoning carries significant mortality and substantial late morbidity and has been known since the 19th century, understanding of its pathogenetic consequence of tissue hypoxia remains surprisingly incomplete. Thus, although carbon monoxide displaces oxygen from haemoglobin, having a more than 200-fold greater affinity than oxygen for haemoglobin, anaemic hypoxia does not explain carbon monoxide's toxicity, because oxygen transport and even oxygen consumption are increased due to a compensatory rise in cardiac output. Direct tissue toxicity is also an unsatisfactory explanation, and it is more likely that carbon monoxide alters a number of intracellular enzymes.

Nevertheless, the level of carboxyhaemoglobin is a guide to severity, in that levels up to 20% represent mild poisoning and 30–50% severe poisoning, with >50% often associated with fatality, especially if there is associated metabolic acidosis. These levels should be seen in the context of 5–10% in heavy smokers and up to 6% in some industries and in some cities. Levels below 5% are considered safe. However, a low level does not exclude the possibility of a previously high level, so that (as for any drug) the time from the initial exposure should be taken into account when interpreting a blood level (the T1/2 of COHb is 5 hr). Moreover, even levels of 3–6% may impair exercise tolerance and increase arrhythmias in cardiac patients, and levels of 5–8% reduce vigilance in healthy subjects.

> Pulse oximetry cannot distinguish between oxyhaemoglobin and carboxyhaemoglobin, so that the SpO_2 is unaffected.
> The PaO_2 is of course also unaffected, though modern blood gas analyzers incorporate co-oximetry which provides a direct measurement of dyshaemoglobins, such as carboxyhaemoglobin.

Several clinical patterns of poisoning may be seen.
- If the onset of poisoning is gradual, the patient may present with a flu-like illness, comprising headache, dizziness, weakness, nausea and finally coma. If a number of people are so affected, a mistaken diagnosis of food poisoning may be made.
- If the onset is sudden, rapid coma occurs with fitting, arrhythmias, shock and then death.

- The classical cherry-red appearance of the skin is in fact uncommon, though the presence of retinal haemorrhages is a useful diagnostic clue.
- Cardiac arrhythmias are common, especially in patients with associated heart disease.
- Exposure during pregnancy (q.v.) may cause fetal damage.

> The clinical course is variable and unpredictable.
> A biphasic response is common, with up to 20% of severely affected patients having a late recovery on the one hand and on the other hand about 10% of patients suffering a late deterioration which may be severe. This delayed relapse may occur up to one month after hospital discharge and after seemingly full recovery. It is primarily neurological with a fluctuating mental state and tremor, dysphasia, ataxia and incontinence, though most of these features disappear again within the next year.
> In patients who survive, permanent neurological and neuropsychiatric damage may result, especially disorders of personality and cognition. Infarction of skin, heart, peripheral nerve and bowel may be seen.

Treatment modalities are as follows.
- **100% oxygen** should be promptly administered. 100% oxygen increases the elimination of carbon monoxide 5-fold compared with room air, the half-life of carboxyhaemoglobin being shortened about 4-fold from its normal 5 hr. Mechanical ventilation may assist optimal oxygenation.
- **Hyperbaric oxygen** (HBO), though not definitively confirmed as effective in controlled studies, is commonly recommended in severe cases. Typically, one or two treatments are given within the first 12 hr. This form of treatment may be useful up to 16 hr after the initial event, but beyond 24 hr it does not appear to influence outcome. HBO shortens the half-life of carboxyhaemoglobin by a further 4-fold compared with 100% oxygen.
- Other measures, such as exchange transfusion, hypothermia and barbiturate or other sedation have been found to be ineffective.
  See also
- Inhalation injury,
- Warfare agents – Phosgene.

Bibliography

Annane D, Chadda K, Gajdos P, et al. Hyperbaric oxygen therapy for acute domestic carbon monoxide poisoning: two randomized controlled studies. *Intens Care Med* 2011; 37: 486.

Blumenthal I. Carbon monoxide poisoning. *J R Soc Med* 2001; 94: 270.

Caravanti EM, Adams CJ, Joyce SM, et al. Fetal toxicity associated with maternal carbon monoxide poisoning. *Ann Emerg Med* 1988; 17: 714.

Choi IS. Delayed neurologic sequelae in carbon monoxide intoxication. *Arch Neurol* 1983; 40: 433.

Cobb N, Etzel RA. Unintentional carbon monoxide-related deaths in the United States, 1979 through 1988. *JAMA* 1991; 266: 659.

Ernst A, Zibrak JD. Carbon monoxide poisoning. *N Engl J Med* 1998; 339: 1603.

Hampson NB. Pulse oximetry in severe carbon monoxide poisoning. *Chest* 1998; 114: 1036.

Hampson NB, Hauff NM. Risk factors for short-term mortality from carbon monoxide poisoning treated with hyperbaric oxygen. *Crit Care Med* 2008; 36: 2523.

Hampson NB, Rudd RA, Hauff NM. Increased long-term mortality among survivors of acute carbon monoxide poisoning. *Crit Care Med* 2009; 37: 1941.

Hardy KR, Thom DR. Pathophysiology and treatment of carbon monoxide poisoning. *Clin Toxicol* 1994; 32: 613.

Mokhlesi B, Leikin JB, Murray P, et al. Adult toxicology in critical care: part II: specific poisonings. *Chest* 2003; 123: 897.

Myers RAM, Britten JS. Are arterial blood gases of value in treatment decisions for carbon monoxide poisoning? *Crit Care Med* 1989; 17: 139.

Raphael JC, Elkharrat D, Jars-Guincestre MC, et al. Trial of normobaric and hyperbaric oxygen for acute carbon monoxide intoxication. *Lancet* 1989; 2: 414.

Rose JJ, Wang L, Xu Q, et al. Carbon monoxide poisoning: pathogenesis, management, and future directions of therapy. *Am J Respir Crit Care Med* 2017; 195: 596.

Runciman WW, Gorman DF. Carbon monoxide poisoning: from old dogma to new uncertainties. *Med J Aust* 1993; 158: 439.

Scheinkestel CD, Bailey M, Myles PS, et al. Hyperbaric or normobaric oxygen for acute carbon monoxide poisoning: a randomised controlled clinical trial. *Med J Aust* 1999; 170: 203.

Shimazu T. Half-life of blood carboxyhemoglobin. *Chest* 2001; 119: 661.

Smith SJ, Brandon S. Morbidity from acute carbon monoxide poisoning at three-year follow-up. *BMJ* 1973; 1: 318.

Tibbles PM, Edelsberg JS. Hyperbaric-oxygen therapy. *N Engl J Med* 1996; 334: 1642.

Walden SM, Gottlieb SO. Urban angina, urban arrhythmias: carbon monoxide and the heart. *Ann Intern Med* 1990; 113: 337.

Weaver LK, Hopkins RO, Chan KJ, et al. Hyperbaric oxygen for acute carbon monoxide poisoning. *N Engl J Med* 2002; 347: 1057.

Winter PM, Miller JN. Carbon monoxide poisoning. *JAMA* 1976; 236: 1502.

Zimmerman JL. Poisonings and overdoses in the intensive care unit: general and specific management issues. *Crit Care Med* 2003; 31: 2794.

Ziser A, Shupak A, Halpern P, et al. Delayed hyperbaric oxygen treatment for acute carbon monoxide poisoning. *BMJ* 1984; 289: 960.

Carbon tetrachloride

Carbon tetrachloride (tetrachormethane) is a heavy, colourless, volatile (boiling point 77°C), non-flammable, water-insoluble, toxic liquid with a characteristic odour. It is an organic halogen compound (a chlorinated hydrocarbon), first prepared in 1839 from combining chloroform with chlorine. It has been used as a refrigerant, a solvent and a dry-cleaning agent until replaced by **tetrachloroethylene**, a more stable and less toxic agent. It was even used as an anaesthetic, although the industrial solvent, **trichloroethylene**, became much more commonly used than carbon tetrachloride for this latter purpose, until recognized to be a potential carcinogen.

Carbon tetrachloride is well absorbed from the lungs and the gut. Poisoning may thus result from
- inhalation as a result of either industrial exposure or sniffing (solvent abuse),
- accidental or deliberate ingestion.

Clinical features include local irritation, gastrointestinal symptoms which may be severe, neurological features of headache, convulsions and coma, cardiovascular findings of hypotension and arrhythmias, and most importantly hepatorenal damage which is often delayed for at least 2 days after exposure. In particular, hepatic necrosis with later fatty infiltration may be produced. Other organ damage may involve the lungs, adrenals, pancreas, bone marrow, cerebellum and optic nerve.

Treatment comprises removal from further exposure, gastric lavage if there has been recent ingestion and symptomatic support.

Subsequent exposure must be avoided, as even low concentrations may then produce fever, fatigue and depression.

Bibliography
Wartenberg D, Reyner D, Scott CS. Trichlorethylene and cancer: epidemiological evidence. *Environ Health Perspect* 2000; 108: 161.

Carbonic anhydrase inhibitors

The prototype **carbonic anhydrase inhibitor** is **acetazolamide**, a non-bacteriostatic sulphonamide with a molecular weight of 222 Da. It is a potent reversible inhibitor of the enzyme, carbonic anhydrase.

Its potential therapeutic uses have been
- as a diuretic, though not nowadays since its diuretic effect is mild and comparable only with that of thiazides,
- to alkalinize the urine in glaucoma,
- in acute mountain sickness (see High altitude),
- in some convulsive disorders,
- in periodic paralysis (even in the presence of hypokalaemia) (q.v.),
- in sleep apnoea syndromes (see Sleep disorders of breathing).

In Intensive Care, acetazolamide has been used in the management of severe metabolic alkalosis, since it enhances the urinary excretion of bicarbonate 5-fold and thus produces metabolic acidosis.

However, if carbon dioxide excretion is limited, as in some patients with chronic lung disease, increased hypercapnia may result. On the other hand, it has sometimes been used as an adjunct to weaning from mechanical ventilation of patients with chronic airways obstruction and severe metabolic alkalosis.

It is given in a dose of 500 mg 8 hrly, but only short-term use is recommended as tolerance rapidly develops.

Among many occasional adverse reactions, hypokalaemia can be important. Toxic effects include
- drowsiness,
- paraesthesiae,
- rare hypersensitivity, including erythema multiforme (q.v.),
- teratogenicity.

It is contraindicated in
- hyponatraemia (q.v.),
- hypokalaemia,
- hyperchloraemia,
- metabolic acidosis (q.v.),
- severe liver or renal disease,
- hypersensitivity to sulphonamides.

Bibliography
Faisy C, Mokline A, Sanchez O, et al. Effectiveness of acetazolamide for reversal of metabolic alkalosis in weaning COPD patients from mechanical ventilation. *Intens Care Med* 2010; 36: 859.

Hanley T, Platts MM. Acetazolamide (Diamox) in the treatment of congestive heart failure. *Lancet* 1956; 270: 357.

Preisig PA, Toto RD, Alpern RJ. Carbonic anhydrase inhibitors. *Renal Physiol* 1987; 10: 136.

Carboxyhaemoglobin See

- Carbon monoxide.

Carcinoembryonic antigen

Carcinoembryonic antigen (CEA), like alpha-fetoprotein (q.v.), is a glycoprotein which behaves as an oncofetal antigen. It is a commonly used **tumour marker/biomarker** (q.v.).

The normal level is <3 µg/L, and its half-life is about 2 weeks.

It is a useful marker in a number of conditions, namely,
- gastrointestinal cancers,
- some non-gastrointestinal cancers,
- some non-malignant gastrointestinal diseases.

In **gastrointestinal cancers** (originally colorectal cancer), CEA is increased only when the bowel wall has become penetrated, so that it is not a useful screening test. Although not quantitatively related to tumour bulk, it becomes particularly increased with liver metastases, even if they are small. On the other hand, it can be normal if the cancer is poorly differentiated.

It may provide some preoperative guide to operability and more usefully a postoperative indication of the completeness of resection, the presence of recurrence or the response of metastatic disease to treatment.

Cancers of the stomach and pancreas may also be associated with an elevated CEA level.

Non-gastrointestinal cancers include particularly adenocarcinoma of the lung (see Lung tumours). This is especially so if there has been extrathoracic spread and more particularly if there are liver metastases from squamous cell carcinoma. Cancer of the breast may also be associated with an elevated CEA level.

Non-malignant gastrointestinal diseases comprise conditions such as inflammatory bowel disease (q.v.), alcoholic liver disease, heavy smoking and pancreatitis (q.v.).

Bibliography

Fletcher RH. Carcinoembryonic antigen. *Ann Intern Med* 1986; 104: 66.

Locker GY, Hamilton S, Harrus J, et al. ASCO 2006 update of recommendations for the use of tumor markers in gastrointestinal cancer. *J Clin Oncol* 2006; 24: 5313.

Carcinoid syndrome

Carcinoid tumours are neuroendocrine tumours (NETs) with a carcinoma-like appearance histologically (hence the name carcinoid). They are the most common endocrine-secreting tumours of the gut, though most such tumours do not secrete sufficient quantities of mediators to produce the overt clinical features referred to as the **carcinoid syndrome**.

The tumours may arise anywhere in the gut and occasionally in the bronchial tree. The appendix is the commonest site (40%), followed by the small intestine (24%, half in the ileum), rectum (14%) and lung (10%). Gut tumours metastasize to the liver, but lung tumours tend to metastasize to bone. Carcinoid tumours can be associated with the **multiple endocrine neoplasia** (type I) condition (q.v.). The taxonomy of these tumours has recently been revised to emphasize histological differentiation and any degree of malignant behaviour.

Most silent carcinoid tumours occur in the appendix and most secretory tumours occur in the ileum. To provide enough tumour mass to produce symptoms, clinically apparent tumours are usually associated with hepatic metastases.

The tumours contain argentaffin cells, which secrete a number of biologically active substances, characteristically serotonin but also histamine, bradykinin, catecholamines, prostaglandins, growth hormone releasing factor, adrenocorticotropic hormone and pancreatic polypeptide.

Symptoms are mostly, though not solely, attributable to serotonin. Given the subtlety of symptoms in many patients, diagnostic delays for many years are common. The classical clinical feature (seen in only 15% of cases) is of paroxysmal vasomotor disturbance, seen in 90% of these patients as red-purple cyanotic flushing of the face and neck, which is triggered by alcohol, food, emotion or exertion. The episode lasts for a few minutes and is associated with tachycardia and hypotension. Eventually, many patients (40%) develop large purple telangiectases.

Since bronchial carcinoids secrete directly into the systemic circulation, they can produce much more severe and prolonged flushing episodes (up to 2 weeks), which spread to the trunk and are associated with lacrimation, rhinorrhoea, salivation and even facial oedema.

Sometimes, a full **carcinoid storm** may occur with
- tachycardia,
- hypotension,
- oliguria,
- tremor,
- coma,
- even death.

Many other clinical features may also be seen in the carcinoid syndrome, namely

- **cardiac**
  - endocardial fibrosis may occur with a resultant murmur,
  - oedema is frequent,
  - tricuspid valve regurgitation may be seen.
- **cutaneous**
  - the rash of pellagra is seen in 10% of patients, being caused by the diversion of tryptophan to 5-hydroxytryptamine (serotonin),
  - hyperpigmentation may also occur (see Pigmentation disorders).
- **endocrine** (q.v.)
  - occasionally Zollinger–Ellison, Cushing's or MEN syndromes may be seen.
- **gastrointestinal**
  - diarrhoea (q.v.) from increased peristalsis occurs in most patients (90%),
  - abdominal cramps are frequent (40%),
  - there is an increased prevalence of peptic ulceration (14%).
  - hepatomegaly, ascites and an abdominal mass are common.
- **general**
  - fever (q.v.), night sweats (q.v.), mental changes and bone pain are sometimes seen.
- **respiratory**
  - dyspnoea due to bronchoconstriction occurs in up to 50% of patients.

The diagnosis is made from the measurement of increased 5-hydroxyindoleacetic acid (5-HIAA) in urine to >125 μmol per day and usually to >250–500 μmol per day. False-positive results may occur from many foods, including avocados, bananas, mushrooms, pineapples, plums and walnuts and from guaiacolate in cough medicines. False-negative results may occur from phenothiazines. Histopathology is important, because immunochemical staining is positive for chromogranin A (CgA), which may also be identified in plasma samples. Since most tumours are initially quite small (<2 cm), they can be difficult to localize, even with sophisticated imaging techniques (ultrasound, CT, MRI, and nuclear methods including SPECT and PET). Unfortunately, most patients have multiple liver metastases at the time of diagnosis, and complex imaging is unnecessary.

Treatment is surgical if possible. **Resection** *is performed if the tumour can be identified and there are no metastases (about 20% of cases). Liver metastases may sometimes be amenable to resection and embolization. Otherwise, surgical debulking is performed if feasible, and liver transplantation has even been reported.*

- Diarrhoea is improved with **cyproheptadine** or with an H_1–H_2 combination, e.g. diphenhydramine and ranitidine, if histamine is a major contributor.
- **Somatostatin** (and especially the synthetic analog, **octreotide**, 50–100 mcg SC bd) blocks the release of mediators, although refractoriness commonly eventuates (see also Acromegaly). In these cases, **telotristat** (a tryptophan hydroxylase inhibitor) 250 mg tds may be an effective addition.
- **Interferon** is probably helpful in some patients.
- Conventional **chemotherapy** is disappointing, but newer agents such as **everolimus** appear promising.
- New techniques include **radionuclide therapy** with an isotopically labelled somatostatin analog (SSA) which targets tumour cells containing SSA receptors. These techniques have shown promise in selected cases.

*In **carcinoid storm**, fluids and inotropes are required, though adrenaline (epinephrine) should be used with care as it may aggravate hypotension, due to the release of tumour mediators which it may provoke.*

The prognosis is good in the short term, since the tumours are very slowly growing. The average 5-year survival is 60%, though it is greater for tumours in the appendix, rectum and lung.

See also
- Mastocytosis,
- Serotonin syndrome.

Bibliography

Coupe M, Levi S, Ellis M, et al. Therapy for symptoms in the carcinoid syndrome. *Q J Med* 1989; 73: 1021.

Godwin JD. Carcinoid tumors: an analysis of 2837 cases. *Cancer* 1975; 36: 560.

McCaughan BC, Martini N, Bains MS. Bronchial carcinoids. *J Thorac Cardiovsc Surg* 1985; 89: 8.

Modlin IM, Moss SF, Oberg K, et al. Gastrointestinal neuroendocrine (carcinoid) tumours: current diagnosis and management. *Med J Aust* 2010; 193: 46.

Plockinger U, Rindi G, Arnold R, et al. Guidelines for the diagnosis and treatment of neuroendocrine gastrointestinal tumours: a consensus statement on behalf of the European Neuroendocrine Tumour Society (ENETS). *Neuroendocrinology* 2004; 80: 394.

Wolin EM. Advances in the diagnosis and management of well-differentiated and intermediate-differentiated neuroendocrine tumors of the lung. *Chest* 2017; 151: 1141.

Yao JC, Hassan M, Phan A, et al. One hundred years after 'carcinoid': epidemiology of and prognostic factors for neuroendocrine tumors in 35,825 cases in the United States. *J Clin Oncol* 2008; 26: 3063.

Cardiac tumours

Cardiac tumours are relatively common, though most are asymptomatic and the diagnosis is often difficult.

Cardiac tumours may be primary or secondary.

- **Primary tumours** are generally histologically benign (80%) and most found at autopsy are **myxomas** (see below), but occasionally a fibroma, lipoma or hamartoma (as in tuberous sclerosis) may be identified. On the other hand, most cardiac tumours found antemortem are **papillary fibroelastomas** (PFEs). Rarely, primary tumours may be malignant, in which case they are usually sarcomas.
- **Secondary tumours** comprise at least 95% of cardiac neoplasms at autopsy and are found in about 10% of patients with terminal malignant disease. They usually arise from haematogenous spread and derive primarily from cancers of the lung or breast, from melanoma and from lymphoma.

Cardiac tumour should be suspected if there is otherwise unexplained
- arrhythmia,
- cardiac failure,
- murmur,
- syncope,
- systemic embolization,
- pericardial effusion,
- abnormal cardiac silhouette.

Diagnosis is confirmed by non-invasive imaging with echocardiography, CT scanning or MRI.

Cardiac myxoma arises from the endothelium, usually in the left atrium on the fossa ovalis. Occasionally, it may arise in the right atrium. The tumour is often very mobile during the cardiac cycle, because it is attached to the endocardium by a stalk or pedicle.

Clinical features are due to local obstruction, systemic symptoms or systemic embolization.

- **Local obstruction** of the mitral valve or pulmonary veins may give rise to dyspnoea, cardiac failure and fatigue. Syncope may occur and is typically positional. There may be a varying murmur.
- **Systemic symptoms** are due to the production of 'toxic' products (such as interleukin 6 (IL-6)) and include fever, weight loss, malaise and even myalgia and Raynaud's phenomenon (q.v.).
- **Systemic embolization** occurs in one third of cases, in whom it is an important cause of stroke. Although the tumours are histologically benign, they can occasionally continue to grow in sites of distal implantation.

A **'myxoma complex'** may sometimes be seen, in which there are multicentric tumours, which are prone to recurrence and which are associated with skin pigmentation (q.v.), endocrine hypersecretion (especially Cushing's syndrome – q.v.), and testicular tumour in men or breast fibroadenoma in women. The myxoma complex (or Carney complex) is familial, and an underlying genetic mutation has been identified.

Laboratory investigations typically show anaemia, leukocytosis, thrombocytopenia, raised ESR, increased IgG and often increased IL-6.

The chief differential diagnosis is mitral valve disease and bacterial endocarditis (q.v.). Definitive diagnosis is by echocardiography.

Treatment is with **surgical removal**, *but recurrence is sometimes seen.*

Bibliography

Acebo E, Val-Bernal JF, Gomez-Roman JJ, et al. Clinicopathologic study and DNA analysis of 37 cardiac myxomas: a 28-year experience. *Chest* 2003; 123: 1379.

Casey MC, Vaughn CJ, He J, et al. Mutations in the protein kinase A R1alpha regulatory subunit cause familial cardiac myxomas and Carney complex. *J Clin Invest* 2000; 106: R31.

Goodwin JF. Diagnosis of left atrial myxoma. *Lancet* 1963; 1: 464.

Hancock EW. Malignant pericardial disease. *Cardiol Clin* 1990; 8: 673.

Klatt EL, Heitz DR. Cardiac metastases. *Cancer* 1990; 65: 1456.

McGregor GA, Cullen RA. The syndrome of fever, anaemia and high sedimentation rate with an atrial myxoma. *BMJ* 1959; 2: 991.

Meng Q, Lai H, Lima J, et al. Echocardiographic and pathologic characteristics of primary cardiac tumors; a study of 149 cases. *Int J Cardiol* 2002; 84: 69.

Pimede L, Duhaut P, Loire R. Clinical presentation of left atrial myxomas: a series of 112 consecutive cases. *Medicine* 2001; 80: 159.

Reynan K. Cardiac myxomas. *N Engl J Med* 1995; 333: 1610.

Salcedo EE, Cohen GI, White RD, et al. Cardiac tumors: diagnosis and management. *Curr Probl Cardiol* 1992; 17: 73.

Tazelaar HD, Locke TJ, McGregor CGA. Pathology of surgically excised primary cardiac tumors. *Mayo Clin Proc* 1992; 67: 957.

Welch TD, Shafi S, Oh JK. Diseases of the pericardium, cardiac tumors, and cardiac trauma. In: *Scientific American Medicine. Cardiovascular Medicine.* Hamilton: Dekker Medicine. 2020.

Cardiomyopathies

Cardiomyopathies are a heterogeneous group of myocardial diseases, specifically separate from hypertensive, valvular or ischaemic cardiac disease.

> Cardiomyopathies are traditionally classified into four (or three) types, namely,
> - dilated,
> - hypertrophic,
> - restrictive,
> - obliterative (regarded by some as a variant of restrictive).
>
> Transient stress-induced cardiomyopathy (**Takotsubo cardiomyopathy** – q.v.) can also be relevant in the critically ill.

Dilated cardiomyopathy is nowadays usually idiopathic. Many of these cases are familial and are associated with a variety of recently described mutations, involving actin, dystrophin or nuclear envelope proteins. Asymptomatic relatives commonly have echocardiographic abnormalities.

Dilated cardiomyopathy may also be seen
- in alcoholism,
- in malnutrition
  - beriberi (q.v.), selenium deficiency (q.v.),
- post-partum (see Pregnancy),
- in post-infective states (septic cardiomyopathy, SCM)
  - viral, diphtheritic, parasitic, systemic septic,
- with toxic agents
  - cocaine (q.v.), anti-cancer drugs of the anthracycline group, zidovudine,
- in a variety of diseases
  - collagen-vascular diseases, sarcoidosis, thyrotoxicosis, myxoedema, phaeochromocytoma, acromegaly, muscular dystrophy (see these separate conditions).

The most common virus involved is probably coxsackie B, and the main parasitic form is Chagas' disease (due to *Trypanosoma cruzi*) seen in South America.

There is dilatation of both the left and right ventricles with cardiac failure, arrhythmias, dyspnoea, fatigue and embolization. Acute pulmonary oedema may be much less than otherwise expected because of concomitant right ventricular failure. The failure is of the hyperdynamic type in beriberi (q.v.) and thyrotoxicosis (q.v.). Clinical examination shows heart failure, gallop rhythm and mitral regurgitation.

The chest X-ray shows marked cardiomegaly and pulmonary congestion. The ECG shows a variety of changes, including LVH, often LBBB, abnormal P waves, first degree heart block, a variety of arrhythmias, and ST-T abnormalities which may mimic acute myocardial infarction. Cardiac catheterization is not commonly performed nowadays but shows a decreased cardiac output with reduced ejection fraction and increased LVEDP (i.e. HFrEF). The diagnosis is confirmed by echocardiography and/or radionuclide studies.

> The differential diagnosis of dilated cardiomyopathy is
> - myocarditis, or
> - advanced hypertensive, valvular or ischaemic disease.

Treatment is of the underlying disorder if identified.
- *Cardiac therapy includes digitalis, diuretics, vasodilators, salt restriction and rest.* **Digoxin** *has now been confirmed to be both symptomatically and functionally helpful, even in patients in sinus rhythm.*
- *Hypokalaemia and hypomagnesaemia should be avoided.*
- *Warfarin is indicated for systemic or pulmonary embolism.*
- *Sometimes, parenteral inotropes (dobutamine, milrinone or levosimendan) may be used for a few days to stabilize a difficult situation.*
- *Cardiac transplantation may be indicated in advanced cases.*

Hypertrophic cardiomyopathy (HCM) is mostly (60%) hereditary, being inherited as an autosomal dominant. It has been shown to be a genetic disease of the cardiac muscle sarcomere. About one third of such cases have an abnormality on chromosome 14 of the gene which codes for the beta heavy chain of cardiac myosin, transcripts of which may be detectable in peripheral blood lymphocytes, thus providing a convenient screening test. Other cases have a variety of mutations (over 100 having now been described), involving chromosomes 1, 2, 11, 15, 16 or 18, giving single amino acid substitutions. The same defect occurs in all affected members of the same family.

There are variable patterns of ventricular hypertrophy without dilatation, mostly involving the septum, which may be massive and cause a pressure gradient from the apex of left ventricle to the aorta, with frank obstruction in about 25% of cases. Histologically, the individual myofibrils are hypertrophied and disordered.

Hypertrophic cardiomyopathy is commonly associated with obstruction of the left ventricular outflow tract (LVOT), and it is then referred to as **hypertrophic obstructive cardiomyopathy** (HOCM) or its variants, asymmetrical septal hypertrophy (ASM) or systolic anterior movement of the mitral valve (SAM). It used to be referred to as idiopathic hypertrophic subaortic stenosis (IHSS).

Clinical features include angina, syncope, arrhythmias, left heart failure and systemic embolization. On examination, there is an abnormal carotid pulse in obstructed cases, raised jugular venous pressure, gallop rhythm, and systolic murmur either from left ventricular outflow obstruction or mitral regurgitation.

The abnormal clinical findings are exacerbated by agents which cause
- tachycardia or increased myocardial contractility
  - e.g. beta agonists, digitalis,
- decreased preload or afterload
  - e.g. vasodilators, hypovolaemia, tachycardia, standing, Valsalva manoeuvre.

The chest X-ray is non-specific. The ECG shows LVH, sometimes with extensive Q waves due to the massive septal hypertrophy (and thus resembling AMI).

Definitive diagnosis is made initially by echocardiography and occasionally by cardiac catheterization, which typically shows normal systolic performance, with normal cardiac output and LVEDP, increased contractility with increased ejection fraction, but markedly decreased left ventricular compliance. The haemodynamic problem is thus obstruction and/or abnormal diastolic performance, so that the failure occurs even when the ejection fraction is as high as 80% (i.e. HFpEF). Cardiac MRI is currently the preferred imaging modality for detailed examination.

The differential diagnosis of hypertrophic cardiomyopathy is
- aortic stenosis, or
- subvalvular membranous stenosis.

---

*Treatment is medical with **beta blockers** (and sometimes calcium channel blockers) in moderate to high doses.*
- *Digitalis, nitrates and diuretics are contraindicated.*
- *Arrhythmias can be difficult to treat.*
- *Strenuous sport should be avoided.*

- *__Atrioventricular pacing__ with a dual chamber sequential device may favourably alter the pattern of ventricular depolarization and decrease obstruction.*
- *Surgery is indicated in about 10% of cases in due course, with myotomy or myectomy usually achieving a satisfactory symptomatic result, though the incidence of sudden death is not changed.*
- *Successful chemical septal ablation has been recently described.*
- *In general, the treatment of HCM is complex and is ideally conducted in a specialized centre.*

The prognosis is very variable, with a mortality of 2–3% per year due to sudden cardiac death (SCD), though the condition often becomes more stable in older patients. The mortality has reduced nearly 10-fold in recent years with modern therapy. It is the commonest cause of sudden cardiac death in patients under 35 years of age, including athletes, in whom the condition may have previously been entirely silent. Some of the variability in prognosis relates to the different mutations that may give rise to the condition. Family screening is recommended.

Restrictive cardiomyopathy
- may occasionally be familial,
- may sometimes be idiopathic,
- is usually due to myocardial infiltration in malignancy, amyloidosis, haemochromatosis or glycogen storage diseases (see these separate conditions).

The clinical features include cardiac failure, especially right heart failure, gallop rhythm and Kussmaul's sign (i.e. paradoxical increase in JVP on inspiration).

The chest X-ray only sometimes shows cardiomegaly. The ECG typically shows low voltages. Echocardiography (or cardiac catheterization) shows the findings of a rigid and incompliant ventricle, with impaired diastolic filling and a picture somewhat resembling constrictive pericarditis. The LVEDP is increased, and the cardiac output and ejection fraction may be decreased. However, unlike constrictive pericarditis in which the pressures tend to be equalized from the LVEDP to the right atrium, the LVEDP is much higher than the RVEDP and there is often pulmonary hypertension.

There is no satisfactory treatment, except sometimes that of the primary disease.

Obliterative cardiomyopathy is sometimes regarded as variant of restrictive cardiomyopathy. It is due to massive endocardial fibrosis, and it is usually seen only in developing countries, especially in Africa where it is common. It is probably hypereosinophilic in origin. There is associated intracardiac thrombosis, as well as endocardial hypertrophy.

Clinical features include cardiac failure, arrhythmias and embolization. Mitral and tricuspid regurgitation are usual.

Treatment is not effective, except for surgery in some cases.

The mortality is 25% within 1 year and two thirds within 5 years.

Bibliography

Beesley SJ, Weber, G, Sarge T, et al. Septic cardiomyopathy. *Crit Care Med* 2018; 46: 625.

Cannon RO, Tripodi D, Dilsizian V, et al. Results of permanent dual-chamber pacing in symptomatic nonobstructive hypertrophic cardiomyopathy. *Am J Cardiol* 1994; 73: 571.

Cherian KM, John TA, Abraham KA. Endomyocardial fibrosis. *Am Heart J* 1983; 105: 706.

Fatkin D, MacRae C, Sasaki T, et al. Missense mutations in the rod domain of the lamin A/C gene as causes of dilated cardiomyopathy and conduction-system disease. *N Engl J Med* 1999; 341: 1715.

Gheorghiade M, Zarowitz BJ. Review of randomized trials of digoxin therapy in patients with chronic heart failure. *Am J Cardiol* 1992; 69: 48G.

Gupta PN, Valiathan MS, Balakrishnan KG, et al. Clinical course of endomyocardial fibrosis. *Br Heart J* 1989; 62: 450.

Homans DC. Peripartum cardiomyopathy. *N Engl J Med* 1985; 312: 1432.

Katritsis D, Wilmshurst PT, Wendon JA, et al. Primary restrictive cardiomyopathy: clinical and pathologic characteristics. *J Am Coll Cardiol* 1991;18: 1230.

Kelly DP, Strauss AW. Inherited cardiomyopathies. *N Engl J Med* 1994; 330: 913.

Maron B, Maron M. Hypertrophic cardiomyopathy. *Lancet* 2013; 381: 242.

Maron BJ, Bonow RO, Cannon RO. Hypertrophic cardiomyopathy. *N Engl J Med* 1987; 316: 780 & 844.

Maron BJ, Shirani J, Poliac LC, et al. Sudden death in young competitive athletes – clinical, demographic and pathological profiles. *JAMA* 1996; 276: 199.

Nishimura R, Trusty JM, Hayes DL, et al. Dual-chamber pacing for hypertrophic cardiomyopathy. A randomized double-blind crossover trial. *J Am Coll Cardiol* 1997; 29: 435.

Seggewiss H, Geichmann U, Faber L, et al. Percutaneous transluminal septal myocardial ablation in hypertrophic cardiomyopathy. *J Am Coll Cardiol* 1998; 31: 252.

Spirito P, Seidman CE, McKenna WJ, et al. The management of hypertrophic cardiomyopathy. *N Engl J Med* 1997; 336: 775.

Sugrue DD, Rodeheffer RJ, Codd MB, et al. The clinical course of idiopathic dilated cardiomyopathy. *Ann Intern Med* 1992; 117: 117.

Cardiopulmonary bypass *See*

- Coagulation disorders – cardiopulmonary bypass coagulopathy.

See also

- Adrenal insufficiency,
- Anaemia – 2. Anaemia due to haemolysis (Extracorpuscular defects),
- Anticoagulants – 2. Hirudin and derivatives (Bivalirudin),
- Hypothermia,
- Methaemoglobinaemia,
- Platelet function disorders – 2. Acquired.

Cardiorenal syndrome(s)

The **cardiorenal syndrome** (CRS), or more correctly syndromes, refers to the clinical consequence of the interaction of the heart (or circulation) and the kidneys in severe illness. In clinical practice, the context of CRS is generally within the overall setting of multiorgan failure (q.v.). Thus, the focus on two organs in this situation is somewhat artificial, though it may help clinical understanding of the relevant pathophysiology.

The kidneys may be damaged in either acute or chronic heart failure, referred to as CRS types 1 and 2, respectively. In acute situations, the kidney damage takes the form of acute kidney injury (AKI), whereas in more chronic situations, the kidney damage is generally fibrosis.

Conversely, the heart may be damaged in either acute or chronic renal failure, referred to as CRS types 3 and 4, respectively. In AKI, heart failure is due to volume overload and metabolic insult, whereas in chronic kidney disease, the heart failure is due to left ventricular dysfunction.

Finally, both the heart and the kidney may be simultaneously damaged in many forms of systemic illness (e.g. sepsis), referred to as CRS type 5.

See also

- Fabry's disease.

Bibliography

Cruz DN, Bagshaw SM. Heart-kidney interaction: epidemiology of cardiorenal syndromes. *Int J Nephrol* 2010; 2011: 351291.

Li X, Hassoun HT, Santora R, et al. Organ crosstalk: the role of the kidney. *Curr Opin Crit Care* 2009; 15: 481.

Rangaswami J, Bhalla V, Blair JEA, et al. Cardiorenal syndrome: classification, pathophysiology, diagnosis, and treatment strategies: a scientific statement from the American Heart Association. *Circulation* 2019; 139: e840.

Ricci Z, Romagnoli S, Ronco C. Cardiorenal syndrome. *Crit Care Clin* 2021; 37: 335.

Ronco C, Haapio M, House AA, et al. Cardiorenal syndrome. *J Am Coll Cardiol* 2008; 25: 1527.

Cardiovascular disorders

Many **cardiovascular disorders** are encountered so commonly in Intensive Care that they are regarded as 'core' to the specialty. These conditions include myocardial ischaemia and infarction, heart failure, arrhythmias, shock and hypertension.

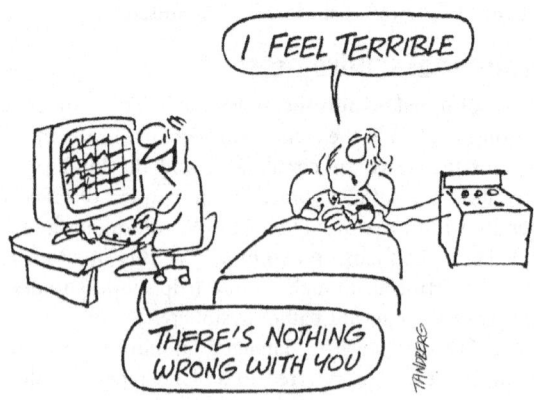

However, numerous other cardiovascular disorders are less commonly seen, and it is these which are considered in this book. They include

- Aortic coarctation,
- Aortic dissection,
- Arteriovenous malformations,
- Arteritis,
- Atrial natriuretic factor,
- Autonomic dysreflexia,
- Brugada syndrome,
- Cardiac tumours,
- Cardiomyopathies,
- Cardiopulmonary bypass,
- Dextrocardia,
- Digoxin-specific antibody,
- Eisenmenger syndrome,
- Endocarditis,
- Hereditary haemorrhagic telangiectasia,
- Hyperdynamic state,
- Kawasaki disease,
- Marfan's syndrome,
- Microcirculation,
- Microvascular dysfunction,
- Mycotic aneurysms,
- Multisystem inflammatory syndrome in children,
- Pericarditis,
- Raynaud's phenomenon/disease,
- Takotsubo cardiomyopathy,
- Telangiectasia,
- Temporal arteritis,
- Tetralogy of Fallot,
- Toxic shock syndrome,
- Vasculitis.

Bibliography

Becker RC, Meade TW, Berger PB, et al. The primary and secondary prevention of coronary artery disease. *Chest* 2008; 133: (suppl. 6): 776S.

Burakoff R, ed. Cardiovascular Medicine. In: *Scientific American Medicine*. Hamilton: Dekker Medicine. 2020.

Calhoun DA, Oparil S. Treatment of hypertensive crisis. *N Engl J Med* 1990; 323: 1177.

Creager MA, Beckman J, Loscalzo J, eds. *Vascular Medicine*. 2nd edition. Philadelphia: Saunders (Elsevier). 2012.

Gheorghiade M, Zarowitz BJ. Review of randomized trials of digoxin therapy in patients with chronic heart failure. *Am J Cardiol* 1992; 69: 48G.

Goodman SG, Menon V, Cannon CP, et al. Acute ST-segment elevation myocardial infarction. *Chest* 2008; 133: (suppl. 6): 708S.

Guyton AC. Blood pressure control: special role of the kidney and body fluids. *Science* 1991; 252: 1813.

Harrington RA, Becker RC, Cannon CP, et al. Antithrombotic therapy for non-ST-segment elevation acute coronary syndromes. *Chest* 2008; 133: (suppl. 6): 670S.

Heusch G, Schulz R. Characterization of hibernating and stunned myocardium. *Eur Heart J* 1997; 18 (suppl. D): 102.

Libby P, Zipes DP, eds. *Braunwald's Heart Disease*. 11th edition. Philadelphia: Saunders (Elsevier). 2018.

Marik P, Varon J. The obese patient in the ICU. *Chest* 1998; 113: 492.

Muller DWM. Gene therapy for cardiovascular disease. *Br Heart J* 1994; 72: 309.

Nora JJ. Causes of congenital heart disease: old and new modes, mechanisms, and models. *Am Heart J* 1993; 125: 1409.

Salem DN, O'Gara PT, Madias C, et al. Valvular and structural heart disease. *Chest* 2008; 133: (suppl. 6): 593S.

Singer DE, Albers GW, Dalen JE, et al. Antithrombotic therapy in atrial fibrillation. *Chest* 2008; 133: (suppl. 6): 546S.

Wilson NJ, Neutze JM. Adult congenital heart disease: principles and management guidelines. *Aust NZ J Med* 1993; 23: 498 & 697.

CAR T-cell therapy

Chimeric antigen receptor T-cell (CAR T-cell) therapy is a new technique of cancer immunotherapy, introduced for the treatment of B-cell haematological malignancies, including B-cell acute lymphoblastic leukaemia (B-ALL), diffuse large B-cell lymphoma (DLBCL, the most common form of non-Hodgkin's lymphoma), and most recently multiple myeloma.

CAR T-cell therapy is one form of **immune effector cell** (IEC) therapy, whereby autologous T cells are modified to recognise a tumour antigen (either a specific receptor (e.g. CD-19) or a major histocompatibility complex) – see Cancer complications.

This complex and expensive procedure involves harvesting the patient's own T lymphocytes via apheresis and then inserting a gene in them in a specialized laboratory, so that they now express on their surface a chimeric antigen receptor which recognizes the CD19 antigen. This surface antigen is uniquely expressed by B cells, whether normal or malignant. The new (chimeric) cells are multiplied in culture, and the resultant product is then reinjected into the patient. The total time from harvest to delivery is currently about 1 month, but faster techniques are in development. Products produced commercially include **tisagenlecleucel** and **axicabtagene ciloleucel**, but there are others, including some produced at specialist oncology centres.

The consequent binding of the autologous CAR T-cells to the CD-19 positive tumour B cells induces an inflammatory response which destroys the tumour cells. This therapy is used in refractory or relapsed cases, in whom the usual prognosis has been very poor and in whom very high success rates have now been reported. However, the response may take several months to take full effect, after which long-term and even complete remission commonly occurs.

This technology is of relevance to Intensive Care, because two serious but potentially reversible complications may require ICU support in up to one third of cases, namely,
- **cytokine release syndrome** (CRS) and
- **immune-effector cell-associated neurotoxicity syndrome** (ICANS).

CRS is a common complication, and it ranges in severity from mild (grade 1) to life-threatening (grade 4). It is manifest by fever and hypotension due to a capillary leak syndrome. Coagulopathy (q.v.) and multiorgan failure (q.v.) may result. Vasopressors rather than fluid administration are preferred for circulatory support, and corticosteroids are helpful in severe cases. CRS occurs after an average of about 3 days, with a duration of about 1 week. Risk factors include high tumour burden and concomitant infection.

ICANS is manifest by headache, impaired consciousness, confusion, seizures and focal paralysis. The EEG and MRI may show abnormalities. This complication occurs after an average of about 5 days, but it may occur as late as 2 months after infusion. It typically lasts for about 2 weeks.

In both settings, the specific anti-IL-6 receptor antibody, **tocilizumab** *(q.v.), is given in severe cases, usually with concomitant corticosteroids (e.g. methylprednisolone 1 mg/kg IV bd).* **Siltuximab** *(an interleukin 6 (IL-6) monoclonal antibody) and* **anakinra** *(a recombinant IL-1 receptor antagonist) may also be used in refractory cases.*

Febrile neutropenia and infections are also common complications due to prior immunosuppression, and importantly they can mimic CRS and ICANS. Other complications, such as tumour-lysis syndrome (q.v.), macrophage activation syndrome (q.v.) and anaphylaxis (q.v.), may sometimes be seen. Potential loss of normal B cells is an off-tumour (but targeted) effect which may lead to severe or recurrent infections, a complication which can be treated with immunoglobulin replacement.

CAR T-cell therapy may also offer future potential in autoimmune conditions and in some infectious diseases.

Bibliography

Azoulay E, Darmon M, Valade S. Acute life-threatening toxicity from CAR T-cell therapy. *Intens Care Med* 2020; 46: 1723.

Boll B, Subklewe M, von Bergwelt-Baildon M. Ten things the haematologist wants you to know about CAR-T cells. *Intens Care Med* 2020; 46: 1243.

Gutierrez C, Brown ART, May, HP, et al. Critically ill patients treated for chimeric antigen receptor-related toxicity: a multicenter study. *Crit Care Med* 2022; 50: 81.

Gutierrez C, McEvoy C, Munshi L, et al. Critical care management of toxicities associated with targeted agents and immunotherapies for cancer. *Crit Care Med* 2020; 48: 10.

Maude SL, Laetsch TW, Buechner J, et al. Tisgenlecleucel in children and young adults with B-cell lymphoblastic leukaemia. *N Engl J Med* 2018; 378: 439.

Schuster SJ, Bishop MR, Tam CS, et al. Tisgenlecleucel in adult relapsed or refractory diffuse large B-cell lymphoma. *N Engl J Med* 2019; 380: 45.

Selim AG, Tam CS. Chimeric antigen receptor T-cell therapy for haematological malignancies. *Med J Aust* 2020; 213: 404.

Cat bites *See*
- Bites and stings.

Cat-scratch disease

Cat-scratch disease (CSD) is still a disease of incompletely defined cause.

The first organism to be clearly associated with this disease was a small pleomorphic Gram-negative bacillus initially identified in 1988 and designated *Afipia felis* in 1992. Subsequently, the novel α-proteobacterium, *Rochalimaea henselae*, was identified by PCR in bacillary angiomatosis, particularly in immunocompromised patients, and is now thought to be the actual causative agent of cat-scratch disease. This organism is related to rickettsiae (q.v.) and to bartonella and brucella (q.v.). Indeed, the genus designation Bartonella has replaced the former name Rochalimaea, so that the aetiological agent of CSD is now referred to as *B. henselae*.

The apparent reservoir for these organisms is the domestic cat, in which they reside asymptomatically, but they can cause a variety of lesions in humans (and in armadillos). The cat flea is the likely vector for transmission of the organism between animals.

Usually the scratch from an infected cat gives rise to a self-limited local lymphadenitis, which in up to 10% may suppurate. At the site of the scratch, an inflammatory lesion appears within 3–14 days and is followed in 1–3 weeks by the lymphadenopathy, which can last a very variable time from 2 weeks to 8 months. Mild systemic symptoms are common. The illness lasts 6–12 weeks.

In immunocompromised patients, disseminated disease may sometimes occur. This may comprise pneumonitis with hilar lymphadenopathy (q.v.), encephalitis (q.v.) retinitis, hepatitis (q.v.), splenomegaly (q.v.), thrombocytopenia (q.v.) or metastatic abscess.

Bacillary angiomatosis (BA) is an angioproliferative response, in which atypical endothelial cells form numerous poorly structured capillary channels. BA and the related **bacillary peliosis hepatis** arise in the skin and viscera in response to the presence of *B. henselae* (and probably other similar organisms, such as *B. quintana* in louse-infested or homeless environments). These complications occur particularly in immunocompromised patients, such as those with AIDS (q.v.). In the skin, small angiomatous nodules are seen. The viscera affected include the liver, spleen, lymph nodes, bone marrow, lungs and brain.

Laboratory tests are generally unhelpful, and the diagnosis is traditionally made clinically and by exclusion. A positive skin test has been reported but is non-specific. Serology has a low sensitivity and moreover does not distinguish between past exposure and current disease. Culture of the organism is difficult because bacteraemia is infrequent and the organism is fastidious and slowly growing. Recently, PCR testing of biopsy tissue has been reported to have a sensitivity of up to 100%, though the test so far has limited availability. BA is diagnosed histologically.

The differential diagnosis includes
- other infections
  - infectious mononucleosis (see Epstein–Barr virus),
  - pyogenic bacteria,
  - brucellosis (q.v.),
  - toxoplasmosis (q.v.),
  - fungal disease,
  - tuberculosis (q.v.),
  - lymphogranuloma venereum,
- sarcoidosis (q.v.),
- Hodgkin's disease.

Treatment is symptomatic only, as antibiotics are not helpful, though gentamicin or ciprofloxacin often with corticosteroids may be helpful in immunocompromised patients. BA is treated with erythromycin or doxycycline for 4 weeks.

The course is benign and self-limited, though it may run for several months. Disseminated BA may be fatal. A single episode of cat-scratch disease gives rise to immunity.

Bibliography

Anderson B, Sims K, Regnery R, et al. Detection of *Rochalimaea henselae* DNA in cat scratch disease patients by PCR. *J Clin Microbiol* 1994; 32: 942.

Bergmans AM, Peeters MF, Schellkens JF, et al. Pitfalls and fallacies of cat scratch disease serology. *J Clin Microbiol* 1997; 35: 1931.

Karim AA, Cockerell CJ, Petri WA. Cat scratch disease, bacillary angiomatosis, and other infections due to *Rochalimaea*. *N Engl J Med* 1994; 330: 1509.

Regnery RL, Martin M, Olson J. Naturally occurring '*Rochalimaea henselae*' infection in domestic cat. *Lancet* 1992; 340: 557.

Regnery R, Tappero J. Unraveling mysteries associated with cat-scratch disease, bacillary angiomatosis, and related syndromes. *Emerg Infect Dis* 1995; 1: 1.

Relman DA, Falkow S, LeBoit PE, et al. The organism causing bacillary angiomatosis, peliosis hepatis, and fever and bacteremia in immunocompromised patients. *N Engl J Med* 1991; 324: 1514.

Slater LN, Welch DF, Hensel D, et al. A newly recognized fastidious gram-negative pathogen as a cause of fever and bacteremia. *N Engl J Med* 1990; 323: 1587.

Zangwill KM, Hamilton DH, Perkins BA, et al. Cat scratch disease in Connecticut – epidemiology, risk factors, and evaluation of a new diagnostic test. *N Engl J Med* 1993; 329: 8.

Cathinones See

- Amphetamines.

Cavitation

The chief causes of one or more **lung cavities** are
1. necrotizing pneumonia (see below)
   - often leading to lung abscess and/or empyema,
2. cancer (see Lung tumours)
   - bronchogenic carcinoma, metastases,
3. tuberculosis (q.v.)
   - or fungal or parasitic infection,
4. septic infarct,
5. infected cysts or bullae,
6. vasculitis (q.v.)
   - rheumatoid, Wegener's granulomatosis (q.v.),
7. lymphomatoid granulomatosis (q.v.),
8. angiocentric lymphoma.

Necrotizing pneumonia, **lung abscess** and **empyema** represent the extreme of pyogenic infections in the lung. Empyema is one of the causes of failure of resolution of chest infection.

The responsible organisms are usually klebsiella, staphylococci, pseudomonas or mixed anaerobic organisms, and they may follow aspiration (q.v.).

The clinical features of empyema are those of
- persistent infection (fever, cough, dyspnoea, chest pain),
- signs of pleural effusion (either a single loculus or multiloculated) (see Pleural disorders),
- finger clubbing (if the diagnosis is delayed).

Rupture through the skin (empyema necessitans) or into the bronchial tree (bronchopleural fistula) may occur.

Diagnosis is established by chest X-ray and aspiration of pleural fluid.

*Treatment of necrotizing pneumonia, lung abscess and/or empyema consists of prolonged **antibiotic therapy**.*
- *An empyema should be drained, either by traditional chest tube or by image-guided catheter.*
- *Intrapleural fibrinolytic therapy (e.g. streptokinase 250,000 U in 20 mL of saline, or alteplase 2–10 mg in 10–50 mL of sterile water, left to dwell for 60 min) may be of value if the empyema is loculated, though this recommendation has been challenged. A similar technique may be used to clear an obstructed chest tube or pleural catheter being used to drain a purulent or recurrent effusion.*
- *If loculation still causes difficulty in drainage, video-assisted thoracoscopic surgery (VATS) is indicated for this task.*
- *Surgical resection, including decortication of organized, thickened pleura, is rarely required nowadays.*

The prognosis nowadays is generally good, since the responsible infection is likely to respond well to antibiotics.

Bibliography

Angelillo Mackinlay TA, Lyons GA, Chimondeguy DJ, et al. VATS debridement versus thoracotomy in the treatment of loculated postpneumonia empyema. *Ann Thorac Surg* 1996; 61: 1626.

Bryant RE, Salmon CJ. Pleural empyema. *Clin Infect Dis* 1996; 22: 747.

Davies RJO, Traill ZC, Gleeson FV. Randomised controlled trial of intrapleural streptokinase in community acquired pleural infection. *Thorax* 1997; 52: 416.

Janda S, Swiston J. Intrapleural fibrinolytic therapy for treatment of adult parapneumonic effusions and empyema: a systematic review and meta-analysis. *Chest* 2012; 142: 401.

Jerjes-Sanchez C, Ramirez-Rivera A, Elizalde JJ, et al. Intrapleural fibrinolysis with streptokinase as an adjunctive treatment in hemothorax and empyema: a multicenter trial. *Chest* 1996; 109: 1514.

Landreneau RJ, Keenan RJ, Hazelrigg SR, et al. Thoracoscopy for empyema and hemothorax. *Chest* 1995; 109: 18.

Leatherman JW, Mcdonald FM, Niewohner DE. Fluid-containing bullae in the lung. *South Med J* 1985; 78: 708.

Maskel NA, Davies CW, Nunn AJ, et al. UK controlled trial of intrapleural streptokinase for pleural infection. *N Engl J Med* 2005; 352: 865.

Muers MF. Streptokinase for empyema. *Lancet* 1997; 349: 1491.

Sahn SA. Management of complicated parapneumonic effusions. *Am Rev Respir Dis* 1993; 148: 813.

Silverman SC, Mueller PR, Saini S, et al. Thoracic empyema: management with image-guided catheter drainage. *Radiology* 1988; 169: 5.

Temes RT, Follis F, Kessler RM, et al. Intrapleural fibrinolysis in management of empyema thoracis. *Chest* 1996; 110: 102.

Walt MA, Sharma S, Hohn J, et al. A randomized trial of empyema therapy. *Chest* 1997; 111: 1548.

Weissberg D, Refaelyb Y. Pleural empyema: 24-year experience. *Ann Thorac Surg* 1996; 62: 1026.

Cellulitis *See*

- Gangrene.

Central pontine myelinolysis

Central pontine myelinolysis (CPM) refers to demyelination primarily in the pons, though this process is also apparent in the basal ganglia, thalamus, internal capsule and cerebellum on sensitive MRI examination. Thus, the newer name of **osmotic demyelination syndrome** has been suggested.

> Central pontine myelinolysis was originally described in 1959 in alcoholism and malnutrition.
>
> Nowadays, it is most commonly reported in patients who have been hyponatraemic, in whom it is thought to have been produced by osmotic injury from over-zealous correction of the hyponatraemia (especially correction which is too rapid). Although it has a reported prevalence of up to 25% under such circumstances, it can still occur even when careful guidelines are followed (see below). In such cases, there has commonly been associated hypokalaemia, hypomagnesaemia or hypophosphataemia.
>
> It may also be seen after liver transplantation and in patients with normonatraemia but other electrolyte or vitamin deficiencies.

Clinical features include
- spastic quadriparesis or paraparesis,
- corticobulbar signs of dysarthria and dysphagia,
- mutism and possibly the locked-in state.

The process may be irreversible and may sometimes be fatal. It can also be delayed for up to 1 week or more after commencement of treatment of hyponatraemia, though typically it becomes manifest on about the 3rd day after the start of sodium replacement. Improvement commences after about 2 weeks but is often incomplete, especially in alcoholics.

> *Treatment is **preventative**.*
>
> *Repair of **hyponatraemia** should be not >0.5 mmol/L per hr, unless the hyponatraemia is associated with encephalopathy, in which case the sodium should be corrected by up to 2 mmol/L per hr but by not more than 10 mmol/L in total over the first 24 hr. However, the plasma sodium concentration may be difficult to control due to unpredictable volume shifts and concomitant diuresis, so that it should be measured at frequent intervals for target guidance. Given its complexities, the treatment of significant hyponatraemia is best undertaken in an ICU.*
>
> *In general, a plasma concentration of about 120 mmol/L is a symptomatically safe goal. Above this, further normalization can be more leisurely until a level of 130 mmol/L is reached.*
>
> *Thus, if for example the plasma sodium concentration is 105 mmol/L, the amount of sodium required for acute repair in a 70 kg person is (120 − 105) × 60% × 70 kg = 630 mmol, which should be given as 4 L of N saline (or preferably 1.2 L of 3% saline) to achieve the target increase at the recommended rate (as above). In severe cases, 3% saline may be commenced as 100 mL boluses given up to three times in the first 30 min, with each 100 mL bolus expected to increase the plasma sodium concentration by about 2 mmol/L. More simply, 500 mL of 3% saline may be safely given at 100 mL per hr in symptomatic cases.*
>
> *However, if the originating process has been acute (i.e. <48 hr), symptoms of hyponatraemia may be seen at higher levels, sometimes up to 130 mmol/L. In this case, the treatment goals need to be shifted up accordingly.*
>
> *On the other hand, if the process has been chronic, the patient is asymptomatic and there is no hypovolaemia, fluid restriction alone can be appropriate.*
>
> *If treatment results in an overshoot of the target, the plasma sodium concentration may be relowered by giving either an IV infusion of 1 L of 5% dextrose over 2 hr or a single dose of desmopressin (q.v.) 1–2 mcg IV.*

See also
- Syndrome of inappropriate antidiuretic hormone.

Bibliography

Adrogue HJ, Madias NE. Hyponatremia. *N Engl J Med* 2000; 342: 1581.

Arieff AI, Guisado R. Effects on the central nervous system of hypernatremic and hyponatremic states. *Kidney Int* 1976; 10: 104.

Ayus JC, Krothapalli RK, Arieff AI. Treatment of symptomatic hyponatremia and its relation to brain damage: a prospective study. *N Engl J Med* 1987; 317: 1190.

Berl T. Treating hyponatremia: damned if we do and damned if we don't. *Kidney Int* 1990; 37: 1006.

Brown WD. Osmotic demyelination disorders: central pontine and extrapontine myelinolysis. *Curr Opinion Neurol* 2000; 13: 691.

Brunner JE, Redmond JM, Haggar AM, et al. Central pontine myelinolysis and pontine lesions after rapid correction of hyponatremia: a prospective magnetic resonance imaging study. *Ann Neurol* 1990; 27: 61.

Laureno R, Karp BI. Pontine and extrapontine myelinolysis following rapid correction of hyponatraemia. *Lancet* 1988; 1: 1439.

Pirzada NA, Ali II. Central pontine myelinolysis. *Mayo Clin Proc* 2001; 76: 559.

Soupart A, Decaux G. Therapeutic recommendations for management of severe hyponatremia: Current concepts on pathogenesis and prevention of neurologic complications. *Clin Nephrol* 1996; 46: 149.

Sterns RH, Cappuccio JD, Silver SM, et al. Neurologic sequelae after treatment of severe hyponatremia: a multicenter perspective. *J Am Soc Nephrol* 1994; 4: 1522.

Sterns RH, Riggs JE, Schochet SS. Osmotic demyelination syndrome following correction of hyponatremia. *N Engl J Med* 1986; 314: 1535.

Strange K. Regulation of solute and water balance and cell volume in the central nervous system. *J Am Soc Nephrol* 1992; 3: 12.

Tien R, Arieff AI, Kucharczyk W, et al. Hyponatremic encephalopathy: is central pontine myelinolysis a component? *Am J Med* 1992; 92: 513.

Worthley LIG. Chronic hyponatraemia and risk of myelinolysis: why is it so difficult to control the change in plasma sodium? *Crit Care Resusc* 2006; 8: 368.

Young GB. Central pontine myelinolysis: a lesson in humility. *Crit Care Med* 2012; 40: 1026.

Cerebellar degeneration

Cerebellar degeneration occurs in a number of forms.

1. **Hereditary, spinocerebellar degenerative disorders**

These are neurodegenerative conditions, which are unrelated except for the marked clinical feature of ataxia. A number of different mutational mechanisms and inheritance patterns have recently been identified, leading to considerable phenotypic heterogeneity within the overall group of ataxias.

The best known of these conditions is **Friedreich's Ataxia**, which is manifest by areflexia and loss of proprioception as well as ataxia. There is associated cardiomyopathy (q.v.) and skeletal abnormality, particularly of the chest wall. The patient is generally wheelchair-bound by early adulthood and has died by middle age.

2. **Subacute cerebellar degeneration**

This is a paraneoplastic condition (q.v.), especially in carcinoma of the lung or ovary. In addition to ataxia, there may be sensory symptoms and mental changes.

Plasmapheresis is ineffective, even though circulating antibodies to cerebellar Purkinje cells have been found.

3. **Cerebellar degeneration due to alcoholism or nutritional deficiency**

Cerebellar degeneration is most commonly caused by alcohol. Myxoedema (q.v.) may sometimes be implicated.

Deficiency of vitamin E, which arises from fat malabsorption (q.v.), has also been reported as a rare cause.

Bibliography

Campuzano V, Montermini L, Molto MD, et al. Friedreich's ataxia: autosomal recessive disease caused by intronic GAA triplet repeat expansion. *Science* 1996; 271: 1423.

Delatycki M, Williamson R, Forrest S. Friedrich ataxia: update on pathogenesis and possible therapies. *J Med Genet* 2000; 37: 1.

Durr A, Cossee M, Agid Y, et al. Clinical and genetic abnormalities in patients with Friedreich's ataxia. *N Engl J Med* 1996; 335: 1169.

Gotoda T, Arita M, Arai H, et al. Adult-onset spinocerebellar dysfunction caused by a mutation in the gene for the α-tocopherol-transfer protein. *N Engl J Med* 1995; 333: 1313.

Cerebral arterial gas embolism *See*

- Diving.

Cerebral arteritis *See*

- Arteritis.

Cerebral salt wasting

Cerebral salt wasting (CSW) refers to a transient condition of hyponatraemia due to excess sodium loss in the urine and associated with severe acute neurological disease (e.g. subarachnoid haemorrhage). Nowadays, it is commonly thought to be a misnomer and to be probably a form of the **syndrome of inappropriate antidiuretic hormone** (SIADH) (q.v.).

Hyponatraemia in CNS disease is generally due to SIADH, in which excess renal salt loss can potentially occur if there has been associated volume overload (as in protocols for preventing or treating vasospasm in subarachnoid haemorrhage). Nevertheless, it is theoretically possible for acute brain injury itself to cause excessive renal salt loss via either release of brain natriuretic peptide (BNP, see Atrial natriuretic factor) or stimulation of the sympathetic nervous system which could then promote renin release.

If CSW really occurs,
- there will be consequent hypovolaemia, which would be the only clinical or biochemical distinguishing feature between it and SIADH, and
- concomitant SIADH could be present anyway.

The treatment of patients in this setting is complex, in that volume status and fluid needs can be difficult to assess reliably. Volume repletion required in putative CSW would be in conflict with fluid restriction recommendations in SIADH, though these latter recommendations need to be tempered in cases of subarachnoid haemorrhage where fluid restriction would be harmful due to exacerbation of cerebral ischaemia. When in doubt, the careful administration of isotonic saline may be the safest option, together with careful monitoring of circulatory, fluid and electrolyte parameters.

See
- Diabetes insipidus,
- Hyponatraemia,
- Syndrome of inappropriate antidiuretic hormone.

Bibliography
Singh S, Bohn D, Carlotti AP, et al. Cerebral salt wasting: truths, fallacies, theories, and challenges. *Crit Care Med* 2002; 30: 2575.

Charcot–Marie–Tooth disease

Charcot–Marie–Tooth disease (CMT, peroneal muscular atrophy) is the most common hereditary polyneuropathy (q.v.). It is usually an autosomal dominant condition, though several separate gene loci have been identified.

There is segmental demyelination (with local nerve hypertrophy) and consequent distal weakness and atrophy of the legs, often with pes cavus. Sensory as well as motor impairment occurs, and the hands may eventually be involved.

It is a benign condition with no major morbidity and no mortality.

Gene therapy is undergoing trials in this disease, as in a number of other neuromuscular conditions.

See also
- Neuropathy.

Chelating agents

A **chelate** is a complex compound with a central metal atom attached to a larger molecule (a ligand) in a ring structure. A **chelating agent** refers to the ligand which can attach to the metal ion at two or more points, thus forming a ring. Chelates are more stable than non-chelated compounds of comparable composition. Haemoglobin and chlorophyll are examples of chelate compounds in nature. Chelates are widely used in industrial and laboratory processes.

In clinical medicine, chelating agents are used in the treatment of **heavy metal poisoning** (q.v.), because they bind the metal more strongly than do the vulnerable components of the living organism.

Although humans have always had environmental exposure to heavy metals in food, water and cooking utensils, this exposure increased markedly after industrialization. These metals cannot be metabolized but persist in the body, where they produce prolonged toxic effects by combining with a reactive group (a ligand) thereby affecting chemical function.

Chelating agents are heavy metal antagonists, since they compete with these reactive groups in the body for the metal and therefore they can prevent or treat toxic effects by permitting excretion. Clearly, a selective chelator is required so as not to bind the body's own essential metals, though it must distribute in the same body spaces. It must also have a greater affinity than the body's own ligands, it must produce non-toxic complexes pending excretion and it must be able to mobilize the metal after binding so as to permit excretion.

The heavy metals of most relevance in this setting are
- arsenic (q.v.),
- cadmium (q.v.),
- iron (q.v.),
- lead (q.v.),
- mercury (q.v.).

There are four important chelating agents for clinical use, namely
- calcium disodium edetate (EDTA),
- dimercaprol (BAL),
- penicillamine,
- desferrioxamine (DFO).

Calcium disodium edetate (sodium calcium edetate, ethylene-diaminetetraacetate, EDTA) is chiefly used in lead poisoning, though it is also of value in enhancing the clearance of cadmium (and also chromium, cobalt, copper, magnesium, nickel, selenium, uranium, vanadium, zinc) and (in double dosage) of the radioactive products from nuclear accidents (e.g. plutonium). The toxic metal displaces calcium from the chelator. It has also been used in atherosclerosis but without evidence to support this indication.

Since it is poorly absorbed from the gut, it is given intravenously; 2 g (two 5 mL ampoules of 200 mg/mL each) are diluted to 500–1000 mL in isotonic dextrose or saline and are administered daily for 5 days in two divided doses each over 1 hr. If combined with BAL for lead poisoning, there should be a 4 hr delay between the administration of the two agents, with BAL given first.

EDTA has a half-life of about 40 min, distributes in the extracellular fluid and is excreted in the urine (50% in the first hour), so that it is contraindicated in anuria.

The side-effects of EDTA include
- fever,
- thirst,
- nausea,
- myalgia,
- hypotension,
- reversible renal tubular damage,
- T-wave inversion on ECG,
- increased intracranial pressure,
- increased prothrombin time,
- dermatitis,
- phlebitis.

Dimercaprol (2,3-dimercaptopropanol, British anti-Lewisite, BAL) was designed to combat arsenic-containing war gas in World War II. Later, its use was extended to heavy metal poisoning, particularly from lead and mercury. It is an oily pungent liquid, which is given intramuscularly and metabolized and excreted within 4–6 hr.

A less toxic analog of BAL is available, as meso-2,3-dimercaptosuccinic acid (**DMSA**, succimer), which is given orally in a dose of 500 mg 8 hrly. In some countries, another BAL analog (2,3-dimercapto-1-propanesulfonic acid, **DMPS**, or unithiol) with possibly greater efficacy is available.

The individual doses of BAL are 3–5 mg/kg (3 mg/kg for arsenic, 4 mg/kg for lead and 5 mg/kg for mercury). The urine should be alkalinized concomitantly to decrease the breakdown of chelate complex.
- In arsenic poisoning, it is given 4 hrly until abdominal symptoms subside.
- In lead poisoning, it is given 4 hrly for 48 hr, 6 hrly for 48 hr and then 12 hrly for 5–7 days, usually in combination with EDTA.
- It may also be of use in gold, bismuth, antimony and thallium poisoning.
- It is not of use in cadmium poisoning.
- DMPS is also being studied in the treatment of some forms of snake bite (q.v.), as viper venom contains toxic metalloproteinases which use zinc (q.v.) as a cofactor, and the zinc may then be captured and neutralized by the chelate.

The side-effects of BAL can be dramatic, though they are reversible and not usually serious. They reach their peak within 20 min of injection and disappear by 2 hr. They include
- tachycardia,
- hypertension,
- nausea,
- sweating,
- lacrimation,
- anxiety,
- generalized burning and tingling, particularly of the mouth and penis,
- chest and abdominal pain.

They are probably reduced by the administration of ephedrine, 30–60 mg orally, 30 min beforehand.

Penicillamine, a characteristic degradation product of penicillins, was first found in 1953 in the urine of patients with liver disease given penicillin. It is the D-isomer of β,β-dimethylcysteine (D-3-mercaptovaline).

It is used in poisoning from antimony, copper, gold, lead, mercury and zinc (and also arsenic, cadmium, cobalt, nickel), but it is a second choice after BAL. It is also commonly used in Wilson's disease (q.v.), cystinuria and rheumatoid arthritis. It may possibly be of value in scleroderma (q.v.) and in primary biliary cirrhosis (q.v.).

It is well absorbed from the gut and is given orally in a dose of 0.5–2 g per day in four divided doses. The usual course of therapy for heavy metal poisoning is 5 days.

Although there is a theoretical risk of penicillin anaphylaxis, there are no traces of penicillin in the preparations nowadays available, but care should be taken in patients who are allergic to penicillin.

Elective surgery is contraindicated for 6 weeks after administration because of impaired collagen cross-linking.

The side-effects of penicillamine are common.
- About 30% of patients get fever and itch, perhaps because of cross-reactivity with penicillin.
- Skin lesions are common during long-term administration and consist of
  - friability,
  - maculopapular rash,
  - pemphigoid (q.v.),
  - even systemic lupus erythematosus (q.v.).
- Anorexia, nausea, abdominal discomfort and diarrhoea are also common.
- Rarer reactions include
  - marrow aplasia, which can occasionally be fatal,

- haemolytic anaemia (see Anaemia),
- nephrotic syndrome (q.v.),
- bronchoalveolitis,
- myasthenia gravis (q.v.).

Desferrioxamine (deferoxamine, DFO) is isolated initially as an iron chelate from *Streptomyces pilosus* from which the iron is then removed chemically to produce a ligand with a high affinity for ferric iron.

DFO is able to remove iron from haemosiderin and ferritin and to a lesser extent from transferrin, but not from haemoglobin, myoglobin, cytochromes and other iron-containing enzymes. The chelate complex produced is excreted in the urine and is also dialyzable.

DFO is used
- in the treatment of acute iron poisoning (q.v.),
- in transfusion haemosiderosis, e.g. in the chronic treatment of thalassaemia (q.v.),
- in the diagnosis and treatment of iron storage disease (q.v.),
- sometimes in the treatment of aluminium toxicity (q.v.) in dialysis patients,
- never in haemochromatosis (q.v.).

Since iron overload conditions probably predispose to infection, sometimes with exotic microorganisms (e.g. *Yersinia*), careful microbiological surveillance is recommended.

It is given parenterally, preferably intravenously if the patient has circulatory impairment, in which case a dose of up to 1 g/hr or 4 g over 12 hr and up to 16 g per day may be given. In acute iron poisoning, the need for further doses depends on the serum iron level. During iron elimination in this way, the urine becomes orange-red in colour.

Oral chelating agents of a similar nature, **deferiprone** and **deferasirox**, were more recently introduced, and they may be used in patients unable to tolerate DFO.

Bibliography

Burns CB, Currie B. The efficacy of chelation therapy and factors influencing mortality in intoxicated petrol sniffers. *Aust NZ J Med* 1995; 25: 197.

Jackson TW, Ling LJ, Washington V. The effect of oral deferoxamine in iron absorption in humans. *J Toxicol Clin Toxicol* 1995; 33: 325.

Mathieu D, Mathieu-Nolf M, Germain-Alonso M, et al. Massive arsenic poisoning: effect of haemodialysis and dimercaprol on arsenic kinetics. *Intens Care Med* 1992; 18: 47.

Mills KC, Curry SC. Acute iron poisoning. *Emerg Clin North Am* 1994; 12: 397.

Proper R, Shurn S, Nathan D. Reassessment of the use of deferoxamine B in iron overload. *N Engl J Med* 1976; 294: 1421.

Proudfoot AT, Simpson D, Dyson EH. Management of acute iron poisoning. *Med Toxicol* 1986; 1: 83.

Chemical exposures *See*

- Chemical poisoning.

Chemical poisoning

Chemical poisoning due to drug overdosage is a commonly encountered problem in Intensive Care and its management principles are well known. However, many other chemical agents, generally of a non-therapeutic nature, may cause uncommon forms of poisoning following ingestion or other exposure. In particular, **chemical exposure** is a common environmental hazard in many parts of the world and in many industrial or accidental situations.

Important poisonings or exposures described in this book are those involving
- Aluminium,
- Arsenic,
- Asbestos,
- Beryllium,
- Cadmium,
- Carbon monoxide,
- Carbon tetrachloride,
- Cathinones,
- Chlorine,
- Cocaine,
- Cyanide,
- Dioxins,
- Ergot,
- Ethylene glycol,
- Formaldehyde,
- Gamma-hydroxybutyric acid,
- Heavy metals,
- Herbicides,
- Hydrogen sulphide,
- Insecticides,
- Lead,
- Lewisite,
- 'Mad Hatter' causes,
- Mercury,
- Methanol,
- Monosodium glutamate,
- Organophosphates,
- Paraquat,
- Pesticides (i.e. insecticides and herbicides),
- Phosgene,
- Prussic acid,

- Strychnine,
- Tetrachlorethylene,
- Tetrachlormethane,
- Thallium,
- Toxic gases and fumes,
- Trichlorethylene,
- Warfare agents.

Some uncommon drug poisonings (e.g. amphetamines) are also considered under the headings of the individual drugs themselves (see Drugs).

Bibliography

Alapat PM, Zimmerman JL. Toxicology in the critical care unit. *Chest* 2008; 133: 1006.

American College of Physicians. Occupational and environmental medicine: the internist's role. *Ann Intern Med* 1990; 113: 974.

Bascom R, Bromberg PA, Costa DL, et al. Health effects of outdoor pollution. *Am J Respir Crit Care Med* 1996; 153: 3 & 477.

Cugell DW. The hard metal diseases. *Clin Chest Med* 1992; 13: 269.

Kales SN, Christiani DC. Current concepts: acute chemical emergencies. *N Engl J Med* 2004; 350: 800.

Mokhlesi B, Garinella, PS, Joffe A, et al. Street drug abuse leading to critical illness. *Intens Care Med* 2004; 30: 1526.

Mokhlesi B, Leiken JB, Murray P, et al. Adult toxicology in critical care: part I: general approach to the intoxicated patient. *Chest* 2003; 123: 577.

Mokhlesi B, Leikin JB, Murray P, et al. Adult toxicology in critical care: part II: specific poisonings. *Chest* 2003; 123: 897.

Nemery B. Metal toxicity and the respiratory tract. *Eur Respir J* 1990; 3: 202.

Nriagu JO, Pacyna JM. Quantitative assessment of worldwide contamination of air, water and soils by trace metals. *Nature* 1988; 333: 134.

Olson KR, ed. *Poisoning & Drug Overdose*. 7th edition. New York: McGraw-Hill (Appleton & Lange). 2017.

Redlich CA, Sparer JS, Cullen MR. Sick building syndrome. *Lancet* 1997; 349: 1013.

Rosenstock L, Cullen M, Brodkin C, et al., eds. *Textbook of Clinical Occupational and Environmental Medicine*. 2nd edition. Philadelphia: Saunders. 2004.

Roxe DM, Krumlovsky FA. Toxic interstitial nephropathy from metals, metabolites, and radiation. *Semin Nephrol* 1988; 8: 72.

Shannon MW, Borron SW, Burns MJ, eds. *Haddad and Winchester's Clinical Management of Poisoning and Drug Overdose*. 4th edition. Philadelphia: WB Saunders. 2007.

Trujillo MH, Guerrero J, Fragachan C, et al. Pharmacologic antidotes in critical care medicine: a practical guide for drug administration. *Crit Care Med* 1998; 26: 377.

Wiegand TJ, Patel MM, Olson KR. Management of poisoning and drug overdose. In: *Scientific American Medicine. Interdisciplinary Medicine.* Hamilton: Decker Medicine. 2020.

Chest wall disorders

Chest wall disorders include
1. congenital conditions
    - pectus carinatum ('pigeon chest'),
    - pectus excavatum ('sunken chest') (q.v.),
2. kyphoscoliosis (q.v.),
3. ankylosing spondylitis (q.v.),
4. old thoracoplasty,
5. obesity,
6. neuromuscular disorders,
7. inflammation
    - costochondritis, i.e. Tietze's syndrome,
8. trauma,
9. tumour
    - primary, which are uncommon and usually benign,
    - secondary, which are more common.

Bibliography

Bergofsky EH. Respiratory failure in disorders of the thoracic cage. *Am Rev Respir Dis* 1979; 119: 643.

Coruh B, Benditt JO. Chest wall and neuromuscular disorders. In: *Scientific American Medicine. Pulmonary & Critical Care Medicine*. Hamilton: Dekker Medicine. 2020.

Davies D. Ankylosing spondylitis and lung fibrosis. *Q J Med* 1972; 41: 395.

Eisinger RS, Islam S. Caring for people with untreated pectus excavatum. *Chest* 2020; 157: 590.

Libby DM, Briscoe WA, Boyce B, et al. Acute respiratory failure in scoliosis or kyphosis: prolonged survival and treatment. *Am J Med* 1982; 73: 532.

Ray CS, Sue DY, Bray G, et al. Effects of obesity on respiratory function. *Am Rev Respir Dis* 1983; 128: 501.

Chest X-ray

Chest X-ray is a routine investigation in Intensive Care, as it is in much of medical practice. Indeed, it has been considered an essential extension of clinical examination. In ICU, it is used routinely to assess pulmonary problems, other intrathoracic and chest wall issues, inserted tubes and lines and some extrathoracic features (e.g. neck, upper abdomen). More sophisticated imaging may then be prompted.

> A useful ICU aphorism is that a normal chest X-ray in a patient with hypoxaemia suggests one of three diagnoses, namely,
> - acute pulmonary embolism,
> - non-cardiac right-to-left shunting (e.g. hepatopulmonary syndrome – q.v.), or
> - early pulmonary infiltrate (e.g. idiopathic pulmonary fibrosis, berylliosis, byssinosis – see these separate conditions).

Bibliography
Cade JF, Pain MCF. *Essentials of Respiratory Medicine.* Oxford: Blackwell. 1988.

Cheyne–Stokes respiration *See*
- Sleep disorders of breathing.

Chikungunya

Chikungunya is a febrile illness that resembles dengue fever (q.v.). It is a mosquito-borne disease, first described in Africa and now encountered throughout tropical regions. It has become an important consideration in the diagnosis of fever in returned travellers from areas which have recently suffered outbreaks of the disease.

The incubation period can range from 2–12 days. Many cases are mild and pass unrecognized. Typical symptoms include the sudden onset of fever, with headache, myalgia and sometimes a rash. Polyarthralgia occurs a few days later and can be debilitating. Although most patients recover fully within a week or more, in some patients the joint pains can last for months and in patients with comorbidities the illness can be more severe. However, death from chikungunya is rare.

The differential diagnosis is clearly wide (see Dengue fever), but the specific diagnosis can be confirmed serologically or by PCR.

There is no specific treatment, and only symptomatic measures are available (primarily analgesia).

There is no vaccine, but standard mosquito-protection measures should be implemented in risk areas.
See
- Mosquitoes.

Chlorine

Chlorine (Cl, atomic number 17, atomic weight 35) is the second lightest halogen after fluorine. It is a corrosive, pungent, greenish-yellowish gas, 2.5 times heavier than air and with a boiling point of –34°C. It was first isolated in 1774 and is the main anion in salt water. The chlorine molecule, which consists of two atoms of chlorine (i.e. Cl_2), is a very reactive substance, readily giving rise to chlorides and various oxidative species, including ions and oxides.

Chlorine is widely used as an industrial bleach and disinfectant, and because of its toxicity it has been used as a military poison (see Warfare agents). The maximum recommended exposure levels are not >3 mg/m^3 (1 ppm).

Levels above this cause eye and respiratory irritation, with higher levels causing suffocation and pulmonary oedema. Levels 1000-fold higher cause death within minutes.

Treatment of chlorine poisoning is symptomatic and supportive.
See also
- Acute lung irritation.

Bibliography
Adelson L, Kaufman J. Fatal chlorine poisoning: report of two cases with clinicopathologic correlation. *Am J Clin Pathol* 1971; 56: 430.
Centers for Disease Control and Prevention. Chlorine gas toxicity from mixture of bleach with other cleaning products. *JAMA* 1991; 256: 2529.
Schonhofer B, Voshaar T, Kohler D. Long-term lung sequelae following accidental chlorine gas exposure. *Respiration* 1996; 63: 155.

Cholangitis

Cholangitis is usually associated with biliary obstruction, and this in turn is most commonly due to choledocholithiasis (i.e. stones in the common bile duct).

Acute cholangitis (ascending cholangitis) is generally a complication of acute cholecystitis, which is due to cystic duct obstruction. This in turn is virtually always caused by cholelithiasis (i.e. stones in the gall bladder). However, most gallstones remain silent. Their precursor, biliary sludge, is a mucous mixture of cholesterol crystals and bilirubin granules. It can be associated with pregnancy, fasting and weight loss, liver disease, parenteral nutrition and some drugs (e.g. ceftriaxone, ciclosporin, octreotide).

The clinical features of acute cholangitis are dominated by biliary colic, i.e. severe pain in the right upper quadrant, rapid in onset, constant in nature (and thus not true colic), lasting up to 1 hour and associated with nausea, vomiting and often a high fever.

> The differential diagnosis includes
> - pancreatitis (q.v.),
> - ureteric colic,

- acute myocardial infarction,
- hepatitis (q.v.),
- other causes of biliary obstruction at the porta hepatis,
- acute intermittent porphyria (q.v.).

The diagnosis is made most conveniently on ultrasonography.

*Treatment is with **antibiotics** and urgent endoscopic or surgical **removal** of the obstructing stone.*

Chronic cholangitis is also usually due to biliary duct obstruction, but the causes include stricture or carcinoma as well as stones.

- **Recurrent pyogenic cholangitis** may also occur. This is occasionally secondary to intestinal parasites.
- **Primary sclerosing cholangitis** (PSC) may sometimes be seen, involving both intrahepatic and extrahepatic bile ducts. This is an immunologically mediated condition of unknown aetiology but commonly associated with ulcerative colitis (q.v.). It carries a 30% mortality over 5 years due to complicating hepatic failure or cholangiocarcinoma.

The clinical features of chronic cholangitis include jaundice, fever, anorexia, weight loss and fatigue.

Liver function tests, particularly the alkaline phosphatase and gamma GT, are abnormal. The causative lesion is best defined by ERCP.

*The obstruction should be dealt with on its surgical merits, because without **mechanical relief** chronic cholangitis may lead to biliary cirrhosis (q.v.). Endoscopic stricture dilatation may be helpful in selected patients.*

- *__Ursodeoxycholic acid__ (ursodiol) (see Biliary cirrhosis) provides symptomatic and biochemical benefit but no survival advantage.*
- *There is no effective treatment for primary sclerosing cholangitis apart from **liver transplantation** in advanced cases.*

Bibliography

Angulo P, Lindor KD. Primary sclerosing cholangitis. *Hepatology* 1999; 30: 325.

Berger MY, van der Velden JJ, Lijmer JG, et al. Abdominal symptoms: do they predict gallstones? A systematic review. *Scand J Gastroenterol* 2000; 35: 70.

Johnston DE, Kaplan MM. Pathogenesis and treatment of gallstones. *N Engl J Med* 1993; 328: 412.

Lai EC, Mok FP, Tan ES, et al. Endoscopic biliary drainage for severe acute cholangitis. *N Engl J Med* 1992; 326: 1582.

LaRusso NF, Wiesner RH, Ludwig J, et al. Primary sclerosing cholangitis. *N Engl J Med* 1984; 310: 899.

Lavillegrand J-R, Mercier-Des-Rochettes E, Baron E, et al. Acute cholangitis in intensive care units: clinical, biochemical, microbiological spectrum and risk factors for mortality: a multicentre study. *Crit Care* 2021; 25: 49.

Lazaridis KN, LaRusso NF. Primary sclerosing cholangitis. *N Engl J Med* 2016; 375: 1161.

Miura F, Okamoto K, Takada T, et al. Tokyo Guidelines 2018: initial management of acute biliary infection and flow-chart for acute cholangitis. *J Hepatobiliary Pancreat Sci* 2018; 25: 31.

Vennes JA, Bond JH. Approach to the jaundiced patient. *Gastroenterology* 1983; 84: 1615.

Cholera

Cholera is an acute diarrhoeal disease caused by the Gram-negative bacillus *Vibrio cholerae*. The usual pathogen was the 01 strain, mostly confined until 1961 to Asia. Subsequently, the 7th world pandemic was caused by the El Tor biotype. Later, the 8th world pandemic which started in Southern and Eastern India in 1992 was caused by a new serogroup, 0139-Bengal.

As humans are the only natural host, infection arises from faecal contamination of water or food. The organisms multiply in the proximal small bowel, where they secrete enterotoxin but do not invade the bowel wall. The molecular mechanisms of the pathogenesis of cholera have been particularly well studied.

Clinically, there is painless, acute, severe, watery diarrhoea after an incubation period of a few days (range 2 hr to 5 days). Up to a litre per hour of isotonic fluid is lost in this way, with resultant hypovolaemia. The illness lasts from 1 to 7 days.

The diagnosis is made clinically and from microscopic examination of the stool, in which the organism is easily seen and from which it can be readily grown.

*Treatment is with **fluid resuscitation**, including rapid restoration of the circulation and continuing maintenance. The latter may require up to 10 L in the first 24 hr, preferably of half-normal saline, with 50 mmol/L of $NaHCO_3$ and 12.5 mmol/L of KCl.*

Tetracycline *(e.g. doxycycline 100 mg bd for 2 days) eradicates the organism and reduces the severity and duration of illness. In areas where the organisms have become tetracycline-resistant, single doses of 1 g orally of **ciprofloxacin** and more recently of **azithromycin** have been effective.*

The mortality is 50%, if hypovolaemia is severe and simple resuscitative measures are not available. Natural infection gives long-lasting immunity, but available vaccines have been only of limited and temporary efficacy, although older parenteral or newer oral vaccines are of value in controlling outbreaks. However, clean water and sanitation remain the most important preventative measures at the societal level.

Other tetracycline-sensitive **vibrio species** can also give clinical disease, including
- diarrhoea,
- cellulitis,
- sepsis.
See also
- Diarrhoea.

Bibliography
Lucas ME, Deen JL, von Seidlein L, et al. Effectiveness of mass oral cholera vaccination in Beira, Mozambique. *N Engl J Med* 2005; 352: 757.
Popovic T, Fields PL, Olsvik O, et al. Molecular subtyping of toxigenic *Vibrio cholerae* O139 causing epidemic cholera in India and Bangladesh, 1992-1993. *J Infect Dis* 1995; 171: 122.

Cholestasis

Cholestasis occurs in a number of settings. These include
- biliary tract obstruction,
- benign postoperative intrahepatic cholestasis,
- pregnancy,
- drugs,
- critical illness.

1. **Biliary tract obstruction**
See Cholangitis.
2. **Benign postoperative intrahepatic cholestasis**
This is usually seen after major surgery, in which there have been operative difficulties entailing undue prolongation, hypotension or massive transfusion. This entity probably overlaps that seen in critical illness (see below).

The liver function tests are normal, apart from increased conjugated bilirubin.

The process appears within 1–2 days of surgery and lasts 2–4 weeks.
3. **Pregnancy**
Cholestasis is sometimes seen in late pregnancy (q.v.), but it disappears after delivery, though it may recur with oral contraceptives (q.v.).
4. **Drugs**
These include particularly phenothiazines, erythromycin estolate, oral contraceptives (q.v.), and the anti-staphylococcal antibiotics, flucloxacillin and dicloxacillin (especially the former drug).
5. **Critical illness**
Abnormal liver function tests are frequently observed in critically ill patients. Either **cholestatic liver dysfunction** (CLD) or **ischaemic hepatitis** (see Hepatitis) may be seen.

It has now been appreciated that CLD is not due to mechanical obstruction of bile (whether extrahepatic or intrahepatic) but rather to non-obstructive hepatocyte dysfunction. Although often related to factors such as inflammation and medications, the mechanism of CLD is uncertain. Interestingly, the resultant hyperbilirubinaemia has been suggested to represent a possible adaptive or protective response rather than a pathophysiological complication, but any survival benefit has not so far been demonstrated.

Bibliography
Chandrasekhara V, Ginsberg GG. Gallstones and biliary tract disease. In: *Scientific American Medicine. Gastroenterology*. Hamilton: Dekker Medicine. 2020.
Jenniskens M, Langouche L, Vanwijngaerden Y-M, et al. Cholestatic liver (dys)function during sepsis and other critical illnesses. *Intens Care Med* 2016; 42: 16.
Johnston DE, Kaplan MM. Pathogenesis and treatment of gallstones. *N Engl J Med* 1993; 328: 412.
LaMont JT, Isselbacher KJ. Postoperative jaundice. *N Engl J Med* 1973; 288: 305.
Vennes JA, Bond JH. Approach to the jaundiced patient. *Gastroenterology* 1983; 84: 1615.

Cholinergic agonists

Cholinergic agonists include

- acetylcholine,
- methacholine,
- bethanechol, carbachol,
- choline esters,
- cholinomimetic alkaloids (pilocarpine, muscarine),
- mushroom poisons (mycetism)(q.v.).

The traditional pharmacology of cholinergic agonists is well known, comprising both muscarinic and nicotinic effects.

The **muscarinic effects** occur in autonomic ganglia, CNS, heart, secretory glands and smooth muscle (and are antagonized by atropine).

The **nicotinic effects** are exerted
- at the neuromuscular junction (and antagonized by curare),

in the autonomic ganglia, adrenal gland and CNS (all antagonized by trimethaphan).

However, cholinergic pharmacology has been recognized as more complex in recent times because of new data derived from the molecular cloning of receptors and from the pharmacology of **pirenzepine**.

Cholinergic crisis

A **cholinergic crisis** may occur
- during the treatment of myasthenia gravis (q.v.),
- from exposure to nerve agents in chemical warfare (q.v.).

In myasthenia gravis, it arises from the excess dosage of anticholinesterase drugs which increase weakness because of depolarization of muscle. Although the differentiation of overtreatment from undertreatment with such drugs can be difficult, cholinergic excess
- typically occurs at the time of the peak effect of the drug,
- is associated with muscarinic side-effects of salivation, sweating, gastrointestinal distress, bradycardia and constricted pupils.

If necessary, the diagnosis can be confirmed by giving **edrophonium** 1–2 mg/IV, though in this case muscle weakness will be temporarily worsened and brief respiratory support may be required.

Atropine should thus not be given routinely to such patients, as it could mask these important (muscarinic) markers of cholinergic overdose (see Cholinergic agonists).

Cholinolytic agents See
- Anticholinergic agents.

Christmas disease See
- Haemophilia.

Chromium

Chromium (Cr, atomic number 24, atomic weight 52) is a hard grey metal, discovered in 1797 and so named because of its multi-coloured compounds (e.g. in gem stones), because while abundant in nature it is always present as a compound. Its main industrial use is to increase the strength and corrosion resistance of alloys. Chromium in trivalent form as present in meat, eggs and dairy foods is one of the body's essential **trace elements** (q.v.). Chromium in hexavalent form as used in industrial processes is potentially toxic, though it is poorly absorbed orally.

Chromium deficiency is clinically uncommon. It is seen following poor oral intake over an extended period and especially with prolonged total parenteral nutrition administration, unless specific replacement is given.

The clinical manifestations of chromium deficiency have been reported to include glucose intolerance (with a syndrome indistinguishable from non-insulin-dependent diabetes mellitus) and neuropathy (q.v.).

An increased blood chromium (and cobalt) level has been reported in some patients following hip replacement with certain types of metal-on-metal prostheses. Clinical toxicity in this setting has included anorexia, malaise and a metallic taste in the mouth, but this has been attributed primarily to the concomitantly increased cobalt levels (see Cobalt). More severe toxicity (in other settings) includes dermatitis, gastritis, hepatic necrosis, renal tubular damage, lung cancer and fetal abnormalities.

The average daily requirement is 10–50 mcg orally, and the recommended IV dose is 0.2–0.4 µmol per day. The normal whole blood level is 10–100 nmol/L (0.5–5 mcg/L), with levels >135 nmol/L suggesting a failing metal implant. The normal urinary excretion is <50 nmol/24 hr (or <3 nmol/mmol creatinine).

Bibliography
Barceloux DG. Chromium. *J Toxicol Clin Toxicol* 1999; 37: 173.
Langley A, Dameron CT. Modern metal implant toxicity and anaesthesia. In: Riley R, ed. *Australasian Anaesthesia*. Melbourne: ANZCA. 2015; 57.
Mertz W. Chromium in human nutrition: a review. *J Nutr* 1993; 123: 626.

Chronic fatigue syndrome

Chronic fatigue syndrome (CFS), sometimes referred to as **myalgic encephalomyelitis**, is a complex condition with multiple differential diagnoses, no specific confirmatory tests, no established therapy and an unpredictable course. It is a common and enigmatic condition of disabling physical and cognitive function, making it frustrating for both clinicians and patients.

Although typical cases have no currently identifiable aetiology, chronic fatigue is also a known aftermath of a number of specific conditions, including
- ciguatera (q.v.),
- iron deficiency (q.v.), even if not anaemic,
- 'long COVID' complication of COVID-19 (see Coronavirus),
- Epstein–Barr virus infection (q.v.),
- dengue (q.v.),
- Lyme disease (q.v.),
- post-viral syndromes in general,
- Q fever (see Rickettsial diseases),
- Ross River virus disease (q.v.).

Bibliography

Clayton EW. Beyond myalgic encephalomyelitis/chronic fatigue syndrome: an IOM report on redefining an illness. *JAMA* 2015; 313: 1101.

Prins JB, van der Meer JW, Bleijenberg G. Chronic fatigue syndrome. *Lancet* 2006; 367: 346.

Sandler CX, Lloyd AR. Chronic fatigue syndrome: progress and possibilities. *Med J Aust* 2020; 212: 428.

Churg–Strauss syndrome

Churg–Strauss syndrome comprises
- asthma (q.v.),
- eosinophilia (q.v.),
- systemic vasculitis (q.v.).

Its prevalence is about 2 per million of the population. It may be a subtype of polyarteritis nodosa (q.v.), with extravascular granulomas and eosinophilic vasculitis affecting both small arteries and venules. It may be related to Wegener's granulomatosis (q.v.), i.e. it is one of the anti-neutrophil cytoplasmic antibody (ANCA)-associated systemic vasculitides.

Several cases have been reported following the use of the leukotriene antagonists zafirlukast and later montelukast in patients with asthma. The probable mechanism is the unmasking of an underlying but hitherto unrecognized vasculitis.

> Clinical features include fever, anorexia, weight loss, arthralgia (q.v.), polyneuropathy (q.v.), and lung and renal involvement.

Investigations often show an increased ANCA, an autoantibody found especially in Wegener's granulomatosis (q.v.) but also in polyarteritis nodosa (q.v.) and in idiopathic crescentic glomerulonephritis. The class of ANCA found is usually p-ANCA, unlike the c-ANCA typically found in Wegener's granulomatosis.

Diagnosis is confirmed by biopsy.

*Treatment is with **corticosteroids** and possibly with **cyclophosphamide**. There have been reports of the successful use in this condition of **interferon alpha**, **rituximab** (q.v.) and **omalizumab** (an anti-IgE antibody used in atopic asthma – q.v.).*

The outlook is limited.

A variant is **allergic granulomatosis and angiitis**, which is seen in patients with prior asthma and allergy for many years.

> Clinical features include fever, dyspnoea, purpura (q.v.), skin nodules, polyneuropathy (q.v.) and sometimes acute myocardial infarction.

> Pulmonary involvement occurs in 25% of cases and includes peripheral infiltrate, non-cavitating nodules and pleural effusion.
> It may sometimes be fulminating.

There is anaemia and leukocytosis with marked eosinophilia (q.v.). The diagnosis is made clinically and histologically.

*Treatment is with **corticosteroids** and added cyclophosphamide if refractory.*

Bibliography

Choi YH, Im J-G, Han, BK, et al. Thoracic manifestations of Churg–Strauss syndrome. *Chest* 2000; 117: 117.

Chumbley LC, Harrison EG, DeRemee RA. Allergic granulomatosis and angiitis (Churg–Strauss syndrome). *Mayo Clin Proc* 1977; 52: 477.

Churg J, Strauss L. Allergic granulomatosis, allergic angiitis, and periarteritis nodosa. *Am J Pathol* 1951; 27: 277.

Gatenby PA. Anti-neutrophil cytoplasmic antibody-associated systemic vasculitis: nature or nurture? *Intern Med J* 2012; 42: 351.

Guillevin L, Cohen P, Gayraud M, et al. Churg–Strauss syndrome: clinical study and long-term follow-up of 96 patients. *Medicine* 1999; 78: 26.

Lanham JG, Elkon KB, Pusey CD, et al. Systemic vasculitis with asthma and eosinophilia: a clinical approach to the Churg–Strauss syndrome. *Medicine* 1984; 63: 65.

Sable-Fourtassou R, Cohen P, Mahr A, et al. Antineutrophil cytoplasmic antibodies and the Churg–Strauss syndrome. *Ann Intern Med* 2005; 143: 632.

Salama AD. Pathogenesis and treatment of ANCA-associated systemic vasculitis. *J R Soc Med* 1999; 92: 456.

Wechsler ME, Finn D, Gunawardena D, et al. Churg–Strauss syndrome in patients receiving montelukast as treatment for asthma. *Chest* 2000; 117: 708.

Wechsler ME, Garpestad E, Kocher O, et al. Pulmonary infiltrates, eosinophilia, and cardiomyopathy following corticosteroid withdrawal in patients with asthma receiving zafirlukast. *JAMA* 1998; 279: 455.

Chylothorax *See*
- Pleural effusion.

Ciguatera

Ciguatera arises from a toxin produced by algae, which are ingested by small fish, which in turn are consumed by larger bottom-dwelling fish which concentrate the toxin. Such fish are most common around coral reefs. The toxin is lipid-soluble and heat-stable, but there is no practical laboratory test for it in human samples. Its half-life is unknown.

The onset of symptoms is usually within a few hours and consists of gastrointestinal symptoms, sweating (q.v.), itching and abnormal sensory perception. There is occasional circulatory failure. It generally lasts for only a few days and is rarely fatal. Initially, the differential diagnosis includes tetrodotoxin poisoning (q.v.).

Uncommonly, there is prolonged convalescence, referred to as chronic ciguatera poisoning. This condition is one of the differential diagnoses of **chronic fatigue syndrome** (myalgic encephalomyelitis)(q.v.).

Treatment is with **emesis** *and resuscitation if necessary.* **Atropine** *may improve some symptoms, and* **mannitol** *25–50 g IV has been reported to be very helpful.*

See also
- Food poisoning,
- Paralytic shellfish poisoning,
- Tetrodotoxin.

Bibliography

Gillespie NC, Lewis RJ, Pearn JH, et al. Ciguatera in Australia: occurrence, clinical features, pathophysiology and management. *Med J Aust* 1986; 145: 584.

Lehane L. Ciguatera update. *Med J Aust* 2000; 172: 176.

Morris JG. Ciguatera fish poisoning. *JAMA* 1980; 244: 273.

Pearn JH. Chronic fatigue syndrome: chronic ciguatera poisoning as a differential diagnosis. *Med J Aust* 1997; 166: 309.

CINMA *See*
- Critical illness neuromuscular abnormality.

Circadian rhythm

A **circadian rhythm** refers to the synchronization of a central biological clock to the Earth's day–night cycle. Such rhythms are widely distributed in nature, from plants to animals. This diurnal rhythm determines not just the body's sleep–wake cycle but also a wide range of physiological functions, including endocrine, immune, metabolic, temperature (see Pyrexia), cardiovascular, autonomic and psychic responses. It is adaptive in coordinating important bodily functions with the natural environment, but its loss (as in serious illness) is deleterious to homeostasis and thus to health. The central pacemaker for this rhythm lies in the hypothalamus with projections to the pineal gland to regulate the secretion of **melatonin** (q.v.), which is involved in synchronizing tissue responses and which is the best-known marker of the circadian rhythm.

Bibliography

Boots R, Mead G, Rawashdeh O, et al. Circadian hygiene in the ICU environment (CHIE) study. *Crit Care Resusc* 2020; 22: 361.

Chan MC, Spieth PM, Quinn K, et al. Circadian rhythms: from basic mechanisms to the intensive care unit. *Crit Care Med* 2012; 40: 246.

Saper CB, Scammell TE, Lu J. Hypothalamic regulation of sleep and circadian rhythms. *Nature* 2005; 437: 1257.

Telias I, Wilcox ME. Sleep and circadian rhythm in critical illness. *Crit Care* 2019; 23: 82.

Climate change

Climate change has been referred to as the greatest global health threat of the present century. Climate change in this context refers to anthropogenic causation, as opposed to naturally occurring climate variability.

Climate change is chiefly manifest as a global temperature rise due to the increase in greenhouse gases (particularly carbon dioxide and methane) in the atmosphere, but it also involves greater climatic instability. This process has adverse consequences for many aspects of human (and other biological) health, including food shortage, unsafe water, poor air quality, socioeconomic disadvantage, increased extreme weather events and natural ecosystem destruction.

Some clinical diagnoses may also be impacted (e.g. mosquito-borne diseases – q.v.), for it has been said that global climate change appears to be altering many previously accepted epidemiological and geographical principles underpinning a clinician's expectations of encountering a particular infectious disease in a particular area. In Intensive Care, clinicians will need to be prepared for previously uncommon conditions, e.g. rare infections, heat injury (q.v.).

Climate change is one of the elements of the new broad-ranging discipline of **planetary health**, which also includes other features of environmental degradation, such as pollution, loss of biological diversity, deforestation and desertification.

Bibliography

Atwole L, Baqui AH, Benfield T, et al. Call for emergency action to limit global temperature increases, restore biodiversity and protect health. *J R Soc Med* 2021; 114: 422.

Bein T, Karagiannidis C, Quintel M. Climate change, global warming, and intensive care. *Intens Care Med* 2020; 46: 485.

Capon AG, Talley NJ, Horton RC. Planetary health: what is it and what should doctors do? *Med J Aust* 2018; 208: 296.

Haines A, Ebi K. The imperative for climate action to protect health. *N Engl J Med* 2019; 380: 263.

Hanna EG, McIver LJ. Climate change: a brief overview of the science and health impacts for Australia. *Med J Aust* 2018; 208: 311.

Rocque RJ, Beaudoin C, Ndjaboue R, et al. Health effects of climate change: an overview of systematic reviews. *BMJ Open* 2021; 11: e046333.

Salas RN, Malina D, Solomon CG. Prioritizing health in a changing climate. *N Engl J Med* 2019; 381: 773.

Watts N, Amann M, Arnell N, et al. The 2020 report of the Lancet Countdown on health and climate change: responding to converging crises. *Lancet* 2021; 397: 129.

Clopidogrel *See*
- Antiplatelet agents.

Clostridial infections

Clostridia are anaerobic spore-forming Gram-positive bacilli which secrete potent exotoxins. These organisms are undergoing taxonomic reclassification based on new genetic studies.

There are three major disease groups of clostridial infections, namely,
1. Histotoxic (chiefly *C. perfringens*),
2. Enterotoxigenic (*C. perfringens* and *C. difficile*),
3. neurotoxic (*C. tetani* and *C. botulinum*).

1. Histotoxic

C. perfringens is found in the lower gut and in the soil, and it can enter a new site such as a wound, uterus or burn following appropriate trauma. The disease so produced is **gas gangrene**, an uncommon condition which requires in addition to the presence of the organism, associated necrosis, avascularity and/or a foreign body. The alpha toxin produced gives rise to haemolysis, necrosis and myocardial depression.

There is an incubation period of 8–72 hr, followed by
- local symptoms
  - pain, swelling, skin discolouration, crepitus, and foul-smelling, brown discharge,
- systemic features
  - fever, hypotension, oliguria, haemolysis, myonecrosis.

Uterine infection is usually post-abortal.

Sometimes, a benign and localized gas abscess, i.e. a Welch abscess, only is formed.

> The differential diagnosis of a gas-forming or crepitant cellulitis includes
> - Gram-negative infection
>   - especially in diabetics,
> - mixed anaerobic infection
>   - e.g. perineal phlegmon from a peri-rectal abscess,
> - trapped air
>   - see Gas in soft tissues.

Treatment of gas gangrene is with
- resuscitation,
- extensive surgical clearance,
- **penicillin** 7.2–14.4 g (12–24 million U) IV per day in divided doses for 2 weeks,
- antitoxin, although this has never been formally proven to be useful,
- hyperbaric oxygenation as an adjunct.

The average mortality is 15–30% and up to 50% if the abdominal wall or uterine cavity is severely infected.

2. Enterotoxigenic

Food poisoning (q.v.) caused by *C. perfringens* is second only to staphylococcal in incidence. The organisms are usually ingested from rewarmed meat and multiply in the small intestine, where they produce enterotoxin and thus diarrhoea (q.v.).

There is an incubation period of about 12 hr. There are no systemic symptoms, and the condition subsides within 24 hr.

Pig-bel (necrotic jejunitis) seen in New Guinea is probably caused by the same organism.

Colitis can be produced by *C. difficile*, which is found in soil and in normal faecal flora and which may overgrow when the normal flora are altered by antibiotic therapy (see *Clostridium difficile*, see Colitis).

3. Neurotoxic

The neurotoxic organisms *C. tetani* and *C. botulinum* give rise to the specific diseases, respectively, of
- tetanus (q.v.),
- botulism (q.v.).

Bibliography

Loewenstein MS. Epidemiology of Clostridium perfringens food poisoning. *N Engl J Med* 1972; 286: 1026.

Murrell TGC, Roth L, Egerton J, et al. Pig-bel: enteritis necroticans, a study in diagnosis and management. *Lancet* 1966; 1: 217.

Rechner PM, Agger WA, Mruz K, et al. Clinical features of clostridial bacteremia: a review from a rural area. *Clin Infect Dis* 2001; 33: 349.

Unsworth IP, Sharp PA. Gas gangrene: an 11-year review of 73 cases managed with hyperbaric oxygen. *Med J Aust* 1984; 140: 256.

Weinstein L, Barza MA. Gas gangrene. *N Engl J Med* 1973; 289: 1129.

Clostridium difficile

Clostridium difficile **infection** (CDI) has been referred to as antibiotic-associated colitis, originally pseudomembranous colitis, more recently *Clostridium difficile*-associated diarrhoea (CDAD) and most recently *Clostridioides difficile* infection. See Colitis.

It was originally described after the use of clindamycin, though it is now recognized to follow the use of many different antibiotics, especially fluoroquinolones and cephalosporins. There appears to be an increased risk with the use of proton pump inhibitors (PPIs) and NSAIDs.

CDI is thus an important nosocomial infection, with a faecal–oral route of transmission. It may be at least in part a zoonosis (q.v.), since pigs and cattle harbour related strains of the culprit organism.

It is due to the overgrowth of the toxin-producing *C. difficile* following the suppression by antibiotics of the normal bowel flora (see Microbiome). At least two toxins are produced, referred to as A (enterotoxic) and B (cytotoxic), with the latter being much the more potent. A number of ribotypes (RTs) have been described, with resistant strains identified over the past two decades in a number of countries, driven perhaps by the widespread use of fluoroquinolone antibiotics. The ribotype 027 strain produces toxins A and B and an additional binary toxin, and it has caused severe infections in Europe and North America.

In patients who are negative for *C. difficile* infection and who have haemorrhagic colitis, a toxin producing *Klebsiella oxytoca* may sometimes be to blame.

The 'incubation period' of typical new-onset diarrhoea is usually 4–9 days after the commencement of the culprit antibiotic regimen, but it can be as short as 2 days or as long as 6 weeks.

The condition is most frequent in seriously ill patients and is commonly nosocomial (when it is not necessarily antibiotic-related). Because of this, enteric precautions are required in affected hospital patients. Infection control measures of importance include hand hygiene, barrier protection of staff, isolation of infected patients, the use of a sporicidal disinfectant such as hypochlorite, and careful antibiotic prescribing.

About 50% of cases have the characteristic pseudomembranous changes evident on endoscopy, though only 20% get diarrhoea (often of a variable nature) and only 10% have severe symptoms of blood-stained diarrhoea with abdominal pain, fever and leukocytosis.

Toxic megacolon is a rare complication.

Diagnosis requires the demonstration of toxin by assay in the faeces, since culture, though sensitive, is non-specific, as up to 25% of hospital patients have been reported to have positive cultures anyway. Molecular and antigen testing methods are also available in some laboratories. The measurement of faecal lactoferrin (q.v.) may be a useful screening test for inflammatory diarrhoea (such as CDI) in hospitalized patients. Abdominal CT scanning commonly shows a thickened colonic wall, but this finding is non-specific.

Treatment consists of removing the potentially offending antibiotics where possible and giving oral **vancomycin** *(125 mg qid) for 7–10 days. Oral* **metronidazole** *(400 mg tds) may also be used, but it is less effective. In more severe cases, higher doses of oral* **vancomycin** *(500 mg qid) together with IV* **metronidazole** *(500 mg tds) improve outcome. The expensive new antibiotic* **fidaxomicin** *(200 mg bd) may be used for recurrent or refractory disease.*

Recent studies suggest that **probiotic therapy** *with lactobacilli may be of benefit, particularly for primary prevention and possibly also for prevention of recurrence.*

Faecal transplantation *(q.v.) has been found to be effective in about 90% of refractory or recurrent cases, but the procedure is complex, expensive and as yet non-standardized.*

Surgery *may be considered in fulminant cases which have not responded to medical therapy, particularly if there is concern about bowel wall integrity. Either total colectomy or more recently loop ileostomy with colonic lavage has been reported to decrease mortality, but the surgery can be challenging and the perioperative risk itself is high.*

Bezlotoxumab*, a human monoclonal antibody to C. difficile toxin, can prevent recurrence by enhancing passive immunity to the toxin and preventing the organism from binding to host cells in the colon. It is not indicated for treatment, but it can be used together with an appropriate antibiotic regimen in patients being treated but at high risk of recurrence.*

Relapse is common and is not prevented by more prolonged therapy. Recurrence may be due to either persistence or new acquisition of *C. difficile* spores. A fatal outcome is sometimes seen.

Bibliography
Adelman MW, Woodworth MH, Shaffer VO, et al. Critical care management of the patient with Clostridioides difficile. *Crit Care Med* 2021; 49: 127.

Antonelli M, Martin-Loeches I, Dimopoulos G, et al. Clostrdioides difficile (formerly *Clostridium difficile*) infection in the critically ill: an expert statement. *Intens Care Med* 2020; 46: 215.

Blaser MJ, Smith PD, Ravdin JL, et al., eds. *Infections of the Gastrointestinal Tract*. 2nd edition. New York: Raven Press. 2002.

Bobo LD, Dubberke ER, Kollef M. *Clostridium difficile* in the ICU. *Chest* 2011; 140: 1643.

Chauhan A, Apostolov R, van Langenberg D, et al. Faecal microbiota transplantation for recurrent Clostridioides difficile infection: an Australian perspective – effective, safe, yet room for improvement. *Intern Med J* 2021; 51: 106.

Dial S, Alrasadi K, Manoukian C, et al. Risk of *Clostridium difficile* diarrhea among hospital inpatients prescribed proton pump inhibitors. *CMAJ* 2004; 171: 33.

Elliott B, Chang BJ, Golledge CL, et al. *Clostridium difficile*-associated diarrhoea. *Intern Med J* 2007; 37: 561.

Fehily SR, Basnayake C, Wright EK, et al. The gut microbiota and gut disease. *Intern Med J* 2021; 51: 1594.

Guery B, Galperine T, Barbut F. Clostridioides difficile: diagnosis and treatments. *BMJ* 2019; 366: 14609.

Guy AY, Kutty PK. Clostridioides difficile infection. *Ann Intern Med* 2018; 169: ITC49.

Hempel S, Newberry SJ, Maher AR, et al. Probiotics for the prevention and treatment of antibiotic-associated diarrhea: a systematic review and meta-analysis. *JAMA* 2012; 307: 1959.

Hickson M, D'Souza AL, Muthu N, et al. Use of probiotic *Lactobacillus* preparation to prevent diarrhoea associated with antibiotics: randomized double blind placebo controlled trial. *BMJ* 2007; 335: 80.

Hvas CL, Jorgensen SMD, Jorgensen SP, et al. Fecal microbiota transplantation is superior to fidaxomicin for treatment of recurrent *Clostridium difficile* infection. *Gastroenterology* 2019; 156: 1324.

Johnson S, Clabots CR, Linn FV, et al. Nosocomial *Clostridium difficile* colonization and disease. *Lancet* 1990; 336: 97.

Jones EM, MacGowan AP. Back to basics in management of *Clostridium difficile* infections. *Lancet* 1998; 351: 505.

Kelly CP, Pothoulakis C, La Mont JT. *Clostridium difficile* colitis. *N Engl J Med* 1994; 330: 257.

Leffler DA, Lamont JT. *Clostridium difficile* infection. *N Engl J Med* 2015; 372: 1539.

Loo VG, Bourgault AM, Poirier L, et al. Host and pathogen factors for *Clostridium difficile* infection and colonization. *N Engl J Med* 2011; 365: 1693.

Lyerly DM, Krivan HC, Wilkins TD. *Clostridium difficile*: its disease and toxins. *Clin Microbiol Rev* 1988; 1: 1.

Moayyedi P, Yuan Y, Baharith H, et al. Faecal microbiota transplantation for *Clostridium difficile*-associated diarrhoea: a systematic review of randomised controlled trials. *Med J Aust* 2017; 207: 166.

Mylonakis E, Ryan ET, Calderwood SB. *Clostridium difficile*-associated diarrhea. *Arch Intern Med* 2001; 161: 525.

Pochapin M. The effect of probiotics in *Clostridium difficile* diarrhea. *Am J Gastroenterol* 2000; 95: S11.

Riley TV. Epidemic *Clostridium difficile*. *Med J Aust* 2006; 185: 133.

Trubiano JA, Cheng AC, Korman TM, et al. Australasian Society of Infectious Diseases updated guidelines for the management of *Clostridium difficile* infection in adults and children in Australia and New Zealand. *Intern Med J* 2016; 46: 479.

van Langenberg DR, Gearry RB, Wong H-L, et al. The potential value of faecal lactoferrin as a screening test in hospitalized patients with diarrhoea. *Intern Med J* 2010; 40: 819.

Young GP, Bayley N, Ward P, et al. Antibiotic-associated colitis caused by *Clostridium difficile*: relapse and risk factors. *Med J Aust* 1986; 144: 303.

Coagulation disorders

Coagulation and **inflammation** are two intertwined pathways that respond to bodily injury and thus provide physiological defence to both local and systemic insults. The cross-talk between these two systems is considerable, with many substrates, proteases, activators and inhibitors in common. The integrated pathological process is referred to as **thromboinflammation** or sometimes **immunothrombosis**, involving activation of endothelial cells, coagulation, platelets, leukocytes and cytokines. This balanced system of responses to adverse stimuli can be overwhelmed in serious infections, which probably explains why many such infections are complicated by thrombosis or bleeding.

The plasma **contact system** consisting of factor XII, prekallikrein (PK), kininogen and C1 esterase inhibitor is the major driver of both the proinflammatory and the procoagulant responses, with resultant activation of the intrinsic **coagulation, kinin, complement, fibrinolysis** and **innate immune** systems. Bacterial (and fungal and viral) activation of factor XII is an important initiating step in this process. This surface defence mechanism provided by the contact activation system against foreign proteins also extends to the artificial surfaces so common in modern interventional medical practice.

Thus, the contact (or intrinsic) pathway of coagulation appears to be more involved in pathological processes than in normal haemostasis, which instead is dominated by the tissue factor stimulation of factor VII (and the extrinsic pathway). This difference suggests that factor XII or factor XI might be future targets for safe anticoagulation without bleeding consequences (see Anticoagulants).

Tissue factor is classically expressed on endothelial cells, but its presence in microvesicles in monocytes and in some tumour cells and its identification in bodily secretions, such as saliva, semen and breast milk, point to additional roles other than in haemostasis and these further roles may relate to other aspects of the host response to injury (e.g. inflammation and healing).

Coagulation disorders comprise a group of conditions within the broader group of disorders of **haemostasis** (q.v.). They may be hereditary or acquired.

Hereditary coagulation disorders can comprise a deficiency of any of the individual coagulation factors. Each deficiency (except for factor XII deficiency, which is generally asymptomatic) gives rise to a specific coagulopathy. Combined defects are rare, but they have provided the opportunity to gain new insights into a number of biological mechanisms, including cell protein transport and vitamin K dependence.

The better known and most common hereditary coagulation disorders are
- von Willebrand's disease (q.v.),
- the haemophilias (q.v.).

Acquired coagulation disorders on the other hand usually demonstrate deficiency of multiple coagulation factors.

These disorders include
- disseminated intravascular coagulation (q.v.),
- liver disease,
- vitamin K deficiency (q.v.),
- trauma-induced coagulopathy (TIC)
  - more correctly termed a haemostatic disorder (see above), as it includes thrombocytopenia and enhanced fibrinolysis as well complex coagulation factor deficiency related to tissue damage, shock and dilution,
- cardiopulmonary bypass (CPB) coagulopathy
  - multifactorial in aetiology, including haemodilution, coagulation factor losses from procedural bleeding, both contact and extrinsic pathway activation, platelet depletion and dysfunction, increased fibrinolysis, hypofibrinogenaemia and residual heparinization,
  - associated with increased transfusion needs and adverse clinical outcomes,
  - assessed by point-of-care viscoelastic as well as laboratory testing,
- iatrogenic acquired coagulopathy
  - especially drug-induced, e.g. following administration of anticoagulant or antiplatelet agents,
  - with aggravation of an existing local or systemic haemostatic defect as the usual finding in this setting.

For most coagulation factors, a plasma concentration of at least 30–40% of the normal level is required for effective haemostasis, with the exception that a deficiency of factor XII is not associated with any bleeding tendency. Indeed, in some mammalian species such as dolphins, factor XII is naturally absent.

Coagulation factors are of course plasma proteins, and most are proteases (i.e. proteolytic enzymes), except for fibrinogen and for factors V and VIII (which are cofactors). They are referred to as serine proteases because serine provides their active catalytic site, and thus they have considerable homology with the broad proteolytic enzyme, trypsin. They circulate in an inactive form (referred to as a zymogen or proenzyme) until activation via a conformation change reveals their active catalytic site. The activation of the members of the coagulation sequence is sequential, referred to originally in the 1960s as a cascade or waterfall.

The characteristics of the individual coagulation factors are shown in the Table below. In addition, their gene structures have been recently defined, thus permitting better understanding of their abnormalities, improved diagnostic techniques and the development of recombinant forms for human use.

Coagulation factors

Coagulation factor	Molecular weight (kDa)	Plasma concentration (mcg/mL)	Plasma concentration (µM)	Half-life (hr)
Fibrinogen (I)	340	3000	9.0	90
Prothrombin (II)	72	90	1.4	65
Factor V	330	10	0.03	15
Factor VII	50	0.5	0.01	3
Factor VIII	330	0.1	0.0003	10
Factor IX	56	5	0.09	25
Factor X	59	8	0.135	40
Factor XI	160	5	0.03	45
Factor XII	80	30	0.375	50
Factor XIII	326	10	0.03	200

Bibliography

Aschnoune K, Faraoni D, Brohi K. What's new in management of traumatic coagulopathy. *Intens Care Med* 2014; 40: 1727.

Barton C. Treatment of coagulopathy related to hepatic insufficiency. *Crit Care Med* 2016; 44: 1927.

Bartoszko J, Karkouti K. Managing the coagulopathy associated with cardiopulmonary bypass. *J Thromb Haemost* 2021; 19: 617.

Chakraverty R, Davidson S, Peggs K, et al. The incidence and cause of coagulopathies in an intensive care population. *Br J Haematol* 1996; 93: 460.

Conway EM. Reincarnation of ancient links between coagulation and complement. *J Thromb Haemost* 2015; 13: S121.

Flier JS, Underhill LH. Molecular and cellular biology of blood coagulation. *N Engl J Med* 1992; 326: 800.

Foley JH, Conway EM. Cross-talk pathways between coagulation and inflammation. *Circ Res* 2016; 118: 1392.

Greenberg CS, Sane DC. Coagulation problems in critical care medicine. In: Lumb PD, Shoemaker WC, eds. *Critical Care: State of the Art*, Chapter 9. Fullerton: Society of Critical Care Medicine. 1990; p 187.

Iba T, Levy JH. Inflammation and thrombosis: roles of neutrophils, platelets and endothelial cells and their interactions in thrombus formation during sepsis. *J Thromb Haemost* 2017; 16: 231.

Kornblith LZ, Moore HB, Cohen MJ. Trauma-induced coagulopathy: the past, present, and future. *J Thromb Haemost* 2019; 17: 852.

Leung LLK. Hemostasis and its regulation. In: *Scientific American Medicine. Hematology*. Hamilton: Dekker Medicine. 2020.

Levi M, ten Cate H. Disseminated intravascular coagulation. *N Engl J Med* 1999; 341: 586.

Long AT, Kenne E, Jung R, et al. Contact system revisited: an interface between inflammation, coagulation, and innate immunity. *J Thromb Haemost* 2016; 14: 427.

Marder VJ, Aird WC, Bennett JS, et al., eds. *Hemostasis and Thrombosis: Basic Principles and Clinical Practice.* 6th edition. Philadelphia: Lippincott Williams & Wilkins. 2012.

Mavrommatis AC, Theodoridis T, Economou M, et al. Activation of the fibrinolytioc system and utilization of the coagulation inhibitors in sepsis: comparison with severe sepsis and septic shock. *Intens Care Med* 2001; 27: 1853.

Moore HB, Gando S, Iba T, et al. Defining trauma-induced coagulopathy with respect to future implications for patient management: communication from the SSC of the ISTH. *J Thromb Haemost* 2020; 18: 740.

Najem MY, Couturaud F, Lemarie CA. Cytokine and chemokine regulation of venous thromboembolism. *J Thromb Haemost* 2020; 18: 1009.

Oldenburg J, Schwaab R. Molecular biology of blood coagulation. *Semin Thromb Hemost* 2001; 27: 313.

Peyvandi F, Mannucci PM. Rare coagulation disorders. *Thromb Haemost* 1999; 82: 1207.

Posma JJN, Posthuma JJ, Spronk HMH. Coagulation and non-coagulation effects of thrombin. *J Thromb Haemost* 2016; 14: 1908.

Rapaport SI. Preoperative hemostatic evaluation: which tests, if any? *Blood* 1983; 61: 229.

Roberts HR, ed. Seventh Novo Nordisk symposium on haemostasis management. *Semin Haematol* 2004; 41(1): suppl. 1.

Schmaier AH. The contact system and kallikrein/kinin systems: pathophysiologic and physiologic activities. *J Thromb Haemost* 2016; 14: 28.

Shamanaev A, Emsley J, Gailani D. Proteolytic activity of contact factor zymogens. *J Thromb Haemost* 2021; 19: 330.

Spahn DR, Bouillon B, Duranteau J, et al. The European guideline on management of major bleeding and coagulopathy following trauma: fifth edition. *Crit Care* 2019; 23: 98.

Tripodi A, Mannucci PM. The coagulopathy of chronic liver disease. *N Engl J Med* 2011; 365: 147.

Zhang B, Ginsburg D. Familial multiple coagulation factor deficiencies: new biologic insight from rare genetic bleeding disorders. *J Thromb Haemost* 2004; 2: 1564.

Coagulation factors *See*

- Coagulation disorders.

Cobalt

Cobalt (Co, atomic number 27, atomic weight 59) is a hard grey metal, discovered in 1735 but known in compounds since antiquity as a valued source of blue pigment. Its main industrial use is in smelting and the production of special metal alloys. Cobalt is present in certain foods, and it is one of the body's essential **trace elements** (q.v.). It is best known clinically as a key element in vitamin B_{12}.

Cobalt toxicity is referred to as cobaltism, and it adversely affects a number of cardiac, endocrine and neurological functions. Increased cobalt intake has been used illegally to enhance performance in racehorses, in which there is an increase in red blood cells but at the expense of later serious adverse effects.

An increased blood cobalt (and chromium) level has been reported in some patients following hip replacement with certain types of metal-on-metal prostheses. Clinical toxicity has included anorexia, malaise and a metallic taste in the mouth, and this has been attributed primarily to the concomitantly increased cobalt levels (see also Chromium).

The RDA of cobalt has not been well defined, since its normal intake is mostly via vitamin B_{12}. However, the minimum daily requirement is probably about 1 mcg, though the average intake is several-fold higher than this. An intake >10 mg/kg is toxic. The total body cobalt is only about 1 mg. The normal plasma level is <20 nmol/L (<1.2 mcg/L), with levels >120 nmol/L suggesting a failing metal implant. The normal urinary excretion is <3 nmol/mmol creatinine, but it is increased in occupationally exposed subjects, with levels >30 nmol/mmol creatinine indicating significant absorption.

Bibliography
Langley A, Dameron CT. Modern metal implant toxicity and anaesthesia. In: Riley R, ed. *Australasian Anaesthesia*. Melbourne: ANZCA. 2015; p57.
Mao X, Wong AA, Crawford RW. Cobalt toxicity – an emerging clinical problem in patients with meta-on-metal hip prostheses. *Med J Aust* 2011; 194: 649.

Cocaine

Cocaine is a white, crystalline alkaloid (q.v.) derived from the leaves of the South American coca plant. It has the composition of $C_{17}H_{21}NO_4$. The usual form is cocaine hydrochloride, a powder which may be inhaled or sniffed but is poorly absorbed and cannot be smoked. It is an irritant and gives chronic rhinitis or even nasal ulceration. It is a mucous membrane anaesthetic, hence its application in clinical medicine. It produces rapid euphoria and alertness, which last for up to 90 min, and is addictive. The most rapid and massive effects are seen when a packet ruptures in a 'body-packer'.

The freebase form (crack), which appeared in the 1980s, is well absorbed and may be smoked or injected. It produces even more intense euphoria, but its action is brief and it is more addictive.

Clinical features of toxicity are numerous.
- **Acute toxicity** is manifest neurologically by headache, dizziness, dysphoria, formication, focal signs, fits and coma. Prolonged use may give rise to depression, irritability, disordered sleep, confusion, paranoia and fits. These neurological effects are due to excess dopaminergic neurotransmission.
- **Cardiovascular effects** of arrhythmias (including cardiac arrest), myocardial infarction, hypertension or stroke may be seen, even in the absence of high doses or concomitant cardiac disease. These effects are due to excess noradrenaline (norepinephrine) action. Long-term use may produce premature atherosclerosis.
- **Respiratory effects** include upper respiratory tract damage, pulmonary oedema (which may be haemorrhagic) and spontaneous barotrauma (q.v.). When inhaled with smoke, it may cause permanent lung damage.
- **Systemic effects** such as hyperthermia (q.v.), rhabdomyolysis (q.v.), renal failure, liver failure, disseminated intravascular coagulation (q.v.) and bowel ischaemia may be seen.
- **Fetal damage** can occur.

*Acute treatment is with **benzodiazepines** and if necessary a calcium antagonist and/or antiarrhythmic agent. **Vigabatrin** (γ-vinyl-GABA, GVG), an anticonvulsant, showed promise in early studies in treating cocaine addiction, but this benefit was not borne out in later studies.*

Mechanical or even surgical removal of cocaine-filled packages may be required in 'body packers'. Dialysis and haemoperfusion are not effective in eliminating cocaine.

However, medical care attends clearly to only a small part of a much wider societal problem.

Bibliography
Benowitz NL. Clinical pharmacology and toxicology of cocaine. *Pharmacol Toxicol* 1993; 72: 3.
Cregler LL, Mark H. Medical complications of cocaine abuse. *N Engl J Med* 1986; 315: 1495.
Dellinger RP, Zimmerman JL. Management of the critically ill cocaine abuser. In: Lumb PD, Shoemaker WC, eds. *Critical Care: State of the Art*, Chapter 6. Fullerton: Society of Critical Care Medicine. 1990; p 115.
de Prost N, Lefebvre A, Questel F, et al. Prognosis of body packers. *Intens Care Med* 2005; 31: 955.
Dewey SL, Morgan AE, Ashby CR, et al. A novel strategy for the treatment of cocaine addiction. *Synapse* 1998; 30: 119.
Forrester JM, Steele AW, Waldron JA, et al. Crack lung: an acute pulmonary syndrome with a spectrum of clinical and histopathologic findings. *Am Rev Respir Dis* 1990; 142: 462.
Gawin FH. Cocaine addiction: psychology and neurophysiology. *Science* 1991; 251: 1580.
Hollander JE. The management of cocaine-associated myocardial ischaemia. *N Engl J Med* 1995; 333: 1267.

Karch SB. Cocaine: history, use, abuse. *J R Soc Med* 1999; 92: 393.

Kloner RA, Razkalla SH. Cocaine and the heart. *New Engl J Med* 2003; 348: 487.

Lange RA, Hillis LD. Medical progress: cardiovascular complications of cocaine. *N Engl J Med* 2001; 345: 351.

Levine SR, Brust JCM, Futrell N, et al. Cerebrovascular complications of the use of the 'crack' form of alkaloidal cocaine. *N Engl J Med* 1990; 323: 699.

Mokhlesi B, Garinella, PS, Joffe A, et al. Street drug abuse leading to critical illness. *Intens Care Med* 2004; 30: 1526.

Mokhlesi B, Leikin JB, Murray P, et al. Adult toxicology in critical care: part II: specific poisonings. *Chest* 2003; 123: 897.

Shanti CM, Lucas CE. Cocaine and the critical care challenge. *Crit Care Med* 2003; 31: 1851.

Vasica G, Tennant CC. Cocaine use and cardiovascular complications. *Med J Aust* 2002; 177: 260.

Coeliac disease

Coeliac disease (CD, gluten-sensitive enteropathy, non-tropical sprue) is an autoimmune disorder (q.v.) in which the ingestion of wheat gluten triggers an immune response and consequent small bowel inflammation. Its prevalence is about 1% of the population and may be increasing. Formerly believed to affect primarily children of Northern European ancestry, it is now known to affect people of all ages in most countries.

Gluten is the principal protein in wheat, and similar proteins are found in barley and rye. In genetically predisposed people, gluten triggers an IgA antibody to tissue transglutaminase (tTG), the enzyme which degrades gluten peptides in the small bowel. Antibodies are also produced to the deamidated gliadin peptides (DGPs), gliadin being the soluble protein component in gluten. Virtually all affected patients carry the histocompatibility antigens HLA DQ2 or DQ8. The immune response targets the small bowel mucosa, with consequent chronic inflammation, villous atrophy and mucosal dysfunction.

Classical coeliac disease is manifested by gastrointestinal symptoms. However, it is now recognized that the disease can also be non-classical, with predominantly extra-gastrointestinal symptoms. Subclinical forms may occur with antibodies and intestinal damage but no symptoms, and latent forms may occur with just antibodies but no intestinal damage (or symptoms). Untreated refractory coeliac disease (RCD) can predispose to small bowel T-cell lymphoma or adenocarcinoma.

Thus, coeliac disease can present with a wide range of clinical features, including

- chronic or intermittent diarrhoea (the most typical symptom),
- irritable bowel syndrome (q.v.),
- features of malabsorption (q.v.),
- consequences of malabsorption (q.v.),
- weight loss,
- fatigue (the most common non-classical symptom),
- skin rash (e.g. dermatitis herpetiformis – q.v.),
- other autoimmune disorders (q.v.),
- positive family history.

Diagnosis is supported by testing for coeliac-specific tTG and DGP antibodies, provided the patient is on a gluten-containing diet at the time. The total IgA levels are increased. Negative genetic testing effectively excludes the diagnosis. Definitive diagnosis requires histological confirmation of villous atrophy and mucosal inflammation in a duodenal biopsy taken at endoscopy. In patients with a confirmed diagnosis, tests of small bowel function (e.g. iron and vitamin assays) should be performed.

A similar condition called **sprue-like enteropathy** caused by the selective angiotensin II receptor antagonists, especially olmesartan, should be excluded (see Malabsorption, see Renin–angiotensin–aldosterone).

*The core of treatment is a **gluten-free diet** (GFD) for life. Vitamins, micronutrients and fibre need to be replaced in the diet. A number of new therapies are in prospect, including gluten-specific proteases (glutenases), vaccination and immunomodulation (q.v.).*

Current 'gluten-free' standards in foods require a laboratory measurement of <1 ppm, which protects virtually all patients with CD. This equates to only about 0.5 g (about 1/10 of a teaspoonful) in an average daily total food intake of about 500 g. As an approximate calculation, 0.5 g of gluten is the amount in about one quarter of a slice of bread.

The term **non-coeliac gluten sensitivity** (NCGS) refers to patients with typical symptoms of coeliac disease but with negative diagnostic tests, and it may be caused by other food intolerance (e.g. to FODMAPs – q.v.) or irritable bowel syndrome (q.v.). Many patients with NCGS have adopted a gluten-free diet, though satisfactory results have varied in degree and in duration. Although a gluten-free diet has become popular with many people for various personal reasons (including NCGS), its health benefits have been convincingly shown only in patients with coeliac disease.

Wheat allergy is a separate condition from coeliac disease and typically causes skin or respiratory symptoms, e.g. baker's asthma (see Occupational lung diseases – 2. Occupational asthma). It can be formally diagnosed with an IgE-mediated allergy test, though most cases are self-diagnosed based on improvement following a gluten-free diet.

See
- Malabsorption.

Bibliography

Anderson RP. Coeliac disease: current approach and future prospects. *Intern Med J* 2008; 38: 790.

Campbell CB, Roberts RK, Cowen AE. The changing clinical presentation of coeliac disease in adults. *Med J Aust* 1977; 1: 89.

Duggan JM. Recent developments in our understanding of adult coeliac disease. *Med J Aust* 1997; 166: 312.

Duggan JM. Coeliac disease: the great imitator. *Med J Aust* 2004; 180: 524.

Fasano A, Catassi C. Celiac disease. *N Engl J Med* 2012; 367: 2419.

Feighery C. Coeliac disease. *BMJ* 1999; 319: 236.

Green PH, Cellier C. Celiac disease. *N Engl J Med* 2007; 357: 1731.

Matysiak-Budnik T, Candalh C, Dugave C, et al. Alteration of the intestinal transport and processing of gliadin peptides in celiac disease. *Gastroenterolgy* 2003; 125: 696.

Niland B, Cash BD. Health benefits and adverse effects of a gluten-free diet in non-celiac disease patients. *Gastroenterol Hepatol* 2018; 14: 82.

Potter MDE, Walker MM, Talley NJ. Non-coeliac gluten or wheat sensitivity: emerging disease or misdiagnosis? *Med J Aust* 2017; 207: 211.

Reeves GEM. Coeliac disease: against the grain. *Intern Med J* 2004; 34: 521.

Walker MM, Ludvigsson JF, Sanders DS. Coeliac disease: review of diagnosis and management. *Med J Aust* 2017; 207: 173.

Colchicine

Colchicine is a plant alkaloid (q.v.) with a unique and specific anti-inflammatory effect in gout (q.v.), in which it was first used in 1763. It is also used 'off-label' in some cases of familial Mediterranean fever (q.v.) and primary biliary cirrhosis (q.v.). Recent trials have further suggested that low-dose colchicine may be effective in the secondary prevention of ischaemic heart disease.

It is a toxic and antimitotic agent with a narrow therapeutic margin. Most of the drug is eliminated via the gut. Its toxic effects are thus chiefly gastrointestinal, with nausea, vomiting, diarrhoea and abdominal pain.

On the other hand, colchicine inhibits macrophage migration inhibitory factor (MIF), which can be cardiotoxic in sepsis, at least experimentally. Thus, colchicine might theoretically assist mitochondrial function in critical illness.

Since it is metabolized mainly by the enzyme CYP344, the concurrent use of other drugs which inhibit this enzyme, such as clarithromycin, has been associated with an increased risk of colchicine toxicity, including fatalities.

In overdose, profuse and bloody diarrhoea occurs, and the patient may present with an acute abdomen. There is extensive vascular injury, particularly affecting the kidneys, and there may be multiorgan failure (q.v.). Ascending paralysis can lead to fatal respiratory paralysis. After a few days, bone marrow depression and alopecia (q.v.) may be produced.

A dose as small as 7 mg has been reported to be fatal, though ingestion of <30 g is not generally fatal, whereas >60 mg is commonly lethal.

Treatment consists of supportive measures, particularly with fluids and electrolytes in the early stages. Later, circulatory and multiorgan support may be required.

Abdominal pain may be relieved by atropine and morphine. Gastrointestinal decontamination with activated charcoal is recommended.

See
- Behcet's syndrome,
- Diarrhoea,
- Drugs,
- Idiopathic pulmonary fibrosis,
- Malabsorption – Maldigestion,
- Megaloblastic anaemia – Vitamin B_{12} deficiency,
- Multiorgan failure,
- Multiple myeloma – 6. Amyloidosis,
- Myopathy – Secondary myopathy,
- Neuropathy – 2. Toxic neuropathies.

Bibliography

Folpini A, Furfori P. Colchicine toxicity: clinical features and treatment. *J Toxicol Clin Toxicol* 1995; 33: 71.

Imazio M, Nidorf M. Colchicine and the heart. *Eur Heart J* 2021; 42: 2745.

Maxwell MJ, Muthu P, Pritty PE. Accidental colchicine overdose: a case report and literature review. *Emerg Med J* 2002: 19: 265.

Murray SS, Kramlinger KG, McMichan JC, et al. Acute toxicity after excessive ingestion of colchicine. *Mayo Clin Proc* 1983; 58: 523.

Putterman C, Ben-Chetrit E, Caraco Y, et al. Colchicine intoxication: clinical pharmacology, risk factors, features and management. *Semin Arthritis Rheum* 1991; 21: 143.

Stemmermann GN, Hayashi T. Colchicine intoxication: a reappraisal of its pathology based on study of three fatal cases. *Human Pathol* 1971; 2: 321.

Cold

Cold is one of the important physical exposures (q.v.) and is represented by
- Frostbite (q.v.),
- Hypothermia (q.v.).

Other cold-induced injuries occur following prolonged exposure to temperatures which are low but greater than freezing. These injuries include
- chilblains,
- trench foot,
- immersion injury,
- cold urticaria (see Urticaria).

Cold intolerance is seen in iron deficiency (q.v.) and in hypothyroidism (q.v.).
See also
- Cold agglutinin disease,
- Multiple myeloma – 5. Cryoglobulinaemia.

Cold agglutinin disease

Cold agglutinin disease is produced by a temperature-sensitive complement-fixing antibody. This occurs in a number of infections and in certain oncological disorders (in which it can represent a primary clonal lymphoproliferative disorder). The highest titres occur during *Mycoplasma pneumoniae* infections, in which an IgM antibody is produced to the red blood cell membrane glycoprotein, IAg. Presumably the antigen is altered by the microorganism (or malignant mutation) so as to become immunogenic. It is thus an autoimmune disorder (q.v.).

Laboratory testing for the cold agglutinin titre for type O red blood cells shows either a 4-fold rise or a titre >1:128. The thermal amplitude of the antibody is usually 30–34°C.

The antibody production is related to the severity of illness and is seen in about 60% of patients with pneumonia due to *M. pneumoniae*. Although antibiotics decrease the duration and severity of infection, they do not clear the microorganism which usually persists for 3–8 weeks. The production of antibody is a self-limited process, and it usually lasts for a few weeks.

The measurement of the titre of cold agglutinins is no longer used as a diagnostic test for pneumonia due to *M. pneumoniae*, since the more modern techniques of PCR and immunoassays are both highly specific and sensitive.

> The clinical consequence of cold agglutinin production is **haemolysis**.
> Although there is a very high rate (80%) of reticulocytosis and a positive direct Coombs test, overt haemolysis is much less common.
> Clinical haemolysis when it occurs typically does so in the second and third week of illness and is associated with jaundice and even haemoglobinuria.
> Its extent is related to the height of titre.
> If clinical haemolysis occurs, the environmental temperature should be kept above the thermal amplitude of the antibody.
> *Treatment in chronic cases includes* **corticosteroids** *and more recently* **rituximab** *(q.v.)*.

Bibliography
Berentsen S, Roth A, Randen U, et al. Cold agglutinin disease: current challenges and future prospects. *J Blood Med* 2019; 10: 93.
Dowd PM. Cold-related disorders. *Prog Dermatol* 1987; 21: 1.
Frank M, Atkinson JP, Gadek J. Cold agglutinins and cold agglutinin disease. *Annu Rev Med* 1977; 28: 291.

Colitis

Colitis or enterocolitis occurs in a number of forms.
1. **Ulcerative colitis** and **Crohn's disease** (granulomatous colitis)
   See Inflammatory bowel disease.
2. **Ischaemic colitis**

This most commonly affects the distal colon in elderly patients, in whom it presents as blood-stained diarrhoea without mucus.

The process may resolve within 48 hr (though subsequent stricture may occur), or it may progress very rapidly to a fatal outcome, often despite surgery.

3. ***Clostridium difficile* infection** (q.v.).

This is typically an antibiotic-associated colitis. It was originally named pseudomembranous colitis. More recently, it has been called *Clostridium difficile*-associated diarrhoea (CDAD) and most recently *Clostridioides difficile* infection.

4. **Infective enterocolitis**

This may be due to
- campylobacter,
- staphylococci,
- *Escherichia coli* (e.g. O157:H7 strain which can cause haemorrhagic diarrhoea) (see Enteropathogenic *E. coli*).

See Diarrhoea.

5. **Irritable bowel syndrome**

Irritable bowel syndrome (IBS) has sometimes been referred to as mucous colitis or spastic colitis. It is a form of visceral hypersensitivity (see Microbiome).

IBS may be distinguished from syndromes associated with bowel inflammation by a negative faecal

calprotectin test (q.v.), negative coeliac serology (see Coeliac disease) and validated clinical criteria. Non-pharmacological therapies are generally effective, including dietary modification (e.g. restricting FODMAPS – q.v.), some forms of psychotherapy, some types of complementary medicines (e.g. peppermint oil and the herbal preparation, iberogast) and possibly probiotics.

Bibliography

Antonelli M, Martin-Loeches I, Dimopoulos G, et al. Clostrdioides difficile (formerly *Clostridium difficile*) infection in the critically ill: an expert statement. *Intens Care Med* 2020; 46: 215.

Blaser MJ, Smith PD, Ravdin JL, et al., eds. *Infections of the Gastrointestinal Tract*. 2nd edition. New York: Raven Press. 2002.

Bobo LD, Dubberke ER, Kollef M. *Clostridium difficile* in the ICU. *Chest* 2011; 140: 1643.

Field M, Rao MC, Chang EB. Intestinal electrolyte transport and diarrheal disease. *N Engl J Med* 1989; 321: 800 & 879.

Guery B, Galperine T, Barbut F. Clostridioides difficile: diagnosis and treatments. *BMJ* 2019; 366: l4609.

Guy AY, Kutty PK. Clostridioides difficile infection. *Ann Intern Med* 2018; 169: ITC49.

Hickson M, D'Souza AL, Muthu N, et al. Use of probiotic *Lactobacillus* preparation to prevent diarrhoea associated with antibiotics: randomized double blind placebo controlled trial. *BMJ* 2007; 335: 80.

Johnson S, Clabots CR, Linn FV, et al. Nosocomial *Clostridium difficile* colonization and disease. *Lancet* 1990; 336: 97.

Leffler DA, Lamont JT. *Clostridium difficile* infection. *N Engl J Med* 2015; 372: 1539.

Linedale EC, Andrews JM. Diagnosis and management of irritable bowel syndrome: a guide for the generalist. *Med J Aust* 2017; 207: 309.

Loo VG, Bourgault AM, Poirier L, et al. Host and pathogen factors for *Clostridium difficile* infection and colonization. *N Engl J Med* 2011; 365: 1693.

Moayyedi P, Yuan Y, Baharith H, et al. Faecal microbiota transplantation for *Clostridium difficile*-associated diarrhoea: a systematic review of randomised controlled trials. *Med J Aust* 2017; 207: 166.

Pochapin M. The effect of probiotics in *Clostridium difficile* diarrhea. *Am J Gastroenterol* 2000; 95: S11.

Schlager TA, Guerrant RL. Seven possible mechanisms for Escherichia coli diarrhea. *Infect Dis Clin North Am* 1988; 2: 607.

Soo WT, Bryant RV, Costello SP. Faecal microbiota transplantation: indications, evidence and safety. *Aust Prescriber* 2020 43: 36.

Trubiano JA, Cheng AC, Korman TM, et al. Australasian Society of Infectious Diseases updated guidelines for the management of *Clostridium difficile* infection in adults and children in Australia and New Zealand. *Intern Med J* 2016; 46: 479.

van Rheenen PF, van de Vijver E, Fidler V. Faecal calprotectin for screening of patients with suspected inflammatory bowel disease: diagnostic meta-analysis. *BMJ* 2010; 341: c3369.

van Langenberg DR, Gearry RB, Wong H-L, et al. The potential value of faecal lactoferrin as a screening test in hospitalized patients with diarrhoea. *Intern Med J* 2010; 40: 819.

Collagen-vascular diseases See

- Connective tissue diseases.

Complement deficiency

The **complement** system is one of the four plasma enzyme cascades (with the coagulation, fibrinolysis and kinin systems) which together are involved in the bodily responses to injury (see also Coagulation disorders).

In particular, the complement system provides the major link between the process of inflammation and the immune system. It is thus involved not only in host resistance to infection, both immunological and non-specific, but also in the mechanisms of tissue injury.

The 18 plasma proteins of the complement system produce components which kill viruses and bacteria and which regulate white cell chemotaxis and phagocytosis, mediator release, solubilization of immune complexes, smooth muscle contraction and cell lysis. There is a complex nomenclature.

Activation occurs via either the **classical** or the **alternative** pathway, each resulting in the cleavage of C3 and the initiation of a common terminal sequence which results in the lytic complex (C5b67 with C8 and C9, i.e. C5b-9).

- The **classical pathway** is activated by immune complexes (containing IgG or IgM antibody). Deficiencies of this pathway thus predispose to immune complex disease (q.v.).
- The **alternative pathway** (or properdin) is activated directly by bacteria or other cells. Deficiencies of this pathway thus predispose to bacterial infection.

As with coagulation, the components of the two pathways undergo a controlled but amplified cascade of limited proteolysis leading to the production of active fragments, many of which have biological activity in their own right, most notably C5a. C5a produces neutrophil chemotaxis, activation and aggregation, a process which can occur to excess in some conditions and give rise to cell damage, e.g. pulmonary endothelial cell damage and acute respiratory distress syndrome (ARDS).

> Like other immune processes both humoral and cellular and indeed other biological responses to injury, complement is a classical double-edged sword which, while geared to provide defence against infection, can cause host damage under certain circumstances of excessive local or systemic activation. The C5 monoclonal antibody, *eculizumab* (q.v.), is effective in blocking the adverse effects of pathological activation of complement in a number of conditions.

Complement deficiency may be inherited or acquired.

Inherited deficiencies in general predispose to either immune complex disease (the classical pathway) or bacterial infection (the alternative pathway).

There are 15 described abnormalities of complement, 14 associated with disease.
- C1–INH with HAE, i.e. hereditary angioedema (q.v.),
- C1, C4, C2 with autoimmune disease (q.v.), especially systemic lupus erythematosus (q.v.),
- C3, factor D, control proteins I and H with bacterial infections,
- properdin, C5–9 with *Neisseria* infections.

Acquired complement deficiency is secondary to overt activation. This form of hypocomplementaemia is associated with, and perhaps related to, some cases of
- adult respiratory distress syndrome (q.v.),
- septic shock,
- cellular damage from extracorporeal circuits,
- haemolysis,
- vasculitis (q.v.).

The laboratory assessment of complement deficiency is most commonly by antigenic assay of C3 and C4 levels and by functional assay of the entire classical pathway as total haemolytic complement (THC).

Bibliography
Colten HR, Rosen FS. Complement deficiencies. *Annu Rev Immunol* 1992; 10: 809.
Conway EM. Reincarnation of ancient links between coagulation and complement. *J Thromb Haemost* 2015; 13: S121.
Schifferli JA, Ng YC, Peters DK. The role of complement and its receptors in the elimination of immune complexes. *N Engl J Med* 1986; 315: 488.
Tomlinson S. Complement defense mechanisms. *Curr Opin Immunol* 1993; 5: 83.
Van de Meer JWM, Kullberg BJ. Defects in host-defense mechanisms. In: Rubin RH, Young LS, eds. *Clinical Approach to Infections in the Compromised Host*. 4th edition. New York: Plenum. 2002.

Conjunctivitis

> **Conjunctivitis** and keratoconjunctivitis may be
> - allergic,
> - infective,
> - associated with specific diseases.

Allergic conjunctivitis is a common condition and is the eye equivalent of allergic rhinitis. It is thus a seasonal, IgE-mediated condition, with bilateral redness, swelling and itch.

The differential diagnosis from herpetic conjunctivitis is important because corticosteroids are contraindicated in the latter condition. The other differential diagnoses include other infective or contact-induced inflammation.

Treatments shown to be effective, apart from **local corticosteroids**, *include* **topical NSAIDs** *(e.g. ketorolac) and* **intranasal corticosteroids**.

Infective conjunctivitis may be caused by viruses, bacteria or *Chlamydia trachomatis* (when typically there is associated genital infection).
- The common viruses are adenovirus or herpes simplex virus. Enterovirus 70, the Newcastle disease virus of poultry, can give a haemorrhagic conjunctivitis in humans.
- The common bacteria are gonococci, haemophilus, meningococci and staphylococci.
- Infective conjunctivitis may also occur in systemic infectious diseases, such as measles and typhus.

Specific diseases associated with conjunctivitis include several systemic disorders, including
- Behcet's syndrome (q.v.),
- exophthalmos (q.v.),
- Reiter's syndrome (q.v.),
- Stevens–Johnson syndrome (q.v.),
- toxic shock syndrome (q.v.).

In addition, keratoconjunctivitis is a major local feature of the sicca syndrome (Sjogren's syndrome – q.v.).

Bibliography
Owen CG, Shah A, Henshaw K, et al. Topical treatment for seasonal allergic conjunctivitis: systematic review and meta-analysis of efficacy and effectiveness. *Br J Gen Pract* 2004; 54: 451.

Connective tissue diseases

Connective tissue diseases (or **collagen-vascular diseases**) are terms commonly used to describe a group of disparate clinical syndromes with certain features in common, such as widespread inflammation and fibrinoid deposition in connective tissue, involvement of joints, blood vessels, skin, muscles and other organs, and commonly systemic symptoms. They are usually presumed to have an autoimmune basis.

These conditions may nowadays be referred to as **diffuse undifferentiated systemic rheumatic disease**. This is typically manifest by Raynaud's phenomenon (q.v.), polyarthritis (q.v.) and rash, and it comprises about 25% of all rheumatic diseases.

The umbrella of connective tissue diseases also used to include more specific rheumatic diseases, including rheumatoid arthritis, systemic lupus erythematosus, scleroderma, polyarteritis nodosa, polymyositis/dermatomyositis, Sjogren's syndrome, Behcet's syndrome, mixed connective tissue disease and overlap syndromes. These conditions are considered separately in this book.

In addition, there are a number of **hereditary connective tissue disorders**, including Ehlers–Danlos syndrome, Marfan's syndrome (q.v.) and pseudoxanthoma elasticum.

See
- Autoimmune disorders,
- Rheumatic diseases.

Conn's syndrome

Conn's syndrome comprises hypertension and hypokalaemia due to excess adrenal production of aldosterone (q.v.). It is often referred to as **primary aldosteronism**.

It is caused by any one of five conditions, namely,
- **benign unilateral adrenal adenoma** (most commonly). Up to 10% of cases are now recognized to be due to a gene mutation.
- **bilateral adrenal hyperplasia** (less commonly). This condition is probably pituitary in origin.
- **adrenal carcinoma** (rarely). This is usually an aggressive cancer.
- **genetic variant** (rarely). This is inherited as an autosomal dominant, in which an abnormal gene product presumably has combined synthetic enzyme activities, so that excess aldosterone is dependent on ACTH and not on angiotensin. This variant responds paradoxically to corticosteroids.
- **liquorice** ingestion in excess (>0.5 kg per week). This occurs because glycyrrhizic acid inhibits the renal inactivation of aldosterone and is thus salt-retaining (see Liquorice). This condition is sometimes called **pseudo primary aldosteronism**.

Conn's syndrome is thus an uncommon (but not rare) cause of secondary hypertension. While aldosterone causes salt and water retention and thus acute hypervolaemic hypertension, the mechanism for sustained hypertension in this setting is unknown. Nevertheless, Conn's syndrome is usually discovered from screening hypertensive patients who have a borderline or low serum potassium level or who have difficult blood pressure control.

The hypokalaemia may be asymptomatic, though it may be associated with cardiac arrhythmias, muscle weakness, insulin-resistant glucose intolerance and polyuria due to a renal tubular defect. There is also an excessive proneness to hypokalaemia following diuretic therapy.

Investigations should be performed with the patient off any medication containing diuretics, beta blockers, calcium channel blockers and ACE inhibitors.
- There is a high 24-hr urinary potassium excretion (at least 30 mmol despite hypokalaemia).
- Provided the patient is not hypokalaemic at the time of testing (since hypokalaemia can suppress aldosterone biosynthesis), there is a high plasma aldosterone level (>450 pmol/L) and a suppressed plasma renin activity (<1 mcg/L). Autonomous aldosterone secretion is demonstrated by failure of its suppression by sodium loading (2 L of isotonic saline over 4 hr), by fludrocortisone (0.4 mg per day for 3 days) or by captopril (25 mg).
- The specific lesion should be localized with CT scanning, adrenal vein sampling if necessary and occasionally adrenal scintigraphy.

*Treatment is with **adrenalectomy**. Spironolactone should be used preoperatively and also for continuing medical treatment of bilateral hyperplasia.*

*Recently, the aldosterone receptor antagonist, **eplerenone**, has been used successfully in patients unable to tolerate spironolactone.*

Bibliography
Blumenfeld JD, Sealey JE, Schlussel Y, et al. Diagnosis and treatment of primary hyperaldosteronism. *Ann Intern Med* 1994; 121: 877.

Editorial. Corticosteroids and hypothalamic-pituitary-adrenocortical function. *BMJ* 1980; 280: 813.

Gittler RD, Fajans SS. Primary aldosteronism (Conn's syndrome). *J Clin Endocrinol Metab* 1995; 80: 3438.

Melby JC. Diagnosis of hyperaldosteronism. *Endocrinol Metab Clin North Am* 1991; 20: 247.

Quinn SJ, Williams GH. Regulation of aldosterone secretion. *Ann Rev Physiol* 1988; 50: 409.

Yang J, Fuller PJ, Stowasser M. Is it time to screen all patients with hypertension for primary aldosteronism? *Med J Aust* 2018; 209: 57.

Constipation

Constipation is the opposite of diarrhoea, and like diarrhoea it is also a common finding in seriously ill patients. It is usually due to drugs (particularly opioids) or to lack of enteral food intake (particularly fibre). On the Bristol Stool Form Scale, it is represented by types 1 and 2. Its management requires good bowel care planning and is part of sound Intensive Care practice.

See also
- Diarrhoea.

Bibliography

Black CJ, Ford AC. Chronic idiopathic constipation in adults: epidemiology, pathophysiology, diagnosis and clinical management. *Med J Aust* 2018; 209: 86.

Copper

Copper (Cu, atomic number 29, atomic weight 64) is a red ductile metal. Since it is found free in nature, it was used as the first metal substitute for stone implements from about 8000 BC and was subsequently combined with tin to form bronze. It may also be combined with zinc to form brass and with zinc and nickel to form nickel silver. Since it is a very good conductor of heat and electricity, its greatest use is in the electrical industry and in alloys.

Copper is chiefly ingested from shellfish or animal organs. Most of the body's copper (100–150 mg) is found in the liver, where it is attached to copper-binding proteins or present in metalloenzymes. These play a key role in mitochondrial function, collagen and elastin cross-linking, and melatonin production. It is thus one of the body's essential trace elements (q.v.).

In the plasma, copper is mostly bound to caeruloplasmin, and the normal serum copper is 11–24 µmol/L. The normal daily requirements are 300–1000 mcg per day orally and the recommended IV dose is 5–20 µmol per day. These doses should be increased if there are excessive gastrointestinal losses and decreased if there is hepatobiliary disease.

The serum copper level is increased by oestrogens, since they increase caeruloplasmin. Increased serum copper is also seen in lymphoma and Wilson's disease (see below).

Caeruloplasmin (CP) is an enzyme which is synthesized in the liver. In addition to its role in the transport of copper (as above), it is also an acute phase reactant, and it may participate in processes which underlie a host of serious illnesses, particularly cardiovascular disease.

Copper deficiency is uncommon. It occurs primarily with prolonged gastrointestinal losses, since it is normally excreted via the bile. Copper deficiency gives rise to anaemia and leukopenia, and rarely to myelopathy (q.v.).

Acute **copper toxicity** is uncommon. It results either from ingestion of contaminated water or food or from deliberate overdose. A dose of 10 g or more can be lethal if untreated, and severe toxicity is seen at serum levels of 80 µmol/L or more.

Clinical features include nausea, vomiting, salivation, abdominal pain and diarrhoea. Haemolysis, jaundice and acute renal failure are commonly seen. Hypotension, arrhythmias and coma may occur.

*Treatment with a **chelating agent** (q.v.) is recommended, as there are reports of the effective use of EDTA and penicillamine.*

Wilson's disease is a rare autosomal recessive disorder with a prevalence of about 1 in 30,000 of the population. It is due to a defect on chromosome 13, resulting in impaired excretion of copper into the bile. Copper thus accumulates in the tissues, especially in the liver and brain, giving rise to 'hepatolenticular degeneration'.

Clinical manifestations are usually apparent by early adulthood with
- hepatosplenomegaly,
- abnormal liver function tests,
- haemolysis,
- neurological deterioration (clumsiness, tremor, rigidity, dysarthria and personality changes),
- pathognomonic Kayser–Fleischer corneal rings, which are thin, brown and peripheral.

Investigations show a low or absent serum caeruloplasmin, increased urinary copper and increased hepatic copper.

*Treatment is with **penicillamine** (see Chelating agents). This binds copper and enhances its urinary excretion up to 3-fold. The usual dose is 1–3 g per day.*
- Concomitant **pyridoxine** 50 mg/week is required.
- *If penicillamine is not tolerated, oral zinc (which reduces copper absorption) or tetrathiomolybdate may be used.*

- *Treatment should be commenced gradually, as too rapid mobilization of copper can lead to acute encephalopathy or hepatotoxicity.*

Bibliography
Barcelouz DG. Copper. *J Toxicol Clin Toxicol* 1999; 37: 217.
Chelly J, Monaco AP. Cloning the Wilson disease gene. *Nature Genetics* 1993; 5: 317.
Ferenci P. Wilson's disease. *Clin Liver Dis* 1998; 2: 31.
Gaetke LM, Chow CK. Copper toxicity, oxidative stress, and antioxidant nutrients. *Toxicology* 2003; 189: 147.
Gitlin N. Wilson's disease: the scourge of copper. *J Hepatol* 1998; 28: 734.
Lazarchick J. Update on anaemia and neutropenia in copper deficiency. *Curr Opin Hematol* 2012; 19: 58.
Scheinberg IH, Sternlieb I. Wilson's disease. *Annu Rev Med* 1965; 16: 119.
Schilsky ML. Wilson disease: genetic basis of copper toxicity and natural history. *Semin Liver Dis* 1996; 16: 83.
Sternlieb I. Perspectives on Wilson's disease. *Hepatology* 1990; 12: 1234.
Strickland GT, Leu M. Wilson's disease – clinical and laboratory manifestations in 40 patients. *Medicine* 1975; 54: 113.
Wilson SAK. Progressive lenticular degeneration. A familial nervous disease associated with cirrhosis of the liver. *Brain* 1912; 34: 295.
Yarze JC, Martin P, Munoz SJ, et al. Wilson's disease: current status. *Am J Med* 1992; 92: 643.

Coronavirus

Coronavirus infection is ubiquitous, as it is one of the commonest causes of the common cold. The responsible virus is named HCoV.

However, more pathogenic forms of this virus have in recent years been responsible for the **severe acute respiratory syndrome** (SARS) (q.v.), the **Middle East respiratory syndrome** (MERS) (q.v.) and currently the **COVID-19** epidemic. The responsible coronaviruses have been named, respectively, SARS-CoV, MERS-CoV and SARS-CoV-2 (originally 2019 nCoV).

These pathogens all originated most probably in bats. The consequent infections have many clinical features in common with influenza (q.v.).

Within 2 yr of the onset of the present pandemic, there have been over 300 million confirmed cases and 6 million deaths worldwide, and there have also been over 100,000 published studies (including nearly 600 RCTs and over 6000 systematic reviews) – a truly monumental human experience.

Bibliography
Bond K, Williams E, Howden BP, et al. Serological tests for COVID-19. *Med J Aust* 2020; 213: 397.
Fischetti M, ed. Inside the coronavirus. *Sci Am* 2020; 323: 28.
Iba T, Levy JH, Levi M, et al. Coagulopathy of coronavirus disease 2019. *Crit Care Med* 2020; 48: 1358.
Jevremovic V, Ison MG. Coronaviruses: HCOV, SARS-COV, MERS-COV, and COVID-19. In: *Scientific American Medicine. Infectious Diseases*. Hamilton: Dekker Medicine. 2020.
Thevarajan I, Buising KL, Cowie BC. Clinical presentation and management of COVID-19. *Med J Aust* 2020; 213: 134.
Tsang JLY, Binnie A, Fowler RA. Twenty articles that critical care clinicians should read about COVID-19. *Intens Care Med* 2021; 47: 337.
Various. COVID-19: implications for health care. *Med J Aust* 2020; 212: no. 10.
Various. The coronavirus pandemic. *Sci Am* 2020; 322: no. 6.
Various. Special section on COVID-19. *Intens Care Med* 2020; 46: no. 6.
Various. Multiple articles on COVID-19. *Intens Care Med* 2020; 46: no. 8.
Various. How COVID changed the world. *Sci Am* 2022; 326: no. 3.

Costochondritis *See*
- Chest wall disorders.

Coturnism

Coturnism is a rare syndrome of muscle damage with weakness and rhabdomyolysis (q.v.) caused by eating the common quail (*Coturnix* species) which have fed on plants that are poisonous to humans but not to the bird itself.

See also
- Food poisoning.

Cough

Cough is a complex but common event which can be viewed in differing ways:
- as a mechanism of airway defence,
- as a symptom of varying severity and significance,
- as a mechanism for the spread of infection, and even
- as an auto-resuscitation manoevre in serious acute arrhythmias.

In Intensive Care practice, the failure of intubated patients to be able to clear their tracheobronchial secretions by coughing requires appropriate suctioning and may be a factor in some cases of delayed extubation.

In non-intubated patients, although persistent cough is often unexplained and can present particular treatment challenges, consensus guidelines have been published concerning its management, although these have been criticized for their variability and low evidence base.

See also
- Angiotensin-converting enzyme.

Bibliography

Canning BJ, Chang AB, Bolser DC, et al. Anatomy and neurophysiology of cough: CHEST guideline and expert panel report. *Chest* 2014; 146: 1633.

Gibson P, Wang G, McGarvey L, et al. Treatment of unexplained chronic cough: CHEST guideline and expert panel report. *Chest* 2016; 149: 27.

Irwin RS, French CT, Lewis SZ, et al. Overview of the management of cough: CHEST guideline and expert panel report. *Chest* 2014; 146: 885.

Jiang M, Guan W-j, Fang Z-f, et al. A critical review of the quality of cough clinical practice guidelines. *Chest* 2016; 150: 777.

Lee KK, Davenport PW, Smith JA, et al. Global physiology and pathophysiology of cough: part 1: cough phenomenology – CHEST guideline and expert panel report. *Chest* 2021; 159: 282.

COVID-19 *See*
- Coronavirus.

C-reactive protein

C-reactive protein (CRP) is a plasma protein of the pentraxin type, with a stable ring structure of five monomers and a molecular weight of about 115 kDa. It is the originally described 'acute phase' reactant and was given its name in 1930 because of the serological reaction with the polysaccharide C fraction of pneumococci noted in patients with pneumonia.

As CRP is highly conserved across vertebrate species, it presumably has a useful role in host defence, and indeed it is the only acute phase protein involved in the clearance of microorganisms, a process which it assists by its ability to bind to microbial polysaccharide and activate complement. Its plasma level is genetically determined, and several polymorphisms have been described (though without identified clinical implications).

Like other acute phase proteins, it is rapidly synthesized in the liver in response to cytokine stimulation, particularly by interleukin 6 (IL-6). Its level can rise 100-fold within 36–48 hr. In normal subjects, the plasma concentration is <10 mg/L, with a mean of about 1 mg/L. In patients with sepsis, it can rise to 500 mg/L or more, with the best discrimination between the presence and absence of infection found at about 50 mg/L. Since its half-life is about 6 hours, its level rapidly declines with resolution of inflammation. Its response may be reduced in liver disease and increased in renal disease.

There has been a great resurgence of interest in CRP as a marker of sepsis, since its biochemical characterization permitted the development of fast, accurate and cheap immunoassays. It is currently regarded as one of the best of the non-specific markers of sepsis (like procalcitonin – q.v.), having displaced the role of ESR measurement in this setting. In particular, serial changes reflect resolution or otherwise of the underlying process, and thus may assist decisions about antibiotic response, duration of therapy and prognosis.

Of course, while CRP is elevated in most infections from any microorganism, it is also expected to be increased in cases of major trauma, necrosis, malignancy and non-infective inflammation (e.g. pancreatitis).

Its level when assayed by high sensitivity methods has also been found to be predictive of acute coronary events in patients with cardiovascular disease. Presumably, this phenomenon reflects the increasingly recognized role of inflammation in the genesis of cardiovascular disease and of the metabolic syndrome in particular. However, the utility of CRP measurements in this area is so far confined to population studies and not to individual assessment.

See
- Biomarkers,
- Pyrexia.

See also
- Calcitonin – Procalcitonin.

Bibliography

Black S, Kushner I, Samols D. C-reactive protein. *J Biol Chem* 2004; 279: 48487.

Gabay C, Kushner I. Acute phase proteins and other systemic responses to inflammation. *N Engl J Med* 1999; 340: 448.

Harrison M. Erythrocyte sedimentation rate and C-reactive protein. *Aust Prescriber* 2015; 38: 93.

Ho KM, Lipman J. An update on C-reactive protein for intensivists. *Anaesth Intens Care* 2009; 37: 234.

Pepys MB. C-reactive protein fifty years on. *Lancet* 1981; I: 653.

Pepys MB, Berger A. The renaissance of C-reactive protein. *BMJ* 2001; 322: 4.

Povoa P. C-reactive protein: a valuable marker of sepsis. *Intens Care Med* 2002; 28: 235.

Reny J-L, Vuagnat A, Ract C, et al. Diagnosis and follow-up of infections in intensive care patients: value of C-reactive protein compared with other clinical and biological variables. *Crit Care Med* 2002; 30: 529.

Ridker PM, Bassuk SS, Toth PP. C-reactive protein and risk of cardiovascular disease. *Curr Atherosclerosis Rep* 2003; 5: 341.

CREST syndrome *See*
- Scleroderma.

Creutzfeldt–Jakob disease

Creutzfeldt–Jakob disease (CJ disease, CJD) is an encephalopathy due to infection with a small transmissible proteinaceous particle called a prion. It is the human form of transmissible dementia, generally transmitted in nature by ingestion of infected animal tissues. It is related to the human disease, **kuru**, and to the animal diseases, **scrapie** and **bovine spongiform encephalopathy** (BSE, 'mad cow disease'). Its incidence is 1–2 in 1 million of the population per year.

It is still a mystery how a variant of a normal cell membrane protein (albeit as yet with no known function) without RNA or DNA can be an infectious agent. Moreover, there is no detectable serological response. At all events, insoluble aggregates of misfolded prion protein (PrP) appear responsible for the amyloid plaques and fibrils seen in the brains of infected subjects. Presumably, there has been a mutation in the PrP gene on chromosome 20 in non-iatrogenic cases.

Most cases are sporadic, but a few cases are familial (about 10%). Some are iatrogenic (perhaps 200 cases worldwide) and have occurred particularly in middle-aged patients who have had surgery (especially neurosurgery) or trauma. It has also been reported in patients formerly given the human pituitary-derived hormones, growth hormone for short stature or gonadotrophin for infertility, between 1960 and 1985. It may possibly occur after ingestion of animal brains (and perhaps other tissues of infected animals), since ritualistic cannibalism of human brains was the practice which used to lead to kuru.

A variant form (nvCJD) was reported in a cluster of cases among young patients in the UK, with 95 cases by 2001. It followed the epidemic of BSE which commenced in 1986 in that country (and reached its peak in 1992) and has been shown to be caused by the same strain of transmissible agent as BSE. There was concern about its potential transmission from apparently healthy persons incubating the disease to others via blood, blood products, organ donation or instrumentation, and there is epidemiological evidence that this may have occurred in a patient after blood transfusion, with a latent period of 6.5 years.

The incubation period has been reported to be 1–3 years in patients with a single definable culprit event, but it is perhaps much longer in some patients. The patient is infectious during this time.

Clinical features comprise rapidly progressive dementia, together with myoclonus and pyramidal, extrapyramidal and cerebellar signs. Cerebellar signs are dominant in the familial variant referred to as Gerstmann–Straussler syndrome.

The CSF is normal on routine examination, but more sophisticated testing may show an abnormal 14–3–3 protein. The CT scan shows cerebral atrophy, and the EEG may show triphasic forms. The diagnosis can only be made histologically, with the demonstration of spongiform changes (neuronal vacuolation), astrocyte proliferation, neuronal loss and amyloid plaques, but no inflammatory response. Genetic screening for PrP gene variants (and thus susceptibility to exogenous prion infection) is now possible.

There is no effective treatment.

The outcome is always fatal, after a clinical illness of about 6 months.

The following points are of importance in Intensive Care practice.
- Special care needs to be taken in handling potentially infectious material.
  - The infectious agent may be present widely throughout the body.
  - Importantly, it is not inactivated by routine techniques used to destroy nucleic acids, namely boiling, irradiation, ethylene oxide, glutaral (glutaraldehyde), formalin, alcohol or iodine.
  - It is however inactivated by prolonged autoclaving or by sodium hydroxide or hypochlorite.
- Due to difficulties in diagnosis, the human prion diseases may be more common than previously thought.
  - Moreover, most body tissues and fluids may be infectious for prolonged periods.
  - This has adverse implications for blood, tissue and organ donation and transplantation.

Detailed updated infection control guidelines have been published, with a particular focus on potential iatrogenic transmission.

Bibliography

Andrews NJ, Farrington CP, Cousens SN, et al. Incidence of variant Creutzfeldt-Jakob disease in the UK. *Lancet* 2000; 356: 481.

Beale AJ. BSE and vCJD: what is the future? *J R Soc Med* 2001; 94: 207.

Beale AJ. More on BSE/vCJD. *J R Soc Med* 2001; 94: 611.

Brown P, Cervenakova L, Goldfarb LG, et al. Iatrogenic Creutzfeldt-Jakob disease: an example of the interplay between ancient genes and modern medicine. *Neurology* 1994; 44: 291.

Brown P, Will RG, Bradley R, et al. Bovine spongiform encephalopathy and variant Creutzfeldt-Jakob disease: background, evolution and current concerns. *Emerg Infect Dis* 2001; 7: 1.

Bruce ME, Will RG, Ironside JW, et al. Transmissions of mice indicate that 'new variant' CJD is caused by the BSE agent. *Nature* 1997; 389: 448.

Collins SJ, Lawson VA, Masters CL. Transmissible spongiform encephalopathy. *Lancet* 2004; 363: 51.

Collins S, Masters CL. Iatrogenic and zoonotic Creutzfeldt-Jakob disease. *Med J Aust* 1996; 164: 598.

DeArmond SJ. Overview of the transmissible spongiform encephalopathies: prion protein disorders. *Br Med Bull* 1993; 49: 725.

Edney ATB. Spongiform encephalopathies: still many unanswered questions. *J R Soc Med* 1996; 89: 423.

Hill AF, Butterworth RJ, Joiner S, et al. Investigation of variant Creutzfeldt-Jakob disease and other prion diseases with tonsil biopsy samples. *Lancet* 200; 353: 183.

Holman RC, Khan AS, Belay ED, et al. Creutzfeldt-Jakob disease in the United States, 1979–1994: using national mortality data to assess the possible occurrence of variant cases. *Emerg Infect Dis* 1996; 2: 4.

Ironside JW, Head MW. Variant Creutzfeldt-Jakob disease and its transmission by blood. J *Thromb Haemost* 2003; 1: 1479.

Koehler AP, Athan E, Collins SJ. Updated Creutzfeldt-Jakob disease infection control guidelines: sifting facts from fiction. *Med J Aust* 2013; 198: 245.

Llewelyn CA, Hewitt PE, Knight RS, et al. Possible transmission of variant Creutzfeldt-Jakob disease by blood transfusion. *Lancet* 2004; 363: 417.

Masters CL. The emerging European epidemic of variant Creutzfeldt-Jakob disease and bovine spongiform encephalopathy. *Med J Aust* 2001; 174: 160.

Mitchell AR. Creutzfeldt-Jakob disease. *Lancet* 1996; 347: 1704.

Parchi P, Castellani R, Capellari S, et al. Molecular basis of phenotypic variability in sporadic Creutzfeldt-Jakob disease. *Ann Neurol* 1996; 39: 767.

Pattison J. The emergence of bovine spongiform encephalopathy and related diseases. *Emerg Infect Dis* 1998; 4: 3.

Prusiner SB. Molecular biology of prion disease. *Science* 1991; 252: 1515.

Prusiner SB, Hsiao KK. Human prion diseases. *Ann Neurol* 1994; 35: 385.

Venters GA. New variant Creutzfeldt-Jakob disease: the epidemic that never was. *BMJ* 2001; 323: 858.

Will RG. Gene influence on Creutzfeldt-Jakob disease. *Lancet* 1994; 344: 1310.

Will RG, Ironside JW, Zeidler M, et al. A new variant of Creutzfeldt-Jakob disease in the UK. *Lancet* 1996; 347: 921.

Wilson K, Code C, Ricketts MN. Risk of acquiring Creutzfeldt-Jakob disease from blood transfusions. *BMJ* 2000; 321: 17.

Zerr I, Schulz-Schaeffer WJ, Giese A, et al. Current clinical diagnosis in Creutzfeldt-Jakob disease: identification of uncommon variants. *Ann Neurol* 2000; 48: 323.

Cricoarytenoid arthritis

The cricoarytenoid joints may be affected in rheumatoid arthritis, as may the temporomandibular joints. The condition is often mild and asymptomatic.

Cricoarytenoid arthritis, if severe, is one of the causes of upper airway obstruction and can thus be especially relevant in Intensive Care.
- Acutely,
  - there is stridor, hoarseness and dysphagia,
  - sometimes, there is pain radiating to the ear,
  - the larynx is tender, and the arytenoids are red and swollen at laryngoscopy.
- Chronically,
  - there may also be stridor or hoarseness due to ankylosis of these joints.

See
- Asthma – Stridor.

Bibliography
Montgomery WW. Cricoarytenoid arthritis. *Laryngoscope* 1963; 73: 801.

Critical illness myopathy *See*
- Myopathy.

Critical illness neuromuscular abnormality

Critical illness neuromuscular abnormality (CINMA) is also referred to as **ICU-acquired weakness.**

Weakness acquired in the ICU is generally multifactorial, with critical illness, immobility and certain medications recognized as precipitating factors. The weakness can persist long after discharge from ICU, and the consequent physical deconditioning is one of the important complications leading to delayed functional recovery in some patients. It thus forms part of the condition sometimes referred to as **post–Intensive Care syndrome** (q.v.).

CINMA is a global term, and its components can include both **critical illness myopathy** (q.v.) and **critical illness polyneuropathy** (q.v.), as well as overlap syndromes. Weakness in ICU patients may also be due to an underlying or primary condition, such as myasthenia gravis (q.v.), motor neuron disease (q.v.), myelopathy (q.v.), neuropathy (e.g. Guillain–Barré syndrome) (q.v.).

See
- Myopathy – Acute necrotizing myopathy, Critical illness myopathy,
- Neuropathy – Polyneuropathy (5. Critical illness neuropathy).

Bibliography

Jolley SE, Bunnell AE, Hough CL. ICU-acquired weakness. *Chest* 2016; 150: 1129.

Kress JP, Hall JB. ICU-acquired weakness and recovery from critical illness. *N Engl J Med* 2014; 370: 1626.

Vanhorebeek I, Latronico N, Van den Berghe G. ICU-acquired weakness. *Intens Care Med* 2020; 46: 637.

Critical illness polyneuropathy See
- Neuropathy.

Crohn's disease See
- Inflammatory bowel disease.

Crustaceans

Crustaceans are one of the main groups of arthropods (q.v.). They have five pairs of legs. They are important in human disease because they may harbour pathogenic organisms involved in hepatitis (q.v.), norovirus (q.v.), paragonimiasis (q.v.) and paralytic shellfish poisoning (q.v.).

Cryoglobulinaemia See
- Multiple myeloma.

Cryptococcosis

Cryptococcosis (torulosis) is a systemic disease caused by the yeast-like organism *C. neoformans*. The organism is found worldwide, usually in avian excreta, especially from pigeons. Exposure to inhaled particles and thus asymptomatic infection is probably very common, with clinical infection occurring mostly from either massive exposure or in compromised hosts, especially those with impaired cell-mediated immunity. Nowadays therefore the condition is mostly seen in patients with AIDS (q.v.). The pathogenesis is probably similar to that of tuberculosis (q.v.) or other mycoses, and the pulmonary effects are chiefly due to a mass rather than to the virulence of the microorganism.

Perhaps up to a third of documented cases and presumably a higher proportion of total cases are asymptomatic, despite even extensive X-ray changes. In the others, there are chest symptoms which are chronic and rarely progressive. Occasionally, there may be dissemination to the meninges in compromised hosts. Chronic meningitis or the symptoms of a space-occupying lesion then become apparent. Dissemination elsewhere in the body may also occur, particularly to the skin where ulcerated papules may occur.

The diagnosis is made by demonstrating the presence of the organism or its antigen in blood or CSF. The demonstration of the organism in sputum is non-specific. The CSF in cases of meningitis additionally shows a positive India ink stain in 50% of cases and increased pressure, lymphocytes and protein, and decreased glucose. Biopsy of appropriate material is also diagnostic. Chest X-ray typically shows a mass with or without cavitation, sometimes multiple and occasionally diffuse. Hilar lymphadenopathy is sometimes seen, as is pleural effusion (q.v.).

Treatment is required for extrapulmonary disease in all cases. For pulmonary disease, treatment is required only if the involvement is extensive or the patient is immunocompromised.

- Treatment is with **amphotericin B** to a total of 2–3 g over 6 weeks. If renal function and bone marrow function are normal, the addition of **flucytosine** 10 g per day in divided doses permits a lower dose of amphotericin B and results in fewer failures.
- If pulmonary resection is to be performed, **fluconazole** should be used to prevent associated meningitis, for which there is a 5% risk.

The mortality of cryptococcal meningitis is always 100% without treatment, but it is reduced to about 40% with treatment.

Bibliography
Chang CC, Hall V, Cooper C, et al. Consensus guidelines for the diagnosis and management of cryptococcosis and rare yeast infections in the haematology/oncology setting, 2021. *Intern Med J* 2021; 51: 118.
Nadrous HF, Antonios VS, Terrell CL, et al. Pulmonary cryptococcosis in nonimmunocompromised patients. *Chest* 2003; 124: 2143.

Cushing's syndrome

Cushing's syndrome refers to adrenal cortical hyperactivity.

> Cushing's syndrome is caused by
> - excess adrenal stimulation,
> - intrinsic adrenal overactivity,
> - iatrogenic administration of corticosteroids in pharmacological doses.

1. **Excess adrenal stimulation** arises from excess adrenocorticotropic hormone (ACTH), which may be secreted either by the pituitary (Cushing's disease) or ectopically.
   - Excess pituitary secretion of ACTH causes bilateral adrenal hyperplasia and is responsible for two thirds of the cases of Cushing's syndrome. The original pituitary cause is often unclear because, although there is sometimes an adenoma, some cases are postulated to be due to excess hypothalamic secretion of CRH, causing in turn a hyperplastic response in the pituitary.
   - Ectopic production of ACTH is either from a carcinoma (lung, pancreas, kidney, thymus) or a carcinoid tumour (which can also secrete CRH) (see Paraneoplastic syndromes).
2. **Intrinsic adrenal overactivity** may be due to neoplasia or hyperplasia.
   - Adrenal adenomas usually secrete cortisol only, whereas the uncommon carcinomas if secretory usually release androgens as well.
   - Bilateral non-ACTH-dependent hyperplasia is an unusual entity with several forms, namely
     - macronodular,
     - probably originally pituitary in origin but with nodular autonomy later developing,
     - micronodular,
     - occasionally familial, and thought by some to be due to autoantibodies to ACTH receptors,
     - a food-dependent form, in which adrenal cells inappropriately express gastric inhibitory peptide, GIP, which stimulates cortisol release.
3. The **iatrogenic causes** of Cushing's syndrome are well recognized, but these overt changes are much less common than the subclinical effects of the invariable hypothalamic–pituitary–adrenal suppression which is seen in all patients receiving any but small doses of corticosteroids. This is clearly an important phenomenon in the seriously ill (see Adrenal insufficiency).

The clinical features of Cushing's syndrome include facial plethora, skin fragility with easy bruising and poor wound healing, and susceptibility to infections. Diabetes, hypertension, obesity, osteoporosis, depression, amenorrhoea (q.v.), hirsutism (q.v.), cataracts, glaucoma, pancreatitis (q.v.), oedema, renal calculi, benign intracranial hypertension (q.v.) and hypokalaemia may also occur. Proximal myopathy (q.v.) is also seen and together with osteoporosis and skin fragility represent catabolic changes.

As is well known, many of the clinical features of Cushing's syndrome, such as diabetes, hypertension, obesity and hirsutism, are common in a variety of other settings (e.g. alcoholism).

> An explosive onset of hypokalaemic alkalosis, pigmentation and severe weakness may result from ectopic ACTH produced by a small cell lung carcinoma.

The most usual screening test is the dexamethasone suppression test, in which following dexamethasone 1 mg orally at midnight, the serum cortisol level at 9 a.m. is >140 nmol/L. Apart from Cushing's syndrome, the level may also be increased (i.e. fail to be suppressed to the normal level by dexamethasone 1 mg) in association with stress, alcohol, oestrogens, depression or Intensive Care. A 24-hr basal urinary free cortisol should also be measured (normal <200 nmol). If both tests are normal, no further testing is required.

Abnormal screening tests have traditionally been confirmed with a 2-day low-dose dexamethasone suppression test, which if normal excludes Cushing's syndrome. More recently, abnormal screening tests have been followed by a high-dose dexamethasone (8 mg) suppression test, with the ACTH level measured before and after.
- If the ACTH level is low (<2 pmol/L), the Cushing's syndrome is of adrenal origin.
- If the ACTH level is normal or more usually high-normal (10–20 pmol/L) and suppressed, the Cushing's syndrome is of pituitary origin.

- If the ACTH level is high (>20 pmol/L) and not suppressed, the Cushing's syndrome is of ectopic origin. However, the plasma ACTH level may be normal even if there is ACTH-dependence, since ACTH precursor or fragments may be responsible, especially in ectopic production.

Following biochemical confirmation of Cushing's syndrome, the primary site should be localized by CT scanning or MRI.

*Treatment is primarily **surgical**.*

- *Pituitary tumours are removed by transphenoidal adenomectomy, which for small tumours has a 90% cure rate, though there is a small risk of postoperative diabetes insipidus or meningitis.*
- *Primary adrenal disorders require unilateral or bilateral adrenalectomy, depending on the nature of the pathology. In the presence of excess pituitary ACTH, bilateral adrenalectomy carries a 10–40% postoperative risk of **Nelson's syndrome** (markedly increased skin pigmentation and pituitary chromophobe tumour with visual defects), though this complication can be prevented by postoperative pituitary irradiation.*
- *After even limited pituitary or adrenal surgery, endocrine function may take up to 2 years to recover, during which time replacement therapy is required.*
- *Since the progesterone antagonist, **mifepristone (RU486)**, also shows glucocorticoid antagonism, it has been used in cases of Cushing's syndrome with reported success. Mifepristone is best known for its use in **medical abortion** (cf. Pregnancy), but it has also been used successfully in settings where progesterone receptors may be pathologically active, as in some cases of **meningioma**.*

See
- Adrenocorticotropic hormone.

See also
- Carcinoid syndrome,
- Cardiac tumours,
- Lung tumours,
- Paraneoplastic syndromes.

Bibliography

Al-Kurd A, Mazeh H. The endocrine system: adrenal glands. In: *Scientific American Medicine. Organ Systems: Anatomy & Physiology.* Hamilton: Dekker Medicine. 2020.

Aron DC, Findling JW, Tyrrell JB. Cushing's disease. *Endocrinol Metab Clin North Am* 1987; 16: 705.

Bertagna X. New causes of Cushing's syndrome. *N Engl J Med* 1992; 327: 1024.

Editorial. Corticosteroids and hypothalamic-pituitary-adrenocortical function. *BMJ* 1980; 280: 813.

Jeffcoate WJ. Treating Cushing's disease. *BMJ* 1988; 296: 227.

Johanssen S, Allolio B. Mifepristone (RU 486) in Cushing's syndrome. *Eur J Endocrinol* 2007; 157: 561.

Kaye TB, Crapo L. The Cushing syndrome: an update on diagnostic tests. *Ann Intern Med* 1990; 112: 434.

Nieman L. Cushing syndrome. In: *Scientific American Medicine. Endocrinology & Metabolism.* Hamilton: Dekker Medicine. 2020.

Odell WD. Ectopic ACTH secretion: a misnomer. *Endocrinol Metab Clin North Am* 1991; 20: 371.

Cyanide

A **cyanide** is a compound containing the monovalent group, CN. Inorganic salts derived from hydrocyanic acid (such as sodium cyanide) are very toxic. Hydrogen cyanide (HCN, Prussic acid – q.v.) itself is a very volatile liquid. Organic cyanides are called nitriles and include acrylonitrile, which is used in the manufacture of plastics. Cyanides are widely used in a variety of industrial processes. In nature, cyanide is found most notably in the pit of the wild cherry but also in very low concentrations in some other plants (e.g. stone fruits, almonds).

Toxicity occurs from reversible inhibition of oxidative phosphorylation due to blocking of cytochrome oxidase, with consequent reduced energy production, anaerobic metabolism, tissue hypoxia and metabolic acidosis. The type of hypoxia is classically referred to as 'histotoxic', which is characterized by poor tissue oxygen extraction and consequent arterialization of venous blood.

> **Cyanide poisoning** occurs traditionally from suicidal, accidental or homicidal ingestion, or from occupational exposure, though it may also occur from smoke inhalation (see Inhalation injury) and more recently it has been observed after prolonged use of sodium nitroprusside (see below).

Concentrations as low as 200 parts per million for 30 min or ingestion of 300 mg of salt or 100 mg of HCN are usually fatal within a few minutes.

The onset of poisoning is very rapid and requires prompt treatment. In non-fatal cases, complete recovery is the rule even without treatment, because of natural detoxification by hepatic rhodanase with the production of non-toxic sulphocyanides.

Since the circumstances of potential exposure are usually apparent, acute poisoning can generally be clinically suspected well before its biochemical confirmation. Clinical features include neurological dysfunction with impaired consciousness, headache, dizziness, agitation, confusion and fits, and systemic signs with tachycardia and tachypnoea.

Investigations show increased venous oxygen saturation, metabolic acidosis and increased blood lactate. Blood cyanide levels, if available, of >1 mg/L are toxic and >3 mg/L are fatal. A lactate level of 8 mmol/L has been associated with a cyanide level of >1 mg/L.

Treatment is with 100% oxygen, mechanical ventilation, fluid resuscitation, anticonvulsants and especially an appropriate antidote in more severe cases.

Antidotes include
- **nitrites** *(amyl nitrite by inhalation, sodium nitrite by IV injection of 5 mg/kg over 3 min), followed by sodium thiosulphate (50 mL of 25% solution IV), or*
- *a cobalt-containing compound, such as* **cobalt edetate** *or* **hydroxycobalamin**. *These latter agents are the antidotes of choice and are given in a dose of 10.5 mg/kg and 70 mg/kg, respectively, in 200 mL over 15 min. The usual pharmaceutical preparation, cobalt edetate, can cause vomiting and hypotension.*

Hydroxycobalamin can cause maroon-coloured urine. Dialysis or haemoperfusion are not effective.

In Intensive Care practice, the potential cyanide toxicity of **sodium nitroprusside** (SNP) was not widely appreciated.

This toxicity occurs because SNP contains 44% cyanide which is degraded to thiocyanate in the liver, from where it is excreted in the urine. Toxicity is related to both the total dose and the rate of administration. Neurological damage, including neuropathy (q.v.), encephalopathy (q.v.), coma and focal signs may occur and can be irreversible. Unexplained cardiac arrest or death can occur.

The greatest occurrence was after open-heart surgery, where it was estimated that perhaps 1000 deaths per year may have occurred from SNP in the USA in previous years, though this number should be put in context of the large total usage of SNP of about 500,000 patient-days per year in that country at that time.

This is a difficult subject to clarify, as most cases are probably unrecognized because of difficulties in measurement. Thus, increased levels of thiocyanate and even cyanide usually occur as late phenomena, as does metabolic (lactic) acidosis (q.v.).

See also
- Acute lung irritation,
- Retrobulbar neuritis,
- Warfare agents.

Bibliography
Curry SC, Arnold-Capell P. Nitroprusside, nitroglycerin, and angiotensin-converting enzyme inhibitors. *Crit Care Clin* 1991; 7: 555.
Freeman AG. Optic neuropathy and chronic cyanide intoxication: a review. *J R Soc Med* 1988; 81: 103.
Kulig K. Cyanide antidotes and fire toxicology. *N Engl J Med* 1991; 325: 1801.
Mokhlesi B, Leikin JB, Murray P, et al. Adult toxicology in critical care: part II: specific poisonings. *Chest* 2003; 123: 897.
Robin ED, McCauley R. Nitroprusside-related cyanide poisoning. *Chest* 1992; 102: 1842.
Vick JA, Froehlich H. Treatment of cyanide poisoning. *Milit Med* 1991; 156: 330.
Zerbe NF, Wagner BK. Use of vitamin B_{12} in the treatment and prevention of nitroprusside-induced cyanide toxicity. *Crit Care Med* 1993; 21: 465.

Cystic fibrosis

Cystic fibrosis (CF) is a common genetic disorder transmitted as an autosomal recessive trait. It occurs in about 1 in 3500 live births. The persistence of the cystic fibrosis trait despite its obviously adverse clinical effect may in part be due to a beneficial offset from an historic reduction in bacterial infections of the gastrointestinal tract, such as cholera.

The abnormal gene is on the long arm of chromosome 7, a region which codes for a 1480 amino acid protein, 'CF transmembrane regulator' (CFTR). This protein functions as a cAMP-activated ion channel regulating the physiological properties of mucosal epithelial cells. Over 2000 CFTR mutations have now been described. These genetic polymorphisms lead to some phenotypic variability. However, in about 70% of patients with cystic fibrosis, amino acid no. 508 on this protein is missing, giving the F508del mutation. The resultant protein is abnormal in that it cannot be glycosylated, so that it is misfolded and retained in the Golgi apparatus rather than being transferred to the cell membrane. The lungs and pancreas are particularly affected.

The cell membrane then has an increased sodium absorption and decreased chloride transfer, with the result that exocrine gland secretions are abnormally viscid. Consequently, there is impaired clearance of respiratory secretions, with mucus plugging and secondary infection, especially due to *Staphylococcus aureus* and *Pseudomonas aeruginosa*. CF-related organisms also include *H. influenzae*, *Burkholderia cepacia* and *Stenotrophomonas maltophilia*. Typical infections are neutrophil-driven and polymicrobial with multiple resistance patterns, and they are either chronic or recurrent.

Although bronchiectasis, atelectasis and fibrosis are produced, the lesions rarely cavitate.

Airway CFTR activity has also been found to be decreased in smokers without CF, and this may explain some of the similarity of dysfunction between CF and COPD.

> Clinical features of cystic fibrosis are usually present from childhood, though some variants first appear in adult life.
> - There is progressive, chronic airways obstruction,
>   - with cough, sputum, dyspnoea and wheeze.
> - Physical examination shows cyanosis, clubbing and hyperinflation.
> - Haemoptysis (q.v.) and pneumothorax (q.v.) are common early complications.
> - Cor pulmonale frequently occurs subsequently.
> - Extrapulmonary manifestations include
>   - pancreatic insufficiency, always exocrine but sometimes also endocrine with resultant insulin-dependent diabetes,
>   - recurrent bowel obstruction,
>   - biliary cirrhosis (q.v.),
>   - infertility due to aspermia.

The diagnosis is made on the basis of increased sodium and chloride levels in sweat, as follows:
- chloride >60 mmol/L is found in all patients and is diagnostic if the patient is <20 yr,
- chloride >80 mmol/L is not seen in any other condition and is diagnostic if the patient is >20 yr.

The differential diagnosis, especially of milder cases in adults, includes primary ciliary dyskinesia (q.v.).

*Treatment is with **physiotherapy** (postural drainage and breathing exercises), **nebulized mist therapy**, **bronchodilators** and **intensive antibiotic therapy**. It is important to note that patients with CF have increased clearance of most antibiotics, and thus the dosage of these needs to be adjusted upwards accordingly.*
- **Pancreatic enzyme replacement** *is required, as is adequate salt and water balance and protection from proneness to heat exhaustion. Optimal nutrition includes supplementation with fat-soluble vitamins.*
- *Inhaled **amiloride** has been reported to be helpful, as it blocks membrane sodium channels.*
- **DNase** *(dornase alpha) has been shown to reduce the incidence of chest infections but at considerable cost and thus uncertain cost-effectiveness. Subsequently, inhaled hypertonic saline and mannitol have been found to have a probably similar effect.*
- *Antifibrinolytic therapy with **tranexamic acid** given systemically has been reported to be helpful in haemoptysis.*
- **Ivacaftor**, *a CFTR channel modulator specific to a particular mutation (G551D), has shown considerable benefit in patients with that uncommon mutation (i.e. only about 10% of patients with CF). Ivacaftor (a 'potentiator') may also be used in combination with **lumacaftor** or **tezacaftor** ('correctors') for moderate effect in patients with more common mutations.*
- **Lung transplantation** *has been available since the 1980s for advanced cases, and **liver transplantation** may also be indicated in some cases.*
- *Future prospects clearly include **gene therapy**, as well as a broad range of other novel therapeutics.*
- *The management of patients with CF who require **Intensive Care** can be particularly challenging, especially if mechanically ventilated.*

With recent improvements in treatment, patients with cystic fibrosis generally now survive into adulthood. The median life expectancy at birth is currently over 40 yr, at least in developed countries where the health care systems can afford the necessarily expensive modern programs of sophisticated CF care.

See also
- Asthma,
- Bronchiectasis,
- Situs inversus.

Bibliography

Bell SC, Mall MA, Gutierrez H, et al. The future of cystic fibrosis care: a global perspective. *Lancet Respir Med* 2020; 8: 65.

Brock DJH. Prenatal screening for cystic fibrosis. *Lancet* 1996; 347: 148.

Davidson DJ, Porteous DJ. The genetics of cystic fibrosis lung disease. *Thorax* 1998; 53: 389.

Editorial. What is cystic fibrosis? *N Engl J Med* 2002; 347: 439.

Edmondson C, Davies JC. Current and future treatment options for cystic fibrosis lung disease: latest evidence and clinical implications. *Ther Adv Chronic Dis* 2016; 7: 170.

Elborn JS. Cystic fibrosis. *Lancet* 2016; 388: 2519.

Elborn JS, Shale DJ, Britton JR. Cystic fibrosis: current survival and population estimates to the year 2000. *Thorax* 1991; 46: 881.

Elkins MR, Robinson M, Rose BR, et al. A controlled trial of long-term inhaled hypertonic saline in patients with cystic fibrosis. *N Engl J Med* 2006; 354: 229.

Flume PA, Mogayzel PJ, Robinson KA, et al. Cystic fibrosis pulmonary guidelines: pulmonary complications of haemoptysis and pneumothorax. *Am J Respir Crit Care Med* 2010; 182: 298.

Frizzell RA. Functions of the cystic fibrosis transmembrane conductance regulator protein. *Am J Respir Crit Care Med* 1995; 151: S54.

Fuchs HJ, Borowitz DS, Christiansen DH, et al. Effect of recombinant human DNase on exacerbations of respiratory symptoms and on pulmonary function in patients with cystic fibrosis. *N Engl J Med* 1994; 331: 637.

Hilman BC. Genetic and immunologic aspects of cystic fibrosis. *Ann Allergy Asthma Immunol* 1997; 79: 379.

Hoffman LR, Ramsey BW. Cystic fibrosis therapeutics: the road ahead. *Chest* 2013; 143: 207.

King CS, Brown AW, Aryal S, et al. Critical care of the adult patient with cystic fibrosis. *Chest* 2019; 155: 202.

Knowles MR, Church NL, Waltner WE, et al. A pilot study of aerosolized amiloride for the treatment of lung disease in cystic fibrosis. *N Engl J Med* 1990; 322: 1189.

Masel P. Management of cystic fibrosis in adults. *Aust Prescriber* 2012; 35: 118.

Merlo CA, Boyle MP. Modifier genes in cystic fibrosis lung disease. *J Lab Clin Med* 2003; 141: 237.

Mills CE. Nutrition and lung disease in cystic fibrosis. *Clin Chest Med* 2007; 28: 319.

Orenstein DM. Diagnosis of cystic fibrosis. *Semin Respir Med* 1985; 6: 252.

Pittman JE, Ferkol TW. The evolution of cystic fibrosis care. *Chest* 2015; 148: 533.

Robinson M, Regnis JA, Bailey DL, et al. Effect of hypertonic saline, amiloride, and cough on mucociliary clearance in patients with cystic fibrosis. *Am J Respir Crit Care Med* 1996; 153: 1503.

Rosenstein BJ, Zeitlin PL. Cystic fibrosis. *Lancet* 1998; 351: 277.

Rowe SM, Clancy JP, Sorscher EJ. A breath of freash air. *Sci Am* 2011; 305: 49.

Rowe SM, Miller S, Sorscher EJ. Cystic fibrosis. *N Engl J Med* 2005; 352: 1992.

Rubin BK. Emerging therapies for cystic fibrosis lung disease. *Chest* 1999; 115: 1120.

Sawyer SM, Robertson CF, Bowes G. Cystic fibrosis: a changing clinical perspective. *Aust NZ J Med* 1997; 27: 6.

Stoltz DA, Meyerholz DK, Welsh MJ. Origins of cystic fibrosis lung disease. *N Engl J Med* 2015; 372: 351.

The Cystic Fibrosis Genotype-Phenotype Consortium. Correlation between genotype and phenotype in patients with cystic fibrosis. *N Engl J Med* 1993; 329: 1308.

Tsui L-C. The cystic fibrosis transmembrane conductance regulator gene. *Am J Respir Crit Care Med* 1995; 151: S47.

Wallis G. Diagnosing cystic fibrosis: blood, sweat, and tears. *Arch Dis Child* 1997; 76: 85.

Welsh MJ, Smith AE. Cystic fibrosis. *Sci Am* 1995; 273: 36.

Yankaskas JR, Mallory GB. Lung transplantation in cystic fibrosis: consensus conference statement. *Chest* 1998; 113: 217.

Yankaskas JR, Marshall BC, Sufian B, et al. Cystic fibrosis adult care: consensus conference report. *Chest* 2004; 125: 1S.

Cytomegalovirus

Cytomegalovirus (CMV) is a ubiquitous DNA virus and one of the eight human herpesviruses (q.v.). It is present in many bodily fluids and is transmitted from person to person across the placenta, in breast milk, in child care centres, from communal living, from close personal contact, in blood transfusion and in transplanted organs.

Following initial infection, the virus is carried for life in many different cells in many different organs. It remains dormant until reactivation and replication during periods of immunocompromise, especially during T-cell dysfunction. Severe disease is uncommon in immunocompetent patients.

Although CMV infection is usually asymptomatic, it can cause the following disease states.

- Mononucleosis may be produced at any age but especially in young adults. It is similar to that produced by Epstein–Barr virus infection, except that there is no heterophile antibody (see Epstein–Barr virus). Symptoms are typically mild.
- It is the most common viral pathogen in patients after organ transplantation, especially bone marrow transplantation. After a latent period of 1–4 months, there is fever, neutropenia (q.v.), pneumonitis and occasionally disseminated disease. Prolonged viraemia is associated with poorer outcomes.
- It is the most frequent and important pathogen in patients with AIDS (q.v.). CMV and HIV potentiate each other's replication. Disseminated disease may include pneumonitis, gastrointestinal ulceration, encephalitis (q.v.), polyradiculopathy, retinitis.

Laboratory testing has multiple components. As serology indicates previous exposure, immune monitoring requires tests such as Quantiferon or similar assays. Assays for viral load involve nucleic acid tests. Immunochemistry is used to detect CMV invasion in tissue specimens. Specific testing can be made for drug resistance and therapeutic drug monitoring.

*Treatment is with **ganciclovir** IV (q.v.) or **valganciclovir** (the prodrug of ganciclovir) as first line or with **foscarnet** as second line. Oral ganciclovir may be used for prophylaxis or suppression in seropositive transplant recipients. Novel agents include **letermovir** for prophylaxis and **maribavir** for refractory cases. **Immunotherapy** with virus-specific T cells has been investigated both for prophylaxis and treatment. **Vaccination** may offer future promise.*

The mortality is up to 90% in CMV pneumonitis.

Bibliography
Goodgame, RW. Gastrointestinal cytomegalovirus disease. *Ann Intern Med* 1993; 119: 924.
Jacobson MA, Mills J. Serious cytomegalovirus disease in acquired immunodeficiency syndrome (AIDS): clinical findings, diagnosis, and treatment. *Ann Intern Med* 1988; 108: 585.
Lancini D, Faddy HM, Flower R, et al. Cytomegalovirus disease in immunocompetent adults. *Med J Aust* 2014; 201: 578.
Merigan TC, Renlund DG, Keay S, et al. A controlled trial of ganciclovir to prevent cytomegalovirus disease after heart transplantation. *N Engl J Med* 1992; 326: 1182.
Yong MK, Gottlieb D, Lindsay J, et al. New advances in the management of cytomegalovirus in allogenic haemopoietic stem cell transplantation. *Intern Med J* 2020; 50: 277.

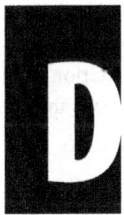

Dantrolene *See*
- Amphetamines,
- Baclofen,
- Heat stroke,
- Malignant hyperthermia,
- Neuroleptic malignant syndrome,
- Rhabdomyolysis,
- Serotonin syndrome,
- Tetanus.

Decompression sickness *See*
- Diving.

Defibrotide *See*
- Anticoagulants,
- Budd–Chiari syndrome.

Delirium

Delirium (acute encephalopathy – q.v., acute confusional state, or sometimes formerly 'acute brain syndrome', or even 'ICU psychosis') describes a syndrome of acute cerebral dysfunction, which commonly occurs during any acute severe illness. It is manifest by disordered
- consciousness,
- orientation,
- expression,
- perception,
- attention span,
- memory,
- motor activity (commonly with agitation which may cause harm to self or others).

Several tools have been validated for delirium assessment in Intensive Care patients, but they generally have limited sensitivity and specificity (e.g. the Confusion Assessment Method for the Intensive Care Unit, CAM-ICU).

> More promising perhaps has been a later tool referred to as Intensive Care Delirium Screening Checklist (ICDSC) listing eight items, of which the presence of four or more correlates with a specialist diagnosis of delirium.
> These eight symptoms comprise
> - alteration of consciousness,
> - disorientation,
> - fluctuation of symptoms,
> - hallucinations and/or delusions,
> - inattention,
> - inappropriate mood or speech,
> - psychomotor agitation (or slowing),
> - sleep cycle disturbance.

It has also been appreciated that some patients may develop the less dramatic features of a chiefly hypoactive state, sometimes referred to as 'quiet delirium', with a flat affect and paradoxically a worse prognosis. This state may be included in the broader category of 'acute apathy syndromes', which have multiple neuropsychiatric causes, many of which occur outside the ICU setting.

Delirium typically has a rapid onset. It usually lasts only hours to days, during which time it may fluctuate in severity, being typically worse at night and improving even as far as lucidity during the day.

Since delirium is reported to occur in about 30% of postoperative patients admitted to ICU, its recognition is important because it is associated with adverse outcome indices, even when corrected for confounding variables. It thus requires ongoing attention to preventable factors and to appropriate pharmacological management. Sometimes, there may be persisting cognitive impairment, although cognitive impairment itself is a predisposing factor to the development of delirium following a toxic or metabolic insult.

Delirium is often considered in conjunction with the related conditions of pain, agitation, immobility and sleep deprivation, referred to in total as **PADIS** (q.v.), which reflect the constellation of distressful symptoms suffered by critically ill patients in the ICU environment.

Delirium is due to a specific organic or somatic problem.

Most typically, this is a systemic infection (most commonly, pneumonia or urosepsis).

The cause can also include
- hypoxaemia,
- hypotension,
- cardiac failure,
- liver disease,
- metabolic disorders,
- renal disease,
- CNS disease
  - cerebrovascular, infection, trauma,
- the postoperative state,
- drugs
  - narcotics, benzodiazepines, antibiotics, anticholinergics, antihistamines.

It is also commonly seen
- after drug withdrawal
  - especially alcohol but also other sedatives,
- in adverse environmental conditions
  - especially those associated with sleep deprivation, and conflicting, overloaded or deprived sensory input,
  - in these settings, the body's normal circadian rhythm (q.v.) is overwhelmed by intense pathophysiological stimuli.

As the syndrome of delirium is heterogeneous in its pathophysiology and clinical features, it is unrealistic to believe that any single measure may be of general prophylactic or therapeutic value, that treatment other than for distress is necessarily warranted and that the relationship between delirium and adverse outcomes may be other than an association. These concepts are in accord with the multiplicity of negative trials of various management options of delirium in ICU patients.

*Delirium is best managed pharmacologically with a butyrophenone (usually **haloperidol**, commencing at 1–2 mg IV 2–4 hrly to a maximum of 10 mg over 24 hr), though one of the newer atypical neuroleptics/antipsychotics (such as **olanzapine**, **risperidone** or **quetiapine**) or **dexmedetomidine** may also be helpful. Reduced doses should be given in elderly or frail patients. However, while useful for managing patient distress, these agents do not alter the clinical course of the delirium. The use of **melatonin** (q.v.) is of unproven value, and **cholinesterase inhibitor** therapy is ineffective (see Anticholinesterases). The use of **benzodiazepines** should be minimized, as their use has been linked to sedation-induced delirium.*

The patient's environment should be optimized, with attention to pain management, normalization of sleep–wake cycles (see Circadian rhythm), assistance with visual orientation and reduction of immobility.

*Detailed **clinical practice guidelines** have recently been published to provide an evidence-based set of recommendations for the management of delirium (as well as pain, agitation, sleep and immobility, i.e. PADIS) in ICU patients.*

Bibliography
Balas MC, Weinhouse GL, Denehy L, et al. Interpreting and implementing the 2018 pain, agitation/sedation, delirium, immobility, and sleep disruption clinical practice guideline. *Crit Care Med* 2018; 46: 1464.
Barr J, Fraser GL, Puntillo K, et al. Clinical practice guidelines for the management of pain, agitation, and delirium in adult patients in the intensive care unit. *Crit Care Med* 2013; 41: 263.
Barr J, Pandharipande PP, eds. Creating and implementing the 2013 ICU pain, agitation, and delirium guidelines for adult ICU patients. *Crit Care Med* 2013; 41: S1.
Bergeron N, Dubois MJ, Dumont M, et al. Intensive Care Delirium Screening Checklist: evaluation of a new screening tool. *Intens Care Med* 2001; 27: 859.
Bienvenu OJ, Neufeld KJ, Needham DM. Treatment of four psychiatric emergencies in the intensive care unit. *Crit Care Med* 2012; 40: 2662.
Brown CH, Dowdy D. Risk factors for delirium: are systemic reviews enough? *Crit Care Med* 2015; 43: 232.

Brown TM. Drug-induced delirium. *Semin Clin Neuropsychiatry* 2000; 5: 113.

Burry LD, Cheng W, Williamson DR, et al. Pharmacological and non-pharmacological interventions to prevent delirium in critically ill patients: a systematic review and network meta-analysis. *Intens Care Med* 2021; 47: 943.

Devlin JW, Fong JJ, Fraser GL, et al. Delirium assessment in the critically ill. *Intens Care Med* 2007; 33: 929.

Devlin JW, Skrobik Y, Gelinas C, et al. Executive summary: clinical practice guidelines for the prevention and management of pain, agitation/sedation, delirium, immobility, and sleep disruption in adult patients in the ICU. *Crit Care Med* 2018; 46: 1532.

Dubois M-J, Bergeron N, Dumont M, et al. Delirium in an intensive care unit: a study of risk factors. *Intens Care Med* 2001; 27: 1297.

Ely EW, Gautam S, Margolin R, et al. The impact of delirium in the intensive care unit on hospital length of stay. *Intens Care Med* 2001; 27: 1892.

Figueroa-Ramos MI, Arroya-Novoa CM, Lee KA, et al. Sleep and delirium in ICU patients: a review of mechanisms and manifestations. *Intens Care Med* 2009; 35: 781.

Honarmand K, Rafay H, Le J, et al. A systematic review of risk factors for sleep disruption in critically ill adults. *Crit Care Med* 2020; 48: 1066.

Jones D, Hodgson CL, Shehabi Y, et al. Reducing confusion about post-cardiotomy delirium. *Crit Care Resusc* 2017; 19: 5.

Kronzer VL, Avidan MS. Preventing postoperative delirium: all that glisters is not gold. *Lancet* 2016; 388: 1854.

Luetz A, Heymann A, Radtke FM, et al. Different assessment tools for intensive care unit delirium: which score to use? *Crit Care Med* 2010; 38: 409.

Neto AS, Nassar AP, Cardoso SO, et al. Delirium screening in critically ill patients: a systematic review and meta-analysis. *Crit Care Med* 2012; 40: 1946.

Ouimet S, Kavanagh BP, Gottfried SB. Incidence, risk factors and consequences of ICU delirium. *Crit Care Med* 2007; 33: 66.

Pandharipande P, Jackson J, Ely EW. Delirium: acute cognitive dysfunction in the critically ill. *Curr Opin Crit Care* 2005; 11: 360.

Pun BT, Ely EW. The importance of diagnosing and managing ICU delirium. *Chest* 2007; 132: 624.

Riker RR, Fraser GL. Delirium – beyond the CAM-ICU. *Crit Care Med* 2020; 48: 134.

Salluh JI, Wang H, Schneider EB, et al. Outcome of delirium in critically ill patients: systematic review and meta-analysis. *BMJ* 2015: 350: h2538.

Shehabi Y, Howe BD, Bellomo R, et al. Early sedation with dexmedetomidine in critically ill patients. *N Engl J Med* 2019; 380: 2506.

Stollings JL, Kotfis K, Chanques G, et al. Delirium in critical illness: clinical manifestations, outcomes, and management. *Intens Care Med* 2021; 47: 1089.

Weber JB, Coverdale JH, Kunik ME. Delirium: current trends in prevention and treatment. *Intern Med J* 2004; 34: 115.

Dementia

Dementia describes chronic cerebral dysfunction and is manifest by disturbed cognition with impaired

- orientation,
- expression,
- memory (with predominantly anterograde amnesia),
- decision-making.

There is usually no disturbance of consciousness, perception, attention span or motor activity, and no directly associated organic illness.

Dementia may of course occur in association with delirium (q.v.) or with psychiatric illness.

Most such patients have either **Alzheimer's disease** (AD) or **multi-infarct (vascular) dementia** (vascular cognitive impairment, VCI). Less commonly, Lewy body dementia, Parkinson's disease with dementia and frontotemporal dementia may be diagnosed.

Many other conditions (some treatable) may also cause dementia, including

- myxoedema (q.v.),
- thiamine deficiency (see Beriberi),
- vitamin B_{12} deficiency (q.v.),
- syphilis (q.v.),
- aluminium toxicity (including dialysis dementia) (q.v.),
- toxic encephalopathy (e.g. from alcohol),
- quinidine,
- Whipple's disease (q.v.),
- occult hydrocephalus (q.v.),
- cerebral tumour,
- Creutzfeldt–Jakob disease (q.v.),
- post-traumatic state (after head injury).

Depression and drug effects need to be specifically excluded.

Ten per cent of the population over the age of 65 yr and 20% over 80 yr develop some degree of dementia, making dementia the third most common (but the most expensive) disorder in the elderly after cardiovascular disease and cancer. Genetic testing for Alzheimer's disease, especially for the apolipoprotein E gene (APOE) as a risk factor, is clinically and ethically controversial. The most common tool for assessing dementia has been the (now recently copyrighted) 'Mini-Mental State Examination' (MMSE), though other screening tests and scales are also valid and are being increasingly used. Diagnostic clarification requires brain imaging, preferably with MRI scanning.

Alzheimer's disease is associated with the accumulation of amyloid plaque (amyloid β-peptide, Aβ) in the brain. Since Aβ is prothrombotic (although its precursor has anticoagulant properties), it is possible that Alzheimer's disease has a thrombohaemorrhagic component to its development, and this finding may have future therapeutic implications.

The centrally acting anticholinesterase, **THA**, was initially thought to provide therapeutic benefit in Alzheimer's disease, but this benefit was not confirmed in subsequent studies. The newer anticholinesterases, **donepezil**, **rivastigmine** and **galantamine**, have been licensed for the symptomatic relief of Alzheimer's dementia on the basis of more convincing trial evidence. However, the symptomatic benefits are only modest, improvement may require doses which produce adverse effects, there has been no evidence of decreased disease progression, and long-term efficacy is unknown. See Anticholinesterases.

In patients unable to tolerate a cholinesterase inhibitor, **memantine** (an NMDA antagonist) may be of benefit.

The efficacy of the complementary medicines, **ginkgo biloba** and **vitamin E**, in treating dementia is controversial, as the studies suggesting efficacy have been criticized on methodological grounds. However, there is limited indirect evidence that the lipid-lowering agents of the **statin** group may help prevent dementia.

Recent major trials of **solanezumab** (an antibody which can bind to and thus clear amyloid protein) and **verubecestat** (an antibody which can inhibit the cleavage of amyloid precursor protein) have failed to show therapeutic efficacy, throwing into doubt some of the more simplistic views of the role of amyloid protein in the causation of the dementia in Alzheimer's disease. On the other hand, **aducanumab** (an antibody that binds to and clears amyloid β aggregates) has had recent approval by the US Food and Drug Administration amid much controversy. These negative or problematic trial results illustrate the general disappointment which has followed the enormous research investment to date in seeking a useful drug for dementia.

On the other hand, a major Finnish study has shown prophylactic benefit in high-risk patients from a lifestyle regimen combining healthy diet, physical exercise and cognitive training.

Bibliography
Arie T. Pseudodementia. *BMJ* 1983; 286:1301.
Bryson HM, Benfield P. Donepezil. *Drugs & Aging* 1997; 10: 234.
Chong TWH, Macpherson H, Schaumberg MA, et al. Dementia prevention: the time to act is now. *Med J Aust* 2021; 214: 302.
Fischman J, ed. A new era for Alzheimer's. *Sci Am* 2020; 322: 22.
Guttman R, Seleski M, eds. *Diagnosis, Management and Treatment of Dementia*. Chicago: American Medical Association. 1999.
Harvey K, Stough C. Caution with complementaries for cognitive impairment. *Aust Prescriber* 2011; 34: 19.
Katzman R. Alzheimer's disease. *N Engl J Med* 1986; 314: 964.
LoGiudice D. Dementia: an update to refresh your memory. *Intern Med J* 2002; 32: 535.
Mayeux R, Saunders AM, Shea S, et al. Utility of the apolipoprotein E genotype in the diagnosis of Alzheimer's disease. *N Engl J Med* 1998; 338: 506.
Morantz RA, Walsh JW, eds. *Brain Tumors*. New York: Marcel Dekker. 1994.
Panegyres PK, Goldblatt J, Walpole I, et al. Genetic testing for Alzheimer's disease. *Med J Aust* 2000; 172: 339.
Saunders AM, Hulette C, Welsh-Bohmer KA, et al. Specificity, sensitivity, and predictive value of apolipoprotein-E genotyping for sporadic Alzheimer's disease. *Lancet* 1996; 348: 90.
Schmaier AH. Alzheimer disease is in part a thrombohaemorrhagic disorder. *J Thromb Haemost* 2016; 14: 991.
Shah A, Royston MC. Donepezil for dementia. *J R Soc Med* 1997; 90: 531.
Smith JS, Kiloh LG. The investigation of dementia. *Lancet* 1981; 1: 824.
Wells CE, ed. *Dementia*. Philadelphia: F.A. Davis. 1977.

Demyelinating diseases

Demyelinating diseases are seen in several forms.
1. **Multiple sclerosis (q.v.)**
2. **Transverse myelitis**

Transverse myelitis refers to the acute onset of motor and sensory impairment of the legs with hyporeflexia. There is associated bladder dysfunction, and the process may extend up to the chest or even neck. The aetiology is unknown, though some cases are post-viral.

Usually, the condition is an initial manifestation of **multiple sclerosis** (q.v.), but occasionally it occurs in patients with already known multiple sclerosis. It is sometimes associated with the antiphospholipid syndrome (q.v.) or systemic lupus erythematosus (SLE) (q.v.).

If associated with bilateral optic neuritis (q.v.), the condition is called **neuromyelitis optica** (Devic's disease). This disorder is autoimmune and generally separate from multiple sclerosis.

The differential diagnosis of transverse myelitis includes
- epidural abscess (q.v.),
- Guillain–Barré syndrome (q.v.),
- spinal cord infarction or compression.

The CSF typically contains lymphocytes. MRI of the brain and spinal cord is useful in diagnosis. The demonstration of a specific autoantibody may separate neuromyelitis optica from multiple sclerosis.

*Treatment for acute episodes includes **corticosteroids** parenterally and **plasmapheresis**. **Corticosteroids** orally with **immunosuppression** and possibly **rituximab** (q.v.) may prevent relapses.*

*For patients with neuromyelitis optica who have AQP4 autoantibodies, the new monoclonal antibody to interleukin 6 (IL-6), **satralizumab**, reduces the relapse rate,*

The outlook is often one of permanent neurological damage.

3. **Acute (post-infectious) disseminated encephalomyelitis (ADEM)**

This is a serious though fortunately rare complication of acute exanthematous viral infection (especially measles) or vaccination. It is probably an autoimmune response against myelin from cross-reaction with viral protein.

It is associated with the rapid onset of
- headache,
- stupor,
- fits,
- focal neurological signs.

Recovery is usual and commences within a few weeks. *There may be a useful response to plasmapheresis.*

4. **Progressive multifocal leukoencephalopathy (PML)**

This is an uncommon opportunistic infection of oligodendroglia due to a polyoma virus of the papovavirus family, called JC virus after the first identified patient (John Cunningham), though originally it was thought to be due to the monkey virus, SV40. It is a progressive demyelinating neurodegenerative condition, but many aspects of its mode of transmission and pathways of pathogenicity remain unclear.

It is usually associated with systemic immunological disorders, such as
- AIDS (q.v.),
- chronic granulomatous disease,
- lymphoma,
- myeloproliferative disorders.

Some cases were reported after the administration of the new drug **natalizumab**, introduced to prevent relapse in multiple sclerosis. In 2005, this promising new therapeutic agent was withdrawn after only 4 months on the market. However, it was later reintroduced, with the strict caveat of careful monitoring and avoidance of use in combination regimens (e.g. with interferon beta) that may have been responsible for the PML or other opportunistic infections previously reported.

Cases were occasionally reported following the use of **efalizumab** for psoriasis, and this drug was later withdrawn from the market.

Rare cases have now been also reported following the use of the immunosuppressant agent, **rituximab** (q.v.), in (q.v.).

Clinical features include a variety of neurological deficits with mental, visual and motor dysfunction.

The virus may be detected in peripheral blood lymphocytes, though its identification in brain biopsy is diagnostic. Viral identification in CSF by PCR may obviate the need for biopsy. The most useful imaging is with MRI.

*There is no reliably effective therapy, though **cidofovir** may complement antiretroviral therapy in AIDS patients with PML. Anecdotal reports have suggested that the antidepressant drug, **mirtazapine**, may be of benefit, and some response has been described with **pembrolizumab**.*

It is always fatal, with a mortality of 80% within 1 yr and an average survival of only 4 months in patients with AIDS.

5. **Other demyelinating conditions**

These include
- **Central pontine myelinolysis** (osmotic demyelination syndrome) (q.v.).
- **Reversible posterior leukoencephalopathy** (q.v.).
- **Toxic leukoencephalopathy**, which may occur either acutely or subacutely following drug overdose, chronic opiate abuse or acute hypoxia.

Bibliography

Brooks BR, Walker DL. Progressive multifocal leukoencephalopathy. *Neurol Clin* 1984; 2: 299.

Cortese I, Muranski P, Enose-Akahata Y, et al. Pembrolizumab treatment for progressive multifocal leukoencephalopathy. *N Engl J Med* 2019; 380: 1597.

Lennon VA, Wingerchuk DM, Kryzer TJ, et al. A serum autoantibody marker of neuromyelitis optica: distinction from multiple sclerosis. *Lancet* 2004: 364: 2106.

Lindsey JW. Multiple sclerosis and related disorders. In: *Scientific American Medicine. Neurology.* Hamilton: Dekker Medicine. 2020.

Tippett DS, Fishman PS, Panitch HS. Relapsing transverse myelitis. *Neurology* 1991; 41: 703.

Tormochlen LM. Toxic leukoencephalopathies. *Neurol Clin* 2011; 29: 591.

Tselis A. Acute disseminated encephalomyelitis. *Curr Treat Options Neurol* 2001; 3: 537.

Wingerchuk DM, Weinshenker BG. Neuromyelitis optica. *Curr Treat Options Neurol* 2005; 71: 173.

Yamamura T, Kleiter I, Fujihara K, et al. Trial of satralizumab in neuromyelitis optica spectrum disorder. *N Engl J Med* 2019; 381: 2114.

Dengue

Dengue is produced by a group B arborvirus, indistinguishable in appearance from the Yellow Fever virus (q.v.). It is caused by one of four related but antigenically distinct serotypes within the genus *Flavivirus*. It is transmitted by *Aedes aegypti* mosquitoes and is endemic in many tropical regions of Asia, the Pacific, Central America and West Africa, with epidemics after severe rainy seasons.

The first epidemics were reported in 1779, and a global pandemic began after World War II, particularly in South-East Asia. In temperate countries, it is seen only in travellers. Nowadays, it is primarily an urban disease of the tropics, with humans as the primary reservoir. It is the second most important tropical infection after malaria (q.v.), with up to 100 million cases occurring per year worldwide. Global climate change has been predicted to extend the regions where dengue is endemic.

Two forms of clinical illness are seen, in addition to subclinical infection and mild, non-specific disease.

- **Dengue fever** (DF) is a mild to moderate non-fatal illness which follows an incubation period of 5–7 days (range 3–14 days). There is the sudden onset of fever, severe headache, myalgia, backache, bone pain, facial flush and profound weakness. A morbilliform rash later involves the trunk and extremities and may desquamate. Neutropenia (q.v.) is typical. The illness subsides in 5–7 days, but it may be followed by prolonged asthenia.
- **Dengue haemorrhagic fever** (DHF) is a much more serious condition, usually confined to South-East Asia and only 1/200th as common as DF. Because of increased vascular permeability, it is additionally associated with thrombocytopenia (q.v.), petechiae (q.v.), multiple haemorrhages and shock. The platelet count is $<100 \times 10^9$/L and there is haemoconcentration. It is possible that this form of illness may arise from a more virulent strain of the organism.

The clinical diagnosis of dengue is confirmed by serology or viral PCR.

The differential diagnosis, particularly in the returned traveller with shock, includes various other infections, such as

- viral haemorrhagic fever (q.v.),
- severe malaria (q.v.),
- yellow fever (q.v.),
- rickettsial disease (q.v.),
- toxic shock syndrome (q.v.).

Rarely, a non-infectious condition, such as drug-induced Stevens–Johnson syndrome (q.v.), may mimic dengue.

*Treatment is **symptomatic** with analgesics, fluids and electrolytes. Clearly, avoidance of mosquito exposure is an important prophylactic measure. NSAIDs are best avoided as they are associated with an increased risk of haemorrhage in this setting.*

A live attenuated vaccine has been introduced, but initial trials have suggested potential paradoxical responses in seronegative patients, especially children, so that it is not currently recommended for the prevention of primary infection. Vector control measures are important in endemic areas.

Bibliography

Bhatt S, Gething PW, Brady OJ, et al. The global distribution and burden of dengue. *Nature* 2013; 496: 504.

Gubler DJ, Clark GG. Dengue/dengue hemorrhagic fever: the emergence of a global health problem. *Emerg Infect Dis* 1995; 1: 2.

Halstead SB. Dengue. *Lancet* 2007; 370: 1644.

Rigau-Perez JG, Clark GG, Gubler DJ, et al. Dengue and dengue haemorrhagic fever. *Lancet* 1998; 352: 971.

Simmons CP, Farrar JJ, Nguyen vV, et al. Dengue. *New Engl J Med* 2012; 366: 1423.

Webster DP, Farrar J, Rowland-Jones S. Progress towards a dengue vaccine. *Lancet Infect Dis* 2009; 9: 678.

Wilder-Smith A. The expanding geographic range of dengue in Australia. *Med J Aust* 2021; 215: 171.

Dermatitis

Dermatitis is a very general term encompassing a number of more specific skin conditions.

1. **Atopic dermatitis** (atopic eczema) is well known. It is caused by a complex interplay of genetic, immunological and environmental factors.

   It may have a complication called Kaposi's varicelliform eruption due to dissemination of herpes simplex virus (HSV) or varicella-zoster virus (VZV) infection.

   *Treatment of severe refractory disease includes several options. Both **immunosuppression** with a variety of agents and **traditional Chinese medicinal herbs** have been reported to be helpful. **Probiotics** given to high-risk mothers during pregnancy have been shown to decrease markedly the subsequent frequency of the disease in their infants.*

2. **Contact dermatitis** may be due to allergy, irritation or photosensitization.

   The allergic form may be striking and is referred to as **acute, allergic, eczematous, contact dermatitis** (AECD). It encompasses the entity, **dermatitis medicamentosa**, which is produced by a variety of drugs, including transdermal patches, as well as preservatives and cosmetics.

   *Treatment with topical **tacrolimus** (a calcineurin inhibitor) may be more effective and safer than that with traditional topical corticosteroids.*

   Photosensitization is also often drug-induced, especially with tetracyclines and thiazides.

   Contact dermatitis is the commonest occupational skin disease, though its elucidation can often be challenging. It is also increasingly recognized following exposure to metallic objects, including implants, especially those containing nickel.

3. **Exfoliative dermatitis** (q.v.).
4. **Dermatitis herpetiformis**.
5. **Seborrhoeic dermatitis**.
6. **Stasis dermatitis** is associated with pigmentation and is due to venous hypertension and varicose veins.
7. **Flagellate dermatitis** (flagellate erythema) has been reported after eating undercooked shiitake mushrooms, after receiving bleomycin (q.v.) or in dermatomyositis (q.v.).

   The term 'flagellate' derives from the associated linear scratch marks due to itching. The erythematous pruritic rash lasts about one week, and it may be improved with topical corticosteroids.

Bibliography

Aneja S, Taylor JS. Contact dermatitis and related disorders. In: *Scientific American Medicine. Dermatology.* Hamilton: Dekker Medicine. 2020.

Hanifin JM. Atopic dermatitis: new therapeutic considerations. *J Am Acad Dermatol* 1991; 24: 1097.

Kalliomaki M, Salminen S, Poussa T, et al. Probiotics and prevention of atopic disease: 4-year follow-up of randomized placebo-controlled trial. *Lancet* 2003; 361: 1869.

Katz SI, Hall RP, Lawley TJ, et al. Dermatitis herpetiformis: the skin and the gut. *Ann Intern Med* 1980; 93: 857.

Krob HA, Fleischer AB, D'Agostino R, et al. Prevalence and relevance of contact dermatitis allergens. *J Am Acad Dermatol* 2004; 51: 349.

LeBrec H, Bachot N, Gaspard I, et al. Mechanisms of drug-induced allergic contact dermatitis. *Cell Biol Toxicol* 1999; 15: 57.

Nicolis GD, Helwig EB. Exfoliative dermatitis: a clinicopathologic study of 135 cases. *Arch Dermatol* 1973; 108: 788.

Rietschel RL, Fowler JF, eds. *Fisher's Contact Dermatitis.* 6th edition. Hamilton: BC Dekker. 2008.

Simpson EI, Basco M, Hanifin J. A cross-sectional survey of complementary and alternative medicine in patients with atopic dermatitis. *Am J Contact Dermat* 2003; 14: 144.

Stevens SR. Eczematous disorders, atopic dermatitis, and ichthyosis. In: *Scientific American Medicine. Dermatology.* Hamilton: Dekker Medicine. 2020.

Wollenberg A, Kraft S, Oppel T, et al. Atopic dermatitis: pathogenetic mechanisms. *Clin Exp Dermatol* 2000; 25: 530.

Dermatology

The care of skin disorders is mostly undertaken in the ambulatory setting, and it is rare for a dermatological condition to be the cause of an admission to an ICU. However, their frequency in the population means that many seriously ill patients have a concomitant skin disorder. Moreover, the skin is an important target organ for a variety of complications of serious illnesses, especially drug reactions. In addition, the skin has been regarded as providing a 'view' of internal diseases in some cases. Yet dermatological problems retain perhaps a greater air of mystery for the non-specialist than almost any other organ-system disorder. The current availability of online atlases of dermatology (see Bibliography below) has added a valuable new aid in diagnostic assistance.

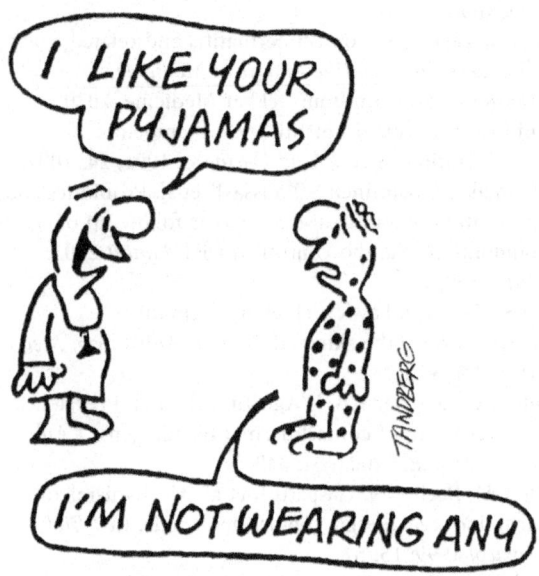

In Intensive Care, the most important differential diagnoses are probably exfoliative dermatitis, skin necrosis and urticaria.

Many other less common dermatological conditions may sometimes be encountered and those also considered in this book include

- Alopecia,
- Blisters,
- Bullae,
- Cellulitis,
- Conjunctivitis,
- Dermatitis,
- Ecthyma,
- Epidermolysis bullosa,
- Erysipelas,
- Erythema marginatum,
- Erythema migrans,
- Erythema multiforme,
- Erythema nodosum,
- Erythromelalgia,
- Exfoliative dermatitis,
- Fasciitis,
- Flushing,
- Folliculitis,
- Furunculosis,
- Hirsutism,
- Hyperhidrosis,
- Hypertrichosis,
- Leukocytoclastic vasculitis,
- Lichenoid skin reaction,
- Livedo reticularis,
- Nail abnormalities,
- Necrolytic migratory erythema,
- Neurofibromatosis,
- Palmar erythema,
- Pediculosis,
- Pemphigus,
- Petechiae,
- Pigmentation disorders,
- Porphyria,
- Pruritus,
- Pseudoporphyria,
- Psoriasis,
- Purpura,
- Pyoderma gangrenosum,
- Raynaud's phenomenon/disease,
- Scalded skin syndrome,
- Scleredema,
- Skin necrosis,
- Skin signs of internal malignant disease,
- Staphylococcal scalded skin syndrome,
- Stevens–Johnson syndrome,
- Sweating,
- Sweet's syndrome,
- Toxic epidermal necrolysis,
- Toxic erythemas,
- Ulcers,
- Urticaria,
- Vesiculobullous diseases,
- Vitiligo,
- Von Recklinghausen's disease,
- Yellow nail syndrome.

Bibliography

Badia M, Trujillano J, Gasco E, et al. Skin lesions in the ICU. *Intens Care Med* 1999; 25: 1271.

Champion RH. Generalised pruritus. *BMJ* 1984; 289: 751.

Denman ST. A review of pruritus. *J Am Acad Dermatol* 1986; 14: 375.

Dowd PM. Cold-related disorders. *Prog Dermatol* 1987; 21: 1.

Fox BJ, Odom RB. Papulosquamous diseases: a review. *J Am Acad Dermatol* 1985; 12: 597.

Gerull R, Nelle M, Schaible T. Toxic epidermal necrolysis and Stevens-Johnson syndrome: a review. *Crit Care Med* 2011; 39: 1521.

Hirschmann JV. Antimicrobial prophylaxis in dermatology. *Semin Cutan Med Surg* 2000; 19: 2.

Johnson RA, Wolff K, eds. *Fitzpatrick's Color Atlas and Synopsis of Clinical Dermatology.* 6th edition. New York: McGraw-Hill. 2009.

Lebwohl MG, ed. Dermatology. In: *Scientific American Medicine.* Hamilton: Dekker Medicine. 2020.

Peter RU. Cutaneous manifestations in intensive care patients. *Intens Care Med* 1998; 24: 997.

Rietschel RL, Fowler JF, eds. *Fisher's Contact Dermatitis.* 6th edition. Hamilton: BC Dekker 2008.

Roujeau JC, Stern RS. Severe adverse cutaneous reactions to drugs. *N Engl J Med* 1994; 10: 1272.

Sehgal VN, Gangwani OP. Fixed drug eruption: current concepts. *Int J Dermatol* 1987; 26: 67.

Wolff K, Goldsmith L, Katz S, et al., eds. *Fitzpatrick's Dermatology in General Medicine.* 7th edition. New York: McGraw-Hill. 2007.

Some online dermatology atlases: www.dermis.net, www.dermatlas.net.

Dermatomyositis *See*

- Polymyositis.

Desferrioxamine *See*

- Chelating agents.

Desmopressin

Desmopressin (1-desamino-8-D-arginine vasopressin, DDAVP) is a synthetic analog of vasopressin (q.v.). It has an antidiuretic to pressor ratio of about 3000:1, compared with the usual 1:1 ratio for vasopressin. It has only minor oxytocic effects. Conversely, other synthetic preparations are available for obstetric use with primarily oxytocic but minimal vasopressor activity (e.g. **syntocinon**).

Desmopressin is the agent of choice for therapeutic use in this group. It has three main uses.
- **Antidiuretic agent**
  This effect is exerted in the kidney by decreasing water reabsorption in the collecting tubule. The chief such use is in diabetes insipidus. This antidiuretic effect is inhibited by glibenclamide.
- **Haemostatic agent**
  In bleeding disorders associated with a platelet function defect (including von Willebrand's disease, haemophilia, renal disease, aspirin use) (q.v.), desmopressin increases factor VIII levels and decreases bleeding time. It has been shown to decrease blood loss after cardiac surgery.
- **Splanchnic vasoconstrictor**
  In portal hypertension with bleeding varices, it decreases portal blood pressure and so assists in controlling haemorrhage.

Desmopressin has a half-life of 8–80 min. It is given either intravenously or intranasally. As an antidiuretic in diabetes insipidus, it is given in a dose of 1–4 mcg IV. In bleeding, it is given in a dose of 20 mcg (i.e. 0.3 mcg/kg) diluted in 50 mL and given over 30 min. This dose may be repeated in 6–12 hr if necessary. If used prophylactically for anticipated bleeding, it should be given 30 min before the planned procedure.

Overhydration, with water intoxication and hyponatraemia, may occur with excess use.

Terlipressin is a prodrug, which is converted gradually in the body after IV injection into lysine-vasopressin. The resultant controlled vasopressin effect has been reported to be useful in variceal bleeding, where its efficacy is similar to that of **octreotide** (q.v.).

See
- Antidiuretic hormone.

Bibliography

Cattaneo M, Harris AS, Stromberg U, et al. The effect of desmopressin on reducing blood loss in cardiac surgery – a meta-analysis of double-blind placebo-controlled trials. *Thromb Haemost* 1995; 74: 1064.

Gordon AC, Russell JA, Walley KR, et al. The effects of vasopressin on acute kidney injury in septic shock. *Intens Care Med* 2010; 36: 83.

Fogel MR, Knauer CM, Andres LL, et al. Continuous intravenous vasopressin in active upper gastrointestinal bleeding: a placebo-controlled trial. *Ann Intern Med* 1982; 96: 565.

Mannucci PM. Desmopressin: a nontransfusional form of treatment for congenital and acquired bleeding disorders. *Blood* 1988; 72: 1449.

Richardson DW, Robinson AG. Desmopressin. *Ann Intern Med* 1985; 103: 228.

Dextrocardia *See*

- Situs inversus.

Diabetes insipidus

Diabetes insipidus (DI) is a syndrome of polyuria due to deficiency of antidiuretic hormone (ADH) (q.v.) secretion by the brain (see Pituitary – posterior pituitary). In the Intensive Care setting, it is generally an acute manifestation of severe brain injury, which may be either global (with raised intracranial pressure) or localized (involving the hypothalamus or pituitary). In the more chronic setting, it may be either congenital or acquired (e.g. after pituitary pathology or surgery, or in histiocytosis – q.v.).

Diabetes insipidus as described above is termed central, as opposed to **nephrogenic diabetes insipidus**, which is due to failure of the renal response to ADH. This in turn is due either to congenital biochemical abnormalities or to acquired tubular pathology, e.g. following treatment with lithium (q.v.).

> Typically in DI, there is polyuria with dilute urine and a raised plasma sodium concentration.
> - Polyuria refers to a urine volume >200 mL/hr.
> - Dilute urine refers to a low urinary specific gravity (<1005), urinary osmolality (<200 mOsm/kg) and urinary sodium concentration (<15 mmol/L).
> - Raised plasma sodium concentration refers to a value >145 mmol/L.

These findings differentiate DI from other causes of polyuria in this setting, such as previous volume loading, induced hypertension or perhaps cerebral salt wasting (q.v.) (see also – Syndrome of inappropriate antidiuretic hormone).

The treatment of DI requires careful monitoring of fluid and electrolyte balance. Fluid losses need to be replaced and ADH needs to be given (as described below). Delayed treatment can lead to hypovolaemic shock and hypernatraemia. Water deficit is treated with 5% dextrose.

ADH replacement is given as **desmopressin** *(DDAVP)(q.v.) in a dose of 1–4 mcg IV. Although DDAVP has a half-life of <1.5 hr, in this setting its dose needs to be repeated only every few hours, i.e. when polyuria recurs. The dramatic response of the polyuria to DDAVP is diagnostically as well as therapeutically important.*

Bibliography
Baylis PH. Posterior pituitary function in health and disease. *Clin Endocrinol Metab* 1983; 12: 747.
Baylis PH, Cheetham T. Diabetes insipidus. *Arch Dis Child* 1998; 79: 84.
Ober KP. Endocrine crises: diabetes insipidus. *Crit Care Clin* 1991; 7: 109.
Richardson DW, Robinson AG. Desmopressin. *Ann Intern Med* 1985; 103: 228.
Singer I, Oster JR, Fishman LM. The management of diabetes insipidus in adults. *Arch Intern Med* 1997; 157: 1293.
Wright WL. Sodium and fluid management in acute brain injury. *Curr Neurol Neurosci Rep* 2012; 12: 466.

Diaphragm

Diaphragmatic disorders include
1. congenital conditions
    - hernia, eventration (commonly congenital and usually left-sided),
2. inflammation
    - subdiaphragmatic abscess, trichiniasis,
3. paralysis,
4. neuromuscular disorders
    - bilateral phrenic nerve injury, due to neuropathy, surgery, trauma,
    - unilateral paralysis, which is commonly asymptomatic and is due either to damage to a phrenic nerve from aneurysm, cardioplegia, lymphadenopathy, malignancy, neuropathy, surgery or trauma, or to direct damage to a hemidiaphragm,
    - critical illness neuromuscular abnormality (q.v.) may cause weakness of the diaphragm as well as of other skeletal muscles,
5. postoperative
    - irritation,
6. spasmodic disorders
    - hiccup, tonic spasm, flutter,
7. trauma,
8. tumour.

Bibliography
Dres M, Goligher EC, Heunks LMA, et al. Critical illness-associated diaphragm weakness. *Intens Care Med* 2017; 43: 1441.
Markand ON, Moorthy SS, Mahomed Y, et al. Postoperative phrenic nerve palsy in patients with open-heart surgery. *Ann Thorac Surg* 1985; 39: 68.
Riley EA. Idiopathic diaphragmatic paralysis. *Am J Med* 1962; 32: 404.
Supinski GS, Morris PE, Dhar S, et al. Diaphragm dysfunction in critical illness. *Chest* 2018; 153: 1040.

Diarrhoea

Diarrhoea is a common condition, but it is worth having a classification, as it includes some uncommon causes. It should be remembered, however, that in about 50% of cases of chronic diarrhoea, no diagnosis is made. Acute diarrhoeal illnesses are even more elusive, as they are usually brief (up to 1–2 days), self-limited, caused by agents not detected by routine laboratory tests and not amenable in any event to specific therapy.

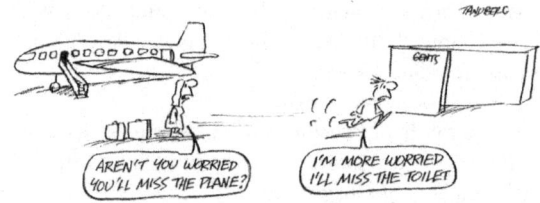

The presence of diarrhoea may be diagnosed on several different criteria related to the frequency, volume or fluidity of stools, but is commonly quantified as a stool output >200 g per day. It is frequently seen in seriously ill patients, in whom it may be related either to the primary cause of the patient's illness or to a complication during their hospital admission. On the Bristol Stool Form Scale, it is represented by types 6 and 7.

A practical subdivision of diarrhoea is into
- large stools, which are usually of small bowel origin,
- small stools, which are usually of large bowel origin and associated with inflammation (and thus blood, mucus and tenesmus).

> Diarrhoea is commonly classified on an aetiological basis into five groups, namely
> - osmotic,
> - secretory,
> - exudative,
> - due to rapid transit time,
> - due to drugs.

1. **Osmotic diarrhoea**

This is caused by
- magnesium-, phosphate- or sulphate-containing medications
  - i.e. antacids or laxatives,
- carbohydrate malabsorption
  - e.g. lactose and sucrose in disaccharidase or lactase deficiency (q.v.),
- mannitol or sorbitol
  - i.e. sugar alcohols,
- lactulose
  - an indigestible disaccharide, commonly given as a laxative,
- excess legumes
  - these contain raffinose or stachyose.

2. **Secretory diarrhoea**

This occurs with
- some bacterial infections
  - a number of bacteria, such as enteropathogenic *Escherichia coli* (q.v.), *Vibrio cholerae*, *Clostridium botulinum*, *Staphylococcus aureus*, may produce an enterotoxin which stimulates excess intestinal excretion and thus toxigenic gastroenteritis.
- irritative fatty acids
  - e.g. non-absorbable fatty acid laxatives, such as castor oil, or in malabsorption or bacterial overgrowth,
- bile acids
  - following ileal resection,
- hormone-producing tumours
  - including carcinoid (q.v.), gastrinoma, and vasoactive intestinal peptide tumour (VIPoma) of pancreas.
  - VIPoma may give 'pancreatic cholera', i.e. watery diarrhoea, hypokalaemia and alkalosis (the WDHA or Verner–Morrison syndrome).
  - Hormonally produced secretory diarrhoea may respond to octreotide.
- other tumours
  - e.g. villous adenoma, colon cancer and mastocytosis (see Urticaria).

3. **Exudative diarrhoea**

This is usually seen following
- invasive bacterial infection with direct damage to the bowel wall.
- In specific infections, the bacteria involved are typically campylobacter, salmonella (both typhoidal and especially nontyphoidal), shigella and yersinia.
- A variety of non-bacterial organisms are also commonly seen, including
  - viruses (norovirus, rotavirus, enterovirus, adenovirus),
  - protozoa (giardia, entamoeba),
  - parasites (helminths),
  - fungi (candida).

These conditions thus give rise to a form of gastroenteritis, manifest particularly by bacterial dysentery.
- A similar condition is seen in
  - inflammatory bowel disease (q.v.),
  - antibiotic-associated or pseudomembranous colitis (see Colitis – *Clostridium difficile* infection).

4. **Rapid transit time**

A rapid transit time in the bowel may cause diarrhoea.

This is seen following bowel resection and with entero-enteral fistulae. It may also contribute to the irritable bowel syndrome (q.v.).

Rapid intestinal transit may also be part of the mechanism by which hormone-secreting tumours cause diarrhoea (see above).

5. **Drugs**

These are common causes of diarrhoea.
- Some may cause osmotic diarrhoea (see above).
- Some (e.g. antibiotics, beta blockers, colchicine, cytotoxics, digitalis, ethanol, nonsteroidal anti-inflammatory agents, quinidine) may cause secretory diarrhoea via direct effects.
- Some antibiotics may lead to antibiotic-associated colitis (see Colitis – *Clostridium difficile* infection).

Bibliography
Beers M, Cameron S. Hemolytic uremic syndrome. *Emerg Infect Dis* 1995; 1: 4.
Blaser MJ, Smith PD, Ravdin JL, et al., eds. *Infections of the Gastrointestinal Tract*. 2nd edition. New York: Raven Press. 2002.
Cappell M. Colonic toxicity of administered drugs and chemicals. *Am J Gastroenterol* 2004; 99: 1175.
Dionne JC, Mbuagbaw L, Devlin JW, et al. Diarrhea during critical illness: a multicenter cohort study. *Intens Care Med* 2022; 48: 570.
Fairchild PG, Blacklow NR. Viral diarrhea. *Infect Dis Clin North Am* 1988; 2: 677.
Field M, Rao MC, Chang EB. Intestinal electrolyte transport and diarrheal disease. *N Engl J Med* 1989; 321: 800 & 879.
Goldberg MB, Paras M. Gastrointestinal tract infections. In: *Scientific American Medicine. Gastroenterology*. Hamilton: Dekker Medicine. 2020.
Hellard ME, Fairley CK. Gastroenteritis in Australia: who, what, where, and how much? *Aust NZ J Med* 1997; 27: 147.
Kelly CP, Pothoulakis C, La Mont JT. *Clostridium difficile* colitis. *N Engl J Med* 1994; 330: 257.
Krejs GJ. VIPoma syndrome. *Am J Med* 1987; 82: 37.
Linedale EC, Andrews JM. Diagnosis and management of irritable bowel syndrome: a guide for the generalist. *Med J Aust* 2017; 207: 309.
Lyerly DM, Krivan HC, Wilkins TD. *Clostridium difficile*: its disease and toxins. *Clin Microbiol Rev* 1988; 1: 1.
Phillips SF. Diarrhea: a current view of the pathophysiology. *Gastroenterology* 1972; 63: 495.
Schlager TA, Guerrant RL. Seven possible mechanisms for *Escherichia coli* diarrhea. *Infect Dis Clin North Am* 1988; 2: 607.
Slutsker L, Ries AA, Greene KD, et al. *Escherichia coli* O157:H7 diarrhea in the United States: clinical and epidemiologic features. *Ann Intern Med* 1997; 126: 505.
Van Langenberg DR, Gearry RB, Wong H-L, et al. The potential value of faecal lactoferrin as a screening test in hospitalized patients with diarrhoea. *Intern Med J* 2010; 40: 819.
Wanke CA, Guerrant RL. Viral hepatitis and gastroenteritis transmitted by shellfish and water. *Infect Dis Clin North Am* 1987; 1: 649.
Wong CS, Jelacic S, Habeeb RL, et al. The risk of the hemolytic-uremic syndrome after antibiotic treatment of *Escherichia coli* O157-H7 infections. *N Engl J Med* 2000; 342: 1930.
Young GP, Bayley N, Ward P, et al. Antibiotic-associated colitis caused by *Clostridium difficile*: relapse and risk factors. *Med J Aust* 1986; 144: 303.

DIC *See*

- Disseminated intravascular coagulation.

Differentiation syndrome

Differentiation syndrome refers to a constellation of clinical features, including fever, hypotension, pulmonary infiltrates, pulmonary haemorrhage, pleural effusions and renal dysfunction, seen in patients who have received **all-trans retinoic acid** (ATRA) instead of chemotherapy for acute promyelocytic leukaemia. The differentiation syndrome has also been reported after the use of **arsenic trioxide** (q.v.) in the treatment of relapsed acute promyelocytic leukaemia and after the use of ATRA in other conditions, including myelodysplastic syndrome, lung cancer (NSCLC with metastases), prostate cancer and neural tumours.

The differentiation syndrome and associated leukocytosis are thought to be related to the ability of ATRA and arsenic trioxide to cause differentiation of the leukaemia cells into maturing myeloid cells, which accumulate in the lungs and other organs. Lung biopsy may be necessary to confirm the diagnosis.

It occurs in about 15% of patients treated with these agents, usually within the first month. The syndrome is reversible if recognized promptly and the culprit drug withdrawn. Interestingly, ATRA can generally be resumed safely once the syndrome has subsided.

*Treatment with high-dose **corticosteroids** is recommended, provided infection has been excluded. Diuretic therapy is probably helpful.*

Bibliography
Frankel SR, Eardley A, Lauwers G, et al. The 'retinoic acid syndrome' in acute promyelocytic leukemia. *Ann Intern Med* 1992; 117: 292.
Nicholls MR, Terada LS, Tuder RM, et al. Diffuse alveolar hemorrhage with underlying pulmonary capillaritis in the retinoic acid syndrome. *Am J Respir Crit Care Med* 1998; 158: 1302.

Diffuse alveolar haemorrhage

Diffuse alveolar haemorrhage (DAH) refers to parenchymal lung bleeding with consequent haemoptysis (q.v.) and pulmonary infiltrates (q.v.). Systemic coagulopathy, local causes (particularly malignancy), left heart failure and aspiration of blood need to be specifically excluded.

The condition may present with respiratory failure and a clinical picture of ARDS (q.v.).

Its pathogenesis is considered to be an **immune-mediated pulmonary capillaritis** in most cases. Thus, it may be caused by

- collagen-vascular diseases (especially systemic lupus erythematosus – q.v.),
- drugs (e.g. cocaine – q.v.),
- Goodpasture's syndrome (q.v.),
- idiopathic pulmonary haemosiderosis (q.v.),
- idiopathic rapidly progressive glomerulonephritis (see Glomerular diseases),
- vasculitis (including Wegener's granulomatosis) (q.v.).

Bibliography
Green RJ, Ruoss SJ, Kraft SA, et al. Pulmonary capillaritis and alveolar hemorrhage: update on diagnosis and management. *Chest* 1996; 110: 1305.
Lara AR, Schwarz M. Diffuse alveolar hemorrhage. *Chest* 2010; 137: 1164.
Leatherman JW, Davies SF, Hoidal JR. Alveolar hemorrhage syndromes: diffuse microvascular lung hemorrhage in immune and idiopathic disorders. *Medicine* 1984; 63: 343.
Schwarz MI, Albert RK. 'Imitators' of the ARDS: implications for diagnosis and treatment. *Chest* 2004; 125: 1530.
Specks U. Diffuse alveolar hemorrhage syndromes. *Curr Opinion Rheumatol* 2001; 13: 12.
Young KR. Diagnostic pitfalls in alveolar hemorrhage syndromes. *Pulmonary Perspectives* 2000; 17: 11.

Diffuse fibrosing alveolitis See

- Idiopathic pulmonary fibrosis.

Diffuse parenchymal lung diseases See

- Interstitial lung diseases.

Digoxin-specific antibody

Digoxin-specific immune antigen-binding Fab fragment (digoxin FAB antibody) is derived from antibodies made in sheep to digoxin conjugated with human albumin. It has a molecular weight of 50 kDa. It binds to and thus decreases the concentration of free digoxin (and digitoxin) in plasma, and the complex thus formed is excreted in the urine. Since digoxin has greater affinity for the exogenous antibody than for tissue receptors, not only is less free drug available to interact with cardiac and other cell membranes but the drug is progressively removed from tissue receptors. It is very expensive, i.e. about $1000 per vial or $10,000 per treatment.

Its chief indication is life-threatening digoxin overdosage, usually associated with ventricular arrhythmias.

Typically, more than 10 mg of digoxin has been taken orally and plasma levels are greater than 10 ng/mL.

The dose is calculated as follows.
- Firstly, the body's digoxin load (in mg) is calculated as plasma level (ng/mL), multiplied by volume of distribution (5.6 l/kg), multiplied by body weight (kg), divided by 1000. Alternatively, the body load may be estimated based on the numbers of tablets taken, if known, as mg ingested divided by 0.8.
- Secondly, the number of vials required equals load (in mg) divided by 0.6 (the no. of mg of digoxin able to be bound per vial).

An average dose is 10 vials, though 20 vials should be given if the clinical situation is life-threatening and no levels or dosage are known. A vial containing 40 mg of powder is reconstituted to 4 mL and binds 0.6 mg of digoxin (or digitoxin). The drug is administered IV over 30 min using a 0.22 μm cyclovir filter.

Clinical improvement should be seen within 30 min. The plasma level of digoxin will increase markedly after administration of the antibody but almost all is bound and awaiting urinary excretion. A new steady state plasma level is not achieved for 5–6 hr.

The antibody may be used in renal failure, although excretion is delayed in that setting. Since digoxin overdose can cause hyperkalaemia, the serum potassium level must be monitored. Anaphylaxis associated with the antibody's use has not so far been reported, perhaps partly because no cases of re-challenge have yet been described. Re-emergence of digoxin toxicity has not been reported. As might be expected, any re-digitalization needs to be deferred for several days.

The successful use of digoxin-specific immune antigen-binding Fab fragment has been reported in **toad venom poisoning**, since this venom may a contain digitalis-like substance (see Bites and stings).

Bibliography
Antman EM, Wenger TL, Butler VP, et al. Treatment of 150 cases of life-threatening digitalis intoxication with digoxin-specific Fab antibody fragments. *Circulation* 1990; 81: 1744.
Brubacher JR, Ravikumar PR, Bania T, et al. Treatment of toad venom poisoning with digoxin-specific Fab fragments. *Chest* 1996; 110: 1282.
Kelly RA, Smith TW. Recognition and management of digitalis toxicity. *Am J Cardiol* 1992; 69: 1186.
Pincus M. Management of digoxin toxicity. *Aust Prescriber* 2016; 39: 18.

Smith TW, Haber E, Yeatman L, et al. Reversal of advanced digoxin intoxication with Fab fragments of digoxin-specific antibodies. *N Engl J Med* 1976; 294: 797.

Taboulet P, Baud FJ, Bismuth C. Clinical features and management of digitalis poisoning – rationale for immunotherapy. *J Toxicol Clin Toxicol* 1993; 31: 247.

Dimercaprol *See*
- Chelating agents.

Dioxins

A **dioxin** is a chemical compound consisting of two benzene rings connected by a pair of oxygen atoms. Since each ring contains 8 carbon atoms which can each bind to a hydrogen or other atom (the most concerning to health being chlorine), up to 75 isomers are possible. Dioxins are usually formed as a by-product of the manufacture of herbicides based on 2,4,5-trichlorophenol and are the most toxic of artificial substances.

The term 'dioxin' particularly refers to one specific dioxin (2,3,7,8-tetrachlorodibenzo-p-dioxin, TCDD), a very stable substance which is insoluble in water but soluble in oils, so that it is not diluted environmentally but accumulates in animal tissues. It is not a useful substance but a by-product in the manufacture of chlorophenoxyacetic acid derivatives, both of 2,4,5-trichlorophenoxyacetic acid (2,4,5-T), a major ingredient in the defoliant, Agent Orange, and of the antiseptic, hexachlorophene. Agent Orange also includes 2,4-dichlorophenoxyacetic acid (2,4-D) and is likely to be contaminated with dioxin (TCDD).

There is no safe level of TCDD, which is lethal for some animal species at five parts per billion, i.e. as little as 60 mcg can kill a mouse. It is a potential carcinogen. Agent Orange itself may increase the incidence of non-Hodgkin's lymphoma and soft tissue sarcoma. Other late toxic effects include chloracne, neurological disorders, muscle dysfunction, impotence, birth defects and mutations. Industrial accidents since the 1970s have been associated with extensive loss of nearby animal life and the forced evacuation sometimes permanently of whole communities.

Chlorophenoxyacetic acid derivatives are cellular toxins and their ingestion whether accidental or via the food chain can cause severe poisoning. Clinical features include acute gastrointestinal symptoms (nausea, vomiting, diarrhoea and abdominal pain), profound muscle weakness, rhabdomyolysis (q.v.), metabolic acidosis and hypotension. Death may occur within 24 hr. Survivors may develop liver and renal failure and peripheral neuropathy. Long-term toxic effects are described above.

There is no specific antidote, and treatment of acute poisoning is supportive, particularly for coma, hypotension, metabolic acidosis and rhabdomyolysis (q.v.).

Related compounds include the PCBs (polychlorinated biphenols) and PCDFs (polychlorinated dibenzofurans).

- PCBs in particular are produced by electrical fires, which can cause widespread contamination of buildings. These substances give skin, liver and reproductive effects, and they are potential carcinogens.
- PCDFs have caused outbreaks of disease following contamination of cooking oil. The reproductive consequences of a generalized ectodermal disorder in offspring have been well documented.

Glyphosate is the least toxic chlorophenoxyacetic acid derivative and is widely used as a general herbicide.

Diphtheria

Diphtheria is caused by the dumbbell-shaped Gram-positive bacillus, *Corynebacterium diphtheriae*, which produces a potent exotoxin. It is spread by droplets and thus primarily affects the pharynx, though sometimes primary sites elsewhere are seen. Bacterial multiplication occurs locally, and the exotoxin but not the bacteria become disseminated.

A characteristic grey, leathery and adherent local membrane is also produced by the toxin. The size of the membrane correlates with the extent of toxin produced.

The illness follows an incubation period of 2–5 days. Although the pharyngitis is generally mild, cervical lymphadenopathy can be marked, and there may be purpura and shock.

Cutaneous diphtheria is seen
- in the tropics (jungle sore),
- after trauma (wound diphtheria),
- in association with poor hygiene (e.g. in poor alcoholics).

There are three important complications of diphtheria.
1. **Upper airway obstruction**
   Obstruction from the pharyngeal membrane may give rise to a medical emergency.
2. **Myocarditis**
   This occurs in 10–25% and is the usual cause of death. Cardiac involvement becomes apparent in the second week of illness, with ST abnormalities and then arrhythmias, complete heart block, bundle branch block, cardiac failure and shock.

> An AV conduction defect may persist after recovery.
> 3. **Peripheral neuritis**
> This occurs in 10% of patients 2–6 weeks after the initial illness. It particularly involves the cranial nerves (III, VI, VII, IX and X) and peripheral motor nerves, including the phrenic nerve (see Neuropathy).
> Sometimes, a Guillain–Barré syndrome-like condition (q.v.) may be seen.

The diagnosis is made clinically and confirmed by culture or fluorescent antibody detection of swab material.

A 'diphtheria-membrane', though less adherent, may also be seen in pharyngitis due to
- group A streptococci,
- infectious mononucleosis (see Epstein–Barr virus),
- viruses,
- candida.

*Treatment is with **diphtheria antitoxin** (DAT), if diagnosed within 48 hr, in a dose of 20,000–100,000 U (50% IM and 50% IV 1 hr later).*
- *Antibiotics (erythromycin, penicillin or clindamycin) are indicated in the acute illness, and they may also help eradicate a carrier state.*
- *Rest, isolation and treatment of complications are required.*

Prevention is with immunization, and the disease occurs only in the unimmunized, so that it is rarely seen in developed countries. A 75% herd immunity is required to prevent community outbreaks, which are now seen in adults as well as in children in circumstances where there has been waning community immunity. Immunization does not prevent the carrier state. The Schick test was used in the past for assessment of immunity. Separately from immunization, there can be a changing community incidence due to the natural cycling of the disease, such as has been observed historically.

Bibliography
Boyer NH, Weinstein L. Diphtheritic myocarditis. *N Engl J Med* 1948; 239: 913.
Doble RA, Tobey DN. Clinical features of diphtheria in the respiratory tract. *JAMA* 1979; 242: 2197.
Farizo KM, Strebel PM, Chen RT, et al. Fatal respiratory disease due to Corynebacterium diphtheriae: case report and review of guidelines for management, investigation, and control. *Clin Infect Dis* 1993; 16: 59.
Galazka AM, Robertson SE, Oblapenko GP. Resurgence of diphtheria. *Eur J Epidemiol* 1995; 11: 95.
Harmisch JP, Tronca E, Nolan CM, et al. Diphtheria among alcoholic urban adults. *Ann Intern Med* 1989; 111: 71.
Mofred A, Guerin JM, Falfoul-Borsali N, et al. Cutaneous diphtheria. *Rev Med Interne* 1994; 15: 515.

Dipyridamole See
- Antiplatelet agents.

Dissecting aneurysm See
- Aortic dissection.

Disseminated intravascular coagulation

Disseminated intravascular coagulation (DIC) is the archetypal thrombohaemorrhagic disorder. It is the most common of the **thrombotic microangiopathies** (TMAs) (q.v.), and it needs to be differentiated from the other TMAs in any relevant clinical setting. It is a life-threatening complication which is commonly encountered in Intensive Care practice.

DIC has been defined by the International Society on Thrombosis and Haemostasis (ISTH) as 'an acquired syndrome characterized by the intravascular activation of coagulation with loss of localization arising from different causes that can originate from and cause damage to the microvasculature, which if sufficiently severe can produce organ dysfunction'.

> DIC has been referred to as the response of the blood to injury.
> It is not a primary condition, but rather a complication or marker of other serious illness, especially sepsis, trauma, malignancy and obstetric disasters.
> - Sepsis may be due to bacterial, viral, fungal or protozoal infection.
> - Trauma may be blunt, penetrating, thermal or hypoxic.
> - Malignancy includes both solid tumours and haematological neoplasia.
> - Obstetric disasters include acute fatty liver of pregnancy, amniotic fluid embolism, placental abruption, post-partum haemorrhage and pre-eclampsia (see these separate conditions).
> - Other causes include envenomation (see Bites and Stings), giant haemangioma (q.v.), incompatible blood transfusion and rhabdomyolysis (q.v.).

However, DIC can cause significant clinical problems in its own right. These problems include

- **microthrombosis** (leading to organ dysfunction) and
- **consumption coagulopathy** (leading to haemorrhage).

In this sense, DIC is perhaps akin to other entities in the Intensive Care Unit like shock, acidosis and fever, which are all complications of some other primary illness, but which can then cause problems in their own right.

Laboratory diagnosis requires the demonstration of **coagulopathy** (prolonged prothrombin time), **consumption** (decreased platelet count and fibrinogen) and **secondary fibrinolysis** (increased fibrin degradation products, e.g. D-dimer).

Its chief treatment is that of the underlying condition or trigger process, as described above.

Supportive treatment includes
- **platelet transfusion**, to a platelet count above $50 \times 10^9/L$ if bleeding, and
- **thromboprophylaxis**, especially in septic patients (if not already receiving such prophylaxis for venous thromboembolism).

In some countries, **recombinant thrombomodulin** (q.v.) is used as a specific anticoagulant in managing DIC. See
- Amniotic fluid embolism,
- Anaemia – Intravascular haemolysis,
- Antithrombin III deficiency,
- Cancer complications,
- Coagulation disorders,
- Diving – Decompression sickness,
- Fibrinolysis,
- Haemangioma,
- Heat stroke,
- Microangiopathic haemolysis,
- Protein C,
- Serotonin syndrome,
- Thrombohaemorrhagic disorders,
- Trauma-induced coagulopathy.

Bibliography

Bick RL. Disseminated intravascular coagulation; a review of etiology, pathophysiology, diagnosis and management. *Clin Appl Thromb Hemost* 2002; 8: 1.

Iba T, Levy JH, Warkentin TE, et al. Diagnosis and management of sepsis-induced coagulopathy and disseminated intravascular coagulation. *J Thromb Haemost* 2019; 17: 1989.

Levi M, ed.. Disseminated intravascular coagulation. *Semin Thromb Hemost* 2001; 27: 565.

Levi M, Schultz MJ. What do sepsis-induced coagulation test result abnormalities mean to intensivists. *Intens Care Med* 2017; 43: 581.

Levi M, ten Cate H. Disseminated intravascular coagulation. *N Engl J Med* 1999; 341: 586.

Rabinovich A, Abdul-Kadir R, Thachil J, et al. DIC in obstetrics: Diagnostic score, highlights in management, and international registry – communication from the DIC and Women's Health SSCs of the International Society of Thrombosis and Haemostasis. *J Thromb Haemost* 2019; 17: 1562.

Squizzato A, Gallo A, Levi M, et al. Underlying disorders of disseminated intravascular coagulation: communication from the ISTH SSC subcommittees on Disseminated Intravascular Coagulation and Perioperative and Critical Care Thrombosis and Haemostasis. *J Thromb Haemost* 2020; 18: 2400.

Squizzato A, Hunt BJ, Kinasewitz GT, et al. Supportive management strategies for disseminated intravascular coagulation: an international consensus. *Thromb Haemost* 2016; 203: 896.

Zeerleder S, Hack E, Wuillemin WA. Disseminated intravascular coagulation in sepsis. *Chest* 2005; 128: 2864.

Disulfiram *See*

- Amoebiasis,
- Flushing,
- Mushroom poisoning.

Diving

Diving accidents have become common because of the proliferation of diving activities both professional and recreational worldwide. Because of the availability of modern transport, diving sequelae may be seen well away from the original geographical site of the dive itself.

> The most important diving accidents are **gas embolism** and **decompression sickness**.
> - The most common, however, are ear or sinus damage due to barotrauma.
> - Diving-induced damage may also relate to pre-existing diseases, some of which are contraindications to diving, such as many respiratory, cardiovascular and neurological disorders.
> - Diving may also be a cause of drowning (q.v.).

Diving accidents are usually associated with well-defined risk factors, such as multiple dives, exceeding 'tables', rapid ascent, alcohol or subsequent air travel. A patent foramen ovale is an important risk factor in some patients. Clearly, other factors such as accidents, environmental problems, equipment failure, carelessness and inexperience may also be involved.

Cerebral arterial gas embolism (CAGE) is responsible for about 15% of major problems. It occurs because of rapid ascent with the head up and is due to alveolar overdistension and rupture giving rise to pulmonary barotrauma (q.v.) with embolization to the systemic circulation, if there is a direct communication with the pulmonary vasculature.

Neurological changes occur rapidly and may be either dramatic (coma) or subtle (paraesthesiae or mood changes).

Decompression sickness is due to formation of nitrogen bubbles from too rapid an ascent. The nitrogen was dissolved in tissues, especially lipids at depth, and appropriate staged decompression is therefore essential to prevent its unduly rapid release during ascent. Using sensitive Doppler tests, some bubbles in fact may be detected in virtually all divers, regardless of the care taken with the dive. Intravascular changes of disseminated intravascular coagulation (q.v.) and complement activation (q.v.) may be produced.

Symptoms can appear as soon as 1 hr or as late as 36 hr after the ascent.

- In type 1 (25% of diving accidents), the skin and joints are affected, and the condition is thus called the bends.
- In type 2 (more than half of all major diving accidents), there are neurological changes, including focal and spinal cord signs and respiratory distress (the chokes).

Bone necrosis may occur if the process is repeated. There is commonly headache, lethargy and altered sensation.

*Treatment priorities are positioning on the left side, oxygen (especially for CAGE) and **recompression** in a hyperbaric facility. This may usefully be undertaken even up to several hours later.*

Bibliography
Charles MJ, Wirjosemito SA. Flying and diving: still a real hazard. *J Hyperbaric Med* 1989; 4: 23.
Elliot DH, Hallenbeck LM, Bove AA. Acute decompression sickness. *Lancet* 1974; 2: 1193.
Emerson GM. What you need to know about diving medicine but won't find in a textbook. *Emergency Med* 2002; 14: 371.
Francis J. Decompression sickness. *Emergency Med* 2002; 14: 358.
Gorman D. Accidental arterial gas embolism. *Emergency Med* 2002; 14: 364.
Lundgren CEG, Miller JN, eds. *The Lung at Depth*. New York: Marcel Dekker. 1999.

Melamed Y, Shupak A, Bitterman H. Medical problems associated with underwater diving. *N Engl J Med* 1992; 326: 30.
Moon RE, Camporesi EM, Kisslo JA. Patent foramen ovale and decompression sickness in divers. *Lancet* 1989; 1: 513.
Tetzlaff K, Reuter M, Leplow B, et al. Risk factors for pulmonary barotrauma in divers. *Chest* 1997; 112: 654.
Weathersby PK, Survanshi SS, Homer LD, et al. Predicting the time of occurrence of decompression sickness. *J Appl Physiol* 1992; 72: 1541.
Weinmann M, Tuxen D, Scheinkestel C, et al. Decompression illnesses. *SPUMS J* 1991; 21: 135.

Dog bites *See*

- Bites and stings.

Drowning

Drowning is a common accident due to a wide variety of activities at all ages in most societies. Drowning is a major cause of accidental death, calculated variously as an average incidence of 1 in 30,000 of the population per year or as 500,000 deaths worldwide per year. For every case of fatal drowning, there are four further cases of non-fatal drowning (formerly called near drowning). By far the majority of cases of drowning are potentially preventable. This particularly applies to cases of hypoxic blackout due to deliberate hyperventilation prior to diving or to prolonged breath-holding during submersion.

The WHO definition of drowning is respiratory impairment due to submersion in liquid.

In general, the lungs become flooded, though in 10% of patients the lungs are dry and have been protected by intense laryngospasm. The changes in blood volume and composition depend on the amount and tonicity of fluid aspirated. Usually the volume of water aspirated is not large, and serum electrolyte changes are minimal. Fresh water gives hypervolaemia and haemodilution. Salt water (5% saline) gives hypovolaemia and haemoconcentration. However, these differences are not always clear-cut, and the pathological changes after fatal drowning and the clinical and investigational findings after non-fatal drowning are similar for both fresh and sea water.

After non-fatal drowning, the patient is comatose and apnoeic, and may even have fixed dilated pupils until resuscitated.

Even after resuscitation, central nervous system derangement with confusion, restlessness, delirium (q.v.) and convulsions may persist for some time, due to hypoxic damage with cerebral oedema and even infarction.

Investigations show arterial hypoxaemia, metabolic acidosis (q.v.), variable serum electrolyte levels, and albuminuria, haematuria (q.v.) and sometimes haemoglobinuria (q.v.). The chest X-ray generally shows perihilar densities initially, though more florid pulmonary oedema commonly becomes apparent some hours later. An assessment should be made of any associated injuries.

Treatment of non-fatal drowning comprises the following.
- Aspiration of the upper airway for fluid and foreign bodies should be promptly made, but not aspiration of the tracheobronchial tree as this is ineffective.
- The stomach should be aspirated, as the stomach is full and vomiting is common because of the large amount of water that has often been swallowed.
- Cardiopulmonary resuscitation is usually required. Even if the resuscitative needs on site are minimal, the patient should be transferred to hospital, because respiratory failure may occur up to 12 hr later, with tachypnoea, cough, frothy blood-stained sputum, chest pain and wheeze.
- Intensive Care treatment is required for respiratory failure (due to acute pulmonary oedema early or acute respiratory distress syndrome later), cardiac arrhythmias, metabolic acidosis, cerebral oedema, gastric distension, coagulopathy, hypothermia (see below) and infections.
- Extracorporeal life support should be considered in cases of prolonged cardiac arrest, if promptly available.
- Corticosteroids are of unproven value.
- Prophylactic antibiotics are not indicated.

Hypothermia (q.v.) is usual, because the temperature of even tropical waters is less than that of the body and only a few minutes are required for temperature equilibration. Hypothermia probably has some neuroprotective effect.

If the body temperature is <30°C, there is severe depression of the circulation and the patient may appear lifeless; if the temperature is <28°C, ventricular fibrillation occurs. Ventricular fibrillation may also be precipitated by the necessary procedure of intubation, and defibrillation is usually unsuccessful if the temperature is <30°C. At this temperature also, the activity and clearance of drugs is impaired.

Passive or even active external warning is often inadequate, and core rewarming may then be required. Rewarming should pause at about 33°C for 12 hr, because moderate hypothermia to this degree is currently recommended for normothermic adult patients being treated for non-fatal drowning.

The outlook is excellent for victims of non-fatal drowning who have not suffered a cardiac arrest. The survival rate is still 90% if the period of arrest is <5 min, but it is 0% if the period of arrest is >25 min. On average, there is a two thirds mortality if cardiopulmonary resuscitation is required. Children have a better outcome than adults. The prognosis is also more favourable if there has been hypothermia (core temperature <35°C), but this prognostic criterion is inexact, perhaps since cardiac arrest may have happened during normothermia with cooling occurring only subsequently. There are several reported predictive indices of outcome in general, but they are unhelpful in the individual patient.

Bibliography

Bierens JJ, Modell J, Pepe P, et al., eds. *Handbook on Drowning: Prevention, Rescue, Treatment.* Berlin: Springer. 2005.

Dix J. *Asphyxia and Drowning: An Atlas.* Boca Raton: CRC Press. 2000.

Edwards ND, Timmins AC, Randalls B, et al. Survival in adults after cardiac arrest due to drowning. *Intens Care Med* 1990; 16: 336.

Golden FS, Tipton MJ, Scott RC. Immersion, near-drowning and drowning. *Br J Anaesthesia* 1997; 79: 214.

Hasibeder WR. Near-drowning. *Int J Intens Care* 2003; 10: 166.

Markarian T, Loudou A, Heyer V, et al. Drowning classification: a reappraisal of clinical presentation and prognosis for severe cases. *Chest* 2020; 158: 596.

Modell JH. Serum electrolyte changes in near-drowning victims. *JAMA* 1985; 253: 557.

Modell JH. Drowning. *N Engl J Med* 1993; 328: 253.

Moon RE, Long RJ. Drowning and near-drowning. *Emerg Med* 2002; 14: 377.

Orlowski JP. Drowning, near-drowning, and ice-water drowning. *JAMA* 1988; 260: 390.

Sachdeva RC. Near drowning. *Crit Care Clin* 1999; 15: 281.

Szpilman D. Near-drowning and drowning classification. *Chest* 1997; 112: 660.

Szpilman D, Bierens JJLM, Handley AJ, et al. Drowning. *N Engl J Med* 2012; 366: 2102.

Szpilman D, Morgan PJ. Management for the drowning patient. *Chest* 2021; 159: 1473.

Thom O, Roberts K, Devine S, et al. Treatment of the lung injury of drowning: a systematic review. *Crit Care* 2021; 25: 253.

Williamson JP, Illing R, Gertler P, et al. Near-drowning treated with therapeutic hypothermia. *Med J Aust* 2004; 181: 500.

Drug allergy

Drug allergy is uncommon and comprises only 6% of all adverse drug reactions (ADRs), which overall are of course common.

Importantly, drug allergy can occur with only small doses of drug. However, most drug reactions of a seemingly allergic nature are not in fact immune-mediated (i.e. true allergy) but due to other effects often of a chemical nature, e.g. mast cell release.

Drug allergy is separate from
- **drug intolerance**, which is an adverse pharmacological effect of a drug even at low dose,
- **drug idiosyncrasy**, which is a non-pharmacological effect due to biochemical alteration in drug metabolism at any dose.

The most common drug allergy is to **penicillin**. This occurs in 1–5% of recipients and is responsible for 90% of all cases of drug allergy and for 90% of cases of fatal anaphylaxis.

Other important drug allergies are seen following
- anaesthetic agents (mostly neuromuscular blocking agents (NMBAs) and especially suxamethonium, but not volatile agents),
- aspirin (q.v.),
- diagnostic contrast agents (especially those containing iodine),
- antibiotics (especially beta-lactams, but also glycopeptides), sulphonamides,
- hormones,
- gelatin and dextran,
- opiates,
- chlorhexidine,
- echinacea, a popular complementary medicine for cold and flu symptoms.

Serious reactions to selective cyclo-oxygenase-2 (COX-2) inhibitors (particularly parenteral parecoxib) have been reported in patients with prior sensitivity to sulphonamides.

Most allergic drug reactions take the form of a mild systemic illness, similar to serum sickness (q.v.), with
- fever (q.v.),
- urticaria (q.v.),
- arthralgia (q.v.),
- lymphadenopathy (q.v.).

The typical onset occurs after 6–12 days and disappears several days after drug cessation.

Anaphylaxis is the potentially fatal manifestation of drug allergy with an onset within minutes. It usually follows parenteral drug administration, but it can follow oral dosage. It occurs in about 1 in 10,000 general anaesthetics, and it causes death in about 1 in 2 million general anaesthetics.

Its clinical features include one or more of the following:
- pruritus (q.v.),
- flushing (q.v.),
- angioedema of any region but especially of the face and larynx (q.v.),
- hypovolaemia with hypotension and shock.

Perioperative anaphylaxis, especially to NMBAs, has been associated with the widespread use in some communities of pholcodine in over-the-counter cough remedies and is due to cross-sensitivity.

Drug allergy may be diagnosed when
- the clinical manifestations are not those of any known pharmacological effect of the drug,
- the drug doses are very small,
- there are allergic symptoms,
- the same reaction occurs with rechallenge,
- it occurs with related drugs.

Skin tests are of most diagnostic value, though less so for **penicillin**.

In practice,
- patients with a history of anaphylaxis or urticaria after penicillin should be skin tested;
- following an immediate reaction, 50% of patients have negative skin tests after 5 years, because patients with IgE reactions tend to lose their sensitivity with time since exposure;
- patients with a history of a maculopapular rash after penicillin are not at risk of a subsequent immediate reaction;
- patients who previously developed a Stevens–Johnson syndrome (q.v.) after penicillin should never receive the drug again and skin tests are not indicated in them;
- a positive family history is not related to personal risk of penicillin allergy;
- penicillin may be safely given to patients with negative skin tests and desensitization is unnecessary, though it would be wise to give a small test dose initially.

The preferred in vitro test is the serum tryptase, which reflects the release of mast cell contents. It may be shown to be elevated in blood taken shortly after a major systemic allergic event, though not after food-induced anaphylaxis. Levels generally peak within 1 hr of mast cell degranulation and decline thereafter with a half-life of about 2 hr. Sometimes, IgE antibodies to a specific drug may be detected, but tests involving other immunoglobulins or cell-mediated immunity do not correlate with symptoms.

Treatment includes
- cessation of the drug,
- specific measures for anaphylaxis, particularly adrenaline (epinephrine) together with IV fluids,
- corticosteroids for an Arthus-type reaction (i.e. serum sickness) or other delayed hypersensitivity reaction (e.g. symptomatic rash),
- desensitization which should be considered if the drug is needed to be given again, or alternatively a drug alert bracelet should be offered.

Detailed clinical management guidelines, especially for anaphylaxis, have been published and widely distributed.

Bibliography

Baldwin JL, Speck AL. Drug allergies. In: *Scientific American Medicine. Allergy & Immunology.* Hamilton: Dekker Medicine. 2020.

Gorevic P. Drug allergy. In: Kaplan AP, ed. *Allergy.* New York: Churchill Livingstone. 1985; p 473.

Katelaris CH, Smith WB. 'Iodine allergy' label is misleading. *Aust Prescriber* 2009; 22: 125.

Kolawole H, Marshall SD, Crilly H, et al. Australian and New Zealand Allergy Group/Australian and New Zealand College of Anaesthetists perioperative anaphylaxis management guidelines. *Anaesth Intens Care* 2017; 45: 151.

Papadopoulos J, Kane-Gill S, Cooper B, eds. Identification and prevention of common adverse drug events in the intensive care unit. *Crit Care Med* 2010; 36: 6 (suppl.).

Rosenberg J, Pentel P, Pond S, et al. Hyperthermia associated with drug intoxication. *Crit Care Med* 1986; 14: 964.

Shear NH, Knowles S, Shapiro L. Cutaneous adverse drug reactions. In: *Scientific American Medicine. Dermatology.* Hamilton: Dekker Medicine. 2020.

Solensky R, Earl HS, Gruchalla RS, et al. Lack of penicillin resensitization in patients with a history of penicillin allergy after receiving repeated penicillin courses. *Arch Intern Med* 2002; 162: 822.

Weiss ME. Drug allergy. *Med Clin North Am* 1992; 76: 857.

Drug–drug interactions

A **drug–drug interaction** refers to a clinically significant effect which is different from the effects seen when the same drugs are given individually. Such interactions may be clinically adverse, favourable or neutral.

In hospital practice, 10–20% of all drug reactions are due to drug–drug interactions. In addition, adverse reactions are more frequent if multiple drugs are administered, even when such an incidence is discounted for the actual number of drugs. Since the number of drugs that may be properly prescribed concomitantly, especially in an Intensive Care Unit, is enormous and since it is impossible to remember them all, most drug–drug interactions are probably undetected.

Comprehensive compendia are now available covering the interactions of specific drugs. However, it is best to use an automated monitoring system (especially if built in to an electronic medical record and prescribing system), but even then the clinical significance of a potential interaction is not necessarily clear.

> The number of drug combinations in a particular patient can be calculated as:
>
> no. = $n! \div 2(n-2)!$,
>
> where n is the number of drugs and n! is factorial n (see Figure below).
>
> Thus, if 7 drugs are concomitantly prescribed, there are 21 drug combinations, each with their own potential to display an interaction.
>
> The prevalence of drug–drug interactions has been reported to be 20% if 10 or more drugs are concomitantly prescribed.

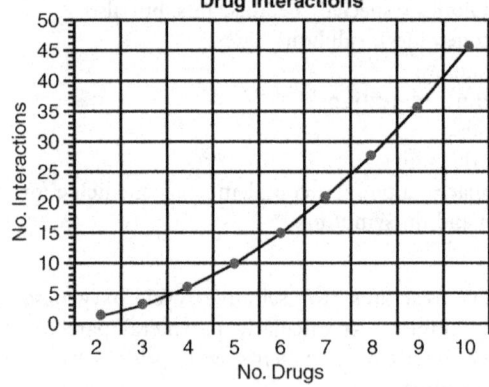

The types of drug–drug interaction include
- pharmacological antagonism or synergy,
- pharmacokinetic changes (e.g. absorption, binding, metabolism, excretion),

- pharmacodynamic changes (e.g. interference at receptor sites).

Clearly multiple drug prescription is inevitable in Intensive Care practice, but combinations should be routinely checked.

A drug–drug interaction is not necessarily a cause for cessation of the drugs involved, as appropriate dosage adjustment may be possible.

Drugs should always be remembered as a potential cause of unusual events. Even new events may occur. Some events may be predicted from in vitro or experimental evidence, some information is available from case reports, and online services can be valuable (e.g. the Liverpool drug interaction website).

The most important drug–drug interactions are those which diminish drug efficacy or increase drug toxicity, especially in the seriously ill.

Bibliography
Chrispin PS, Park GR. Unexpected drug reactions and interactions in the critical care unit. *Curr Opin Crit Care* 1997; 3: 262.
Hansten PB, Horn JR. *Drug Interactions*. Philadelphia: Lippincott Williams and Wilkins. 2006.
Leape LL, Brennan TA, Laird N, et al. The nature of adverse events in hospitalized patients: results from the Harvard Medical Practice Study II. *N Engl J Med* 1991; 324: 377.
Papadopoulos J, Kane-Gill S, Cooper B, eds. Identification and prevention of common adverse drug events in the intensive care unit. *Crit Care Med* 2010; 36: 6 (suppl.).
Peck CC, Temple R, Collins JM. Understanding consequences of concurrent therapies. *JAMA* 1993; 269: 1550.
Snyder BD, Polasek TM, Doogue MP. Drug interactions: principles and practice. *Aust Prescriber* 2012; 35: 85.
Zarowitz BJ. Drug-drug interactions in ICU. In: Parker MM, Shapiro MJ, Porembka DT, eds. *Critical Care: State of the Art*, Chapter 4. Anaheim: Society of Critical Care Medicine. 1995; p 91.

Drug fever

Drug fever usually occurs without the diagnostic assistance of other typical signs of drug hypersensitivity, such as rash or eosinophilia.

Drug fever is especially seen with the use of
- antimicrobials (particularly beta-lactams),
- antihypertensives (methyldopa, hydralazine),
- anticonvulsants (phenytoin),
- allopurinol,
- isoniazid.

In some cases, the onset of fever may be delayed for weeks or even months after the drug is first administered, e.g. methyldopa, phenytoin, isoniazid.

In the Intensive Care setting, other drugs which may also produce drug fever include
- amphotericin B,
- dexmedetomidine,
- diuretics,
- procainamide,
- propranolol,
- quinidine.

Bibliography
Johnson DH, Cunha BA. Drug fever. *Infect Dis Clin North Am* 1996; 10: 85.
Mackowiak PA, LeMaistre CF. Drug fever. *Ann Intern Med* 1987; 106: 728.
Olson KR, Benowitz NL. Environmental and drug-induced hyperthermia: pathophysiology, recognition and management. *Emerg Med Clin North Am* 1984; 2: 459.

Drugs

The use of **drugs** as therapeutic agents is one of the cornerstones of the treatment of the seriously ill, as it is in most medical specialties. Yet adverse drug reactions (ADRs) are frequent, they contribute greatly to hospital costs and to patient morbidity, and they are one of the leading causes of death.

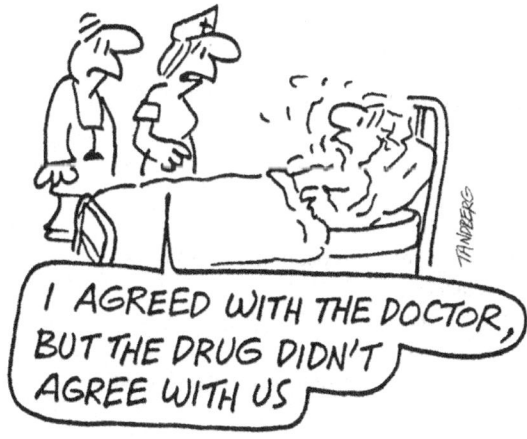

The non-therapeutic use of drugs is separately considered as **poisoning** (q.v.).

The drugs considered in this book are selected from those which have uncommon but important uses or those whose use may present particular problems. These discussions involve the following:

1. **General issues related to drug usage**, including
   - Alkaloids,
   - Autacoids,
   - Cholinergic crisis,
   - Drug allergy,
   - Drug–drug interactions,
   - Drug fever,
   - Malignant hyperthermia,
   - Neuroleptic malignant syndrome,
   - Serotonin syndrome.
2. **Uncommon problems with common drugs**, including
   - Acyclovir (aciclovir),
   - Adenosine,
   - Angiotensin-converting enzyme inhibitors,
   - Anticoagulants,
   - Antiplatelet agents,
   - Aspirin,
   - Bismuth,
   - Bleomycin,
   - Carbonic anhydrase inhibitors,
   - Colchicine,
   - Desmopressin,
   - Ergotamine,
   - Gamma-hydroxybutyric acid,
   - Heparin(s),
   - Lithium,
   - Methysergide,
   - Nitric oxide,
   - Nitrous oxide,
   - Octreotide,
   - Olmesartan,
   - Oral contraceptives,
   - Oxytocin,
   - Propofol,
   - Prostacyclin,
   - Sodium nitroprusside,
   - Statins,
   - Sucralfate,
   - Tetrahydroaminoacridine (THA),
   - Valerian,
   - Valproate,
   - Vaptans.
3. **Uncommon but important drugs**, including
   - Amphetamines,
   - Anticholinergic agents,
   - Anticholinesterases,
   - Baclofen,
   - Bacitracin,
   - Bromocriptine,
   - Cathinones,
   - Chelating agents,
   - Cholinergic agonists,
   - Dantrolene,
   - Desferrioxamine,
   - Digoxin-specific antibody,
   - Disulfiram,
   - Leflunomide,
   - Liquorice,
   - Methylene blue,
   - Prussian blue
   - Rituximab.
4. **Specific organ-related drug issues**, including
   - Drugs and the kidney,
   - Drugs and the lung.

Bibliography

Adedoyin A, Branch RA. The effect of liver disease on drugs. *Curr Opin Crit Care* 1997; 3: 255.

Alapat PM, Zimmerman JL. Toxicology in the critical care unit. *Chest* 2008; 133: 1006.

Brunton L, Hila-Dandan R, Knollmann BC, eds.-in-chief. *Goodman & Gilman's The Pharmacological Basis of Therapeutics.* 13th edition. New York: McGraw-Hill. 2017.

Carruthers S, Hoffman B, Melmon K, et al., eds. *Melmon and Morrelli's Clinical Pharmacology.* 4th edition. New York: McGraw-Hill. 2000.

Chernow B, ed. *The Pharmacological Approach to the Critically Ill Patient.* 3rd edition. Baltimore: Williams & Wilkins. 1994.

Chrispin PS, Park GR. Unexpected drug reactions and interactions in the critical care unit. *Curr Opin Crit Care* 1997; 3: 262.

Classen D, Pestonik S, Evans, R, et al. Adverse drug events in hospitalized patients: excess length of stay, extra costs and attributable mortality. *JAMA* 1997; 277: 301.

Crowe AV, Griffiths RD. Nutritional failure and drugs. *Curr Opin Crit Care* 1997; 3: 268.

Gora-Harper ML, in conjunction with the Society of Critical Care Medicine. *The Injectable Drug Reference.* Princeton: Bioscientific Resources. 1998.

Karch FE, Lasagna L. Adverse drug reactions: a critical review. *JAMA* 1975; 234: 1236.

Kennedy D. Classifying drugs in pregnancy. *Aust Prescriber* 2014; 37: 38.

Koch-Weser J. Definition and classification of adverse drug reactions. *Drug Information Bulletin* 1968; July/September: 72.

Koch-Weser J. Bioavailability of drugs. *N Engl J Med* 1974; 291: 233 & 503.

Lazarou J, Pomeranz B, Corey P. Incidence of adverse drug reactions in hospitalized patients: a meta-analysis of prospective studies. *JAMA* 1998; 279: 1200.

Ling L, Clark RF, Erickson T, et al., eds. *Toxicology Secrets*. Philadelphia; Hanley & Belfus. 2001.

Marik P, Varon J. The obese patient in the ICU. *Chest* 1998; 113: 492.

Naranjo CA, Shear NH, Lanctot KL. Advances in the diagnosis of adverse drug reactions. *J Clin Pharmacol* 1992; 32: 897.

Nigen S, Knowles SR, Shear NH. Drug eruptions: approaching the diagnosis of drug-induced skin diseases. *J Drugs Dermatol* 2003; 2: 278.

Papadopoulos J, Kane-Gill S, Cooper B, eds. Identification and prevention of common adverse drug events in the intensive care unit. *Crit Care Med* 2010; 36: 6 (suppl.).

Paw HGW, Shulman R. *Handbook of Drugs in Intensive Care*. 6th edition. Cambridge: Cambridge University Press. 2019.

Rossi S, ed.-in-chief. *Australian Medicines Handbook*. Adelaide: AMH. 2020.

Shann F. *Drug Doses*. 17th edition. Melbourne: Royal Children's Hospital. 2017.

Shannon MW, Borron SW, Burns MJ, eds. *Haddad and Winchester's Clinical Management of Poisoning and Drug Overdose*. 4th edition. Philadelphia: WB Saunders. 2007.

Shear NH, Knowles S, Shapiro L. Cutaneous adverse drug reactions. In: *Scientific American Medicine. Dermatology*. Hamilton: Dekker Medicine. 2020.

Susla GM, Suffredini AF, McAreavey D, et al., eds. *The Handbook of Critical Care Drug Delivery*. 3rd edition. Baltimore: Williams & Wilkins. 2006.

Thompson DF, Pierce DR. Drug-induced nightmares. *Ann Pharmacother* 1999; 33: 93.

Trujillo MH, Guerrero J, Fragachan C, et al. Pharmacologic antidotes in critical care medicine: a practical guide for drug administration. *Crit Care Med* 1998; 26: 377.

Vargas E, Terleira A, Hernando F, et al. Effect of adverse drug reactions on length of stay in surgical intensive care units. *Crit Care Med* 2003; 31: 694.

Drugs and the kidney

In Intensive Care practice, drug-induced acute renal damage has been calculated to occur in about 15% of patients. Drugs should thus be remembered as potentially contributing to any case of renal failure in the seriously ill, particularly if the cause is not otherwise readily apparent.

Separately of course, drug dosing itself needs to be adjusted in many cases of renal disease, particularly with those many drugs that accumulate in renal failure.

There are several mechanisms and manifestations of drug-induced nephrotoxicity.

1. **Acute pre-renal renal failure**

Glomerular filtration rate (GFR) is vulnerable to local as well as systemic circulatory changes. Such local changes may be produced by several groups of drugs.

- **Noradrenaline** (norepinephrine) is a renal vasoconstrictor and can thus reduce GFR, although its effect in this regard can be difficult to distinguish from the effect of the underlying hypotension for which it is being given in the first place. Low-dose dopamine was commonly given in this setting in an attempt to offset the potentially adverse direct effects on the kidney of potent vasoconstrictors like noradrenaline (norepinephrine), but this previously popular strategy has not been shown to confer any renal or survival benefit.

- **Angiotensin-converting enzyme (ACE) inhibitors** (q.v.) cause reversible renal impairment in patients in whom renal autoregulation is active. This autoregulation is driven by efferent arteriole constriction, is produced by angiotensin II (q.v.) and is required to preserve GFR. Clearly ACE inhibitors interfere with this mechanism, which is active in patients with hypovolaemia or with renal artery stenosis (if bilateral or if unilateral with a poorly functioning contralateral kidney). Renal failure in this setting is not structural (i.e. it is not associated with proteinuria, an abnormal urinary sediment or histological changes), but there can be striking hyperkalaemia. Rapid reversal occurs with cessation of the ACE inhibitor and with rehydration.

- **Non-steroidal anti-inflammatory agents (NSAIDs)** can also cause acute renal dysfunction, especially in patients with some degree of underlying renal insufficiency. This occurs because NSAIDs inhibit the synthesis of prostaglandins and because prostaglandins in turn are required to maintain afferent arteriole dilatation and thus GFR in the face of impaired renal blood flow. The adverse effect of NSAIDs in this situation is compounded by any concomitant administration of methotrexate or triamterene.

- **Ciclosporin** causes afferent arteriole constriction and thus the potential for acute renal dysfunction. This effect is increased when NSAIDs or ACE inhibitors are also given.

2. **Acute kidney injury**
Acute kidney injury (AKI), formerly called **acute tubular necrosis** (ATN), is the commonest type of drug-induced renal damage in seriously ill patients as well as the commonest type of renal impairment due to circulatory failure. Several drugs are particularly implicated.
- **Aminoglycosides**, especially gentamicin, are the cause of most cases of drug-induced AKI (ATN). Although the pathogenetic mechanism is unclear, the risk is increased by hypovolaemia, hypokalaemia, hypomagnesaemia, hyperbilirubinaemia and other nephrotoxic drugs, as well as by the duration and total dose of aminoglycoside given.
- **Amphotericin B** causes renal impairment in most patients given large doses, either daily or cumulative. The risk is increased with diuretics and decreased with added sodium (e.g. 300 mmol per day). The newer liposomal preparations of amphotericin B are much less nephrotoxic, though they are more expensive.
- **Ciclosporin** can cause AKI (ATN) as well as reduced GFR. Nephrotoxicity is one of its main side-effects and is generally manifest as slowly progressive but reversible acute renal failure with hyperkalaemia. As the risk is dose-related, it is increased by drugs which increase blood ciclosporin levels, such as calcium channel blockers (especially diltiazem), ketoconazole, erythromycin.
- **Radiocontrast agents**, either ionic or non-ionic, may cause AKI (ATN) in patients who are old or dehydrated and especially in patients with diabetes and existing renal impairment. The damage is usually mild, except in patients with severe existing renal impairment. Some protection was previously claimed for acetylcysteine, but this benefit was not confirmed in subsequent large trials. Bicarbonate was found to be no better than saline, but calcium channel blockers and prostaglandin E_1 could possibly be helpful. Adequate hydration is the most important prophylactic measure.

3. **Acute interstitial nephritis**
See Tubulointerstitial diseases.

4. **Chronic interstitial nephritis**
See Tubulointerstitial diseases.

5. **Glomerular injury**
Drug-induced glomerular injury is an important cause of the nephrotic syndrome (see Glomerular diseases).

Bibliography
Aronoff GR, Bennett WM, Berns JS, et al. eds. *Drug Prescribing in Renal Failure: Dosing Guidelines for Adults and Children*. 5th edition. Philadelphia: American College of Physicians. 2007.

Hoitsma AJ, Wetzels JFM, Koene RAP. Drug-induced nephrotoxicity: aetiology, clinical features and management. *Drug Safety* 1991; 6: 131.
Olyaei AJ, Bennett WM. Pharmacologic approach to renal insufficiency. In: *Scientific American Medicine. Nephrology*. Hamilton: Dekker Medicine. 2020.
Papadopoulos J, Kane-Gill S, Cooper B, eds. Identification and prevention of common adverse drug events in the intensive care unit. *Crit Care Med* 2010; 36: 6 (suppl.).
Rossert J. Drug-induced acute interstitial nephritis. *Kidney Int* 2001; 60: 804.
Weisbord SD, Gallagher M, Jneid H, et al. Outcomes after angiography with sodium bicarbonate and acetylcysteine. *N Engl J Med* 2018; 378: 603.

Drugs and the lung

Many different pulmonary reactions involving a large variety of drugs and poisons may occur.

> Although pulmonary reactions are less common than drug-induced reactions involving other organs and systems, they are important because
> - they can be severe and life-threatening,
> - they are often reversible if the responsible drug is ceased,
> - they can mimic other more common respiratory diseases.

The mechanisms of drug-induced reactions are probably many, and among others they include immunological (allergic) and pharmacological (idiosyncratic, facultative, toxic) processes.

The diagnosis of a drug-induced pulmonary reaction is usually presumptive.

Clinical suspicion is complemented by a careful history rather than laboratory tests. Even in allergic reactions, serum antibody levels and skin tests are not usually helpful. Rechallenge with the responsible drug would be diagnostically confirmatory but is usually unsafe.

> *The suspected offending drug should be stopped and most reactions then subside, though some pulmonary infiltrates may take weeks to resolve.*
>
> *Corticosteroid therapy may hasten the resolution of infiltrative reactions, but other reactions should be treated on their symptomatic merits.*

Many reactions are such that the patient should be warned about possible future exposure to the drug.

The types of pulmonary reactions to drugs are as follows.

1. **Bronchospasm**
   - Type 1 hypersensitivity
     - antibiotics (especially penicillin),
     - antisera,
     - iodides (especially older contrast media),
     - iron-dextran (formerly),
   - Irritant reflexes
     - acetylcysteine,
     - aerosols (especially cromoglycate),
     - beta-adrenergic blockers,
   - Smooth muscle contraction
     - histamine,
     - methacholine,
     - $PGF_2\alpha$,
   - Prostaglandin inhibition
     - aspirin (q.v.),
     - other NSAIDs.
2. **Interstitial infiltration**
   - Acute (usually with eosinophilia)
     - azathioprine,
     - gold,
     - imatinib,
     - isoniazid,
     - leflunomide (q.v.),
     - nitrofurantoin,
     - para-aminosalicylic acid (PAS),
     - penicillin,
     - sulphonamides,
     - tricyclic antidepressants,
   - Chronic
     - bleomycin (q.v.),
     - busulphan,
     - cyclophosphamide,
     - gold,
     - hexamethonium (formerly),
     - melphalan,
     - methysergide,
     - nitrofurantoin,
     - oxygen,
   - Systemic lupus erythematosus–like
     - digitalis,
     - gold,
     - griseofulvin,
     - hydralazine,
     - isoniazid,
     - methyldopa,
     - oral contraceptives,
     - penicillin,
     - phenytoin,
     - procainamide,
     - reserpine (formerly),
     - sulphonamides,
     - tetracyclines,
     - thiazides.
3. **Pulmonary oedema**
   - Increased hydrostatic pressure
     - adrenaline (epinephrine),
     - IV fluids,
     - propranolol,
   - Increased capillary permeability
     - blood transfusion,
     - dextropropoxyphene,
     - heroin,
     - salicylates,
     - thiazides.
4. **Pulmonary vascular changes**
   - Pulmonary hypertension
     - aminorex (formerly),
     - talc,
   - Vasculitis
     - hydralazine,
     - penicillin,
     - phenytoin,
     - promazine,
     - quinidine,
     - sulphonamides.
5. **Respiratory failure**
   - CNS depression
     - alcohol,
     - anaesthetics,
     - opiates,
     - sedatives,
   - Neuromuscular blockade
     - aminoglycosides,
     - muscle relaxants.
6. **Pulmonary haemorrhage**
   - anticoagulants (q.v.),
   - antiplatelet agents (q.v.),
   - thrombolytic agents.
7. **Hilar lymphadenopathy**
   - phenytoin.

In addition, a few drugs are occasionally associated with various pleural disorders, particularly eosinophilic effusions.

Bibliography

Albertson TE, Walby WF, Derlet RW. Stimulant-induced pulmonary toxicity. *Chest* 1995; 108: 1140.

Cooper JA, White DA, Matthay RA. Drug-induced pulmonary disease. *Am J Respir Dis* 1986; 133: 321 & 488.

Foucher P, Biour M, Blayac JP, et al. Drugs that may injure the respiratory system. *Eur Respir J* 1997; 10: 265.

Heffner JE, Harley RA, Schabel SI. Pulmonary reactions from illicit substance abuse. *Clin Chest Med* 1990; 11: 151.

Morelock SY, Sahn SA. Drugs and the pleura. *Chest* 1999; 116: 212.

Parsons PE. Respiratory failure as a result of drugs, overdoses, and poisonings. *Clin Chest Med* 1994; 15: 93.

Dysentery See
- Diarrhoea.

Dysphagia

Dysphagia or difficulty in swallowing is a common symptom, and it is most commonly due to gastro-oesophageal reflux disease (GORD, GERD).

Other important causes of dysphagia include
- achalasia,
- oesophageal ring, including multiple rings, as in eosinophilic oesophagitis,
- oesophageal stricture (often associated with GORD),
- oropharyngeal dysfunction due to neurological (bulbar) disease
  - typically associated with cough and nasal regurgitation,
- oesophagitis
  - drugs (especially an NSAID tablet lodged in the oesophagus for >5 min),
  - infections (especially due to candida but also cytomegalovirus (CMV) or herpes simplex virus (HSV)),
  - caustic chemical ingestion.
- local mechanical obstruction,
- carcinoma,
- Plummer–Vinson (or Paterson–Kelly) syndrome
  - associated with mucosal atrophy and iron deficiency (q.v.),
- diffuse oesophageal spasm,
- oesophageal diverticulum,
- collagen-vascular disease, typically scleroderma (q.v.),
- external oesophageal compression,
- post-extubation following mechanical ventilation in ICU
  - associated with impaired laryngeal function,
  - resulting in the risk of aspiration pneumonia.

The chief investigation for dysphagia is endoscopy, which also provides treatment options in many cases. Manometry and barium studies may also be diagnostically helpful.

Bibliography

Brodsky MB, Pandian V, Needham DM. Post-extubation dysphagia: a problem needing multidisciplinary efforts. *Intens Care Med* 2020; 46: 93.

DeVault KR. Symptoms of esophageal disease. In: Feldman M, Friedman L, Brandt L, eds. *Sleisenger and Fordtran's Gastrointestinal and Liver Disease*. 11th edition. Philadelphia: Elsevier. 2020.

Duncan S, McAuley DF, Walshe M, et al. Interventions for oropharyngeal dysphagia in acute and critical care: a systematic review and meta-analysis. *Intens Care Med* 2020; 46: 1326.

Katzka DA. Eosinophilic esophagitis. *Curr Opin Gastroenterol* 2006; 22: 429.

Macht M, White D, Moss M. Swallowing dysfunction after critical illness. *Chest* 2014; 146: 1681.

Macht M, Wimbish T, Bodine C, et al. ICU-acquired swallowing disorders. *Crit Care Med* 2013; 41: 2396.

Selvanderan S, Wong S, Holloway R, et al. Dysphagia: clinical evaluation and management. *Intern Med J* 2021; 51: 1021.

Dysproteinaemias

Dysproteinaemias comprise **multiple myeloma** (q.v.) and its variants, namely
- benign monoclonal gammopathy,
- cryoglobulinaemia,
- heavy chain disease,
- Waldenstrom's macroglobulinaemia.

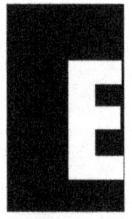

Eating disorders See
- Anorexia nervosa.

Eaton Lambert syndrome See
- Myasthenia gravis.

Ebola haemorrhagic fever

Ebola haemorrhagic fever (Ebola virus disease, EVD) is a severe acute viral illness of tropical Africa. It can also occur in travellers who have visited this region. It is a **viral haemorrhagic fever** (VHF)(q.v.) and is thus related to a number of other types of similar infections, due to Lassa (q.v.), Marburg and Crimean-Congo viruses.

The primary animal reservoir has been identified as probably the fruit bat, but once a human outbreak has occurred, it is perpetuated by transmission from person to person via both direct and indirect contact, including air-borne spread. Since primates can also be infected, they remain an important additional animal reservoir for the virus.

In retrospect, Ebola has been postulated to have possibly been the cause of the famous plague of Athens in 430 BC (see Plague). However, the first recognized outbreak occurred in 1976 in Central Africa (near the Ebola River in the Congo) and several later outbreaks have occurred in equatorial Africa. A major outbreak occurred between 2013 and 2016 in West Africa, prompting a WHO declaration of a public health emergency of international concern. Before it was controlled, more than 28,000 people were infected, 11,000 people died, national health systems were overwhelmed, there was worldwide panic and the cost to the local and international community was several billion dollars. Although there was a small mutation which increased the virulence and transmissibility of the virus, the major factors in the severity and extent of the outbreak were related to its location in a group of poor countries with contiguous and porous borders and with limited public health infrastructure.

The latest outbreak commenced in 2018 in the Democratic Republic of the Congo, with some spread to adjacent countries. It lasted about two years and caused over 2000 deaths, with the case fatality rate being two thirds.

Following an average incubation period of 6–10 days (and possibly up to 21 days), there is an acute onset of fever, headache, myalgia, abdominal pain, diarrhoea (q.v.), rash, bleeding, shock and multiorgan failure (q.v.). Like the other VHFs, the underlying pathogenetic mechanism is extensive endothelial cell damage.

Diagnosis is made by isolation of viral RNA in blood or body fluids, by demonstration of viral antigen (by ELISA) or by PCR. IgG and IgM antibodies are found in convalescent serum.

Treatment is supportive, with strict isolation precautions to protect staff. Corticosteroids, immunoglobulin and fresh frozen plasma have been reported to be helpful in some cases. **Monoclonal antibody** *treatment improves survival in infected patients. The new antiviral agent,* **remdesivir**, *was developed for this condition, but its efficacy has been disappointing. An effective* **vaccine** *(rVSV-ZEBOV) has recently been produced, providing a success rate of over 97% and epidemic control when given early.*

The mortality has been reported to have ranged between 53 and 88%, including among infected health care workers, though it is about 20% where advanced care is available.

Special precautionary guidelines have been published, including specific infection control measures.

Bibliography

Baseler L, Chertow DS, Johnson KM, et al. The pathogenesis of Ebola virus disease. *Annu Rev Pathol* 2017; 12: 387.

Bennet D, Brown D. Ebola virus. *BMJ* 1995; 310: 1344.

Bouree P, Bergman J-F. Ebola virus infection in man. *Am J Trop Med Hyg* 1983; 32: 1465.

CDC documents: www.cdc.gov/ebola.

Howard CR. Viral hemorrhagic fevers: properties and prospects for treatment and prevention. *Antiviral Res* 1984; 4: 169.

Kiiza P, Mullin S, Teo K, et al. Treatment of Ebola-related critical illness. *Intens Care Med* 2020; 46: 285.

Leroy EM, Kumulunqui B, Pourrut X, et al. Fruit bats as reservoirs of Ebola virus. *Nature* 2005; 438: 575.

Leroy EM, Rouquet P, Formenty P, et al. Multiple Ebola virus transmission events and rapid decline of central African wildlife. *Science* 2004; 303: 387.

Li YH, Chen SP. Evolutionary history of Ebola virus. *Epidemiol Infect* 2014; 142: 1138.

Martin P, Laupland KB, Frost EH, et al. Laboratory diagnosis of Ebola virus disease. *Intens Care Med* 2015; 41: 895.

Mulangu S, Dodd LE, Davey RT, et al. A randomized controlled trial of Ebola virus disease therapeutics. *N Engl J Med* 2019; 381: 2293.

Parkes-Ratanshi R, Ssekabira U, Crozier I. Ebola in West Africa: be aware and prepare. *Intens Care Med* 2014; 40: 1742.

Piot P. Ebola's perfect storm. *Science* 2014; 345: 1221.

Sanchez A, Ksiazek TG, Rollin PE, et al. Reemergence of Ebola virus in Africa. *Emerg Infect Dis* 1995; 1: 3.

Suresh V. The enigmatic haemorrhagic fevers. *J R Soc Med* 1997; 90: 622.

Tattevin P, Durante-Mangoni E, Massaquoi M. Does this patient have Ebola virus disease? *Intens Care Med* 2014; 40: 1738.

Echinacea *See*

- Angioedema,
- Drug allergy.

Echinococcosis

Echinococcosis (hydatid disease) refers to human infection with the cysts of the dog tapeworm, *Echinococcus granulosus* (see Helminths). The disease is endemic in Australia, India and the Middle East. Other forms of echinococcus are found in other animals, e.g. foxes, in some parts of the world. It is thus a zoonosis (q.v.).

The adult cestode lives in the dog's intestine, and eggs passed in the faeces are ingested by intermediate hosts, usually sheep but occasionally incidentally humans. The cycle is normally completed when dogs eat an infected carcass or offal of one of the intermediate hosts. Hydatid disease is thus most commonly found in sheep-raising countries.

- Following ingestion by humans, the parasites circulate to any part of the body but especially the liver and the lungs.
- The cysts then gradually enlarge and can be many centimetres in diameter before giving symptoms of a space-occupying nature.
- Cyst rupture can give rise to allergic symptoms, including urticaria, bronchospasm or even anaphylaxis (q.v.). Expectorated sputum may appear to contain grape skins.
- Since the cysts are infective, the rupture can also give rise to disseminated infection and thus new cysts from the contained scolices.

The diagnosis is suggested by X-ray, since the cysts are often calcified. A fluid level may be seen and daughter cysts either free or attached may be identified within the main cyst. Positive serology is sensitive for liver though not lung involvement, but it is not specific.

Treatment is generally with **surgery** and/or the **antihelminthic agents**, mebendazole or albendazole, though the cure rate from one month of pharmacological treatment is only 30%.

A successful alternative to surgery is percutaneous ultrasound-guided needle aspiration and instillation of a scolicidal solution, such as alcohol or hypertonic saline.

Bibliography
Eckert J, Deplazes P. Biological, epidemiological, and clinical aspects of echinococcosis, a zoonosis of increasing concern. *Clin Microbiol Rev* 2004; 17: 107.
Kammerer WS, Schantz PM. Echinococcal disease. *Infect Dis Clin North Am* 1993; 7: 605.
McCullagh PJ. Hydatid disease: medical problems, veterinary solutions, political obstacles. *Med J Aust* 1996; 164: 7.
McManus DP, Zhang W, Li J, et al. Echinococcosis. *Lancet* 2003; 362: 1295.

Ecstasy *See*
- Amphetamines.

Ecthyma
Ecthyma is a skin infection due to group A streptococci and resembling impetigo, except that it is deeper and ulcerated.

Ecthyma gangrenosum (see Gangrene) is a severe local pseudomonal infection.

It is seen in critically ill patients who are immunocompromised, usually with haematological malignancy, neutropenia or burns.

While typically caused by pseudomonas, it may sometimes be caused by other Gram-negative bacilli or even fungi.

The organisms are present in the adventitia of local vessels.

It presents as a small, round, red, painless macule on the arms, buttocks or groin. This macule then vesiculates and finally sloughs to give a black gangrenous ulcer, with a red halo up to 5 cm in diameter.

If extensive, the condition carries a high mortality despite antibiotic therapy.

Bibliography
Greene SL, Su WP, Muller SA. Ecthyma gangrenosum. *J Am Acad Dermatol* 1984; 11: 781.
Hirschmann JV. Fungal, bacterial, and viral infections of the skin. In: *Scientific American Medicine. Dermatology.* Hamilton: Dekker Medicine. 2020.

Ectopic hormone production
Ectopic hormone production may arise in a variety of malignancies but most commonly in lung cancer, especially small cell carcinoma (see Lung tumours). Renal, pancreatic, thymic and carcinoid tumours also commonly produce ectopic hormones.

Such hormones are polypeptides and may include
- ACTH (q.v.),
- calcitonin (q.v.),
- glucagon (q.v.),
- hCG (see Pregnancy),
- luteinizing hormone,
- parathyroid hormone (q.v.),
- somatostatin (q.v.),
- vasopressin (q.v.).
  See also
- Paraneoplastic syndromes.

Bibliography
Mallette LE. The parathyroid polyhormones: new concepts in the spectrum of peptide hormone action. *Endocr Rev* 1991; 12: 110.

Eculizumab

Eculizumab is a humanized recombinant monoclonal antibody to the complement factor C5, which blocks its cleavage to C5a. Thus, complement-mediated cytotoxic and inflammatory processes may be reduced.

It has been shown to be highly effective in a number of rare diseases, including paroxysmal nocturnal haemoglobinuria (q.v.), catastrophic antiphospholipid syndrome (q.v.), atypical haemolytic uraemic syndrome (q.v.) and possibly refractory Guillain–Barré syndrome (q.v.).

Its main side-effect is headache, and there is the need for meningococcal vaccination prior to its use because it increases susceptibility to meningococcal infection.

A new analog, **ravulizumab**, has recently been introduced, with the advantage of a longer half-life and thus less frequent administration, i.e. infusions every 2 months instead of every 2 weeks.

EDTA *See*

- Chelating agents.

Eisenmenger syndrome

Eisenmenger syndrome arises from congenital cardiac defects in which progressive pulmonary vascular obstruction has caused a predominant right-to-left shunt. These cyanotic congenital heart defects are not treatable surgically, except by transplantation, once pulmonary vascular disease has become irreversible and the Eisenmenger syndrome is established.

Eisenmenger syndrome typically develops when left-to-right shunts (atrial septal defect (ASD), ventricular septal defect (VSD), patent dutus arteriosus (PDA)) reverse. This most commonly occurs in ASDs in older patients and is associated with an irreversible plexiform pulmonary arteriopathy, similar to that seen in primary pulmonary hypertension (q.v.).

Bibliography

Borow KM, Karp R. Atrial septal defect: lessons from the past, directions for the future. *N Engl J Med* 1990; 323: 1698.

Nora JJ. Causes of congenital heart disease: old and new modes, mechanisms, and models. *Am Heart J* 1993; 125: 1409.

Wilson NJ, Neutze JM. Adult congenital heart disease: principles and management guidelines. *Aust NZ J Med* 1993; 23: 498 & 697.

Embolism, air *See*

- Diving – Gas embolism.

Emphysema

Emphysema literally means puffed up, and the term is most commonly encountered as pulmonary emphysema, i.e. a well-recognized component of chronic obstructive lung disease. However, abnormal air collections occur in other settings, as in **interstitial emphysema** and **subcutaneous emphysema** (see Barotrauma).

Empyema *See*

- Cavitation,
- Pleural disorders.

Encephalitis

Encephalitis refers to an inflammatory encephalopathy (q.v.). It is most commonly caused by an acute viral infection of the brain, in which case there is viral replication and consequent inflammation in the brain parenchyma and sometimes in adjacent structures. Encephalitis is typically a severe and rapidly progressive neurological syndrome.

There is commonly associated meningeal involvement, i.e. **meningoencephalitis**. Sometimes, there is associated spinal cord involvement, i.e. **encephalomyelitis**.

> Clinical features of encephalitis include
> - delirium (q.v.),
> - fits,
> - coma.
>
> If there is associated meningitis, there is also
> - headache,
> - neck stiffness,
> - fever.
>
> Temporal lobe involvement suggests that the virus is herpes simplex virus (HSV).
>
> Coexisting sepsis suggests a bacterial infection, e.g. meningococcal or pneumococcal.

The differential diagnosis includes bacterial, fungal or protozoal infections or non-infectious conditions, such as an autoimmune, toxic, neoplastic or paraneoplastic process. The specific diagnosis may be made by viral isolation or serology, though this is successful in only about one third of cases. It is however important, since some viral infections, most notably due to HSV, are treatable. Even a delayed diagnosis can be epidemiologically useful.

Examination of the cerebrospinal fluid (CSF) shows lymphocytes, moderately increased protein and normal glucose. The CSF should also be tested by PCR for specific viral nucleic acid, but no identifiable agent is found in about one third of cases. Neuroimaging with CT or preferably MRI scanning and EEG examination are important adjunctive investigations.

The viruses most frequently involved are the herpes group (HSV, Epstein–Barr virus (EBV), cytomegalovirus (CMV), varicella-zoster virus (VZV)) (q.v.), HIV (q.v.), arborvirus (e.g. Ross River virus – q.v., West Nile virus – q.v., Japanese encephalitis virus), enterovirus, picornavirus, measles and mumps. The most common virus is **HSV type 1**, and it generally responds well to treatment with acyclovir (q.v.).

'Australian encephalitis' is usually caused by the mosquito-borne flavivirus (an arborvirus), **Murray Valley encephalitis** (MVE) virus, which despite its name most commonly occurs in Northern Australia. Diagnosis is serological. Although most infections are asymptomatic, it causes death in about 20% of affected victims and residual neurological sequelae in another 40%.

There is no specific treatment, but Intensive Care support is recommended.

An encephalitic picture may also be seen in some **paraneoplastic syndromes** (q.v.) and **autoimmune disorders** (q.v.).

- **N-methyl-D-aspartate receptor encephalitis** (NMDARE) is due to anti-NMDA-receptor antibodies in the cerebrospinal fluid and may be triggered by ovarian teratoma in young women or by HSV encephalitis. Neuropsychiatric features are typically prominent with the resultant limbic encephalitis.
- **Acute** (post-infectious) **disseminated encephalomyelitis** (ADEM) (see Demyelinating diseases) is a rare early complication of acute exanthematous viral infection (especially measles) or vaccination It is due to an autoimmune response and is usually reversible. It is separate from **subacute sclerosing panencephalitis** (SSPE), which is a rare later complication of measles infection or vaccination. This is due to persistence of mutated virus and is usually fatal.
- Encephalitis can be associated with thyroid antibodies in Hashimoto's disease (see Autoimmune diseases, see Hypothyroidism).

Treatment includes surgery (for cancer) and immunotherapy (corticosteroids, immunoglobulin, plasmapheresis, rituximab, cyclophosphamide, bortezomib). Antiepileptic and antipsychotic drugs are commonly required. Tramadol (which is an NMDA receptor antagonist) has been reported to be helpful in cases of refractory dyskinesia in NMDARE.

Bibliography

Britton PN, Eastwood K, Brew BJ, et al. Consensus guidelines for the investigation and management of encephalitis. *Med J Aust* 2015; 202: 576.

Burrow JNC, Whelan PI, Kilburn CJ, et al. Australian encephalitis in the Northern Territory: clinical and epidemiological features, 1987–1996. *Aust NZ J Med* 1998; 28: 590.

Dalmau J, Gleichman AJ, Hughes EG, et al. Anti-NMDA-receptor encephalitis: case series and analysis of the effects of antibodies. *Lancet Neurol* 2008; 7: 1091.

Dalmau J, Graus F. Antibody-mediated encephalitis. *N Engl J Med* 2018; 378: 840.

Ho KM. Use of tramadol to attenuate severe dyskinesia in anti-N-methyl-D-aspartate receptor encephalitis. *Anaesth Intens Care* 2010; 47: 561.

Honarmand S, Glaser CA, Chow E, et al. SSPE in the differential diagnosis of encephalitis. *Neurology* 2004; 63: 1489.

Knox J, Cowan RU, Doyle JS, et al. Murray Valley encephalitis: a review of clinical features, diagnosis and treatment. *Med J Aust* 2012; 196: 322.

Meyfroidt G, Kurtz P, Sonneville R. Critical care management of infectious meningitis and encephalitis. *Intens Care Med* 2020; 46: 192.

Neyens RR, Gaskill GE, Chalela JA. Critical care management of anti-N-methyl-D-aspartate receptor encephalitis. *Crit Care Med* 2018; 46: 1514.

Sonneville R, Venkatesan A, Honnorat J. Understanding auto-immune encephalitis in the ICU. *Intens Care Med* 2019; 45: 1795.

Varvat J, Lafond P, Page Y, et al. Acute psychiatric syndrome leading young patients to ICU: consider anti-NMDA-receptor antibodies. *Anaesth Intens Care* 2010; 38: 748.

Whitley RJ. Viral encephalitis. *N Engl J Med* 1990; 323: 242.

Encephalomyelitis See

- Encephalitis.

Encephalopathy

Encephalopathy refers to acute diffuse cerebral dysfunction. It is typically due to toxic or metabolic causes. If due to an inflammatory cause, it is referred to as **encephalitis** (q.v.).

Encephalopathy is manifest by impaired consciousness, often with fitting or myoclonus. The fitting may be generalized or focal and may be continual, as in epilepsia partialis continua.

Focal neurological signs can also of course be associated with an intracranial mass lesion, which should be excluded if such signs are found. Associated signs of meningeal irritation suggest meningitis or subarachnoid haemorrhage.

There is typically
- metabolic flap,
- coarse tremor,
- involuntary movements and mouthings,
- abnormal tone.

Treatment of fitting or myoclonic jerks is most usefully effected in most cases with a **benzodiazepine** *(e.g. clonazepam IV). Any reversible cause should clearly be treated also if possible (e.g. uraemia, sepsis, hypoglycaemia, opioid toxicity). As with any unconscious patient, respiratory and circulatory safety must be ensured.*

The prognosis is determined partly by the reversibility of the underlying cause and partly by the extent of neurological damage. For example, the encephalopathy of uraemia is usually totally reversible after effective dialysis, whereas the encephalopathy which follows a major hypoxic event such as cardiac arrest may not recover at all. Loss of the pupillary response to light for more than 24 hr is an ominous prognostic sign.

It has been increasingly recognized that repeated minor head trauma, as occurs in contact sports, can also cause long-term cerebral damage, a condition referred to as **chronic traumatic encephalopathy** (CTE).

See also
- Demyelinating diseases – 3. Progressive multifocal leukoencephalopathy,
- Wernicke–Korsakoff syndrome.

Bibliography
Bolton CF, Young GB, Zochodne DW. The neurological complications of sepsis. *Ann Neurol* 1993; 33: 94.
Brooks BR, Walker DL. Progressive multifocal leukoencephalopathy. *Neurol Clin* 1984; 2: 299.
Celesia GG, Grigg MM, Ross E. Generalized status myoclonicus in acute anoxic and toxic-metabolic encephalopathies. *Arch Neurol* 1988; 45: 781.
Edgren E, Hedstrand U, Kelsey S, et al. Assessment of neurological prognosis in comatose survivors of cardiac arrest. *Lancet* 1994; 343: 1055.
Fraser CL, Arieff AI. Nervous system complications in uremia. *Ann Intern Med* 1988; 109: 143.

Endarteritis *See*
- Arteritis.

Endocarditis

Endocarditis refers to inflammatory lesions on the heart valves or endocardium.

- As the organisms involved are usually bacteria, the term 'bacterial endocarditis' is commonly used, though the organisms can sometimes be fungal, rickettsial or chlamydial. The term **infective endocarditis** (IE) is thus often preferred.
- Non-infective endocarditis (NIE) may also be seen and may be referred to as non-bacterial, thrombotic, verrucous or Loeffler's endocarditis.

Infective endocarditis is an uncommon condition, with an incidence of only about 1 per 10,000 of the population per year. Its pathogenesis remains poorly understood, but the basic lesion comprises a blood clot sheltering bacteria and attached to a cardiac valve. It is an example of thromboinflammation or immunothrombosis (see Coagulation disorders).

Non-infective endocarditis is less commonly diagnosed clinically, though it is more commonly found at autopsy. Its causes include malignancy, hypercoagulable states (see Thrombophilia) and autoimmune disorders, such as the antiphospholipid syndrome (q.v.). Systemic embolism occurs frequently.

Acute endocarditis of duration up to 6 weeks is usually caused by an aggressive pathogen, which has infected normal endocardium following metastatic suppuration from an original pyogenic infection elsewhere.

The organisms involved are usually *Staphylococcus aureus* (especially in hospital patients) but also *Streptococcus pneumoniae* and Gram-negative bacilli (especially in drug addicts).

Acute endocarditis presents as the sudden onset of
- fever,
- petechiae (q.v.)
  - including Janeway lesions and Olser's nodes, which are either autoimmune or embolic and from which organisms may sometimes be cultured,
- a new or changing cardiac murmur,
- disseminated intravascular coagulation (q.v.),
- systemic emboli, especially to the brain and kidney,
- meningismus.

In drug addicts, the tricuspid valve is commonly involved and the course of the illness is very acute.

Subacute endocarditis (or subacute bacterial endocarditis, SBE) is caused by relatively avirulent organisms, which are often endogenous and are disturbed by instrumentation so as to infect an endocardium previously rendered abnormal by congenital or rheumatic lesions. However, it has been appreciated that bacteraemia is much more likely to occur with common daily activities than after (say) a dental procedure.

The organisms usually involved are *S. viridans*, enterococci, and other streptococcal species, which reside in the mouth, urogenital system or gut.

In subacute endocarditis, the features are more insidious and non-specific than in acute endocarditis.
- There has been a previous 'culprit' procedure in two thirds of cases and a prior cardiac lesion with a murmur in over 90%.
- Systemic features include fever, anorexia and malaise.
- Systemic emboli are common and particularly involve the brain, gut, retina, kidney and periphery. Systemic emboli which are large suggest either paradoxical embolization or cardiac emboli from thrombi, tumour or fungal material. Peripheral emboli are manifest as petechiae (q.v.), lineal subungual splinter haemorrhages, Janeway lesions on the palms, and Olser's nodes on the pulp of the fingers.
- There is anaemia (q.v.), focal or diffuse glomerulonephritis may occur (see Glomerular diseases), and sometimes the emboli may cause a mycotic aneurysm (q.v.).

Prosthetic valve endocarditis occurs on both mechanical valves and bioprostheses, with an incidence of 3% in the first year and 1% per year thereafter.
- Early endocarditis is usually associated with other perioperative complications.
- Late endocarditis is usually procedurally related.

Valvular dysfunction, particularly regurgitation, commonly results.

Investigations for endocarditis show anaemia, leukocytosis (in the acute phase), raised ESR, increased IgG, decreased complement (q.v.), circulating immune complexes (q.v.), and commonly positive rheumatoid factor and renal abnormalities. Blood cultures are important and should include specific culture methods to detect more fastidious microorganisms. Cultures taken from arterial blood may sometimes reveal microorganisms not identified in blood taken by more routine venepuncture. Even so, about 10% of patients remain culture-negative, especially if antibiotics have been previously given, but also if the organism is one that is technically difficult to isolate in the laboratory. Thus, infections due to some of these less common organisms may be best diagnosed serologically. Transoesophageal echocardiography is the diagnostic imaging technique of choice, especially for prosthetic valve endocarditis.

The differential diagnosis of endocarditis may sometimes be difficult and includes
- non-bacterial thrombotic endocarditis,
- rheumatic fever,
- atrial myxoma (see Cardiac tumours),
- post-bypass syndromes,
- malignancy (especially carcinoma of the kidney),
- collagen-vascular diseases (q.v.).

Complications include
- valvular damage,
- abscess-induced myocardial dysfunction,
- septal invasion with conduction abnormalities,
- cardiac failure,
- pericarditis,
- systemic embolization.

Treatment is with high-dose parenteral antibiotics for 4–6 weeks in native valve endocarditis or 6–8 weeks in prosthetic valve endocarditis.
- *The most commonly used antibiotic is **penicillin** in a dose of 7.2–10.8 g (12–18 million U) IV per day in divided doses for sensitive organisms and in twice that dose for less sensitive organisms.*
- ***Gentamicin** should be added for synergistic treatment of enterococci (in which case, ampicillin may also be substituted for penicillin).*
- ***Vancomycin** 2 g per day should be used if the patient is sensitive to penicillin or if the responsible organism is methicillin-resistant S. aureus (MRSA).*
- *For sensitive S. aureus, **flucloxacillin** or **dicloxacillin** 12 g per day or cefalothin in the same dose should be used.*
- *For Gram-negative organisms, a **third-generation cephalosporin**, sometimes with gentamicin, should be given.*
- ***Amphotericin B** 1 mg/kg per day, preferably with **flucytosine** 10 g per day, is given for fungal endocarditis, but there is still an 80% mortality, so that early surgery is indicated, especially if the lesions are bulky.*
- *For **culture-negative endocarditis**, gentamicin plus flucloxacillin or ampicillin (depending on the likely organism) is given, except in prosthetic valve endocarditis when vancomycin should also be added.*

An antibiotic response should be seen within 2 days and always within 1 week. Cultures should become negative, but even if therapy is effective, embolization can still occur for some weeks.

Antithrombotic therapy is sometimes considered in bacterial endocarditis. However, it does not prevent embolization of vegetations and increases the risk of cerebral haemorrhage. It should therefore be used only if such therapy would have been indicated in its own right in the absence of the current endocarditis (e.g. with many types of prosthetic valves).

Surgical repair or replacement of the damaged valve is indicated if there is significant circulatory compromise or if the endocarditis is bulky, invasive, staphylococcal, pseudomonal or fungal. In such cases, early surgery is preferred. There is nowadays a low risk of infection of a new prosthesis.

The recommendations for **prophylactic antibiotics** for patients with structural heart disease subjected to a risk procedure were revised in 2007 and generally relaxed compared to the American Heart Association guidelines of 1997 (see Dajani et al. 1997 in the Bibliography). Based on overall patient benefit, the emphasis was shifted to those cardiac conditions with the highest risk of complications from IE rather than on those procedures with the highest risk of causing bacteraemia.

It is perhaps of interest that the National Institute for Health and Clinical Excellence (NICE) in the UK has published even more relaxed recommendations, i.e. no prophylaxis for any cardiac patient for any procedure except at an infected site. These controversial recommendations were based on the poor relationship between IE and procedures, the uncertain efficacy of prophylactic antibiotics in this setting and the risk of anaphylaxis from beta-lactam antibiotics. However, the evidence-base for the NICE recommendations has been criticized, and they have not been widely accepted, even in the UK.

Structural heart disease includes for this purpose
- all congenital and valvular heart disease,
- mitral valve prolapse,
- prosthetic valves,
- hypertrophic cardiomyopathy,
- prior endocarditis (regardless of whether an overt lesion was demonstrated or not),
- but not generally ASD (whether corrected or not) and corrected PDA.

Only congenital heart disease (cyanotic or repaired), prosthetic valves and previous IE represent the highest risk for IE and thus warrant prophylactic antibiotics after dental, gastrointestinal and urogenital procedures.

Risk procedures include
- major dental work,
- surgery or invasive investigation of the respiratory, gastrointestinal or urogenital tracts,
- surgery of infected lesions,
- obstetric procedures in the presence of infection.

Prophylaxis is not required for **low-risk procedures**, such as
- dental work without gingival bleeding or mucosal perforation,
- endotracheal intubation,
- fibreoptic bronchoscopy,
- GI endoscopy without biopsy,
- barium enema,
- liver biopsy,
- urinary catheterization,
- gynaecological examination,
- uncomplicated vaginal or Caesarean delivery, or uterine curettage,
- body piercing or tattooing.

For **procedures 'above the diaphragm'**,
- the recommended antibiotic prophylaxis is amoxicillin 2–3 g orally 1 hr before the procedure (and 1.5 g 6 hr after the procedure if the procedure lasts more than 3 hr).

- If the patient is sensitive to penicillin or is already on low-dose penicillin prophylaxis for rheumatic fever, erythromycin (1 g oral or IV) (or azithromycin 500 mg oral or IV or clarithromycin 500 mg oral) or clindamycin (600 mg oral or IV/IM) or cefalexin (2 g oral) or cefazolin or ceftriaxone (1 g IV/IM) should be used instead of amoxicillin 2–3 g. However, the cephalosporins should not be used if the penicillin sensitivity involved anaphylaxis.
- If oral intake is not possible, ampicillin (2 g) or cefazolin or ceftriaxone (1 g) should be given IV/IM 30 min before the procedure.
- In very high risk patients, ampicillin 2 g IV and gentamicin 120 mg IV or vancomycin 1 g IV should be used.

For **procedures 'below the diaphragm'**,
- oral or IV amoxicillin (as above) may be used alone if the procedure is low risk and with IV gentamicin if it is high risk.

- Vancomycin should be substituted for amoxicillin in patients sensitive to penicillin.

Since as discussed above many cases of endocarditis are not in fact related to a defined precipitating event and are probably related to normal activities, such as chewing, it is important that careful dental health be maintained in patients at risk.

The prognosis from endocarditis remains unsatisfactory. There is still a 25% overall mortality, rising to 30% if a prosthetic valve is involved and to 50% if the responsible organism is *S. aureus*. The mortality in untreated patients is virtually 100%. The chief causes of death are cardiac failure, embolization and mycotic aneurysms (q.v.).

Bibliography

Alpert JS, Krous HF, Dalen JE, et al. Pathogenesis of Osler's nodes. *Ann Intern Med* 1976; 85: 471.

Bayer AS, Bolger AF, Taubert KA, et al. Diagnosis and management of infective endocarditis and its complications. *Circulation* 1998; 98: 2936.

Calderwood SB, Swinski LA, Karchmer AW, et al. *Prosthetic valve endocarditis. J Thorac Cardiovasc Surg* 1986; 92: 776.

Chambers JB, Shanson D, Hall R, et al. Antibiotic prophylaxis of endocarditis: the rest of the world and NICE. *J R Soc Med* 2011; 104: 138.

Dajani AS, Taubert KA, Wilson W, et al. Prevention of bacterial endocarditis: recommendations by the American Heart Association. *JAMA* 1997; 277: 1794.

DiNubile MJ. Surgery in active endocarditis. *Ann Intern Med* 1982; 96: 650.

Houpikian P, Raoult D. Diagnostic methods: current best practices and guidelines for identification of difficult-to-culture pathogens in infective endocarditis. *Cardiol Clin* 2003; 21: 207.

Kaye D. Changing pattern of infective endocarditis. *Am J Med* 1985; 79 (suppl. 6B): 157.

Lerner PI, Weinstein L. Infective endocarditis in the antibiotic era. *N Engl J Med* 1966; 274: 199, 259, 323 & 388.

Levin HJ, Paulker SG, Salzman EW, et al. Antithrombotic therapy in valvular heart disease. *Chest* 1992; 102: S434.

Liesenborghs L, Meyers S, Vanassche T, et al. Coagulation: at the heart of infective endocarditis. *J Thromb Haemost* 2020; 18: 995.

Mansur AJ, Grinberg M, Lemos da Luz P, et al. The complications of infective endocarditis. *Arch Intern Med* 1992; 152: 2428.

O'Gara PT. Infective endocarditis. In: *Scientific American Medicine. Infectious Diseases*. Hamilton: Dekker Medicine. 2020.

Pierotti LC, Baddour LM. Fungal endocarditis, 1995–2000. *Chest* 2002; 122: 302.

Stein PD, Alpert JS, Copeland J, et al. Antithrombotic therapy in patients with mechanical and biological prosthetic heart valves. *Chest* 1992; 102: S445.

Tornos P, Almirante B, Olona M, et al. Clinical outcome and long-term prognosis of late prosthetic valve endocarditis: a 20-year experience. *Clin Infect Dis* 1997; 24: 381.

Tunkel AR, Kaye D. Endocarditis with negative blood cultures. *N Engl J Med* 1992; 326: 1215.

Weinstein L, Rubin RH. Infective endocarditis. *Progr Cardiovasc Dis* 1973; 16: 239.

Wilson W, Taubert KA, Gewitz M, et al. Prevention of infective endocarditis: guidelines from the American Heart Association. *Circulation* 2007; 116: 1736.

Wolff M, Mourvillier B, Sonnerville R, et al. My paper 10 years later: infective endocarditis in the intensive care unit. *Intens Care Med* 2014; 40: 1843.

Yau JWY, Lee P, Wilson A, et al. Prosthetic valve endocarditis: what is the evidence for anticoagulant therapy? *Intern Med J* 2011; 41: 795.

Endocrinology

Some endocrine disorders are frequently managed in Intensive Care and are well understood there, such as diabetic ketoacidosis, diabetic hyperosmolar non-ketosis, hypoglycaemia and diabetes insipidus.

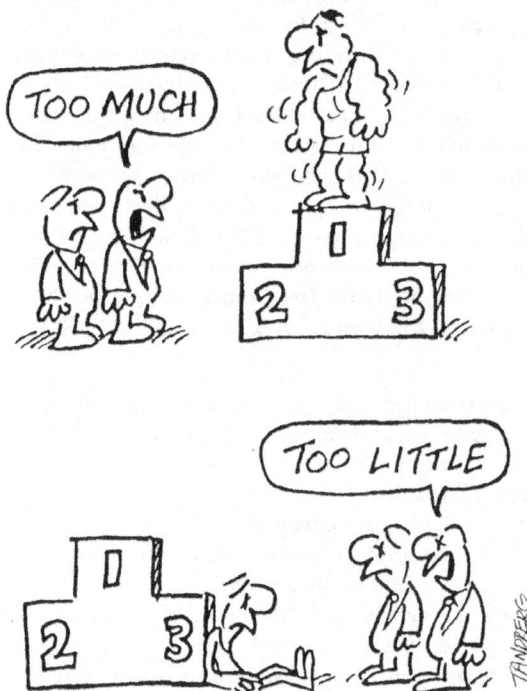

However, many endocrine conditions and issues are less commonly encountered, and they are therefore considered in this book, including

- Acromegaly,
- Adrenal insufficiency,
- Adrenocorticotropic hormone,
- Aldosterone,
- Angiotensin-converting enzyme,
- Antidiuretic hormone,
- Calcitonin,
- Calcium,
- Cerebral salt wasting,
- Conn's syndrome,
- Cushing's syndrome,
- Desmopressin,
- Diabetes insipidus,
- Ectopic hormone production,
- Euthyroid sick syndrome,
- Familial hypocalciuric hypercalcaemia,
- Ghrelin,
- Glucagonoma,
- Graves' disease,
- Growth hormone,
- Hirsutism/hypertrichosis,
- Hypercalcaemia,
- Hyperparathyroidism,
- Hyperphosphataemia,
- Hyperthyroidism,
- Hypocalcaemia,
- Hypoglycaemia,
- Hypokalaemia,
- Hyponatraemia,
- Hypoparathyroidism,
- Hypophosphataemia,
- Hypothalamic–pituitary–adrenal axis,
- Hypothyroidism,
- Insulinoma,
- Islet cell tumour,
- Leptin,
- Multiple endocrine neoplasia,
- Myxoedema,
- Octreotide,
- Osteomalacia,
- Paraganglioma,
- Parathyromatosis,
- Phaeochromocytoma,
- Pseudohyperkalaemia,
- Pseudohyponatraemia,
- Pseudohypoparathyroidism,
- Pseudo primary aldosteronism,
- Pituitary,
- Renin–angiotensin–aldosterone,
- Sheehan's syndrome
- Somatomedin C,
- Somatostatin,
- Syndrome of inappropriate antidiuretic hormone,
- Thyroid function,
- Thyroid storm,
- Vasopressin,
- Waterhouse–Friderichsen syndrome,
- Whipple's triad,
- Zollinger–Ellison syndrome.

However, it may be worth remembering that the largest endocrine organ in the body is the **gastrointestinal tract**. Indeed, the gut was the first structure to be recognized as an endocrine organ, when the gut peptides, gastrin and secretin, were discovered over 100 yr ago, and the fundamental concept of blood-borne communication between cells (the basis of endocrinology) became understood. Nowadays, over 100 peptides have been identified as hormones produced by different types of gut cells, though similar peptides are often expressed by cells outside the gut. Within the gut, peptide hormones are involved in absorption, motility, growth and repair, and immune function. Outside the gut, the same peptides may have functions as diverse as growth factors, neurotransmitters or hunger regulators (see Ghrelin, see Leptin).

In addition, a wide range of **local hormones** provide humoral regulation at local sites throughout the body and are referred to as autacoids (q.v.). Autacoids, neurotransmitters and cytokines are chemical messengers which normally act near to their site of synthesis and are separate entities from the blood-borne hormones of classic endocrinology.

Bibliography
Axelrod L. Glucocorticoid therapy. *Medicine* 1976; 55: 39.
Berl T. Treating hyponatremia: damned if we do and damned if we don't. *Kidney Int* 1990; 37: 1006.
Chernow B, ed. *The Pharmacological Approach to the Critically Ill Patient*. 3rd edition. Baltimore: Williams & Wilkins. 1994.
Chrousos GP. The hypothalamic-pituitary-adrenal axis and immune-mediated inflammation. *N Engl J Med* 1995; 332: 1351.
Cook DM, Loriaux DL. The incidental adrenal mass. *Endocrinologist* 1996; 6: 4.
Curry SC, Arnold-Capell P. Nitroprusside, nitroglycerin, and angiotensin-converting enzyme inhibitors. *Crit Care Clin* 1991; 7: 555.
Deane A, Chapman MJ, Fraser RJL, et al. Bench-to-bedside: the gut as an endocrine organ in the critically ill. *Crit Care* 2010; 14: 228.
Editorial. Corticosteroids and hypothalamic-pituitary-adrenocortical function. *BMJ* 1980; 280: 813.
Editorial. The function of adrenaline. *Lancet* 1985; 1: 561.

Ekins R. The free hormone hypothesis and measurement of free hormones. *Clin Chem* 1992; 38: 1289.

Grinspoon SK, Bilezikian JP. HIV disease and the endocrine system. *N Engl J Med* 1992; 327: 1360.

Ligtenberg JJM, Girbes ARJ, Beentjes JAM, et al. Hormones in the critically ill patient: to intervene or not to intervene? *Intens Care Med* 2001; 27: 1567.

Loriaux DL. The polyendocrine deficiency syndromes. *N Engl J Med* 1985; 312: 1568.

McMahon GT, Dluhy RG. Approach to the patient with endocrine disorders. In: *Scientific American Medicine. Endocrinology & Metabolism*. Hamilton: Dekker Medicine. 2020.

Melmed S, Koenig R, Rosen C, et al., eds. *Williams Textbook of Endocrinology*. 14th edition. Philadelphia: Elsevier. 2019.

Oster JR, Singer I, Fishman LM. Heparin-induced aldosterone suppression and hyperkalemia. *Am J Med* 1995; 98: 575.

Reichlin S. Neuroendocrine-immune interactions. *N Engl J Med* 1993; 329: 1246.

Rose BD. New approach to disturbances in the plasma sodium concentration. *Am J Med* 1986; 81: 1033.

Salem M, Tainsh RE, Bromberg J, et al. Perioperative glucocorticoid coverage: a reassessment 42 years after emergence of a problem. *Ann Surg* 1994; 219: 416.

Tonner DR, Schlechte JA. Neurologic complications of thyroid and parathyroid disease. *Med Clin North Am* 1993; 77: 251.

Energy expenditure

Energy expenditure is one of the key parameters on which nutrition prescriptions are based in the Intensive Care Unit. Energy expenditure per time is referred to as the **metabolic rate,** which is generally expressed as kCal or kJ per day. The most practical measurement of energy expenditure is that made during the resting state, when it is referred to as the **resting energy expenditure** (REE).

Energy expenditure may be either measured or calculated.

- Measurement of energy expenditure is the gold standard, but it is complex and requires the bedside use of a metabolic cart. This machine measures the patient's CO_2 production (the end-product of energy-producing oxidation) and O_2 consumption (because varying substrates give varying energy), from which energy expenditure is calculated using the known calorific values of substrate metabolism. More recently, simple breath-by-breath monitoring of respiratory gases has become incorporated into some bedside monitors in ICU, and this new technology may provide a useful measurement tool when validated.

- Calculation of energy expenditure is a more practical method and involves the use of a predictive equation, such as the classic Harris–Benedict equation or one of many later equations (e.g. Schofield, Ireton-Jones, Faisy, Frankenfield, Fusco, Mifflin, Owen, Penn State or Swinamer). The simplest equation is body weight × 25 (recommended by the American College of Chest Physicians). Unfortunately, all equations are poorly predictive of actual energy expenditure in critically ill patients.

However, even if the prescription of nutrition in ICU patients is perfectly matched to actual energy expenditure, the energy practically delivered is typically incomplete (75–80%), the energy absorption then in the gut is variable, and finally the relationship between energy absorption and clinical outcome has not been established. Thus, it should be no surprise that, despite the incorporation of optimal nutrition into the routine care of critically ill patients, clinical trials of ICU nutrition have had difficulty in demonstrating unequivocal outcome benefits.

Bibliography

Parikh HG, Miller A, Chapman M, et al. Calorie delivery and clinical outcomes in the critically ill: a systematic review and meta-analysis. *Crit Care Resusc* 2016; 18: 17.

Phelan G. Determination of energy expenditure. In: *Scientific American Medicine. Nutrition*. Hamilton: Dekker Medicine. 2020.

Taylor BE, McClave SA, Martindale RG, et al. Guidelines for the provision and assessment of nutrition support therapy in the adult critically ill patient: Society of Critical Care Medicine (SCCM) and American Society for Parenteral and Enteral Nutrition (ASPEN). *Crit Care Med* 2016; 44: 390.

Enterocolitis *See*

- Colitis.

Enteropathogenic *E. coli*

Enteropathogenic (enterotoxigenic, enterohaemorrhagic) *E. coli* (ETEC, EHEC), especially serotype O157:H7, has a reservoir in cattle and was recognized as a human pathogen only in 1982. It produces a Shiga-like toxin and is thus referred to as Shiga toxin producing *E. coli* (STEC). It is the commonest cause of traveller's diarrhoea. It is spread from either contaminated food (especially from undercooked beef) or via the oral–faecal route.

An outbreak in South Australia is estimated to have cost about A$20 million and has prompted reassessment of surveillance programs of meat processing.

A later outbreak occurred in Europe, particularly in Germany, commencing in May 2011. On this occasion, the particular STEC strain was O104:H4 and appeared to have originated in fenugreek seeds imported from Egypt as a spice. About 4000 cases were reported, with a mortality of about 10%.

The infection is usually mild, though it can occasionally be severe and haemorrhagic and even cause **haemolytic–uraemic syndrome** (q.v.), most commonly in children. Variation in disease severity appears to be related to genetic diversity of the organism.

Antibiotics are contraindicated, because they induce the release of the Shiga toxin and thus increase the risk of this potentially devastating complication. However, a subunit of the oral killed cholera vaccine (WC/rBS) may provide some cross-protection.

See also
- Diarrhoea.

Bibliography
Beers M, Cameron S. Hemolytic uremic syndrome. *Emerg Infect Dis* 1995; 1: 4.
Blaser MJ, Smith PD, Ravdin JL, et al., eds. *Infections of the Gastrointestinal Tract*. 2nd edition. New York: Raven Press. 2002.
Hellard ME, Fairley CK. Gastroenteritis in Australia: who, what, where, and how much? *Aust NZ J Med* 1997; 27: 147.
Phillips SF. Diarrhea: a current view of the pathophysiology. *Gastroenterology* 1972; 63: 495.
Schlager TA, Guerrant RL. Seven possible mechanisms for *Escherichia coli* diarrhea. *Infect Dis Clin North Am* 1988; 2: 607.
Slutsker L, Ries AA, Greene KD, et al. *Escherichia coli* O157:H7 diarrhea in the United States: clinical and epidemiologic features. *Ann Intern Med* 1997; 126: 505.
Wong CS, Jelacic S, Habeeb RL, et al. The risk of the hemolytic-uremic syndrome after antibiotic treatment of *Escherichia coli* O157-H7 infections. *N Engl J Med* 2000; 342: 1930.

Enteropathy See
- Coeliac disease,
- Malabsorption,
- Olmesartan.

Envenomation See
- Bites and stings.

Environment

Although environmental contact is an inevitable part of human existence, most such contact is not hazardous to health or survival. However, in a variety of uncommon settings, the **environment** can present particular dangers and some of these will come to the attention of Intensive Care clinicians.

In particular, serious illness may be caused by
- **Chemical exposures**, which can cause chemical poisoning (q.v.),
- **Physical exposures** (q.v.).

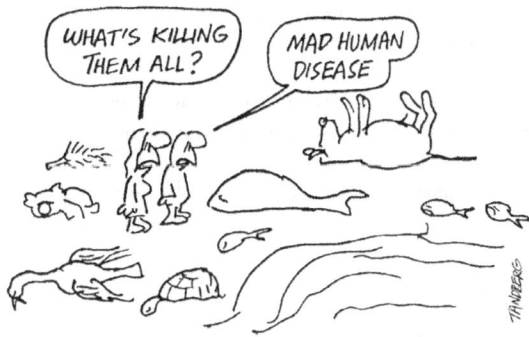

Bibliography
American College of Physicians. Occupational and environmental medicine: the internist's role. *Ann Intern Med* 1990; 113: 974.
Bascom R, Bromberg PA, Costa DL, et al. Health effects of outdoor pollution. *Am J Respir Crit Care Med* 1996; 153: 3 & 477.
Cugell DW. The hard metal diseases. *Clin Chest Med* 1992; 13: 269.
Nriagu JO, Pacyna JM. Quantitative assessment of worldwide contamination of air, water and soils by trace metals. *Nature* 1988; 333: 134.
Redlich CA, Sparer JS, Cullen MR. Sick building syndrome. *Lancet* 1997; 349: 1013.
Rosenstock L, Cullen M, Brodkin CA, et al., eds. *Textbook of Clinical Occupational and Environmental Medicine*. 2nd edition. Philadelphia: Saunders. 2005.
Roxe DM, Krumlovsky FA. Toxic interstitial nephropathy from metals, metabolites, and radiation. *Semin Nephrol* 1988; 8: 72.

Eosinopenia See
- Eosinophilia.

Eosinophilia

Eosinophils arise from the granulocyte–macrophage–eosinophil progenitor, which is stimulated by eosinophilopoietin to differentiate into eosinophilic myelocytes, metamyelocytes and finally mature eosinophils.

Most eosinophils (99%) reside in the tissues, especially in the gut mucosa. Eosinophils have prominent granules which contain peroxidase and other proteins such as neurotoxin. They also have a unique membrane enzyme (lysophospholipase), which forms Charcot–Leyden crystals when eosinophils coalesce and fragment.

Eosinophils are attracted by substances (e.g. ECF-A) released from mast cells. They are stimulated by T cells and activated by monocytes, their presumed role being to kill multicellular parasites, an action which is enhanced by interleukin 3 (IL-3).

Despite this role, **eosinopenia** (which occurs in some infections and following corticosteroids) is not associated with any specific clinical consequence.

Eosinophilia on the other hand (absolute eosinophil count $>0.44 \times 10^9$/L) is associated with a large variety of clinical disorders.

These include
- allergic disorders
  - especially those involving the lungs or the skin,
- drug reactions
  - especially to chlorpromazine, iodides, sulphonamides,
- infections
  - especially parasitic but occasionally fungal,
- malignancy
  - especially myeloproliferative disorders (including eosinophilic leukaemia),
  - but also other leukaemias and lymphoma,
- pulmonary infiltrates (q.v.),
- systemic disorders
  - including connective tissue diseases and granulomatoses,
- **hypereosinophilic syndrome.**

This is an uncommon condition of no known aetiology but with an eosinophil count $>1.5 \times 10^9$/L. It is a chronic multiorgan disorder, with cardiomyopathy, recurrent thromboembolism, and central nervous system and sometimes lung and skin involvement.

It responds to **corticosteroids**, but sometimes **cytotoxics** (e.g. hydroxycarbamide) or **leukapheresis** may be indicated. **Interferon alfa** has been reported to be of benefit and to be steroid-sparing, and other later agents, including **ciclosporin** and **infliximab**, have also been found to be effective in some cases.

Eosinophil maturation, activation and survival are promoted by the cytokine, IL-5. Thus, inhibition of IL-5 by the anti-IL-5 monoclonal antibodies, mepolizumab and reslizumab, has shown clinical efficacy in conditions of persistent eosinophilic inflammation, such as some cases of severe asthma (q.v.).

Bibliography
Fauci A, Harley J, Roberts W, et al. The idiopathic hypereosinophilic syndrome. *Ann Intern Med* 1982; 97: 278.
Gleich GJ, Loegering DA. Immunobiology of eosinophils. *Annu Rev Immunol* 1984; 2: 429.
Kalac M, Quintas-Cardama A, Vrhovac R, et al. A critical appraisal of conventional and investigational drug therapy in patients with hypereosinophilic syndrome and clonal eosinophilia. *Cancer* 2007; 110: 955.
Kita H. The eosinophil: a cytokine-producing cell? *J Allergy Clin Immunol* 1996; 97: 889.
Salter BM, Sehmi R. Hematopoietic processes in eosinophilic asthma. *Chest* 2017; 152: 410.

Eosinophilia and lung infiltration

Pulmonary infiltration with eosinophilia (PIE) includes
- Loeffler's syndrome,
- asthmatic pulmonary eosinophilia,
- tropical eosinophilia,
- eosinophilic pneumonia.

These four conditions are not always clinically discrete, as overlapping patterns may occur and investigations may be non-specific.

Other conditions which may also give rise to pulmonary infiltration in association with blood eosinophilia include
- drug-induced pulmonary syndromes (see Drugs and the lung),
- eosinophilic granuloma (q.v.),
- eosinophilic leukaemia,
- Hodgkin's disease,
- hydatid disease (q.v.),
- polyarteritis nodosa (q.v.),
- Churg–Strauss syndrome (q.v.).

Loeffler's syndrome (simple pulmonary eosinophilia) consists of transient and variable pulmonary infiltrates, associated with a high white cell count (up to 20×10^9/L) and eosinophil count (up to 20% or more). It is probably an allergic reaction to a variety of potential allergens, particularly helminths (q.v.).

It generally lasts less than a month, but it may occasionally last up to 6 months or more. Most cases are clinically silent, but cough and systemic symptoms sometimes occur. Recovery is invariable.

Treatment is generally not indicated. However, if there is a culprit parasitic infection which is active, this will need to be treated on its usual merits, e.g. ascaris and hookworm (ancylostoma) with albendazole, and strongyloides with ivermectin or albendazole.

Asthmatic pulmonary eosinophilia is characterized by asthma with recurrent, variable and changing shadows on chest X-ray and variable eosinophilia. Most cases are associated with *Aspergillus fumigatus* colonization, and the fungus acts as an antigen. The condition is thus also called **allergic bronchopulmonary aspergillosis** (see Aspergillosis).

Typically, the patient is febrile during acute exacerbations and coughs up brown plugs or bronchial casts containing eosinophils and fungal mycelia. Mucoid impaction may occur with bronchial obstruction due to inspissated mucus. Bronchiectasis and lobar shrinkage may be found.

Precipitins for *A. fumigatus* are usually present in serum. The course is generally chronic.

Treatment is as for asthma, with **corticosteroids** *usually required. Specific antifungal therapy has been generally unhelpful, except for* **itraconazole** *in steroid-dependent cases of aspergillosis (q.v.).*

Tropical pulmonary eosinophilia (TPE) is an allergic reaction to degenerating mosquito-borne filaria, particularly *Wuchereria bancrofti* but also *Brugia malayi* (see Helminths). Given the frequency of lymphatic filariasis in tropical countries, this allergic response is uncommon, occurring in <1% of infected patients.

The patient presents with episodic fever, cough (especially at night), wheeze, dyspnoea and often systemic symptoms. Particularly in travellers, it may masquerade as refractory asthma. Untreated, alternating recurrences and remissions may persist for years and eventually lead to pulmonary fibrosis.

The eosinophil count is $>3 \times 10^9$/L, and the serum IgE level is raised. There is an increased antibody titre to filaria (though cross-reactions to other helminth antigens may confuse this picture), but the microfilariae are never themselves found.

Treatment is with **diethylcarbamazine** *(DEC), 6 mg/kg per day for 3 weeks. This generally leads to rapid recovery, though relapse may occur. Spontaneous recovery may sometimes be seen.*

Eosinophilic pneumonia (EP) is a rare syndrome comprising very marked eosinophilia with fever, night sweats, malaise, weight loss, dyspnoea, cough and wheeze. Sometimes, however, it may be asymptomatic.

The aetiology is unknown. It mostly affects middle-aged women, many of whom have a past history of atopy. Cases have also been reported associated with recent commencement of or increase in cigarette smoking or after unusual exposure during military service or firefighting.

Chest X-ray characteristically shows bilateral, symmetrical, peripheral pulmonary infiltrates with perihilar sparing (the 'photonegative' picture of acute pulmonary oedema), though commonly there are less characteristic findings, such as patchy interstitial infiltration, lobar consolidation or cavitation.

Diagnosis is made by transbronchial lung biopsy.

The condition responds dramatically to **corticosteroids**, *though relapse after steroid withdrawal may sometimes occur. However, the condition usually resolves rapidly and completely.*

Bibliography

Allen JN, Davis WB. Eosinophilic lung diseases. *Am J Respir Crit Care Med* 1994; 150: 1423.

Allen JN, Magro CM, King MA. The eosinophilic pneumonias. *Semin Respir Crit Care Med* 2002; 23: 127.

Janz DR, O'Neal HR, Ely EW. Acute eosinophilic pneumonia: a case report and review of the literature. *Crit Care Med* 2009; 37: 1470.

Jederlinic PJ, Sicilian L, Gaensler EA. Chronic eosinophilic pneumonia: a report of 19 cases and a review of the literature. *Medicine* 1988; 67: 154.

Johkoh T, Muller NL, Akira M, et al. Eosinophilic lung diseases: diagnostic accuracy of thin-section CT in 111 patients. *Radiology* 2000; 216: 773.

Naughton M, Fahy J, FitzGerald MX. Chronic eosinophilic pneumonia. *Chest* 1993; 103: 162.

Ong RKC, Doyle RL. Tropical pulmonary eosinophilia. *Chest* 1998; 113: 1673.

Ottesen EA, Nutman TB. Tropical pulmonary eosinophilia. *Annu Rev Med* 1992; 43: 417.

Ricketti AJ, Greenberger PA, Mintzer RA, et al. Allergic bronchopulmonary aspergillosis. *Arch Intern Med* 1983; 143: 1553.

Rosenberg CE, Khoury R. Approach to eosinophilia presenting with pulmonary symptoms. *Chest* 2021; 159: 507.

Salter BM, Sehmi R. Hematopoietic processes in eosinophilic asthma. *Chest* 2017; 152: 410.

Schatz M, Wasserman S, Patterson R. Eosinophils and immunologic lung disease. *Med Clin North Am* 1981; 65: 1055.

Schuyler MR. Allergic bronchopulmonary aspergillosis. *Clin Chest Med* 1983; 4: 15.

Eosinophilic fasciitis See

- Fasciitis.

Eosinophilic granuloma See

- Histiocytosis.

Eosinophilic pneumonia See

- Eosinophilia and lung infiltration.

Epidermolysis bullosa

Epidermolysis bullosa is a group of over 20 rare genetic and acquired disorders of adhesion molecules of the epidermis and epidermal-dermal junction.

They typically appear as blistering after minor trauma. Some conditions are autoimmune and also affect mucosal as well as skin integrity.

Treatment with fluid and electrolyte **resuscitation** *may be required. since blistering can be extensive and cause dehydration and subsequent infection. Gene therapy has been successfully used in some cases.*

Bibliography
Fine J-D. Epidermolysis bullosa: clinical aspects, pathology, and recent advances in research. *Int J Dermatol* 1986; 25: 143.

Epididymitis

Epididymitis can be due to a variety of microorganisms. These particularly include
- chlamydia,
- gonococci,
- meningococci,
- haemophilus,
- salmonella,
- cryptococcus,
- mycobacteria,
- filaria,
- mumps virus.

> - In young heterosexual men,
>   - it is usually associated with urethritis and conjunctivitis (q.v.),
>   - it is chiefly due to *Neisseria gonorrhoeae* or *Chlamydia trachomatis*.
> - In homosexual men,
>   - it is often associated with urethritis,
>   - it is usually due to coliforms or haemophilus.

The differential diagnosis is
- testicular infection, i.e. orchitis (q.v.),
- testicular torsion,
- testicular tumour.

Epidural abscess

An **epidural abscess** may arise anywhere throughout the length of the epidural space, though it is most usefully classified as cranial or spinal.

Cranial epidural abscess arises from direct spread of infection due to
- cranial injury,
- wound infection,
- adjacent sinus or mastoid infection.

Since the dura adheres closely to the skull, the size of such an abscess is limited.

The most commonly involved organisms are *Staphylococcus aureus*, enteric Gram-negative bacilli or anaerobes (the latter particularly if the abscess follows sinus or mastoid infection).

The clinical features are those of the underlying condition, together with neck stiffness. Because of its small size, focal neurological signs are uncommon. The exception is cranial V and VI nerve involvement from petrous extension from mastoid disease, with paralysis of the lateral rectus muscle and facial pain (Gradenigo's syndrome).

Examination of the CSF shows lymphocytes but no organisms.

Treatment is with **antibiotics** *and surgical* **drainage**.

Spinal epidural abscess is uncommon and is mostly due to bacteraemia (when it is often associated with vertebral osteomyelitis). Sometimes, it may be due to adjacent infection, as of a wound.

The thoracic region is more often involved than the cervical or lumbar regions. The abscess is usually posterior involving an average of 4–5 spaces.

The organisms most commonly involved are *S. aureus*, followed by Gram-negative bacilli.

Clinical manifestations are described as typically occurring in four phases, namely
- in the first 1–2 days
  - there is back pain and meningismus,
- in the next 4–5 days
  - there is nerve root pain and fever,
- over the next day
  - there is weakness, numbness and incontinence,
- subsequently
  - irreversible paralysis occurs.

> The differential diagnosis of a spinal epidural abscess is
> - spinal cord compression, due to tumour or vertebral body disease,
> - spinal cord ischaemia,
> - transverse myelitis (q.v.).

The diagnosis is confirmed and its extent delineated by spinal MRI or CT-myelography. Lumbar puncture should not be performed if there is lumbar involvement because of the risk of producing meningitis.

Treatment is with urgent spinal cord **decompression** *and* **antibiotics** *for 3–4 weeks.*

Bibliography
Baker AS, Ojemann RG, Swartz MN, et al. Spinal epidural abscess. *N Engl J Med* 1975; 293: 463.
Jefferson AA, Keogh AJ. Intracranial abscesses. *Q J Med* 1977; 46: 389.

Epstein–Barr virus

Epstein–Barr virus (EBV) is one of the eight human **herpesviruses** (q.v.). Infection is limited to nasopharyngeal epithelial cells, B cells and cervical cells in humans. It is well known as the cause of **infectious mononucleosis** (glandular fever), and it may also be involved in a variety of other conditions, including nasopharyngeal carcinoma in Asians, Burkitt's lymphoma in Africans and several B-cell lymphoproliferative disorders. Meningoencephalitis may sometimes occur (see Encephalitis).

The virus first infects the cells of the nasopharynx, where it replicates and subsequently infects B cells, within which it is disseminated to other parts of the body. Although B cells carry the viral genome, the virus is not replicated but remains latent for long periods. These B cells can produce a variety of antibodies, including the heterophile antibody, a diagnostic marker of EBV infection, though not in fact an antibody directed to viral antigen but coincidentally to red blood cell antigens of several animals.

About half the population seroconvert by 5 years of age due to asymptomatic infection. When primary infection occurs between 10 and 20 years of age, the condition of infectious mononucleosis results. About 15% of seropositive adults shed the virus from the oropharynx, and it is transmitted to others by close contact.

> Clinically, infectious mononucleosis is manifest as fever, pharyngitis and lymphadenopathy (q.v.), often with associated rash (especially if given ampicillin), hepatosplenomegaly and jaundice.
>
> Although the acute illness typically lasts 1–3 weeks, fatigue may last for months (see Chronic fatigue syndrome).
>
> Haemolytic anaemia (q.v.), meningoencephalitis (q.v.) and Guillain–Barré syndrome (q.v.) occasionally occur.
>
> Chronic EBV infection may occur in some patients. Occasionally, overwhelming infection gives rise to a lymphoproliferative syndrome in immunocompromised hosts.

The diagnosis is traditionally confirmed by the typical full blood examination and the presence of serum heterophile antibody which may last for several months. There is an increased number of lymphocytes with >10% being atypical, and often neutropenia (q.v.) and thrombocytopenia (q.v.). Liver function tests are commonly abnormal.

EBV serology testing provides greater accuracy in immunocomptent patients. In immunocompromised patients who may have an EBV-driven malignancy, it can be useful to quantify the EBV viral load by PCR.

*Treatment is **supportive**. Acyclovir (q.v.) provides only minimal clinical benefit, but corticosteroids are occasionally useful for complications.*

Bibliography
Tynell E, Aurelius E, Brandell A, et al. Acyclovir and prednisolone treatment of acute infectious mononucleosis: a multicenter, double-blind, placebo-controlled study. *J Infect Dis* 1996; 174: 324.

Eptifibatide See

- Antiplatelet agents.

Equine morbilliform virus See

- Hendra virus.

Ergot

Ergot is derived from *Claviceps purpurea*, a fungus affecting grasses, especially rye. Infected grain appears large and hard and has brown-black discolouration. Poisoning occurs from the ingestion of affected flour and is referred to as **ergotism** (St Anthony's fire).

The chief features of this condition are peripheral gangrene due to vascular smooth muscle constriction and fits, possibly leading to death.

*Treatment is **symptomatic**.*

Ergot is a complex alkaloid (q.v.) from which a variety of significant natural and synthetic substances have been derived for therapeutic use, including **ergotamine**, **ergometrine**, **methysergide**, **bromocriptine**.

Ergotamine even in normal doses for migraine has been reported to have caused ergotism when combined with drugs which inhibit hepatic CYP3A4 metabolism (e.g. erythromycin and other macrolide antibiotics, azole antifungals such as ketoconazole, verapamil, and more recently HIV protease inhibitors).

Some ergot-derived alkaloids are dopaminergic, most notably **bromocriptine** (q.v.), but also **pergolide** and **cabergoline** used in the treatment of Parkinson's disease and of prolactinoma (see Pituitary). These drugs have been reported to cause occasional cases of pulmonary and/or retroperitoneal fibrosis and of cardiac valvulopathy with consequent valvular regurgitation (since 5HT2B receptors are richly expressed on heart valve tissue and are stimulated by dopamine agonists).

Methysergide has been reported to cause cardiac valvulopathy, as well as the better-known side-effect of retroperitoneal fibrosis. These effects appear to be similar to those which occur in the carcinoid syndrome (q.v.).

It is of interest that ergot is the source of the synthetic hallucinogen, **lysergic acid diethylamide** (LSD).

Bibliography
Ogilvie CM, Milsom SR. Dopamine agonists in the treatment of prolactinoma: are they still first choice? *Intern Med J* 2011; 41: 156.
Redfield MM, Nicholson WJ, Edwards WD, et al. Valve disease associated with ergot alkaloid use. *Ann Intern Med* 1992; 117: 50.

Ergotamine See
- Ergot.

Erysipelas

Erysipelas is a superficial cellulitis caused usually by group A β-haemolytic streptococci. There is a characteristic red and oedematous appearance, especially of the face, that is demarcated, spreads peripherally and may vesiculate. It is associated with fever and local discomfort.

It has sometimes been reported after coronary artery bypass graft surgery as affecting the leg from which the saphenous vein has been removed.

In chronic oedematous states, erysipelas may be recurrent.

The diagnosis is made clinically and is supported if possible by culture of fluid from the lesion.

Treatment is with **penicillin**, which results in improvement within 2 days, though complete resolution requires several days.

The main differential diagnosis is 2-fold:
1. **erysipeloid**

    This is a non-febrile condition with painful, purple lesions on the hand a few days after handling animal or fish products infected with *Erysipelothrix insidiosa* (or *rhusiopathia*), a Gram-positive bacillus resembling listeria (q.v.). It may occasionally be complicated by sepsis.

    It is treated with **penicillin**.
2. **acute allergic contact dermatitis** (AECD, see Dermatitis)

    This may affect the face or limbs, in which case it has often been induced by plants.

Bibliography
Eriksson B, Jorup-Ronstrom C, Karkkoonen K, et al. Erysipelas: clinical and bacteriologic spectrum and serological aspects. *Clin Infect Dis* 1996; 23: 1091.
Grieco MH, Sheldon C. *Erysipelothrix rhusiopathiae*. *Ann NY Acad Sci* 1970; 174: 523.
Hirschmann JV. Fungal, bacterial, and viral infections of the skin. In: *Scientific American Medicine. Dermatology*. Hamilton: Dekker Medicine. 2020.

Erythema marginatum

Erythema marginatum is the characteristic rash of rheumatic fever, though it occurs in only 5% of cases and even then, being transient, it is often missed.

It is an evanescent and asymptomatic rash affecting the limbs and trunk, and though it lasts only a few hours it may recur.

Erythema migrans See
- Lyme disease.

Erythema multiforme

Erythema multiforme is one of the toxic erythemas.

It is an acute hypersensitivity reaction of skin and mucous membranes, following infections, drugs and some other stimuli.
- Infections may be bacterial (streptococcal, TB), viral (herpes simplex virus (HSV), influenza, mumps), fungal or due to mycoplasma.
- Drugs most commonly include allopurinol, barbiturates, NSAIDs, penicillin, phenytoin, sulphonamides.
- Other stimuli include collagen-vascular diseases (q.v.), malignancy, graft-versus-host reaction.

There is a characteristic inner lesion of a red macule that may vesiculate, ulcerate and in some cases become infected. Surrounding this inner lesion but separated from it by an area of normal skin is an erythematous halo. The entire complex looks like a target. Involvement of the outer lip mucosa is characteristic.

In its severe, disseminated and multisystem form, it is called the **Stevens–Johnson syndrome** (see Exfoliative dermatitis).

Treatment should include that of any triggers (e.g. HSV).
- The use of corticosteroids is debatable, though used early they may be helpful.
- Severe cases need supportive care, including fluid resuscitation and adequate nutrition.

Bibliography

Auquier-Dunant A, Mockenhaupt M, Naldi L, et al. Correlations between clinical patterns and causes of erythema multiforme majus, Stevens-Johnson syndrome, and toxic epidermal necrolysis: results of an international prospective study. *Arch Dermatol* 2002; 138: 1019.

Struck MF, Hilbert P, Mockenhaupt M, et al. Severe cutaneous adverse reactions: emergency approach to non-burn epidermolytic syndromes. *Intens Care Med* 2010; 36: 22.

Tonnesen MG, Soter NA. Erythema multiforme. *J Am Acad Dermatol* 1979; 1: 357.

Erythema nodosum

Erythema nodosum is possibly a delayed hypersensitivity reaction to inflammatory or pharmacological stimuli.

- Inflammatory triggers include streptococcal infection, especially of the upper respiratory tract, TB (q.v.), sarcoidosis (q.v.) and inflammatory bowel disease (q.v.).
- Pharmacological triggers include particularly sulphonamides and oral contraceptives (q.v.).

The condition usually occurs in young women. It appears as red, tender nodules, especially on the legs. It is associated with systemic symptoms of fever, malaise and arthralgia and usually lasts for 3–6 weeks.

The clinical diagnosis is clear-cut, but it should prompt a search for an underlying disease.

*Treatment is **symptomatic** and should especially include rest.*
- *Corticosteroids and potassium iodide are helpful in chronic cases.*

Erythrocytosis

Erythrocytosis refers to an increased red blood cell (erythrocyte) count, i.e. $>5.80 \times 10^{12}$/L.

More valid indices of increased total red cell mass (i.e. polycythaemia) are
- increased haemoglobin (>180 g/L),
- increased haematocrit (>0.52) – a better index,
- direct isotopic measurement of red cell mass (>36 mL/kg) – probably the best index.
  See
- Polycythaemia.

Erythromelalgia See
- Thrombocytosis.

Erythropoietin

Erythropoietin (EPO) is a glycoprotein secreted by the kidney in response to anaemia or other causes of cellular hypoxia. Although the feedback sensor mechanism for detecting the relevant oxygenation signal is uncertain, EPO clearly acts as an essential hormone. Its normally low levels in the circulation are adequate to maintain a constant red blood cell mass in the face of usual red cell turnover, which is about 1% per day. These low levels of circulating EPO can then increase up to 1000-fold to provide stimulation of red cell precursors in the bone marrow when increased red cell replenishment is required. As a consequence, red cell production can increase 2-fold in blood loss and up to 8-fold in severe chronic haemolysis. EPO is the body's primary erythropoietic factor, but it acts in cooperation with a number of other growth factors, such as interleukin 6 (IL-6), and with required haematinic factors, such as iron, folic acid and vitamin B_{12}.

While EPO is stimulated physiologically in anaemia (q.v.), it can also be stimulated pathologically, as in secondary polycythaemia (q.v.). Pathological sources of EPO can include tumours of the kidney, adrenal gland, liver, ovary and cerebellum. However, in polycythaemia vera (q.v.), the red cell increase is autonomous, so that the EPO level is actually decreased. EPO levels are also decreased (rather than increased) in some anaemias, such as pure red cell aplasia and anaemia of chronic disease. In these anaemias, the paradoxically low levels of EPO are pathogenetic.

EPO receptors are also present in a number of non-erythroid cells, and this may explain its range of non-haematopoietic functions, such as anti-inflammatory, anti-apoptotic, angiogenetic, immunomodulatory and neuroprotective effects.

Since EPO levels are decreased in critical illness, many clinical trials of EPO have been conducted in non-haematological problems in ICU patients. Unfortunately, the results have not identified any clearly favourable outcome, but the general direction of effect has been promising and supports the need for further specific research in this area.

Recombinant human erythropoietin (rhEPO) has been available for clinical use since the 1980s, following the purification of EPO, its sequencing, its gene isolation and finally the genetic engineering of stable preparations, epoetins. These are collectively referred to as erythropoiesis-stimulating agents (ESAs). They are used clinically in the treatment of some anaemias, such as those in chronic renal disease, in myelodysplasia, after cancer chemotherapy and in paroxysmal nocturnal haemoglobinuria (q.v.). Their potential utility is being explored in non-haematological settings, as described above, and they were popular performance-enhancing drugs in athletes until this form of blood-doping was banned.

The reported side-effects of ESAs include thromboembolism, stroke, tumour progression and death.

See
- Anaemia.

Bibliography

Corwin HL, Gettinger A, Fabian TC, et al. Efficacy and safety of epoetin alfa in critically ill patients. *N Engl J Med* 2007; 357: 965.

Finch CA. Erythropoiesis, erythropoietin, and iron. *Blood* 1982; 60: 1241.

Henry DH, Spivak JL. Clinical use of erythropoietin. *Curr Opinion Hematol* 1995; 2: 118.

Krafte-Jacobs B, Levetown ML, Bray GL, et al. Erythropoietin responses to critical illness. *Crit Care Med* 1994; 22: 821.

Krantz SB. Erythropoietin. *Blood* 1991; 77: 419.

Litton E, Latham P, Inman J, et al. Safety and efficacy of erythropoiesis-stimulating agents in critically ill patients admitted to the intensive care unit: a systematic review and meta-analysis. *Intens Care Med* 2019; 45: 1190.

Nichol A, French C, Little L, et al. Erythropoietin in traumatic brain injury (EPO-TBI): a double-blind randomised controlled trial. *Lancet* 2015; 386: 2499.

Ethylene glycol

Ethylene glycol (1,2-ethanediol, $C_2H_4(OH)_2$ or $HOCH_2.CH_2OH$) is a colourless, odourless, but sweet-tasting and oily liquid. It is the simplest of the glycols, which are organic compounds of the alcohol family but with $(OH)_2$ attached to a carbon structure. It has been widely used since the 1920s as an antifreeze, a brake fluid and in synthetic fibre manufacture.

It may be ingested accidentally or suicidally, but it is most commonly taken deliberately as a cheap substitute for alcohol. Although not toxic itself, its metabolism via alcohol dehydrogenase gives several toxic products, including aldehydes, glycolate, oxalate and lactic acid. Its half-life is about 3 hr. Poisoning from ethylene glycol has many similarities with that from methanol (q.v.).

The minimum lethal dose is about 100 mL in an adult, though recovery has been reported following the ingestion of up to 1 L. A significantly toxic plasma level is >200 mg/L or 3.2 mmol/L.

The clinical features of ethylene glycol poisoning are seen in three stages.
- **early (4–12 hr)**
- There are gastrointestinal disturbances
  - with nausea and vomiting.
- There are neurological (meningoencephalitic) disturbances
  - with intoxication (without the smell of alcohol), nystagmus, ophthalmoplegia (q.v.), myoclonus, decreased reflexes, convulsions and coma.
- **intermediate (12–24 hr)**
- There is cardiorespiratory failure
  - with tachycardia, hypertension, tachypnoea and pulmonary oedema (q.v.).
- **late (1–3 days)**
- There is renal impairment
  - with kidney pain and acute kidney injury (AKI, acute tubular necrosis).

Death occurs at this time from multiorgan failure (q.v.) in severely poisoned patients if untreated.

The diagnosis should be suspected in a patient who is inebriated or comatose with a metabolic acidosis and increased anion gap.

There may be an associated neutrophilia, hyperkalaemia and hypocalcaemia (q.v.).

Urinalysis may show oxalate crystals, as well as haematuria (q.v.) and proteinuria (q.v.). The presence of calcium oxalate crystals in the urine is characteristic and is more the renal reflection of massive oxalate crystal deposition in tissues throughout the body rather than a manifestation solely of renal clearance of toxic metabolites.

*Treatment is similar to that for **methanol poisoning** (q.v.) and comprises*
- *gastric lavage,*
- *cardiorespiratory support,*
- *correction of metabolic acidosis (often requiring up to 1000 mmol or more of bicarbonate),*
- *correction of hypocalcaemia,*
- *administration of **ethyl alcohol** to compete for alcohol dehydrogenase (as for methanol poisoning – q.v.),*
- *administration of **fomepizole** (4-methylpyrazole, 4-MP), an expensive agent shown to inhibit alcohol dehydrogenase and thus prevent the production of toxic metabolites, its dosage being 15 mg/kg IV initially, followed by 10 mg/kg each 12 hr for 48 hr, followed by 15 mg/kg each 12 hr until the plasma ethylene glycol level is <200 mg/L or 3.2 mmol/L,*
- *dialysis or haemofiltration (if the plasma ethylene glycol concentration is >500 mg/L or >8 mmol/L).*

Early diagnosis and treatment are important, because the mortality is high without treatment but virtually nil with treatment.

Bibliography

Barceloux DG, Krenzelok EP, Olson K, et al. American Academy of Clinical Toxicology practice guidelines on the treatment of ethylene glycol poisoning. *J Toxicol Clin Toxicol* 1999; 37: 537.

Brent J, McMartin K, Phillips S, et al. Fomepizole for the treatment of ethylene glycol poisoning. *N Engl J Med* 1999; 340: 832.

DaRoza R, Henning RI, Sunshine I, et al. Acute ethylene glycol poisoning. *Crit Care Med* 1984; 12: 103.

Gabow PA. Ethylene glycol intoxication. *Am J Kidney Dis* 1988; 11: 277.

Hantson Ph, Hassoun A, Mahieu P. Ethylene glycol poisoning treated by intravenous 4-methylpyrazole. *Intens Care Med* 1998; 24: 736.

Jacobsen D, McMartin KE. Methanol and ethylene glycol poisoning: mechanism of toxicity, clinical course, diagnosis and treatment. *Med Toxicol* 1986; 1: 309.

Jacobsen D, McMartin KE. Antidotes for methanol and ethylene glycol poisoning. *J Toxicol Clin Toxicol* 1997; 35: 127.

Karlson-Stiber C, Persson H. Ethylene glycol poisoning: experience from an epidemic in Sweden. *J Toxicol Clin Toxicol* 1992; 30: 565.

Kulig K, Duffy JP, Lenden CH, et al. Toxic effects of methanol, ethylene glycol and isopropyl alcohol. *Topics in Emerg Med* 1984; 6: 14.

Megarbane B, Borron, SW, Baud FJ. Current recommendations for treatment of severe toxic alcohol poisonings. *Intens Care Med* 2005; 31: 189.

Megarbane B, Borron, SW, Trout H, et al. Treatment of acute methanol poisoning with fomepizole. *Intens Care Med* 2001; 27: 1370

Mokhlesi B, Leikin JB, Murray P, et al. Adult toxicology in critical care: part II: specific poisonings. *Chest* 2003; 123: 897.

Parry MF, Wallach R. Ethylene glycol poisoning. *Am J Med* 1974; 57: 143.

Shannon M. Toxicology reviews: fomepizole - a new antidote. *Pediatr Emerg Care* 1998; 14: 170.

Zimmerman JL. Poisonings and overdoses in the intensive care unit: general and specific management issues. *Crit Care Med* 2003; 31: 2794.

Euthyroid sick syndrome

The assessment of thyroid function is difficult in the seriously ill patient. This is because a variety of abnormalities of thyroid function tests may be found which seemingly reflect hypothyroidism, even in the absence of intrinsic thyroid disease. This state has thus been referred to as the **euthyroid sick syndrome** (or, more recently, the **nonthyroidal illness syndrome**, NTIS), and it may reflect the neuroendocrine effects of cytokines. It can occur very early in the course of serious illness, especially sepsis.

Many aspects of serious illness affect thyroid function tests, including

- systemic illness
  - perhaps mediated by TNF-α,
- some specific conditions
  - especially starvation and diabetes mellitus,
- several commonly used drugs
  - notably dopamine, which decreases all thyroid function indices,
  - also corticosteroids, amiodarone and radiographic contrast media, which decrease total T3,
- selenium deficiency (q.v.)
  - related to the impaired peripheral deiodination of T4 to form T3.

In the euthyroid sick syndrome, abnormalities of most thyroid function tests are found.

- **Total T4**
  - is typically low, because of low thyroxine-binding globulin (TBG) or impaired protein binding,
  - occasionally, it may even be increased, because of increased TBG.
- **Free T4**
  - is normal if directly measured,
  - though if calculated it can be misleadingly low.
- **Total T3** and **free T3**
  - are typically also low, because of decreased peripheral conversion of T4 to T3.
- **TSH**
  - is normal or low, even in the presence of a low T4 and T3.
  - This may be due to euthyroidism, to hypothalamic or pituitary depression or to dopamine, which impairs the thyroid-stimulating hormone (TSH) response to TRH.
  - The TSH is of course low if there is secondary hypothyroidism.
  - It is also decreased by starvation and corticosteroids, as well as by dopamine.
  - The TSH may be abnormally increased for several weeks before returning to normal following recovery from serious illness.

The clinical significance of these abnormalities of thyroid function tests is uncertain. While the low T3 may be homeostatic and thus possibly beneficial, a low T4 is associated with an increased mortality, though it is presumably only a marker as replacement therapy does not improve survival.

In general, the normal ranges for thyroid function tests which have been established in well subjects are inappropriate for the assessment of seriously ill patients.

Nevertheless, the diagnosis of genuine hypothyroidism (q.v.) is important because it is curable, though the erroneous treatment of a euthyroid patient is potentially dangerous.

> The most practical approach is to rely on the TSH level, which if elevated generally indicates hypothyroidism and if low generally indicates euthyroidism.
>
> While hypothyroidism will not be over-diagnosed in this way, it may be underdiagnosed if one of the other causes of a low TSH is present, as described above. Laboratory tests thus need to be complemented by clinical features, including past history, goitre, hypothermia or associated autoimmune disorders.
>
> If there is clinical hypothyroidism, especially if the TSH is high, levothyroxine should be given.

See also
- Hypothyroidism.

Bibliography

Berger MM, Reymond MJ, Shenkin A, et al. Influence of selenium supplements on the post-traumatic alterations of the thyroid axis. *Intens Care Med* 2001; 27: 91.

Docter R, Krenning EP, De Jong M, et al. The sick euthyroid syndrome: changes in thyroid hormone serum parameters and hormone metabolism. *Clin Endocrinol* 1993; 39: 499.

Kaptein EM, Spencer CA, Kamiel MB, et al. Prolonged dopamine administration and thyroid hormone economy in normal and critically ill subjects. *J Clin Endocrinol Metab* 1980; 51: 387.

Ramsay I. Drug and non-thyroid induced changes in thyroid function tests. *Postgrad Med J* 1985; 61: 375.

Surks MI, Chopra IJ, Mariash CN, et al. American Thyroid Association guidelines for use of laboratory tests in thyroid disorders. *JAMA* 1990; 263: 1529.

Wartofsky L, Burman KD. Alterations in thyroid function in patients with systemic illness: 'The euthyroid sick syndrome'. *Endocrinol Rev* 1982; 3: 164.

Young R, Worthley LIG. Diagnosis and management of thyroid disease and the critically ill patient. *Crit Care Resusc* 2004; 6: 295.

Exfoliative dermatitis

Exfoliative dermatitis (erythroderma) can complicate a number of dermatological and systemic problems, including psoriasis (especially following steroid withdrawal), atopic dermatitis, contact dermatitis, ichthyosis, drug eruptions and lymphoma. Its most generalized form is called the **Stevens–Johnson syndrome** (see Erythema multiforme), in which up to 10% of the body surface may have epidermal detachment.

> The **staphylococcal scalded skin syndrome** (SSSS) is a form of exfoliative dermatitis, which is produced by the exfoliative toxin of *Staphylococcus aureus*. It is sometimes called **toxic epidermal necrolysis** (TEN) type I. The toxin produces an intraepidermal cleavage plane.
>
> There is a diffuse tender scarlatiniform rash with bullae and an associated fever.
>
> *Treatment of SSSS is with **flucloxacillin** or **dicloxacillin** (or **vancomycin** or perhaps preferably **linezolid**, if the organism is methicillin-resistant) and resuscitation. Corticosteroids are possibly helpful in some cases.*
>
> *The mortality is less than 5%.*

SSSS needs to be distinguished from **toxic epidermal necrolysis** (TEN) type II, which is usually a drug reaction and probably autoimmune-mediated. It is a rare but severe form of Stevens–Johnson syndrome (q.v.), and is thus the most severe cutaneous drug reaction. Its initial report by Lyell in 1956 described it as a 'scalded skin syndrome', and subsequently it was sometimes referred to as **Lyell's syndrome**.

TEN type II is a severe epidermal necrosis with blistering and a burns-like appearance. The cleavage plane is at the epidermal-dermal junction, i. e. deeper than for type I (i.e. SSSS). It typically affects >30% of the body surface.

It is usually associated with allopurinol, anticonvulsants, minocycline, NSAIDs, or sulphonamides, though it can also occur in graft-versus-host disease and in mycoplasma infection.

Differential diagnoses include purpura fulminans (q.v.) and pemphigus vulgaris (q.v.).

*Treatment of TEN type II is as a **burn**, and corticosteroids should be avoided. **Immune globulin** has been reported to be effective if given early. Plasmapheresis (q.v.) has sometimes been recommended, but there is doubt about its efficacy.*

The mortality is 25–50%, and death is due either to sepsis or to organ involvement (especially the gut or lungs).

Bibliography

Auquier-Dunant A, Mockenhaupt M, Naldi L, et al. Correlations between clinical patterns and causes of erythema multiforme majus, Stevens-Johnson syndrome, and toxic epidermal necrolysis: results of an international prospective study. *Arch Dermatol* 2002; 138: 1019.

Gerull R, Nelle M, Schaible T. Toxic epidermal necrolysis and Stevens-Johnson syndrome: a review. *Crit Care Med* 2011; 39: 1521.

Kim P, Goldfarb P, Gaisford T, et al. Stevens-Johnson syndrome and toxic epidermal necrolysis. *J Burn Care Rehabil* 1983; 4: 93.

Lin M-S, Dai Y-S, Pwu R-F, et al. Risk estimates for drugs suspected of being associated with Stevens-Johnson syndrome and toxic epidermal necrolysis. *Intern Med J* 2005; 35: 188.

Lyell A. A review of toxic epidermal necrolysis in Britain. *Br J Dermatol* 1967; 79: 662.

Melish ME, Glasgow LA, Turner MD. The staphylococcal scalded-skin syndrome: isolation and partial purification of the exfoliative toxin. *J Infect Dis* 1972; 125: 129.

Nicolis GD, Helwig EB. Exfoliative dermatitis: a clinicopathologic study of 135 cases. *Arch Dermatol* 1973; 108: 788.

Roujeau JC, Kelly JP, Naldi L, et al. Medication use and the risk of Stevens-Johnson syndrome or toxic epidermal necrolysis. *N Engl J Med* 1995; 333: 1600.

Schwartz RA. Toxic epidermal necrolysis. *Cutis* 1997; 59: 123.

Sehgal VN, Gangwani OP. Fixed drug eruption: current concepts. *Int J Dermatol* 1987; 26: 67.

Stanley JR, Amagai M. Pemphigus, bullous impetigo and staphylococcal scalded skin syndrome. *N Engl J Med* 2006; 355: 1800.

Struck MF, Hilbert P, Mockenhaupt M, et al. Severe cutaneous adverse reactions: emergency approach to non-burn epidermolytic syndromes. *Intens Care Med* 2010; 36: 22.

Thestrup-Pedersen K, Halkier-Sorensen L, Sogaard H, et al. The red man syndrome: exfoliative dermatitis of unknown etiology. *J Am Acad Dermatol* 1988; 18: 1307.

Wolff K, Tappeiner G. Treatment of toxic epidermal necrolysis. *Arch Dermatol* 2003; 139: 85.

Exophthalmos *See*

- Hyperthyroidism.

Exotic pneumonia

Exotic pneumonia is the term applied to pulmonary infection due to an unusual organism.

This unusual organism may be either
- **common**, though not as a respiratory pathogen, or
- **uncommon**, but infectious by virtue of an unusual environment.

The '**common**' organisms include
- some viruses and rickettsiae (q.v.),
- bacteria, such as atypical mycobacteria and actinomyces (q.v.),
- fungi, such as aspergillus (q.v.) and cryptococcus (q.v.),
- protozoa, such as toxoplasma (q.v.).

These organisms cause pneumonia mainly in compromised hosts. In these patients, the diagnostic net has to be cast somewhat wider than usual if one of the more expected organisms is not readily isolated.

The '**uncommon**' organisms include
- bacteria giving rise to melioidosis (q.v.), nocardiosis (q.v.), plague (q.v.), anthrax (q.v.), tularaemia,
- many fungi which have restricted geographical distribution, such as *Histoplasma* (see Histoplasmosis), *Coccidioides* and *Blastomyces*.

These organisms are generally identifiable, provided there is a high level of clinical suspicion of unusual pathogens in patients who may have acquired their infection in an unfamiliar environment, usually as travellers.

Extrinsic allergic alveolitis *See*

- Hypersensitivity pneumonitis.

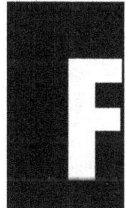

Fabry's disease

Fabry's disease (Fabry disease) is one of the **inborn errors of metabolism** (q.v.). It is characterized by the accumulation of glycosphingolipid (specifically Gb3 or GL-3) in cells, particularly in the vascular endothelium. It is the second commonest **lysosomal storage disorder** after Gaucher's disease (see Storage disorders).

It is due to an X-linked deficiency of alpha-galactosidase A (α-Gal A), a lysosomal hydrolase. Over 800 mutations have so far been described in the relevant gene. It is an uncommon condition, with a prevalence of about 1 in 100,000 of the population. It is incurable, and it results in a greatly reduced life expectancy. Although female heterozygotes are generally asymptomatic, some may show overt disease due to the process of X-inactivation.

Clinical manifestations are primarily renal, but also cardiac and neurological. By adolescence, affected males typically have neuropathic limb pain, telangiectases, renal impairment and corneal deposits. Later, cardiac and cerebrovascular involvement is apparent. End-stage renal disease (ESRD) occurs in all patients who have survived to middle age. Renal biopsy shows characteristic abnormalities.

Diagnosis requires the demonstration of reduced enzyme activity in leukocytes. It is confirmed by genetic analysis. Family testing is then undertaken.

*Treatment with **enzyme replacement (agalsidase)**, given by IV infusion, is recommended to reduce both the progression and severity of the disease, although its impact on long-term outcome remains uncertain.*

***Migalastat** is a recently introduced oral agent, which binds to the active site of the enzyme in the third of patients who have suitable mutations, since even defective enzymes can retain some activity. The stabilized enzyme is thus 'chaperoned', so that it can now enter the lysosome and catabolise the accumulated substrate. Its effectiveness may be similar to enzyme replacement therapy.*

*ESRD requires **dialysis**, and **renal transplantation** has been successful.*

Bibliography

Brady RO, Gal AE, Bradley RM, et al. Enzymatic defect in Fabry's disease: ceramide trihexosidase deficiency. *N Engl J Med* 1967; 276: 1163.

Brady RO, Schiffmann R. Clinical features and recent advances in therapy for Fabry disease. *JAMA* 2000; 284: 2771.

Desnick RJ, Brady R, Barranger J, et al. Fabry disease, an under-recognized multisystemic disorder: expert recommendations for diagnosis, management, and enzyme replacement therapy. *Ann Intern Med* 2003; 138: 338.

Garman SC, Garboczi DN. The molecular defect leading to Fabry disease: structure of human alpha-galactosidase. *J Mol Biol* 2004; 337: 319.

Germain DP, Hughes DA, Nicholls K, et al. Treatment of Fabry's disease with the pharmacologic chaperone migalastat. *N Engl J Med* 2016; 375: 545.

Nicholls K. Fabry disease: an X-linked cause of cardiorenal syndrome. *Intern Med J* 2020; 50 (suppl 4): 11.

Factitious disorders

A **factitious** (i.e. artificial) **disorder** is one which generally mimics a known disease state but which is self-inflicted, usually in a conscious and manipulative way. The related psychiatric disorder is sometimes referred to as **Munchausen syndrome**. It is thus related to but separate from other self-inflicted problems, such as drug overdose or trauma (self-mutilation). These latter conditions are not only much more common but usually also much more readily identifiable.

A number of factitious disorders may sometimes be encountered in seriously ill patients, particularly in those with personality disorders. There is often associated drug abuse, but the separation from real specific disease can sometimes be difficult.

The most important factitious disorders include
- bleeding (e.g. from surreptitious anticoagunat self-administration),
- dermatitis (q.v.),
- diarrhoea (q.v.),
- fever (q.v.),
- hyperthyroidism (q.v.),
- hypoglycaemia (q.v.).

Factor V *See*

- Coagulation disorders,
- Haemophilia – Parahaemophilia,
- Protein C – Activated protein C resistance,
- Thrombophilia.

Factor VIII *See*

- Coagulation disorders,
- Desmopressin,
- Haemophilia,
- Haemostasis,
- Thrombophilia,
- Von Willebrand's disease.

Faecal calprotectin

Faecal calprotectin (FCP) is a neutrophil protein which is released during inflammation and which may be measured in faeces. Faecal calprotectin testing has been found to be useful in distinguishing organic from functional gastrointestinal disorders.

See
- Colitis – 5. Irritable bowel syndrome.

Bibliography

An Y-K, Prince D, Gardiner F, et al. Faecal calprotectin testing for identifying patients with organic gastrointestinal disease: systematic review and meta-analysis. *Med J Aust* 2019; 211: 461.

Burri E, Beglinger C. The use of fecal calprotectin as a biomarker in gastrointestinal disease. *Expert Rev Gastroenterol Hepatol* 2014; 8: 197.

van Rheenen PF, van de Vijver E, Fidler V. Faecal calprotectin for screening of patients with suspected inflammatory bowel disease: diagnostic meta-analysis. *BMJ* 2010; 341: c3369.

Wright EK. Calprotectin or lactoferrin: do they help? *Dig Dis* 2016; 34: 98.

Faecal lactoferrin

Lactoferrin, like calprotectin, is a neutrophil protein released during inflammation. Its measurement in faeces, like faecal calprotectin (q.v.), has also been used in distinguishing between organic and functional intestinal disorders.

See
- Colitis – 3. *Clostridium difficile* infection.

Bibliography

van Langenberg DR, Gearry RB, Wong H-L, et al. The potential value of faecal lactoferrin as a screening test in hospitalized patients with diarrhoea. *Intern Med J* 2010; 40: 819.

Wright EK. Calprotectin or lactoferrin: do they help? *Dig Dis* 2016; 34: 98.

Faecal transplantation

Faecal transplantation or more correctly **faecal microbiota transplantation** (FMT) is a procedure designed to restore the gut microbiome (q.v.) in cases of dysbiosis due to a variety of illnesses. These conditions have included severe, refractory or recurrent *C. difficile* infection (q.v.) in particular, but also cases of inflammatory bowel disease (q.v.), irritable bowel syndrome (q.v.), hepatic encephalopathy and autism.

Although a faecal enema was first reported in 1958 in the treatment of pseudomembranous colitis, as *C. difficile* infection was then called, it is only in recent years that this technique has been shown in clinical trials to be effective enough to have become recommended treatment in severe cases. In these cases, a 90% success rate has been reported. Its efficacy in the other conditions referred to above remains to be clearly established.

The technique is still complex and non-standardized, with the requirement for careful donor screening, suitable preparation and choice of delivery method. Administration can be either from below (via colonoscopy or enema) or from above (via nasogastric tube or capsules, i.e. 'crapsules'). Rare adverse effects have been recorded acutely, such as resistant Gram-negative bacteraemia and possibly immune-mediated disease, but long-term data are still few, and confirmation of microbiome restoration can be temporary in chronic diseases.

Similar techniques have been used in veterinary medicine for many decades, particularly in ruminants like cattle.

Bibliography

Chauhan A, Apostolov R, van Langenberg D, et al. Faecal microbiota transplantation for recurrent *Clostridioides difficile* infection: an Australian perspective – effective, safe, yet room for improvement. *Intern Med J* 2021; 51: 106.

Costello SP, Bryant RV. Faecal microbiota transplantation in Australia: bogged down in regulatory uncertainty. *Intern Med J* 2019; 49: 148.

Costello SP, Hughes PA, Waters O, et al. Effect of fecal microbiota transplantation on 8-week remission in patients with ulcerative colitis: a randomized clinical trial. *JAMA* 2019; 321: 156.

Hvas CL, Jorgensen SMD, Jorgensen SP, et al. Fecal microbiota transplantation is superior to fidaxomicin for treatment of recurrent *Clostridium difficile* infection. *Gastroenterology* 2019; 156: 1324.

Soo WT, Bryant RV, Costello SP. Faecal microbiota transplantation: indications, evidence and safety. *Aust Prescriber* 2020 43: 36.

Van Nood E, Vrieze A, Nieuwdorp M, et al. Duodenal infusion of donor feces for recurrent *Clostridium difficile*. *N Engl J Med* 2013; 368: 407.

Familial hypocalciuric hypercalcaemia See
- Hyperparathyroidism.

Familial Mediterranean fever

Familial Mediterranean fever (FMF) is a rare condition which presents with recurrent attacks of abdominal pain and polyserositis, as well as fever and leukocytosis, but the patient is well between attacks. It was the first described **periodic fever** and it remains the commonest. It is a chief member of the heterogeneous group of conditions referred to as **autoinflammatory disease**, in which various genetic forms of immune dysregulation occur.

It is inherited as an autosomal recessive condition and affects mostly patients of Mediterranean descent, usually Arabs, Armenians, or Sephardic Jews. The responsible gene (*MEFV*) has been cloned. It normally encodes a protein, pyrin, which triggers the inactivation of neutrophil chemotaxis. Several mutations of this gene have been described, leading to dysfunctional pyrin and thus clinically to FMF attacks. The persistence of this genetic abnormality in certain populations may have been due to possibly improved survival during historic plague epidemics.

There is an increased incidence of amyloidosis (q.v.) with nephrotic syndrome and of polyarteritis nodosa (q.v.).

The differential diagnosis is wide and includes diabetic ketoacidosis, acute porphyria (q.v.), systemic lupus erythematosus (SLE) (q.v.), lead colic (q.v.), tabetic crisis (see Syphilis), and perhaps common intrathoracic conditions, such as AMI or pneumonia.

Treatment is with **colchicine** *(q.v.).*

See
- Pyrexia.

Bibliography
Akar S, Yuksel F, Tunca M, et al. Familial Mediterranean fever: risk factors, causes of death, and prognosis in the colchicine era. *Medicine* 2012; 91: 131.
Ben-Chetrit E, Levy M. Familial Mediterranean fever. *Lancet* 1998; 351: 659.
Drenth JPH, van der Meer JWM. Hereditary periodic fever. *New Engl J Med* 2001; 345: 1748.
Editorial. Familial Mediterranean fever. *BMJ* 1980; 281: 2.
Eliakim M, Levy M, Ehrenfeld M. *Recurrent Polyserositis (Familial Mediterranean Fever, Periodic Disease)*. Amsterdam: Elsevier. 1981.
Gattorno M, Hofer M, Federici S, et al. Classification criteria for autoinflammatory recurrent fevers. *Ann Rheum Dis* 2019; 78: 1025.
Moghaddas F. Monogenic autoinflammatory disorders: beyond the periodic fever. *Intern Med J* 2020; 50: 151.
Sohar E, Gafni J, Heller H. Familial Mediterranean fever. *Am J Med* 1967; 43: 227.

Fanconi's syndrome

Fanconi's syndrome consists of increased renal excretion of glucose, amino acids (see Aminoaciduria), phosphate and uric acid, due to abnormal proximal renal tubular reabsorption.

It occurs in
- tubulointerstitial diseases (q.v.)
  - especially allergic interstitial nephritis, such as that due to beta-lactam antibiotics or outdated tetracycline,
- heavy metal poisoning (q.v.)
  - such as from lead or cadmium,
- Sjogren's syndrome occasionally (q.v.).

The Fanconi syndrome can lead to osteomalacia.

The serum phosphate, bicarbonate and often calcium are low, and the alkaline phosphatase increased, while levels of vitamin D and parathyroid hormone (PTH) are normal.

Treatment is with **vitamin D**, **phosphate** *and* **bicarbonate**.

Bibliography
Brenton DP, Isenberg DA, Cusworth DC, et al. The adult presenting Fanconi syndrome. *J Inh Metab Dis* 1981; 4: 211.

Farmer's lung See
- Hypersensitivity pneumonitis.

Fasciitis

There are a number of forms of **fasciitis**.
1. **Necrotizing fasciitis**
   See Gangrene.
2. **Eosinophilic fasciitis**
   This superficially resembles scleroderma (q.v.). The skin is actually normal, but the subcutaneous fascia contains an inflammatory infiltrate.
   The aetiology is unknown, but it has been reported following severe muscular exertion. There is marked eosinophilia (q.v.) with a raised erythrocyte sedimentation rate (ESR). Rheumatoid serology is negative.
   The condition is self-limited, though improvement is hastened by low-dose **corticosteroids**. **Ciclosporin** *and/or other* **cytotoxic agents** *(e.g. azathioprine, methotexate) may be helpful in refractory cases.*
3. **Local fasciitis**
   These include Dupuytren's, plantar fasciitis and diabetic stiff hand syndrome.
4. **Fournier's gangrene**
   See Gangrene.
5. **Cervical necrotizing fasciitis** (CNF)
   See Lemierre's syndrome.

Favism See
- Glucose-6-phosphate dehydrogenase deficiency.

Feeding intolerance See
- Gastric emptying.

Felty's syndrome

Felty's syndrome consists of
- seropositive rheumatoid arthritis, with
- splenomegaly (q.v.) and
- neutropenia (q.v.).

Clinical manifestations often also include fever (q.v.), weight loss, hepatomegaly, lymphadenopathy (q.v.), skin pigmentation (q.v.) and ulceration (q.v.).

> Investigations typically show a white cell count of 1.5–2.0 × 10^9/L with a neutropenia of 0.5–1.0 × 10^9/L.
>
> Neutropenia due to other rheumatic diseases, such as systemic lupus erythematosus (SLE) (q.v.), or to marrow depressant therapy, such as gold, needs to be excluded.
>
> Sometimes the neutropenia is severe (i.e. <0.5 × 10^9/L). It may thus be associated with recurrent infections, especially of the lungs and skin, and particularly with Gram-negative bacilli, staphylococci and streptococci.
>
> The pathogenetic mechanisms of neutropenia are probably multiple and include impaired granulopoiesis, which may be T-cell mediated, increased peripheral destruction and increased margination.
>
> Thrombocytopenia (q.v.) is common, but it is not usually marked.

Treatment is required if the condition is severe.
- *While **corticosteroids** may be useful symptomatically, they may exacerbate infection.*
- ***Splenectomy** may be considered, but continued improvement in the neutrophil count occurs in only about 30% of patients after such surgery.*
- *Disease-modifying drugs such as **gold** have traditionally been useful.*
- *Cytokine therapy with **granulocyte-colony stimulating factor** (G-CSF) offers new potential.*

Bibliography
Goldberg J, Pinals RS. Felty syndrome. *Semin Arthritis Rheum* 1980; 10: 52.
Spivak JL. Felty's syndrome: an analytical review. *Johns Hopkins Med J* 1977; 141: 156.

Ferritin

Ferritin is best known as the protein responsible for iron storage. The serum ferritin level is normally >100 μg/L, but it is decreased in iron deficiency and increased in iron overload conditions (see Iron).

Ferritin is also an **acute phase reactant**, and its level can be of relevance in critically ill patients as a biomarker (q.v.). Thus, it is increased in inflammation (particularly sepsis) and in malignancy. Its highest levels (typically >1000 μg/L) may be seen in the haemophagocytic syndrome (q.v.), in which such high levels can be diagnostically suggestive.

In general, the level of serum ferritin correlates with the outcome in critically ill patients.

Bibliography
Bobbio-Pallavicni F, Verde G, Spirano P, et al. Body iron status in critically ill patients: significance of serum ferritin. *Intens Care Med* 1989; 15: 171.
Cullis JO, Fitzsimons EJ, Griffiths WJ, et al. British Society of Haematology: investigation and management of a raised serum ferritin. *Br J Haematol* 2018; 181: 331.
Lachmann G, Knaak C, Vorderwulbecke G, et al. Hyperferritinemia in critically ill patients. *Crit Care Med* 2020; 48: 459.

Fetal haemoglobin

Fetal haemoglobin (HbF) contains 2-alpha and 2-gamma chains (i.e. it is designated alpha-2 gamma-2). In normal adult haemoglobin, the gamma chains have changed to beta chains, and there is usually only <2% of residual fetal haemoglobin.

Its persistence in larger amounts is chiefly seen in thalassaemia (q.v.).

HbF is also seen in the syndrome of 'hereditary persistence of fetal haemoglobin', an autosomal dominant condition resulting from several gene abnormalities. Homozygotes have 100% HbF and heterozygotes 50%. Whereas traditionally this condition was considered to be asymptomatic, more recently some cases have been found to be anaemic.

Fetomaternal haemorrhage See
- Trauma in pregnancy.

Fever See
- Pyrexia.

Fever of unknown origin See
- Pyrexia.

Fibrinolysis

Fibrinolysis is the process which removes thrombotic material in blood vessels and remodels acute lumenal obstruction, thus restoring vascular patency. Therapeutic fibrinolysis is referred to as **thrombolysis** (q.v.).

Like other plasma enzyme cascades, the fibrinolytic sequence comprises
- an inactive precursor,
- an active enzyme,
- stimulatory and inhibitory influences,
- substrate,
- end-products.

Fibrinolysis is one of the four inter-related enzyme cascades (the other three being the coagulation, kinin and complement systems) which are responsible for integrating many of the bodily responses to injury and which are all triggered by activation of factor XII. See Coagulation disorders.

Plasminogen activator is released as tissue plasminogen activator (t-PA) locally from damaged endothelial cells and also from a variety of other tissues. Activator converts the inactive circulating precursor, **plasminogen**, to the active enzyme, **plasmin**, a broad protease but with a special appetite for **fibrin** (and also to a lesser extent fibrinogen and other coagulation factors). Plasmin also cleaves other proteins, such as matrix proteins and misfolded or necrotic proteins. Other substances may also activate plasminogen, including natural agents, such as **urokinase** (the plasminogen activator in urine) or exogenous products (such as bacteria-derived **streptokinase**).

The effects of plasminogen activator and of plasmin are modulated by the circulating inhibitors, **plasminogen activator inhibitor** (PAI, especially PAI-1) and by **antiplasmin** (especially α_2-antiplasmin, α_2-AP), respectively.

Plasmin then lyses fibrin (and other proteins) by combining with its lysine-binding site, a site which may be blocked by α_2-AP and by substances resembling lysine, such as tranexamic acid (q.v.) (or formerly epsilon aminocaproic acid). When fibrin is laid down in a thrombus, circulating plasminogen is incorporated into the clot. It is this plasminogen which is preferentially activated to plasmin by t-PA, partly because it is protected from circulating inhibitors. The end-products of the lysis of fibrin by plasmin are the **fibrin degradation products** (FDPs), measured conveniently as D-dimer. The end-products of the lysis by plasmin of non-fibrin proteins (such as those noted above) are not identified by current laboratory tests.

Clinical disease arises from disturbed fibrinolysis, either thrombosis from impaired fibrinolysis or haemorrhage from enhanced fibrinolysis. In addition, fibrinolysis is secondarily disturbed in sepsis, with early activation and late exhaustion.

Impaired fibrinolysis may be due to
- decreased t-PA synthesis and/or release,
- increased PAI-1, which is a multifunction protein, best known for its inhibition of plasminogen activator, but more recently recognized as being involved in either mediating or inhibiting (depending on the particular disease) the proliferation, adhesion, migration, signalling and apoptosis of endothelial and smooth muscle cells,
- abnormal or deficient plasminogen (rarely).

Impaired fibrinolysis is one the potential causes of a **hypercoagulable state** (see Thrombophilia).

Enhanced fibrinolysis is uncommon. Its presence is reflected in raised levels of fibrin/fibrinogen degradation products (FDPs).

It gives rise to a haemorrhagic diathesis which is treatable with **tranexamic acid** (TXA)(q.v.) or formerly with epsilon aminocaproic acid (EACA).
- **Primary fibrinolysis** is rare and may include congenital α_2-AP deficiency. It is systemic.
- **Secondary fibrinolysis** is the more common pathological abnormality and may be either systemic or local.
Systemic secondary fibrinolysis may be seen
- in acute promyelocytic leukaemia,
- after congenital heart surgery,
- in primary amyloidosis (q.v.),
- in disseminated intravascular coagulation (the most common situation and one in which it is often compensatory) (q.v.),
- in cardiopulmonary bypass (CPB) coagulopathy (see Coagulation disorders),
- in early traumatic bleeding due to the release of tissue plasminogen activator (tPA), which is the likely mechanism underlying the clinical efficacy of the antifibrinolytic agent **tranexamic acid** (q.v.), in severe acute haemorrhage, specifically after road traffic accidents and after delivery (see Pregnancy).

Local secondary fibrinolysis is most frequently seen after prostatectomy. It may also be involved in some cases of bleeding from the gums, stomach, large bowel, uterus and perhaps subarachnoid space.

Studies have shown that some pathogens may also activate plasminogen to produce plasmin, a process which can enhance infection either by the cleavage of particular surface proteins required for cell entry or by affecting the host's immune response. Thus, theoretically, fibrinolytic inhibition could be of value in the early treatment of infection, whereas fibrinolytic enhancement could be of value in removing fibrin deposits in the later stages of infection.

Recent evidence also suggests that fibrinolysis, specifically the presence of t-PA, may have a role in the brain by regulating neuronal activity and the blood-brain barrier. This phenomenon, which is not plasmin-mediated, may have implications for a number of conditions, including brain injury, stroke and possibly some neurodegenerative disorders.

Bibliography

Balsara RD, Ploplis VA. Plasminogen activator inhibitor-1: the double-edged sword in apoptosis. *Thromb Haemost* 2008; 100: 1029.

Cap AP. CRASH-3: a win for patients with traumatic brain injury. *Lancet* 2019; 394: 1687.

Collen D, Lijnen HR. Basic and clinical aspects of fibrinolysis and thrombolysis. *Blood* 1991; 78: 3114.

CRASH-2 trial collaborators, Shakur H, Roberts I, Bautista R, et al. Effects of tranexamic acid on death, vascular occlusive events, and blood transfusion in trauma patients with significant haemorrhage (CRASH-2): a randomised, placebo-controlled trial. *Lancet* 2010; 376: 23.

Mavrommatis AC, Theodoridis T, Economou M, et al. Activation of the fibrinolytioc system and utilization of the coagulation inhibitors in sepsis: comparison with severe sepsis and septic shock. *Intens Care Med* 2001; 27: 1853.

Medcalf RL. Fibrinolysis: from blood to brain. *J Thromb Haemost* 2017; 15: 2089.

Prins MH, Hirsh J. A critical review of the evidence supporting a relationship between impaired fibrinolytic activity and venous thromboembolism. *Arch Intern Med* 1991; 151: 1721.

Saes JL, Schols SEM, Van Herde WL, et al. Hemorrhagic disorders of fibrinolysis: a clinical review. *Thromb Haemost* 2018; 16: 1498.

Fish envenomation *See*

- Bites and stings – Marine vertebrates.

Fleas

Fleas are insects (see Arthropods) which are common ectoparasites of a number of animals. They are also common vectors for the transmission to humans of disease from their primary host.

See
- Cat-scratch disease,
- Plague,
- Rickettsial diseases – Endemic typhus.

Bibliography

Elston D. Infestations. In: *Scientific American Medicine. Dermatology*. Hamilton: Dekker Medicine. 2020.

Flushing

The causes of **flushing** include the following.

1. **Acne rosacea**

   This is an acneiform eruption on the face, associated with flushing and sometimes with rhinophyma. It is of unknown cause. Eventually, the erythema can be persistent. It is aggravated by heat, cold, sun and wind and may be associated with gastritis.

   *Treatment is with an oral **tetracycline** for several months.*
   - *Isotretinoin may be used in severe cases, though occasionally severe depression and rarely hearing loss have been reported in young patients receiving this drug. Dapsone gel has been shown to be effective.*

2. **Alcohol**

   This is because acetaldehyde, the metabolite produced by alcohol dehydrogenase, is a vasodilator.

3. **Anaphylaxis** (q.v.)
4. **Carcinoid tumour** (q.v.)
5. **Cluster headache**
6. **Drugs**

   These include especially calcitonin (q.v.), disulfiram (with alcohol), desmopressin (DDAVP)(q.v.) in high dose, nifedipine, pentamidine.

7. **Fever** (q.v.)
8. **Food**

   This occurs with some types of food poisoning, including mushrooms (q.v.) and scombroid (q.v.),

9. **Mastocytosis**

   see Urticaria.

10. **Menopause**

    In this, flushing (or flashing) is associated with declining oestrogen levels in about 80% of women. The flushing is probably hypothalamic in origin and is associated with a feeling of heat, then sweating and a rise in surface temperature but a fall in core temperature.

Bibliography

Pochi PE. Hormones, retinoids and acne. *N Engl J Med* 1983; 308: 1024.

FODMAPs

FODMAPs is an acronym for the group of 'Fermentable, Oligo, Di, Mono saccharides And Polyols' which have been reported to be relevant in certain functional bowel conditions. FODMAPs are naturally occurring substances in many vegetables and fruits, and they are ingested as part of a normal diet. They are poorly absorbed and become fermented by the resident bacteria in the colon. Although they are beneficial for the gut microbiota, they may cause bloating in some people. Thus, their dietary restriction may reduce the symptoms of abdominal discomfort experienced by some patients with irritable bowel syndrome (q.v.) and non-coeliac gluten sensitivity (see Coeliac disease).

See
- Microbiome.

Folic acid deficiency

Folic acid together with vitamin B_{12} is required for the metabolism of single carbon units and thus for DNA synthesis.

Folic acid deficiency arises from
- a poor or unusual diet,
- small bowel disease (because 80% of folic acid is absorbed in the small intestine),
- alcoholism,
- chronic renal failure,
- haemolysis (q.v.),
- pregnancy (q.v.),
- drugs which interfere with folic acid metabolism (e.g. anti-tuberculous agents, ethanol, methotrexate, phenytoin, sulphasalazine, trimethoprim).

Folic acid deficiency is associated with a **megaloblastic anaemia** (q.v.), often with thrombocytopenia (q.v.) but without the features of pernicious anaemia (q.v.).

Concomitant iron deficiency (q.v.) is frequent, thereby blocking megaloblastosis, but typical hypersegmented neutrophils are still apparent.

There is an increased incidence of **neural tube defects** (q.v.) in babies of mothers who are either folic acid deficient or who fail to take folic acid supplementation during pregnancy.

Since the serum folate may fall rapidly, e.g. within 2 weeks, in the absence of intake, but the body stores are not yet depleted, the RBC folate level best reflects overall folic acid deficiency. The serum B_{12} level should always be measured, as concomitant deficiency of vitamin B_{12} is frequent.

Treatment is usually with a daily oral dose of 1 mg of folic acid, though as little as 200 mcg is in fact generally adequate. If the diagnosis is correct, treatment gives haematological improvement within a few days.

See also
- Megaloblastic anaemia,
- Neural tube defects.

Bibliography
Dansky LV, Rosenblatt DS, Andermann E. Mechanisms of teratogenesis: folic acid and antiepileptic therapy. *Neurology* 1992; 42 (suppl. 5): 32.
McPartin J, Halligan A, Scott JM, et al. Accelerated folate breakdown in pregnancy. *Lancet* 1993; 341: 148.
Wald NJ, Bower C. Folic acid, pernicious anaemia, and prevention of neural tube defects. *Lancet* 1994; 343: 307.

Folliculitis

Folliculitis is inflammation of the hair follicle giving rise to a small pustule. Unlike acne, which occurs chiefly on the face, chest and back, folliculitis can also affect the trunk and limbs.

It is usually caused by *Staphylococcus aureus* or occasionally by *Pseudomonas aeruginosa*. It can also be caused by the Gram-positive yeast *Malassezia*.

Treatment is local, unless the process is extensive, in which case antibiotics are indicated.

Bibliography
Hirschmann JV. Fungal, bacterial, and viral infections of the skin. In: *Scientific American Medicine. Dermatology.* Hamilton: Dekker Medicine. 2020.

Food poisoning

Although **food poisoning** is a very common condition, its presentation in Intensive Care is uncommon and moreover it may take a number of unusual forms. The types of food poisoning considered in this book include
- Botulism,
- Ciguatera,
- Clostridial infection due to enterotoxigenic *Clostridium perfringens*,
- Coturnism,
- Enteropathogenic *Escherichia coli*,
- Monosodium glutamate ingestion,
- Mushroom poisoning,
- Norovirus,
- Paralytic shellfish poisoning,
- Scombroid,
- Star fruit poisoning.

In addition, some aspects of food poisoning are of an infectious nature and are considered more generally (see Diarrhoea).

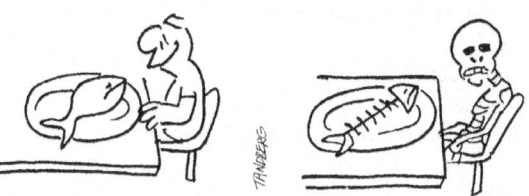

Bibliography
Hughes JM, Merson MH. Fish and shellfish poisoning. *N Engl J Med* 1976; 295: 1117.
Mead PS, Slutsker L, Dietz V, et al. Food-related illness and death in the United States. *Emerg Infect Dis* 1999; 5: 607.
Morse DL, Guzewich JJ, Hanrahan JP, et al. Widespread outbreaks of clam- and oyster-associated

gastroenteritis: role of Norwalk virus. *N Engl J Med* 1986; 314: 678.

Olson KR, ed. *Poisoning and Drug Overdose*. 5th edition. Norwalk: Appleton & Lange. 2006.

Shannon MW, Borron SW, Burns MJ, eds. *Haddad and Winchester's Clinical Management of Poisoning and Drug Overdose*. 4th edition. Philadelphia: WB Saunders. 2007.

Trujillo MH, Guerrero J, Fragachan C, et al. Pharmacologic antidotes in critical care medicine: a practical guide for drug administration. *Crit Care Med* 1998; 26: 377.

Formaldehyde

Formaldehyde (methanal, HCHO) is a colourless, flammable, pungent and irritating gas. It is the simplest aldehyde and is derived from the oxidation of methanol. It is an organic compound extensively used in the chemical industry, in which it is the base for some explosives, tanning agents and disinfectants.

Formalin is a 37% aqueous solution of formaldehyde and is well known as a tissue preservative in pathology laboratories.

Local damage and systemic toxicity result from its ingestion.

There is no specific treatment.

Fournier's gangrene See
- Gangrene.

Frailty

Frailty is by definition a weak and easily damaged state, and it is more commonly encountered in older people. While it would be obvious that frailty in general terms must be a risk factor both for developing critical illness and for poorer outcome after critical illness, recent interest has focussed on more formally quantifying frailty and its consequent relationship to critical illness.

Thus, an 8-point Clinical Frailty Scale is commonly used as one of the assessment parameters of patients admitted to ICU. By this definition, nearly half of the ICU patients over 80 yr of age have some degree of frailty and this is associated with poorer health outcomes, increased health care use and diminished quality of life. Specifically, frailty in critically ill patients increases about 2-fold both the risk of hospital death and the likely subsequent admission of survivors to new nursing home care.

Bibliography
Bagshaw SM, Stelfox HT, McDermid RC, et al. Association between frailty and short- and long-term outcomes among critically ill patients: a multicentre prospective cohort study. *CMAJ* 2014; 186: E95.

Darvall JN, Bellomo R, Paul E, et al. Frailty in very old critically ill patients in Australia and New Zealand: a population-based cohort study. *Med J Aust* 2019; 211: 318.

Friedreich's ataxia See
- Cerebellar degeneration.

Frostbite

When the environmental temperature is less than freezing, atmospheric water vapour becomes ice-crystals (i.e. frost) without first becoming a liquid (i.e. dew).

Frostbite refers to the freezing of tissues, with intracellular ice formation giving rise to mechanical disruption of cells, cellular dehydration, deranged cellular metabolism, haemolysis, thrombosis and gangrene. The tissues start to freeze from about −2°C.

Frostbite arises from cold environmental temperature, often with wind, and usually with various risk factors. Risk factors include
- lack of food or clothing,
- excess exercise,
- illness,
- injury,
- dehydration,
- psychosis,
- alcohol,
- mechanical constriction.

It affects mainly the extremities, which appear cold, white, hard, waxy and pulseless and are affected to a varying depth. The process begins with stinging and is followed by aching and finally numbness.

Reperfusion injury during rewarming may contribute to some of the damage of frostbite.

> The complications of frostbite are
> - local or systemic infection,
> - gangrene (q.v.),
> - local neurological damage,
> - pain, stiffness, wasting, scarring, loss of the subcutaneous fat pad and deformity in the affected part.

*Treatment consists of **emergency rewarming**. The core temperature should be restored if necessary and the affected part thawed rapidly (e.g. with water warmed to 42°C). This may give rise to blistering, which is associated with skin hyperaemia and can be painful and lead to necrosis. Movement should be avoided.*
- *Tetanus toxoid and perhaps antibiotics should be given.*

- *Many forms of adjuvant pharmacological therapy, including vasodilators, antithrombotics, anti-inflammatory agents and free radical scavengers, have been explored, but they have not been subjected to formal clinical trial.*

The prognosis is worse if the cold injury has been of long duration, if the thawing process is slow and in particular if refreezing occurs. Refreezing is such a serious issue because of resultant enhanced tissue damage that rewarming should be deferred if there is any risk of refreezing occurring.

Prevention of frostbite comprises measures both to maintain core temperature and to prevent local exposure, though these simple but effective principles may not always be achievable. The risk is particularly increased in winter sports and especially if exercise is curtailed because of exhaustion, injury or equipment breakdown.

See also
- Hypothermia.

Furunculosis

Furunculosis (boils) refers to deep, inflammatory nodules around hair follicles. They are staphylococcal and can lead to bacteraemia and even metastatic abscesses, endocarditis (q.v.) and/or shock, especially in immunocompromised patients. They may be associated with nasal carriage of the organism or with poor hygiene.

Treatment is by **drainage** *if the lesion is fluctuant and with* **antibiotics** *if there is associated cellulitis or systemic features.*

Bibliography
Hirschmann JV. Fungal, bacterial, and viral infections of the skin. In: *Scientific American Medicine.* Dermatology. Hamilton: Dekker Medicine. 2020.

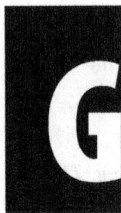

Gamma-hydroxybutyric acid

Gamma-hydroxybutyric acid (GHB) occurs naturally in the central nervous system and was synthesized in the 1960s. It has been variously used or studied as an anaesthetic, an adjunct in alcohol or opiate withdrawal, a treatment for narcolepsy, an agent to reduce tissue oxygen demand in resuscitation and sepsis and a stimulator of growth hormone (particularly for body builders). Because of its ability to impair consciousness and to provide associated relaxation, euphoria, disinhibition and increased sensuality, it has become a popular but illegal drug of abuse particularly at parties and has been labelled in the press as the 'date rape' drug or 'fantasy'.

Intoxication can cause profound unconsciousness, with flaccid paralysis, hypothermia (q.v.), bradycardia, hypotension and respiratory depression. Recovery occurs within a few hours.

Laboratory tests are normal, except that other drugs may have also been taken concomitantly.

Treatment is generally **supportive**, *with particular care to protect the airway.*
- **Atropine** *is useful for bradycardia.*
- *Neither naloxone nor flumazenil have any reversal effect, but* **physostigmine** *(2 mg IV) may be effective.*

Bibliography
Chin RL, Sporer KA, Cullison B, et al. Clinical course of γ-hydroxybutyrate overdose. *Ann Emerg Med* 1998; 31: 716.
Henderson RS, Holmes CM. Reversal of the anaesthetic action of sodium gamma-hydroxybutyrate. *Anaesth Intens Care* 1976; 4: 351.
Li J, Stokes SA, Wockener A. A tale of novel intoxication: a review of the effects of gamma-hydroxybutyric acid with recommendations for management. *Ann Emerg Med* 1998; 31: 729.
Mokhlesi B, Garinella, PS, Joffe A, et al. Street drug abuse leading to critical illness. *Intens Care Med* 2004; 30: 1526.
Mokhlesi B, Leikin JB, Murray P, et al. Adult toxicology in critical care: part II: specific poisonings. *Chest* 2003; 123: 897.
Viera AJ, Yates SW. Toxic ingestion of gamma-hydroxybutyric acid. *South Med J* 1999; 92: 404.

Ganciclovir See
- Acyclovir.

Gangrene

Most cases of **gangrene** (tissue death) involve the lower limb and are due to peripheral ischaemia from atherosclerotic disease. However, some are due to
- embolism,
- infection (see below),
- thromboangiitis obliterans (Buerger's disease),

- trauma,
- vasculitis (q.v.).

> **Infectious gangrene** (gangrenous cellulitis) is a severe type of skin infection that takes a number of forms, which are considered below. These include
> - necrotizing fasciitis, both streptococcal and non-streptococcal,
> - progressive bacterial synergistic gangrene,
> - pyoderma gangrenosum,
> - pseudomonal gangrenous cellulitis,
> - necrotizing cutaneous mucormycosis.

1. **Necrotizing fasciitis** (necrotizing soft-tissue infection, NSTI) is a severe deep tissue infection which typically spreads rapidly along subcutaneous planes. Although it may present with a variety of features including cellulitis and myositis as well as fasciitis, a useful subdivision can be based on either a **streptococcal** (monomicrobial) or **non-streptococcal** (polymicrobial) aetiology, and these have an approximately equal prevalence.
   - **Streptococcal infection** is caused by group-A streptococci (GAS) which may uncommonly cause a rapid-onset and rapidly spreading cellulitis, with skin necrosis and subcutaneous gangrene. It usually affects a limb and typically follows surgical or traumatic injury, though diabetes, varicella infection (q.v.) and immunosuppression are also important predisposing factors. Haematogenous spread can occur from a local site (e.g. streptococcal sore throat) to a distant site (e.g. one of recent trauma). It has been reported as an uncommon complication following the use of **bevacizumab**, an antineoplastic agent which blocks human vascular endothelial growth factor (VEGF) and is used in some metastatic cancers.

   Necrotizing fasciitis due to streptococcal infection is sometimes referred to as **necrotizing soft-tissue infection (NSTI) type II**.

   Invasive group A streptococcal infections occur in about 1 in 10,000 of the population per year in developed countries and are complicated by necrotizing fasciitis in 5–10% of cases. A spate of such cases in the UK received much dramatic publicity, with detailed descriptions of the destruction caused by the 'new, flesh-eating' germ. The resurgence of such infections does not appear to have a clonal basis, as the responsible strains are genetically heterogeneous.

   The affected part is initially blue, but then dark fluid-filled bullae appear, which subsequently rupture revealing non-crepitant gangrene. The lesion is painful and appears like a deep burn. There is also associated systemic toxicity, usually phlebitis, commonly bacteraemia and/or myositis, and often the 'toxic strep syndrome' (see Toxic shock syndrome).

   The mortality is high (about 30%) despite penicillin and surgery, so that early diagnosis is important. The extent and depth of the necrosis can best be determined by CT or MRI.

   A similar clinical picture may sometimes be seen in cutaneous infection with strains of methicillin-resistant *Staphylococcus aureus* (MRSA) which produce the potent toxin Panton–Valentine leukocidin.
   - **Non-streptococcal infection** is usually polymicrobial and is seen after abdominal infection, in diabetics or in fishermen in tropical waters. The usual organisms involved include Gram-negative bacilli, anaerobes and enterococci (i.e. enteric pathogens), or vibrio from tropical seas. This condition is sometimes referred to as **necrotizing soft-tissue infection (NSTI) type I**.

   The intra-abdominal process tends to extend rapidly to the abdominal wall, with local pain and crepitus and systemic toxicity.

   The chief differential diagnosis is a clostridial infection (q.v.) (i.e **NSTI type III**) or perhaps a spider bite (q.v.).

   If the male genitalia are involved, the condition is called **Fournier's gangrene** (described by Jean Alfred Fournier in France in 1883). Previous literature had sometimes referred to the condition as **scrotal fire**. Additional risk factors for this variant include obesity, alcoholism and body piercing of the genitals.

   Treatment of necrotizing fasciitis is with broad-spectrum **antibiotics** *(aminoglycoside and metronidazole, or carbapenem), early and extensive surgical* **debridement**, *general* **support**, *and probably* **hyperbaric oxygen**. *For streptococcal infections,* **clindamycin** *should be added to the β-lactam antibiotic chosen, because of the former's additional antitoxin effect (even if some organisms are resistant to it in vitro).*

2. **Progressive bacterial synergistic gangrene** (Meleney's progressive synergistic gangrene) is usually associated with a pre-existing lesion, including a colostomy.

   There is a painful non-crepitant ragged ulceration, with an inner rim of gangrene, a middle rim of purple erythema and an outer rim of pink oedematous skin. The process tends to extend only slowly.

   The infection is usually polymicrobial and involves microaerophilic streptococci, together with either Gram-negative bacilli or *S. aureus*.

*Treatment usually requires extensive surgical **debridement** and systemic **antibiotics**.*
4. **Pyoderma gangrenosum** (q.v.).
5. **Pseudomonal gangrenous cellulitis** comprises a circumscribed non-crepitant largely painless lesion, with a necrotic centre and erythematous halo.

It is seen in patients with burns or immunocompromise. It has a rapid onset and produces systemic toxicity.
6. **Necrotizing cutaneous mucormycosis** is a non-painful, non-crepitant lesion consisting of a necrotic centre with a purple heaped margin.

It is usually found in diabetics as a slowly progressive lesion which does not produce systemic toxicity. The responsible fungus is sensitive to amphotericin.

Bibliography

Anaya D, Dellinger E. Necrotizing soft-tissue infection: diagnosis and management. *Clin Infect Dis* 2007; 44: 705.

Bessman AN, Wagner W. Nonclostridial gas gangrene. *JAMA* 1975; 233: 958.

Bisno AL, Stevens DL. Streptococcal infections of skin and soft tissue. *N Engl J Med* 1996; 334: 240.

Brown RD, Davis NL, Lepawski M, et al. A multicentre review of the treatment of major truncal necrotising infections with and without hyperbaric oxygen therapy. *Am J Surg* 1994; 167: 483.

Dahl PR, Perniciaro C, Holmkvist KA, et al. Fulminant group A streptococcal necrotizing fasciitis: clinical and pathologic findings in 7 patients. *J Am Acad Dermatol* 2002; 47: 489.

Davies HD, McGeer A, Schwartz B, et al. Invasive group A streptococcal infections in Ontario, Canada. *N Engl J Med* 1996; 335: 547.

Devaney B, Frawley G, Frawley J, et al. Necrotising soft tissue infections: the effect of hyperbaric oxygen on mortality. *Anaesth Intens Care* 2015; 43: 685.

Eke N. Fournier's gangrene: a review of 1726 cases. *Br J Surg* 2000; 87: 718.

Elliott DC, Kufera JA, Myers RAM, et al. Necrotizing soft tissue infections: risk factors for mortality and strategies for management. *Ann Surg* 1996; 224: 672.

Giuliano A, Lewis F, Hadley K, et al. Bacteriology of necrotizing fasciitis. *Am J Surg* 1977; 134: 52.

Green RJ, Dafoe DC, Raffin TA. Necrotizing fasciitis. *Chest* 1996; 110: 219.

Hirschmann JV. Fungal, bacterial, and viral infections of the skin. In: *Scientific American Medicine. Dermatology.* Hamilton: Dekker Medicine. 2020.

Jarrett P, Rademaker M. Duffill M. The clinical spectrum of necrotising fasciitis. *Aust NZ J Med* 1997; 27: 29.

Kaul R, McGeer A, Low DE, et al. Population-based surveillance for group A streptococcal necrotizing fasciitis: clinical features, prognostic indicators, and microbiological analysis of seventy-seven cases. *Am J Med* 1997; 103: 18.

Lille ST, Sato TT, Engray LH, et al. Necrotizing soft tissue infections: obstacles in diagnosis. *J Am Coll Surg* 1996; 182; 7.

Morpurgo E, Galandiuk S. *Fournier's gangrene. Surg Clin N Am* 2002; 82: 1213.

Phan HH, Cocanour CS. Necrotizing soft tissue infections in the intensive care unit. *Crit Care Med* 2010; 38 (suppl.): S460.

Riegels-Nielsen P, Hesselfeldt-Nielsen J, Bang-Jensen E, et al. Fournier's gangrene. *J Urol* 1984; 132: 918.

Seal DV. Necrotizing fasciitis. *Curr Opin Infect Dis* 2001; 14: 127.

Short B. Fournier gangrene: an historical perspective. *Intern Med J* 2018; 48: 1157.

Stevens DL. Invasive group A *Streptococcus* infections. *Clin Infect Dis* 1992; 14: 2.

Stevens DL. The flesh-eating bacterium. *J Infect Dis* 1999; 179 (suppl. 2): S366.

Stevens DL, Bryant AE. Necrotizing soft-tissue infections. *N Engl J Med* 2017; 377: 2253.

Stone HH, Martin JJ. Synergistic necrotizing cellulitis. *Ann Surg* 1972; 175: 702.

Unsworth IP, Sharp PA. Gas gangrene: an 11-year review of 73 cases managed with hyperbaric oxygen. *Med J Aust* 1984; 140: 256.

Urbina T, Madsen MB, de Prost N. Understanding necrotizing soft tissue infections in the intensive care unit. *Intens Care Med* 2020; 46: 1739.

Ustin JS, Malangoni MA. Necrotizing soft-tissue infections. *Crit Care Med* 2011; 39: 2156.

Weinstein L, Barza MA. Gas gangrene. *N Engl J Med* 1973; 289: 1129.

Gas gangrene *See*

- Clostridial infections.

Gas in soft tissues

Gas in soft tissues may be due to a number of conditions.
1. **Anaerobic cellulitis**

This is due to clostridial infection, usually produced by *Clostridium perfringens* (see *Clostridial infections*).
2. **Necrotizing fasciitis** (see *Gangrene*)

This is usually polymicrobial cellulitis and is seen particularly in diabetics or perineal infection. Gram-negative enteric bacilli (especially *Escherichia coli* and klebsiella) are usually present, and anaerobes (bacteroides) are common.

3. **Trapped air**

This usually arises from a procedural, surgical or traumatic injury, though it may sometimes be caused by a compressed gas injury or by deep hydrogen peroxide irrigation. Gas from trapped air does not spread, unless it connects with a tension pneumothorax (see Pleural disorders).

See also
- Emphysema.

Bibliography
Bessman AN, Wagner W. Nonclostridial gas gangrene. *JAMA* 1975; 233: 958.
Giuliano A, Lewis F, Hadley K, et al. Bacteriology of necrotizing fasciitis. *Am J Surg* 1977; 134: 52.
Unsworth IP, Sharp PA. Gas gangrene: an 11-year review of 73 cases managed with hyperbaric oxygen. *Med J Aust* 1984; 140: 256.
Weinstein L, Barza MA. Gas gangrene. *N Engl J Med* 1973; 289: 1129.

Gastric emptying

For solid food, the normal half-time of **gastric emptying** is <1 hr.

For liquids, the half-life in the stomach is normally about 20 min, but this can be greatly increased in the seriously ill.

> In Intensive Care patients, **gastroparesis** (i.e. delayed gastric emptying in the absence of mechanical obstruction) of varying degree occurs in a large of number of conditions, though it is most typically seen in diabetes. It is manifest by bloating, regurgitation and abdominal pain.
>
> *Gastroparesis may respond to treatment with **prokinetic** drugs, such as metoclopramide (10 mg qid), erythromycin (200 mg bd), domperidone (20 mg qid), or most recently ulimorelin (600–1200 mcg/kg tds). These prokinetic medications represent several different classes of drugs, e.g. metoclopramide is a 5-HT4 agonist, erythromycin is a motilin receptor agonist, domperidone is a dopamine receptor antagonist, and ulimorelin is a ghrelin (q.v.) receptor agonist.*

Delayed gastric emptying is one of the markers of gastric intolerance to enteral feeding in Intensive Care patients, in whom a gastric residual volume (GRV) of 200 mL has traditionally been used as the upper limit of normal. More recently, it has been shown that a GRV up to 500 mL is not associated with adverse outcomes. While the finding of increased GRV suggests feeding intolerance, other useful findings may include vomiting, diarrhoea, abdominal distention and discomfort.

On the other hand, while the use of prokinetic agents has been reported to improve gastric emptying and to reduce feeding intolerance, more substantive clinical benefit related to bowel function, complicating pneumonia, length of stay or mortality has not been shown.

Bibliography
Heyland D, Cook DJ, Winder B, et al. Enteral nutrition in the critically ill patient: a prospective study. *Crit Care Med* 1995; 23: 1055.
Lewis K, Alqahtani Z, Mcintyre L, et al. The efficacy and safety of prokinetic agents in critically ill patients receiving enteral nutrition: a systematic review and meta-analysis of randomized trials. *Crit Care* 2016; 20: 259.
Montejo JC, Minambres E, Bordeje L, et al. Gastric residual volume during enteral nutrition in ICU patients: the REGANE study. *Intens Care Med* 2010; 36: 1386.

Gastrinoma See

- Zollinger–Ellison syndrome.

Gastroenteritis See

- Diarrhoea.

Gastroenterology

Gastrointestinal dysfunction of a general nature is very common in the seriously ill, and some would say it is virtually invariable. On the one hand, the gut is a target organ of many systemic insults, and on the other hand, the gut may itself contribute to adverse systemic responses by mechanisms such as cytokine release, enzyme spill or bacterial translocation.

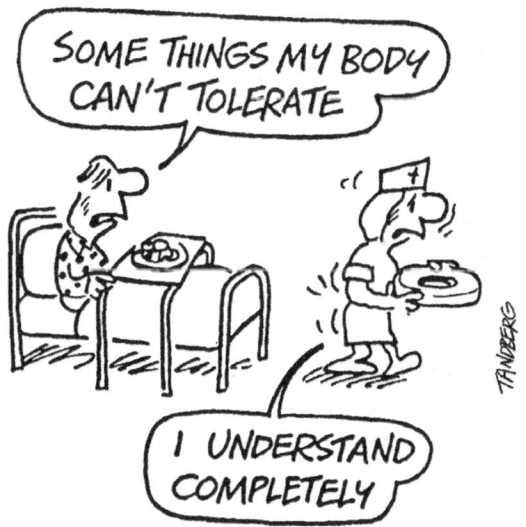

Less common specific gastrointestinal disorders and issues are also sometimes encountered, and those considered in this book include
- Abdominal compartment syndrome,
- Achlorhydria,
- Angiodysplasia,
- Anorectal infections,
- Boerhaave's syndrome,
- Cholangitis,
- Cholestasis,
- *Clostridium (Clostridioides) difficile*,
- Coeliac disease,
- Colitis,
- Crohn's disease,
- Constipation,
- Diarrhoea,
- Dysphagia,
- Eating disorders,
- Enterocolitis,
- Enteropathy,
- Faecal calprotectin,
- Faecal lactoferrin,
- Faecal transplantation,
- Feeding intolerance,
- FODMAPs,
- Food poisoning,
- Gastric emptying,
- Gastrinoma,
- Gastroenteritis,
- Gastrointestinal tumours,
- Gastroparesis,
- Ghrelin,
- Gingivitis,
- Glossitis,
- Inflammatory bowel disease,
- Intra-abdominal hypertension,
- Irritable bowel syndrome,
- Leptin,
- Malabsorption,
- Mallory–Weiss syndrome,
- Microbiome,
- Mouth diseases,
- Pancreatic stone protein,
- Pancreatitis,
- Parotitis,
- Peutz–Jeghers syndrome,
- Plummer–Vinson syndrome,
- Pneumatosis coli,
- Probiotics,
- Proctitis,
- Pseudomembranous colitis,
- Pseudo-obstruction of the colon,
- Retroperitoneal fibrosis,
- Short bowel syndrome,
- Sprue-like enteropathy,
- Stomatitis,
- Tongue,
- Ulcerative colitis,
- VIPoma,
- WDHA syndrome,
- Whipple's disease.

In addition, the gastrointestinal tract is the largest endocrine organ in the body, and interestingly it was the first structure to be recognized as an endocrine organ (see Endocrinology). The gut peptides, gastrin and secretin, were discovered more than 100 yr ago, and over 100 peptides produced by different types of gut cells have since been identified as hormones. Gut hormones are involved in gastrointestinal absorption, motility, growth and repair, and immune function. Outside the gut, the same peptides may have quite different blood-borne functions (see Endocrinology).

Bibliography

Abraham E, ed. Acid suppression in a critical care environment. *Crit Care Med* 2002; 30: no.6, suppl.

Barie PS, Fischer E, Eachempati SR. Acute acalculous cholecystitis. *Curr Opin Crit Care* 1999; 5: 144.

Berger HG, Matsuno S, Cameron JL, eds. *Diseases of the Pancreas*. Berlin: Springer. 2008.

Blaser MJ, Smith PD, Ravdin JL, et al., eds. *Infections of the Gastrointestinal Tract*. 2nd edition. New York: Raven Press. 2002.

Doe WF. The immunology of the gut. In: Peters PJ, Rosen FS, Walport M, eds. *Clinical Aspects of Immunology*. 4th edition. Oxford: Blackwell. 1993; p 2079.

Dooley J, Lok ASF, Garcia-Tsao G, et al., eds. *Sherlock's Diseases of the Liver and Biliary System*. 13th edition. Hoboken: Wiley. 2018.

Fehily SR, Basnayake C, Wright EK, et al. The gut microbiota and gut disease. *Intern Med J* 2021; 51: 1594.

Feldman M, Friedman L, Brandt L. *Sleisenger and Fordtran's Gastrointestinal and Liver Disease*. 11th edition. Philadelphia: Elsevier. 2020.

Go VLW, et al., eds. *The Pancreas: Biology, Pathobiology and Diseases*. New York: Raven Press. 1993.

Johnston DE, Kaplan MM. Pathogenesis and treatment of gallstones. *N Engl J Med* 1993; 328: 412.

Mutlu GM, Mutlu EA, Factor P. GI complications in patients receiving mechanical ventilation. *Chest* 2001; 119: 1222.

Powell LW, Piper DW, eds. *Fundamentals of Gastroenterology*. 6th edition. Sydney: McGraw-Hill. 1995.

Shearman DJC, Finlayson NDC. *Diseases of the Gastrointestinal Tract and Liver*. 2nd edition. Edinburgh: Churchill Livingstone. 1989.

Various. Gastroenterology. In: *Scientific American Medicine*. Hamilton: Dekker Medicine. 2020.

Gastrointestinal tumours

Gastrointestinal tumours (GISTs) are rare mesenchymal tumours of the gut. Thus, they involve the smooth muscle rather than the epithelial cells and are sarcomas rather than carcinomas. They primarily involve the stomach and are potentially malignant. Most tumours have an underlying gene abnormality, most commonly of the c-KIT gene, but very few are hereditary.

In tumours which are not resectable, treatment with the tyrosine kinase inhibitor, **imatinib**, *is effective in those with the KIT-positive gene mutation. The newer agent,* **sunitinib**, *may be helpful in refractory cases.*

See also
- Lymphangioleiomyomatosis.

Gastroparesis See
- Gastric emptying.

Gaucher's disease

Gaucher's disease (Gaucher disease, GD) is one of the **inborn errors of metabolism** (q.v.). It is characterized by the accumulation of glucosylceramide in cells. It is the commonest **lysosomal storage disorder** (see Storage disorders).

It is a recessive disorder due to a deficiency of glucocerebrosidase (beta-glucosidase, GBA), a lysosomal enzyme. Several hundred mutations have so far been described in the relevant gene. It is an uncommon condition, occurring in about one per 75,000 births worldwide, but especially in Ashkenazi Jews. Phenotypic expression is variable, but progression is usual, resulting in premature death.

Clinical features result from the widespread accumulation of lipid-laden macrophages, resulting typically in hepatosplenomegaly, bone marrow disease and bone disease.

Diagnosis is confirmed by the finding of Gaucher cells in the bone marrow, enzyme analysis in peripheral leukocytes and mutation analysis.

Treatment with **enzyme replacement** *is successful in preventing irreversible complications. Recombinant glucocerebrosidases, initially* **alglucerase** *or later* **imiglucerase**, **taliglucerase** *and* **velaglucerase**, *are currently used, though such therapy is complex and very expensive. Substrate reduction therapy can be given for maintenance, using an inhibitor of glucocerebrosidase,* **miglustat** *or* **eliglustat**.

Bone marrow transplantation *has the potential to be curative.* **Splenectomy** *is no longer recommended except in refractory disease.* **Gene therapy** *is expected to provide definitive management in the future.*

Bibliography

Beutler E. Gaucher's disease. *N Engl J Med* 1991; 325: 1354.

Charrow J, Esplin JA, Gribble TJ, et al. Gaucher disease: recommendations on diagnosis, evaluation and monitoring. *Arch Intern Med* 1998; 158: 1754.

Jmoudiak M, Futerman AH. Gaucher disease: pathological mechanisms and modern management. *Br J Haematol* 2005; 129: 178.

Meikle PJ, Hopwood JJ, Clague AE, et al. Prevalence of lysosomal storage disorders. *JAMA* 1999; 281: 249.

Szer J, Peters H. Gaucher disease: a multi-organ disorder with a heterogeneous phenotype. *Intern Med J* 2020; 50 (suppl 4): 7.

Genomics See
- Haemostasis.

Germ warfare

Germ warfare has been banned by international treaty and national stockpiles of such agents have been destroyed, but the technology remains widely known and the consequent potential for bioterrorism (q.v.) is thus of worldwide concern.

See
- Anthrax,
- Botulism,
- Melioidosis,
- Plague,
- Warfare agents.

Bibliography

Breman JG, Henderson DA. Diagnosis and management of smallpox. *N Engl J Med* 2002; 346: 1300.

Rotz LD, Khan AS, Lillibridge SR, et al. Public health assessment of potential bioterrorism agents. *Emerg Infect Dis* 2002; 8: 225.

Whitby M, Ruff TA, Street AC, et al. Biological agents as weapons 2: anthrax and plague. *Med J Aust* 2002; 176: 605.

Ghrelin

Ghrelin is a peptide hormone secreted by the gastrointestinal tract. Ghrelin is stimulated by gastric emptying and has thus been referred to as the 'hunger hormone'. It has the opposite effect of **leptin** (q.v.), which has been referred to as the 'satiety hormone'. Ghrelin also stimulates growth hormone (see Acromegaly) and has anti-inflammatory effects.

Ulimorelin is a synthetic ghrelin agonist which can act as a prokinetic in delayed gastric emptying (q.v.). This condition is most obviously manifested by an increased gastric residual volume (typically >500 mL). Delayed gastric emptying is a frequent problem in critically ill patients and is clinically important because it is associated with intolerance of enteral feeding.

Bibliography
Deane A, Chapman MJ, Fraser RJL, et al. Bench-to-bedside: the gut as an endocrine organ in the critically ill. *Crit Care* 2010; 14: 228.

Giant cell arteritis *See*
- Arteritis.

Gingivitis *See*
- Mouth diseases.

Glomerular diseases

Glomerular diseases are mostly immunological in origin, and their distinction is made on renal biopsy. They are responsible for either nephritic and/or nephrotic clinical pictures.

> The **nephritic response** comprises
> - haematuria (q.v.),
> - proteinuria (q.v.),
> - hypertension,
> - renal impairment.
> There is an active urine sediment, with red cell, white cell and granular casts, including abnormal or dysmorphic red blood cell shapes.

The nephritic picture may be produced by either focal or diffuse glomerular disease.
- **Focal disease** involves <50% of glomeruli. It includes
  - IgA nephropathy,
  - thin basement membrane disease,
  - systemic lupus erythematosus (SLE) (q.v.),
  - Alport's syndrome (hereditary nephritis with deafness and cataracts).
- **Diffuse disease** involves >50% of glomeruli. It includes
  - rapidly progressive or crescentic glomerulonephritis (including Goodpasture's syndrome – q.v.),
  - membrano-proliferative (mesangiocapillary) glomerulonephritis,
  - fibrillary glomerulonephritis,
  - post-infectious glomerulonephritis,
  - SLE (q.v.),
  - vasculitis (q.v.).

> The **nephrotic response** comprises
> - marked proteinuria (q.v.) (>3 g per day), due to podocyte damage,
> - hypoalbuminaemia,
> - oedema,
> - hypercoagulability (see Thrombophilia),
> - hyperlipidaemia.
> The urine sediment shows fatty casts, sometimes with haematuria.

The nephrotic picture may be produced by
- **membranous nephropathy** (30%),
- **minimal change disease** (20%),
- **focal segmental glomerulosclerosis** (FSGS) (15%),
- **systemic disorders** (25%), including
  - diabetes,
  - amyloid (q.v.),
  - pre-eclampsia (q.v.),
  - autoimmune diseases (especially SLE – q.v.),
  - infection,
  - malignancy,
  - drugs (NSAIDs, captopril, gold, lithium – q.v., mercury – q.v., penicillamine – q.v.),
- **membrano-proliferative glomerulonephritis** (occasionally),
- **post-infectious glomerulonephritis** (occasionally).

Bibliography
Abraham PA, Keane WF. Glomerular and interstitial disease induced by nonsteroidal anti-inflammatory drugs. *Am J Nephrol* 1984; 4: 1.
Balow J. Renal vasculitis. *Kidney Int* 1985; 27: 954.
Balow JE, Austin HA, Tsokos GC, et al. Lupus nephritis. *Ann Intern Med* 1987; 106: 79.
Bonegio RGB, Salant DS. Glomerular diseases. In: *Scientific American Medicine*. Nephrology. Hamilton: Dekker Medicine. 2020.
Kincaid-Smith P. Analgesic abuse and the kidney. *Kidney Int* 1980; 17: 250.
Llach F. Hypercoagulability, renal vein thrombosis, and other thrombotic complications of the nephrotic syndrome. *Kidney Int* 1985; 28: 429.
Morgan DB, Dillon S, Payne RB. The assessment of glomerular function: creatinine clearance or plasma creatinine? *Postgrad Med J* 1978; 54: 302.

Muirhead N. Management of idiopathic membranous nephropathy: evidence-based recommendations. *Kidney Int* 1999; 70 (suppl.): S47.

Nolin L, Courteau M. Management of IgA nephropathy: evidence based recommendations. *Kidney Int* 1999; 70 (suppl.): S56.

Ronco PM, Flahault A. Drug-induced end-stage renal disease. *N Engl J Med* 1994; 331: 1711.

Turner NN, Lamiere N, Goldsmith DJ, et al., eds. *Oxford Textbook of Clinical Nephrology*. 4th edition. Oxford: Oxford University Press. 2018.

Glossitis *See*

- Mouth diseases.

Glucagonoma

Glucagonoma is an alpha-cell tumour of the pancreas, which gives rise to a characteristic syndrome of hyperglycaemia with weight loss, anaemia and a distinct dermatitis. Most such tumours occur in the tail of the pancreas, most are malignant and most occur in older women. Hepatomegaly is common because of metastases, and sometimes there is associated **multiple endocrine neoplasia** (MEN) (q.v.).

The dermatitis is referred to as **necrolytic migratory erythema** and is sufficiently characteristic for dermatologists to be responsible for most diagnoses of glucagonoma. The initial skin lesion is a reddish macule which then vesiculates and finally sloughs, leaving an area of local hypopigmentation. These lesions are seen especially on the buttocks, groin and distal extremities. Sometimes the entire sequence of lesions can be found simultaneously. There is a characteristic histology, with inflammatory cells in clefts. The skin lesions occur early in the course of the disease, even before metastases, and disappear within a few days of successful resection. A generalized decrease in serum amino acid levels may be responsible for this unusual dermatitis.

Investigations show a plasma glucagon level usually 10–20 times normal.

Surgical **resection** *is often possible, as the tumour is slowly growing.*
- Otherwise, **cytotoxic** therapy is appropriate.
- **Octreotide** may be dramatically helpful in some patients.
- Successful **liver transplantation** has been reported.

Bibliography

Leichter SB. Clinical and metabolic aspects of glucagonoma. *Medicine* 1980; 59: 100.

Glucose-6-phosphate dehydrogenase deficiency

Glucose-6-phosphate dehydrogenase (G6PD) deficiency is one of the most common worldwide disorders, perhaps because it may originally have given some protection against malaria. The gene for the G6PD isoenzymes is on the X chromosome; therefore, the disease affects especially men. However, even heterozygote women may have a significant deficiency, explained by the Lyon–Beutler hypothesis of random X inactivation in different cells. This phenomenon has also provided the theoretical basis for the use of G6PD as a valuable marker in confirming the monoclonal pathobiology of most cancers.

G6PD is a dimer, with each component having a molecular weight of 55 kDa. There are over 200 molecular variants, which increases the proportion of inactive monomers and thus gives rise to the biochemical defect.

G6PD catalyzes the conversion of NADP+ to NADPH, a potent reducing agent and protector of red blood cells against oxidative damage. G6PD deficiency is thus associated with vulnerability to haemolysis (q.v.). Severe disease is also associated with impaired neutrophil function and thus proneness to infection.

The clinical picture (referred to as **favism**, because of its classical precipitation by the ingestion of fava beans) may take one of three forms, namely,
- **Class 1** (the least common) with chronic haemolytic anaemia,
- **Class 2** (of intermediate frequency) with episodic haemolysis and associated with severe deficiency,
- **Class 3** (the commonest) with haemolysis following a significant oxidative insult and associated with moderate deficiency.

The usual screening test for G6PD deficiency is a qualitative point-of-care or spot test, but this detects only severe deficiency, i.e. <30% activity. The detection of intermediate deficiency, as in heterozygote women with <70% activity (i.e. below the lower limit of normal), requires a more sophisticated quantitative test using a spectrophotometric assay. G6PD activity may be expressed as percentage of activity or as IU/g of Hb.

Treatment comprises
- **avoidance of culprit drugs**, *namely, antimalarials (classically primaquine, but also the newer analog, tafenoquine), chloramphenicol, nitrofurantoin, sulphonamides, high-dose aspirin, high IV doses of vitamin C,*

- **resuscitation** and circulatory support, including transfusion in the event of acute favism, which is manifest by severe disseminated intravascular coagulation (q.v.) and haemolysis (q.v.),
- possibly high-dose **vitamin E**.
  See
- Anaemia – Haemolysis.

Bibliography
Beutler E. The genetics of glucose-6-phosphate dehydrogenase deficiency. *Semin Hematol* 1990; 27: 137.

Glycocalyx

The **glycocalyx** is a gel-like layer that coats the vascular endothelial surface. Because of its fragility, it was difficult to study using conventional histological techniques, so that understanding of its structure and function is relatively recent.

This complex layer is composed of protein and carbohydrate and comprises multiple components. There is an inner layer of membrane-bound proteoglycan and an outer layer of glycosaminoglycans (hyaluronic acid and heparan sulphate) with plasma proteins (albumin and antithrombin). The inner layer also penetrates the intercellular clefts. Apart from the plasma proteins, the components of the glycocalyx are secreted by the endothelial cells.

The glycocalyx has antithrombotic and anti-inflammatory functions and helps maintain vascular integrity.
- As an antithrombotic guardian, it contributes via its glycosaminoglycans to the anticoagulant properties of the intact endothelium, which additionally secretes prostacyclin and tissue factor pathway inhibitor (TFPI) to complement these properties.
- An anti-inflammatory agent, it inhibits leukocyte adhesion which is involved in host defence against infection.
- As a vascular regulator, it is responsible for the modifier (membrane reflection coefficient, σ) in the current version of the Starling equation describing the movement of fluids across semipermeable membranes due to hydrostatic and oncotic forces.

However, its fragility renders it vulnerable to damage, particularly by leukocyte interactions, leading to **microcirculatory dysfunction** (q.v.). Glycocalyx damage is a hallmark of sepsis, with consequent capillary leak, oedema, microthrombosis and loss of vascular responsiveness. This process is exacerbated by a variety of other insults, including hypervolaemia and hyperglycaemia.

Shedding of the glycocalyx may be reflected by increased levels of its components in plasma and urine, and tests for these may become useful laboratory markers of microcirculatory (microvascular) dysfunction in future Intensive Care practice.

A number of therapeutic approaches may tend to provide protection of the glycocalyx, including careful fluid balance, albumin, antithrombin, heparin(s), corticosteroids and glycaemic control. However, such modalities are yet to confirmed as effective in this way in appropriate clinical trials.

Bibliography
Ait-Outfella H, Maury E, Lehoux S, et al. The endothelium: physiological functions and role of microcirculatory failure during sepsis. *Intens Care Med* 2010; 36: 1286.
Iba T, Levy JH. Derangement of the endothelial glycocalyx in sepsis. *J Thromb Haemost* 2019; 17: 283.
Reitsma S, Slaaf DW, Vink H, et al. The endothelial glycocalyx: composition, functions, and visualization. *Pflugers Arch* 2007; 454: 345.
Weinbaum S, Tarbell JM, Damiano ER. The structure and function of the endothelial glycocalyx layer. *Annu Rev Biomed Eng* 2007; 9: 121.

Glycogen storage diseases

Glycogen storage diseases (GSD) are some of the **inborn errors of metabolism** (q.v.). GSDs are of several types, all associated with a positive family history and a specific biochemical defect giving rise to impaired glycogenolysis (and thus pyruvate shortage and poor exercise performance). There are 10 identified GSDs.

The best-known example is **McArdle's disease** (GSD type V), an autosomal recessive condition, which is due to muscle phosphorylase deficiency and is associated with weakness, poor exercise tolerance and myoglobinuria (q.v.). The genetic defect can also be detected in leukocytes, but diagnosis relies on muscle biopsy.

There is no specific treatment, but exercise training, dietary supplementation (added protein, pyridoxine and creatine) and sucrose loading before exercise have all been reported to be helpful.

Biochemical defects in other GSDs affect different organs, especially the brain, heart and liver. There may be hepatomegaly, hypoglycaemia, hyperlipidaemia, hyperuricaemia, lactic acidosis (q.v.), impaired growth, cyclical neutropenia (q.v.) and bacterial infection. If dietary compliance is poor, chronic renal disease, inflammatory bowel disease (q.v.), hepatic adenoma, amyloid (q.v.), gout (q.v.) or osteoporosis may result.

Bibliography
Layzer RB. McArdle's disease in the 1980s. *N Engl J Med* 1985; 312: 370.
Pears JS, Jung RT, Hopwood D, et al. Glycogen storage disease diagnosed in adults. *Quart J Med* 1992; 82: 207.
Talente GM, Coleman RA, Alter C, et al. Glycogen storage disease in adults. *Ann Intern Med* 1994; 120: 218.

Goodpasture's syndrome

Goodpasture's syndrome comprises pulmonary haemorrhage and glomerulonephritis associated with autoantibodies to basement membranes of alveoli and glomeruli. Since the renal component can sometimes occur alone, an additional pulmonary injury may be required for full expression of the symptom-complex, such as viral infection or toxic exposure (including smoking).

Clinical features are usually seen in young men, and the initial presentation is usually haemoptysis (q.v.). The interstitial and alveolar haemorrhage may be considerable enough to cause anaemia (q.v.). There is an active nephritic picture (see Glomerular diseases) with rapidly progressive renal failure.

Chest X-ray shows a patchy and variable pulmonary infiltrate (q.v.), initially due to haemorrhage and later to fibrosis. Renal biopsy shows a necrotizing proliferative glomerulonephritis, commonly with crescentic formation. Occasionally, the renal involvement is only mild and focal.

The diagnosis is based on the demonstration of anti-GBM antibodies in serum and on biopsy of the lung or more commonly kidney, the latter showing the characteristic immunofluorescent finding of IgG deposition along the glomerular basement membrane.

Treatment with corticosteroids even in high dose is ineffective. The mainstay of current treatment is **plasma pheresis** *(q.v.) (which removes antibodies), with or without immunosuppression with corticosteroids and cytotoxics, usually cyclophosphamide (to prevent new antibody formation). Plasmapheresis is typically conducted with 4 L exchanges daily for 1 week. Plasmapheresis interrupts both the haemoptysis and the impending renal failure. However, it does not reverse renal failure if oliguria is established, and it is reported to carry a substantially increased risk of superinfection.*

Until recently, the mortality was high with fatal pulmonary haemorrhage commonly occurring early and end-stage renal disease supervening in 80% of survivors within 1 yr. This is because although anti-GBM antibodies disappear spontaneously within 1 yr and recurrence is unusual, irreversible damage has occurred during this time unless there is effective treatment. For the same reason, any consideration of transplantation should be deferred until the antibodies have disappeared.

Idiopathic pulmonary haemosiderosis (IPH) is a rare disease indistinguishable from the pulmonary component of Goodpasture's syndrome and occurring mainly in children and young adults. There may be associated coeliac disease (q.v.). It is often fatal, although the prognosis appears very variable.

There is no clearly effective therapy. Corticosteroids may reduce recurrences, and associated iron deficiency (q.v.) should be treated. Lung transplantation has been disappointing.

Bibliography
Green RJ, Ruoss SJ, Kraft SA, et al. Pulmonary capillaritis and alveolar hemorrhage: update on diagnosis and management. *Chest* 1996; 110: 1305.
Joachimescu OC, Sieber S, Koch A. Idiopathic pulmonary haemosiderosis revisited. *Eur Respir J* 2004; 24: 162.
Kefalides NA. The Goodpasture antigen and basement membranes: the search must go on. *Lab Invest* 1987; 56: 1.
Kelly PT, Haponik EF. Goodpasture syndrome: molecular and clinical advances. *Medicine* 1994; 73: 171.
Leatherman JW, Davies SF, Hoidal JR. Alveolar hemorrhage syndromes: diffuse microvascular lung hemorrhage in immune and idiopathic disorders. *Medicine* 1984; 63: 343.
Pacheo A, Casanova C, Fogue L, et al. Long-term clinical follow-up of adult idiopathic pulmonary hemosiderosis and celiac disease. *Chest* 1991; 99: 1525.
Specks U. Diffuse alveolar hemorrhage syndromes. *Curr Opin Rheumatol* 2001; 13: 12.
Turner N, Mason PJ, Brown R, et al. Molecular cloning of the human Goodpasture antigen demonstrates it to be the α3 chain of type IV collagen. *J Clin Invest* 1992; 89: 592.
Young KR. Diagnostic pitfalls in alveolar hemorrhage syndromes. *Pulmonary Perspectives* 2000; 17: 11.

Gout

Gout is a crystal-induced synovitis. It is characterized by recurrent attacks of acute arthritis, usually associated with an increased plasma urate. The mechanism of inflammation is neutrophil ingestion of sodium urate crystals with consequent release of inflammatory mediators. The prevalence of gout appears to have been increasing in recent years in most countries and is currently about 2% of the population.

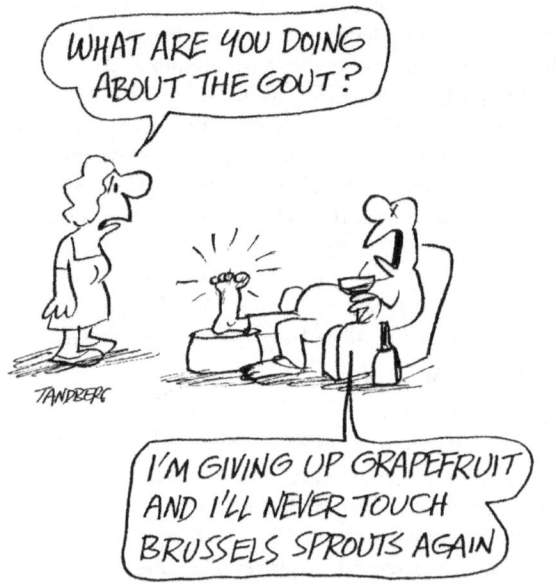

Uric acid has no known biological function but is an end-product of purine metabolism, i.e. nucleic acid breakdown.

The mechanisms for hyperuricaemia are
- **metabolic** (with increased uric acid production)
  - primary (sometimes associated with a specific enzyme defect of purine metabolism),
  - secondary (especially associated with increased nucleic acid turnover, e.g. in the tumour-lysis syndrome – q.v.).
- **renal** (with decreased excretion of uric acid)
  - primary,
  - secondary (including chronic renal disease, lead nephropathy, drug-induced renal disease due to ciclosporin, diuretics, low-dose salicylates).

Uric acid completely dissociates at a normal pH to give urate anion. If the plasma concentration is >400 µmol/L, there is supersaturation with sodium urate, which therefore precipitates, the crystals then being ingested by neutrophils. The normal plasma urate concentration is 100–400 µmol/L. While virtually all patients with gout have hyperuricaemia, for reasons which are not clear only about 10% of patients with hyperuricaemia develop gout.

The clinical features of gout are well known. A typical attack consists of the sudden onset of pain in a single joint, usually in the lower extremity. Within a few hours, the joint becomes red, hot, swollen and extremely painful. The process is self-limited and usually subsides within a few days. Half of the cases occur at the first metatarsophalangeal joint (podagra), but the process is polyarticular in 10–15% of cases. Acute gout may be associated with fever.

The disease may then enter an interval period, with recurrent attacks at variable intervals. The next attack usually occurs within 2 yr. In some patients, a chronic phase subsequently occurs, perhaps after 10–20 yr, with persistent symptoms. In chronic gout, there may be a polyarthritis involving both upper and lower limbs, with urate deposits (tophi) on tendons, around joints, in the ear and sometimes in deeper structures.

There is a high incidence of renal disease associated with chronic tophaceous gout, even greater than that associated with diabetes mellitus.

However, the renal disease is usually due to associated hypertension, and gouty nephropathy is usually mild, though tubulointerstitial urate deposits may be found.

There is a 10–25% prevalence of renal calculi, though it is worth noting that most uric acid stones are in fact from acid urine and not from gout, hyperuricaemia or hyperuricuria.

In renal disease due to lead nephropathy, the gout is referred to as saturnine gout.

Concomitant diseases are also common, including
- diabetes mellitus, in up to 80% of cases,
- obesity,
- hyperlipidaemia,
- cardiovascular disease,
- metabolic syndrome (insulin-resistance syndrome).

Associated cardiovascular disease is thus very frequent.

The diagnosis of gout is usually readily made on the basis of the clinical features, together with an increased plasma urate. However, the plasma urate is an insensitive test, and the level may even fall to some extent during the acute attack. The urinary urate (even >6 mmol per day) is non-specific. Acutely there may be leukocytosis. The diagnosis may be confirmed if necessary by examination of synovial fluid or of a tophus for urate crystals. Histological examination of tophi shows that the chalky material consists of crystal masses.

If there is any suspicion of septic arthritis, examination of synovial fluid is mandatory. This is particularly important to consider, since septic arthritis may precipitate an acute attack of gout in that joint and cause diagnostic confusion.

Treatment of **acute disease** *traditionally has been with* **colchicine** *(q.v.), 0.5 mg orally hrly until relief or a total of 3–5 mg has been given or side-effects have occurred, though it is no longer acceptable to use doses which cause severe gastrointestinal distress. Despite its efficacy, colchicine has been largely superseded because of its potential in traditional doses to cause marked gastrointestinal side-effects. However, low-dose regimens where the initial dosage is kept below 3 mg in the first 24 hr are still recommended,*

- **Indometacin** is in fact just as effective, 50–75 mg being given initially, followed by 25–50 mg tds for 5–7 days. Other NSAIDs are also effective. Cyclo-oxygenase-2 (COX-2) inhibitors have been considered useful improvements to this class of agents.
- **Corticosteroids** either oral or intra-articular may be considered if NSAIDs or colchicine are contraindicated or ineffective, but the diagnosis should always be reviewed before their use in case septic arthritis has been overlooked.

In **chronic disease**, *the plasma urate should be decreased either by*

- enhancing urinary excretion with a uricosuric agent (e.g. **probenecid**, 500 mg qid, or sulphinpyrazone, 100 mg qid), or more usually by
- inhibiting biosynthesis with a xanthine oxidase inhibitor (e.g. **allopurinol**, 50–100 mg per day initially, increasing over several weeks to 100–300 mg per day or more in divided doses, depending on the plasma urate level which should be reduced below a saturating concentration – see above). Allopurinol occasionally produces marked side-effects, including drug fever (q.v.), rash, hepatitis (q.v.), vasculitis (q.v.) and rarely a severe toxic syndrome comprising all these features, together with eosinophilia (q.v.) and renal dysfunction, especially in East Asian patients.

  The goal of the long-term reduction of plasma urate levels is both to eliminate further acute attacks and to promote the dissolution of tophi. The target is a normal plasma urate level, i.e. <400 μmol/L, though lower levels (e.g. <300 μmol/L) are recommended if tophi are present.
- An alternative xanthine oxidase inhibitor, **febuxostat**, has become available for use in patients intolerant of allopurinol, especially if there is associated chronic kidney disease. Given in the usual dose of 80 mg per day, it is effective and safe but expensive.
- An alternative uricosuric agent, **benzbromarone**, has also been recently introduced for hospital use.
- New preparations of **uricase** (e.g. rasburicase) markedly reduce uric acid levels and tophi by further oxidizing uric acid to allantoin, an end-product more common in other animals. These agents can be useful in the short term, but they are not suitable for maintenance therapy (see Tumour-lysis syndrome).
- Low doses of colchicine (e.g. 0.5 mg bd) may also be used in maintenance therapy.
- Renal calculi should be treated with enhanced urine flow and alkalinization.
- Treatment of predisposing factors (especially obesity and excess alcohol intake) and of concomitant disease (e.g. hypertension) is important.

Hyperuricaemia if asymptomatic (see above) probably does not require treatment.

Pseudogout is due to the deposition of crystals containing calcium pyrophosphate dihydrate (CPPD, apatite).

This can give a syndrome resembling gout, though it can also mimic osteoarthritis and even rheumatoid arthritis. It requires examination of synovial fluid for its definitive diagnosis.

Bibliography

Beck LH. Requiem for gouty nephropathy. *Kidney Int* 1986; 30: 280.

Boss GR, Seegmiller JE. Hyperuricemia and gout: classification, complications and management. *N Engl J Med* 1979; 300: 1459.

Dalvi SR, Pillinger MH. Saturnine gout, redux: a review. *Am J Med* 2013; 126: 450.

Dieppe PA, Huskisson EC, Crocker P, et al. Apatite deposition disease: a new arthropathy. *Lancet* 1976; 1: 266.

Edwards Nl. Crystal-induced joint disease. In: *Scientific American Medicine*. Rheumatology. Hamilton: Dekker Medicine. 2020.

Emmerson BT. The management of gout. *N Engl J Med* 1996; 334: 445.

Fam AG. Treating acute gouty arthritis with selective COX 2 inhibitors. *BMJ* 2002; 325: 980.

Galassi FM, Borghi C. A brief history of uric acid from gout to cardiovascular risk factor. *Eur J Intern Med* 2015; 26: 373.

Gupta MN, Sturrock RD, Field M. Prospective comparative study of patients with culture proven and high suspicion of adult onset septic arthritis. *Ann Rheum Dis* 2003; 62: 327.

Hadler NM, Franck WA, Bress NM, et al. Acute polyarticular gout. *Am J Med* 1974; 56: 715.

Hui M, Carr A, Cameron S, et al. The British Society for Rheumatology guidelines for the management of gout. *Rheumatology* 2017; 56: e1.

McGill NW. Gout and other crystal arthropathies. *Med J Aust* 1997; 166: 33.

McGill NW. Management of gout: beyond allopurinol. *Intern Med J* 2010; 40: 545.

Mikula TR, Sang KG. New insights into gout epidemiology. *Curr Opin Rheumatol* 2006; 18: 199.

Pascual E. Gout update: from lab to the clinic and back. *Curr Opin Rheumatol* 2000; 12: 213.

Simkin PA. The pathogenesis of podagra. *Ann Intern Med* 1977; 86: 230.

Stamp LK, O'Donnell JL, Chapman PT. Emerging therapies in the long-term management of hyperuricaemia and gout. *Intern Med J* 2007; 37: 258.

Ting K, Graf SW, Whittle SL. Update on the diagnosis and management of gout. *Med J Aust* 2015; 203: 86.

Yu KH, Luo SF, Liou LB, et al. Concomitant septic and gouty arthritis: an analysis of 30 cases. *Rheumatology* 2003; 42: 1062.

Graft-versus-host disease

Graft-versus-host disease (GVHD) is a systemic immune complication of transplantation when the graft includes some donor immune cells, as in bone marrow transplantation (BMT). GVHD is an expected immune reaction, since these donor cells recognize some host cells as 'not self', and at the time the host is unable to mount an immune defence against the graft (i.e. rejection). The process is mainly T-cell mediated.

GVHD is arbitrarily referred to as acute if occurring within 100 days of grafting and as chronic if occurring after 100 days, though in fact it is more a continuum of reactions. Patients with GVHD may come to the attention of intensivists for resuscitation, treatment of concomitant infections and multiorgan support.

Acutely, GVHD affects primarily
- **skin** (with rash and at its most extreme toxic epidermal necrolysis – q.v.),
- **liver** (with obstruction of bile canaliculi giving cholestasis and of sinusoids giving Budd–Chiari syndrome – q.v.),
- **gastrointestinal tract** (giving pain and diarrhoea).

Later disease affects similar organs but with varying severity and with marked autoimmune features (as in many collagen-vascular diseases – q.v.).

During the entire course of GVHD, the patient has severe immunodeficiency due to the combination of the disease itself and its necessary treatment.

*Regimens for both prevention and treatment comprise complex combinations of **immunomodulation** (q.v.), and these programs require highly specialized oversight and ongoing research.*

The mortality of transplantation is greatly increased by this complication, which is not necessarily treatable in any currently successful way if it is severe.

See
- Autoimmune disorders.

Granulomatosis with polyangiitis See
- Wegener's granulomatosis.

Graves' disease See
- Hyperthyroidism.

Growth hormone See
- Acromegaly.

Guillain–Barré syndrome

Guillain–Barré syndrome (GBS) is an acute progressive polyneuropathy (see Neuropathy). It is the most common type of acute neuromuscular paralysis. Its occurrence is worldwide, and its incidence is about 2 per 100,000 of the population per year.

Although formerly considered a discrete entity, it is nowadays regarded as a heterogeneous syndrome with several variants. These include
- **acute inflammatory demyelinating polyneuropathy** (AIDP), by far the most common form,
- the **Miller Fisher syndrome** (MFS), with ophthalmoplegia, ataxia and areflexia but limited peripheral weakness,
- **acute motor axonal neuropathy** (AMAN),
- **acute motor and sensory axonal neuropathy** (AMSAN),
- **Bickerstaff encephalitis**, with brainstem encephalitis and associated MFS, and
- **rare variants** with isolated abnormalities, e.g. pure sensory or dysautonomic features.

The aetiology of GBS is presumably immunological, with an immune response to an antecedent infection within the previous 2 months targeting peripheral nerve components (particularly myelin, but sometimes the axonal membrane) via molecular mimicry. The most common antecedent infection is with *Campylobacter jejuni*, especially in severe cases, but viral infections (cytomegalovirus (CMV), Epstein–Barr virus (EBV), HIV) have also been associated with the development of GBS. There is an increased incidence of GBS in systemic conditions, such as trauma, Hodgkin's disease, bone marrow transplantation and systemic lupus erythematosus (SLE) (q.v.), and also rarely following vaccination, especially for influenza.

Pathologically, there is widespread but patchy inflammation and demyelination of peripheral nerves – motor, sensory, cranial and autonomic. There is direct axonal degeneration in the uncommon but severe variants, AMAN or AMSAN.

> Clinical features comprise the acute onset of predominantly motor dysfunction commencing usually in the legs and ascending to the trunk, arms, face and even bulbar muscles over a few days. The weakness is symmetrical, and it varies in severity from mild difficulty to complete paralysis. There is areflexia.
>
> Most patients develop some concomitant sensory changes, particularly paraesthesiae and pain. Dysautonomia is common, with arrhythmias, labile blood pressure and ileus.
>
> Typically, the condition progresses for 1–4 weeks and is followed by gradual improvement over weeks to months, except when there has been axonal degeneration.
>
> Complications particularly include
> - respiratory failure,
> - inappropriate antidiuretic hormone (ADH) syndrome (q.v.),
> - the consequences of prolonged Intensive Care with associated instrumentation.

The diagnosis is made clinically and is supported by nerve conduction studies and by CSF findings of a raised protein level but usually no increased white cells. A variety of glycolipid antibodies may be found, most notably anti-GQ1b in the Miller Fisher variant.

The differential diagnosis of GBS includes
- other acute polyneuropathies (see Neuropathy),
- spinal cord disorders (see Myelopathy),
- neuromuscular junction disorders (botulism – q.v., myasthenia gravis – q.v.),
- muscle disorders (see Myopathy),
- for MFS, brainstem stroke or Wernicke's encephalopathy (q.v.).

A discrete sensory level, markedly asymmetrical features or white cells in the CSF suggest either an inflammatory or neoplastic condition.

The most difficult differential diagnosis can be from **chronic inflammatory demyelinating polyneuropathy** (CIDP), which is a more prolonged and usually relapsing condition. This condition is distinguishable from classical GBS by its time-course, though there is temporal (and possibly aetiological) overlap. It too is probably a heterogeneous condition, and it generally has a poorer prognosis than GBS.

The treatment of patients affected by GBS requires complex and prolonged care, with Intensive Care management in more severe cases (20–30% of patients).

*Corticosteroids are not helpful, except in CIDP. However, **plasmapheresis** (q.v.) and **immune globulin** have both been shown in clinical trials to be effective if given early, presumably because they modulate the inflammatory process responsible for the nerve injury rather than promote nerve regeneration or remyelination. They are of similar efficacy and have no demonstrable additive benefit when combined.*

- *Plasmapheresis should be commenced early, with 3.5 L exchanges every second day for 5 occasions. The course may need be repeated after 2 weeks if there is a relapse.*
- *Immune globulin is given in a dose 0.5 g/kg per day for 5 days. As it is less complicated than plasmapheresis, it is generally the preferred treatment.*
- *Either treatment may be repeated if there is no response or a relapse (as in 10% of cases). Alternatively, eculizumab (q.v.) may be considered in this setting.*

The overall mortality is now <5%, but recovery is slow and some patients have persistent weakness (especially those with preceding *Campylobacter jejuni* infection). Most patients (about 80%) have recovered full muscle strength by one year. Recurrent disease is rare, except occasionally in association with neurofibromatosis (q.v.) and with some HLA types.

See
- Neuropathy.

See also
- Bell's palsy,
- Botulism,
- Demyelinating diseases – Transverse myelitis,
- Diphtheria,
- Epstein–Barr virus,
- Lyme disease,
- Varicella.

Bibliography

Ashbury AK, Cornblath DR. Assessment of current diagnostic criteria for Guillain–Barre syndrome. *Ann Neurol* 1990; 27 (suppl.): S21.

Bromberg MB, Feldman EL, Albers JW. Chronic inflammatory demyelinating polyradiculoneuropathy. *Neurology* 1992; 42: 1157.

Dalakas MC, Engel WK. Chronic relapsing (dysimmune) polyneuropathy: pathogenesis and treatment. *Ann Neurol* 1981; 9 (suppl.): 134.

Feasby TE, Hughes RA. Campylobacter jejuni, antiganglioside antibodies, and Guillain–Barré syndrome. *Neurology* 1998; 51: 340.

Fisher M. An unusual variant of acute idiopathic polyneuritis (syndrome of ophthalmoplegia, ataxia and areflexia). *N Engl J Med* 1956; 255: 57.

Fuller GN, Jacobs JM, Guiloff RJ. Nature and incidence of peripheral neuropathy syndromes in HIV infection. *J Neurol Neurosurg Psychiatry* 1993; 56: 372.

Haber P, DeStafano F, Angulo FJ, et al. Guillain-Barré syndrome following influenza vaccination. *JAMA* 2004; 292: 2478.

Hahn AF. Guillain-Barré syndrome. *Lancet* 1998; 352: 635.

Hughes RAC. Ineffectiveness of high-dose intravenous methylprednisolone in Guillain-Barré syndrome. *Lancet* 1991; 338: 1142.

Hughes RA, van der Meche FG. Corticosteroids for treating Guillain-Barré syndrome. *Cochrane Database Systematic Review* 2000; 2: CD001446.

Lasky T, Terracciano GJ, Magder L, et al. The Guillain-Barré syndrome and the 1992–1993 and 1993–1994 influenza vaccines. *N Engl J Med* 1998; 339: 1797.

Misawa S, Kuwahara S, Sato Y, et al. Safety and efficacy of eculizumab in Guillain-Barré syndrome: a multicentre, double-blind, randomised phase 2 trial. *Lancet Neurol* 2018; 17: 519.

Moore P, Owen J. Guillain-Barré syndrome: incidence, management and outcome of major complications. *Crit Care Med* 1981; 9: 549.

Plasma Exchange/Sandoglobulin Guillain-Barré Syndrome Trial Group. Randomised trial of plasma exchange, intravenous immunoglobulin, and combined treatments in Guillain-Barré syndrome. *Lancet* 1997; 349: 225.

Rees JH, Soudain SE, Gregson NA, et al. *Campylobacter jejuni* infection and Guillain-Barré syndrome. *N Engl J Med* 1995; 333: 1374.

Ropper AH. Campylobacter diarrhea and Guillain-Barré syndrome. *Arch Neurol* 1988; 45: 655.

Ropper AH. The Guillain-Barré syndrome. *N Engl J Med* 1992; 326: 1130.

Ropper AH, Victor M. Influenza vaccination and the Guillain-Barré syndrome. *N Engl J Med* 1998; 339: 1845.

Shahrizaila N, Yuki N. Bickerstaff brainstem encephalitis and the Fisher syndrome: anti-CQ1b antibody syndrome. *J Neurol Neurosurg Psychiatry* 2013; 84: 576.

van der Meche FGA, Schmitz PIM. The Dutch Guillain-Barré Study Group: A randomized trial comparing intravenous immune globulin and plasma exchange in Guillain-Barré syndrome. *N Engl J Med* 1992; 326: 1123.

van Doorn PA, Ruts L, Jacobs BC. Clinical features, pathogenesis, and treatment of Guillain-Barré syndrome. *Lancet Neurol* 2008; 7: 939.

Wijdicks EF, Klein CJ. Guillain-Barré Syndrome. *Mayo Clin Proc* 2017; 92: 467.

Winer JB. Bickerstaff's encephalitis and the Miller Fisher syndrome. *J Neurol Neurosurg Psychiatry* 2001; 71: 433.

Yuki N, Hartung HP. Guillain-Barré syndrome. *N Engl J Med* 2012; 366: 2294.

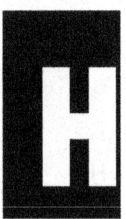

Haemangioma

Haemangioma is a benign vascular tumour, either congenital or acquired. It may occur at virtually any site, and because of its vascular fragility it is subject to easy bleeding, either spontaneously or as a result of minor trauma.

Giant haemangiomas or angiosarcomas (as in the liver, i.e. Kasabach–Merritt syndrome) may cause disseminated intravascular coagulation (q.v.), haemolysis (q.v.) and thrombocytopenia (q.v.).

See
- Telangiectasia.

See also
- Mediastinal diseases,
- Pulmonary hypertension.

Bibliography

Alliot C, Tribout B Barrios M, et al. Angiosarcoma variant of Kasabach-Merritt syndrome. *Eur J Gastroenterol Hepatol* 2001; 13: 731.

Haematology

The general principles related to bleeding, thromboembolism, anticoagulation, the use of blood products and the complications of haematological malignancies are well understood in Intensive Care practice.

On the other hand, although specific individual haematological disorders are usually uncommon in Intensive Care patients, the great frequency with which haematological problems are encountered in general is reflected in the large variety of such conditions which needs to be considered by Intensive Care clinicians. These conditions and issues include

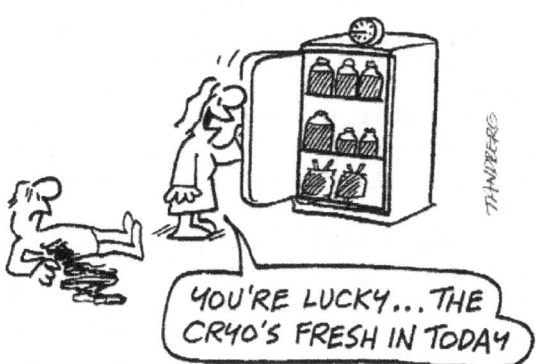

- Abciximab,
- Agranulocytosis,
- Aminocaproic acid,
- Anaemia,
- Anticardiolipin antibody,
- Anticoagulants.
- Antiphospholipid syndrome,
- Antiplatelet agents,
- Antithrombin III,
- Argatroban,
- Basophilia,
- Bivalirudin,
- Bleeding,
- Brodifacoum,
- Christmas disease,
- Clopidogrel,
- Coagulation disorders,
- Coagulation factors,
- C-reactive protein,
- Cryoglobulinaemia,
- Defibrotide,
- Disseminated intravascular coagulation,
- Dysproteinaemias,
- Eosinopenia,
- Eosinophilia,
- Eptifibatide
- Erythrocytosis,
- Erythropoietin,
- Factor V,
- Factor VIII,
- Ferritin,
- Fetal haemoglobin,
- Fibrinolysis,
- Glycocalyx,
- Haemoglobin disorders,
- Haemoglobinopathy,
- Haemolysis,
- Haemophilia,
- Haemostasis,
- Heparin(s),
- Heparin-induced thrombocytopenia,
- Hirudin(s),
- Hypersplenism,
- Idiopathic thrombocytopenic purpura,
- Immune thrombocytopenic purpura,
- Immunothrombosis,
- ITP,
- Lupus anticoagulant,
- Lymphadenopathy,
- lymphocytosis,
- Lymphopenia,
- Mast cells,
- May–Thurner syndrome,
- Megaloblastic anaemia,
- Methaemoglobinaemia,
- Microangiopathic haemolysis,
- Neutropenia,
- Neutrophilia,
- Pancytopenia,
- Parahaemophilia,
- Paroxysmal nocturnal haemoglobinuria,
- Pernicious anaemia,
- Petechiae,
- Plasminogen,
- Platelet function disorders,
- Platelets,
- Polycythaemia,
- Post-transfusion purpura,
- Protein C,
- Protein S,
- Protein Z,
- Prothrombin G20210A abnormality,
- Prothrombin complex concentrate,
- Purpura,
- Reticulocytes,
- Serpins,
- Sickle cell anaemia,
- Sideroblastic anaemia,
- Splenomegaly,
- Storage disorders,
- Thalassaemia,
- Thrombasthenia,
- Thrombocytopenia,
- Thrombocytosis/thrombocythaemia,
- Thromboembolism,
- Thrombohaemorrhagic disorders,

- Thromboinflammation,
- Thrombolysis,
- Thrombomodulin,
- Thrombophilia,
- Thrombopoietin,
- Thrombotic microangiopathy,
- Thrombotic thrombocytopenic purpura,
- Tirofiban,
- Tranexamic acid,
- Trauma-induced coagulopathy,
- Vitamin K deficiency,
- Von Willebrand's disease,
- Warfarin.

Bibliography

Arya S, Hong R, Gilbert EF. Reactive hemophagocytic syndrome. *Pediatr Pathol* 1985; 3: 129.

Barrett-Connor E. Anemia and infection. *Am J Med* 1972; 52: 242.

Berliner N, ed. Hematology. In: *Scientific American Medicine*. Hamilton: Dekker Medicine. 2020.

Bohnsack JF, Brown EJ. The role of the spleen in resistance to infection. *Annu Rev Med* 1986; 37: 49.

Bolan CD, Alving BM. Pharmacologic agents in the management of bleeding disorders. *Transfusion* 1990; 30: 541.

Collen D, Lijnen HR. Basic and clinical aspects of fibrinolysis and thrombolysis. *Blood* 1991; 78: 3114.

Colman N, Herbert V. Hematologic complications of alcoholism: overview. *Semin Hematol* 1980; 17: 164.

Copeman PW. Livedo reticularis: signs in the skin of disturbance of blood viscosity and blood flow. *Br J Dermatol* 1975; 93: 519.

Dexter TM. Stem cells in normal growth and disease. *BMJ* 1987; 295: 1192.

Doll DC, List AF. Myelodysplastic syndromes. *Semin Oncol* 1992; 19: 1.

Editorial. Nitrous oxide and acute marrow failure. *Lancet* 1982; 2: 856.

Editorial. Peripheral stem cells made to work. *Lancet* 1992; 339: 648.

Goodnough LT, ed. RFVIIa: potential treatment of critical bleeding in the future ICU. *Intens Care Med* 2002; 28 (suppl. 2): S221.

Greenberg CS, Sane DC. Coagulation problems in critical care medicine. In: Lumb PD, Shoemaker WC, eds. *Critical Care: State of the Art*, Chapter 9. Fullerton: Society of Critical Care Medicine. 1990; p 187.

Guyatt G, Akl EA, Crowther M, et al., eds. Antithrombotic therapy and prevention of thrombosis, 9th ed: ACCP evidence-based clinical practice guidelines. *Chest* 2012; 141: no. 2 (suppl.).

Hirsh J, Levine MN. Low molecular weight heparin. *Blood* 1992; 79: 1.

Kushner I, Rzewnicki DL. The acute phase response: general aspects. *Baillieres Clin Rheumatol* 1994; 8: 513.

Lieschke GJ, Burgess AW. Granulocyte colony-stimulating factor and granulocyte-macrophage colony-stimulating factor. *N Engl J Med* 1992; 327: 28 & 99.

Marder VJ, Aird WC, Bennett JS, et al., eds. *Hemostasis and Thrombosis: Basic Principles and Clinical Practice*. 6th edition. Philadelphia: Lippincott Williams & Wilkins. 2012.

Metcalf D. Hematopoietic regulators: redundancy or subtlety? *Blood* 1993; 82: 3515.

Moake JL. Common hemostatic problems and blood banking in critical care medicine. In: Lumb PD, Shoemaker WC, eds. *Critical Care: State of the Art*, Chapter 8. Fullerton: Society of Critical Care Medicine. 1990; p 161.

Nachman RL. Thrombosis and atherogenesis: molecular connections. *Blood* 1992; 79: 1897.

Ogawa M. Differentiation and proliferation of hemopoietic stem cells. *Blood* 1993; 81: 2844.

Provan D, ed. *ABC of Clinical Haematology*. 4th edition. London: BMJ Publishing. 2018.

Rapaport SI. Preoperative hemostatic evaluation: which tests, if any? *Blood* 1983; 61: 229.

Rose WF. The spleen as a filter. *N Engl J Med* 1987; 317: 704.

Salama A, Mueller-Eckhardt C. Immune-mediated blood cell dyscrasias related to drugs. *Semin Hematol* 1992; 29: 54.

Schafer AI. Bleeding and thrombosis in the myeloproliferative disorders. *Blood* 1984; 64: 1.

Shram AM, Berliner N. Nonmalignant disorders of leukocytes. In: *Scientific American Medicine. Hematology*. Hamilton: Dekker Medicine. 2020.

Silverstein RL, Nachman RL. Cancer and clotting – Trousseau's warning. *N Engl J Med* 1992; 327: 1163.

Sox HC, Liang MH. The erythrocyte sedimentation rate: guidelines for rational use. *Ann Intern Med* 1986; 104: 515.

Weitz JI. Low-molecular-weight heparins. *N Engl J Med* 1997; 337: 688.

Haematuria

Haematuria is a striking clinical finding, but in fact as little as 1 mL/L can cause a visible colour change, and much lower concentrations can be detected chemically (by dipstick test), though its quantification is not generally of significant diagnostic or prognostic value.

Urinary tract blood loss is considered to be abnormal if there are
- >1 red blood cell (RBC) per high-power field on urine microscopy (>3 RBCs in women), or
- >10,000 RBCs per mL of urine.

Haematuria is usually without clots, perhaps because of the local action of urokinase.

> Haematuria needs to be distinguished from other causes of red or red-brown urine.
> These include most importantly
> - **haemoglobinuria** (from haemolysis – q.v.),
> - **myoglobinuria** (from rhabdomyolysis – q.v.),
>   but in these the colour remains in the supernatant after standing or centrifugation.
>   Red urine may also be caused by
> - drugs
>   - such as phenothiazines, rifampicin, sulphasalazine,
> - porphyria (q.v.),
> - ingestion of some vegetables
>   - e.g. beetroots,
> - ingestion of some food dyes.
>   More brownish urine
> - may contain bilirubin or melanin,
> - may be caused by drugs
>   - such as methyldopa, metronidazole, nitrofurantoin.

Haematuria
- with marked proteinuria suggests glomerulonephritis,
- with pyuria suggests urinary tract infection.

Macroscopic haematuria, with a urinary red cell count of $>10^6$ per mL of glomerular origin (i.e. with dysmorphic red cells), is often indicative of a rapidly progressive glomerulonephritis with crescent formation.

The causes of isolated haematuria may be either renal or extra-renal.
- **Renal causes** may be
  - glomerular,
  as in glomerulonephritis or following heavy exercise,
  - extra-glomerular,
  as with calculi, carcinoma, trauma, vascular disease, haemorrhagic disease, cystic disease.
- **Extra-renal causes** are the most common and include disorders of the
  - ureter (calculi),
  - bladder (infection, tumour, trauma, cyclophosphamide),
  - prostate (benign hypertrophy, carcinoma),
  - urethra (infection, trauma).

Many instances of haematuria, especially if transient, have no demonstrable cause in younger patients.

Appropriate investigations include examination of the urine and urinary sediment, renal ultrasound examination, possibly intravenous pyelography and possibly cystoscopy.

See
- Glomerular diseases,
- Tubulointerstitial diseases.

See also
- Drowning,
- Ethylene glycol,
- Heat stroke,
- Nephrolithiasis,
- Polyarteritis nodosa,
- Renal artery occlusion,
- Renal cortical necrosis,
- Renal cystic disease,
- Renal vein thrombosis,
- Schistosomiasis,
- Systemic lupus erythematosus.

Bibliography

Cronin RE, Kaehny WD, Miller, PD, et al. Renal cell carcinoma: unusual systemic manifestations. *Medicine* 1976; 55: 291.

Froom P, Ribak J, Benbassat J. Significance of microhaematuria in young adults. *BMJ* 1984; 288: 20.

Haemochromatosis

Haemochromatosis is a common inherited disease, with a prevalence of 12% of the population for heterozygotes or carriers and of 3.6 per 1000 of the population for homozygotes. Some heterozygotes (25%) have minor abnormalities of iron metabolism but no clinical disease. Even many homozygotes (50%) do not have clinical disease.

It is an autosomal recessive disease with the abnormal gene located close to the HLA region on chromosome 6. The abnormal gene is referred to as HFE (derived from High Fe). The HFE gene has been identified and cloned, and its C282Y mutation has been found to be responsible for most familial cases of the disease. The defect gives rise to decreased **hepcidin** (see Iron) and thus excess iron absorption, with greatly increased iron stores in the body and deposition in parenchymal cells, particularly of the liver, heart, pancreas and testes.

> Haemochromatosis is the primary, idiopathic or hereditary form of **iron overload disease**.

> Secondary iron overload syndromes occur in the iron-loading anaemias (q.v.), such as thalassaemia and hereditary spherocytosis.
> Mild iron overload also occurs in alcoholism.

Symptoms usually commence between 30 and 60 years of age. They occur later and much less frequently in women because of menstruation and pregnancy. The classical tetrad comprises diabetes, liver disease, pigmentation and gonadal failure. There is lethargy, weakness, arthralgia (and later arthritis) (q.v.), abdominal pain, loss of libido and impotence.

On examination, there is hepatomegaly, greyish skin pigmentation, arthropathy and testicular atrophy. Advanced disease may be complicated by diabetes mellitus, cirrhosis, hepatocellular carcinoma (q.v.) and cardiac failure.

> The diagnosis should be considered
> - in any case of liver disease of unknown cause,
> - in the presence of a positive family history,
> - when there is a syndrome of fatigue, diabetes, arthritis (q.v.) and cardiac failure.

Appropriate laboratory investigations are as follows.
- The serum iron level is not helpful, since it may be already increased in the presence of hepatic cell destruction from any cause.
- The serum iron to iron-binding capacity ratio (i.e. transferrin saturation) is the earliest and most useful abnormal test, as it is increased, often to 80–90% (normal <55%).
- The serum ferritin may be increased (>400 μg/L in men and >200 μg/L in women) if there is clinical disease (but see Ferritin).
- If either the serum transferrin saturation or the serum ferritin is abnormal, liver biopsy should be performed even in asymptomatic patients to
  - confirm the diagnosis,
  - assess the presence of cirrhosis,
  - measure the iron concentration (hepatic iron index is increased >2.0).
- Liver function tests are often abnormal, but there is usually no jaundice.
- Imaging of the liver with CT or MRI may be helpful.

While population screening is not cost-effective, all first and second degree relatives of any index case should be tested. Clearly, siblings have a 25% chance of being homozygous. HLA typing while not diagnostically useful may be helpful in family studies, because the case is probably normal if neither HLA haplotype is shared with the index case. Testing should be commenced at the age of 10 years and continued three yearly until the age of 70 years. HFE genetic testing is now available.

Treatment is with lifelong **venesection** which removes iron via haemoglobin (500 mL of blood contains 250 mg of iron). Since the patient often has 10–20 g of excess iron in the body, 50 units of blood may have to be removed (i.e. one unit each 1–2 weeks for 1–2 years). Thereafter, 3–5 venesections per year will maintain the iron stores at a low level without inducing iron deficiency (q.v.), for which the best end-points are haemoglobin of 110 g/L and low-normal ferritin levels.

Dietary restriction of iron intake is unhelpful, but alcohol intake should be minimized, and care should be taken with vitamin C intake since this enhances iron absorption.

Liver transplantation has been shown to restore hepcidin levels and thus prevent recurrence of iron overload.

There is a 50% average mortality within 20 years. With treatment
- the prognosis is normal if there is no cirrhosis,
- skin pigmentation and cardiac failure improve,
- diabetes mellitus improves but does not disappear,
- gonadal failure and arthritis may sometimes improve,
- cirrhosis does not regress entirely, and indeed primary liver cancer may still occur. Its development is best screened for with an alpha-fetoprotein level (q.v.) and annual imaging of the liver with ultrasound.

See also
- Iron.

Bibliography

Adams PC, Kertesz AE, Valberg LS. Clinical presentation of hemochromatosis. *Am J Med* 1991; 90: 445.

Bassett ML. Haemochromatosis: iron still matters. *Intern Med J* 2001; 31: 237.

Bomford A. Genetics of haemochromatosis. *Lancet* 2002; 360: 1673.

Burke W, Thomson E, Khoury MJ, et al. Hereditary hemochromatosis: gene discovery and its implications for population-based screening. *JAMA* 1998; 280: 172.

Burt MJ, George DK, Powell LW. Haemochromatosis – a clinical update. *Med J Aust* 1996; 164: 348.

Challoner T, Briggs C, Rampling MW, et al. A study of the haematological and haemorrheological consequences of venesection. *Br J Haematol* 1986; 62: 671.

Editorial. Serum-ferritin. *Lancet* 1979; 1: 533.

Finch CA. The detection of iron overload. *N Engl J Med* 1982; 307: 1702.

Finch CA, Huebers H. Perspectives in iron metabolism. *N Engl J Med* 1992; 306: 1520.

Gertig DM, Hopper JL, Allen KJ. Population genetic screening for hereditary haemochromatosis. *Med J Aust* 2003; 179: 517.

Olynyk JK. Hereditary haemochromatosis: diagnosis and management in the gene era. *Liver* 1999; 19: 73.

Powell LW, Bassett ML. Haemochromatosis: diagnosis and management after the cloning of the HFE gene. *Aust NZ J Med* 1998; 28: 159.

Radford-Smith DE, Powell EE, Powell LW. Haemochromatosis: a clinical update for the practicing physician. *Intern Med J* 2018; 48: 509.

Valberg LS, Ghent CN. Diagnosis and management of hereditary hemochromatosis. *Annu Rev Med* 1985; 36: 27.

Haemodilution See

- Anaemia.

Haemoglobin disorders

Haemoglobin disorders (haemoglobinopathies) are a diverse group of disorders providing one mechanism of red blood cell (RBC) abnormality and thus anaemia due to increased RBC destruction (i.e. haemolysis – see Anaemia). There are over 100 types of haemoglobinopathy and many are asymptomatic.

Haemoglobin requires the complex globin assembly of 2 alpha and 2 beta chains, which must then be coordinated with haem synthesis. The alpha genes are on chromosome 16 and the non-alpha genes are on chromosome 11. As well as two alpha chains, haemoglobin A (HbA) contains two beta chains, HbF contains two gamma chains and HbA_2 contains two delta chains.

Genetic defects may cause amino acid substitution (as in sickle cell anaemia) or incoordinated assembly (as in thalassaemia). The resultant abnormal haemoglobin may be unstable, bind oxygen incorrectly, oxidize or crystallize.

1. **Thalassaemia**

Thalassaemia is encountered worldwide, perhaps because heterozygotes had some survival advantage, e.g. enhanced malarial resistance (as with sickle cell anaemia – see below, and with glucose 6-phosphate dehydrogenase deficiency – q.v.). Thalassaemia arises from a variety of genetic defects which cause mismatching of globin chains with resultant molecular aggregation, cell deformity and metabolic and immunological abnormalities of the RBC membrane.

Beta thalassaemia is the common form of the disease and is due to impaired beta chain production. The chains are thus unmatched and there is a compensatory increase in gamma and delta chains, so that haemoglobin HbF and HbA_2 are also present.

Thalassaemia major (**Cooley's anaemia**) is usually homozygous and is associated with severe disease, consisting of haemolytic anaemia (q.v.), hepatosplenomegaly, growth retardation and susceptibility to infections. **Iron overload** (q.v.) results from the inevitable multiple transfusions and may be prevented or treated by desferrioxamine (deferoxamine, DFO) (see Chelating agents), or if DFO is not tolerated by one of the new oral iron chelators, deferiprone or deferasirox, though in turn their side-effects can be a concern. Bone marrow transplantation from HLA-identical donors has been performed in over 1000 patients worldwide and has been reported to give an 80% cure rate.

Thalassaemia minor (thalassaemia trait) is usually heterozygous and presents with mild disease.

There are many genetic variants, with abnormalities clinically resembling beta thalassaemia. In alpha thalassaemia, there are excess beta chains and no substitute chains available in the adult for the deficient alpha chains.

The differential diagnosis of thalassaemia is chiefly iron deficiency anaemia (q.v.), but in thalassaemia the RBC count is normal.

The diagnosis of thalassaemia is made on the basis of anaemia, decreased mean corpuscular volume (MCV), normal RBC count, peripheral blood film showing hypochromia and microcytosis but with basophilic stippling and nucleated erythrocytes, increased HbA_2 and HbF, and specifically abnormal haemoglobin electrophoresis.

Gene therapy (with Zynteglo) has recently been approved for use in patients with beta thalassaemia who are transfusion-dependent.

2. **Sickle cell anaemia**

Sickle cell anaemia (sickle cell disease, SCD) occurs in many countries around the world, especially in West Africa (and thus also in African Americans), the Eastern Mediterranean and India. Like thalassaemia, its wide prevalence and persistence are possibly due to some protection by the trait against malaria. In developed countries, the median survival of adults with sickle cell disease (SCD) has risen to about 50 yr.

Sickle cell anaemia is due to the presence of HbS, which has a glutamate residue replaced by valine in the sixth position of the beta chain. A number of other genotypes have also been described. HbS in deoxy form has reduced solubility and polymerizes, so that the red blood cell becomes distorted into an inflexible sickle shape, leading to increased blood viscosity. This process of sickling occurs especially in the microvasculature and is aggravated by hypoxia, acidosis and increased 2,3-DPG. The process is at least partly irreversible, so that the cells remain damaged even after re-oxygenation and are then prematurely removed by the reticuloendothelial system, giving rise to haemolytic anaemia. The problem of hyperviscosity is compounded by endothelial dysfunction and haemostatic activation, so that all components of Virchow's triad for thrombosis are in fact affected.

Heterozygotes have 30–50% HbS (i.e. they have HbAS) and are asymptomatic. Homozygotes have 70–98% HbS (i.e. they have HbSS) and have symptomatic disease, with

- chronic haemolytic anaemia,
- acute vaso-occlusive crises.

These two complications are responsible for the majority of the morbidity and mortality of the disease.

Clinical features are those of chronic haemolytic anaemia. There is jaundice, and about 50% of patients have pigment gallstones. There is hyposplenism and increased susceptibility to infection. The kidneys show loss of concentrating ability. The central nervous system, eyes, lungs, liver, kidneys, bone marrow and penis may be affected by acute vascular occlusion.

Two clinical problems related to sickle cell disease are of importance to Intensive Care practice. These are especially noteworthy because about 50% of all deaths in patients with sickle cell disease occur in ICU.
1. The **'acute chest syndrome'** (ACS) is associated with pulmonary vascular occlusion and perhaps local infection, and an extensive but asymmetrical 'white-out' on chest X-ray. Clinical features include chest pain, tachypnoea, cough and wheeze. There is typically an increased plasma level of phospholipase A_2. ACS is responsible for most ICU admissions in patients with sickle cell disease.
2. **Sickle cell crisis** is an acute, life-threatening and painful vaso-occlusive process, leading to local ischaemia or even infarction. The initiating event is often not apparent. The target organs are especially the kidney and the bone marrow, and multiorgan failure (q.v.) may occur.

The diagnosis is based on the typically abnormal blood film and confirmed by haemoglobin electrophoresis. The white cell count and platelet count are usually elevated.

Treatment of a sickle cell crisis includes rest, hydration, oxygenation, alkali, analgesia and antibiotics (in ACS).
- Since severe **pain**, especially that of avascular necrosis in bone marrow, may last for over a week, there is a risk of narcotic addiction.

- The frequency of the acute chest syndrome is reduced by **hydroxycarbamide**, and the severity of an individual episode may be attenuated by inhaled **nitric oxide** (NO).

General **anaesthesia** is normally recommended to be deferred until the HbS level has been lowered to about 50% by transfusion (or exchange transfusion, so that the haematocrit is not >0.35). In fact, however, there have been reported series of general anaesthetics without complications despite no specific precautions. Pregnancy (q.v.) and even oral contraceptives (q.v.) add to the anaesthetic risk.

Blood transfusions, either simple transfusion or exchange transfusion, are frequently required, but extended cross-matching procedures are mandated to avoid the severe complications which can flow from RBC alloimmunization.

In the future, **gene therapy** offers prospect for cure, and in the meantime **bone marrow (stem cell) transplantation** has been successful in some patients with an HLA-identical donor.

Haemoglobin C disease results from the replacement of glutamate by lysine at the sixth position on the beta chain. It is thus a variant of sickle cell anaemia, except that it is mild. Heterozygotes are asymptomatic, while homozygotes have mild anaemia with splenomegaly.

Haemoglobin E disease is a further variant in which lysine replaces glutamate at the 26 position on the beta chain. The trait is particularly common in some South-East Asian populations. The clinical features are similar to those of HbC disease. Drugs with oxidizing properties such as dapsone should be avoided.

Compound haemoglobinopathies may also be seen, with heterozygote combinations of HbS, β-thalassaemia, HbC and HbE. Many other amino acid substitutions have been reported, which give unstable haemoglobins associated with chronic haemolytic anaemia without spherocytosis.

Some haemoglobin variants confer abnormal oxygen binding.
- **Left shift of the haemoglobin oxygen dissociation curve**
  - i.e. increased oxygen affinity is produced by haemoglobin Chesapeake, Rainier or Yakima.
- **Right shift of the haemoglobin oxygen dissociation curve**
  - i.e. decreased oxygen affinity is produced by haemoglobin Kansas and can cause cyanosis.

Bibliography

Bunn HF. Pathogenesis and treatment of sickle cell disease. *N Engl J Med* 1997; 337: 762.

Charache S, Terrin ML, Moore RD, et al. Effect of hydroxyurea on the frequency of painful crises in sickle cell anaemia. *N Engl J Med* 1995; 332: 1317.

Cohen AR, Galanello R, Piga A. Safety and effectiveness of long-term therapy with the oral iron chelator deferiprone. *Blood* 2003; 102: 1583.

Davies SC, Luce PJ, Win AA, et al. Acute chest syndrome in sickle-cell disease. *Lancet* 1984; 1: 36.

Dessap AM, Fartoukh M, Machado RF. Ten tips for managing critically ill patients with sickle cell disease. *Intens Care Med* 2017; 43: 80.

Embury SH. The clinical pathophysiology of sickle cell disease. *Annu Rev Med* 1986; 37: 361.

Francis RB, Johnson CS. Vascular occlusion in sickle cell disease: current concepts and unanswered questions. *Blood* 1991; 77: 1405.

Koshy M, Burd L. Management of pregnancy in sickle cell anemia. *Hematol Oncol Clin North Am* 1991; 5: 585.

Novelli EM, Gladwin MT. Crises in sickle cell disease. *Chest* 2016; 149: 1082.

Otis S, Price EA. Hemoglobinopathies and hemolytic anemias. In: *Scientific American Medicine. Hematology*. Hamilton: Dekker Medicine. 2020.

Piomelli S, Loew T. Management of thalassemia major (Cooley's anemia). *Hematol Oncol Clin North Am* 1991; 5: 557.

Platt OS. Easing the suffering caused by sickle cell disease. *N Engl J Med* 1994; 330: 783.

Rice L, Teruya M. Sickle cell patients face death in ICU. *Crit Care Med* 2014; 42: 1730.

Schrier SL. Thalassemia: pathophysiology of red cell shapes. *Annu Rev Med* 1994; 45: 211.

Styles LA, Schalkwijk CG, Aarsman AJ, et al. Phospholipase A2 levels in acute chest syndrome of sickle cell disease. *Blood* 1996; 87: 2573.

Weatherall DJ. The treatment of thalassemia – slow progress and new dilemmas. *N Engl J Med* 1993; 329: 877.

Haemoglobinopathy See

- Haemoglobin disorders.

Haemoglobinuria See

- Anaemia – Haemolysis,
- Cold agglutinin disease,
- Drowning,
- Haematuria,
- Rhabdomyolysis.

Haemolacria

Haemolacria refers to the uncommon symptom of weeping blood. Bloody tears are always due to local conditions, including trauma, infection, vascular tumours (e.g. haemangioma) or retrograde epistaxis. They are never caused by a systemic bleeding disorder.

Haemolysis See

- Anaemia – Haemolysis.
  See also
- Bites and stings – Envenomation,
- Clostridial infections,
- Cold agglutinin disease,
- Complement deficiency,
- Copper – Wilson's disease,
- Disseminated intravascular coagulation,
- Folic acid deficiency,
- Frostbite,
- Glucose-6-phosphate dehydrogenase deficiency,
- Haemangioma,
- Haemoglobinopathy,
- Haemolytic–uraemic syndromes,
- HELLP syndrome,
- Hypophosphataemia,
- Malaria,
- Microangiopathic haemolysis,
- Porphyria,
- Pseudohyperkalaemia,
- Rhabdomyolysis,
- Thrombotic thrombocytopenic purpura.

Bibliography

Boutboul D, Touzot F, Szalat R. Understanding therapeutic emergencies in acute hemolysis. *Intens Care Med* 2018; 44: 482.

Haemolytic–uraemic syndromes

The **haemolytic–uraemic syndromes** comprise childhood and adulthood haemolytic–uraemic syndrome (HUS), as well as atypical HUS. They are members of the group of **thrombotic microangiopathies** (TMAs) (q.v.), which also include the related conditions of thrombotic thrombocytopenic purpura (TTP) (q.v.) and disseminated intravascular coagulation (DIC) (q.v.).

These conditions have the common features of thrombotic microangiopathy, namely,
- microangiopathic haemolysis (q.v.),
- thrombocytopenia (q.v.),
- platelet-fibrin thrombi in small vessels,

- renal involvement (usually reversible, even if dialysis is required acutely),
- other organ involvement sometimes (including brain, liver, lungs, skin).

In more chronic situations, the histology may show concentric vascular thickening as in malignant hypertension or scleroderma (q.v.).

While HUS is usually idiopathic, there is sometimes such marked local clustering as to suggest an epidemic, especially in children. This most commonly follows a few days of diarrhoea due to **enteropathogenic** *Escherichia coli* (q.v. and also see below).

The occurrence of **atypical HUS** (aHUS) within families has led to greater genetic and pathogenetic understanding of the condition, with several mutations now described which give rise to unbridled C3 activation within the complement sequence (see Complement deficiency).

HUS may be associated with
- pregnancy (q.v.)
  - especially the post-partum state, when it may particularly occur if there has been placental abruption (abruptio placentae), retained placenta or pre-eclampsia,
- bone marrow transplantation,
- immunomodulation (q.v.)
  - with ciclosporin and some cancer chemotherapeutic agents, e.g. mitomycin C,
- mucous adenocarcinoma of the gastrointestinal tract,
- antiphospholipid syndrome (q.v.),
- quinine-induced immune thrombocytopenia (see Thrombocytopenia),
- food poisoning (q.v.)
  - due to enteropathogenic (enterotoxigenic, entero-haemorrhagic) *E. coli*, especially serotype O157:H7, and usually in children (see Diarrhoea). This is an important cause of outbreaks of HUS and its risk appears to be increased if antibiotics have been used.

Sometimes, these conditions lead to HUS and sometimes to TTP. Whether its pathogenesis primarily involves endothelial cell or platelet activation is uncertain.

Investigations show thrombocytopenia with increased beta-thromboglobulin (βTG), haemolysis with raised LDH, neutrophilia, and platelet-fibrin thrombi in small arteries in biopsy material (e.g. bone marrow, kidney). Coagulation is normal and there is no disseminated intravascular coagulation, the complement level is normal, the direct Coombs' test is negative, and the urinary sediment is usually normal.

Treatment should be with **plasmapheresis** *(q.v.) if the condition is severe.*
- Traditionally, therapy with aspirin and/or corticosteroids has been used, but aspirin in particular should be used with caution because of the risk of bleeding.
- Platelet transfusion may also give rise to problems (e.g. thrombotic deterioration), and thus should be used only if the patient is bleeding.
- Renal support should be instituted on its normal merits.
- Clearly, any culprit drugs should be stopped.
- New therapeutic potential may be offered by **eculizumab** (q.v.), originally introduced for paroxysmal nocturnal haemoglobinuria (q.v.). It is a recombinant monoclonal antibody which blocks the cleavage of C5 to C5a (see Complement deficiency) and thus the consequent complement-mediated cytotoxic and inflammatory attack, especially in atypical HUS.

There is an 80% response to early treatment and complete remission is usual, though the microangiopathic changes may take some months to subside. However, one third of cases suffer a recurrence, though this is usually mild and often asymptomatic, being demonstrated only by new thrombocytopenia and microangiopathic haemolysis. The renal recovery may sometimes be delayed and incomplete, especially if the patient is untreated. The mortality is worse post-partum, because it is then often associated with cardiomyopathy, but even in this circumstance survival is substantially better than with TTP.

See also
- Thrombotic thrombocytopenic purpura.

Bibliography

Aster RH. Quinine sensitivity: a new cause of hemolytic-uremic syndrome. *Ann Intern Med* 1993; 119: 243.

Azoulay E, Knoebl P, Garnacho-Montero J, et al. Expert statements on the standard of care in critically ill adult patients with atypical hemolytic uremic syndrome. *Chest* 2017; 152: 424.

Beers M, Cameron S. Hemolytic uremic syndrome. *Emerg Infect Dis* 1995; 1: 4.

Caprioli J, Peng L, Remuzzi G. The hemolytic uremic syndromes. *Curr Opin Crit Care* 2005; 11: 487.

Franchini M. Atypical hemolytic uremic syndrome: from diagnosis to treatment. *Clin Chem Lab Med* 2015; 53: 1679.

Hovinger JAK, Heeb SR, Skowronska M, et al. Pathophysiology of thrombotic thrombocytopenic purpura and hemolytic uremic syndrome. *J Thromb Haemost* 2018; 16: 618.

Kaplan B, Drummond K. The hemolytic-uremic syndrome is a syndrome. *N Engl J Med* 1978; 298: 964.

Legendre CM, Licht C, Loirat C. Eculizumab in atypical hemolytic-uremic syndrome. *N Engl J Med* 2013; 369: 1379.

Remuzzi G. HUS and TTP: variable expression of a single entity. *Kidney Int* 1987; 32: 292.

Wehling C, Kirschfink M. Tailored eculizumab regimen for patients with atypical hemolytic uremic syndrome. *J Thromb Haemost* 2014; 12: 1437.

Wong CS, Jelacic S, Habeeb RL, et al. The risk of hemolytic-uremic syndrome after antibiotic treatment of *Escherichia coli* O157:H7 infection. *N Engl J Med* 2000; 342: 1930.

Zipfel P, Naumann HP, Jozsi M. Genetic screening of hemolytic uremic syndrome. *Curr Opin Nephrol Hypertens* 2003; 12: 653.

Haemophagocytic lymphohistiocytosis (HLH) *See*

- Haemophagocytic syndrome.

Haemophagocytic syndrome

Haemophagocytic syndrome is a severe inflammatory disorder characterized by dysregulated macrophages, which display uncontrolled phagocytosis of red blood cells, lymphocytes, platelets and their precursors throughout the reticuloendothelial system. It has also been referred to as **haemophagocytic lymphohistiocytosis** (HLH). It is distinct from malignant histiocytosis and represents an inappropriate and uncontrolled immune response to infection or some other serious disease, with consequently excessive cytokine release. Secondary HLH has also been referred to as **macrophage activation syndrome** (MAS).

Although some cases are familial, most are secondary to
- infection
  - usually viral (particularly due to a herpesvirus, e.g. Epstein–Barr virus – q.v.),
  - sometimes bacterial (occasionally tuberculosis – q.v.) or parasitic (especially histoplasmosis – q.v.),
- malignancy
  - usually lymphoma,
- autoimmune disease
  - usually a connective tissue disease (particularly systemic lupus erythematosus (SLE) – q.v., or Still's disease – q.v.).

Clinically, there is fever, splenomegaly (q.v.), and sometimes lymphadenopathy (q.v.) and even hepatomegaly.

> As multiorgan failure (q.v.) may develop in severe cases, the haemophagocytic syndrome should be remembered as one of the uncommon causes of this complication.

Diagnosis is confirmed by laboratory findings of cytopenias (particularly anaemia and thrombocytopenia) in peripheral blood and cell-laden macrophages in the bone marrow. The C-reactive protein, D-dimer and ferritin levels are increased. The very high serum levels of ferritin (>1000 μg/L and sometimes much higher) typically seen in HLH are due to increased macrophage iron stores, presumably because macrophage secretion is the primary source of serum ferritin (see Ferritin).

Treatment is primarily that of the underlying disorder and supportive care.

- *In severe cases, a combination of **corticosteroids** and the cytotoxic agent, **etoposide** (VP-16), has been found to be helpful.*
- ***Immunoglobulin** IV may be useful in infection-related cases.*
- ***Corticosteroids** and **immunomodulation** (q.v.) (ciclosporin, etanercept, infliximab, rituximab – q.v.) are indicated in cases related to connective tissue disease. The inerleukin 1 (IL-1) receptor antagonist, **anakinra**, has been reported to be helpful in refractory cases. The IL-6 receptor antagonist, **tocilizumab** (q.v.), has been recommended in critically ill patients where sepsis can be excluded.*
- *The only curative treatment for primary HLH is **allogeneic transplantation**.*

Bibliography

Athale J. Challenges in identifying hemophagocytic lymphohistiocytosis in the ICU. *Crit Care Med* 2020; 48: 599.

Creput C, Galicier L, Buyse S, et al. Understanding organ dysfunction in hemophagocytic lymphohistiocytosis. *Intens Care Med* 2008; 34: 1177.

Fisman DN. Hemophagocytic syndromes and infection. *Emerg Infect Dis* 2000; 6: 6.

Gauvin F, Toledano B, Champagne J, et al. Reactive hemophagocytic syndrome presenting as a component of multiple organ dysfunction syndrome. *Crit Care Med* 2000; 28: 3341.

Grom AA. Macrophage activation syndrome and reactive hemophagocytic lymphohistiocytosis: the same entities? *Curr Opin Rheumatol* 2003; 15: 587.

Janka GE. Hemophagocytic syndromes. *Blood Rev* 2007; 21: 245.

Lachmann G, Knaak C, Vorderwulbecke G, et al. Hyperferritinemia in critically ill patients. *Crit Care Med* 2020; 48: 459.

La Rosee P, Horne A, Hines M, et al. Recommendations for the management of hemophagocytic lymphohistiocytosis in adults. *Blood* 2019; 133: 2465.

Otrock ZK, Eby CS. Clinical characteristics, prognostic factors, and outcomes of adult patients with hemophagocytic lymphohistiocytosis. *Am J Hematol* 2015; 90: 220.

Ramos-Casals M, Brito-Zeron P, Lopez-Guillermo A, et al. Adult haemophagocytic syndrome. *Lancet* 2014; 383: 1503.

Haemophilia

Haemophilia (classical haemophilia or haemophilia A) is the best known of the hereditary haemorrhagic disorders, because although uncommon (1 in 5,000 males) its effects are striking. It is due to either a quantitative or qualitative defect of factor VIII: C, the gene for which is on the X chromosome. More than 500 mutations have been described in this gene, which was cloned in 1984. The disease is generally confined to hemizygotic males, and females are typically carriers. However, clinical haemophilia can sometimes occur in women due either to random X-linked inactivation called lyonization or to rare inheritance of an affected X chromosome from both parents.

Acquired haemophilia A (AHA) is a rare but potentially serious bleeding disorder. It is caused by the development of autoantibodies against factor VIII. Most cases are idiopathic, but it may occur in association with autoimmune diseases (q.v.), malignancy or pregnancy (q.v.).

Factor VIII is a large plasma protein of molecular weight 330 kDa, plasma concentration 100 mcg/L (100%) and half-life 10 hr. Unlike the other coagulation factors, it is nowadays understood to be produced in hepatic endothelial cells rather than in hepatocytes. Additional extrahepatic production must also be possible, because in the rare reported case in 2016 in the USA of a recipient of a liver transplanted from a haemophilia A donor, the recipient did not develop haemophilia and indeed maintained normal factor VIII levels.

Factor VIII acts as a coagulation cofactor rather than a zymogen and assists the activation of factor X to Xa. It does this via intrinsic Xase complex, which comprises factor IXa, factor VIIIa, Ca^{++} and platelet anionic membranes and which catalyzes the conversion of factor X to Xa. The active cofactor itself (VIIIa) is produced following limited cleavage of the inactive factor VIII by the small amount of thrombin already present.

The severity of disease is directly related to the plasma concentration, which ranges from virtually undetectable to about 50%. The severity of the disease was also compounded by complicating HIV and hepatitis C virus (HCV) infections until the 1990s when recombinant concentrates were introduced. An increased risk of fractures due to decreased bone density may also be seen in haemophilia.

*Treatment was traditionally with **factor VIII concentrates**, but recombinant factor VIII concentrates became available in 1992, with extended half-life factor concentrates (e.g. turoctocog) now an added bonus. The factor VIII level should be raised to 25–50% before invasive procedures. Replacement therapy is resource intensive. Paradoxically, the use of replacement therapy to prevent bleeding associated with major surgery confers a risk of postoperative venous thromboembolism that is similar to that in the general population after similar surgery.*

*Dramatic new treatment concepts include the use of a recombinant, humanized, bispecific antibody (**emicizumab**) which can bypass factor VIII by directly bridging activated factor IX with factor X. However, it has been reported to cause the occasional complication of thrombotic microangiopathy (q.v.).*

Avoidance of aspirin and administration of tranexamic acid (q.v.) or desmopressin (q.v.) are helpful in cases of active bleeding.

Activated factor VIIa was specifically introduced for the treatment of haemophiliac patients who had developed factor VIII inhibitors, though it is now becoming widely used in previously normal patients with severe refractory bleeding following trauma or surgery. Haemophilia patients with inhibitors may also be successfully treated with factor eight inhibitor bypassing activity (**FEIBA**).

Gene therapy has so far been challenging, unlike in haemophilia B (see below), because the factor VIII molecule is too large to fit conveniently inside the usual viral vector.

Acquired haemophilia is treated by control of bleeding, elimination of the responsible autoantibody and management of any underlying disorder if possible.

Haemophilia B (Christmas disease) is due to factor IX deficiency. Like haemophilia A, it is a congenital sex-linked recessive disorder. DNA studies have shown that the 'Royal Disease' of haemophilia affecting Queen Victoria's family and thus other members of the European aristocracy was in fact haemophilia B, which likely originated as a mutation in Queen Victoria's father.

It is due to any of hundreds of mostly recent mutations in the F9 gene, and it affects about 1 in

30,000 males. Factor IX is a plasma protein of molecular weight 56 kDa and plasma concentration 5 mg/L. It is a zymogen with a half-life of 25 hr.

The management principles are similar to those of **haemophilia**, *except that the concentration required for haemostasis is generally lower (usually 20% is adequate) and the smaller size of factor IX results in a larger distribution volume (being about the size of albumin space).* **Recombinant factor IX concentrate** *became available in 1997, and extended half-life agents were later introduced. Recently, trials of* **gene therapy** *using AAV (adeno-associated virus) vector technology have shown efficacy in elevating factor IX levels and reducing symptom severity for prolonged periods.*

Haemophilia C, the least common haemophilia, is due to factor XI deficiency. Like the other haemophilias, it is congenital, though it has an autosomal recessive inheritance. It is generally a mild disorder, often uncovered only when excessive bleeding is noted after surgery or trauma.

Factor XI is a plasma protein of molecular weight 160 kDa and plasma concentration 5 mcg/L. It is a zymogen with a half-life of 45 hr.

Treatment if necessary is with **fresh frozen plasma**.

Parahaemophilia is a term sometimes given to the rare inherited condition of factor V deficiency. Factors V and VIII are homologous proteins, thought to have descended from a common ancestral protein via gene duplication. They are the two labile clotting factors, which disappear rapidly when blood is stored, so that their clinical replenishment requires the administration of fresh frozen plasma.

Like factor VIII, factor V is a cofactor, but it acts at the following step in the coagulation pathway. Thus it acts via prothrombinase, which comprises factor Xa, factor Va, Ca^{++} and platelet anionic membranes and which catalyzes the conversion of prothrombin to thrombin. The active cofactor itself (Va) is produced following limited cleavage of the inactive factor V by the small amount of thrombin already present.

Factor V is a plasma protein of molecular weight 330 kDa, plasma concentration 10 mcg/L and half-life 15 hr. It is not a zymogen, but like factor VIII it circulates as a pro-cofactor.

Unlike the other haemophilias, factor V deficiency can paradoxically cause a thrombotic as well as a haemorrhagic state, since factor V is required not only for coagulation (as described above) but also for the anticoagulant action of protein C (q.v.).

See also
- Coagulation disorders.

Bibliography

Aledort LM. Economic aspects of haemophilia care in the United States. *Haemophilia* 1999: 5: 282.

Arruda VR. The search for the origin of factor VIII synthesis and its impact on therapeutic strategies for haemophilia A. *Haematologica* 2015; 100: 849.

Berntorp E, ed. Modern management of haemophilia A to prevent bleeding and arthropathy. *Semin Thromb Hemost* 2003; 29: 1.

Bloom AL. Progress in the clinical management of haemophilia. *Thromb Haemost* 1991; 66: 166.

Chuah MK, Collen D, Van den Driessche T. Gene therapy for hemophilia. *J Gene Med* 2001; 3: 3.

Fay PJ. Activation of factor VIII and mechanism of cofactor action. *Blood Rev* 2004; 18: 1.

Franchini M, Mannucci PM. Acquired haemophilia A: a 2013 update. *Thromb Haemost* 2013; 110: 1087.

Furie B, Furie BC. Molecular basis of hemophilia. *Semin Hematol* 1990; 27: 270.

Gitschier J, Wood WI, Goralka TM, et al. Characterization of the human factor VIII gene. *Nature* 1984; 312: 326.

Green P. The 'Royal Disease'. *J Thromb Haemost* 2010; 8: 2214.

Hoyer LW. Haemophilia A. *N Engl J Med* 1994; 330: 38.

Klinge J, Ananyeva NM, Hauser CAE, et al. Hemophilia A – from basic science to clinical practice. *Semin Thromb Hemost* 2002; 28: 309.

Mann KG, Kalafatis M. Factor V: a combination of Dr Jekyll and Mr Hyde. *Blood* 2002 101: 20.

Mannucci PM. Hemophilia: treatment options in the twenty-first century. *J Thromb Haemost* 2003; 1: 1349.

Mannucci PM, Tuddenham EGD. The hemophiliac – from royal genes to gene therapy. *N Engl J Med* 2001; 344: 1773.

Oldenburg J, Schwaab R. Molecular biology of blood coagulation. *Semin Thromb Hemost* 2001; 27: 313.

Sommer SS, Scaringe WA, Hill KA. Human germline mutation in the factor IX gene. *Mutat Res* 2001; 487: 1.

Srivastava AWFH, Santagostino E, Dougall A, et al. Guidelines for the management of haemophilia. *Haemophilia* 2020; 26: 1.

Haemoptysis

Haemoptysis, or the expectoration of blood, should always be regarded as potentially serious.

Haemoptysis may range from minor blood-streaking of the sputum to the expectoration of large amounts of frank blood. Most haemoptysis is minor, but even relatively small amounts of blood can be quite startling when mixed with expectorated sputum. On the other hand, an amount of blood of only 150 mL can fill the entire conducting airway system and thus cause significant clinical problems which would not be seen if such a volume arose from bleeding at most other sites. Thus, if death occurs from haemoptysis, it is from respiratory failure and not from haemorrhagic shock. In fact, massive haemoptysis is uncommon. It can be defined as more than 200 mL per day, but factors more relevant to outcome include ability to clear the airway, speed of bleeding, underlying respiratory reserve and access to emergency care.

The source of expectorated blood is not always clear from the history. Blood from the mouth, nose or throat, or the upper gastrointestinal tract, may well into the throat and then be coughed up. Patients, and even clinicians, may also have difficulty sometimes in distinguishing between haemoptysis and haematemesis.

Some degree of haemoptysis is common with many acute respiratory infections, though most causes of more than minor haemoptysis are serious chronic diseases, such as carcinoma, tuberculosis (q.v.), bronchiectasis (q.v.) and severe left heart failure (classically in the past due to mitral stenosis).

Although the cause may be apparent from the clinical features and/or chest X-ray, bronchoscopy is usually required to clarify the diagnosis. However, even after extensive investigation, some episodes of haemoptysis are not satisfactorily explained.

The chief causes of haemoptysis are (in approximate order of frequency)
1. acute chest infection, i.e. bronchitis, pneumonia,
2. carcinoma or rarely bronchial adenoma (see Lung tumours),
3. chronic bronchitis,
4. pulmonary infarction,
5. acute pulmonary oedema, i.e. left heart failure (q.v.),
6. foreign body,
7. bronchiectasis (q.v.) or lung abscess (see Cavitation),
8. tuberculosis (q.v.),
9. systemic bleeding disorder (see Haemostasis),
10. drug reaction (see Drugs and the lung),
11. Goodpasture's syndrome (q.v.),
12. Wegener's granulomatosis (q.v.),
13. lymphomatoid granulomatosis (see Wegener's granulomatosis).

Haemoptysis may also be occasionally iatrogenic, such as after transbronchial lung biopsy, insertion of a chest tube, overinflation of a balloon-tipped pulmonary artery catheter or other invasive pulmonary procedure.

Treatment is primarily that of the underlying condition. In all cases, a patent airway must be ensured. A skilled respiratory team is required to manage patients with life-threatening haemoptysis.

*In refractory cases, **bronchial artery embolization, endobronchial tamponade** or even **surgery** may be indicated if the responsible lesion can be localized.*

Bibliography
Andrejak C, Parrot A, Bazelly B, et al. Surgical lung resection for severe hemoptysis. *Ann Thorac Surg* 2009; 88: 1556.
Bobrowitz ID, Ramakrishna S, Shim Y-S. Comparison of medical v surgical treatment of major hemoptysis. *Arch Intern Med* 1983; 143: 1343.
Davidson K, Shojaee S. Managing massive haemoptysis. *Chest* 2020; 157: 77.
Jean-Baptiste E. Clinical assessment and management of massive hemoptysis. *Crit Care Med* 2000; 28: 1642.
Ong T-H, Eng P. Massive hemoptysis requiring intensive care. *Intens Care Med* 2003; 29: 317.
Remy J, Arnaud A, Fardou H, et al. Treatment of hemoptysis by embolization of bronchial arteries. *Radiology* 1977; 122: 33.
Swanson KL, Johnson CM, Prakash UB, et al. Bronchial artery embolization. *Chest* 2002; 121: 789.
Valipour A, Kreuzer A, Koller H, et al. Bronchoscopy-guided topical hemostatic tamponade therapy for the management of life-threatening hemoptysis. *Chest* 2005; 127: 2113.

Haemostasis

Disorders of **haemostasis** (i.e. bleeding disorders) comprise five groups of conditions. These are

1. coagulation disorders (q.v.),
2. thrombocytopenia (q.v.),
3. platelet function disorders (q.v.),
4. abnormally enhanced fibrinolysis (q.v.),
5. vascular fragility (see Purpura).

Disorders of haemostasis (and thrombosis) have been at the forefront of discoveries in **genomic science** since the genes for factor VIII, factor IX and vWF were among the first to be characterized and cloned in the 1980s. Molecular genetic testing and recombinant clotting factors then followed. Currently, there is a list of 91 tier 1 genes which may be inherited as germline mutations, of which 21 result in coagulation factor deficiencies and 61 in platelet abnormalities (with the remaining

9 resulting in thrombotic disorders). In addition, many hundreds of diagnostic grade tier 2 or 3 genes have possible linkages with bleeding or thrombosis, but these relationships are yet to be supported by the requisite robustness of epidemiological and laboratory evidence. These scientific advances have many obvious benefits, including assistance with therapeutic decision-making, disease prognosis and family counselling.

While the cause of a **major bleeding disorder** is either well known previously (e.g. haemophilia) or is readily identifiable at the time of clinical encounter, **mild bleeding disorders** are both more common and more challenging to elucidate. The mild bleeding disorders are manifest clinically by mucocutaneous bleeding or by seemingly excessive postoperative or post-traumatic bleeding in a patient with no previously recognized bleeding tendency. Although the most common identifiable causes of mild bleeding disorders are von Willebrand's disease, platelet function disorders, coagulation factor deficiencies or various combinations of these conditions, laboratory confirmation of a particular disorder can be challenging, and indeed most cases remain undiagnosed (and are probably multifactorial).

Bibliography
Boender J, Kruip MJ, Leebeek FW. A diagnostic approach to mild bleeding disorders. *J Thromb Haemost* 2016; 14: 1507.
Mezzano D, Quiroga T. Diagnostic challenges of inherited mild bleeding disorders: a bait for poorly explored clinical and basic research. *J Thromb Haemost* 2019; 17: 257.

Hamman–Rich syndrome See
- Interstitial pneumonia.

Hand–Schuller–Christian disease See
- Histiocytosis.

Hantavirus

In 1993, a small epidemic of unusual cases of severe acute respiratory failure was reported in the Southwestern USA. Within a month, the causative agent had been identified on serological and genetic evidence as a hitherto unrecognized species of **hantavirus** (Sin Nombre virus), transmitted to humans via contact with infected deer mice and without human-to-human passage. Within 8 months, 48 cases in that area had been confirmed, with a mortality of about one third even in young previously healthy patients, and the geographic distribution of cases had begun to widen. Hantavirus had previously only been known as a rodent-borne cause of haemorrhagic fever with renal failure in the Eastern Hemisphere.

Clinical features commence with the features of a non-specific viral illness, after a probable incubation period of 9–33 days. There is fever, malaise, headache, myalgia and gastrointestinal disturbance. It then progresses to an acute respiratory distress syndrome (q.v.), with acute pulmonary oedema due to increased capillary permeability – the hantavirus pulmonary syndrome (HPS). There is associated septic shock, lactic acidosis (q.v.) and thrombocytopenia (q.v.). During recovery, there is a diuretic phase, followed generally by prolonged convalescence.

*Treatment with **mechanical ventilation** appears to be required in about half the cases, together with haemodynamic monitoring and inotropic support.*

The putative antihantavirus drug, ribavirin, is not effective in HPS.

Bibliography
Duchin JS, Koster FT, Peters CJ, et al. Hantaviral pulmonary syndrome: clinical description of disease caused by a newly recognized hemorrhagic fever virus in the Southwestern United States. *N Engl J Med* 1994; 330: 949.
Hallin GW, Simpson SQ, Crowell RE, et al. Cardiopulmonary manifestations of hantavirus pulmonary syndrome. *Crit Care Med* 1996; 24: 252.
Hughes JM, Peters CJ, Cohen ML, et al. Hantavirus pulmonary syndrome: an emerging infectious disease. *Science* 1993; 262: 850.
Khan AS, Young JC. Hantavirus pulmonary syndrome: at the crossroads. *Curr Opin Infect Dis* 2001; 14: 205.
Schmaljohn C, Hjelle B. Hantaviruses: a global disease problem. *Emerg Infect Dis* 1997; 3: 2.
Shope RE. A midcourse assessment of hantavirus pulmonary syndrome. *Emerg Infect Dis* 1999; 5: 1.

Heat

Heat injury results from adverse environmental exposure (see Environment). It occurs if the body's thermoregulatory processes are overwhelmed.
- This occurs particularly in association with a high environmental temperature.
- It is aggravated by direct sunlight and high humidity.
- Increased risk occurs with
  - exercise,
  - dehydration,
  - old age,
  - excess clothing,
  - some drugs, such as phenothiazines and anticholinergics.

The heat-related issues discussed in this book are
- Heat cramps,
- Heat exhaustion/stress,
- Heat rash,
- Heat shock proteins,
- Heat stroke,
- Hot tubs,
- Hyperthermia.
  See also
- Pyrexia.

Bibliography
Lugo-Amador NM, Rothenhaus T, Moyer P. Heat-related illness. *Emerg Med Clin North Am* 2004; 22: 315.
Marr JJ, Geiss PT. Management of heat injury syndromes. In: Shoemaker WC, Thompson WL, eds. *Critical Care: State of the Art*. Fullerton: Society of Critical Care Medicine. 1982; p K1.

Heat cramps

Heat cramps are painful muscular spasms, which can occur even in the presence of a normal body temperature.

They may be prevented with adequate hydration and are treated with massage and stretching.

Heat exhaustion/stress

Heat exhaustion (or heat stress) is a more severe form of heat injury than heat cramps. It is associated with a moderate increase in body temperature up to 40°C.

There is fatigue, headache, nausea, thirst, cramps, irritability and hyperventilation. Dehydration and postural hypotension occur, and the patient, though sweating freely, feels cold, often with associated piloerection.

Treatment consists of **rest** *in a cool and preferably dry environment, with* **hydration** *and external* **cooling**.

Heat rash

Heat rash is due to occlusion of sweat ducts, which gives rise to
- small, clear, asymptomatic vesicles (miliaria crystallina) on exposed skin,
- red, pruritic vesicles (miliaria rubra) on covered skin,
- friction blisters at sites of pressure.

Heat shock proteins

Since adverse environmental exposure may jeopardize the survival of any living organism by producing the major acute changes referred to as stress, a common pattern of defence is set in train, resulting in multiple structural and functional changes in the organism. This stress response is often referred to as the heat shock response, because the original and best studied stressor was hyperthermia. This response is associated with the rapid elaboration of a set of proteins, called **heat shock proteins** (HSPs), and a decrease in other cellular proteins. This response is rapid and reversible and is geared to protecting the essential cellular machinery from irreversible injury, thus promoting both survival during the stress and rapid recovery thereafter.

HSPs are members of a larger family of intracellular proteins which maintain the integrity of the cell's structure and are sometimes referred to as 'molecular chaperones'. HSPs are important in regulating protein homeostasis, including multi-protein complexes, and client proteins that are protected include kinases, integrins, transcription factors and toll-like receptors.

HSPs are classified as either large (68–100 kDa) or small (15–30 kDa). Hsp90, Hsp70 and Hsp40 are the most studied members of the stress protein family. HSPs are synthesized not only typically after a brief increase in temperature of 3–5°C, but also after other insults such as hypoxia, hypoglycaemia, infection and acute chemical exposure. They have been identified in all major cell structures and are also present at low levels in unstressed cells, so that they thus have a background function, probably in maintaining membrane integrity.

Following the cloning of the first gene in 1978, all have now been cloned. Extensive amino acid homology has been found, even between humans and bacteria, even though these two species diverged more than 1.5 billion years ago. The response is thus presumed to be of great antiquity. HSPs appear to bind to denatured elements and thus prevent their aggregation and resultant cell damage. In general, the process is protective, because there is a correlation between HSP induction on mild stress and the development of tolerance to thermal or other stress.

The development of HSPs may have relevance in fever (q.v.) and/or sepsis. Thus, the failure to mount a fever is associated with an increased mortality in infections, although any benefit of fever itself has not been demonstrated. In addition, thermal pretreatment (and probably also post-treatment) has been shown to protect experimentally against pulmonary and neurological damage and consequent mortality in sepsis.

On the other hand, HSPs may also provide a mechanism for the induction of autoimmunity (q.v.) via molecular mimicry and for cancer migration and metastasis. Thus, targeting HSPs by the use of specific HSP inhibitors has also become an important research field in a number of pathological conditions.

Bibliography
Bruemmer-Smith S, Stuber F, Schroeder S. Protective functions of intracellular heat-shock protein (HSP)

70-expression in patients with severe sepsis. *Intens Care Med* 2001; 27: 1835.

Buchman TG. Manipulation of stress gene expression: a novel therapy for the treatment of sepsis? *Crit Care Med* 1994; 22: 901.

Chu EK, Ribeiro SP, Slutsky AS. Heat stress increases survival rates in polysaccharide-stimulated rats. *Crit Care Med* 1997; 25: 1727.

Delogu G, Bosco LL, Marandola M, et al. Heat shock protein (HSP70) expression in septic patients. *J Crit Care* 1997; 12: 188.

Lindquist S. The heat shock response. *Annu Rev Biochem* 1986; 55: 1151.

Schopf FH, Biebl MM, Buchner J. The HSP90 machinery. *Nat Rev Mol Cell Biol* 2017; 18: 345.

Trepel J, Mollapour M, Giaccone G, et al. Targeting the dynamic HSP90 complex in cancer. *Nat Rev Cancer* 2010; 10: 537.

van Eden W, ed. *Heat shock proteins and inflammation.* Basel: Birkhauser. 2003.

van Eden W, Young DB, eds. *Stress Proteins in Medicine.* New York: Dekker. 1996.

Villar J, Ribeiro SP, Mullen JBM, et al. Induction of the heat shock response reduces mortality rate and organ damage in a sepsis induced acute lung injury model. *Crit Care Med* 1994; 22: 914.

Heat stroke

Heat stroke (heatstroke) is the most severe form of heat injury and is a dangerous complication. It is diagnosed on the basis of core temperature >40°C and hot but dry skin.

It is seen in both epidemics and sporadically in individuals.

- Epidemics occur during heat waves in urban areas, especially among the elderly, debilitated or alcoholic populations, even if sedentary.
- Individual cases occur in hot environments, either in association with strenuous physical exercise, as in athletes or new military recruits, or in confined areas, such as prisons, military barracks or pilgrim crowds.

Apart from a high environmental temperature often without direct sunlight, the risk increases

- with drug administration (anticholinergics, phenothiazines, tricyclic antidepressants, monoamine oxidase inhibitors, beta blockers, diuretics),
- with impairment of the body's ability to dissipate heat (as in a humid environment or with dehydration, cardiac failure or inability to sweat).

Heat stroke has a variable onset. It may develop over many hours in the elderly or sick exposed to increased environmental temperatures. In the young and healthy who exercise heavily in high ambient temperatures, the onset is sudden. There is a rise in body temperature, usually to at least 41°C and typically with the cessation of sweating, so that the skin appears flushed and dry. The upper temperature limit for survival is generally about 44°C. Heat stroke represents a major failure of thermoregulation, though the mechanism of damage is more than direct thermal injury and probably includes the elaboration of mediators such as nitric oxide.

- **Neurological dysfunction** occurs with delirium (q.v.), coma, fits and decerebrate posture.
- **Circulatory failure** is seen, with marked tachycardia and eventually the abrupt onset of hypotension, pulmonary oedema (especially in the elderly) and shock.
- **Dehydration** and **hypovolaemia** are usual.
- **Associated features** include
  - hyperventilation,
  - hypokalaemia,
  - metabolic acidosis (q.v.), which may be severe,
  - haemoconcentration,
  - leukocytosis,
  - disseminated intravascular coagulation (q.v.),
  - hypophosphataemia (q.v.),
  - renal failure, with proteinuria and microscopic haematuria and possibly subsequent acute kidney injury (AKI, acute tubular necrosis),
  - hepatocellular damage of varying severity,
  - rhabdomyolysis (q.v.),
  - vomiting and diarrhoea (q.v.).

There is thus widespread cellular damage and the presence of a medical emergency.

*Treatment consists of urgent **active cooling** to 39°C within 30 min. Cooling should then be tapered to prevent an overshoot in the process. Effective external cooling may be achieved by the use of either ice-packs or a cooling blanket. Internal cooling techniques include cold IV fluids, cold stomach or bladder lavage, and extracorporeal devices.*

Requisite supportive therapy includes fluids, electrolytes, circulatory and respiratory support, and attention to any metabolic, haematological and renal dysfunction.

The value of heparin is unsubstantiated, and the efficacy of dantrolene has not been confirmed in clinical trials. Antipyretics are of little value in this setting.

The condition has a high mortality (with reports from 10% to 80%), but it is preventable by avoiding the risk factors referred to above and by the provision of appropriate first-aid. In established heat stroke, even prompt Intensive Care may not prevent death. Important complications in survivors include acute renal failure and neurological damage.

A similar condition occurring after exposure to triggering agents (classically during general anaesthesia) is referred to as **malignant hyperthermia** (q.v.).

Bibliography
Bouchama A, al-Sedairy S, Siddiqui S, et al. Elevated pyrogenic cytokines in heat stroke. *Chest* 1993; 104: 1498.
Bouchama A, Cafege A, Devol EB, et al. Ineffectiveness of dantrolene sodium in the treatment of heatstroke. *Crit Care Med* 1991; 19: 176.
Bouchama A, Knochel JP. Heat stroke. *N Engl J Med* 2002; 346: 1978.
Clowes GHA, O'Donnell TF. Heat stroke. *N Engl J Med* 1974; 291: 564.
Costrini A. Emergency treatment of exertional heatstroke and comparison of whole body cooling techniques. *Med Sci Sports Exerc* 1990; 22: 15.
Knochel JP. Heat stroke and related heat stress disorders. *Dis Mon* 1989; 35: 301.
Lugo-Amador NM, Rothenhaus T, Moyer P. Heat-related illness. *Emerg Med Clin North Am* 2004; 22: 315.
Marr JJ, Geiss PT. Management of heat injury syndromes. In: Shoemaker WC, Thompson WL, eds. *Critical Care: State of the Art*. Fullerton: Society of Critical Care Medicine. 1982; p K1.
Pease S, Bouadma L, Kermarrec N, et al. Early organ dysfunction course, cooling time and outcome in classic heatstroke. *Intens Care Med* 2009; 35: 1454.
Simon HB. Hyperthermia. *N Engl J Med* 1993; 329: 483.

Heavy chains *See*
- Multiple myeloma.

Heavy metal poisoning *See*
- Chelating agents.
  See
- Arsenic,
- Cadmium,
- Iron,
- Lead,
- Mercury.
  See also
- Fanconi's syndrome,
- Neuropathy,
- Pigmentation disorders.

HELLP syndrome

The **HELLP syndrome** comprises h̲aemolysis, e̲levated l̲iver enzymes and l̲ow p̲latelet count. It is a pregnancy-related disease of unknown aetiology, first described in 1982 as a separate subgroup of pre-eclampsia (q.v.). It has been reported to occur in 2–12% of cases of pre-eclampsia, usually in the more severe cases. It usually occurs in the third trimester, though 30% of patients present within the first 48 hr of the post-partum period. In these cases, many have had no evidence of pre-eclampsia prior to delivery.

The clinical features include upper abdominal pain and malaise in virtually all patients. Weight gain, oedema and hypertension are commonly present, but these are not necessarily diagnostic for pre-eclampsia at the time.

A severe illness can follow, with associated
- shock,
- acute respiratory distress syndrome (ARDS) (q.v.),
- acute renal failure,
- ascites and pleural effusions,
- subcapsular haematoma of the liver, which may even lead to hepatic rupture,
- generalized haemorrhage,
- convulsions,
- blindness due to retinal detachment,
- placental abruption (abruptio placentae) (q.v.), especially if there is acute renal failure,
- disseminated intravascular coagulation (q.v.).

These complications occur in 1–15% of cases, and they are more frequent in the post-partum state (except of course for placental abruption).

There is a microangiopathic haemolysis (q.v.) with thrombocytopenia (q.v.) but no laboratory evidence initially of disseminated intravascular coagulation (q.v.), though this eventually occurs in about 20% of cases. The liver function tests are abnormal.

The differential diagnosis includes
- acute fatty liver of pregnancy (q.v.),
- other causes of thrombotic microangiopathy (q.v.), e.g. thrombotic thrombocytopenic purpura (TTP), haemolytic–uraemic syndrome (HUS), severe antiphospholipid syndrome (CAPS), malignancy,
- mild and asymptomatic gestational thrombocytopenia, seen in 5–8% of normal pregnancies.

HELLP may not always be distinguishable from some of the other thrombotic microangiopathies, especially HUS and APS.

*Treatment is with **emergency delivery**, usually by Caesarean section, and Intensive Care management.*
- *The liver should be treated as for **hepatic trauma**, with great care with palpation, etc. Difficult hepatic bleeding*

may require hepatic artery embolization. Laparotomy is sometimes indicated if there appears to be an acute abdominal crisis.
- **Plasmapheresis** (q.v.) should be considered for persistent haematological abnormality.

The condition clearly confers added maternal and fetal risk.

See also
- Pre-eclampsia.

Bibliography

Burrows RF, Kelton JG. Thrombocytopenia at delivery: a prospective survey of 6715 deliveries. *Am J Obstet Gynecol* 1990; 162: 731.

Jayawardena L, Mcnamara E. Diagnosis and management of pregnancies complicated by haemolysis, elevated liver enzymes and low platelets syndrome in the tertiary setting. *Intern Med J* 2020; 50: 342.

Martin JN, Files FC, Blake PG. Plasma exchange for preeclampsia: I. Postpartum use for persistently severe preeclampsia with HELLP syndrome. *Am J Obstet Gynecol* 1990; 162: 126.

Pousti TJ, Tominaga GT, Scannell G. Help for the HELLP syndrome. *Intens Care World* 1994; 11: 62.

Sibai B. Diagnosis, controversies, and management of the syndrome of hemolysis, elevated liver enzymes, and low platelet count. *Obstet Gynecol* 2004; 103: 981.

Sibai BM, Ramadan MK, Usta I, et al. Maternal morbidity and mortality in 442 pregnancies with hemolysis, elevated liver enzymes and low platelets (HELLP syndrome). *Am J Obstet Gynecol* 1993; 169: 1000.

Van Dam PA, Renier M, Baekelandt M, et al. Disseminated intravascular coagulation and the syndrome of hemolysis, elevated liver enzymes, and low platelets in severe preeclampsia. *Obstet Gynecol* 1989; 73: 97.

Weinstein L. Syndrome of hemolysis, elevated liver enzymes and low platelet count: a severe consequence of hypertension. *Am J Obstet Gynecol* 1982; 142: 159.

Helminths

Helminths are multicellular organisms with complex extra-human life-cycles. Many have the ability to cause **parasitic infections** in humans. These include
- cestodes (tapeworms),
  - those important in human disease include *Echinococcus* (q.v.),
  - see also Megaloblastic anaemia – vitamin B_{12} deficiency,
- nematodes (roundworms),
  - those important in human disease include *Ascaris*; *Ancylostoma* and *Necator* (hookworms); *Strongyloides* (roundworms); *Toxocara* (dog roundworms); *Trichinella*; *Wuchereria* (milcrofilaria),
  - see also Eosinophilia and lung infiltration – Loeffler's syndrome and tropical pulmonary eosinophilia,
- trematodes (flatworms or flukes),
  - those important in human disease include *Paragonimus* (see Paragonimiasis) and *Schistosoma* (see Schistosomiasis).

See also
- Parasitic infections.

Bibliography

Khemasuwan D, Farver CF, Mehta AC. Parasites of the airways. *Chest* 2014; 145: 883.

Van Voorhis WC. Helminthic infections. In: *Scientific American Medicine. Infectious Diseases*. Hamilton: Dekker Medicine. 2020.

Hemianopia

Hemianopia refers to loss of half of a visual field. The particular half affected depends on the site of the lesion which has interrupted the optic tract or radiation.

Hemianopia may be caused by
- cerebral tumour (including pituitary tumours),
- stroke (both haemorrhagic and ischaemic),
- cerebral abscess (parietal, subdural),
- meningitis,
- superior sagittal sinus thrombosis,
- migraine (occasionally).

Bibliography

Morantz RA, Walsh JW, eds. *Brain Tumors*. New York: Marcel Dekker. 1994.

Hendra virus

Hendra virus (HeV) is endemic in flying foxes (bats) in Eastern Australia. When originally identified in 1994, it was referred to as **equine morbilliform virus**. It was then named Hendra virus after the Brisbane suburb where the first affected stables were located, adjacent to the city's two main horse-racing tracks. It is related to the Nipah virus found throughout South-East Asia. Although the virus does not cause apparent illness in flying foxes, it can cause serious disease when transmitted to humans via an infected intermediate host, e.g. horses which have ingested feed or water contaminated by bat excreta. It is thus a zoonosis (q.v.).

Infected humans have had close equine rather than bat contact, and there has been no human-to-human transmission, as infectivity appears to be low. The incubation period is 1–3 weeks. Although only a few cases of clinical disease have been reported, with pneumonia or meningitis/encephalitis, the mortality has been over 50%.

Diagnosis is serological.

There is no specific treatment, although a monoclonal antibody has been tried for postexposure prophylaxis.

The development of a vaccine for horses, the intermediate host, was completed in 2015 and is expected to forestall future human outbreaks.

See
- Zoonoses.

Bibliography
Young JR, Selvey CE, Symons R. Hendra virus. *Med J Aust* 2011; 195: 250.

Henoch–Schonlein purpura

Henoch–Schonlein (or Schonlein–Henoch) **purpura** (HSP) is also commonly referred to as **immunoglobulin A vasculitis**. It typically affects small vessels and may be triggered by a respiratory infection, following which cross-reactivity in the immune system leads to large immune complexes that deposit in endothelial cells. It affects children much more commonly than adults.

The clinical features are palpable purpuric rash, haematuria (q.v.), arthritis (q.v.) and abdominal pain. The diagnosis is clinical, but skin biopsy may be required to separate the differential diagnoses. Renal function should be assessed, and blood examination excludes thrombocytopenia as a cause of the purpura.

Treatment is supportive, and corticosteroids are no longer routinely recommended. Immunomodulation (q.v.) may be indicated if renal dysfunction occurs.

The disease is self-limited and generally subsides within 1 month, although later recurrence may commonly be seen, and renal function should be followed up.

See
- Purpura,
- Vasculitis.

Bibliography
Cameron JS. Henoch-Schonlein purpura: clinical presentation. *Contrib Nephrol* 1984; 40: 246.
Hetland LE, Susrud KS, Lindahl KH, et al. Henoch-Schonlein purpura: a literature review. *Acta Derm Venereol* 2017; 97: 1160.
Saulsbury FT. Henoch-Schonlein purpura. *Curr Opin Rheumatol* 2010; 22: 598.
Szer I. Henoch-Schonlein purpura: when and how to treat. *J Rheumatol* 1996; 23: 1661.

Heparin(s)

Heparin is one of the most commonly used drugs in clinical medicine. Standard, unfractionated heparin (UFH) and the newer members of the heparin family (particularly the **low molecular weight heparins**, LMWHs) are the most widely used **anticoagulants** (q.v.), both for prevention and treatment of a wide range of thromboembolic conditions. Their most important complication is bleeding.

An uncommon but important and nowadays well recognized complication is **heparin-induced thrombocytopenia** (HIT) (q.v.).

More uncommon complications of heparin therapy include
- **osteoporosis**
  - associated with prolonged use,
- **hyperkalaemia**
  - due to hypoaldosteronism and usually in the presence of renal failure and/or diabetes,
- **skin necrosis** (q.v.)
  - though this is more commonly seen after warfarin (q.v.), when it occurs in patients with protein C deficiency (see Protein C),
  - see also Heparin-induced thrombocytopenia,
- **increased liver enzymes**
  - transaminitis, with levels that though increased are still usually in the normal range, reach a peak after 1 week and then decrease despite continuing therapy,
- **interaction with intravenous glyceryl trinitrate** (nitroglycerin, GTN)
  - with consequent resistance to heparin.

Although heparin was originally identified and later used because of its anticoagulant properties, there has been recognition of its pleotropic properties, doubtless related to its complex molecular structure. Thus, the various heparin preparations also appear to have anti-inflammatory effects, which may contribute not only to their efficacy in thromboembolism but also to potential utility in sepsis, malignancy and autoimmune disorders (q.v.) (see Coagulation disorders).

Bibliography
Hemker HC. A century of heparin: past, present and future. *J Thromb Haemost* 2016; 14: 2329.
Hirsh J, Bauer KA, Donati MB, et al. Parenteral anticoagulants. *Chest* 2008; 133 (suppl.): 141S.
Hirsh J, Levine MN. Low molecular weight heparin. *Blood* 1992; 79: 1.

Oster JR, Singer I, Fishman LM. Heparin-induced aldosterone suppression and hyperkalaemia. *Am J Med* 1995; 98: 575.

Poteruche TJ, Libby P, Goldhaber SZ. More than an anticoagulant: do heparins have direct anti-inflammatory effects. *Thromb Haemost* 2017; 117: 437.

Schindewolf M, Kroll H, Ackermann H, et al. Heparin-induced non-necrotizing skin lesions: rarely associated with heparin-induced thrombocytopenia. *J Thromb Haemost* 2010; 8: 1486.

Thachil J. The versatile heparin in COVID-19. *J Thromb Haemost* 2020; 18: 1020.

Weitz JI, Hirsh J, Samama MM. New antithrombotic drugs. *Chest* 2008; 133 (suppl.): 234S.

Heparin-induced thrombocytopenia

Heparin-induced thrombocytopenia has become recognized as the most common cause of drug-associated thrombocytopenia. It may take one of two forms, sometimes referred to as
- Type I, which is mild, early, non-immune and very common, and
- Type II, which is severe, delayed, immune and less common.

Type I
Mild thrombocytopenia occurs in up to 30% of patients given heparin and is sometimes referred to as **heparin associated thrombocytopenia** (HAT). It is less common after porcine heparin than after bovine heparin.

It becomes apparent shortly after the commencement of unfractionated heparin and is probably non-immune. It may occur even with small doses of heparin.

It is asymptomatic and self-limited, even if heparin is continued.

No treatment or even cessation of heparin is required.

Type II
A more severe form of thrombocytopenia, called **heparin-induced thrombocytopenia** (HIT, or formerly, heparin-induced thrombocytopenia syndrome, HITS, or heparin-induced thrombocytopenia and thrombosis syndrome, HITTS), is less commonly seen. Although first described over 40 years ago, it is only in subsequent years that its mechanism, diagnosis and treatment have been clarified in detail.

Clearly, HIT is a paradox, in that it is a thrombotic complication of an antithrombotic agent. More specifically, the thrombocytopenia represents a prothrombotic state rather than a haemorrhagic one, an anomaly perhaps reminiscent of the thrombotic propensity in the antiphospholipid syndrome despite the presence of a prolonged activated partial thromboplastin time (APTT). On the other hand, patients with HIT are not protected from major bleeding if the platelet count is sufficiently low (e.g. $<25 \times 10^9$/L)

The traditional prevalence of HIT was 0.5–5% of those given heparin, depending on the patient population and the origin of the heparin given, but this has been reduced by about 90% since the replacement of unfractionated heparin by low molecular weight heparins became widespread. Nowadays, HIT is responsible for only about 1% of the cases of thrombocytopenia seen in Intensive Care practice.

HIT is associated with a heparin-dependent IgG antiplatelet antibody. The antigen recognized is a complex of heparin's glycosaminoglycans (which are negatively charged) and platelet factor 4 (PF-4, a positively charged protein released from the platelet's α granule and capable of binding to heparin). Antibody binding to this complex, which has attached to the platelet's surface Fc receptor, causes platelet activation and procoagulant release and subsequent platelet removal from the circulation. There may also be endothelial cell damage, because heparin and heparin-like material are bound to the endothelial cell surface.

A number of aspects of this process remain mysterious. Thus, since the protein moiety in the antigen is PF-4, the antibody is therefore autoimmune. However, the antibody is transient, having generally disappeared within 3 months. Moreover, there is no anamnestic response in patients inadvertently challenged during this time, and after about 1 year there is no increased incidence of HIT in patients with a previous history of HIT re-exposed to heparin. Since HIT typically occurs in patients not previously exposed to heparin and too early for an IgG response to a new antigen, it follows that some natural antibodies must already be present. It is likely that these have been produced from prior bacterial exposure, since PF4 also binds to bacteria. The platelet/bacterial interaction produces antibodies not just to the original bacteria but also to other bacteria as well. This process enhances bacterial phagocytosis and is part of the body's innate immunity. Thus, HIT appears to be a misdirected immune response, where platelets are mistaken for bacteria when heparin is given.

Further complexity arises from the recent discovery that some patients with seemingly typical HIT based on clinical and laboratory criteria may have autoimmune antibodies that can activate platelets even in the absence of heparin. This condition, referred to as **aHIT**, may explain certain unusual and generally rare syndromes, such as

- spontaneous HIT (i.e. in the absence of heparin exposure),
- delayed or persistent HIT,
- very severe HIT (i.e. with associated DIC – q.v.),
- HIT induced by heparin flush, and
- HIT associated with fondaparinux.

Of those patients (about 15%) who develop antibodies as shown by sophisticated immunoassay, only about half have evidence of platelet activation as shown by functional assays, and less than half of these in turn develop thrombocytopenia, which is usually moderate with an average platelet count of about 60×10^9/L. Most thrombocytopenia is asymptomatic, but if the patient is untreated thrombosis develops in 10% within 2 days and in 50% within 30 days.

The clinical manifestations of HIT typically occur between 5 and 10 days after the commencement of heparin, most commonly seen in the postoperative orthopaedic or cardiovascular patient. Two other time-courses may sometimes be seen, namely a more rapid onset in patients re-exposed to heparin within 3 months, and a delayed onset up to 1 week after cessation of heparin. The skin necrosis occasionally seen at sites of subcutaneous heparin injection is probably a local manifestation of HIT, and the rare systemic reaction occurring within 30 minutes of intravenous heparin is probably a generalized manifestation of HIT. Non-necrotic skin lesions in patients given heparin are generally due to delayed hypersensitivity and not to HIT.

Thrombosis is the feared complication of HIT, but its incidence and severity are not related to the degree of thrombocytopenia. The hypercoagulable state in HIT is more severe than that seen even in congenital AT III deficiency (see Antithrombin III). While thrombosis is usually venous, it may also be arterial or microvascular, and it may affect unusual sites (including grafts and extracorporeal circuits). The presence of a central venous catheter may predispose the patient to a venous thrombus of the upper limb. In general, thrombosis in HIT can be severe and extensive, and it carries a 20% risk of amputation and a 30% mortality.

Diagnostic confirmation is important because of its therapeutic implications. Clearly, it is necessary to exclude as far as possible other causes of thrombocytopenia (q.v.). It should be noted that the thrombocytopenia relevant in HIT may be relative rather than absolute, i.e. a fall of 50% from a previously high platelet count may result in a count of $>150 \times 10^9$/L (i.e. still within the normal range) but would still qualify for a diagnosis of HIT.

Specific laboratory testing for HIT involves either a functional assay to demonstrate heparin-induced platelet activation or an immunoassay to show the presence of the antibody involved. Functional assays, such as platelet aggregation or 14C-serotonin release, are widely available but are subject to considerable technical variability. Immunoassays are more sensitive but can be very expensive. Although required for diagnosis, laboratory tests are not suitable for screening, since the presence of antibodies is very common but clinical manifestations are much less frequent.

Treatment of HIT requires **total cessation of heparin**, *as changing to another animal source or a low molecular weight preparation is mostly ineffective, even if no cross-reactivity can be shown in vitro. Heparin-coated intravascular circuits should also be withdrawn in cases of HIT. On the other hand, occasional cases have been reported of well documented HIT in patients in whom the antibody has waned (seroreversion) and the platelet count has recovered despite continuation of heparin.*

Although some limited antithrombotic protection may be offered by dextran or aspirin, these agents are no longer recommended. Early warfarin should not be given, because of the risk of warfarin necrosis in those patients who may also have protein C deficiency (q.v.) and because the antithrombotic effect of warfarin takes some days to become established. Thus, patients with existing thrombosis would remain untreated during this time, and even those without current thrombosis are at risk because of the high incidence (about 6-fold) of developing thrombosis within the first 2 days if untreated due to the continuing 'thrombin storm' when heparin is stopped.

Urgent **antithrombotic treatment** *is therefore required for optimal management. For this purpose, the following agents have been shown to be effective (though note that the first two agents have become difficult to obtain):*

- **danaparoid**, *a low molecular weight heparinoid (see Anticoagulants),*
  - *given in a dose of 200 U/hr IV following an initial bolus of 2250 U and a loading dose of 400 U/hr for 4 hr and then 300 U/hr for 4 hr,*
- **lepirudin**, *a member of the hirudin family and thus a direct thrombi inhibitor (see Anticoagulants),*
  - *given in a dose of 0.1–0.15 mg/kg/hr IV following an initial bolus of 0.2–0.4 mg/kg,*
- **argatroban**, *a direct thombin inhibitor (see Anticoagulants),*
  - *given in a dose of 2 mcg/kg/min IV.*
- **fondaparinux**, *a synthetic pentasaccharide representing the antithrombin binding site of heparin (see Anticoagulants),*
  - *given in a dose of 7.5 mg SC per day.*
- **bivalirudin**, *a synthetic analog of hirudin and a direct thrombin inhibitor (see Anticoagulants),*

- given in a dose of 0.5–1 mg/kg IV bolus followed by 1.75–2.5 mg/kg/hr.
• **rivaroxaban**, a NOAC or DOAC (see Anticoagulants),
- given in a dose of 15 mg orally bd.

These agents need to be given in therapeutic doses, as prophylactic doses even in patients without current thrombosis have been found to be suboptimal. The duration of treatment should be until the platelet count has become stable, when antithrombotic therapy with warfarin can be continued or not on its usual merits.

Immune globulin has been reported to be successful in severe and protracted cases by producing rapid and persistent ablation of the antibody-heparin-platelet activation process.

Bibliography

Aster RH, Bougie DW. Drug-induced immune thrombocytopenia. *N Engl J Med* 2007; 357: 904.

Aster RH, Curtis BR, McFarland JG, et al. Drug-induced immune thrombocytopenia: pathogenesis, diagnosis, and management. *J Thromb Haemost* 2009; 7: 911.

Bick RL. Heparin-induced thrombocytopenia and paradoxical thromboembolism: diagnostic and therapeutic dilemmas. *Clin Appl Thromb Hemost* 1997; 3: 63.

Chong BH. Heparin-induced thrombocytopenia. *J Thromb Haemost* 2003; 1: 1471.

Chong BH, Ismail F, Cade J, et al. Heparin-induced thrombocytopenia: studies with low molecular weight heparinoid, Org 10172. *Blood* 1989; 73: 1592.

Farag SS, Savoia H, O'Malley CJ, et al. Lack of in vitro cross-reactivity predicts safety of low-molecular weight heparins in heparin-induced thrombocytopenia. *Clin Appl Thromb Hemost* 1997; 3: 58.

Greinacher A. *Heparin-associated thrombocytopenia. Vessels* 1995; 1: 17.

Greinacher A, Selleng K, Warkentin E. Autoimmune heparin-induced thrombocytopenia. *J Thromb Haemost* 2017; 15: 2099.

Hoylaerts MF, Vanassche T, Verhamme P. Bacterial killing by platelets, making sense of (II)IT. *J Thromb Haemost* 2018; 16: 1182.

Kelton JG, Arnold DM, Bates SM. Nonheparin anticoagulants for heparin-induced thrombocytopenia. *N Engl J Med* 2013; 368: 737.

Lewis BE, Wallis DE, Leya F, et al. Argatroban anticoagulation in patients with heparin-induced thrombocytopenia. *Arch Intern Med* 2003; 163: 1849.

Magnani HN, Gallus A. Heparin-induced thrombocytopenia: a report of 1478 clinical outcomes of patients treated with danaparoid (Orgaran) from 1982 to mid 2004. *Thromb Haemost* 2006; 95: 967.

Padmanabhan A, Jones CG, Pechauer SM, et al. IVIg for treatment of severe refractory heparin-induced thrombocytopenia. *Chest* 2017; 152: 478.

Selleng K, Warkentin TE, Greinacher A. Heparin-induced thrombocytopenia in intensive care patients. *Crit Care Med* 2007; 35: 1165.

Schindewolf M, Kroll H, Ackermann H, et al. Heparin-induced non-necrotizing skin lesions: rarely associated with heparin-induced thrombocytopenia. *J Thromb Haemost* 2010; 8: 1486.

Shantsila E, Lip GYH, Chong BH. Heparin-induced thrombocytopenia. *Chest* 2009; 135: 1651.

Shih AW, Sheppard J-AI, Warkentin TE. Platelet count recovery and seroreversion in immune HIT despite continuation of heparin: further observations and literature review. *Thromb Haemost* 2017; 117: 1868.

Various. Drug-induced thrombocytopenia. *Chest* 2005; 127(2): suppl.

Warkentin TE. Heparin-induced thrombocytopenia: yet another treatment paradox. *Thromb Haemost* 2001; 85: 947.

Warkentin TE. Heparin-induced thrombocytopenia: pathogenesis and management. *Br J Haematol* 2003; 121: 535.

Warkentin TE, Chong BH, Greinacher A. Heparin-induced thrombocytopenia: towards consensus. *Thromb Haemost* 1998; 79: 1.

Warkentin TE, Greinacher A, eds. *Heparin-Induced Thrombocytopenia*. 5th edition. London: CRC Press. 2012.

Warkentin TE, Greinacher A, Koster A, et al. Treatment and prevention of heparin-induced thrombocytopenia: ACCP evidence-based clinical practice guidelines *Chest* 2008; 133 (suppl.): 340S.

Warkentin TE, Levine MN, Hirsh J, et al. Heparin-induced thrombocytopenia in patients treated with low-molecular-weight heparin or unfractionated heparin. *N Engl J Med* 1995; 332: 1330.

Warkentin TE, Pai M, Linkins LA. Direct oral anticoagulants for treatment of HIT. *Blood* 2017; 130: 1104.

Warkentin TE, Sheppard J-AI, Heels-Ansdell D, et al. Heparin-induced thrombocytopenia in medical surgical critical illness. *Chest* 2013; 144: 848.

Hepatic diseases

Most **hepatic diseases**/disorders encountered in the Intensive Care Unit are common and well known. They include hepatic failure (such as fulminant hepatic failure, FHF), cirrhosis, portal hypertension, hepatic encephalopathy and hepatorenal syndrome. Similarly, abnormal liver function tests but with an elusive aetiology are very common in Intensive Care patients.

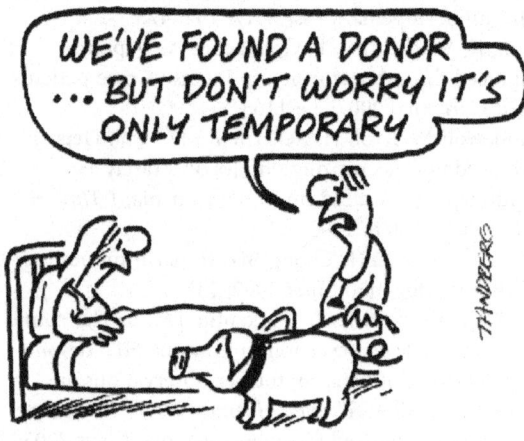

Some conditions and issues of course are less common and are therefore considered in this book, including
- Acute fatty liver of pregnancy,
- Biliary cirrhosis,
- Black cohosh,
- Budd–Chiari syndrome,
- Hepatic necrosis,
- Hepatic vein thrombosis,
- Hepatitis,
- Hepatocellular carcinoma,
- Hepatoma,
- Hepatopulmonary syndrome,
- Hepatorenal syndrome,
- Hyperammonaemia,
- Khat,
- Liver abscess,
- Non-alcoholic fatty liver disease,
- Non-alcoholic steatohepatitis,
- Portopulmonary hypertension,
- Wilson's disease.

As many drugs are cleared primarily by the liver, undesirably increased levels and thus adverse effects may be seen in patients with significant liver disease (e.g. with Child–Pugh grade B or C scores) when they are given drugs such as morphine, glyceryl trinitrate, propranolol, calcium channel blockers, antidepressants or tranquillizers.

Finally, as most haemostatic (including coagulation) factors are produced in the liver, significant liver disease can be associated with major haemostatic changes affecting both bleeding and thrombosis (see Coagulation disorders, see Thrombophilia).

Bibliography
Adedoyin A, Branch RA. The effect of liver disease on drugs. *Curr Opin Crit Care* 1997; 3: 255.
Alshamsi F, Alshammari K, Belley-Cote E, et al. Extracorporeal liver support in patients with liver failure: a systematic review and meta-analysis of randomized trials. *Intens Care Med* 2020; 46: 1.
Ambrosino P, Tarantino L, Di Minno G, et al. The risk of venous thromboembolism in patients with cirrhosis: a systematic review and meta-analysis. *Thromb Haemost* 2017; 117: 139.
Bailey B, Amre DK, Gaudreault P. Fulminant hepatic failure secondary to acetaminophen poisoning: a systematic review and meta-analysis of prognostic criteria determining the need for liver transplantation. *Crit Care Med* 2003; 31: 299.
Bauer M, Fuhrmann V, Wendon J. Pulmonary complications of liver disease. *Intens Care Med* 2019; 45: 1433.
Bernal W, Auzinger G, Dhawan A, et al. Acute liver failure. *Lancet* 2010; 376: 190.
Bernal W, Wendon J. Acute liver failure. *N Engl J Med* 2013; 369: 2525.
Bernsmeier C, Antoniades CG, Wendon J. What's new in acute liver failure? *Intens Care Med* 2014; 40: 1545.
Better OS. Renal and cardiovascular dysfunction in liver disease. *Kidney Int* 1986; 29: 598.
Calvo CP, Sipman FS, Caramelo C. Renal and electrolyte abnormalities in patients with hepatic insufficiency. *Curr Opin Crit Care* 1996; 2: 413.
Dooley J, Lok ASF, Garcia-Tsao G, et al., eds. *Sherlock's Diseases of the Liver and Biliary System*. 13th edition. Hoboken: Wiley. 2018.
Eckardt K-U. Renal failure in liver disease. *Intens Care Med* 1999; 25: 5.
Editorial. Hepatic osteomalacia and vitamin D. *Lancet* 1982; 1: 943.
Foreman MG, Moss M. The role of hepatic dysfunction in critical illness. *Pulmonary Perspectives* 2001; 18(4): 8.
Fraser CL, Arieff AI. Hepatic encephalopathy. *N Engl J Med* 1985; 313: 865.
Garcia-Tsao G. Treatment of ascites with single total paracentesis. *Hepatology* 1991; 13: 1005.
LaMont JT, Isselbacher KJ. Postoperative jaundice. *N Engl J Med* 1973; 288: 305.
Larsen FS, Wendon J. Understanding paracetamol-induced liver failure. *Intens Care Med* 2014; 40: 888.
Lee WM. Drug-induced hepatotoxicity. *N Engl J Med* 2003; 349: 474.
Lieber CS. Medical disorders of alcoholism. *N Engl J Med* 1995; 333: 1058.

Ludwig J. The nomenclature of chronic active hepatitis: an obituary. *Gastroenterology* 1993; 105: 274.

McClain CJ. Trace metals in liver disease. *Semin Liver Dis* 1991; 11: 321.

Mills PR, Sturrock RD. Clinical associations between arthritis and liver disease. *Ann Rheum Dis* 1982; 41: 295.

Nanchal R, Subramanian R, Karvellas CJ, et al. Guidelines for the management of adult acute and acute-on-chronic liver failure in the ICU: cardiovascular, endocrine, hematologic, pulmonary and renal considerations. *Crit Care Med* 2020; 48: 415.

Raschke RA, Curry SC, Rempe S, et al. Results of a protocol for the management of patients with fulminant liver failure. *Crit Care Med* 2008; 36: 2244.

Riordan SM, Williams R. Current management of fulminant hepatic failure. *Curr Opin Crit Care* 1999; 5: 136.

Romero-Gomez M, Montagnese S, Jalan R. Hepatic encephalopathy in patients with acute decompensation of cirrhosis and acute-on-chronic liver failure. *J Hepatol* 2015; 62: 437.

Runyon BA. Care of patients with ascites. *N Engl J Med* 1994; 330: 337.

Starzl TE, Demetris AJ, Van Thiel D. Liver transplantation. *N Engl J Med* 1989; 321: 1014 & 1092.

Stravitz RT. Critical management decisions in patients with acute liver failure. *Chest* 2008; 134: 1092.

Stravitz RT, Kramer AH, Davern T, et al. Intensive care of patients with acute liver failure: recommendations of the US Acute Liver Failure Study Group. *Crit Care Med* 2007; 35: 2498.

Thomson SJ, Cowan ML, Johnston I, et al. 'Liver function tests' on the intensive care unit: a prospective, observational study. *Intens Care Med* 2009; 35: 1406.

Vennes JA, Bond JH. Approach to the jaundiced patient. *Gastroenterology* 1983; 84: 1615.

Warrilow, S, Bailey M, Pilcher D, et al. Characteristics and outcomes of patients with acute liver failure admitted to Australian and New Zealand intensive care units. *Intern Med J* 2019; 49: 874.

Warrilow SJ, Bellomo R. Preventing cerebral oedema in acute liver failure: the case for quadruple H therapy. *Anaesth Intens Care* 2014; 42: 78.

Weiss N, Jalan R, Thabout D. Understanding hepatic encephalopathy. *Intens Care Med* 2018; 44: 231.

Wilkinson GR. Drug metabolism and variability among patients in drug response. *N Engl J Med* 2005; 352: 2211.

Wright TL. Etiology of fulminant hepatic failure: is another virus involved? *Gastroenterology* 1993; 104: 640.

Hepatic necrosis See
- Hepatitis.

Hepatic vein thrombosis See
- Budd–Chiari syndrome.

Hepatitis

Hepatitis is inflammation of the liver cells. It is produced
- usually by viral infection (especially hepatitis viruses A–G, cytomegalovirus (CMV), Epstein–Barr virus (EBV)),
- sometimes by drugs, toxins, ischaemia or autoimmune disease.

Hepatitis may thus be a final common pathway for a variety of different liver insults.

Sometimes, fulminant hepatitis occurs with no definable cause, so that it is likely that there are other as yet unidentified viruses, mutant viruses or toxins capable of producing this syndrome. About 5–20% of cases of acute and chronic hepatitis have no currently identifiable cause, prompting in particular continuing search for viruses other than the main known seven (A–G).

Clinical features of hepatitis are variable and often extensive.

Typically, there are systemic inflammatory symptoms affecting the gut, joints and central nervous system for 1–2 weeks prior to the onset of more specific local features.

The more specific local features include
- dark urine (in over 90%),
- light stools (in over 50%),
- abdominal discomfort,
- tender smooth hepatomegaly,
- jaundice,
- hepatic fetor (fetor hepaticus), which has a musty odour.

Investigations show abnormal liver function tests with high transaminase levels as the initial finding. The serum bilirubin rises to a maximum of about 350 µmol/L by 2 weeks, and then decreases over the following 2–4 weeks. The alkaline phosphatase is usually moderately elevated, and there are both hypoalbuminaemia and a prolonged prothrombin time in severe cases. The full blood examination is mildly abnormal.

Treatment is frustrating because no modalities alter the course of disease.
- *Bed rest is warranted on the clinical merits of the symptoms, but measures such as diet and vitamins are*

ineffective and even alcohol is not necessarily contraindicated.
- Trials involving corticosteroids, immune globulin, cimetidine and exchange transfusion have shown no efficacy.
- Lactulose (30 mL 4 hrly) is commonly given, but its benefit is uncertain.
- Transplantation is indicated in severe disease with encephalopathy, except in chronic hepatitis B and C because of the high rate of recurrent viraemia and severe hepatitis.
- Predisposition to bacterial infection and coagulopathy need to be attended to.
- Specific treatment is required for hyperammonaemia (q.v.), if present.

The outlook after hepatitis is usually favourable, with an uncomplicated course and complete recovery.
Occasionally, however,
- the disease may **relapse** or become **prolonged**
  - especially with hepatitis B and hepatitis C,
  - also in the elderly,
- there may be an **acute fulminant course** (acute liver failure)
  - leading to hepatic coma and even death,
  - usually seen in hepatitis B and hepatitis C,
  - sometimes in hepatitis E in pregnancy,
- **chronic hepatitis**
  - may occur in hepatitis B or C, predisposing to hepatocellular carcinoma (q.v.),
  - may occur in hepatitis C, predisposing to a carrier state,
  - is manifest by raised serum alanine aminotransferase (ALT) for more than 6 months and progresses slowly to hepatic fibrosis,
  - may be autoimmune, when it is most commonly antinuclear antibody-positive and corticosteroid-responsive,
  - may be cryptogenic.

Many **concomitant extrahepatic syndromes** have also been reported, most commonly in hepatitis B. Thus, there have been associated
- autoimmune haemolytic anaemia (see Anaemia),
- polyarteritis nodosa (q.v.),
- cryoglobulinaemia (q.v.)
  - especially in chronic hepatitis C virus (HCV) infection,
- sicca syndrome (see Sjogren's syndrome)
  - especially in chronic HCV infection,
- immune-mediated renal disease
  - in chronic hepatitis B virus (HBV) and especially HCV infection.

Hepatitis type A virus (HAV, infectious hepatitis virus) is an RNA virus transmitted by faecal contamination. It is chiefly a disease of developing countries, and its occurrence in developed countries is mostly in returned travellers.

The incubation period is usually 3–5 weeks, and there is a viraemia with viral shedding for up to 3 weeks before the appearance of jaundice. The patient is not infectious after 3 weeks of clinical illness unless a relapse occurs. There is no animal reservoir.

Infection gives rise to immunity (an early IgM and a later IgG) and antibodies may be detected in about 50% of the population.

Chronic disease does not occur, and the mortality is <0.2%.

Both passive and active immunization are available. Pooled **immune globulin** *given within 2 weeks of exposure decreases the occurrence of clinical disease. It provides protection for 2–5 months (depending on the dose given) and is recommended for travellers to areas of risk. An inactivated* **vaccine** *provides effective long-term immunity when two doses are given.*

Hepatitis type B virus (HBV, serum hepatitis) is a DNA virus usually transmitted by percutaneous inoculation of infected blood, but the virus in fact is present in many bodily fluids, so that transmission venereally and perinatally is also common. In developed countries, it is nowadays seen mainly in migrants and travellers from developing countries where the infection is endemic.

The incubation period is usually 2–6 months and averages 12 weeks. Antibodies to surface antigen (anti-HBs) and to core antigen (anti-HBc) appear early and persist in the carrier or chronic state, though only anti-HBs is normally seen in convalescent serum or after vaccination.

Chronic disease occurs in about 5% of patients, giving an overall population prevalence of about 1% in developed countries. However, screening studies have shown that about 50% of these patients are unaware that they have been infected. The mortality of chronic disease is 1.5%. Persistent HBs antigen occurs in both carriers and patients with chronic disease, but the latter additionally have abnormal liver function tests and HBc antibodies. A genetic mutation in the viral genome is responsible for some patients with chronic disease being HBe antigen positive and some being negative.

Treatment is with **immune globulin** *if given within 1 week of exposure, but the most appropriate management is prevention with* **recombinant hepatitis B vaccine**.

However, the use of this vaccine has become controversial in some countries following reports of both central and peripheral demyelination after its administration.

Interferon (currently with pegylated preparations) and especially **lamivudine** (or other nucleoside analogs, e.g. entecavir, adefovir, tenofovir) are useful in chronic infection, though progressive resistance over time to **lamivudine** has been reported. Lamivudine may also be helpful in severe acute disease. Inadvertent cessation of therapy even in stable cases has been reported to lead to fulminant hepatic failure. Treatment not only reduces inflammation and thus liver injury but also lessens the potential progression to cirrhosis and hepatocellular carcinoma. Antiviral management is complex and should be supervised by a specialist liver clinic.

Treatment of infected patients who are immunosuppressed or pregnant present special challenges, for which separate protocols have been recommended.

Hepatitis type C virus (HCV, formerly non-A, non-B or post-transfusion hepatitis) is an RNA virus also usually transmitted by percutaneous inoculation or infected blood. It may have originated in dogs before transfer to humans at some time in the last millennium. It was identified in 1989 and is now recognized as the cause of most cases (perhaps 90%) of transfusion hepatitis, but it may also be responsible for up to 25% of sporadic acute community-acquired hepatitis. Most cases are nowadays caused by the use of contaminated injection equipment, related either to illicit drug use in developed countries or to non-sterile medical, dental or traditional practices in developing countries.

The incubation period is usually 5–10 weeks. Anti-HCv antibodies indicate either past or present infection and are present in the acute disease, in the carrier state and in over 50% of cases of hepatocellular carcinoma. Current infection is indicated by the presence of viral RNA on PCR testing. The identification of the specific viral genotype on PCR testing can guide specific antiviral therapy.

Most patients are asymptomatic, even though they are infectious to others. Acute liver failure is virtually never seen with HCV infection. The disease may remain silent and eventual chronic liver impairment may be its first clinical manifestation. Failure of viral clearance is the most important problem following acute infection, and this causes chronic disease in about 75% of cases. Chronic hepatitis in turn commonly leads to cirrhosis or hepatocellular carcinoma (q.v.). There is an increased risk of cardiovascular and cerebrovascular complications in patients with chronic HCV disease. The mortality of hepatitis C is probably similar to that of hepatitis B. The mechanism for its hepatocarcinogenesis is uncertain because, unlike HBV, HCV is not incorporated into the host genome.

Treatment with **immune globulin** acutely and with **interferon alpha** (IFN) in the chronic state is helpful. Combination therapy with **ribavirin** and **IFN** (in both regular and especially pegylated forms) is more effective both initially and after relapse than IFN alone, with response to therapy varying with viral genotype. More recently, triple therapy with the addition of a new antiviral protease inhibitor (e.g. **boceprevir, telaprevir, sofosbuvir, ledipasvir, simeprevir** or **asunaprevir**) to ribavirin and pegylated IFN has increased the virological response rate, though such treatment regimens are complex to manage. IFN-free regimens can be used in patients who are IFN-intolerant, usually because of systemic symptoms, psychiatric disturbance or cytopenia. Somewhat different treatment regimens are indicated for the different HCV genotypes.

End-stage liver disease due to hepatitis C infection is nowadays the most common condition requiring **liver transplantation**. Thus, the goal of treatment even in acute disease is to prevent chronic infection.

HCV infection should now be considered potentially curable, given the new treatment regimens available in specialized centres in developed countries, though these programs are very expensive. In practice, >95% of patients can have viral eradication within 3 months, leading to the possibility of effective community elimination of the virus.

Hepatitis type D virus (HDV, delta-agent) is a small RNA virus that requires hepatitis B virus (HBV) for its expression. Thus, its route of transmission, incubation period and prophylaxis are as for hepatitis B. HDV infection is seen most commonly in Mediterranean countries, but it also occurs in South America, Africa and Asia, with different genotypes found in different geographic regions. Overall, up to 20 million people are infected worldwide with HDV.

About 5% of patients with chronic HBV infection have associated HDV infection. Compared to HBV infection alone, combined infection is associated with more severe disease, more progression to cirrhosis, more hepatocellular carcinoma and a higher acute mortality of up to 20%. Anti-HDV antibodies appear late in the course of disease and reflect exposure rather than ongoing disease.

The only currently available treatment is with **interferon**.

Hepatitis type E virus (HEV) is, like HAV, transmitted via faecal contamination, i.e. it is water-borne. There may be an animal reservoir in swine. It is an important cause of epidemic hepatitis in developing countries. In developed countries, it may be transmitted by blood transfusion, where it is of particular importance in immunocompromised patients.

The immunological status is uncertain, but both IgG and IgM antibodies can be identified after infection. The high incidence of seropositivity suggests that many infections have been mild or misdiagnosed. Viral persistence (i.e. demonstration of HEV RNA in serum) indicates the possibility of chronic infection.

The incubation period is 2–8 weeks. The mortality of acute disease is up to 2% and up to 15% in pregnancy and is due to acute liver failure. HEV infection does not generally lead to identifiable chronic disease.

Trials of two recently developed recombinant HEV vaccines have shown efficacy, but their general availability is limited (except in China).

Hepatitis type F virus (HFV) is a recently described DNA virus. Its role as a formal hepatitis virus remains to be clarified.

Hepatitis type G virus (HGV) is a recently described RNA virus, related to but separate from HCV. It appears to be an important cause of post-transfusion hepatitis, though it may be a coinfection with HCV.

Many **drugs** may cause liver damage, commonly via idiosyncratic reactions (see Drug allergy). This is referred to as **drug-induced liver injury** (DILI), and it is an important cause of liver failure, potentially requiring liver transplantation or causing death.

The clinical and laboratory features are indistinguishable from viral hepatitis.

The 'incubation' period is usually 2–6 weeks, but it can be a short as 1 day or as long as 6 months.

Although this form of liver damage may be predictable for high doses of some drugs (e.g. paracetamol), it is not normally dose-dependent, as with halothane, isoniazid, methyldopa, phenytoin, sulphonamides. It may also follow the use of herbal and dietary supplements or illicit anabolic steroids.

Some promising new drugs were later withdrawn from the market because of reports of serious and sometimes fatal hepatic damage. Examples include tolcapone (an anti-Parkinsonism drug) and trovafloxacin/alatrofloxacin (a 'fourth-generation' quinolone).

Drug-induced hepatitis can persist despite stopping the drug. Continuing the drug may be fatal.

Conversely, in patients with liver disease there is impairment of oxidative drug metabolism, a drug clearance mechanism (e.g. for theophylline) which has been shown to be improved in such patients by supplemental oxygen. Drug clearance by hepatic conjugation (e.g. for paracetamol) is not improved by oxygen.

Toxins producing hepatic damage similar to viral hepatitis may occur with
- mushroom poisoning (q.v.), including Kombucha 'mushroom' tea,
- plant alkaloid poisoning (see Alkaloids),
- ingestion of the herb, black cohosh, for menopausal symptoms,
- chewing the leaves of khat (*Catha edulis*, found in East Africa) as a stimulant,
- use of valerian, a plant remedy used in anxiety and sleep disorders,
- Reye's syndrome (q.v.).

A similar picture, sometimes referred to as **hypoxic or ischaemic hepatitis**, is also commonly seen in critically ill patients. This complication is due to severe hepatic ischaemia and/or congestion, particularly when there is low cardiac output and/or systemic sepsis. There is diffuse hepatocellular necrosis, and liver function tests show marked elevation of transaminases. The prognosis is that of the underlying condition.

Autoimmune hepatitis is an uncommon condition which has features in common with either **primary biliary cirrhosis** (see Biliary cirrhosis) or **primary sclerosing cholangitis** (see Cholangitis).

Bibliography

Ambrosino P, Tarantino L, Di Minno G, et al. The risk of venous thromboembolism in patients with cirrhosis: a systematic review and meta-analysis. *Thromb Haemost* 2017; 117: 139.

Assis DN, Navarro VJ. Human drug hepatotoxicity: a contemporary clinical perspective. *Expert Opin Drug Metab Toxicol* 2009; 5: 463.

Bell SJ, Nguyen T. The management of hepatitis B. *Aust Prescriber* 2009; 32: 99.

Bernal W, Wendon J. Acute liver failure. *N Engl J Med* 2013; 369: 2525.

Chiew AL, Reith D, Pomerleau A, et al. Updated guidelines for the management of paracetamol poisoning in Australia and New Zealand. *Med J Aust* 2020; 212: 175.

Ciesek S, Manns MP. Chronic liver diseases. In: *Scientific American Medicine. Hepatology.* Hamilton: Dekker Medicine. 2020.

Croagh CM, Lubel J. Advances in the management of hepatitis C. *Intern Med J* 2013; 43: 1265.

Davis GL, Esteban-Mur R, Rustgi V, et al. Interferon alfa–2b alone or in combination with ribavirin for the treatment of relapse of chronic hepatitis C. *N Engl J Med* 1998; 339: 1493.

Dienstag JL, Schiff ER, Wright TL, et al. Lamivudine as initial treatment for chronic hepatitis B in the United States. *N Engl J Med* 1999; 341: 1256.

D'Souza R, Foster GR. Diagnosis and management of chronic hepatitis B. *J R Soc Med* 2004; 97: 318.

Farrell GC. Acute viral hepatitis. *Med J Aust* 1998; 168: 565.

Farrell GC. Chronic viral hepatitis. *Med J Aust* 1998; 168: 619.

Froomes PRA, Morgan DJ, Smallwood RA, et al. Comparative effects of oxygen supplementation on theophylline and acetaminophen clearance in human cirrhosis. *Gastroenterology* 1999; 116: 915.

Fuhrmann V, Kneidinger N, Herkner H, et al. Hypoxic hepatitis: underlying conditions and risk factors for mortality in critically ill patients. *Intens Care Med* 2009; 35: 1397.

Gross JB, Persing DH. Hepatitis C: advances in diagnosis. *Mayo Clin Proc* 1995; 70: 296.

Hoofnagle JH. Type D (delta) hepatitis. *JAMA* 1989; 261: 1321.

Hoofnagle JH, Bjornsson ES. Drug-induced liver injury: types and phenotypes. *N Engl J Med* 2019; 381: 264.

Hutin YJ, Pool V, Cramer EH, et al. A multistate, foodborne outbreak of hepatitis A. *N Engl J Med* 1999; 340: 595.

Jackson K, MacLachlan J, Cowie B, et al. Epidemiology and phylogenetic analysis of hepatitis D virus infection in Australia. *Intern Med J* 2018; 48: 1308.

Johnson RJ, Gretch Dr, Yamabe H, et al. Membranoproliferative glomerulonephritis associated with hepatitis C virus infection. *N Engl J Med* 1993; 328: 465.

Kaplowitz N, Aw TY, Simon FR, et al. Drug-induced hepatotoxicity. *Ann Intern Med* 1986; 104: 826.

Keays R, Harrison PM, Wendon JA, et al. Intravenous acetylcysteine in paracetamol fulminant hepatic failure: a prospective controlled trial. *BMJ* 1991; 303: 1026.

Krawczynski K. Hepatitis E. *Hepatology* 1993; 17: 932.

Lau JY, Wright TL. Molecular virology and pathogenesis of hepatitis B. *Lancet* 1995; 342: 1335.

Lee WM. Hepatitis B virus infection. *N Engl J Med* 1997; 337: 1733.

Liang TJ, Rehermann B, Seeff LB, et al. Pathogenesis, natural history, treatment, and prevention of hepatitis C. *Ann Intern Med* 2000; 132: 296.

Linnen J, Wages J, Zhen-Yong ZK, et al. Molecular cloning and disease association of hepatitis G virus: A transfusion-transmissible agent. *Science* 1996; 271: 505.

Lok AS, McMahon BJ. Chronic hepatitis B: update of recommendations. *AASLD Practice Guidelines. Hepatology* 2004; 39: 857.

Lubel JS, Strasser SI, Thompson AJ, et al. Australian consensus recommendations for the management of hepatitis B. *Med J Aust* 2022; 216: 478.

Maddrey WC. Chronic hepatitis. *Dis Mon* 1993; 39: 53.

McCaughan GW, Koorey DJ. Liver transplantation. *Aust NZ J Med* 1997; 27: 371.

McCaughan GW, Strasser SI. Emerging therapies for hepatitis C virus (HCV) infection: the importance of HCV genotype. *Aust NZ J Med* 2000; 30: 644.

McHutchison JG, Gordon SC, Schiff ER, et al. Interferon alfa-2b alone or in combination with ribavirin as initial treatment for chronic hepatitis C. *N Engl J Med* 1998; 339: 1485.

Mitra AK. Hepatitis C-related hepatocellular carcinoma. *Epidem Rev* 1999; 21: 180.

Mohsen W, Levy MT. Hepatitis A to E: what's new? *Intern Med J* 2017; 47: 380.

Moulds RFW, Malani J. Kava: herbal panacea or liver poison. *Med J Aust* 2003; 178: 451.

Navarro VJ, Khan I, Bjornsson E, et al. Liver injury from herbal and dietary supplements. *Hepatology* 2017; 65: 363.

Pak E, Esrason KT, Wu VH. Hepatotoxicity of herbal remedies: an emerging dilemma. *Prog Transplant* 2004; 14: 91.

Perron AD, Patterson JA, Yanofsky NN. Kombucha 'mushroom' hepatotoxicity. *Ann Emerg Med* 1995; 26: 660.

Riordan SM, Williams R. Current management of fulminant hepatic failure. *Curr Opin Crit Care* 1999; 5: 136.

Schaefer EAK, Dienstag JL. Viral hepatitis. In: *Scientific American Medicine. Hepatology.* Hamilton: Dekker Medicine. 2020.

Shapiro CN. Transmission of hepatitis viruses. *Ann Intern Med* 1994; 120: 82.

Shrestha MP, Scott RM, Joshi DM, et al. Safety and efficacy of a recombinant hepatitis E vaccine. *N Engl J Med* 2007; 356: 895.

Teoh NC, Farrell GC. Management of chronic hepatitis C virus infection: a new era of disease control. *Intern Med J* 2004; 34: 324.

Thompson AJV. Australian recommendations for the management of hepatitis C virus infection: a consensus statement. *Med J Aust* 2016; 204: 268.

Thompson AJ, Holmes JA. Treating hepatitis C – what's new? *Aust Prescriber* 2015; 38: 191.

Tsukuma H, Hiyama T, Tanaka S, et al. Risk factors for hepatocellular carcinoma among patients with chronic liver disease. *N Engl J Med* 1993; 328: 1797.

Whiting P, Clouston A, Kerlin P. Black cohosh and other herbal remedies associated with acute hepatitis. *Med J Aust* 2002; 177: 440.

Wright TL. Etiology of fulminant hepatic failure: is another virus involved? *Gastroenterology* 1993; 104: 640.

Zuckerman AJ. The new GB hepatitis viruses. *Lancet* 1995; 345: 1453.

Hepatocellular carcinoma

Hepatocellular carcinoma (HCC, hepatoma) is generally associated with pre-existing liver disease. Typically, this precursor disease is cirrhosis, especially following hepatitis B or C infection (q.v.) or haemochromatosis (q.v.). Sometimes, hepatocellular carcinoma may follow cirrhosis due to alcohol, non-alcoholic fatty liver disease (NAFLD – q.v.), $α_1$-antitrypsin deficiency (q.v.), methotrexate or schistosomiasis (q.v.). Occasionally, it may follow hepatic damage without cirrhosis, e.g. after ingestion of aflatoxins, androgens and possibly oral contraceptives (q.v.). Its prevalence is about 8 per 100,000 of the population and appears to be increasing. However, as most cases of hepatocellular carcinoma are linked to prior liver disease, the condition is potentially preventable.

Hepatocellular carcinoma is seen most commonly in men, typically younger men in Africa, middle-aged men in East Asia and elderly men in developed countries.

Clinical features of hepatocellular carcinoma include
- weight loss,
- painful hepatomegaly,
- hepatic friction rub,
- worsening of portal hypertension.

It is commonly associated with paraneoplastic features (q.v.), such as
- dysfibrinogenaemia,
- hypoglycaemia,
- hypercalcaemia (q.v.),
- polycythaemia (q.v.).

Investigations involving liver function tests are usually unhelpful, as they are typically abnormal beforehand, although the aspartate transaminase and/or alkaline phosphatase may be especially abnormal. Imaging and biopsy are typically required for diagnosis including the extent of the tumour. The optimal imaging modality for diagnosis is contrast enhanced CT or MRI scanning, which are often sufficiently specific to obviate the need for histological confirmation from targeted biopsy material. Angiography can help assess resectability because, unlike hepatic metastases, hepatocellular carcinoma may have increased vascularity. Although the alpha-fetoprotein level (q.v.) is increased in about 70% of patients, it is neither sufficiently specific nor sensitive for diagnosis, though it may assist with the assessment of progress and possibly with the screening of high-risk patients. Ultrasound surveillance of susceptible patients, especially those with cirrhosis, remains the best screening tool and should be offered to these patients every 6 months.

Treatment is best supervised by a multidisciplinary team in a specialized centre guided by an endorsed liver cancer staging system.
- *The optimal treatment is with* **resection** *if technically feasible.*
- *Otherwise, liver transplantation may be considered for early stage disease, following which the 5-yr survival is about 75%. Liver transplantation has the advantage of eliminating the underlying disease as well as the tumour itself.*
- *Useful disease control may be produced by local vascular embolization, percutaneous tumour ablation, selective radiation (internal or stereotactic) or chemotherapy (e.g. with sorafenib)*
- *Patients with incurable disease should supported with palliative care.*

The median survival is only about 12 months and the overall 5-yr survival is about 20%, with death most commonly due to tumour progression, liver failure or spontaneous tumour rupture. The prognosis is worse if there are metastases (usually to lung or bone) or jaundice.

Bibliography

Earl TM, Chapman WC. Hepatocellular carcinoma: resection versus transplantation. *Semin Liver Dis* 2013; 33: 282.

El-Serag HB, Mason AC. Rising incidence of hepatocellular carcinoma in the United States. *N Engl J Med* 1999; 340: 745.

Fan S-T, Lo C-M, Lai ECS, et al. Perioperative nutritional support in patients undergoing hepatectomy for hepatocellular carcinoma. *N Engl J Med* 1994; 331: 1547.

Farmer DG, Rosove MH, Shaked A, et al. Current treatment modalities for hepatocellular carcinoma. *Ann Surg* 1994; 219: 236.

Forner A, Reig M, Bruix J. Hepatocellular carcinoma. *Lancet* 2018; 391: 1301.

Heimbach JK, Kulik LM, Finn RS, et al. AASLD guidelines for the treatment of hepatocellular carcinoma. *Hepatology* 2018; 67: 358.

Koorey D. Hepatocellular carcinoma: prevention, detection and treatment ... in the real world. *Intern Med J* 2007; 37: 513.

Livraghi T, Giorgio A, Marin G, et al. Hepatocellular carcinoma and cirrhosis in 746 patients: long-term results of percutaneous ethanol injection. *Radiology* 1995; 197: 101.

Lubel JS, Roberts SK, Strasser SI, et al. Australian recommendations for the management of hepatocellular carcinoma: a consensus statement. *Med J Aust* 2021; 214: 475.

Margolis S, Homcy C. *Systemic manifestations of hepatoma. Medicine* 1972; 51: 381.

Mazzaferro V, Regalia E, Doci R, et al. Liver transplantation for the treatment of small hepatocellular carcinomas in patients with cirrhosis. *N Engl J Med* 1996; 334: 693.

McCaughan GW, Koorey DJ, Strasser SI. Hepatocellular carcinoma: current approaches to diagnosis and management. *Intern Med J* 2002; 32: 394.

Mitra AK. *Hepatitis C-related hepatocellular carcinoma. Epidem Rev* 1999; 21: 180.

Tsukuma H, Hiyama T, Tanaka S, et al. Risk factors for hepatocellular carcinoma among patients with chronic liver disease. *N Engl J Med* 1993; 328: 1797.

Venook AP. Treatment of hepatocellular carcinoma: too many options? *J Clin Oncol* 1994; 12: 1323.

Wands JR, Blum HE. Primary hepatocellular carcinoma. *N Engl J Med* 1991; 325: 729.

Hepatoma *See*
- Hepatocellular carcinoma.

Hepatopulmonary syndrome

Hepatopulmonary syndrome (HPS or hepatogenic pulmonary angiodysplasia) was described in 1984 as a condition characterized by cirrhosis, cyanosis and clubbing. It comprises impaired arterial oxygenation in association with liver disease.

Its pathogenesis is unknown, but it may be due to failure of the liver to preserve the normal balance of pulmonary vasoconstrictor and vasodilator substances, with resultant excessive pulmonary vasodilatation due to impaired clearance of vasoactive mediators. Histologically, there are diffuse precapillary dilatations, arteriovenous malformations (q.v.) and pleural spider naevi. The associated liver disease is usually severe and accompanied by portal hypertension. Typically, such patients may be on the waiting list for liver transplantation, in whom the occurrence of HPS may be about 10%.

Clinical features of hepatopulmonary syndrome are dominated by hypoxaemia, which can sometimes be severe.

There is dyspnoea, cyanosis and digital clubbing.
In the upright position, the hypoxaemia is paradoxically worse (**orthodeoxia**) and there is tachypnoea (platypnoea) – see Platypnoea–orthodeoxia syndrome.
In mild disease, there are no symptoms.
Examination of the chest is normal.

The chest X-ray is normal, but the dilatations may be apparent on CT scan. Lung function tests show a decreased diffusing capacity and abnormal ventilation–perfusion relationships (typically shunt) manifest by a widened alveolar–arterial oxygen pressure gradient (A-aDO$_2$).

The differential diagnosis includes the many, much more common causes of pulmonary dysfunction in patients with liver disease, namely,
- diaphragmatic disadvantage,
- pleural effusion,
- atelectasis.

*Treatment is uncertain, but **indometacin** or possibly **octreotide** may be helpful.*

Liver transplantation *causes the condition to reverse eventually, provided it has not become chronic.*

In Intensive Care practice, the hepatopulmonary syndrome should be remembered as a cause of hypoxaemia in patients with significant liver disease and a normal chest X-ray.

See also
- Pulmonary hypertension – Portopulmonary hypertension.

Bibliography

Bauer M, Fuhrmann V, Wendon J. Pulmonary complications of liver disease. *Intens Care Med* 2019; 45: 1433.

Herve P, Lebrec D, Brenot F, et al. Pulmonary vascular disorders in portal hypertension. *Eur Respir J* 1998; 11: 1153.

Krowka MJ, Cortese DA. Hepatopulmonary syndrome: current concepts in diagnostic and therapeutic considerations. *Chest* 1994; 105: 1528.

Krowka MJ, Wiseman GA, Burnett OL, et al. Hepatopulmonary syndrome. *Chest* 2000; 118: 615.

Rodriguez-Roisin R, Krowka MJ. Hepatopulmonary syndrome: a liver-induced lung vascular disorder. *N Engl J Med* 2008; 358: 2378.

Schraufnagel DE, Kay JM. Structural and pathological changes in the lung vasculature in chronic liver disease. *Clin Chest Med* 1996; 17: 1.

Hepatorenal syndrome

The **hepatorenal syndrome** (HRS) refers to a particular form of renal dysfunction that occurs in patients with severe liver disease. It is generally triggered by a serious complication, such as gastrointestinal bleeding or sepsis.

It is one of a number of **hepatorenal disorders** (HRD) which are common in seriously ill patients, either because both the liver and kidney have been damaged by a common injury (e.g. toxic insult) or because patients with existing disease in one organ (e.g. liver disease) may then suffer a concomitant complication (e.g. shock) which adversely affects the other organ.

HRS occurs in patients with severe liver disease (manifest by cirrhosis and ascites) but with no pre-existing renal disease. The creatinine has increased to >130 mcmol/L despite treatment of the ascites. This present definition does not accommodate hepatorenal pathophysiology in patients who may have pre-existing renal disease. HRS represents functional renal failure, as there is no histological injury, and it probably results from renal vasoconstriction, triggered as a compensatory response to the splanchnic vasodilatation which occurs in cirrhosis.

Prevention of HRS may to some extent be achieved by albumin infusion (with concomitant diuresis) and by treating any co-existing spontaneous bacterial peritonitis (SBP).

The treatment of HRS includes volume resuscitation, vasopressor support of blood pressure, octreotide (see Somatostatin) and/or terlipressin (see Desmopressin), relief of portal hypertension if possible (e.g. by transjugular intrahepatic portosystemic shunt, TIPS) and renal replacement therapy.

Provided specific treatment is implemented, the prognosis of HRS is primarily that of the underlying liver disease.

Bibliography
Al-Khafaji A, Nadim MK, Kellum JA. Hepatorenal disorders. *Chest* 2015; 148: 550.
Gines P, Schrier RW. Renal failure in cirrhosis. *New Engl J Med* 2009; 361: 1279.
Salerno F, Gerbes A, Gines P, et al. Diagnosis, prevention and treatment of hepatorenal syndrome in cirrhosis. *Gut* 2007; 56: 1310.
Wong F, Nadim MK, Kellum JA. Working party proposal for a revised classification system of renal dysfunction in patients with cirrhosis. *Gut* 2011; 60: 702.

Hepcidin *See*

- Iron.

Herbicides *See*

- Dioxins,
- Paraquat.

Hereditary haemorrhagic telangiectasia *See*

- Arteriovenous malformations.

Herpesviruses

The **herpesviruses** comprise a group of over 100 related DNA viruses, of which eight infect humans. They share a common property of latency and reactivation. Reactivation can occur many years after the initial infection, which itself may be mild and seemingly unrelated.

The eight pathogenic viruses include herpesvirus 1 and 2 (HSV-1, HSV-2), varicella-zoster virus (VZV), cytomegalovirus (CMV), Epstein–Barr virus (EBV), and herpesvirus 6, 7 and 8 (HSV-6, HSV-7 and HSV-8). HSV-8 is referred to as Kaposi sarcoma–associated virus.

Infections due to these individual viruses are considered separately.
See
- Acyclovir,
- Cytomegalovirus,
- Epstein–Barr virus,
- Kaposi's sarcoma,
- Varicella-zoster.

Bibliography
Hirsch MS. Herpesvirus infections. In: *Scientific American Medicine. Infectious Diseases.* Hamilton: Dekker Medicine. 2020.
Whitley RJ, Roizman B. Herpes simplex virus infections. *Lancet* 2001; 357: 1513.

High altitude

Moderate altitude (1500–2500 m) exists in many regions of the world which are either populated or commonly visited. This altitude is of clinical relevance only in patients with existing cardiopulmonary disease and in the occasional particularly susceptible patient who even then has only mild distress. It is the altitude to which commercial airlines are pressurized (i.e. up to 2440 m or 8000 ft).

High altitude (2500–4000 m) is the usual threshold for permanent habitation. The PaO_2 has fallen to 50 mmHg by 4000 m. This region contains the usual threshold for high-altitude medical problems.

Very high altitude (4000–5500 m) encompasses the limits of permanent habitation and acclimatization. At these heights, the barometric pressure is about half

> that at sea level, and the arterial oxygenation is approximately the normal venous level.
>
> **Extreme altitude** (5500–8848 m, the height of Mount Everest) is reached only by mountaineering expeditions.

It has been estimated that up to 150 million people live at high altitude, primarily in Asia and South America. Many others travel to these regions for recreation or work. This hostile environment is one of not only hypoxia, but also low temperatures, dry air and increased solar radiation.

High-altitude medical problems are primarily due to fluid shifts from the intravascular to the extravascular space. The brain and lungs are particularly vulnerable to these changes, which typically occur in otherwise healthy subjects who may visit high altitude areas for a variety of reasons and who require acute physiological adaptation to remain healthy. Chronic physiological adaptation is of course well recognized in those millions of people who have lived successfully for many generations in these often remote areas.

High-altitude medical problems comprise the following entities.

1. Acute mountain sickness

This is especially manifest by headache but also fatigue, dizziness, insomnia and nausea. It is due to cerebral hypoxia (i.e. it is a form of hypoxic encephalopathy). It is experienced by about 70% of subjects at least to some degree and is worse on exercise. It is associated with an impaired ventilatory response to hypoxia. It is not associated with unfitness, but it is assisted by acclimatization. It lasts only a few days.

Its treatment is symptomatic, including **oxygen** *administration. Effective measures include* **acetazolamide** *and* **dexamethasone** *(see below) but not furosemide.* **Descent** *from altitude is required if the illness is severe.*

2. Pulmonary oedema

High-altitude pulmonary oedema (HAPE) is manifest by dyspnoea, fatigue and cough and if severe by cerebral dysfunction. It is associated with exercise and lack of acclimatization. It has an average prevalence of only 0.5%, though this can be increased 10-fold or more if ascent is rapid. It is much more common in those who have suffered a previous episode. It may also be more common in those with polymorphisms of the genes encoding for pulmonary surfactant proteins.

It generally occurs gradually but always within 2–4 days and is commonly preceded by the less severe features of acute mountain sickness. It has a mortality of about 10%, especially if treatment fails.

It is associated with pulmonary hypertension but a normal pulmonary artery wedge pressure. It is thus a high-flow, protein-rich, oedema process, similar to that seen after the relief of acute pulmonary artery obstruction or in hypertensive encephalopathy. It is associated with an irregular hypoxic pulmonary arteriolar constriction, multiple small thrombi, peripheral vasoconstriction and fluid retention due to increased secretion of antidiuretic hormone.

Treatment requires descent from altitude and the administration of oxygen.

- Diuretics are not appropriate.
- **Continuous positive airway pressure/positive end-expiratory pressure** *(CPAP/PEEP) is effective. Interestingly, ancient Chinese merchants crossing high mountains such as the Himalayas were known to use pursed-lip breathing if breathless.*
- *Intubation and mechanical ventilation may occasionally be required.*
- **Nitric oxide** *has been reported to be of benefit.*
- **Nifedipine** *has been found to be useful prophylactically in susceptible people.*
- **Sildenafil** *has been reported to be of benefit in both prevention and treatment of HAPE.*
- *The long-acting β-agonist* **salmeterol** *has also been reported to be useful.*
- *The novel peptide* **solnatide** *has been shown to be highly effective in experimental studies.*

3. Cerebral oedema

High-altitude cerebral oedema (HACE) is manifest by headache, disorientation, ataxia, hallucinations and coma. Papilloedema and retinal haemorrhages are commonly seen. There is increased intracranial pressure and cerebral petechiae. It often follows acute mountain sickness (see above) and may be an extreme form of that condition.

It occurs in about 20% of patients suffering from pulmonary oedema, though its onset may be delayed for several days. It has a mortality of about 15%, and survivors may suffer from prolonged neurological sequelae.

Treatment requires descent from **altitude** *and the administration of* **oxygen**.

- **Corticosteroids** *(dexamethasone 4 mg 6 hrly) are recommended.*
- **Acetazolamide** *(250 mg bd) and corticosteroids (dexamethasone 2 mg tds) provide useful prophylaxis.*

4. Miscellaneous conditions

These include
- chronic mountain sickness (Monge disease),
  - manifest by fatigue, headache, dizziness, poor mental function, dyspnoea, polycythaemia (q.v.), cyanosis and pulmonary hypertension,

- possibly caused by central hypoventilation in the 5–10% of residents at high altitude who develop the condition due to loss of acclimatization,
- now treatable with ACE inhibitors (q.v.),
• thromboembolism,
• peripheral oedema,
• syncope.

5. **Prior conditions adversely affected by altitude**

These include
• heart disease,
• chronic obstructive lung disease,
• hypertension,
• obesity,
• sickle cell disease (q.v.),
• decompression sickness.

Bibliography

Bartsch P, Mairbaurl H, Maggiorini M, et al. Physiological aspects of high-altitude pulmonary edema. *J Appl Physiol* 2005; 98: 1101.

Boyer SJ, Blume FD. Weight loss and changes in body composition at high altitude. *J Appl Physiol* 1984; 57: 1580.

Cottrell JJ. Altitude exposure during aircraft flight: flying higher. *Chest* 1988; 92: 81.

Cramer D, Ward S, Geddes D. Assessment of oxygen supplementation during air travel. *Thorax* 1996; 51: 202.

Frayser R, Houston CS, Bryan AC, et al. Retinal hemorrhage at high altitude. *N Engl J Med* 1970; 282: 1183.

Hackett PH, Rennie D, Levine HD. The incidence, importance and prophylaxis of acute mountain sickness. *Lancet* 1976; 2: 1149.

Hackett PH, Roach RC. High-altitude illness. *N Engl J Med* 2001; 345: 107.

Hock RJ. The physiology of high altitude. *Sci Am* 1970; 222: 2: 52.

Hornbein TF, Schoene RB, eds. *High Altitude: An Exploration of Human Adaptation.* New York: Marcel Dekker. 2001.

Houston CS, Dickinson J. Cerebral form of high-altitude illness. *Lancet* 1975; 2: 758.

Hultgren HN. High-altitude pulmonary edema: current concepts. *Annu Rev Med* 1996; 47: 267.

Johnson TS, Rock PB. Acute mountain sickness. *N Engl J Med* 1988; 319: 841.

Luks AM, Swenson ER. Medication and dosage considerations in the prophylaxis and treatment of high-altitude illness. *Chest* 200; 133: 744.

Menon ND. High altitude pulmonary edema. *New Engl J Med* 1965; 273: 66.

Penaloza D, Sime F. Chronic cor pulmonale due to loss of altitude acclimatization (chronic mountain sickness). *Am J Med* 1971; 50: 728.

Plata R, Cornejo A, Arratia C, et al. Angiotensin-converting-enzyme inhibition therapy in altitude polycythaemia. *Lancet* 2002; 359: 663.

Pollard AJ, Murdoch DR. *High Altitude Medicine.* 3rd edition. Abingdon: Radcliffe. 2003.

Richalet JP. High altitude pulmonary oedema: still a place for controversy? *Thorax* 1995; 50: 923.

Saxena S, Kumar R, Madan T, et al. Association of polymorphisms in pulmonary surfactant protein A1 and A2 genes with high-altitude pulmonary edema. *Chest* 2005; 128: 1611.

Scherrer U, Vollenweider L, Delabays A, et al. Inhaled nitric oxide for high-altitude pulmonary edema. *N Engl J Med* 1996; 334: 624.

Schoene RB. Pulmonary edema at high altitude: review, pathophysiology, and update. *Clin Chest Med* 1985; 6: 491.

Schoene RB. Illnesses at high altitude. *Chest* 2008; 134: 402.

Sutton JR, Reeves JT, Wagner PD, et al. Operation Everest II: oxygen transport during exercise at extreme simulated altitude. *J Appl Physiol* 1988; 64: 1309.

Ward M, Millege J, West J. *High Altitude Medicine and Physiology.* Philadelphia: University of Pennsylvania Press. 1989.

Waterlow JC, Bunje HW. Observations on mountain sickness in the Colombian Andes. *Lancet* 1966; 2: 655.

West JB. The physiologic basis of high-altitude diseases. *Ann Intern Med* 2004; 141: 789.

West JB, Boyer SJ, Graber DJ, et al. Maximal exercise at extreme altitudes on Mount Everest. *J Appl Physiol* 1983; 55: 688.

Hirsutism

Hirsutism refers to increased growth of hair at sites that are normally androgen-dependent, namely, the face, chest and abdomen. The term usually applies to women, in whom it may be one of the manifestations of virilization (together with frontal balding, deepening of the voice, acne, enhanced muscle mass and amenorrhoea). Thus, hirsutism is sometimes referred to as hair in the wrong place.

Excess androgens may be exogenous (e.g. anabolic steroids) or endogenous. Increased endogenous androgen production may be either functional or neoplastic and occurs in either the adrenal gland or ovary (e.g. polycystic ovary syndrome – q.v.).

*Treatment, apart from any that may be available for a specific lesion, is either **cosmetic** or **suppressive**. Suppression may be achieved with*

- *corticosteroids (e.g. dexamethasone) which inhibit ACTH production,*
- *oral contraceptives (q.v.) which inhibit pituitary gonadotrophins, and*
- *androgen blockers (cyproterone acetate and spironolactone are the most commonly used agents of this type).*

*There have been reports of the reduction of unwanted hair in women by the twice daily application of cream containing 13.9% **eflornithine** hydrochloride (a drug used IV for African sleeping sickness).*

Hypertrichosis refers to increased hair growth of a non-endocrine nature. It is sometimes referred to as just too much hair, and it may be local or general in distribution. It may be

- familial,
- racial,
- drug-induced (carbamazepine, minoxidil, phenytoin, ciclosporin),
- idiopathic.

Bibliography

Del Rosso JQ. Disorders of hair. In: *Scientific American Medicine. Dermatology.* Hamilton: Dekker Medicine. 2020.

Ikhena DE, Pal L. Hirsutism and hyperandrogenism. In: *Scientific American Medicine. Women's Health.* Hamilton: Decker Medicine. 2020.

Kvedar JC, Gibson M, Krusinski PA. Hirsutism: evaluation and treatment. *J Am Acad Dermatol* 1985; 12: 215.

McKenna TJ. Screening for sinister causes of hirsutism. *N Engl J Med* 1994; 331: 1015.

Paus R, Cotsarelis G. The biology of hair follicles. *N Engl J Med* 1999; 341: 491.

Rusting RL. Hair: why it grows, why it stops. In: *The Frontiers of Biotechnology.* New York: Scientific American. 2002; p 66.

Wolff K, Goldsmith L, Katz S, et al., eds. *Fitzpatrick's Dermatology in General Medicine.* 7th edition. New York: McGraw-Hill. 2007.

Hirudin(s) *See*

- Anticoagulants.

Histiocytosis

Histiocytosis has been reclassified as **Langerhans cell histiocytosis** (LCH) and was formerly referred to as **Histiocytosis X**. More recently, the term **inflammatory myeloid neoplasia** has been suggested. It comprises three diseases, traditionally considered related because of a common histiocytic cell, namely

- eosinophilic granuloma,
- Hand–Schuller–Christian disease,
- Letterer–Siwe disease.

There is a unique granulomatous infiltration with Langerhans-like cells resembling monocytes and macrophages (i.e. histiocytes) and containing a foamy eosinophilic cytoplasm with characteristic inclusions (X or Birbeck granules) and positive staining with anti-CD1a monoclonal antibody. This cell is a specialized immune cell of the dendritic cell system. There is a high prevalence of somatic mutations in LCH, leading to excess activation of the mitogen-activated protein (MAP) kinase pathway.

The infiltrate is a monoclonal proliferation, and it affects skin, bone, liver and central nervous system, as well as lung.

Eosinophilic granuloma (now called pulmonary Langerhans cell histiocytosis) is the form of histiocytosis which affects the lungs, in which it is an uncommon cause of a **diffuse pulmonary infiltrate** (see Interstitial lung diseases). It mostly occurs in Caucasian adults and is strongly associated with smoking. It may be complicated by tumour formation, both malignant and nonmalignant.

Clinical features generally comprise cough and dyspnoea, though 25% of patients are asymptomatic. Spontaneous pneumothorax (q.v.) occurs in 10–20% of cases. Systemic involvement is common with up to 20% of patients having involvement of bone or pituitary (with diabetes insipidus – q.v.).

The chest X-ray shows a diffuse reticular or fine nodular pattern, with 50% of cases also having honeycombing or cysts, many too small to be detected except by CT scanning. Rupture of such a cyst is the cause of propensity to pneumothorax. Lung function tests show decreased gas exchange and ventilatory capacity, as for most pulmonary interstitial diseases, but unlike them there is also airflow obstruction.

The diagnosis is made definitively by lung biopsy, though it may be suggested by the presence of >5% CD1a-positive cells in bronchoalveolar lavage (BAL) fluid.

*Treatment of local disease is with **curettage** if feasible or with irradiation.*

*Systematic disease is treated with **corticosteroids** with or without cytotoxic agents (e.g. vinblastine, cladribine). However, treatment is often not required, as the condition is relatively benign, is frequently asymptomatic and often remits.*

Hand–Schuller–Christian disease occurs in children as well as adults. It is a multisystem disease affecting bone particularly. Diabetes insipidus (q.v.) is common. Pulmonary involvement may include progressive fibrosis with honeycombing.

Letterer–Siwe disease occurs only in infants.

Bibliography
Cheyne C. Histiocytosis X. *J Bone Joint Surg* 1971; 53: 366.
Coppes-Zantinga A, Egeler RM. Historical review: the Langerhans cell histiocytosis X files revealed. *Br J Haematol* 2002; 116: 3.
Crausman RS, Jennings CA, Tuder RM, et al. Pulmonary histiocytosis X: pulmonary function and exercise physiology. *Am J Respir Crit Care Med* 1996; 153: 426.
Kambouchner M, Valeyre D, Soler P, et al. Pulmonary Langerhans' cell granulomatosis (histiocytosis X). *Annu Rev Med* 1992; 43: 105.
Litchenstein L. Histiocytosis: integration of eosinophilic granuloma of the bone, Letterer-Siwe disease and Hand-Schuller-Christian disease as related manifestations of a single nosologic entity. *Arch Pathol* 1953; 56: 84.
Nezelof C, Basset F. Langerhans cell histiocytosis research: past, present and future. *Hematol Oncol Clin North Am* 1998; 12: 385.
Seigelman SS. Taking the X out of histiocytosis X. *Radiology* 1997; 204: 322.
Steinman RS. Dendritic cell system and its role in immunogenicity. *Annu Rev Immunol* 1991; 9: 271.

Histocompatibility complex

The major **histocompatibility complex** (MHC) contains genes responsible for the production of highly polymorphic cell surface antigens which identify cells as 'self' and which are responsible for presentation of peptide antigens to T lymphocytes. In humans, the MHC is specified by the term 'human leukocyte antigen' (HLA) and resides on the short arm of chromosome 6. HLA matching is an important component of donor selection for organ transplantation.

There are two types of MHC molecules, Class I and II.
- Class I antigens (HLA-A, -B, -C) are expressed on virtually all cell types. They consist of two polypeptide chains, a polymorphic heavy chain (44 kDa), and a non-polymorphic light chain (11.5 kDa), called **beta 2-microglobulin** (q.v.). The Class I proteins present peptide fragments of proteins made within the cell, including usually encoded proteins, to $CD8^+$ T cells (killer cells).
- Class II antigens (HLA-DP, -DQ, -DR) are expressed on only a few cell types, mainly lymphocytes, monocytes and dendritic cells, though in inflammation many other cells can also express these antigens. They consist of two polymorphic polypeptide chains of 34 and 28 kDa. The Class II proteins present extracellular antigen in the form of peptide fragments of endogenous endocytosed proteins to $CD4^+$ T cells (helper cells), which then modulate the immune response.
- On occasion, there may be some cross-presentation of extracellular peptides to $CD8^+$ T cells or cytoplasmic peptides to $CD4^+$ T cells, especially after transplantation.

There may be many different alleles at each of the 7 loci in the HLA system. There is a correlation between specific HLA antigens and the presence of a large number of diseases, with relative risks from 2– to 3-fold up to 90-fold or more. The mechanism of this association is not understood in detail, but it is likely to be related to the ability of different MHC types to bind and present particular peptide antigens to T lymphocytes.

There is a relative risk of 10-fold or more of the following diseases (in descending order of frequency in each group) in patients with specific HLA antigens:
- **dermatological diseases**
  - dermatitis herpetiformis, pemphigus vulgaris (q.v.),
- **endocrine diseases**
  - juvenile insulin-dependent diabetes mellitus, congenital adrenal hyperplasia, subacute thyroiditis, Addison's disease (q.v.),
- **gastrointestinal diseases**
  - coeliac disease (q.v.),
- **haematological diseases**
  - haemochromatosis (q.v.),
- **neurological diseases**
  - narcolepsy,
- **renal diseases**
  - Goodpasture's syndrome (q.v.), gold and penicillamine nephropathy,
- **rheumatic diseases**
  - ankylosing spondylitis (q.v.), Reiter's syndrome (q.v.), reactive arthritis (q.v.), psoriatic arthritis (q.v.).

Note that some of these conditions (e.g. haemochromatosis, narcolepsy and most notably congenital adrenal hyperplasia) are not immune-related, and their HLA association may relate to other, non-HLA genes nearby.

Bibliography
Guillet J-G, Lai M-Z, Briner TJ, et al. Immunological self, nonself discrimination. *Science* 1987; 235: 865.
Lundy SK, Gizinski A, Fox DA. Introduction to clinical immunology: overview of immune response,

autoimmune conditions, and immunosuppressive therapeutics for rheumatic diseases. In: *Scientific American Medicine. Allergy & Immunology*. Hamilton: Dekker Medicine. 2020.

Schlossman SF, Boumsell L, Gilks W, et al. Update: CD antigens 1993. *J Immunol* 1994; 152: 1.

Sheehan NJ. The ramifications of HLA-B27. *J R Soc Med* 2004; 97: 10.

Tiwari JL, Terasaki PI. HLA and Disease Associations. New York: Springer-Verlag. 1985.

Histoplasmosis

Histoplasmosis is a systemic mycosis caused by the fungus *Histoplasma capsulatum*, which is found in soil and bird droppings worldwide. Infection from aerosolized spores thus occurs when soil or bird or bat droppings are disturbed.

Over 90% of infections are asymptomatic, but primary disease if severe gives an influenza-like illness. A chronic progressive cavitary disease of the lungs may occur, particularly in older men. Disseminated disease with multiorgan involvement is seen in occasional patients (one in 50,000) with primary disease, in compromised hosts and as a complication of tumour necrosis factor (TNF) antagonist therapy (e.g. in chronic inflammatory conditions, such as rheumatoid arthritis, sarcoidosis, inflammatory bowel disease, psoriasis, Behcet's disease – see these individual conditions) (see Tumour necrosis factor).

> Histoplasmosis has many similarities in pathogenesis and clinical presentation to **tuberculosis** (q.v.). It can also mimic **sarcoidosis** (q.v.), from which the distinction is crucial to avoid erroneous treatment with adverse consequences.

The diagnosis is based on culture of the organism, but it is slowly growing. A positive skin test is not specific for the disease-state, but positive serology is diagnostically helpful.

Bibliography

Kauffman CA. Mycotic infections. In: *Scientific American Medicine. Infectious Diseases*. Hamilton: Dekker Medicine. 2020.

Wheat LJ. Systemic fungal infections: diagnosis and treatment; I. Histoplasmosis. *Infect Dis Clin North Am* 1988; 2: 841.

HIV (human immunodeficiency virus) See

- Acquired immunodeficiency syndrome.

Horner's syndrome

Horner's (Horner) syndrome describes the phenomenon of unilateral miosis (pupillary constriction) with ptosis (lid droop) and often facial anhydrosis and enophthalmos. It is caused by interruption of the sympathetic fibres in the three-neurone pathway originating in the hypothalamus and innervating the eye. The first neurone in this pathway runs from the hypothalamus to the cervical cord, the second neurone runs from the cervical cord through the brachial plexus to the superior cervical ganglion and the third neurone ascends with the carotid artery to the structures of the eye.

> Horner's syndrome may be caused by
> - carotid disease,
> - vertebrobasilar ischaemia,
> - brachial plexus infiltration (particularly due to carcinoma of the lung or breast),
> - syringomyelia (q.v.),
> - migraine and cluster headache,
> - central venous catheterization.

An ipsilateral Horner's syndrome is seen in the **lateral medullary syndrome**, which is caused by vertebral artery thrombosis. In addition, there is nystagmus, ataxia and dysphagia. Typically, there is also ipsilateral impairment of facial sensation and contralateral loss of the sensation of pain and temperature in the limbs.

Bibliography

Reddy G, Coombes A, Hubbard AD. Horner's syndrome following internal jugular vein cannulation. *Intens Care Med* 1998; 24: 194.

Hot flushes See

- Sweating.

Hot tubs See

- Bathing.

Human bites See

- Bites and stings.

Human immunodeficiency virus See

- Acquired immunodeficiency syndrome.

Hydatid disease See

- Echinococcosis.

Hydrocephalus

Hydrocephalus refers to enlargement of the cerebral ventricles. It is classified as either communicating or non-communicating.

Communicating hydrocephalus is the more common form.

It is due to impaired reabsorption of cerebrospinal fluid by the arachnoid granulations over the dural venous sinuses. This may follow previous haemorrhage, infection or trauma.

Non-communicating hydrocephalus arises from obstruction in the ventricular system (e.g. in the aqueduct of Sylvius). Thus, cerebrospinal fluid flow is impaired and the proximal ventricles become enlarged.

Chronic hydrocephalus gives rise to progressive dementia (q.v.), with ataxia and incontinence.
The diagnosis is made by CT and MR scanning.

Treatment is with **shunting**, usually ventriculoperitoneal but sometimes ventriculoatrial or ventriculovenous.

Complications of ventricular shunting include
- infection,
- shunt occlusion,
- subdural haemorrhage.

Hydrogen sulphide

Hydrogen sulphide (H_2S) is a colourless, flammable, poisonous gas with the characteristic smell of rotten eggs, and it is thus referred to as 'stink damp'. It is produced from the natural decay of organic sulphur-containing substances, and it is also present in the gas from mineral spas and from volcanoes. It is also produced as a by-product of petroleum refining, and it is used extensively in the chemical industry as an analytic agent.

Its accidental inhalation can be fatal, with collapse, unconsciousness and apnoea following exposure to concentrations >1000 ppm. At lower concentrations (e.g. 300 ppm), pulmonary oedema may occur, and at much lower concentrations (e.g. 10 ppm), nausea and irritation of the throat and eyes may occur. The threshold concentration for detection is very much lower again, namely 0.005 ppm.

Interestingly, hydrogen sulphide has been recognized to be a physiological signalling molecule, like two other endogenously synthesized gases, namely nitric oxide and carbon monoxide. It may be involved in inflammation, cell proliferation and metabolic regulation. As a vasodilator and metabolic dampener, it might theoretically be of benefit in ischaemia–reperfusion injury, where it has been postulated to be capable of causing a state of suspended animation.

Treatment of poisoning is **symptomatic**.

Bibliography

Beauchamp RO, Bus JS, Popp JA, et al. A critical review of the literature on hydrogen sulfide toxicity. *Crit Rev Toxicol* 1984; 13: 25.

Drabek T. Hydrogen sulphide – curiouser and curiouser! *Crit Care Med* 2012; 40: 2255.

Kapoor A, Thiemermann C. Hydrogen sulfide, neurogenic inflammation and cardioprotection: a tale of rotten eggs and vanilloid receptors. *Crit Care Med* 2010; 38: 728.

Li L, Bhatia M, Moore PK. Hydrogen sulphide: a novel mediator of inflammation? *Curr Opin Pharmacol* 2006; 6: 125.

Steendijk P. Toward therapeutic use of hydrogen sulfide in critical care. *Crit Care Med* 2010; 38: 725.

Szabo C. Hydrogen sulphide and its therapeutic potential. *Nat Rev Drug Discov* 2007; 6: 917.

Wagner F, Asfar P, Calzia E, et al. Bench-to-bedside review: hydrogen sulfide – the third gaseous transmitter: applications for critical care. *Crit Care* 2009; 13: 213.

Hyperammonaemia

Hyperammonaemia is relatively common in critically ill patients, in whom it can be difficult to manage and may lead to significant neurological damage.

Ammonia is produced primarily in the gut (from enteric organisms and from protein breakdown) and in the kidney (initially as ammonium to bind hydrogen ions and thus facilitate acid secretion). Some ammonia is also produced from intense muscle activity, as in extreme exercise or prolonged seizures.

Ammonia in the circulation is cleared by the liver by metabolism to urea via the urea cycle. Thus, both liver disease and specific defects in the enzymes controlling the urea cycle impair ammonia clearance.

The normal ammonia level in blood is up to 50 µmol/L. Levels over 100 µmol/L warrant treatment, and levels over 200 µmol/L cause encephalopathy (q.v.), with cerebral oedema, intracranial hypertension and seizures being particular consequences of acute hyperammonaemia.

The diagnosis of hyperammonaemia is not difficult in cases of **severe acute liver failure**. However, it may be overlooked when other less common causes are involved.

These uncommon causes include
- **some cancer states**
  - e.g. after leukaemia chemotherapy, after bone marrow transplantation, in multiple myeloma (q.v.),

- **inborn errors of metabolism** (IEMs) – q.v.
  - uncommon inherited defects, in this setting usually involving a urea cycle disorder (UCD).

> The three main causes of hyperammonaemia in the critically ill (i.e. liver disease, some cancer states and IEMs) can be exacerbated by a number of conditions which increase ammonia levels, though not to a symptomatic degree in normal subjects.
> These conditions include
> - increased protein load
>   - e.g. due to gastrointestinal haemorrhage,
> - some infections
>   - e.g. from herpesviruses or urease-splitting organisms, such as *Proteus* and *Klebsiella*,
> - some drugs
>   - e.g. antibiotics, anticonvulsants, antidepressants, carbamazepine, paracetamol,
> - physiological stresses
>   - e.g. pneumonia or pregnancy (relevant mainly in IEMs).

Thus, although most relevant IEMs are apparent in childhood, some may present only in adult life when they are unmasked by one of the precipitants listed above. The ornithine transcarbamylase (OTC) deficiency is the commonest such IEM (occurring in 1 in 14,000 live births), but disorders of any of the other four enzymes in the urea cycle have also been well described, i.e. carbamyl phosphate synthetase 1 deficiency (CPS-1), arginosuccinate aciduria, citrullinaemia type 1 and arginase deficiency.

In brief, the **urea cycle** is the metabolic process in the liver whereby two molecules of toxic ammonia and one molecule of bicarbonate combine to form one molecule of non-toxic urea, which can then be excreted in the urine.

The diagnosis of the specific defect in an IEM requires sophisticated laboratory analysis of amino acid profiles in blood and urine. Genetic studies and liver biopsy may also assist accurate recognition, so that prompt treatment, subsequent prophylaxis and family follow-up are facilitated.

Treatment priorities include
- reduction of ammonia production (by protein restriction, lactulose, rifamixin – an oral, non-absorbable antibiotic),
- enhancement of ammonia removal (by renal replacement therapy, and in IEMs by sodium phenylacetate and sodium benzoate),
- elimination of precipitating factors (especially infection, gastrointestinal bleeding),
- management of increased intracranial hypertension (osmotherapy, hypothermia, sedation).

Liver transplantation is a recognized procedure not only for fulminant hepatic failure but also for serious IEMs.

Bibliography

Bachmann C. Mechanisms of hyperammonemia. *Clin Chem Lab Med* 2002; 40: 653.

Bernal W, Wendon J. *Acute liver failure N Engl J Med* 2013; 369: 2525.

Clay AS, Hainline BE. Hyperammonaemia in the ICU. *Chest* 2008; 132: 1368.

Crosbie DC, Sugamar H, Simpson MA, et al. Late-onset ornithine transcarbamylase deficiency: a potentially fatal yet treatable cause of coma. *Crit Care Resusc* 2009; 11: 222.

Kwan L, Wang C, Levitt L. Hyperammonemic encephalopathy in multiple myeloma. *N Engl J Med* 2002; 346: 1674.

Lockwood AH. Controversies in ammonia metabolism: implications for hepatic encephalopathy. *Metab Brain Dis* 2007; 22: 285.

Summar M, Barr F, Dawling S, et al. Unmasked adult-onset urea cycle disorder in the critical care setting. *Crit Care Clin* 2005; 21 (suppl.): S1.

Warrilow S, Fisher C, Bellomo R. Correction and control of hyperammonemia in acute liver failure: the impact of continuous renal replacement timing, intensity, and duration. *Crit Care Med* 2020; 48: 218.

Hyperbaric oxygen *See*

- Carbon monoxide,
- Diving – Decompression sickness,
- Gangrene – Necrotizing fasciitis.

See also
- Actinomycosis,
- Bites and stings – Spider bites,
- Clostridial infections,
- Methaemoglobinaemia,
- Multiple sclerosis,
- Pneumatosis coli,
- Pyoderma gangrenosum.

Bibliography

Featherstone PJ, Ball CM. The therapeutic use of air under hyperbaric pressure. *Anaesth Intens Care* 2021; 49: 159.

Weaver LK. Hyperbaric oxygen in the critically ill. *Crit Care Med* 2011; 39: 1784.

Hypercalcaemia

Hypercalcaemia is an important phenomenon, since
- it may present a life-threatening crisis, and

- it may also be a marker of significant and potentially treatable underlying disease.

The causes of hypercalcaemia are

1. **Increased gastrointestinal absorption**

Normal absorption of calcium is under vitamin D control and increased absorption thus occurs from excess vitamin D intake, as well as in the milk–alkali syndrome (in which there is associated metabolic alkalosis) and in sarcoidosis (q.v.).

2. **Increased bone reabsorption**

Normal absorption is under parathyroid control and increased reabsorption thus occurs in hyperparathyroidism (q.v.), as well as in hyperthyroidism (q.v.) (in which it is mild and uncommon), metastatic malignancy, multiple myeloma (q.v.), Paget's disease (q.v.), immobility (though usually there is associated disease) and as a paraneoplastic phenomenon (q.v.) (due to ectopic hormone production or to cytokine release, such as of interleukin 1 (IL-1)).

3. **Increased renal absorption**

Normal renal absorption of calcium is under parathyroid hormone control and increased absorption thus occurs in hyperparathyroidism, as well as in adrenal insufficiency and sometimes following thiazide administration.

> If the patient is well, the usual cause of hypercalcaemia is hyperparathyroidism.

In **tumour-associated hypercalcaemia**, the malignancy is usually apparent clinically, when it is generally a manifestation of advanced disease.

- The ectopic hormone produced is parathyroid hormone related protein (PTHrP). Even in bony metastases, there may be a humoral element. PTHrP is synthesized by some squamous cell carcinomas (particularly lung, breast and kidney) but also by some normal tissues, such as the placenta. The intact protein of 173 amino acids can be assayed, though variable fragments are also found. PTHrP may have a morphogenetic role at least in the fetus, because 'knockout' mice show marked developmental defects.
- Vitamin D in the form of the active 1, 25-dihydroxyvitamin D (1, 25 (OH)2D) is also produced ectopically in some tumours (particularly lymphomas) and in some granulomas (particularly sarcoidosis and tuberculosis). This form of vitamin D can now be assayed, though normally the best indicator of vitamin D status is the measurement of 25-hydroxyvitamin D (25OHD) – see Vitamin D.
- Thus, measurement should be made of the PTH level routinely and of the 1, 25 (OH)2D level if lymphoma or sarcoidosis are suspected.

> The major clinical consequence of hypercalcaemia is hypovolaemia from impaired renal reabsorption of salt and water.

Treatment depends on the plasma level.
- If <3.0 mmol/L, no symptoms of dehydration are likely, and no specific treatment is required.
- If >3.0 & <3.5 mmol/L, and there are no significant symptoms, treatment of the underlying disease only is required.
- If >3.5 mmol/L, or if symptoms are present, specific treatment is required.

Treatment priorities are **rehydration** and **lowering of the plasma calcium level**.

- *The most important therapeutic measure is **intravenous saline**, given as 6–8 hrly litres, with furosemide after urine flow is established to promote calciuresis. Since dehydration is the most immediately life-threatening complication of hypercalcaemia, diuretics must be used with great care, and fluid volume should be monitored by measuring the cardiac filling pressures. Hypernatraemia should be avoided by intermittently giving isotonic dextrose. Consequent hypokalaemia or hypomagnesaemia should be avoided.*
- **Corticosteroids** *are effective in some malignancies, in sarcoidosis and following excess vitamin D.*
- **Phosphate** *may be used, provided there is no concomitant hyperphosphataemia, in which case there is the risk of **metastatic calcification**. A dose of 1–1.5 g/24 hr is given IV, but its effect is temporary.*
- **Bisphosphonates** *(biphosphonates) (originally developed as calcium- and phosphate-binding detergents to prevent washing machine scale) are generally regarded as the front-line agents. Disodium **pamidronate** (APD), given in a dose of 90 mg IV over 4 hr, with an onset within 12–24 hr and a duration of up to 2 weeks, is the agent of choice. APD may cause fever, phlebitis, hypomagnesaemia and hypophosphataemia. Sodium etidronate (dose 500 mg orally once to thrice per day) is rarely used now. The newer and more expensive bisphosphonate, **zoledronic acid**, in a dose of 4–8 mg IV over 5 min may have a faster and more prolonged effect and a higher success rate than APD, and it could be usefully considered in those 30% of cases of hypercalcaemia in malignancy with an inadequate response to APD by 10 days. **Osteonecrosis of the jaw** (ONJ) is a serious though uncommon complication of prolonged bisphosphonate treatment, particularly in this setting, with an estimated incidence of about 1 in 1000.*

Because of this complication, a 'drug holiday' is now recommended after 5–10 yr of bisphosphonate therapy.
- **Calcitonin** (q.v.) *produces a rapid though incomplete and transient effect and is only occasionally used. It is given in a dose of 4 U/kg SC 12 hrly.*
- *Plicamycin (mithramycin) is a potent though toxic anticancer agent (dose 25 mcg/kg IV) and is rarely used nowadays for hypercalcaemia.*

Bibliography

Anderson JJB, Toverud SU. Diet and vitamin D: a review with an emphasis on human function. *J Nutr Biochem* 1994; 5: 58.

Beall DP, Scofield RH. Milk-alkali syndrome associated with calcium carbonate consumption. *Medicine* 1995; 74: 89.

Bilerzikian JP. Management of acute hypercalcemia. *N Engl J Med* 1992; 326: 1196.

Cox M, Haddad JG. Lymphoma, hypercalcemia, and the sunshine vitamin. *Ann Intern Med* 1994; 21: 709.

DeLuca HF. Vitamin D metabolism and function. *Arch Intern Med* 1978; 138: 836.

Dickinson M, Prince HM, Kirsa S, et al. Osteonecrosis of the jaw complicating bisphosphonate treatment for bone disease in multiple myeloma: an overview with recommendations for prevention and treatment. *Intern Med J* 2009; 39: 304.

Major P, Lortholary A, Hon J, et al. Zoledronic acid is superior to palmidronate in the treatment of hypercalcaemia of malignancy. *J Clin Oncol* 2001; 19: 558.

Mallette LE. The parathyroid polyhormones: new concepts in the spectrum of peptide hormone action. *Endocr Rev* 1991; 12: 110.

Mundy GR. Hypercalcemia of malignancy revisited. *J Clin Invest* 1988; 82: 1.

Nussbaum SR. Pathophysiology and management of severe hypercalcemia. *Endocrinol Metab Clin North Am* 1993; 22: 343.

Ralston SH, Gallacher SJ, Patel U, et al. Comparison of three intravenous biphosphonates in cancer-associated hypercalcemia. *Lancet* 1989; 2: 1180.

Rodan GA, Fleisch HA. Bisphonates: mechanisms of action. *J Clin Invest* 1996; 97: 2692.

Theriault RL. Hypercalcemia of malignancy: pathophysiology and implications for treatment. *Oncology* 1993; 7: 47.

Wysolmerski JJ, Broadus AE. Hypercalcemia of malignancy: the central role of parathyroid hormone-related protein. *Annu Rev Med* 1994; 45: 189.

Hyperdynamic state

The **hyperdynamic state** comprises generalized vasodilatation and increased blood flow (cardiac output). It is well recognized in clinical medicine as one of the systemic manifestations of inflammation. It is also a prominent feature of exercise, anaemia, pregnancy and thyrotoxicosis.

Despite the increased cardiac output, if the adverse stimuli are sufficiently severe, the hyperdynamic state can become associated with hypotension and sometimes shock, requiring fluid and vasopressor therapy. This situation is typical of early septic shock, as well as of other forms of vasodilatory (i.e. vasoplegic or distributive) shock. It can also be seen after open-heart surgery, anaphylaxis and neurological insults.

> In Intensive Care practice, if the cause of a hyperdynamic state is not apparent, there are a number of uncommon causes which should be considered. These include
> - **adrenal insufficiency** (q.v.),
> - **aspirin toxicity** (q.v.),
> - **beriberi** (q.v.), possibly with associated dilated cardiomyopathy (q.v.),
> - **Paget's disease of bone** (q.v.).
>
> The first three conditions are particularly important, because they require specific therapy without which the circulatory impairment can become refractory.

Bibliography

Levy B, Fritz C, Tahon E, et al. Vasoplegia treatments: the past, the present, and the future. *Crit Care* 2018; 22: 52.

Hypereosinophilic syndrome *See*
- Eosinophilia.

Hyperhidrosis *See*
- Sweating.

Hyperhomocystinaemia *See*
- Thrombophilia.

Hyperparathyroidism

Hyperparathyroidism encompasses several groups of conditions associated with increased circulating levels of parathyroid hormone (PTH).

Primary hyperparathyroidism is usually caused by a single parathyroid adenoma. It can also be caused by diffuse hyperplasia of the chief cells, due either to a parathyrotropic substance or to upwards resetting of the calcium homeostat. Rarely, it may be caused by parathyroid carcinoma. It is one of the important presenting features of multiple endocrine neoplasia (MEN) type I (q.v.).

Persistent hyperparathyroidism may sometimes be due to **parathyromatosis**, which is caused by small nodules of hypersecreting tissue throughout the neck and mediastinum which have been either derived from embryonic rests or seeded from the gland itself (for example, at surgery).

Normally, PTH secretion is controlled by the Ca^{++}-sensing receptor, which comprises a receptor on the cell surface coupled to an intracellular part via transmembrane elements characteristic of the G protein–coupled receptor superfamily. A similar receptor is also present on the thyroid C cells (where it controls calcitonin secretion), in the kidney (where it controls calcium and phosphorus exchange), and in the central nervous system (where its role is currently uncertain).

Clinical features of primary hyperparathyroidism are numerous and variable.
- The classical features of the student's triad ('**bones, stones and abdominal groans**') are in fact uncommon.
- Most patients are asymptomatic, having been discovered during coincidental plasma calcium screening.
- Skeletal features include pain, local tenderness, spontaneous fracture, cystic lesions (osteitis fibrosa cystica) and pseudogout (q.v.).
- Renal features include nephrolithiasis (q.v.), nephrocalcinosis, polyuria and dysfunction.
- Abdominal features include pain, constipation, weight loss and pancreatitis (q.v.).
- Neuromuscular features include weakness, fatigue, apathy, somnolence, depression and hypotonia.
- Cardiovascular features include hypertension and short QT interval.
- Miscellaneous features include calcium deposits in the conjunctiva.

The skeletal features are due to increased PTH, while the other features are chiefly due to the resultant hypercalcaemia.

Diagnosis is based on the demonstration of hypercalcaemia (q.v.) in the presence of an increased serum PTH level. There is associated hypophosphataemia (q.v.) and hyperchloraemia. The urinary calcium is usually increased.

If the urinary calcium is not increased, benign or **familial hypocalciuric hypercalcaemia** (FHH) should be suspected. This is a rare condition inherited as an autosomal dominant and caused by a defect in the Ca^{++}-sensing receptor in the parathyroid (and kidney).

X-ray, especially of the skull and hands, may show typical changes. In some patients, hypercalcaemia may be masked by concomitant renal disease, liver disease, vitamin D deficiency or magnesium deficiency.

Treatment is **surgical**, though successful parathyroidectomy requires particular operative experience and skill. Minimally invasive surgery for this has been developed. There is a risk of **postoperative tetany**, especially if there is significant bony disease, which causes the 'hungry bone phenomenon' and which requires prompt and often vigorous treatment with calcium and 1,25-dihydroxyvitamin D. The subsequent postoperative course may be associated with either hypoparathyroidism or recurrent hyperparathyroidism.

Follow-up alone without surgery is acceptable if the hypercalcaemia is mild (<3 mmol/L), the alkaline phosphatase is not elevated and the patient is truly asymptomatic (i.e. there is an absence of even subtle symptoms, including any of a psychiatric nature).

Secondary hyperparathyroidism is a complication of other diseases, especially chronic renal failure. It arises from stimulation of PTH from hypocalcaemia (q.v.) and hyperphosphataemia (q.v.).

Since the hyperparathyroidism is compensatory, hypercalcaemia is uncommon.

The diagnosis is
- suspected when the serum calcium level in this setting is normal instead of low,
- strengthened if there is specific bone disease (osteitis fibrosa cystica), and
- confirmed if the PTH assay is elevated.

Treatment is of the underlying disease where possible.
- **Phosphate-binding agents** (non-aluminium containing) and small doses of **vitamin D** may be used.
- The new calcimimetic agent, **cinacalcet**, has been found to be useful in this setting, though it is very expensive.

'Tertiary' hyperparathyroidism is seen in the occasional patient with secondary hyperparathyroidism, in whom a hyperplastic gland is presumed to become autonomous and produce an adenoma which then leads to hypercalcaemia.

It is most convincingly documented by persistent hypercalcaemia after renal transplantation, though even then severe secondary disease may take over a year for the hyperplastic glands to regress.

Parathyroidectomy with removal of all glands and autotransplantation is occasionally required for tertiary hyperparathyroidism.

'**Pseudo**' **hyperparathyroidism** is the term used to describe hypercalcaemia presumed to be due to ectopic hormone production in malignancy. Hypercalcaemia in this setting is not in fact commonly due to ectopic PTH production but to parathyroid hormone related protein (PTHrP) (see Hypercalcaemia), and the term is thus usually a misnomer.

Bibliography
Becker C. Diseases of calcium metabolism and metabolic bone disease. In: *Scientific American Medicine. Endocrinology & Metabolism.* Hamilton: Dekker Medicine. 2020.
Bilezikian JP, Potts JT, Fuleihan G-H, et al. Summary statement from a workshop on asymptomatic primary hyperparathyroidism: a perspective for the 21st century. *J Bone Miner Res* 2002; 17 (suppl. 2): N2.
Block GA, Martin KJ, de Francisco ALM, et al. Cinacalcet for secondary hyperparathyroidism in patients receiving hemodialysis. *Ne Engl J Med* 2004; 350: 1516.
Brown EM. Extracellular Ca^{2+} sensing regulation of parathyroid cell function, and role of Ca^{2+} and other ions as extracellular (first) messengers. *Physiol Rev* 1991; 71: 371.
Brown EM, Gamba G, Riccardi D, et al. Cloning and characterization of an extracellular Ca^{2+}-sensing receptor from bovine parathyroid. *Nature* 1993; 366: 575.
Deftos LJ, Parthemore JG, Stabile BE. Management of primary hyperparathyroidism. *Annu Rev Med* 1993; 44: 19.
Fischer JA. 'Asymptomatic' and symptomatic primary hyperparathyroidism. *Clin Invest* 1993; 71: 505.
Glendenning P. Diagnosis of primary hyperparathyroidism: controversies, practical issues and the need for Australian guidelines. *Intern Med J* 2003; 33: 598.
Heath H. Familial benign (hypocalciuric) hypercalcemia: a troublesome mimic of mild primary hyperparathyroidism. *Endocrinol Metab Clin North Am* 1989; 18: 723.
Heath H, Hodgson SE, Kennedy MA. Primary hyperparathyroidism: incidence, morbidity and potential economic impact in a community. *N Engl J Med* 1980; 302: 189.
Mallette LE. The parathyroid polyhormones: new concepts in the spectrum of peptide hormone action. *Endocr Rev* 1991; 12: 110.
Pocotte SL, Ehrenstein G, Fitzpatrick LA. Regulation of parathyroid hormone secretion. *Endocr Rev* 1991; 12: 291.
Slatopolsky E, Delmez JA. Pathogenesis of secondary hyperparathyroidism. *Am J Kidney Dis* 1994; 23: 229.
Tonner DR, Schlechte JA. Neurologic complications of thyroid and parathyroid disease. *Med Clin North Am* 1993; 77: 251.

Hyperphosphataemia

Hyperphosphataemia is associated with
- acute and chronic renal failure,
- hypercalcaemia (q.v.) due to increased gastrointestinal absorption,
- secondary hyperparathyroidism (q.v.),
- pseudohypoparathyroidism (q.v.),
- the tumour-lysis syndrome (see Cancer complications) or other acute cell lysis (as in burns or rhabdomyolysis – q.v.),
- sodium phosphate (e.g. Fleet) used orally as an osmotic laxative for bowel preparation before colonoscopy. These preparations are hypertonic and can cause major fluid and electrolyte disturbances, especially in patients with comorbidities related to cardiovascular, kidney or liver disease.

Treatment is by **restricting phosphate intake**, *which also helps to maintain the serum calcium at a normal level and thus decreases the risks of secondary hyperparathyroidism (q.v.), osteodystrophy and* **metastatic calcification** *in chronic renal failure. Since the necessary dietary restriction to 800–1000 mg per day results in an unpalatable diet, a phosphate-binding antacid may usefully be added, though care should be taken with either magnesium- or aluminium-based antacids. The serum phosphate level should be kept at 1.5–2 mmol/L.*

The new agents **lanthanum** *and* **sevelamer** *have been found to be useful in this setting.*

Bibliography
Coburn JW, Salusky IB. Control of serum phosphorus in uremia. *N Engl J Med* 1989; 320: 1140.
Connor A, Tolan D, Hughes S, et al. Consensus guidelines for the safe prescription and administration of oral bowel-cleansing agents. *Gut* 2012; 61: 1525.
Weisinger JR, Bellorin-Font E. Magnesium and phosphorus. *Lancet* 1998; 352: 391.

Hypersensitivity pneumonitis

Hypersensitivity pneumonitis (extrinsic allergic alveolitis, EAA) is an interstitial lung disease produced by the inhalation of organic dusts.

> **Farmer's lung** (due to a thermophilic *Actinomyces* growing in mouldy hay) used to be the most common example, until recent changes in farming practices.
> Other common examples are
> - **bird fancier's lung**
>   - due to pigeon, budgerigar, hen or parrot proteins,
> - **humidifier fever**
>   - due to organisms similar to those causing farmer's lung but growing in forced air heating, cooling or humidification systems.

There are many other causes of hypersensitivity pneumonitis, but they are quite uncommon and generally associated with unusual occupational, recreational or environmental exposures, as follows
- animal food worker's lung (fish meal),
- bagassosis (mouldy, overheated, sugar cane bagasse),
- bible-printer's lung (mouldy typesetting water),
- blackfat tobacco smoker's lung (blackfat tobacco),
- cheese worker's lung (cheese mould),
- coffee worker's lung (coffee-bean extract or dust),
- corn farmer's lung (corn dust),
- detergent lung (detergents),
- furrier's lung (fox fur),
- hot tub lung (mycobacteria),
- laboratory worker's lung (rat urine),
- malt worker's lung (mouldy barley, malt dust),
- maple bark stripper's lung (mouldy maple bark),
- mummy-handler's lung (mummy wrappings),
- mushroom worker's lung (mushroom compost),
- New Guinea lung (mouldy thatch dust),
- paper mill-worker's lung (mouldy wood pulp),
- paprika splitter's lung (paprika dust),
- pituitary snuff taker's lung (heterologous pituitary powder),
- saxophonist's lung (mouldy reed),
- sequoiosis (mouldy redwood sawdust),
- suberosis (mouldy oak bark, cork dust),
- tea grower's lung (tea plants),
- tobacco grower's/worker's lung (mouldy tobacco),
- wheat weevil disease (infected wheat flour),
- wine grower's lung (mouldy grapes),
- woodworker's lung (mouldy sawdust).

Since the responsible inhaled antigens are small, i.e. $<1\mu$, they penetrate to the distal alveoli, unlike the larger antigens involved with asthma which are deposited more proximally. Since only a minority of exposed subjects develop symptomatic disease, there is clearly marked variation in individual susceptibility to the resultant immune and inflammatory response. It is less common in tobacco smokers.

> Unlike asthma, the clinical features of hypersensitivity pneumonitis include
> - marked systemic upset,
>   - with fever, headache, myalgia and malaise, often of a flu-like nature and resulting in a common misdiagnosis of infection,
> - respiratory features of a restrictive rather than obstructive nature,
>   - with symptoms of cough and dyspnoea but not generally wheeze, and findings of crackles rather than rhonchi.

The course is usually acute, typically occurring within 6–8 hr of exposure to the relevant antigen. It subsides spontaneously if the antigen is removed, but it may be prolonged for weeks if there is continued exposure, as on a farm. In such cases, the onset may sometimes be insidious. Occasionally, a chronic process may be seen with cough and dyspnoea on exertion but no systemic features and often no prior acute episodes identified.

Chest X-ray shows micronodular shadows initially and fibrosis (especially of the upper lobes) later. High-resolution CT scan is more sensitive than plain X-ray in showing the pulmonary structural changes. Lung function tests show a restrictive ventilatory defect and impaired gas exchange in the acute and chronic phases of the disease but not in the intervals between acute episodes.

The diagnosis is particularly dependent on a history of appropriate exposure. Precipitating antibodies to specific antigen are detectable in acute cases, but positive serology indicates only exposure to antigen and not necessarily disease therefrom. Other causes of interstitial disease should be excluded, though separation from idiopathic pulmonary fibrosis (q.v.) or other idiopathic interstitial pneumonias (q.v.) may be difficult. Lung biopsy in such patients will often show granulomas, which then suggest the correct diagnosis. The brochoalveolar lavage (BAL) fluid has >50% lymphocytes, mostly suppressor-cytotoxic T cells, but these findings are of limited diagnostic specificity. International consensus guidelines for the diagnosis of hypersensitivity pneumonitis have recently been published.

Avoidance of the offending antigen usually results in complete symptomatic remission. A short course of *corticosteroids* hastens resolution in acute farmer's lung, but steroid agents are mostly reserved for cases of hypersensitivity pneumonitis which are severe or chronic. *Immunosuppressive therapy*, e.g. with azathioprine or *mycophenolate*, may be useful as steroid-sparing in chronic cases (see Immunomodulation).

Bibliography
Bernardo J, Center DM. Hypersensitivity pneumonia. *Dis Mon* 1981; 27: 1.
Fernandez-Perez ER, Travis WD, Lynch DA, et al. Executive summary: diagnosis and evaluation of hypersensitivity pneumonitis: CHEST guideline and expert panel report. *Chest* 2021; 160: 595.
Fink JN, Ortega HG, Reynolds HY, et al. Needs and opportunities for research in hypersensitivity pneumonitis. *Am J Respir Crit Care Med* 2005; 171: 792.
Glazer C, Rose C, Lynch D. Clinical and radiological manifestations of hypersensitivity pneumonitis. *J Thorac Imaging* 2002; 17: 261.
Ismail T, McSharry C, Royd G. Extrinsic allergic alveolitis. *Respirology* 2006; 11: 262.
Lacasse Y, Girard M, Cornier Y. Recent advances in hypersensitivity pneumonitis. *Chest* 2012; 142: 208.
Mohr LC. Hypersensitivity pneumonitis. *Curr Opin Pulm Med* 2004; 10: 401.
Morell F, Roger A, Cruz M-J, et al. Suberosis: clinical study and new etiologic agents in a series of eight patients. *Chest* 2003; 124: 1145.
Nicholson DP. Extrinsic allergic pneumonias. *Am J Med* 1972; 53: 131.
Salvaggio JE. Extrinsic allergic alveolitis: past, present and future. *Clin Exp Allergy* 1997; 27 (suppl. 1): 18.

Hypersplenism

Hypersplenism refers to a diverse group of conditions associated with **splenomegaly** from any cause and with consequent removal of the formed elements of the blood.

The splenomegaly is most commonly congestive and due to portal or splenic vein obstruction, as in hepatic cirrhosis or cardiac failure.

It may also occur from direct infiltration, as in
- lymphoma,
- myeloproliferative disorders,
- collagen-vascular disorders (q.v.),
- granulomatous disease,
- infectious diseases,
- Felty's syndrome (q.v.).

Clinically, there is haemolytic anaemia (see Anaemia), although even massive splenomegaly does not always cause a decreased red blood cell mass, since there may be considerable haemodilution. Other formed elements, particularly platelets, may also be removed. The bone marrow is typically hyperplastic, unless there is a primary haematological disorder.

Treatment may require **splenectomy**, including any accessory spleen(s), if clinical disease is substantial.
- *Corticosteroids or radiotherapy may sometimes be helpful.*
See also
- Splenomegaly.

Bibliography
Bohnsack JF, Brown EJ. The role of the spleen in resistance to infection. *Annu Rev Med* 1986; 37: 49.
Rose WF. The spleen as a filter. *N Engl J Med* 1987; 317: 704.

Hyperthermia See
- Pyrexia.

Hyperthyroidism

Hyperthyroidism can have a number of causes.
1. **Graves' disease** refers to autoimmune thyroid disease characterized by diffuse toxic goitre and caused by the production of antibodies to thyroid-stimulating hormone (TSH) receptors (and thus loss of endogenous TSH control) (see Autoimmune disorders).

Other associated features of an autoimmune nature may sometimes be seen, particularly including ophthalmopathy and pretibial myxoedema.

> The classical clinical picture of Graves' disease, often seen in a young woman, includes
> **Symptoms** of
> - palpitations,
> - tremor,
> - sweating (q.v.),
> - weight loss,
> - irritability and insomnia;
> **Signs** of
> - smooth non-tender goitre,
> - proptosis and lid lag, with occasionally the more severe eye involvement of exophthalmos or even ophthalmoplegia (see below),
> - hyperdynamic circulatory state (q.v.),
> - tremor,
> - palmar erythema,
> - clubbing (rarely).

Investigations show increased T4 and T3 and suppressed TSH levels. If there is associated hypoproteinaemia and thus decreased thyroxine-binding globulin (TBG), the free T4 level needs to be measured (or calculated). Hyperthyroidism is excluded by a normal TSH level, unless the patient has a TSH-secreting pituitary tumour (see below).

Treatment options include **antithyroid drugs** *(carbimazole, propylthiouracil),* **subtotal thyroidectomy** *or* **radioiodine** *(commonly in a standard dose of 555 MBq or 15 mCi), the choice varying between centres. Some clinicians treat with antithyroid drugs for 12–18 months, following which about 50% of patients are in remission and need no further treatment, while about 50% relapse and need surgery or radioiodine. Some clinicians instead favour initial ablation therapy with radioiodine (except in young women), followed by replacement therapy.*

Beta blockade, sedation, rest, adequate nutrition and long-term follow-up are also important.

2. **Toxic nodular goitre** arises in a pre-existing goitre, in which eventual autonomy of thyroid hormone production occurs.
3. **Toxic adenoma** (Plummer's nodule) may be a variant of toxic nodular goitre but may also occur within an atrophic gland.
4. **Drug-induced hyperthyroidism** can occur following the deliberate ingestion of T4 or T3. More practically, it can follow the administration of iodine-containing medications, especially **amiodarone**, which can produce a variety of abnormalities of thyroid function, including hyperthyroidism (which is reported to occur in 10% of patients on a low iodine intake). In this condition, there is an isolated increase in T4 and not T3.
5. **Excess TSH** from a pituitary tumour can cause hyperthyroidism. In this setting, there may be headache and the eye signs are different, since they include field defects. There are no associated autoimmune phenomena. Rarely, increased TSH may be produced but without resultant hyperthyroidism, because of thyroid hormone resistance.

Hyperthyroidism may sometimes present in a number of less common forms.
1. **Occult hyperthyroidism** is seen especially in elderly patients, in whom its first clinical manifestation is cardiac. Thus, arrhythmias (especially atrial fibrillation), angina and cardiac failure are the usual features.

This is an important phenomenon, because it is one of the specifically treatable causes of cardiac disease.

The diagnosis is confirmed by an elevated T3 and decreased TSH, but the T4 level is not necessarily elevated.

2. **Atypical hyperthyroidism** refers to the condition when one single, perhaps atypical, clinical feature predominates, such as myopathy or personality change.
3. **Pregnancy-associated hyperthyroidism** may occur in a molar pregnancy (see Pregnancy – 5. neoplasia).
4. **Drug-suppressed hyperthyroidism** occurs especially during concomitant beta blocker administration. Beta blockers mask many of the prominent clinical features of hyperthyroidism, including tremor, sweating and circulatory changes, though they do not influence weight loss, personality changes, goitre, eye signs or laboratory tests.

5. **Thyroid storm** refers to a severe exacerbation of hyperthyroidism with fever, dehydration, shock and extreme restlessness. Weakness, seizures, coma, abdominal symptoms and cardiac failure may occur. It was first described by Lahey in 1928.

It is one of the uncommon causes of **multiorgan failure** (q.v.), when it may mimic the features of severe sepsis. It is a rare but important endocrine emergency with life-threatening potential. Even with Intensive Care, the mortality is probably about 20%.

It usually follows concomitant infection, but it may follow trauma or the abrupt withdrawal of antithyroid drugs. It has also been reported following the use of radiographic iodinated contrast media in patients with existing hyperthyroidism.

If the underlying hyperthyroidism was not previously known, it may be difficult to detect in the presence of severe infection or trauma, but it may be suspected if the physiological response to the current insult appears excessive.

It is confirmed by the finding of increased T4 or T3 and suppressed TSH levels.

The condition requires urgent **resuscitation** *and treatment of the precipitating disease. If cardiogenic shock has occurred,* **veno-arterial extracorporeal membrane oxygenation** *(ECMO) has been recommended.*

Treatment of the thyrotoxic component is multifaceted and requires decreasing the synthesis of thyroid hormone, blocking its release and inhibiting its peripheral effects.

- **Antithyroid** *treatment is given as propylthiouracil (100 mg qid nasogastrically, followed by sodium iodide 0.5 g IV bd).*
- **Beta blockers** *should be used and also* **corticosteroids** *in very severe cases.*

- *Plasmapheresis (q.v.) use has been reported in very severe cases, but it has been of doubtful efficacy. Following resolution of the emergency condition, the underlying thyrotoxicosis then requires definitive treatment.*

6. **Malignant exophthalmos** refers to severe sight-threatening eye involvement. It is part of the constellation of features comprising the inflammatory entity, thyroid-associated ophthalmopathy (TAO), which is considered to be an autoimmune complication of Graves' disease.

   The hyperthyroidism is treated on its normal merits, although radioiodine has been reported to exacerbate ophthalmopathy.

   - First-line treatment for exophthalmos is usually with **corticosteroids**, though oral selenium (q.v.) may be helpful in less severe cases. More severe cases require **immunomodulation** (q.v.), such as with ciclosporin, mycophenolate, rituximab (q.v.), immune globulin (**or plasmapheresis – q.v.**) or the insulin-like growth factor 1 receptor (IGF-1R) inhibitor **teprotumumab**.
   - In vision-threatening disease, surgical **decompression** of the orbit is required, together with tarsorrhaphy, high-dose steroids and sometimes orbital radiotherapy.

Bibliography

Bourcier S, Coutrot M, Kimmoun A, et al. Thyroid storm in the ICU: a retrospective multicenter study. *Crit Care Med* 2020; 48: 83.

Burrow GN. The management of thyrotoxicosis in pregnancy. *N Engl J Med* 1985; 313: 562.

Carter JA, Utiger RD. The ophthalmopathy of Graves' disease. *Annu Rev Med* 1992; 43: 487.

Cooper DS. Which anti-thyroid drug? *Am J Med* 1986; 80: 1165.

Cooper DS. Hyperthyroidism. *Lancet* 2003; 362: 459.

DeGroot LJ, Quintans J. The causes of autoimmune thyroid disease. *Endocr Rev* 1989; 10: 537.

El-Kaissi S, Frauman AG, Wall JR. Thyroid-associated ophthalmopathy: a practical guide to classification, natural history and management. *Intern Med J* 2004; 34: 482.

Franklyn J, Sheppard M. Radioiodine for thyrotoxicosis: perhaps the best option. *BMJ* 1992; 305: 727.

Hall AJH, Topliss DJ. Medical and surgical treatment of thyroid eye disease. *Intern Med J* 2022; 52: 14.

Jiang YZ, Hutchinson KA, Bartelloni P, et al. Thyroid storm presenting as multiple organ dysfunction syndrome. *Chest* 2000; 118: 877.

Khir ASM. Suspected thyrotoxicosis. *BMJ* 1985; 290: 916.

Lazar MA. Thyroid hormone receptors: multiple forms, multiple possibilities. *Endocr Rev* 1993; 14: 184.

Magner JA. Thyroid-stimulating hormone: biosynthesis, cell biology, and bioactivity. *Endocr Rev* 1990; 11: 354.

Nayak B, Burman K. Thyrotoxicosis and thyroid storm. *Endocrinol Metab Clin North Am* 2006; 35: 663.

Ramsay I. Drug and non-thyroid induced changes in thyroid function tests. *Postgrad Med J* 1985; 61: 375.

Shupnik MA, Ridgway EC, Chin WW. Molecular biology of thyrotropin. *Endocr Rev* 1989; 10: 459.

Smallridge RC. Metabolic and anatomic thyroid emergencies: a review. *Crit Care Med* 1992; 20: 276.

Smith TJ, Hegedus L. Graves' disease. *N Engl J Med* 2016; 375: 1552.

Stockigt JR. Hyperthyroidism secondary to drugs and acute illness. *Endocrinologist* 1993; 3: 67.

Surks MI, Chopra IJ, Mariash CN, et al. American Thyroid Association guidelines for use of laboratory tests in thyroid disorders. *JAMA* 1990; 263: 1529.

Tonner DR, Schlechte JA. Neurologic complications of thyroid and parathyroid disease. *Med Clin North Am* 1993; 77: 251.

Topliss DJ, Eastman CJ. Diagnosis and management of hyperthyroidism and hypothyroidism. *Med J Aust* 2004; 180: 186.

Waldstein SS, Slodki SJ, Kaganiec GI. A clinical study of thyroid storm. *Ann Intern Med* 1960; 52: 626.

Woeber KA. Thyrotoxicosis and the heart. *N Engl J Med* 1992; 327: 94.

Wong R, Farrell SG, Grossmann M. Thyroid nodules: diagnosis and management. *Med J Aust* 2018; 209: 92.

Hypertrichosis See
- Hirsutism.

Hyperuricaemia See
- Gout.

Hyperviscosity See
- Multiple myeloma.

Hypocalcaemia

The plasma calcium represents <1% of the total body calcium, and of this only the ionized fraction (normally about 50%) influences physiological events. The non-ionized (i.e. protein-bound) fraction is typically low in critically ill patients because hypoalbuminaemia is so common. Thus, the ionized or free calcium level can be normal despite a low total serum calcium in these patients.

On the other hand, the ionized calcium level itself is also frequently abnormal in critically ill patients, in whom it does not necessarily indicate a true calcium abnormality but may be merely a marker (like many other abnormal parameters) of the severity of the patient's illness. In these cases, when the illness resolves, the ionized calcium level returns to normal without specific treatment.

> True **hypocalcaemia** refers to decreased ionized calcium (iCa), which is nowadays measured directly and conveniently by most modern blood gas analyzers.
>
> Alternatively, a corrected total calcium (mmol/L) may be calculated approximately as:
>
> $$\text{ionized Ca}^{++} = \text{measured total Ca}^{++} + (0.02 \times (40-\text{serum albumin})).$$
>
> However, this formula and other similar ones have been criticized for their inaccuracy in the Intensive Care setting.

Hypocalcaemia is classified as due to
1. **Parathyroid deficiency**
This occurs most commonly post-thyroidectomy, but may also be post-parathyroidectomy (the 'hungry bone' syndrome, see Hyperparathyroidism) or idiopathic (see Hypoparathyroidism).
2. **Parathyroid hormone resistance**
This is seen with pseudohypoparathyroidism (q.v.), chronic renal failure, malabsorption (q.v.), hypo- and hyper-magnesaemia (see Magnesium), hyperphosphataemia (q.v.) and drugs (especially phenytoin).
3. **Other conditions**
These include disorders such as pancreatitis (q.v.), rhabdomyolysis (q.v.) and osteoblastic metastases.

In the second two groups of causes (i.e. 2. & 3. above), parathyroid hormone (PTH) levels are increased.

Relative hypocalcaemia may be caused by haemodilution, as in resuscitation of patients with severe trauma and following massive transfusion (due to calcium chelation from the citrate anticoagulant).

The clinical features of hypocalcaemia comprise those of the underlying disease as well as of the low serum calcium level itself. The latter depend on the rate as well as the severity of the deficiency. Although most hypocalcaemia is mild and asymptomatic (especially in critically ill patients), clinical features may include paraesthesiae, especially around the mouth, restlessness and Trousseau's and/or Chvostek's signs. More chronic hypocalcaemia may give rise to fatigue and muscle aches. The ECG typically shows a prolonged QT interval.

Treatment of acute hypocalcaemia (if required) is with **calcium** IV (e.g. 10 mL of 10% calcium gluconate (= 1 g = 2.2 mmol)) or orally (e.g. 1 g of calcium chloride (= 6.8 mmol) tds. The recommended normal daily intake of calcium for maintenance of bone health is 1000 mg per day for men and 1200 mg per day for women.

Clearly, the underlying disease requires treatment, and as indicated above this may be all that is required to correct the hypocalcaemia.

Calcium supplementation (with or without concomitant vitamin D, q.v.) is commonly prescribed in the community in normocalcaemic and otherwise well patients to improve bone health. However, it has not been shown to prevent osteoporosis or fractures, and it may exacerbate constipation, renal calculi and cardiovascular disease.

Bibliography
Aberegg SK. Ionized calcium in the ICU: should it be measured and corrected? *Chest* 2016; 149: 846.
Becker C. Diseases of calcium metabolism and metabolic bone disease. In: *Scientific American Medicine. Endocrinology & Metabolism*. Hamilton: Dekker Medicine. 2020.
Cholst IN, Steinberg SF, Tropper PJ, et al. The influence of hypermagnesemia on serum calcium and parathyroid hormone levels in human subjects. *N Engl J Med* 1984; 310: 1221.
Kelly A, Levine MA. Hypocalcemia in the critically ill patient. *J Intens Care Med* 2013; 28: 166.
Lebowitz MR, Moses AM. Hypocalcemia. *Semin Nephrol* 1992; 12: 146.
Reid IR, Bolland MJ. Controversies in medicine: the role of calcium and vitamin D supplements in adults. *Med J Aust* 2019; 211: 468.
Slomp J, van der Voort PHJ, Gerritsen RT, et al. Albumin-adjusted calcium is not suitable for diagnosis of hyper- and hypocalcemia in the critically ill. *Crit Care Med* 2003; 31: 1389.
Vivien B, Langeron O, Morell E, et al. Early hypocalcemia in severe trauma. *Crit Care Med* 2005; 33: 1946.
Zaloga GP. Hypocalcemia in critically ill patients. *Crit Care Med* 1992; 20: 251.

Hypoglycaemia See
- Islet cell tumour,
- Paraneoplastic syndromes – Ectopic hormone production.
  See also
- Acromegaly,
- Acute fatty liver of pregnancy,
- Adrenal insufficiency,
- Adrenocorticotropic hormone,
- Amnesia,
- Factitious disorders,

- Glycogen storage disorders,
- Heat shock proteins,
- Hepatocellular carcinoma,
- Hypothermia,
- Lung tumours,
- Malaria,
- Sweating.

Hypokalaemia *See*
- Conn's syndrome,
- Cushing's syndrome.

See also
- Anorexia nervosa,
- Carbonic anhydrase inhibitors,
- Cardiomyopathy – Dilated cardiomyopathy,
- Diarrhoea – VIPoma,
- Drugs and the kidney – Acute kidney injury (AKI, acute tubular necrosis),
- Heat stroke,
- Hypercalcaemia,
- Magnesium,
- Myopathy,
- Periodic paralysis,
- Renal tubular acidosis,
- Rhabdomyolysis,
- Syndrome of inappropriate antidiuretic hormone,
- Tubulointerstitial diseases.

Hyponatraemia

Hyponatraemia refers to a plasma sodium concentration <135 mmol/L. It is termed mild if <135 mmol/L, moderate if <130 mmol/L and severe if <125 mmol/L. If it has developed within 48 hr, it is termed acute. It is a common finding in seriously ill patients, in whom it is associated with adverse clinical outcomes.

Hyponatraemia is most frequently associated with
- surgical complications
  - the postoperative or post-traumatic state (due to increased secretion of ADH, see Antidiuretic hormone),
  - transurethral resection of the prostate,
  - bowel preparation,
- systemic disorders
  - congestive cardiac failure,
  - hepatic cirrhosis,
  - endocrine failure (adrenal, thyroid),
  - CNS damage,
- polydipsia
- drugs
  - thiazides especially, but also NSAIDs, opiates, PPIs,
  - ADH-like agents (oxytocin, desmopressin, vasopressin) (see Antidiuretic hormone).

The symptoms of hyponatraemia are due to **brain oedema** (hyponatremic encephalopathy) and include headache, confusion and nausea, together with vomiting, seizures and coma in severe cases. However, these symptoms are non-specific, and they do not necessarily have a good relationship with either the severity or the acuteness of the underlying biochemical defect. Moreover, mild cases are commonly asymptomatic.

Hyponatraemia can be classified in a number of ways, but it is important to remember that optimal treatment cannot follow any single classification based on the key parameters of plasma sodium concentration, the speed of development, the severity of symptoms, the patient's volume status or the serum osmolality. In general, the most useful first step has traditionally been clinical assessment to determine whether the patient is hypovolaemic, euvolaemic or hypervolaemic.

Hypovolaemic hyponatraemia indicates a loss of both sodium and fluid, as with excess gastrointestinal, renal or skin losses. This form of hyponatraemia can lead to a typical resuscitation emergency in Intensive Care practice. The urine sodium concentration is <30 mmol/L (except in renal disease, after diuretics, in adrenal insufficiency or after vomiting) and the urine osmolality is >100 mOsm/kg.

Euvolaemic hyponatraemia typically occurs in syndrome of inappropriate antidiuretic hormone secretion (SIADH) (q.v.) or with polydipsia and is due to water retention rather than sodium deficit. The urine sodium concentration is >30 mmol/L. The urine osmolality is >100 mOsm/kg in SIADH and <100 mOsm/kg in polydipsia.

Hypervolaemic hyponatraemia occurs in congestive cardiac failure, hepatic cirrhosis or some forms of renal failure (e.g. nephrotic syndrome). It is due to both salt and especially water retention, and thus there is associated oedema. The urine sodium concentration is <30 mmol/L and the urine osmolality is >100 mOsm/kg.

True hyponatraemia is always **hypotonic**, with a serum osmolality of <275 mOsm/kg. By contrast, **pseudohyponatraemia** (q.v.) occurs when other osmotically active substances are present, e.g. glucose, mannitol, glycine or radiocontrast media. These may or may not be included in formulae used to calculate osmolality, so that measured osmolality should always be used in such circumstances.

The treatment of hyponatraemia depends on its cause, severity and acuity. Detailed management principles are discussed under **central pontine myelinolysis** (q.v.) and **syndrome of inappropriate antidiuretic hormone** (q.v.). In principle, urgent repair of hyponatraemia is indicated only if there are severe symptoms, in which case the risk from brain oedema is greater than the potential risk of osmotic demyelination (see Central pontine myelinolysis).

See
- Central pontine myelinolysis,
- Cerebral salt wasting,
- Pseudohyponatraemia,
- Syndrome of inappropriate antidiuretic hormone.

See also
- Adrenal insufficiency,
- Aldosterone,
- Amphetamines,
- Atrial natriuretic factor,
- Carbonic anhydrase inhibitors,
- Porphyria.

Bibliography

Achinger SG, Ayus JC. Treatment of hyponatremic encephalopathy in the critically ill. *Crit Care Med* 2017; 45: 1762.

Nigro N, Grossmann M, Chiang C, et al. Polyuria-polydipsia syndrome: a diagnostic challenge. *Intern Med J* 2018; 48: 244.

Spasovski G, Vanholder R, Allolio B, et al. Clinical practice guideline on diagnosis and treatment of hyponatraemia. *Intens Care Med* 2014; 40: 320.

Tee SL, Sindone A, Roger S, et al. Hyponatraemia in heart failure. *Intern Med J* 2020; 50: 659.

Hypoparathyroidism

Hypoparathyroidism refers to the failure of the parathyroid gland to secrete parathyroid hormone (PTH). The condition may be either idiopathic or postoperative (i.e. following parathyroidectomy or more commonly thyroidectomy).

Idiopathic hypoparathyroidism may be an isolated defect, sometimes genetic. More commonly, it is associated with
- antibodies to other endocrine organs
  - and thus often other endocrine failure, especially of the thyroid and adrenal glands,
- mucocutaneous candidiasis
  - when the condition is referred to as polyglandular autoimmunity type I.

A rare type of hypoparathyroidism is the Di George syndrome, with associated lymphopenia (q.v.) and thymic aplasia.

The clinical features of hypoparathyroidism are those of **hypocalcaemia** (q.v.).

Treatment is with **vitamin D**, since it has a similar action to PTH and since PTH has not been to date a practical therapeutic agent. However, trials of recombinant human PTH (**teriparatide**) have been effective in hypoparathyroidism.
- Hypoparathyroidism if acute requires calcium IV (e.g. 10 mL of 10% calcium gluconate) or if less acute calcium chloride 1 g orally tds.
- Synthetic vitamin D analogs may also be used.

Pseudohypoparathyroidism refers to the syndrome of PTH-resistance, first described by Albright, in which there is hypocalcaemia, hyperphosphataemia, parathyroid hyperplasia and the somatic abnormalities of short stature, moon face and obesity.

The occasional case in which there is normocalcaemia is sometimes referred to as **pseudopseudohypoparathyroidism**.

In fact, several other mechanisms may also cause PTH-resistance, including
- chronic renal failure,
- malabsorption (q.v.),
- hypomagnesaemia (see Magnesium),
- drugs (especially phenytoin).

Bibliography

Bilezikian JP, Brandi ML, Cusano NE, et al. Management of hypoparathyroidism: present and future. *J Clin Endocrinol Metab* 2016; 101: 2313.

Loriaux DL. The polyendocrine deficiency syndromes. *N Engl J Med* 1985; 312: 1568.

Pocotte SL, Ehrenstein G, Fitzpatrick LA. Regulation of parathyroid hormone secretion. *Endocr Rev* 1991; 12: 291.

Tonner DR, Schlechte JA. Neurologic complications of thyroid and parathyroid disease. *Med Clin North Am* 1993; 77: 251.

Hypophosphataemia

Hypophosphataemia may have a large variety of causes. These include
- primary hyperparathyroidism (q.v.),
- hypercalcaemia of malignancy (q.v.),
- phosphate-binding antacids,
- hypertonic carbohydrate feeding,
- renal tubular defects,
- dialysis and other forms of renal replacement therapy (RRT),
- correction of diabetic ketoacidosis,
- refeeding syndrome (q.v.),
- liver disease,

- malabsorption (q.v.),
- osteomalacia (except in chronic renal failure),
- post-exercise exhaustion,
- heat stroke (q.v.),
- respiratory alkalosis.

A **phosphate level of <0.5 mmol/L** is associated with
- muscular weakness, including diaphragmatic dysfunction and ventilator dependence,
- rhabdomyolysis (q.v.),
- 2,3-diphosphoglycerate depletion (and thus a left-shifted oxygen dissociation curve),
- impaired neutrophil function.

A **phosphate level of <0.3 mmol/L** is additionally associated with
- impaired red cell glycolysis and thus haemolysis (see Anaemia).

Treatment of significant hypophosphataemia requires **phosphate** *ions IV. This is given as sodium/potassium phosphate (13.4 mmol per 20 mL ampoule, i.e. 0.67 mmol/mL) diluted in saline or dextrose. The usual dose is 1 ampoule given over 4–6 hr, though half this dose is adequate in milder deficiency and 2–4 times this dose is needed in severe deficiency (i.e. <0.3 mmol/L and especially if <0.16 mmol/L).*

Bibliography

Aubier M, Murciano D, Lecocguic Y, et al. Effect of hypophosphatemia on diaphragmatic contractility in patients with acute respiratory failure. *N Engl J Med* 1985; 313: 420.

Charro T, Bernard F, Skrobik Y, et al. Intravenous phosphate in the intensive care unit: more aggressive repletion regimens for moderate and severe hypophosphatemia. *Intens Care Med* 2003; 29: 1273.

Coburn JW, Salusky IB. Control of serum phosphorus in uremia. *N Engl J Med* 1989; 320: 1140.

Kingston M, Al-Siba'l MB. Treatment of severe hypophosphatemia. *Crit Care Med* 1985; 13: 16.

Weisinger JR, Bellorin-Font E. Magnesium and phosphorus. *Lancet* 1998; 352: 391.

Hyposplenism

Hyposplenism, or more commonly complete **asplenia**, is generally caused by splenectomy (often traumatic). It may also be congenital or follow bone marrow transplantation.

The finding of Howell–Jolly bodies (HJBs) on the peripheral blood film reflects the absence of the spleen as a filter for damaged blood cells.

The clinical relevance of anatomical or functional hypersplenism relates to the increased risk of fatal sepsis in such patients, with a recorded mortality of about 50% if overwhelming postsplenectomy infection (OPSI) occurs. Since the population prevalence of patients at risk is about 1 in 1000 and since the risk is probably lifelong, strong international recommendations have been published for prophylactic immunization against the most relevant bacteria, particularly *Streptococcus pneumoniae*, meningococci and *Haemophilus influenzae* type b. Similarly, there are published recommendations for both prophylactic and emergency antibiotic regimens, usually with amoxicillin.

In addition, it has been appreciated that the loss of a functioning spleen may have broad implications for dysregulated coagulation, inflammation, endothelial function and blood filtration.

Bibliography

Kanhutu K, Jones P, Cheng AC, et al. Spleen Australia guidelines for the prevention of sepsis in patients with asplenia and hyposplenism in Australia and New Zealand. *Intern Med J* 2017; 47: 848.

Katz SC, Pachter HL. Indications for splenectomy. *Am Surg* 2006; 72: 565.

O'Neal HR, Niven AS, Karam GH. Critical illness in patients with asplenia. *Chest* 2016; 150: 1394.

Rubin LG, Schaffner W. Clinical practice: care of the asplenic patient. *N Engl J Med* 2014; 371: 349.

Spelman D, Buttery J, Daley A, et al. Guidelines for the prevention of sepsis in asplenic and hyposplenic patients. *Intern Med J* 2008; 38: 349.

Hypothalamic–pituitary–adrenal axis See

- Adrenal insufficiency,
- Pituitary.

Hypothermia

Hypothermia refers to a state of lowered core temperature below 35°C. Since clinical thermometers may not read below 35°C, a reading of 35°C on such a device does not exclude hypothermia and indeed should prompt the measurement of core temperature using a specific low-reading thermometer. Hypothermia, like hyperthermia (q.v.), is a dangerous complication, usually of environmental exposure (see Environment).

Hypothermia may occur even in temperate weather following immersion or wind chill. Patients who are at extremes of age, who are physically or mentally ill or are injured, or who have impaired consciousness (e.g. from alcohol or drugs) are especially predisposed to hypothermia. Hypoglycaemia (q.v.), myxoedema (q.v.), head injury, multiple trauma and drug overdose are commonly encountered causes of secondary hypothermia.

Hypothermia generally has an insidious onset with fatigue, apathy, confusion, incoordination and shivering. Its immediate assessment must include not only its quantification but also its precipitating factors and complications.

It should also be remembered that even modest hypothermia alters the disposition of many drugs commonly used in Intensive Care, both decreasing clearance and decreasing efficacy of many drugs in different ways. The net effect can be complex, with prolonged duration and increased concentration potentially offset by decreased potency (and perhaps toxicity). The final response for most drugs is both poorly documented to date and difficult to predict, so that clinical assessment and monitoring are especially important in this setting.

If the temperature falls to <35°C (**mild hypothermia**), there is
- confusion and disorientation,
- shivering, tachycardia and hypertension.

If the temperature falls to <32°C (**moderate hypothermia**), there is
- muscular rigidity and loss of shivering,
- progressive metabolic acidosis (q.v.),
- hypovolaemia, bradycardia and hypotension,
- coagulopathy (q.v.) and thrombocytopenia (q.v.),
- dilated pupils and drowsiness,
- J waves on ECG and potentially fatal arrhythmias, which can be readily precipitated by minor stimuli including movement.

If the temperature falls to <28°C (**severe hypothermia**), there is
- unconsciousness, areflexia and rigidity,
- shock and cardiac instability or arrest (usually in ventricular fibrillation),
- apnoea.

Treatment is with a warm, dry and sheltered environment and warm fluids by mouth. If the process is severe, passive or even active **rewarming** is required, the latter preferably in hospital.
- **Passive external rewarming** is suitable for only mild cases. It can achieve a rewarming rate of about 1°C per hr.
- Techniques of active rewarming, either external or internal, have not been subject to formal comparative evaluation, though many are available. Active techniques can achieve a rewarming rate of about 2°C per hr if external and up to 12°C per hr if internal. **External (active) rewarming** with an electric blanket may lead to relapse, though this may not apply to external rewarming with warm air or a radiant heater. **Internal (core) rewarming** may be achieved by warmed (i.e. 40°C) enteral, parenteral, peritoneal, pleural or dialysis fluids, or by veno-venous bypass using a haemofiltration system.
- Rewarming may be associated with washout acidosis or hypovolaemia.

Hypothermic **cardiac arrest** can be particularly difficult to treat, since the cold heart is relatively refractory to drugs and electrical stimuli. Normal resuscitation should be continued until the core temperature has been increased to at least 30°C before being deemed unsuccessful. Survival has been reported following CPR for up to 4 hr in patients with an initial temperature of <20°C. Survival with good cerebral function has been achieved in young patients in hypothermic asystole by using cardiopulmonary bypass.

Intubation, mechanical ventilation, invasive monitoring and circulatory resuscitation are always required in cases of more than mild hypothermia.

The outcome of victims of hypothermia clearly varies with its severity, its underlying cause and its treatment. In cases of coma and cardiac arrest, death should not be declared until rewarming has been shown to be fruitless. In survivors, there may be multiorgan failure (q.v.), rhabdomyolysis (q.v.), neurological damage, sepsis and local injury (e.g. frostbite).

Perioperative hypothermia is an important phenomenon and has been reported in up to one third of surgical patients in the operating theatre. It is due to impaired thermoregulation caused by anaesthesia, together with a cool environment, open body cavities and cold IV fluids. Even mild perioperative hypothermia has been shown to be associated with an increased incidence of bleeding, wound infections and cardiac events, and with increased hospital stay. The likely mechanism of this increased morbidity is hypothermia-induced stress response, with the production of greatly elevated levels of catecholamines, cortisol and other counterregulatory hormones. This increased morbidity has been shown in controlled trials to be prevented by maintaining normothermia with active warming using forced air.

Sepsis-induced hypothermia is a seeming paradox which occurs in about 10% of patients with a clinical diagnosis of sepsis. Inability to mount a fever in the presence of severe infection is now known to be associated with a doubling of mortality (see Heat shock proteins). This finding is in contrast to an older view that induced hypothermia might be beneficial in sepsis. Hypothermic patients with sepsis have higher plasma levels of interleukin 6 (IL-6), tumour necrosis factor α

(TNF-α) and eicosanoids (especially thromboxane A_2 and prostacyclin) than do febrile patients and are more acidotic. The cyclo-oxygenase inhibitor, ibuprofen, has been reported to improve the prognosis in hypothermic sepsis.

Therapeutic hypothermia of mild degree (i.e. 32–35°C) has been recommended as providing outcome benefit in patients resuscitated from cardiac arrest, but later studies suggested that this benefit may also be achieved by normothermia and thus by avoiding the frequent hyperthermic response in these patients. Thus, the optimal degree of targeted temperature management (TTM) in this situation remains to be clarified.

Therapeutic hypothermia has also been a commonly recommended component in the management of patients with traumatic brain injury, but formal studies have failed to confirm outcome benefit in these patients. Its potential benefit in mitigating neurological injury in a variety of other settings has also been explored but again without confirmed benefit to date.

Side-effects and technical uncertainties related to the degree and duration of cooling (if used) have provided ongoing clinical controversy. Active cooling may be achieved either non-invasively by cold water-jacketted blankets, cooling pads or cold air, or invasively by cold intravenous, gastric, bladder or rectal fluids, by an intravascular cooling catheter system or by an extracorporeal circuit. In most cases, the normal physiological response of shivering needs to be controlled by sedation and sometimes by neuromuscular relaxants.

The adverse effects caused by perioperative hypothermia necessarily also apply to therapeutic hypothermia (see above). In addition, in a patient who has the rare condition of **cryoglobulinaemia** (q.v.), hypothermia of any type can cause severe ischaemic damage.

See also
- Cold,
- Drowning,
- Frostbite,
- Multiple myeloma – 5. Cryoglobulinaemia.

Bibliography

Alqalyoobi S, Boctor N, Sarkeshik AA, et al. Therapeutic hypothermia and mortality in the intensive care unit: systematic review and meta-analysis. *Crit Care Resusc* 2019; 21: 287.

Arons MM, Wheeler AP, Bernard GR, et al. Effects of ibuprofen on the physiology and survival of hypothermic sepsis. *Crit Care Med* 1999; 27: 699.

Bernard SA, Buist M. Induced hypothermia in critical care medicine: a review. *Intens Care Med* 2003; 31: 2041.

Bernard SA, Gray TW, Buist MD, et al. Treatment of comatose survivors of out-of-hospital cardiac arrest with induced hypothermia. *N Engl J Med* 2002; 346: 557.

Brauer A, Wrigge H, Kersten J, et al. Severe accidental hypothermia: rewarming strategy using a veno-venous bypass system and a convective air warmer. *Intens Care Med* 1999; 25: 520.

Britt LD, Dascombe WH, Rodriguez A. New horizons in management of hypothermia and frostbite injury. *Surg Clin North Am* 1991; 71: 345.

Chen H, Wu F, Yang P, et al. A meta-analysis of therapeutic hypothermia in adult patients with traumatic brain injury. *Crit Care* 2019; 23: 396.

Clemmer TP, Fisher CJ, Bone RC, et al. Hypothermia in the sepsis syndrome and clinical outcome. *Crit Care Med* 1992; 20: 1395.

Clifton GL, Miller ER, Choi SC, et al. Lack of effect of induction of hypothermia after acute brain injury. *N Engl J Med* 2001; 344: 556.

Cooper DJ, Nichol AD, Bailey M, et al. Effect of early sustained prophylactic hypothermia on neurologic outcomes among patients with severe traumatic brain injury: the POLAR randomized clinical trial. *JAMA* 2018; 320: 2211.

Dexter WW. Hypothermia: safe and efficient methods of rewarming the patient. *Postgrad Med* 1990; 88: 55.

Dowd PM. Cold-related disorders. *Prog Dermatol* 1987; 21: 1.

Easterbrook PJ, Davis HP. Thrombocytopenia in hypothermia: a common but poorly recognised complication. *BMJ* 1985; 291: 23.

Frank SM, Fleischer LA, Breslow MJ, et al. Perioperative maintenance of normothermia reduces the incidence of morbid cardiac events: a randomized clinical trial. *JAMA* 1997; 277: 1127.

Hanania NA, Zimmerman JL. Accidental hypothermia. *Crit Care Clin* 1999; 15: 235.

Herr DL, Badjatia N, eds. Therapeutic temperature management: state of the art in the critically ill. *Crit Care Med* 2009; 37 (suppl.): S185.

Kim JH, Nagy A, Putzu A, et al. Therapeutic hypothermia in critically ill patients: a systematic review and meta-analysis of high quality randomized trials. *Crit Care Med* 2020; 48: 1047.

Ku J, Brasel KJ, Baker CC, et al. Triangle of death: hypothermia, acidosis, and coagulopathy. *New Horizons* 1999; 7: 61.

Kurisu K, Yenari MA. Therapeutic hypothermia for ischemic stroke: pathophysiology and future promise. *Neuropharmacology* 2018; 134: 302.

Kurz A, Sessler DI, Lenhardt R. Perioperative normothermia to reduce the incidence of surgical-wound infection and shorten hospitalization. *N Engl J Med* 1996; 334: 1209.

Larach MG. Accidental hypothermia. *Lancet* 1995; 345: 493.

Lefrant J-Y, Muller L, Coussaye JE, et al. Temperature measurement in intensive care patients: comparison of urinary bladder, oesophageal, rectal, axillary, and inguinal methods versus pulmonary artery core method. *Intens Care Med* 2003; 29: 414.

Lloyd EL. Treatment after exposure to cold. *Lancet* 1972; 1: 491.

Perman SM, Goyal M, Neumar RW, et al. Clinical applications of targeted temperature management. *Chest* 2014; 145: 386.

Polderman KH. Application of therapeutic hypothermia in the ICU: opportunities and pitfalls of a promising treatment modality. Part 1: indications and evidence. *Intens Care Med* 2004; 30: 556.

Polderman KH. Application of therapeutic hypothermia in the ICU: opportunities and pitfalls of a promising treatment modality. Part 2: practical aspects and side effects. *Intens Care Med* 2004; 30: 757.

Polderman KH, Herold I. Therapeutic hypothermia and controlled normothermia in the intensive care unit: practical considerations, side effects, and cooling methods. *Crit Care Med* 2009; 37: 1101.

Reuler JB. Hypothermia: pathophysiology, clinical settings, and management. *Ann Intern Med* 1978; 89: 519.

Sessler DI. Mild perioperative hypothermia. *N Engl J Med* 1997; 336: 1730.

Sunjic KM, Webb AC, Sunjic I, et al. Pharmacokinetic and other considerations for drug therapy during targeted temperature management. *Crit Care Med* 2015; 43: 2228.

The Hypothermia after Cardiac Arrest Study Group. Mild therapeutic hypothermia to improve the neurologic outcome after cardiac arrest. *N Engl J Med* 2002; 346: 549.

Tisherman SA, Sterz F, eds. *Therapeutic Hypothermia*. Berlin: Springer. 2005.

Tortorici MA, Kochanek PM, Poloyac SM. Effects of hypothermia on drug disposition, metabolism, and response: a focus on hypothermia-mediated alterations on the cytochrome P450 enzyme system. *Crit Care Med* 2007; 35: 2196.

Varon J, Acosta P. Therapeutic hypothermia: past, present and future. *Chest* 2008; 133: 1267.

Varon J, Sadovnikoff N, Sternbach GL. Hypothermia: saving patients from the big chill. *Postgrad Med* 1992; 92: 47.

Vassal T, Benoit-Gonin B, Carrat F, et al. Severe accidental hypothermia treated in an ICU: prognosis and outcome. *Chest* 2001; 120: 1998.

Walpoth BH, Walpoth-Aslan BN, Mattle HP, et al. Outcome of survivors of accidental deep hypothermia and circulatory arrest treated with extracorporeal blood warming. *N Engl J Med* 1997; 337: 1500.

Woodhouse P, Keatinge WR, Coleshaw SR. Factors associated with hypothermia in patients admitted to a group of inner city hospitals. *Lancet* 1989; 2: 1201.

Hypothyroidism

Hypothyroidism refers to the bodily deficiency of thyroid hormone. **Myxoedema** describes the florid clinical syndrome associated with this. However, most patients with hypothyroidism have only mild symptoms, and indeed many are asymptomatic.

Hypothyroidism has many causes, though more than 95% are due to intrinsic thyroid disease, from
- inflammation, especially Hashimoto's (autoimmune) thyroiditis,
- previous surgery,
- iodine deficiency or excess,
- drugs, e.g. lithium, amiodarone, other iodine-containing medications,
- local irradiation.

A few cases are due to disease of the
- pituitary (with thyroid-stimulating hormone (TSH) deficiency), or
- hypothalamus (with thyrotropin-releasing hormone (TRH) deficiency).

The classical clinical features of myxoedema include
- cold intolerance,
- thick dry skin,
- hoarse voice,
- apathy,
- motor retardation,
- constipation,
- occasionally headache, myalgia, arthralgia (q.v.), oedema.

However, a single feature may at times predominate.

More importantly, the changes may occur so slowly as to be difficult to recognize without assistance (e.g. from an old photograph).

Diagnosis is based on decreased T4 and increased TSH, though marginal abnormalities of these tests commonly occur in asymptomatic patients, in whom diagnosis then remains difficult. The TSH is not elevated if the hypothyroidism is of pituitary or hypothalamic origin. T3 is decreased late in the course of disease and is not a useful test in this setting. Antithyroid antibodies (mainly to thyroid peroxidase, i.e. anti-TPO, and also to thyroglobulin) occur early in autoimmune thyroiditis (see Autoimmune disorders). Elevated thyroglobulin levels may also occur in recurrent papillary thyroid cancer.

Treatment is with **thyroid replacement**, generally levothyroxine 100 mcg per day, though it is usually commenced at lower doses, e.g. 50 mcg per day. The addition of T3 has not been shown to be of clinical value (except in myxoedema coma – see below).

Sometimes higher maintenance doses are needed, in which case they should be achieved over some weeks. Increased doses are particularly required during pregnancy. Increased doses are also required during concomitant therapy with agents which alter the bioavailability of T4, such as sucralfate, colestyramine or soy bean–based feeds (which decrease absorption of T4) and barbiturates, carbamazepine, phenytoin or rifampicin (which increase hepatic metabolism of T4).

On the other hand, in elderly or cardiac patients, initial doses should often be as low as 25 mcg per day.

The euthyroid state is achieved when symptoms have receded and the TSH level is normal, as the T4 level is not a reliable guide to euthyroidism.

> **Myxoedema coma** is a rare but serious complication of hypothyroidism.
>
> It is seen mainly in the elderly and is usually precipitated by infection or exposure. There is hypothermia (q.v.) as well as coma.
>
> Treatment comprises **resuscitation** and administration of **T3** 10 mcg IV qid.
> - *Resuscitation needs to be undertaken with great care, as fluid overload can easily be produced on the one hand, and repair of hypothermia can require considerably increased fluids on the other hand. The complexity of this treatment requires the facilities of an Intensive Care Unit.*
> - *It is wise to administer **corticosteroids** concomitantly, in case there is associated hypopituitarism and thus adrenal insufficiency.*

Bibliography
Bastenie PA, Bonnyns M, Vanhaelst L. Natural history of primary myxedema. *Am J Med* 1985; 79: 91.
DeGroot LJ, Quintans J. The causes of autoimmune thyroid disease. *Endocr Rev* 1989; 10: 537.
Editorial. Subclinical hypothyroidism. *Lancet* 1986; 1: 251.
Jordan RM. Myxedema coma: the prognosis is improving. *Endocrinologist* 1993; 3: 149.
Lazar MA. Thyroid hormone receptors: multiple forms, multiple possibilities. *Endocr Rev* 1993; 14: 184.
Loriaux DL. The polyendocrine deficiency syndromes. *N Engl J Med* 1985; 312: 1568.
Magner JA. Thyroid-stimulating hormone: biosynthesis, cell biology, and bioactivity. *Endocr Rev* 1990; 11: 354.
Mazzaferri EL. Adult hypothyroidism. *Postgrad Med* 1986; 79: 64 & 75.
Ramsay I. Drug and non-thyroid induced changes in thyroid function tests. *Postgrad Med J* 1985; 61: 375.
Roberts CG, Ladenson PW. Hypothyroidism. Lancet 2004; 363: 793.
Shupnik MA, Ridgway EC, Chin WW. Molecular biology of thyrotropin. *Endocr Rev* 1989; 10: 459.
Smallridge RC. Metabolic and anatomic thyroid emergencies: a review. *Crit Care Med* 1992; 20: 276.
Surks MI, Chopra IJ, Mariash CN, et al. American Thyroid Association guidelines for use of laboratory tests in thyroid disorders. *JAMA* 1990; 263: 1529.
Surks MI, Ortiz E, Daniels GH, et al. Subclinical thyroid disease: scientific review and guidelines for diagnosis and management. *JAMA* 2004; 291: 228.
Topliss DJ, Eastman CJ. Diagnosis and management of hyperthyroidism and hypothyroidism. *Med J Aust* 2004; 180: 186.
Vance ML. Hypopituitarism. *N Engl J Med* 1994; 330: 1651.
Tonner DR, Schlechte JA. Neurologic complications of thyroid and parathyroid disease. *Med Clin North Am* 1993; 77: 251.
Walsh JP, Stuckey BGA. What is the optimal treatment for hypothyroidism. *Med J Aust* 2001; 174: 141.

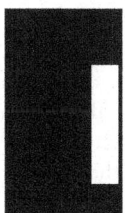

ICU-acquired weakness

ICU-acquired weakness is an important complication of serious illness. However, it is more appropriately referred to as **critical illness neuromuscular abnormality** (q.v.).

See
- Myopathy – Acute necrotizing myopathy, Critical illness myopathy,
- Neuropathy – Polyneuropathy (5. Critical illness neuropathy).

Bibliography
Jolley SE, Bunnell AE, Hough CL. ICU-acquired weakness. *Chest* 2016; 150: 1129.
Kress JP, Hall JB. ICU-acquired weakness and recovery from critical illness. *N Engl J Med* 2014; 370: 1626.
Vanhorebeek I, Latronico N, Van den Berghe G. ICU-acquired weakness. *Intens Care Med* 2020; 46: 637.

Idiopathic inflammatory myopathy (IIM) *See*
- Myopathy,
- Myositis.

Idiopathic interstitial pneumonias *See*
- Interstitial pneumonias.

Idiopathic pulmonary fibrosis

Idiopathic pulmonary fibrosis (IPF, diffuse fibrosing alveolitis, cryptogenic fibrosing alveolitis) is a specific form of chronic progressive diffuse interstitial pulmonary fibrosis. It is the most common of the **idiopathic interstitial pneumonias** (q.v.).

Its prevalence is about 25–30 per 100,000 of the population, and its incidence is about 5–10 per 100,00 of the population per year. It occurs predominantly in patients >40 years of age, particularly men. There is no known racial or geographic preponderance.

Although its aetiology is uncertain and no single pathogenetic mechanism has yet been defined, there are common histological, radiological and clinical features exhibited by most patients with this condition, justifying its consideration as a separate entity. However, it may well represent a group of disorders, and in any event it is not easy to distinguish from similar processes associated with systemic disease (especially collagen-vascular diseases, see Systemic diseases and the lung) or certain drugs (see Drugs and the lung). Currently, it is thought to be associated with an abnormal and persistent response to an initial and then recurrent injury to the alveolar epithelium.

Aetiological factors may be immunological, although no specific antigen has been identifiable and no consistent inflammatory process has been found which precedes the relentless progression of fibrosis. An association with other autoimmune diseases (q.v.) has sometimes been found, and there appears to be some genetic predisposition. No infective agent has been consistently identified, but some association with prior occupational exposure to wood and metal dusts has been reported. The condition is more common in smokers or with environmental pollution or chronic microaspiration.

The pathological changes consist of thickening of alveolar walls, abnormal proliferation of mesenchymal cells, disorganized collagen deposition, fibrosis, subepithelial fibrotic foci and eventually an extensive but patchy distribution of distorted pulmonary architecture with cystic spaces (honeycombing). Inflammation if present is mild. These findings may show considerable temporal inhomogeneity. This process is referred to as 'usual interstitial pneumonitis' (UIP). UIP is not specific to idiopathic pulmonary fibrosis, as it is seen also in other chronic fibrotic lung diseases of known aetiology, such as asbestosis (q.v.), connective tissue diseases (q.v.) and hypersensitivity pneumonitis (q.v.).

> The clinical features of idiopathic pulmonary fibrosis are usually dominated by progressive dyspnoea. The first presentation is sometimes as an apparent acute respiratory infection. A dry cough is common, as is fever and weight loss.
>
> On physical examination, there is frequently cyanosis, clubbing and tachypnoea. Diffuse crackles are heard, particularly at the lung bases. A late finding is cor pulmonale. Extrapulmonary manifestations (if present) suggest a concomitant systemic disorder.
>
> As most patients are >40 years old, comorbidities are common.
>
> Acute exacerbations are common, and they have potentially fatal consequences.

The chest X-ray may initially be normal, even in the presence of dyspnoea. The radiological abnormalities predominantly affect the lower zones and comprise bilateral reticular changes, often with honeycombing. There is no diffuse opacification or nodularity, no hilar lymphadenopathy and no pleural effusion. High-resolution CT scanning (HRCT) is the imaging modality of current choice. In specialist centres, the findings on HRCT of honeycombing (particularly subpleurally and basally), septal thickening, ground glass lesions and traction bronchiectasis can be sufficiently characteristic to support a firm diagnosis even in the absence of histological confirmation.

Lung function tests show changes similar to those described for sarcoidosis (q.v.). Pulmonary hypertension is commonly seen, but it correlates poorly with the degree of fibrosis.

A number of blood biomarkers (q.v.) have been identified in patients with IPF, but firm correlation with either the severity of the disease or its typically unpredictable course has been elusive, though in general increased levels have been associated with increased mortality. Recently, plasma levels of several biomarkers, including CA 125, chitinase-3-like protein-1 (YKL-40), C-X-C motif chemokine 13 (CXCL13), matrix metalloproteinase 7 (MMP7), osteopontin (OPN), surfactant protein D (SP-D) and vascular cell adhesion protein-1 (VCAM-1), have been shown to be associated with transplant-free survival, particularly in patients treated with the new antifibrotic agents.

Although a presumptive diagnosis may be made on the basis of the clinical and radiological features together with the absence of systemic disease, or culprit exposures or drugs, lung biopsy is required for definitive diagnosis. However, a clinical diagnosis may be acceptable if the patient is particularly unwell and/or the features are unequivocal.

The chief differential diagnosis includes
- late sarcoidosis (q.v.),
- cryptogenic organizing pneumonia (formerly called bronchiolitis obliterans organizing pneumonia (BOOP) (q.v.),
- lymphangitis carcinomatosa,
- scleroderma (q.v.),
- hypersensitivity pneumonitis (q.v.),
- lymphangiomyomatosis (q.v.),
- histiocytosis (q.v.).

Biopsy is required to distinguish these diseases.

Treatment of this condition is uniformly disappointing, as no therapeutic modality has shown clear efficacy. Patients should always be considered for clinical trials, and both supportive care and attention to comorbidities or complications should be priorities.

- *Treatment used to comprise chiefly* **corticosteroids**. *However, in most patients there was a continued progression, although a modest symptomatic response was sometimes seen initially. Moreover, there was an adverse steroid response in those cases with patchy fibrosis and honeycombing. Given the absence of an inflammatory process and the lack of any efficacy in most cases, the routine use of corticosteroids is no longer recommended (except in combination regimens – see below).*
- *The place of* **immunosuppressive therapy** *is unresolved, though cytotoxic therapy (azathioprine, cyclophosphamide) particularly in combination may be useful in early stage disease. The combination of prednisone, azathoiprine and N-acetylcysteine (as an antioxidant) has been shown to be helpful. The initial promise of interferon gamma was not borne out in a larger subsequent study. Colchicine, penicillamine, bosentan, etanercept, statins and ACE inhibitors have not been shown to be effective.*
- *New therapeutic modalities specifically targeting fibroblast proliferation (e.g.* **pirfenidone**) *or vascular growth factors (e.g.* **nintedanib**) *have shown efficacy in slowing disease progression.*
- *Targeting protease-activated receptors (PARs) may be a future option, because PARs are involved in the cellular (as opposed to the classic fibrin-forming) activity of coagulation factors and abnormal coagulation activation occurs in and may contribute to IPF.*
- *Long-term oxygen therapy can be symptomatically helpful in most patients.*
- **Lung transplantation** *may be an option for some patients. A 1-year survival of about 80% and 5-year survival of about 45% have been reported.*
- *Mechanical ventilation for acute respiratory failure in such patients is almost always associated with death within about 1 week.*

The course of the disease is very variable. The median time from onset of symptoms to death is about 3 years, though reported survival has ranged from 1 month to over 20 years. The mortality is 50% at 3 years and 80% at 5 years. The duration of survival appears to correlate with the severity of disease at the time of diagnosis.

See also
- Interstitial lung diseases,
- Interstitial pneumonias.

Bibliography

Agusti C, Xaubet A, Roca J, et al. Interstitial pulmonary fibrosis with and without associated collagen vascular disease. *Thorax* 1992; 47: 1035.

Behr J, Kolb M, Cox G. Treating IPF – all or nothing? A PRO-CON debate. *Respirology* 2009; 14: 1072.

Canestaro WJ, Forrester SH, Raghu G, et al. Drug treatment of idiopathic pulmonary fibrosis: systematic review and network meta-analysis. *Chest* 2016; 149: 756.

Carrington CB, Gaensler EA, Coutu RE, et al. Natural history and treated course of usual and desquamative interstitial pneumonia. *N Engl J Med* 1978; 298: 801.

Cherniack RM, Colby TV, Flint A, et al. Correlation of structure and function in idiopathic pulmonary fibrosis. *Am J Respir Crit Care Med* 1995; 151: 1180.

Crystal RG, Bitterman PB, Rennard SI, et al. Interstitial lung diseases of unknown cause. *N Engl J Med* 1984; 310: 154 & 235.

Flaherty KR, Toews GB, Lynch JP, et al. Steroids in idiopathic pulmonary fibrosis: a prospective assessment of adverse reactions, response to therapy, and survival. *Am J Med* 2001; 110: 278.

Fumeaux T, Rothmeier C, Jolliet P. Outcome of mechanical ventilation for acute respiratory failure in patients with pulmonary fibrosis. *Intens Care Med* 2001; 27: 1868.

Gross TJ, Hunninghake GW. Idiopathic pulmonary fibrosis. *N Engl J Med* 2001; 345: 517.

Homma Y, Ohtsuka Y, Tanimura K, et al. Can interstitial pneumonia as the sole presentation of collagen vascular disease be differentiated from idiopathic interstitial pneumonia. *Respiration* 1995; 62: 248.

Hubbard R, Lewis S, Richards K, et al. Occupational exposure to metal or wood dust and aetiology of cryptogenic fibrosing alveolitis. *Lancet* 1996; 347: 284.

International Consensus Statement. Idiopathic pulmonary fibrosis: diagnosis and treatment. *Am J Respir Crit Care Med* 2000; 161: 646.

Jo HE, Troy LK, Keir G, et al. Treatment of idiopathic pulmonary fibrosis in Australia and New Zealand: a position statement from the Thoracic Soociety of Australia and New Zealand and the Lung Foundation Australia. *Respirology* 2017; 22: 1436.

Johnston IDA, Prescott RJ, Chalmers JC, et al. British Thoracic Society study of cryptogenic fibrosing alveolitis: current presentation and initial management. *Thorax* 1997; 52: 38.

Kamp DW. Idiopathic pulmonary fibrosis: the inflammatory hypothesis revisited. *Chest* 2003; 124: 1187.

Klingsberg RC, Mutsaers SE, Lasky JA. Current clinical trials for the treatment of idiopathic pulmonary fibrosis. *Respirology* 2010; 15: 19.

Kottmann RM, Hogan CM, Phipps RP, et al. Determinants of initiation and progression of idiopathic pulmonary fibrosis. *Respirology* 2009; 14: 917.

Lin C, Borensztajn K, Spek CA. Targeting coagulation factor receptors – protease-activated receptors in idiopathic pulmonary fibrosis. *J Thromb Haemost* 2017; 15: 597.

Lynch DA, Godwin JD, Safrin S, et al. High-resolution computed tomography in idiopathic pulmonary fibrosis: diagnosis and prognosis. *Am J Respir Crit Care Med* 2005; 172: 488.

Marinelli WA. Idiopathic pulmonary fibrosis: progress and challenge. *Chest* 1995; 108: 297.

Mason DP, Brizzio ME, Alster JM, et al. Lung transplantation for idiopathic pulmonary fibrosis. *Ann Thorac Surg* 2007; 84: 1121.

Michaelson JE, Aguayo SM, Roman J. Idiopathic pulmonary fibrosis. *Chest* 2000; 118: 788.

Prasad J, Holland AE, Glaspole I, et al. Idiopathic pulmonary fibrosis: an Australian perspective. *Intern Med J* 2016; 46: 663.

Raghu G, Collard HR, Egan JJ, et al. An official ATS/ERS/JRS/ALAT statement: idiopathic pulmonary fibrosis: evidence-based guidelines for diagnosis and management. *Am J Respir Crit Care Med* 2011; 183: 788.

Riches DWH, Worthen GS, eds. Mechanisms of pulmonary fibrosis. *Chest* 2001; 120: suppl. 1.

Schmidt SL, Sundaram B, Flaherty KR. Diagnosing fibrotic lung disease: when is high-resolution computed tomography sufficient to make a diagnosis of idiopathic pulmonary fibrosis? *Respirology* 2009; 14: 934.

Swaminathan AC, Todd JL. That was then, this is now: a fresh look at idiopathic pulmonary fibrosis biomarkers in the antifibrotic era. *Chest* 2020; 158: 1321.

Swigris JJ, Kuschner WG, Kelsey JL, et al. Idiopathic pulmonary fibrosis. *Chest* 2005; 127: 275.

Turner-Warwick M, Burrows B, Johnson A. Cryptogenic fibrosing alveolitis. *Thorax* 1980; 35: 171.

Various. Controversies in the diagnosis and management of idiopathic pulmonary fibrosis. *Chest* 2005; 128 (suppl.): 513S.

Ziesche R, Hofbauer E, Wittmann K, et al. A preliminary study of long-term treatment with interferon gamma-1b and low-dose prednisolone in patients with idiopathic pulmonary fibrosis. *N Engl J Med* 1999; 341: 1264.

Idiopathic pulmonary haemosiderosis *See*

- Goodpasture's syndrome.

Idiopathic thrombocytopenic purpura *See*

- Immune thrombocytopenic purpura.

Immotile cilia syndrome *See*

- Kartagener's syndrome,
- Primary ciliary dyskinesia,
- Situs inversus.

Immune complex disease

Immune complex disease is a heterogeneous condition in which exogenous or endogenous antigens have combined with antibodies to cause either local or systemic tissue damage.

The amount of **immune complex** formed is related to the relative concentrations of antigen and antibody, the largest amount and in general the largest size of immune complexes being formed when antigen and antibody are present in molar equivalence. Their usual clearance is by the reticuloendothelial system following their transport on red blood cell membranes. This clearance is rapid and does not produce damage.

However, if normal clearance is impaired, such as by complement factor deficiency, immune complexes can be deposited in small blood vessels in any organ or tissue in the body but particularly in the kidney and to a lesser extent in the skin and choroid plexus. Vasoactive substances are then released from circulating basophils and later from tissue mast cells and infiltrated neutrophils, platelets are activated, and vascular permeability is enhanced. The immune complexes can then migrate beyond the endothelium to the basement membrane and even into surrounding tissues.

Immune complex disease may be local or systemic.

1. **Localized immune complex disease**

The prime example of this phenomenon is the **Arthus reaction**. This is an acute haemorrhagic and necrotic local reaction usually in the skin and occurring 2–4 hr after the injection of antigen into an immunized animal.

Clinically, such a phenomenon occurs when antigen is localized, so that any reaction with formed antibodies is also localized. This occurs with

- endogenous antigens which are either structural (e.g. basement membrane) or secreted (e.g. thyroglobulin),
- exogenous antigens which are concentrated locally (e.g. inhaled).

Examples with endogenous antigens include Goodpasture's syndrome (q.v.), Hashimoto's thyroiditis and pemphigus vulgaris (q.v.).

Examples with exogenous antigens include hypersensitivity pneumonitis (q.v.).

2. **Systemic immune complex disease**

Serum sickness is the prime example of this phenomenon. This is a condition associated with fever, rash, lymphadenopathy (q.v.), splenomegaly (q.v.) and arthritis (q.v.) about 10 days after a large exposure to foreign antigen. Serum sickness runs a benign and self-limited course over about a week, though occasionally reversible vasculitis (q.v.) or polyneuritis (q.v.) may occur.

A chronic form may develop if the antigen exposure is prolonged or repeated.

Systemic immune complex disease can follow

- infections, e.g. viral (such as hepatitis B – q.v.), bacterial (such as streptococcal) and parasitic,
- administration of many different drugs which can act as haptens (such as aspirin, gold, penicillamine, penicillin, phenytoin, sulphonamides and thiazides). There have been reports of this condition associated with the anti-smoking drug, bupropion.

Immune complex assays can be useful as markers of progress, but the levels are neither sensitive nor specific. Their presence may also be suggested by evidence of complement activation (q.v.), with decreased C3 and C4. A more specific test is the immunohistological examination of biopsy material.

Treatment consists of removal of the offending antigen if possible, anti-inflammatory agents (especially antihistamines), corticosteroids, cytotoxics and possibly plasmapheresis (q.v.). Cephalosporins and methyldopa may offer interesting therapeutic possibilities.

Experimental evidence suggests the potential therapeutic value of the cytokines interleukin 4 and 10, of antibodies to integrins and selectins, and of nitric oxide synthetase inhibition.

Bibliography

Lawley TJ, Bielory L, Gascon P, et al. A prospective clinical and immunologic analysis of patients with serum sickness. *N Engl J Med* 1984; 311: 1407.

Schifferli JA, Ng YC, Peters DK. The role of complement and its receptors in the elimination of immune complexes. *N Engl J Med* 1986; 315: 488.

Wiggins RC, Cochrane CG. Immune-complex-mediated biologic effects. *N Engl J Med* 1981; 304: 518.

Immune thrombocytopenic purpura

Immune (or **idiopathic**) **thrombocytopenic purpura** (ITP) is due to an autoimmune IgG antibody, usually directed against the platelet membrane glycoprotein, GP IIb–IIIa, but sometimes against a variety of other platelet antigens. Its prevalence is about 1 in 10,000 of the population.

Secondary immune thrombocytopenia may also occur (see Thrombocytopenia).

Platelets with bound antibody are vulnerable to trapping and thus destruction via phagocytosis, especially in the spleen. Platelet production in the bone marrow increases by 3- to 4-fold, but this is only about half the known marrow reserve, perhaps because platelet antibodies react also with megakaryocytes.

The clinical features are usually seen in young women, in whom there is often associated immune thyroid disease (q.v.). There is no splenomegaly. Sometimes, there is only purpura (q.v.), but if more severe there is also mucosal bleeding.

The course is usually chronic and relatively benign, except for the occasional occurrence of intracranial haemorrhage. The condition may spontaneously remit, only to relapse in the presence of infection.

Acute ITP typically follows a viral illness and disappears within 3 months.

The peripheral blood film is normal apart from the appearance of large platelets. These are young, metabolically active and highly functional. An increased titre of platelet-associated IgG is usual, but this test for autoantibodies is neither sensitive nor specific. The thrombopoietin (TPO) level is normal. Bone marrow disease, hypersplenism, pseudothrombocytopenia and culprit drugs need to be excluded (see Thrombocytopenia).

Treatment is not required if the platelet count is >30–50 × 10^9/L and there is no bleeding. Aspirin should clearly be avoided.

If treatment is required, **corticosteroids** provide first-line therapy and are usually effective within a few days.

- If relapse or persistence occurs, **splenectomy** produces a remission in 75% of cases, with the platelet count rising by the first postoperative day and commonly exceeding normal levels by the second week. Splenectomy is usually deferred for the first 12 months in order to assess a favourable initial outcome (i.e. remission or response), which occurs in about one third of patients.
- High-dose human **immune globulin** (e.g. 20 g IV per day for 5 days) can be combined with the initial course of steroids in severe cases. Alternatively, **plasmapheresis** (q.v.) may be effective.
- **Cytotoxic** agents (particularly mycophenolate), ciclosporin, azathioprine, vincristine, dapsone or interferon alpha have also been used. **Rituximab** (q.v.) is helpful in refractory cases, with an early response of over 50% but a longer-term response of only about 25%. Immunosuppression should clearly be avoided in patients with AIDS.
- An important frontier is the use of **thrombopoietin receptor agonists** (TPO-RAs), e.g. romiplostim, eltrombopag, which have the potential to increase platelet production markedly, even in otherwise refractory cases. Initial response rates of up to 90% have been reported.
- **Veltuzumab**, an anti-CD20 antibody originally used for B-cell malignancies, has recently been shown to be effective in some otherwise refractory cases.
- A variety of novel therapeutic agents with potential utility in ITP are currently undergoing clinical trials, and some may eventually add to the existing complexity of treatment choices in this condition.
- Interestingly, **eradication therapy for Helicobacter pylori** in seropositive patients has been associated with significantly increased platelet counts in some cases, even to the point of ceasing all other therapy.
- **Platelet transfusions** are recommended if bleeding is severe, because 6–20 U bd-qid confers clinical benefit, even though there is increased platelet destruction and the platelet count itself may not necessarily rise.

In **pregnancy** (q.v.), the diagnosis of ITP should not be made unless pre-eclampsia (q.v.) has been excluded. Splenectomy is contraindicated because it may precipitate abortion. Some degree of maternal thrombocytopenia is common anyway (8% prevalence) and is neither immune-mediated nor clinically significant. Corticosteroids and immune globulin may be required in cases of confirmed ITP, if severe. Specialist supervision is required in refractory cases. A platelet count >50 × 10^9/L is recommended for delivery (either vaginal or Caesarean) and >70 × 10^9/L for neuraxial anaesthesia.

Concomitant **cardiovascular disease** or **venous thromboembolism** are not uncommon in older patients with ITP, and their treatment can present particular challenges. It is a myth to consider that thrombocytopenia may protect against thrombosis.

An **ITP-like syndrome** may also be seen in lymphoma or systemic lupus erythematosus (SLE) (q.v.), but in these conditions it is in fact secondary.

See also
- Thrombocytopenia.

Bibliography

Choi PY, Merriman E, Bennett A, et al. Consensus guidelines for the management of adult immune thrombocytopenia in Australia and New Zealand. *Med J Aust* 2022; 216: 43.

Chong BH. Primary immune thrombocytopenia: understanding pathogenesis is the key to better treatments. *J Thromb Haemost* 2009; 7: 319.

Cines DB, Blanchette VS. Immune thrombocytopenic purpura. *N Engl J Med* 2002; 346: 995.

Ferrara JLM. The febrile platelet transfusion reaction: a cytokine shower. *Transfusion* 1995; 35: 89.

George JN. Management of patients with refractory immune thrombocytopenic purpura. *J Thromb Haemost* 2006; 4: 1664.

Kuter DJ, Bussel JB, Lyons RM, et al. Efficacy of romiplostim in patients with chronic immune thrombocytopenic purpura. *Lancet* 2008; 371: 395.

Lakshmanan S, Cuker A. Contemporary management of primary immune thrombocytopenia in adults. *J Thromb Haemost* 2012; 10: 1988.

Nugent D, McMillan R, Nichol JL, et al. Pathogenesis of chronic immune thrombocytopenia: increased platelet destruction and/or decreased platelet production. *Br J Haematol* 2009; 146: 585.

Provan D, Arnold DM, Russell JB, et al. Updated international consensus report on the investigation and management of primary immune thrombocytopenia. *Blood Adv* 2019; 3: 3780.

Sivapathasingam V, Harvey MP, Wilson RB. *Helicobacter pylori* eradication: a novel therapeutic option in chronic immune thrombocytopenic purpura. *Med J Aust* 2008; 189: 367.

Immunodeficiency

Immunodeficiency diseases arise typically because of a defect in either
- immunoglobulin production (i.e. B-cell deficiency), or
- cell-mediated immunity (i.e. T-cell deficiency).

Immunodeficiency can also occur because of disorders of the innate immune system, due to defects in phagocyte number or function (see Neutropenia) or in the complement system (q.v.).

> Immunodeficiency generally comes to the attention of Intensive Care clinicians because it predisposes to infections in general and to serious sepsis in particular. Specific clues may include recurrence of infection, refractoriness to treatment, unexpectedly severe infection from a generally non-pathogenic organism, infection with an unusual or exotic organism or a positive family history (in primary immunodeficiencies).

1. Immunoglobulin deficiency

The best-known such condition is X-linked **agammaglobulinaemia** (q.v.), but many other specific deficiencies of antibody production have been reported, particularly **common variable immunodeficiency** and **selective immunoglobulin deficiency**.

- **Common variable immunodeficiency** (CVID) is a non-inherited form of hypogammaglobulinaemia which usually appears in adult life. Its prevalence is about 1 in 20,000 of the population. There is a generalized decrease in all immunoglobulins, presumably due to B-cell dysfunction. There may be multiple pathogenetic mechanisms, but the clinical features are similar to those of agammaglobulinaemia with proneness to infection and to autoimmune diseases (q.v.). Additional features include chronic lung damage, lymphoid hyperplasia and giardia-induced diarrhoea.
  Treatment is with **replacement therapy** *(with immune globulin) and* **antibiotics**, *while corticosteroids should be used with caution.*
- **Selective immunoglobulin deficiency** comprises a number of categories, some inherited, and including IgG sub-classes, IgM, IgA and combined defects. Their clinical effects are variable, and they are frequently asymptomatic.

2. Cell-mediated immunodeficiency

This is manifested as impaired delayed hypersensitivity with proneness to infections. Infections are frequent and severe and may be due to many different organisms, especially opportunists (e.g. candida, pneumocystis), Gram-negative bacteria and viruses.

- **Primary deficiencies** are sometimes inherited and include
  - **severe combined immunodeficiency disease** (SCID) and its several variants,
  - the **Wiskott–Aldrich syndrome**, an X-linked disorder with associated eczema, thrombocytopenia (q.v.) and lymphoid cancers,
  - **ataxia–telangiectasia**, the mutant gene for which has been identified as being responsible for greatly increased sensitivity to ionizing radiation, so that there is a propensity for chromosomal damage.
- **Secondary deficiencies** are due to other diseases, such as collagen-vascular, inflammatory (especially HIV infection), neoplastic, nutritional or traumatic disorders, or to drugs. Psychological stress has been reported to be a potential cause of increased susceptibility to viral infections in some patients.

Bibliography

Buckley RH, Schiff RI. The use of intravenous immune globulin in immunodeficiency diseases. *N Engl J Med* 1991; 325: 110.

Gupta S, Pattaniak D, Krishnaswamy G. Common variable immune deficiency and associated complications. *Chest* 2019; 156: 579.

Sneller MC, Strober W, Eisenstein E, et al. NIH conference: new insights into common variable immunodeficiency. *Ann Intern Med* 1993; 118: 720.

Sullivan KE, Jyonoudi S. Deficiencies of innate and adaptive immunity. In: *Scientific American Medicine. Allergy & Immunology.* Hamilton: Dekker Medicine. 2020.

Van de Meer JWM, Kullberg BJ. Defects in host-defense mechanisms. In: Rubin RH, Young LS, eds. *Clinical Approach to Infections in the Compromised Host.* 4th edition. New York: Plenum. 2002.

Yu Z, Lennon VA. Mechanism of intravenous immune globulin therapy in antibody-mediated autoimmune diseases. *N Engl J Med* 1999; 340: 227.

Immunology

Immunology has become a daunting field for the non-specialist, since its knowledge base has been doubling every 5 years and since many even relatively recent concepts have become obsolete. For example, the number of relevant molecules has grown enormously, with now over 100 cytokines and over 350 CD (cell surface) antigens, so that there is new understanding of the processes which both initiate and control inflammation.

While immune deficiency is well known as a cause of refractory infections, it is also recognized that excessive immune responses to infection can be the drivers of adverse consequences, such as septic shock, acute respiratory distress syndrome (ARDS) and multiorgan failure. In addition, paradoxical immune responses to foreign material or self-antigens can lead to allergy and autoimmune disease, respectively. Beyond these classic concepts, it is now appreciated that the immune system has a much broader role in health and disease, for example in cardiovascular disease, neuromuscular disorders, cancer surveillance, obesity and depression. The appreciation that there are so many immune-driven conditions has led to the broadening of therapeutic possibilities deriving from the biological modulation of immune responses.

Disorders with an immunological aetiology or more commonly with an immunological contribution are frequent in Intensive Care, as in medicine generally. While many such disorders are more logically considered under specific organ-system headings, some immunological conditions and principles of a general character are considered in this book as separate topics, including

- Agammaglobulinaemia,
- Angioedema,
- Antinuclear antibodies,
- Autoimmune disorders,
- Cold agglutinin disease,
- Complement deficiency,
- Cryoglobulinaemia,
- Eculizumab,
- Haemophagocytic lymphohistiocytosis (HLH),
- Haemophagocytic syndrome,
- Henoch-Schonlein purpura,
- Histocompatibility complex,
- Human immunodeficiency virus,
- Immune complex disease,
- Immunodeficiency,
- Immunomodulation,
- Jarisch–Herxheimer reaction,
- Latex allergy,
- Macrophage activation syndrome,
- PLAID syndrome,
- Plasmapheresis,
- Serum sickness,
- Tocilizumab,
- Tumour necrosis factor,
- Urticaria.

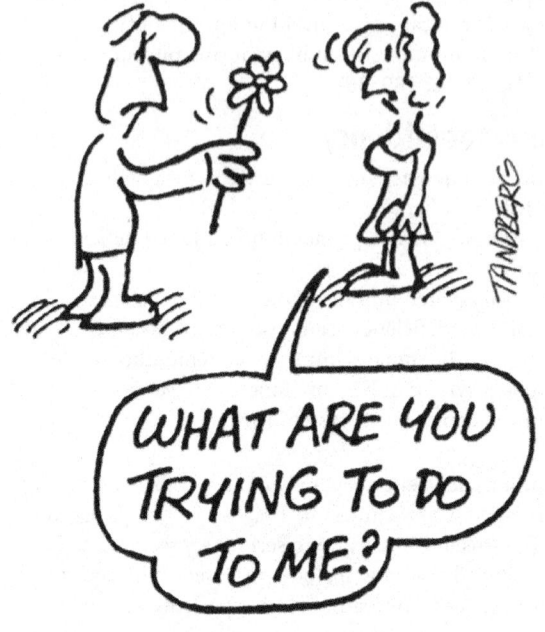

Bibliography

Anderson KC, Weinstein HJ. Transfusion-associated graft-versus-host disease. *N Engl J Med* 1990; 323: 315.

Austen KF, Burakoff SJ, Rosen FS, et al., eds. *Therapeutic Immunology*. 2nd edition. Cambridge: Blackwell. 2001.

Ballow M, Nelson R. Immunopharmacology: immunomodulation and immunotherapy. *JAMA* 1997; 278: 2008.

Barnes PJ, Karin M. Nuclear factor-κβ – a pivotal transcription factor in chronic inflammatory diseases. *N Engl J Med* 1997; 336: 1066.

Chrousos GP. The hypothalamic-pituitary-adrenal axis and immune-mediated inflammation. *N Engl J Med* 1995; 332: 1351.

Clark EA, Ledbetter JA. How B and T cells talk to each other. *Nature* 1994; 367: 425.

Cohen JJ. Apoptosis. *Immunol Today* 1993; 14: 126.

Couriel D, Weinstein R. Complications of therapeutic plasma exchange: a recent assessment. *J Clin Apheresis* 1994; 9: 1.

Davies PJ, Martin SJ, Burton DR, et al. *Roitt's Essential Immunology*. 13th edition. Hoboken: Wiley 2018.

Dwyer JM. Manipulating the immune system with immune globulin. *N Engl J Med* 1992; 326: 107.

Engelhard VH. How cells process antigens. *Sci Am* 1994; 271(2): 54.

Faist E, Wichmann M, Kim C. Immunosuppression and immunomodulation in surgical patients. *Curr Opin Crit Care* 1997; 3: 293.

Fox DA, ed. Allergy & Immunology. *Scientific American Medicine*. Hamilton: Dekker Medicine. 2020.

Guillet J-G, Lai M-Z, Briner TJ, et al. Immunological self, nonself discrimination. *Science* 1987; 235: 865.

Lundy SK, Gizinski A, Fox DA. Introduction to clinical immunology: overview of immune response, autoimmune conditions, and immunosuppressive therapeutics for rheumatic diseases. In: *Scientific American Medicine. Allergy & Immunology*. Hamilton: Dekker Medicine. 2020.

Nossal GJV. Current concepts: immunology: the basic components of the immune system. *N Engl J Med* 1987; 316: 1320.

Nossal GJV. Immunologic tolerance: collaboration between antigen and lymphokines. *Science* 1989; 245: 147.

Nossal GJV. Life, death and the immune system. *Sci Am* 1993; 269(3): 20.

Nossal GJV. Negative selection of lymphocytes. *Cell* 1994; 76: 229.

Pardoll DM. Tumour antigens: a new look for the 1990s. *Nature* 1994; 369: 357.

Parker CW. Allergic reactions in man. *Pharmacol Rev* 1982; 34: 85.

Paul WE. Infectious diseases and the immune system. *Sci Am* 1993; 269(3): 57.

Reichlin S. Neuroendocrine-immune interactions. *N Engl J Med* 1993; 329: 1246.

Reimann PM, Mason PD. Plasmapheresis: technique and complications. *Intens Care Med* 1990; 16: 3.

Roberts NJ. Impact of temperature elevation on immunologic defenses. *Rev Infect Dis* 1991; 13: 462.

Shortman K, Scollay R. Death in the thymus. *Nature* 1994; 372: 44.

Smith RM, Giannoudis PV. Trauma and the immune response. *J R Soc Med* 1998; 91: 417.

Van de Meer JWM, Kullberg BJ. Defects in host-defense mechanisms. In: Rubin RH, Young LS, eds. *Clinical Approach to Infections in the Compromised Host*. 4th edition. New York: Plenum. 2002.

Von Boehmer H. Positive selection of lymphocytes. *Cell* 1994; 76: 219.

Yu Z, Lennon VA. Mechanism of intravenous immune globulin therapy in antibody-mediated autoimmune diseases. *N Engl J Med* 1999; 340: 227.

Zanetti G, Calandra T. Intravenous immunoglobulins and granulocyte colony-stimulating factor for the management of infection in intensive care units. *Curr Opin Crit Care* 1997; 3: 342.

Zweiman B, Levinson AI. Immunologic aspects of neurological and neuromuscular diseases. *JAMA* 1992; 268: 2918.

Immunomodulation

Immunomodulation refers to regulation of the immune system. It is a means of immunotherapy (typically immunosuppression) used in the treatment of autoimmune disorders, transplantation and some refractory inflammatory disorders.

There is a large list of agents with potent immunomodulatory effects currently available for clinical use (see Autoimmune disorders).

Immunothrombosis *See*

- Coagulation disorders.

Inborn errors of metabolism

Inborn errors of metabolism (IEMs) were first recognized by Garrod in 1902. They are genetic disorders resulting from the absence (or abnormality) of a specific enzyme, leading to an accumulation of products prior to, or to a deficiency of products after, that particular enzyme's site of activity. Less commonly, disorders of cofactors can affect multiple enzymes. In general, an IEM results from a single gene mutation, except for cofactors which are composed of multiple subunits and which are therefore encoded for by different genes.

As some patients with an IEM may not show any symptoms until adulthood, the new onset of unusual clinical features should prompt consideration of one of these uncommon conditions.

IEMs are classified according to the type of metabolic disturbance, as follows.
1. amino acid disorders (e.g. phenylketonuria),
2. urea cycle disorders (see Hyperammonaemia),
3. carbohydrate disorders (e.g. galactosaemia, glycogen storage diseases – q.v.),
4. lysosomal storage disorders (see Storage diseases),
5. organic acidaemias,
6. mitochondrial disorders (q.v.),
7. purine and pyrimidine disorders,
8. metal metabolism disorders (e.g. haemochromatosis – q.v., Wilson's disease – q.v.),
9. porphyrias (q.v.).

Bibliography

Bearn AG, Miller ED. Archibald Garrod and the development of the concept of inborn errors of metabolism in the newborn period. *Bull Hist Med* 1979; 53: 315.

Chopra SS, Berry GT. Metabolic disorders: inborn errors of amino acid, ammonia, organic acid, and fatty acid metabolism. In: *Scientific American Medicine. Endocrinology & Metabolism*. Hamilton: Dekker Medicine. 2020.

Wappner RS. Biochemical diagnosis of genetic diseases. *Pediatr Ann* 1993; 22: 282.

Wenger DA, Copploa S, Liu SL. Insights into the diagnosis and treatment of lysosomal storage diseases. *Arch Neurol* 2003; 60: 322.

Infections

Infectious diseases are especially relevant to Intensive Care, because sepsis in its various forms is one of the single largest groups of problems encountered.

Many specific **infections** are therefore commonly encountered and well understood by Intensive Care clinicians, including community-acquired and hospital-acquired pneumonia, classical sepsis (many cases of which are also nosocomial), abdominal sepsis and the systemic inflammatory response in its various guises (and names). The general principles of microbiological diagnosis, antibiotic prescribing and infection control are also part of front-line Intensive Care.

However, the spectrum of infectious diseases that may potentially be encountered in Intensive Care is very large. Moreover, both international travel and global climate change are altering many previously accepted epidemiological and geographical principles underpinning a clinician's expectations of encountering a particular infectious disease in a particular area. Thus, many of the less common specific infections have become of relevance to Intensive Care.

The conditions which are discussed in this book include
- Acquired immunodeficiency syndrome,
- Actinomycosis,
- Amoebiasis,
- Anthrax,
- Aspergillosis,
- Bioterrorism,
- Botulism,
- Bovine spongiform encephalopathy,
- Brucellosis,
- Buruli ulcer,
- Cat-scratch disease,
- Chikungunya,
- Cholera,
- Clostridial infections,
- Coronavirus,
- Creutzfeldt–Jakob disease,
- Cryptococcosis,
- Cytomegalovirus,
- Dengue,
- Diphtheria,
- Ebola haemorrhagic fever,
- Echinococcosis,
- Enteropathogenic *E. coli*,
- Epididymitis,
- Epstein–Barr virus,
- Equine morbilliform virus,
- Fasciitis,
- Fournier's gangrene,
- Gangrene,
- Germ warfare,
- Hantavirus,
- Helminths,
- Hendra virus,
- Herpesviruses,
- Histoplasmosis,
- HIV,
- Human immunodeficiency virus,
- Hydatid disease,
- Influenza,
- Japanese encephalitis,
- Katayama fever,
- Lassa fever,
- Lemierre's syndrome,
- Leprosy,
- Leptospirosis,
- Listeriosis,
- Liver abscess,
- Ludwig's angina,
- Lyme disease,
- Lyssavirus,
- Malaria,
- Meleney's progressive synergistic gangrene,
- Melioidosis,
- Meningococcaemia,
- Middle East respiratory syndrome (MERS),
- Murray Valley encephalitis,
- Mycobacterium ulcerans,
- Mycoplasma hominis,
- *Mycoplasma pneumoniae*,
- Necrotizing fasciitis,
- Necrotizing soft-tissue infection,
- Nocardiosis,
- Norovirus (Norwalk virus),
- Orchitis,
- Pandemics,
- Paragonimiasis,
- Parasitic infections,
- Pediculosis,
- Plague,
- Poliomyelitis,
- Procalcitonin,
- Protozoa,
- Psittacosis,
- Q fever,
- Rabies,

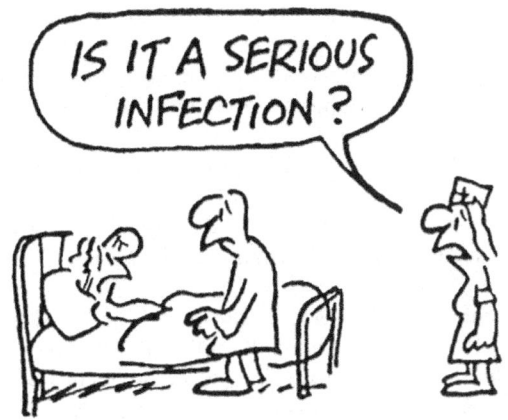

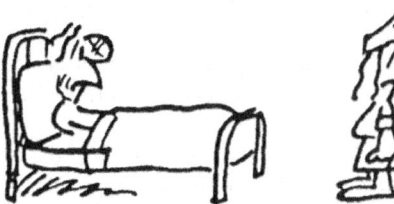
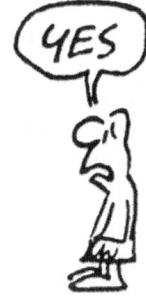

- Relapsing fever,
- Rickettsial diseases,
- Ross River virus,
- Scarlet fever,
- Schistosomiasis,
- Scrotal fire,
- Severe acute respiratory syndrome (SARS),
- Smallpox,
- Spotted fevers,
- Syphilis,
- Tetanus,
- Torulosis,
- Toxoplasmosis,
- Trench fever,
- Tuberculosis,
- Typhoid fever,
- Typhus,
- Varicella-zoster,
- Vincent's angina,
- Viral haemorrhagic fever,
- Waterhouse–Friderichsen syndrome,
- Weil's disease,
- West Nile encephalitis,
- Whipple's disease,
- Yellow fever,
- Zika virus infection,
- Zoonoses,
- Zoster.

Numerous additional issues of more general relevance to infectious diseases are also considered, such as fever, neutropenia, immunocompromise, various drug reactions and mediators.

For sound public health reasons, many infectious diseases must be reported to the local health authorities.

> Although there are inevitable differences between jurisdictions, **urgent public health reporting** would typically include
> - Anthrax (q.v.),
> - Botulism (q.v.),
> - COVID-19 (see Coronavirus),
> - Diphtheria (q.v.),
> - Food-poisoning outbreaks (q.v.),

- Haemolytic–uraemic syndromes (q.v.),
- Legionellosis,
- Listeriosis (q.v.),
- Measles,
- Meningococcal infection (q.v.),
- Middle East respiratory syndrome (MERS) (q.v.),
- Plague (q.v.),
- Poliomyelitis (q.v.),
- Rabies (q.v.),
- Severe acute respiratory syndrome (SARS) (q.v.),
- Smallpox (q.v.),
- Typhoid fever (q.v.),
- Viral haemorthagic fever (q.v.),
- Yellow fever (q.v.).

More routine public health reporting in developed countries would likely also include
- Brucellosis (q.v.),
- Creutzfeldt–Jakob disease (CJD) (q.v.),
- Dengue (q.v.),
- Hepatitis – all types (q.v.),
- Human immunodeficiency virus (HIV) infection (see Acquired immunodeficiency syndrome) (q.v.),
- Leprosy (q.v.),
- Lyssavirus (q.v.),
- Malaria (q.v.),
- Mumps,
- Mycobacterium ulcerans disease (q.v.),
- Pertussis,
- Q fever (see Rickettsial diseases),
- Salmonella infection,
- Shigella infection,
- Syphilis (q.v.),
- Tetanus (q.v.),
- Tuberculosis (q.v.),
- Varicella-zoster infection (see Varicella),
- West Nile virus infection (q.v.).

Bibliography

Azoulay E, ed. Severe infections in the critically ill. *Intens Care Med* 2020; 46: no. 2.

Barrett-Connor E. Anemia and infection. *Am J Med* 1972; 52: 242.

Bennett JE, Dolin R, Blaser MJ, eds. *Mandell, Douglas and Bennett's Principles and Practice of Infectious Diseases.* 9th edition. New York: Elsevier. 2019.

Bion JF, Brun-Buisson C, eds. Infection and critical illness: genetic and environmental aspects of susceptibility and resistance. *Intens Care Med* 2000; 26; suppl. 1.

Bohnsack JF, Brown EJ. The role of the spleen in resistance to infection. *Annu Rev Med* 1986; 37: 49.

Brigden ML, Pattullo AL. Prevention and management of overwhelming postsplenectomy infection – an update. *Crit Care Med* 1999; 27: 836.

Cassell GH, Cole BC. Mycoplasmas as agents of human disease. *N Engl J Med* 1981; 304: 80.

Cohen S, Tyrrell DA, Smith AP. Psychological stress and susceptibility to the common cold. *N Engl J Med* 1991; 325: 606.

Cunha BA, ed. *Infectious Diseases in Critical Care Medicine.* 3rd edition. Boca Baton: CRC Press. 2009.

Durand MI, Calserwood SB, Weber MD, et al. Acute bacterial meningitis in adults. *N Engl J Med* 1993; 328: 21.

Fisman DN. Hemophagocytic syndromes and infection. *Emerg Infect Dis* 2000; 6: 6.

Gilbert GL. Infections in pregnant women. *Med J Aust* 2002; 176: 229.

Gorbach SL, Bartlett JG, Blacklow NR, eds. *Infectious Diseases.* 3rd edition. Philadelphia: WB Saunders. 2004.

Howard CR. Viral hemorrhagic fevers: properties and prospects for treatment and prevention. *Antiviral Res* 1984; 4: 169.

Hughes AJ, Biggs BA. Parasitic worms of the central nervous system. *Intern Med J* 2002; 32: 541.

Keusch GT, Barza MJ, Bennish ML, et al., eds. *Year Book of Infectious Diseases 1998.* St Louis: Mosby-Year Book. 1998.

Manocha S, Walley KR, Russell JA. Severe acute respiratory distress syndrome (SARS): a critical care perspective. *Crit Care Med* 2003; 31: 2684.

Maslin F-X. Global aspects of emerging and potential zoonoses: a WHO perspective. *Emerg Infect Dis* 1997; 3: 2.

Paul WE. Infectious diseases and the immune system. *Sci Am* 1993; 269(3): 57.

Peeling RW, Brunham RC. Chlamydiae as pathogens: new species and new issues. *Emerg Infect Dis* 1996; 2: 4.

Pinder M, Bellomo R, Lipman J. Pharmacological principles of antibiotic prescription in the critically ill. *Anaesth Intens Care* 2002; 30: 134.

Rahall JJ. Antibiotic combinations: the clinical relevance of synergy and antagonism. *Medicine* 1978; 57: 179.

Shafazand S, Weinacker AB. Blood cultures in the critical care unit: improving utilization and yield. *Chest* 2002; 122: 1727.

Sigurdardottir B, Bjornsson OM, Jonsdottir KE, et al. Acute bacterial meningitis in adults. *Arch Intern Med* 1997; 157: 425.

Spach D, Liles W, Campbell G, et al. Tick-borne diseases in the United States. *N Engl J Med* 1993; 329: 936.

Sprung CL, Cohen R, Adini B, eds. Recommendations and standard operating procedures for intensive care unit and hospital preparations for an influenza epidemic or mass disaster. Summary report of the European Society of Intensive Care Medicine's Task Force for intensive care unit triage during an influenza epidemic or mass disaster. *Intens Care Med* 2010; 36 (suppl. 1): S1.

Tomkins L. The use of molecular methods in the diagnosis of infectious diseases. *N Engl J Med* 1992; 327: 1290.

Various. Infectious Diseases. In: *Scientific American Medicine*. Hamilton: Dekker Medicine. 2020.

Whitley RJ. Viral encephalitis. *N Engl J Med* 1990; 323: 242.

Zanetti G, Calandra T. Intravenous immunoglobulins and granulocyte colony-stimulating factor for the management of infection in intensive care units. *Curr Opin Crit Care* 1997; 3: 342.

Zumla A, James DG. Granulomatous infections: etiology and classification. *Clin Infect Dis* 1996; 23: 146.

Inflammatory bowel disease

Non-specific **inflammatory bowel disease** (IBD) comprises ulcerative colitis and Crohn's disease, each with different pathological, clinical and therapeutic aspects, but both requiring distinction from other serious bowel diseases, such as infections or ischaemia. In particular, infections with *Yersinia enterocolitica* or even *Mycobacterium tuberculosis* can provide contemporary challenges in differential diagnosis. In IBD of recent onset, infection with *Clostridium difficile* should be excluded (see Colitis). In older patients, diverticulitis and ischaemic colitis need to be excluded.

It is likely that an altered immune response between the host and the gut microbiota, together with genetic and environmental factors, underpins the intestinal inflammation in these distressing conditions. Thus, biological agents targetting the immuno-inflammatory response may offer new therapeutic opportunities for the IBDs.

Previous fears that combined measles, mumps and rubella (MMR) vaccination in children might predispose to the later development of inflammatory bowel disease were later shown to be unfounded. On the other hand, combined oral contraceptive agents (q.v.) and hormone replacement preparations have been found to be associated with an increased risk of developing IBD, especially in women who are also smokers.

For reasons that are not entirely clear, the global burden of IBD appears to be increasing, especially in developed countries. As the incidence rate of IBD is higher than the mortality rate and as the life expectancy of patients with IBD is relatively normal, the overall prevalence is increased especially among older patients, a phenomenon referred to as 'compounding prevalence' and common to a number of chronic diseases.

1. **Ulcerative colitis** comprises inflammation of colonic epithelium, usually affecting the rectum and distal colon. While there is some minor familial and ethnic clustering, its aetiology is unknown, but it is probable that there are subgroups of separate causation. It is relatively uncommon, with a prevalence of less than 1 in 1000 of the population. Clinical features are seen most commonly in young adults. In the early stages, blood and/or mucus is noted in the stools, and there may even be constipation. In the later stages, there are diarrhoea and systemic features, with fatigue, anorexia, fever and weight loss.

The severity of illness is very variable.

- **Mild disease**

This is seen in most patients (60%), with intermittent diarrhoea (e.g. up to four stools per day) and associated abdominal cramps.

In most such patients (85%), the process remains confined to the rectum (proctitis) or rectum and distal colon (proctosigmoiditis).

There are no systemic features or laboratory abnormalities.

- **Moderate disease**

This occurs in 25% of patients, with involvement of up to half of the colon (left-sided colitis).

There is watery diarrhoea, with blood and mucus (e.g. more than five stools per day), associated with abdominal cramps and rectal urgency.

Some systemic symptoms are usual.

- **Severe disease**

This occurs in 15% of patients, with involvement of the entire colon (extensive or total colitis).

There is constant profuse bloody diarrhoea, with abdominal distension and marked systemic symptoms.

Such patients require hospitalization.

- **Toxic megacolon**

This is the most severe form of the disease and occurs in about 3% of cases.

Since one third of such cases present initially in this way, the differential diagnosis can be difficult, especially as diarrhoea may be minimal at this time and systemic symptoms prominent.

There are signs of an acute abdomen, and the patient may become shocked.

The **local complications** of ulcerative colitis include
- bowel haemorrhage,
- bowel perforation,
- bowel stricture,
- cancer of the colon
  - this is related to the duration, extent and severity of the disease and is responsible for a third of deaths from the disease.

Extra-colonic complications are present in about 40% of cases and are considered due to extraintestinal spill from the dysregulated enteric immune response in IBD. These complications may be prominent and may involve virtually any organ in the body. The most common manifestations involve
- **eyes**
  - with iritis (i.e. uveitis – q.v.) and/or conjunctivitis and/or episcleritis,
- **joints**
  - with migratory monarticular arthritis of large joints (the most common manifestation),
  - with an increased incidence of ankylosing spondylitis (q.v.),
- **liver**
  - with jaundice, sclerosing cholangitis (q.v.), fatty liver,
  - occasionally with cirrhosis,
- **skin**
  - occasionally with erythema nodosum (q.v.),
  - rarely with pyoderma gangrenosum (q.v.).

The diagnosis is made on sigmoidoscopy, at which the mucosa appears friable and granular. Biopsy excludes Crohn's disease or other specific disorders, and microbiological examination excludes amoebae or pathogenic bacteria. Colonoscopy or barium contrast enema shows the extent of disease.

The differential diagnosis is
- Crohn's disease (see below),
- irritable bowel syndrome,
- diverticulitis,
- ischaemic colitis,
- bacterial or amoebic gastroenteritis (see Amoebiasis).

Treatment modalities are several.
- Simple **anti-diarrhoeal** medication (e.g. loperamide, diphenoxylate) may be effective in mild disease, but they should be used with care because of the risk of toxic megacolon.
- **Sulphasalazine** is used primarily for maintenance, but it is also useful for mild exacerbations. Although typically given orally, it may also be used in the form of a retention enema. The frequency of side-effects from sulphasalazine has led to the development of better tolerated compounds derived from its active moiety,

5-aminosalicylic acid (5-ASA, mesalazine, mesalamine). One of the controlled-release forms given topically and/or orally is generally the agent of first choice nowadays for the treatment of mild to moderate disease.
- **Corticosteroids** are used locally in enema form and systemically for moderate or severe disease.
- **Immunosuppressive therapy** (azathioprine, ciclosporin) is indicated for severe or refractory disease. Infliximab, which was originally introduced for Crohn's disease (see below), has been found to be similarly effective in ulcerative colitis. See Immunomodulation.
- **Surgery** (proctocolectomy) may be required.

> - **Toxic megacolon** requires resuscitation, fluids and electrolytes, nasogastric aspiration, intravenous corticosteroids and antibiotics.
> - Anti-diarrhoeal drugs are contraindicated, and indeed they may precipitate this syndrome.
> - As soon as the patient becomes stable, a total proctocolectomy is performed, preferably within 48 hr.

The course of illness is very variable. About 10% of patients experience long remissions of up to 15 years, though most (75%) have intermittent exacerbations over many years. About 10% of patients have continuous disease. The 1-year mortality is 5% overall and up to 15–20% in toxic megacolon.

2. **Crohn's disease** is a granulomatous ileocolitis affecting all layers of the bowel and presenting as an enteritis, enterocolitis, colitis or proctocolitis. Like ulcerative colitis, there is some minor familial and ethnic clustering, but its aetiology remains unknown. The possibility of an infectious cause has long been suspected but never confirmed. In this regard, the organism responsible for the related **Johne's disease** in ruminants, *Mycobacterium avium subspecies paratuberculosis* (MAP), has been implicated in Crohn's disease, though a clinical trial of appropriate antibiotic therapy failed to show sustained improvement in patients.

Clinical features are also seen mainly in young adults, particularly in smokers. Chronic indolent symptomatic disease has been present on average for 5 years before presentation. Mild, watery but not blood-stained diarrhoea and abdominal pain is often diagnosed as irritable bowel syndrome (q.v.). In some patients, there are systemic features of anorexia, fatigue, weight loss, abdominal mass, fistulae, iritis and anaemia.

Complications include
- anal fissure,
- bowel fistulae
  - which occur in 50% of patients at some time during the course of the disease,
- peri-rectal abscess,
- fulminant colitis ('toxic megacolon')
  - this can occur but is uncommon,
- increased incidence of both gallstones and renal oxalate calculi
  - particularly in those patients with severe fat malabsorption (q.v.),
- the eye, joint and skin features seen in ulcerative colitis occur in about 10% of patients (see above).

The differential diagnosis and investigations are as for ulcerative colitis (see above).

Treatment is also similar to that for ulcerative colitis, except that medical therapy is often disappointing and surgery is required in many patients because of either initial disease or its complications. However, there is a high postoperative recurrence rate, and about half of the patients require re-operation.

Infliximab, *a chimeric monoclonal antibody to tumour necrosis factor α (TNF-α) (q.v.), has been shown to enhance greatly the closure of abdominal and perineal fistulae. Potential adverse effects include infection with intracellular organisms and possibly malignancy. Other anti-TNF agents (e.g.* **adalimumab**) *are also effective, both for induction and maintenance in patients with moderate or severe disease, either lumenal or fistulizing. A gut-specific anti-integrin monoclonal antibody,* **vedolizumab**, *has more recently been introduced with similar indications.*

The early promise of **probiotic therapy** *with Lactobacilli in ameliorating the intestinal inflammatory response by modifying the gut flora was not borne out in subsequent clinical trials.*

See also
- Colitis,
- Microbiome,
- Spondyloarthritis.

Bibliography

Black H, Mendoza M, Murin S. Thoracic manifestations of inflammatory bowel disease. *Chest* 2007; 131: 524.

Bongartz T, Sutton AJ, Sweeting MJ, et al. Anti-TNF antibody therapy in rheumatoid arthritis and the risk of serious infections and malignancies: systematic review and meta-analysis of rare harmful effects in randomized controlled trials. *JAMA* 2006; 295: 2275.

Carter MJ, Lobo AJ, Travis SP. Guidelines for the management of inflammatory bowel disease in adults. *Gut* 2004; 53 (suppl. 5): VI.

Colombel JF, Loftus EV, Tremaine WJ, et al. The safety profile of infliximab in patients with Crohn's disease. *Gastroenterology* 2004; 126: 19.

Davis WC, Kuenstner JT, Singh SV. Resolution of Crohn's (Johne's) disease with antibiotics: what are the next steps?. *Expert Rev Gastroenterol Hepatol* 2017; 11: 393.

Fehily SR, Basnayake C, Wright EK, et al. The gut microbiota and gut disease. *Intern Med J* 2021; 51: 1594.

Gibson PR, Anderson RP. Inflammatory bowel disease. *Med J Aust* 1998; 169: 387.

Greenberg GR. Nutritional support in inflammatory bowel disease: current status and future directions. *Scand J Gastroenterol* 1992; 192 (suppl.): 117.

Greenstein RJ. Is Crohn's disease caused by a mycobacterium? Comparisons with leprosy, tuberculosis, and Johne's disease. *Lancet Infect Dis* 2004; 4: 507.

Grimpen F, Pavli P. Advances in the management of inflammatory bowel disease. *Intern Med J* 2010; 40: 258.

Kornbluth A, George J, Sachar DB. Immunosuppressive drugs in Crohn's disease. *Gastroenterologist* 1994; 2: 239.

MacDermott RP, Stenson WF. *Inflammatory Bowel Disease.* New York: Elsevier. 1992.

McNees AL, Markesich D, Zayyani NR, et al. Mycobacterium paratuberculosis as a cause of Crohn's disease. *Expert Rev Gastroenterol Hepatol* 2015; 9: 1523.

Ng SC, Shi HY, Hamidi N, et al. Worldwide incidence and prevalence of inflammatory bowel disease in the 21st century: a systematic review of population-based studies. *Lancet* 2017; 390: 2769.

Podolsky DK. Inflammatory bowel disease. *N Engl J Med* 2002; 347: 417.

Present DH, Rutgeerts P, Targan S, et al. Infliximab for the treatment of fistulas in patients with Crohn's disease. *N Engl J Med* 1999; 340: 1398.

Rachmilewitz D. New forms of treatment for inflammatory bowel disease. *Gut* 1992; 33: 1301.

Sands BE. Biologic therapy for inflammatory bowel disease. *Inflamm Bowel Dis* 1997; 3: 95.

Sands BE, Anderson FH, Bernstein CN, et al. Infliximab maintenance therapy for fistulizing Crohn's disease. *New Engl J Med* 2004; 350: 876.

Shouval DS. Evaluation and treatment of monogenic forms of inflammatory bowel diseases. In: *Scientific American Medicine. Gastroenterology.* Hamilton: Dekker Medicine. 2020.

Schreiber S, Hampe J. Genomics and inflammatory bowel disease. *Curr Opin Gastroenterol* 1999; 16: 297.

Selby WS. Current issues in Crohn's disease. *Med J Aust* 2003; 178: 532.

Thompson NP, Montgomery SM, Pounder RE, et al. Is measles vaccination a risk factor for inflammatory bowel disease? *Lancet* 1995; 345: 1071.

Inflammatory myeloid neoplasia See
- Histiocytosis.

Influenza

Although **influenza** is a commonly encountered infection worldwide, a number of less common aspects of the disease are of special relevance to intensivists. Seasonal influenza is a leading cause of death in all societies, causing about 500,000 deaths worldwide each year. It occurs especially in patients with comorbidities, though for most patients it is only an inconvenience for a few days. Pandemic influenza poses a much greater risk, albeit an intermittent and unpredictable one, and one that would likely overwhelm critical care resources in even the best prepared countries. Overall, the worldwide burden of disease from influenza is greater than that for any other infectious disease. This burden includes not only its well recognized acute respiratory manifestations, but also the potential to precipitate myocardial infarction and stroke, as well as to exacerbate some chronic diseases such as diabetes.

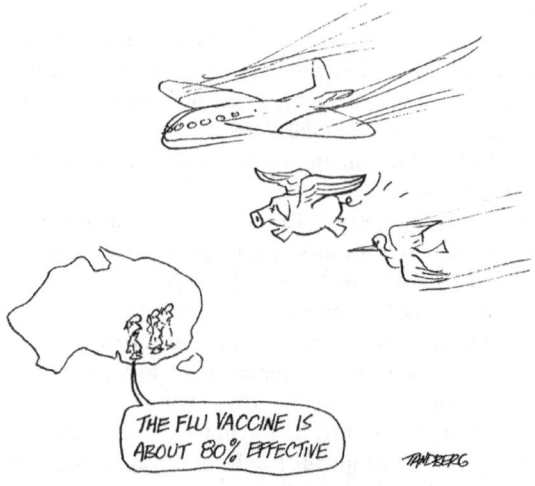

Influenza viruses are classified as A, B and C. Influenza A is found in humans, birds and other animals, and it is responsible for the most common and serious infections and for all recorded pandemics. Influenza B contributes to seasonal disease. Subclassifications of influenza A are based on the virus's surface glycoproteins,

- **haemagglutinin** (H), which mediates viral attachment to cells, and
- **neuraminidase** (N), which promotes the viral release from infected cells.

In total, there are 18 H types and 11 N types, though only a few combinations have caused widespread human disease, namely, H1N1, H2N2 and H3N2.

The surface glycoproteins are the antigens responsible for the host's immune responses, but they are also readily subject to change due to antigenic drift or shift.

- **Antigenic drift** refers to relatively minor changes in H or sometimes N antigenicity due to point mutations that occur frequently due to immune pressure in the population. This drift leads to the need for continuous updating of influenza vaccines.
- **Antigenic shift** refers to major gene changes in H and sometimes N antigenicity due to genetic reassortment during dual infections. Similar major antigenic changes can also occur when an animal virus is transmitted successfully to humans or when a virus is reintroduced after a long absence from humans.

A major new strain of influenza A can lead to a pandemic, as with the 'Spanish' flu (actually from Texas) in 1918–19 (H1N1, with 50–100 million deaths worldwide), the Asian flu in 1957 (H2N2, with 1 million deaths), the Hong Kong flu in 1968 (H3N2, with 1 million deaths) and the brief 'swine flu' pandemic in 2009 (H1N1 09, with half a million deaths). These strains were originally avian viruses which either crossed the species barrier (1918–19) or combined with a human virus in a dual infection in pigs (1957, 1968 and 2009). Avian viruses are particularly important, because asymptomatic water birds (both wild and domestic) are the main natural reservoir for influenza A of all subtypes, with an epicentre in Southern China. Swine are also important, because they are susceptible to infection with both avian and human strains and are therefore a potential mixing vessel for new strains.

The infectivity of influenza is reflected in its basic reproduction number (R_0), which is generally 1–2. Its pathogenicity is reflected in its case fatality rate (CFR), which in recent decades has been <0.02%. See Pandemics.

Influenza management relies primarily on
- *public health measures (for prevention and control),*
- *vaccination (for seasonal prevention, but with only 15–60% effectiveness, depending on the individual year), and*
- *antiviral drugs (the neuraminidase inhibitors, oseltamivir, zanamivir, peramivir and most recently baloxavir for specific treatment). The original antiviral drug, amantadine (an M2 blocker), is no longer*

effective due to acquired viral resistance. If available, rapid molecular testing can guide antiviral treatment.

Several potential universal vaccines are under study to replace the annual quadrivalent vaccine which covers two current strains each of influenza A and B.

Avian influenza ('bird flu') in humans has been caused in recent years by an H5N1 variant. Although this strain was first noted in Hong Kong in 1997 and then widely reported worldwide since 2003 among wild and domestic birds (both sick and well), there have been only a few hundred cases of human infection, since animal–human transmissibility is very low and there has been almost no effective human-human transmission. However, although so far rare in humans, avian influenza clearly has the potential to mutate to a more infectious variant (as in the past). As the H5N1 strain is already highly pathogenic, added infectivity would lead to the potential for a pandemic.

Since 2003, the avian H5N1 strain has spread via migratory water birds from China to the rest of Asia and westwards as far as Europe and Africa. It has infected not only millions of wild and then domestic birds, but it has also since spread to a variety of mammals, both in the wild and in zoos.

In recent years, there have also been sporadic and mild human infections with other avian strains, such as H7N7 and H9N2.

When human infection with the H5N1 strain has occurred, it has generally been severe, with pneumonitis, encephalitis (q.v.), diarrhoea (q.v.) and multiorgan failure (q.v.). The mortality has been over 50%, even in previously healthy young patients.

Treatment with the antiviral agents, oseltamivir and zanamivir, has often been disappointing.

Public health measures are so far the key to prevention and disease control, but the availability of an effective vaccine will also be important.

Pandemic H1N1 09 influenza ('swine flu') first appeared in early 2009 in Mexico and rapidly spread worldwide to over 200 countries as a result of airline travel. This new strain of influenza A represented a complex genetic reassortment of swine, human and avian strains within pigs, a process which may have originated in fact in Asia rather than in Mexico itself.

By the end of the year, there had been an estimated 55 million cases in the USA alone, with 250,000 hospitalizations and over 10,000 deaths, but within a few months, the case numbers had begun to decline markedly worldwide. Unlike seasonal influenza, the new strain infected a disproportionate number of people <25 years old, presumably because older people had some pre-existing immunity, perhaps from prior to 1957. Unusually high rates of infection were also seen in pregnant women (see Pneumonia in pregnancy) and in Indigenous populations.

The incubation period was about 2 days, and viral shedding was reported from the day before symptoms for up to 7 days. The virus was highly infectious, being readily transmitted both by droplet spread and by direct contact

Detailed examination of the pressure which such an epidemic can inflict on Intensive Care resources has been reported from Australia and New Zealand, where 722 patients were admitted to ICUs during the three winter months of 2009. Prolonged ICU stay, complex ventilatory management, multiorgan complications and extracorporeal membrane oxygenation (ECMO) rescue were frequent features. The mortality was nearly 15%, and many of the deaths occurred in young, previously healthy patients.

Following WHO's issuing of a pandemic alert, a complex series of public health measures were implemented, and a specific vaccine was rapidly developed.

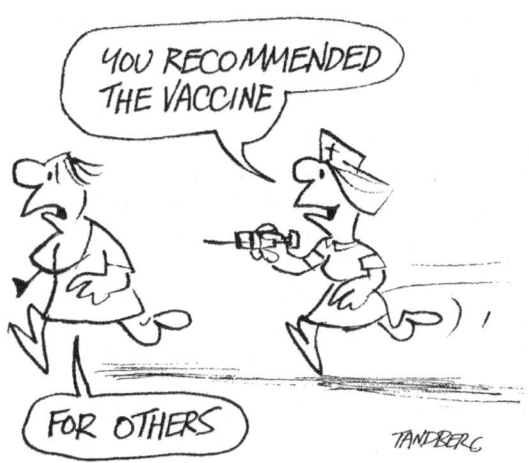

Bibliography

ANZIC Influenza Investigators. Critical care services and 2009 H1N1 influenza in Australia and New Zealand. *N Engl J Med* 2009; 361: 1925.

Arabi Y, Gomersall CD, Ahmed QA, et al. The critically ill avian influenza A (H5N1) patient. *Crit Care Med* 2007; 35: 1397.

Beigel JH. Influenza. *Crit Care Med* 2008; 36: 2660.

Beigel JH, Farrar J, Han AM, et al. Avian influenza A (H5N1) infection in humans. *New Engl J Med* 2005; 353: 1374.

Bishop JF, Murnane MP, Owen R. Australia's winter with the 2009 pandemic influenza A (H1N1) virus. *N Engl J Med* 2009; 361: 2591.

Dawood FS, Jain S, Finelli L, et al. Emergence of a novel swine-origin influenza A (H1N1) virus in humans. *N Engl J Med* 2009; 360: 2605.

Dwyer DE, Emery S, McKinnon M. Preparing for an influenza pandemic. *Med J Aust* 2006; 185 (suppl.): S25.

Gruber PC, Gomersall CD, Joynt GM. Avian influenza (H5N1): implications for intensive care. *Intens Care Med* 2006; 32: 823.

Harrigan PWJ, Webb SAR, Seppelt IM, et al. The practical experience of managing the H1N1 2009 influenza pandemic in Australian and New Zealand intensive care units. *Crit Care Resusc* 2010; 12: 121.

Loh L-C, Hui DS-C, Beasley R, eds. Avian influenza: from basic biology to endemic planning. *Respirology* 2008; 13 (suppl.): S1.

Macfarlane JT, Lim WS. Bird flu and pandemic flu. *BMJ* 2005; 331: 975.

Mitchell MD, Mikkelsen ME, Umscheid CA, et al. A systematic review to inform institutional decisions about the use of extracorporeal membrane oxygenation during the H1N1 influenza pandemic. *Crit Care Med* 2010; 38: 1398.

Smith GJ, Vijaykrishna D, Bahl J, et al. Origins and evolutionary genomics of the 2009 swine-origin H1N1 influenza A epidemic. *Nature* 2009; 459: 1122.

Sprung CL, Cohen R, Adini B, eds. Recommendations and standard operating procedures for intensive care unit and hospital preparations for an influenza epidemic or mass disaster. Summary report of the European Society of Intensive Care Medicine's Task Force for intensive care unit triage during an influenza epidemic or mass disaster. *Intens Care Med* 2010; 36 (suppl. 1): S1.

Torres A, Martin-Loeches I, Sligl W. et al. Severe flu management: a point of view. *Intens Care Med* 2020; 46: 153.

Wong SSY, Yuen K-y. Avian influenza virus infections in humans. *Chest* 2006; 129: 156.

Yang Y, Sugimoto JD, Halloran ME, et al. The transmissibility and control of pandemic influenza A (H1N1) virus. *Science* 2009; 326: 729.

Inhalation injury

Inhalation injury refers to the respiratory complications of **burns**. It can result in significant morbidity and mortality in those initially surviving a fire. Respiratory tract injury results from the inhalation of products of combustion, which may be numerous, and it has an even greater impact on mortality than the two important factors in burn injury of patient age and surface area involved. The immediate assessment of a burns injury thus includes urgent airway examination. This is particularly important in the setting of fires in an enclosed space or affecting victims who were unconscious (e.g. due to drugs, head injury or sleep).

Smoke, the most obvious product of combustion, is a suspension of carbon particles in air and other gases. The particles are often coated with chemicals, such as organic acids and aldehydes. The other gases may include carbon monoxide and toxic fumes, such as sulphur dioxide, nitrogen oxides, ammonia, hydrogen cyanide and hydrochloric acid, these being vaporized chemicals often released from the burning of modern synthetic materials, such as PVC.

Smoke may be hot, but usually it has only a low thermal capacity, so that any burns involve only the upper respiratory tract, in contrast to steam, which has a high thermal capacity (4000 times that of dry air) and can burn as far as the bronchioles. Fortunately, burns due to steam are uncommon.

Respiratory burns (i.e. inhalation injury) may comprise
- direct thermal injury,
- smoke inhalation,
- inhalation of toxic products of combustion,
- later respiratory complications.

Direct thermal injury, particularly of the upper respiratory tract, is common and is usually associated with facial burns. Severe acute upper airways obstruction may result.

As indicated above, thermal injury of the lower respiratory tract and lung parenchyma is difficult to produce except by superheated steam.

Smoke inhalation is also a common thermal injury. More importantly, it gives rise to irritation, sometimes severe, of the entire tracheobronchial tree and usually causes immediate respiratory distress, though this may be delayed for up to 48 hr. There is a chemical bronchitis, with mucosal injury, ciliary dysfunction, mucous plugging, atelectasis and bronchorrhoea. There may also be mucosal oedema and increased vascular permeability.

The upper respiratory tract injury may appear minor at first, but its progress over the next 48 hr needs to be carefully monitored. The patient may develop clinical features of stridor, cough, charcoal-containing sputum, dyspnoea, wheeze, hypoxia and respiratory distress. Bronchial casts may subsequently be coughed. Respiratory and even systemic inflammatory changes may persist for some months.

Inhalation of toxic products of combustion results from fires in confined spaces, e.g. buildings or aircraft.

These products give rise to a severe form of acute lung irritation (q.v.) and are a major cause of fatality.

If the serum lactate level is markedly elevated (e.g. 10 mmol/L or more), carbon monoxide (q.v.) or cyanide (q.v.) toxicity should be considered. Death can occur from tissue hypoxia produced by either of these two gases.

Later respiratory complications are common, such as pulmonary oedema (especially volume overload), acute respiratory distress syndrome (ARDS, q.v.) and secondary bacterial infection (especially pneumonia). Of the burns patients requiring intubation, about 50% develop ARDS, but inhalation injury does not appear to be a major risk factor for this complication. In contrast to other critical care settings, ARDS occurs much later after burns (average time to onset of about 7 days) and confers little added mortality (perhaps since the average underlying mortality is already about 40%).

Hospitalization is required for any person exposed to smoke or fumes or with a singed face, especially if there is cough, stridor, wheeze or dysphonia. Careful observation should continue for at least the first 2 days. Early fibreoptic bronchoscopy provides the best way to assess the extent and severity of respiratory tract injury, with specific search for erythema, oedema, ulceration or carbon deposits.

*Treatment of respiratory burns is with **respiratory support** and with management of any complications on their individual merits.*
- Initial *fluid resuscitation* with IV fluids is based on the calculated total burn size.
- Early **endotracheal intubation** is wise, because of its great technical difficulty due to massive oedema if delayed. **Suxamethonium** can be safely used for intubation only in the initial phase of burn management because of the risk of hyperkalaemia following its use during later phases.
- Repeated **bronchoscopy** and lavage may be required to remove debris and plugs.
- **Bronchodilators** (inhaled β_2 agonists) are helpful if there is bronchospasm.
- *Inhaled **heparin** with **acetylcysteine*** has been reported to reduce cast formation, atelectasis, reintubation and mortality compared with historical controls.

Long-term lung function abnormalities and sometimes significant respiratory complications, such as tracheal or bronchial stenosis and bronchiolitis obliterans (q.v.), have been reported in survivors of respiratory burns.

Bibliography

Baud FJ, Barriot P, Toffis V, et al. Elevated blood cyanide concentrations in victims of smoke inhalation. *N Engl J Med* 1991; 325: 1761.

Crapo RO. Smoke-inhalation injuries. *JAMA* 1981; 246: 1694.

Dancey DR, Hayes J, Gomez M, et al. ARDS in patients with thermal injury. *Intens Care Med* 1999; 25: 1231.

de la Cal MA, Cerda E, Garcia-Hierro P, et al. Pneumonia in patients with severe burns. *Chest* 2001; 119: 1160.

Dennekamp M, Abramson MJ. The effects of bushfire smoke on respiratory health. *Respirology* 2011; 16: 198.

Dietch E. The management of burns. *N Engl J Med* 1990; 323: 1249.

Dyer RF, Esch VH. Polyvinyl chloride toxicity in fires: hydrogen chloride toxicity in firefighters. *JAMA* 1976; 235: 393.

Fogarty PW, George PJM, Solomon M, et al. Long term effects of smoke inhalation in survivors of the King's Cross underground station fire. *Thorax* 1991; 46: 914.

Gueugniaud P-Y, Carsin H, Bertin-Maghit M, et al. Current advances in the initial management of major thermal burns. *Intens Care Med* 2000; 26: 848.

Haponik E, Munster A, eds. *Respiratory Injury: Smoke Inhalation and Burns.* New York: McGraw-Hill. 1990.

Hettiaratchy S, Dziewulski P. ABC of burns. *BMJ* 2004; 328: 1366 et seq.

Holley AD, Reade MC, Lipman J, et al. There is no fire without smoke! Pathophysiology and treatment of inhalational injury in burns: a narrative review. *Anaesth Intens Care* 2020; 48: 114.

Large AA, Owens GR, Hoffman LA. The short-term effects of smoke exposure on the pulmonary function of firefighters. *Chest* 1990; 97: 806.

Mlcak RP, Suman OE, Herndon DN. Respiratory management of inhalation injury. *Burns* 2007; 33: 2.

Park GY, Park JW, Jeong DH, et al. Prolonged airway and systemic inflammatory reactions after smoke inhalation. *Chest* 2003; 123: 475.

Ryan CM, Schoenfeld DA, Thorpe WP, et al. Objective estimates of the probability of death from burn injuries. *N Engl J Med* 1998; 338: 362.

Schulz JT, Ryan CM. The frustrating problem of smoke inhalation injury. *Crit Care Med* 2000; 28: 1677.

Sheridan R. Specific therapies for inhalation injury. *Crit Care Med* 2002; 30: 718.

Walker PF, Buehner MF, Wood LA, et al. Diagnosis and management of inhalation injury: an updated review. *Crit Care* 2015; 19: 351.

Insect bites and stings *See*

- Bites and stings.

Insecticides

Insecticides can also be poisonous in humans. They are either
- **organophosphates**, which irreversibly bind anticholinesterase, penetrate the central nervous system and cause severe poisoning, or
- **carbamates**, which reversibly bind anticholinesterase, do not penetrate the central nervous system and cause less severe poisoning.
 See
- Anticholinesterases,
- Warfare agents – Nerve agents.

Insects

Insects are one of the main groups of **arthropods** (q.v.). They have three pairs of legs. Those insects which are important in human disease, because they are either vectors or directly venomous, include
- ants (see Bites and stings – Insects),
- fleas (q.v.),
- lice (q.v.),
- mosquitoes (q.v.).

Insulinoma See
- Islet cell tumour.

Intensive Care Unit–acquired weakness

Intensive Care Unit–acquired weakness (ICU-AW) is another term for the better-known **critical illness neuromuscular abnormality** (q.v.).

Interstitial lung diseases

The **interstitial lung diseases** (ILDs) are a group of diffuse pulmonary processes, many of unknown aetiology. They are also referred to as **diffuse parenchymal lung diseases** (DPLDs). Their individual diagnoses can sometimes be difficult, and not all cases can be classified with confidence.

The entire spectrum of these conditions, both specific and non-specific, is referred to simply as **pulmonary infiltrates** (q.v.).

Specific interstitial diseases are usually considered separately from the non-specific group listed below. Specific interstitial disease include
- pneumonia,
- pulmonary oedema (q.v.),
- acute respiratory distress syndrome (q.v.),
- aspiration pneumonitis (q.v.),
- malignancy,
- pneumoconioses and other occupational lung diseases (q.v.),
- hypersensitivity pneumonitis (q.v.),
- miliary tuberculosis (q.v.),
- radiation pneumonitis (q.v.),
- uraemia,
- drug reactions (see Drugs and the lung),
- lung involvement in systemic diseases (see Systemic diseases and the lung).

The major interstitial lung diseases (ILDs or DPLDs) are
1. **idiopathic interstitial pneumonias (IIPs)**(q.v.)
   - idiopathic pulmonary fibrosis (IPF),
   - acute interstitial pneumonia (AIP),
   - desquamative interstitial pneumonia (DIP),
   - respiratory bronchiolitis interstitial lung disease (RB-ILD),
   - cryptogenic organizing pneumonia (COP) (formerly bronchiolitis obliterans organizing pneumonia, BOOP),
   - non-specific interstitial pneumonia (NSIP),
   - idiopathic lymphocytic (lymphoid) interstitial pneumonia (LIP),
   - idiopathic pleuroparenchymal fibroelastosis (PPFE),
2. **sarcoidosis** (q.v.)
3. **haemorrhagic infiltrates**
   - Goodpasture's syndrome (q.v.),
   - idiopathic pulmonary haemosiderosis (q.v.),
4. **pulmonary infiltration with eosinophilia (PIE)** (q.v.)
   - Loeffler's syndrome,
   - asthmatic pulmonary eosinophilia,
   - tropical pulmonary eosinophilia,
   - eosinophilic pneumonia,
5. **angiitis and granulomatosis**
   - Wegener's granulomatosis (q.v.),
   - lymphomatoid granulomatosis (q.v.),
   - bronchocentric granulomatosis (q.v.),
6. **rare pulmonary infiltrative conditions**
   - histiocytosis (q.v.),
   - pulmonary alveolar proteinosis (q.v.),
   - pulmonary alveolar microlithiasis,
   - lymphangio(leio)myomatosis (q.v.),
   - pulmonary amyloidosis (see Amyloidosis),

Although listed as a group for comparison, these conditions are considered separately in this book. High-resolution CT scanning (HRCT) is generally the most useful imaging technique in assessing this group of conditions.

Bibliography

Baughman RP, Dent M. Role of bronchoalveolar lavage in interstitial lung disease. *Clin Chest Med* 2001; 22: 331.

Chu SC, Horiba K, Usuki J, et al. Comprehensive evaluation of 35 patients with lymphangioleiomyomatosis. *Chest* 1999; 115: 1041.

Coultas DB, Zumwalt RE, Black WC, et al. The epidemiology of interstitial lung diseases. *Am J Respir Crit Care Med* 1994; 150: 967.

Crystal RG, Bitterman PB, Rennard SI, et al. Interstitial lung diseases of unknown cause. *N Engl J Med* 1984; 310: 154 & 235.

Kitaichi M, Nishimura K, Itoh H, et al. Pulmonary lymphangioleiomyomatosis. *Am J Respir Crit Care Med* 1995; 151: 527.

McCormack FX. Lymphangioleiomyomatosis: a clinical update. *Chest* 2008; 133: 507.

Moss J, ed. *LAM (lymphangioleiomyomatosis) and Other Diseases Characterized by Smooth Muscle Proliferation.* New York: Marcel Dekker. 1999.

Prakash UB, Barham SS, Rosenow EC, et al. Pulmonary alveolar microlithiasis. *Mayo Clin Proc* 1983; 58: 290.

Reynolds HY. Diagnostic and management strategies for diffuse interstitial lung disease. *Chest* 1998; 113: 192.

Skolnik K, Ryerson CJ. Unclassifiable interstitial lung disease: a review. *Respirology* 2016; 21: 51.

Taylor JR, Ryu J, Colby TV, et al. Lymphangioleiomyomatosis. *N Engl J Med* 1990; 323: 1254.

Vij R, Strek ME. Diagnosis and treatment of connective tissue disease-associated interstitial lung disease *Chest* 2013: 143: 814.

Interstitial nephritis See
- Tubulointerstitial diseases.

Interstitial pneumonia

Interstitial pneumonia is the main group of non-specific interstitial lung diseases (ILDs, q.v.). In turn, **idiopathic interstitial pneumonia** (IIP) comprises a number of subgroups, currently classified as
- **idiopathic pulmonary fibrosis** (q.v.), the most frequently seen condition (separately described), and a number of less common entities considered below, namely
- **acute interstitial pneumonia,**
- **desquamative interstitial pneumonia,**
- **respiratory bronchiolitis interstitial lung disease,**
- **cryptogenic organizing pneumonia** (formerly bronchiolitis obliterans organizing pneumonia),
- **non-specific interstitial pneumonia,**
- idiopathic **lymphocytic** (lymphoid) **interstitial pneumonia,**
- idiopathic pleuroparenchymal fibroelastosis.

Acute interstitial pneumonia (AIP) is a rare condition of acute rapidly progressive lung disease, formerly referred to as **Hamman–Rich syndrome**. It behaves as an idiopathic form of **acute respiratory distress syndrome** (ARDS).

There is diffuse alveolar damage (DAD), which is relatively homogeneous. In some cases, it may become organized, with eventual fibrosis, but in other cases, it may resolve completely.

Treatment is as for ARDS from other causes. The usefulness of corticosteroids is uncertain.

The mortality is 60% within 6 months, but survivors generally recover completely.

Desquamative interstitial pneumonia (DIP) is a rare and primarily smoking-related condition. Pathologically, there are evenly distributed changes of alveolar filling with large mononuclear cells, mainly desquamated type II pneumocytes but also macrophages, though without fibrosis and with normal alveolar septa.

DIP was originally considered an early stage of usual interstitial pneumonia (UIP, the pathological finding in idiopathic pulmonary fibrosis – q.v.), but it has more recently been considered a separate and more benign disease, with a mortality of about 30% after 10 years.

Respiratory bronchiolitis interstitial lung disease (RB-ILD) is also a smoking-related condition. Pathologically, pigmented macrophages are found within the respiratory bronchioles, and these lesions are asymptomatic.

The spectrum of disease merges at its more severe end into DIP (see above).

Cryptogenic organizing pneumonia (COP) was formerly called bronchiolitis obliterans organizing pneumonia (BOOP). A number of forms of lung inflammation related to infective, drug-related and systemic inflammatory causes may end in a process of chronic inflammation and organization (rather than healing), with involvement of bronchioles as well as alveoli. Immune insults, such as in graft-versus-host disease and following lung transplantation (in which it is a common form of chronic rejection) can produce a similar end-result.

Clinically, the condition often commences as a flu-like illness, followed by progressive dyspnoea. Lung crackles may be heard.

Inflammatory markers are prominent, and imaging shows a bronchocentric pattern of opacities. The differential diagnosis includes bacterial pneumonia, aspiration or one of the other pulmonary infiltrates (q.v.).

*Treatment with a prolonged course of **corticosteroids** is generally effective.*

Non-specific interstitial pneumonia (NSIP) refers nowadays to the pulmonary component of a variety of systemic disorders, including HIV infection (q.v.), connective tissue diseases (q.v.), and a variety of allergic and environmental exposures.

Pathologically, the inflammatory and later fibrotic changes in the lung are homogeneous in age, unlike those of varying age typical of UIP.

The diagnosis of the underlying condition (which may not be apparent initially) can be challenging, and the distinction from other forms of pulmonary infiltrates requires considerable radiological and pathological expertise.

*Treatment generally comprises **corticosteroids** and **immunosuppression**, with greater efficacy expected in the earlier cellular stage of the disease.*

Idiopathic lymphocytic (lymphoid) interstitial pneumonia (LIP) is a rare condition, originally thought to have been a precursor to low-grade pulmonary lymphoma. In fact, it is the pulmonary accompaniment to a wide variety of systemic inflammatory and autoimmune conditions.

*Treatment involves the combined use of **corticosteroid**, **immunosuppressive** and **cytotoxic** agents.*

Idiopathic pleuroparenchymal fibroelastosis (PPFE) is a rare and recently described condition characterized by bilateral upper lobe pleural thickening with subpleural alveolar fibrosis and elastosis. It is commonly complicated by pneumothorax, respiratory infection and cachexia. The disease is progressive, and the diagnosis is poor.

*Treatment is with **corticosteroids**, but it is of limited benefit.*

> In general, patients with any form of IIP complicated by respiratory failure have a very high acute mortality despite maximum treatment in an ICU.

Bibliography

American Thoracic Society/European Respiratory Society International Multidisciplinary Consensus Classification of the Idiopathic Interstitial Pneumonias, June 2001. *Am J Respir Crit Care Med* 2002; 165: 277.

Boehler A, Kesten S, Weder W, et al. Bronchiolitis obliterans after lung transplantation: a review. *Chest* 1998; 114: 1411.

Cha SI, Fessler MB, Cool CD, et al. Lymphoid interstitial pneumonia: clinical features, associations and prognosis. *Eur Respir J* 2006; 28: 364.

Cordier JF. Cryptogenic organising pneumonia. *Eur Respir J* 2006; 28: 422.

Epler GR, Colby TV, McLoud TC, et al. Bronchiolitis obliterans organizing pneumonia. *N Engl J Med* 1985; 312: 152.

Fischer A, West SG, Swigris JJ, et al. Connective tissue disease-associated interstitial lung disease. *Chest* 2010; 138: 251.

Frankel SK, Cool CD, Lynch DA, et al. Idiopathic pleuroparenchymal fibroelastosis: description of a novel clinicopathologic entity. *Chest* 2004; 126: 2007.

Hamman L, Rich AR. Fulminating diffuse interstitial fibrosis of the lungs. *Trans Am Clin Climatol Assoc* 1935; 51: 154.

Kinder BW, Collard HR, Koth L, et al. Idiopathic nonspecific interstitial pneumonia: lung manifestation of undifferentiated connective tissue disease. *Am J Respir Crit Care Med* 2007; 176: 691.

Ryu JH, Myers JL, Capizzi SA, et al. Desquamative interstitial pneumonia and respiratory bronchiolitis-associated interstitial lung disease. *Chest* 2005; 127: 178.

Travis WD, Costabel U, Hansell DM, et al. An official American Thoracic Society/European Respiratory Society statement: update of the international multidisciplinary classification of idiopathic interstitial pneumonia. *Am J Respir Crit Care Med* 2013; 188: 733.

Vourlekis JS. Acute interstitial pneumonia. *Clin Chest Med* 2004; 25: 739.

Intra-abdominal hypertension

Intra-abdominal hypertension (IAH) and its complication, the **abdominal compartment syndrome** (ACS), are uncommon conditions, usually attributed either to massive interstitial swelling or to a large space-occupying lesion within the abdomen. It has been especially identified after large-volume crystalloid resuscitation. IAH can lead to organ ischaemia and multiorgan dysfunction (ACS), which then carries a significant associated mortality.

IAH is defined as an intra-abdominal pressure >10 mmHg, which is most conveniently measured by a bladder manometer. Pressures >25 mmHg reflect the likelihood of ACS.

*Treatment requires **decompression**, either non-surgically (by paracentesis) or surgically (by laparotomy).*

There has been a marked decrease in the occurrence of IAH and ACS following the widespread adoption of lower-volume regimens of fluid resuscitation in recent years, so that this condition should nowadays be a rare event.

Bibliography

Kirkpatrick AW, Roberts DJ, De Waele J, et al. Intra-abdominal hypertension and the abdominal compartment syndrome: updated consensus definitions and clinical practice guidelines from the World Society of the Abdominal Compartment Syndrome. *Intens Care Med* 2013; 39: 1190.

Maluso P, Olson J, Sarani B. Abdominal compartment hypertension and abdominal compartment syndrome. *Crit Care Clin* 2016; 32: 213.

Rogers WK, Garcia L. Intraabdominal hypertension, abdominal compartment syndrome, and the open abdomen. *Chest* 2018; 153: 238.

Iron

Iron (Fe, atomic number 26, atomic weight 56) comprises 35% of the Earth's composition, being the chief constituent of the Earth's core and a major constituent (5%) of the Earth's crust, in which it is the fourth most common element after oxygen, silicon and aluminium. It has for centuries been the most used and cheapest metal in all societies. As is well known, iron has an important role in biological functions. In addition to its key role in haeme synthesis, iron also regulates the production of cytokines by macrophages and is a cofactor for a number of enzymes involved in inflammation and host defence.

The total body stores of iron are normally about 4.5 g, 65% being present in haemoglobin, a small amount in myoglobin and haeme enzymes, and the remainder in stores in both soluble ferritin (q.v.) and insoluble haemosiderin (in liver, spleen and bone marrow). One mL of blood contains about 0.5 mg of iron. The normal ferritin level is >100 µg/L with a transferrin saturation of >20% (see Ferritin).

Iron absorption is regulated by **hepcidin**, a liver peptide, which inactivates ferroportin and thus limits both iron intake and iron recycling. The level of hepcidin is regulated by iron availability, with downregulation in iron deficiency (q.v.), so that iron absorption is then increased. In haemochromatosis (q.v.), there is a genetic deficiency of hepcidin.

The daily dietary requirement is 10–20 mg, of which about 10% is actually absorbed, with extra requirements for menstruation and pregnancy. The recommended IV dose is 20 µmol per day.

Clinical conditions associated with iron abnormalities include

1. **Iron deficiency**
   See separate entry below,
2. **Iron overload**
   See
   - Haemochromatosis,
   - Haemoglobin disorders,
3. **Iron poisoning**
   See
   - Desferrioxamine.

Bibliography

Bothwell TH, Charlton RW, Cook JD, et al. *Iron Metabolism in Man.* Oxford: Blackwell. 1979.

Conrad ME, Umbreit JN, Moore EG. Iron absorption and cellular uptake of iron. *Adv Exp Med Biol* 1994; 356: 69.

Editorial. Serum-ferritin. *Lancet* 1979; 1: 533.

Finch CA. Erythropoiesis, erythropoietin, and iron. *Blood* 1982; 60: 1241.

Finch CA. The detection of iron overload. *N Engl J Med* 1982; 307: 1702.

Finch CA, Huebers H. Perspectives in iron metabolism. *N Engl J Med* 1992; 306: 1520.

Ganz T, Nemeth E. Iron homeostasis in host defence and inflammation. *Nat Rev Immunol* 2015; 15: 500.

Hershko C, Peto TEA, Weatherall DJ. Iron and infection. *BMJ* 1988; 296: 660.

Huebers HA, Finch CA. The physiology of transferrin and transferrin receptors. *Physiol Rev* 1987; 67: 520.

Kuhn LC. Molecular regulation of iron proteins. *Baillieres Clin Haematol* 1994; 7: 763.

Means RT. Red blood cell function and disorders of iron metabolism. In: *Scientific American Medicine. Hematology.* Hamilton: Dekker Medicine. 2020.

Mills KC, Curry SC. Acute iron poisoning. *Emerg Clin North Am* 1994; 12: 397.

Pieracci FM, Barie PS. Diagnosis and management of iron-related anemias in critical illness. *Crit Care Med* 2006; 34: 1898.

Sayers MH, English G, Finch C. Capacity of the store-regulator in maintaining iron balance. *Am J Hematol* 1994; 47: 194.

Iron deficiency

Iron deficiency is the most common nutritional deficiency worldwide, and it is especially prevalent in developing countries. Even in Western countries, its prevalence may be about 20% of the population, especially women. The specific cause of iron deficiency in an individual patient should be identified and managed. The usual causes include blood loss, poor diet, impaired absorption and increased requirements.

Iron deficiency causes anaemia in only about 25% of cases, and in the remainder there may be non-specific and unexplained symptoms. Thus, in addition to the classic features of anaemia, the non-haematological manifestations of iron deficiency may include

- increased susceptibility to infections in general
  - but paradoxically a probably increased resistance to *Escherichia coli* and malaria (q.v.),
- cold intolerance (see Cold),
- stomatitis and glossistis (see Mouth diseases),
- gastro-oesophageal mucosal atrophy
  - with dysphagia (Plummer–Vinson syndrome) (q.v.) and achlorhydria (q.v.),
- koilonychias (see Nails),
- fatigue (see also Chronic fatigue syndrome), both physical and mental,
- blue sclerae,
- restless legs (q.v.),
- alopecia (q.v.),
- abnormal fetal and childhood development,
- sometimes pica (especially compulsive eating of abnormal material, such as ice).

The diagnosis of iron deficiency is most reliably made by the finding of a low ferritin level (<30 μg/L), but as ferritin is an acute phase reactant, this diagnostic threshold should be increased to <100 μg/L in the presence of inflammation or heart failure (see Iron, see Ferritin). The transferrin saturation is <20%, the red cell mean corpuscular haemoglobin concentration (MCHC) is reduced, and bone marrow examination (if done) shows absent iron stores.

The treatment of iron deficiency without anaemia is the same as that for iron deficiency with anaemia (q.v.), although the response may be less clear-cut.

See
- Anaemia – 1. Anaemia due to blood loss,
- Basophila,
- Ferritin,
- Folic acid deficiency,
- Goodpasture's syndrome – Idiopathic pulmonary haemosiderosis,
- Haemochromatosis,
- Haemoglobin disorders – 1. Thalassaemia,
- Megaloblastic anaemia.

Bibliography
Cook JD, Skikne BS. Iron deficiency: definition and diagnosis. *J Intern Med* 1989; 226: 349.
Hershko C, Peto TEA, Weatherall DJ. Iron and infection. *BMJ* 1988; 296: 660.
Lopez A, Cacoub P, Macdougall IC, et al. Iron deficiency anaemia. *Lancet* 2016; 387: 907.
Low MSY, Grigoriadis G. Iron deficiency and new insights into therapy. *Med J Aust* 2017; 207: 81.
Pasricha SR, Flecknoe-Brown SC, Allen KJ, et al. Diagnosis and management of iron deficiency anaemia: a clinical update. *Med J Aust* 2010; 193: 525.

Iron overload disease See
- Haemochromatosis,
- Haemoglobin disorders.

Irritable bowel syndrome See
- Colitis.

Irukandji syndrome See
- Bites and stings – Marine invertebrates.

Islet cell tumour

Islet cell tumours of the pancreas cause fasting hypoglycaemia (q.v.), which is associated with abnormally high (i.e. non-suppressed) insulin levels and which exhibits Whipple's triad.

Whipple's triad consists of hypoglycaemia, which
- displays typical clinical features (especially neuroglycopenia),
- with an appropriately low blood sugar,
- with relief of symptoms with therapy which restores the blood sugar to normal.

The islet cell tumour is thus an **insulinoma**. Most such tumours (90%) are single, small and benign. Occasionally, they are multiple (as in multiple endocrine neoplasia – q.v.) or even malignant.

> The differential diagnosis includes the other causes of fasting hypoglycaemia, which is also seen in
> - sepsis,
> - liver failure,
> - severe cardiac failure,
> - diffuse malignancy.

The diagnosis is made biochemically by the demonstration of appropriate hypoglycaemia after fasting. The blood glucose level should be <2 mmol/L in men or <1.5 mmol/L in women and not just <3 mmol/L (the lower limit of normal), because this level can occur with normal fasting (falls much greater than this are usually prevented by gluconeogenesis and decreased insulin secretion). The usual fast is overnight (i.e. 12 hr), which has a diagnostic yield of about 65%. If the fast is increased to 24 hr, 48 hr and 72 hr, the diagnostic yields increase accordingly to 71%, 92% and 98%, respectively. At this time also, the ratio of immunoreactive insulin (IRI) to glucose is abnormally increased.

If the diagnosis is still in doubt, a provocative test with exogenous insulin may be administered, in which case there is a failure of proinsulin or C peptide to fall.

Similar findings can also be produced by some oral hypoglycaemic agents, so that the association of profound fasting hypoglycaemia with hyperinsulinaemia should always prompt a urinary drug screen for sulphonylureas (sulfonylureas) in regions where these drugs are still commonly used for diabetes.

If appropriately abnormal fasting hypoglycaemia is associated with a normal IRI: glucose ratio, a non-pancreatic tumour should be sought. Some large mesodermal tumours, such as fibrosarcoma, mesothelioma and rarely haemangiopericytoma, either secrete insulin-like growth factors (IGFs) or metabolize glucose at an excess rate and thus cause marked hypoglycaemia.

A biochemically diagnosed tumour then needs to be localized, and this is most commonly achieved by ultrasound or CT imaging. In cases where localization is difficult, endoscopic ultrasonography, MRI scanning and PET imaging can be useful additional modalities.

Islet cell tumours are potentially curable by surgical resection.

Bibliography
Le Quesne LP, Nabarro JDN, Kurtz A, et al. The management of insulin tumours of the pancreas. *Br J Surg* 1979; 66: 31.

Isolation See
- Quarantine.

ITP See
- Immune thrombocytopenic purpura.

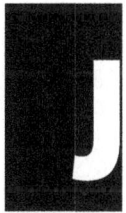

Japanese encephalitis See
- Encephalitis,
- Zoonoses.

Jarisch–Herxheimer reaction

The **Jarisch–Herxheimer reaction** occurs within a few hours of commencing treatment of spirochaetal diseases, particularly leptospirosis (q.v.), relapsing fever (q.v.) and syphilis (q.v.). It is due to the release of lipopolysaccharide products from the organism and resembles an immunological reaction. Like sepsis, it is associated with mediator and cytokine release.

There is fever, tachycardia, hypotension, headache and myalgia. It occurs within 8 hr and lasts about 12–24 hr.

There is no specific treatment, though sometimes supportive care for hypotension may be required. Interestingly, it has been reported to be decreased by inhibition of tumour necrosis factor (q.v.) with anti-TNF antibodies.

Bibliography
Gelfand JA, Elin RJ, Berry FW, et al. Endotoxemia associated with the Jarisch-Herxheimer reaction. *N Engl J Med* 1976; 295: 211.

Jellyfish envenomation See
- Bites and stings – Marine invertebrates.

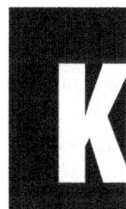

Kaposi's sarcoma See
- Acquired immunodeficiency syndrome,
- Herpesviruses,
- Ulcers.

Kartagener's syndrome

Kartagener's syndrome was described in 1933 as a condition of bronchiectasis (q.v.) with situs inversus (q.v.). Subsequently, the association of chronic sinusitis was recognized, and 40 yr later the further link was made with male infertility associated with live but immotile sperm.

The condition is inherited as an autosomal recessive, with a prevalence of one in 16,000 of the population. Its pathogenesis involves the absence of ATP-ase-containing dynein arms of outer microtubular doublets. This is part of the microtubular machinery required for motility in sperm tails and respiratory cilia. Immotile cilia thus lead to respiratory infection, and immotile sperm lead to infertility. Fertility is also decreased in women, because the oviducts and fimbriae are ciliated.

Kartagener's syndrome has thus been termed **immotile cilia syndrome**, and it is now included among the wider group of cilial motility disturbances generally referred to as **primary ciliary dyskinesia** (q.v.).

The clinical features primarily comprise upper respiratory tract and lower respiratory tract infections commencing in childhood, though associated congenital heart defects may also be seen.

There is thus
- chronic sinusitis,
- secretory otitis media,
- retained tracheobronchial secretions with chronic productive cough,
- bacterial superinfection,
- ultimately bronchiectasis (q.v.),
- occasionally broncholithiasis (q.v.).

The pattern of disability is similar to that seen in cystic fibrosis (q.v.), except that it is milder and without the serious sequelae of pneumonia, cor pulmonale and severe airways obstruction. Also in contrast to cystic fibrosis, the microorganisms involved are chiefly haemophilus, neisseria and streptococci rather than pseudomonas and staphylococci.

Investigations apart from respiratory assessment include examination of the cilia in vitro or their clearance ability in vivo, e.g. by using radioaerosols. Low nasal nitric oxide measurements are typically found. Specific diagnosis of ciliary dyskinesia may be made in specialist centres by high-speed video microscopy analysis.

Bibliography

Afzelius BA. A human syndrome caused by immotile cilia. *Science* 1976; 193: 317.

Corbelli R, Bringolf-Isler B, Amacher A, et al. Nasal nitric oxide measurements to screen for primary ciliary dyskinesia. *Chest* 2004; 126: 1054.

Horani A, Ferkol TW. Advances in the genetics of primary ciliary dyskinesia: clinical implications. *Chest* 2018; 154: 645.

Kennedy MP, Noone PG, Cardon J, et al. Calcium stone lithoptysis in primary ciliary dyskinesia. *Respir Med* 2007; 101: 76.

Marthin JK, Mortensen J, Pressler T, et al. Pulmonary radioaerosol mucociliary clearance in diagnosis of primary ciliary dyskinesia. *Chest* 2007; 132: 966.

Mygind N, Nielsen MH, Pedersen M. Kartagener's syndrome and abnormal cilia. *Eur J Respir Dis* 1983; 64 (suppl. 127): 1.

Noone PG, Leigh MW, Sannuti A, et al. Primary ciliary dyskinesia: diagnostic and phenotypic features. *Am J Respir Crit Care Med* 2004; 169: 459.

Katayama fever *See*
- Schistosomiasis.

Kawasaki disease *See*
- Vasculitis.

Kennedy's disease *See*
- Motor neuron disease.

Khat *See*
- Hepatitis.

Korsakoff syndrome *See*
- Wernicke–Korsakoff syndrome.

Kyphoscoliosis

Kyphoscoliosis refers to a deformity of the vertebral column, with
- kyphosis comprising anterior flexion, and
- scoliosis comprising lateral curvature with rotation.

The two features are usually combined, and distortion of the thoracic cage results.

Kyphoscoliosis is the most common structural abnormality of the thoracic cage (*see* Chest wall disorders). Most cases (80%) are idiopathic, but some are secondary.
- Idiopathic kyphoscoliosis commences in childhood, usually affecting girls, and often becoming severe during the years of rapid skeletal growth.
- Secondary kyphoscoliosis is associated either with neuromuscular diseases, such as poliomyelitis (q.v.) or syringomyelia (q.v.), or sometimes with congenital vertebral defects.

Clinical features may comprise dyspnoea on exertion and increased susceptibility to respiratory tract infections or CNS depressant drugs, in addition to the obvious skeletal deformity.

> If kyphoscoliosis is severe, the mechanical distortion of the chest wall and the mechanical disadvantage of the respiratory muscles lead to ventilatory failure.

Investigations in severely affected patients show markedly impaired ventilatory capacity, with decreased vital capacity and total lung capacity. A vital capacity of <45% is associated with an increased risk of respiratory failure. In contrast to the gas exchange abnormalities seen in parenchymal lung disease, there is hypercapnia and a relatively normal alveolar–arterial oxygen tension difference. Pulmonary hypertension (q.v.) and cor pulmonale are usual.

*Treatment is with **surgical correction**, if possible early in the course of disease.*
- Otherwise, treatment should be directed to those complicating problems which are reversible or preventable (e.g. influenza and pneumococcal vaccination).
- Even after chronic respiratory failure has supervened, the outlook may be favourable for many years with home oxygen therapy and especially mechanical ventilation at night.

Bibliography

Gustafson T, Franklin KA, Midgren B, et al. Survival of patients with kyphoscoliosis receiving mechanical ventilation or oxygen at home. *Chest* 2006; 130: 1828.

Libby DM, Briscoe WA, Boyce B, et al. Acute respiratory failure in scoliosis or kyphosis: prolonged survival and treatment. *Am J Med* 1982; 73: 532.

Lactase deficiency

Lactase deficiency refers to the loss from the intestinal mucosa of the disaccharidase enzyme required to break down the disaccharide, lactose, i.e. glucose–galactose (or sucrose, i.e. glucose–fructose) to monosaccharides which can then be absorbed. Otherwise, these sugars remain in the bowel, where their osmotic load takes up water and produces diarrhoea (q.v.). In the lower bowel, additional bacterial digestion produces even smaller but still non-absorbable fragments, thereby increasing the osmotic effect further.

Lactase deficiency may rarely be congenital, but it is usually acquired in later childhood. It is common in peoples of non–Northern European origin, and its management requires removal of dairy foods from the diet.

In normal subjects without lactase deficiency, ingestion of other saccharides can produce similar gastrointestinal effects, e.g.
- indigestible oligosaccharides from legumes,
- non-absorbable sugar alcohols (mannitol, sorbitol),
- indigestible disaccharides (lactulose).

See
- Diarrhoea – 1. Osmotic diarrhoea,
- FODMAPs

Lactic acidosis

Lactic acidosis is the most common form of metabolic acidosis associated with an increased anion gap, i.e. $[Na^+] - [Cl^-] - [HCO_3^-] > 13$ mmol/L (or about half this if there is severe hypoalbuminaemia). It is a frequent complication of serious illness, and if severe (i.e. pH <7.20) it is associated with a mortality of 60% despite treatment. The cause of this adverse outcome is considered multifactorial, namely a combination of the underlying illness itself and cellular dysfunction induced by the excessively acidic environment.

About 1500 mmol of lactic acid is normally produced per day (primarily in working skeletal muscle), and this load is greatly increased in sepsis, hypotension or other tissue ischaemia. These are conditions which result in impaired oxidation of pyruvate in mitochondria. Pyruvate is normally metabolized aerobically to generate ATP and produce CO_2 and water via the tricarboxylic acid (TCA or Krebs) cycle. In anaerobic conditions, pyruvate is metabolized to lactate.

Decreased lactic acid clearance also occurs in hepatic hypoperfusion, since the liver normally converts lactate back to pyruvate with the consequent regeneration of bicarbonate and more importantly also converts lactate to glucose via gluconeogenesis. Since in exercise lactate production can exceed 300 mmol/hr without significant acidosis, it is apparent that in disease lactic acidosis must arise from impaired clearance as well as from increased production.

The lactate/pyruvate ratio is normally about 10:1. It is increased in lactic acidosis and was formerly the basis of a classification for this condition.

A more practical classification, and one with more therapeutic meaning, is into
- **type A** (with apparent tissue hypoxia). This includes
  - shock and/or trauma (subtype A1),
  - hypoxaemia (subtype A2),
  - probably sepsis.

> This is sometimes referred to as 'shock' lactate, which is an index of tissue hypoxia or hypoperfusion.
> - type B (without apparent tissue hypoxia). This includes
>   - congenital enzyme deficiencies (subtype B3),
>   - acquired diseases, such as renal failure, liver failure, pancreatitis, diabetes, sepsis, malignancy, beriberi (subtype B1),
>   - drugs, such as ethanol, methanol, ethylene glycol, sodium nitroprusside, adrenaline (epinephrine), salicylates, metformin, propofol, and recently linezolid and antiretroviral agents (subtype B2).
>
> This is sometimes referred to as 'stress' lactate, which is an index of hypermetabolism, at least in sepsis.

The clinical features are those of the underlying disease. Particular note must be taken of the presence of tissue hypoxia.

Of course, the serum lactate may also be increased exogenously and thus non-pathologically by the administration of large volumes of lactate-buffered solutions, as formerly in renal replacement therapy. This biochemical abnormality is avoided by using alternative bicarbonate-buffered solutions which later become generally available.

The serum lactate level is increased in lactic acidosis (normal <1–2 mmol/L), but levels >6 mmol/L are required for renal excretion. Levels >2 mmol/L are associated with an adverse outcome in septic shock, and decreasing lactate can be a useful marker of treatment response. Arterial or mixed venous samples should be used, so that global rather than regional changes are assessed. There is no direct relationship between blood lactate and hydrogen ion concentrations.

The serum lactate level is normal (though there is still an increased anion gap) in an unusual form of lactic acidosis due to D-lactate accumulation, as in the short bowel syndrome. D-lactate is produced by some bacteria, whereas mammalian tissues produce L-lactate, the laevo isomer which is measured by most analytical methods.

> In lactic acidosis, the arterial PCO_2 is usually low, but the mixed venous PCO_2 is high.
>
> This venoarterial difference for CO_2 is a better guide to the severity of the problem than the arterial PCO_2 alone. It is due to increased CO_2 production and/or decreased cardiac output.

Treatment is primarily that of the underlying cause, with particular emphasis on improving tissue perfusion. It is important to recognize in any particular case whether increased lactate does or does not indicate hypoperfusion, as it is not only under-resuscitation that has adverse clinical consequences but also over-resuscitation.

The use of **bicarbonate** is controversial, though it is widely prescribed in this setting. It has traditionally been considered reasonable on theoretical grounds to administer it cautiously if the acidosis is severe (i.e. pH <7.20). However, controlled studies have in fact been unable to show either an increased survival following its use or any other outcome evidence to support its administration, apart from a recent substudy analysis suggesting benefit in patients with acute kidney injury.

The **propofol infusion syndrome** (PRIS) is an uncommon but often fatal metabolic acidosis complicating propofol infusion (q.v.). Early recognition is important but can be a challenge.

> While **metabolic acidosis** with a high anion gap is most commonly attributed to lactic acidosis in the critically ill, in some cases unidentified anions appear to be involved.
> - Acquired **pyroglutamic acid** excess, due particularly to paracetamol ingestion, may be one such cause.
> - **Beta-hydroxybutyrate** (BOHB) may be another such cause, particularly in alcoholic patients, since routine tests for ketones identify the presence of acetoacetate and acetone but not BOHB. Similar findings may also be seen with **ketogenic diets** and in **lactation ketoacidosis** (a condition occasionally reported in humans but well recognized in cows).
> - The presence of **methanol** (q.v.), **ethylene glycol** (q.v.), **propylene glycol** (q.v.) and **salicylates** (see Aspirin) should also be excluded in such cases.

Bibliography

Arieff AI. Indications for use of bicarbonate in patients with metabolic acidosis. *Br J Anaesth* 1991; 67: 165.

Bakker J. Blood lactate levels. *Curr Opin Crit Care* 1999; 5: 234.

Bakker J. Lactate: may I have your votes please? *Intens Care Med* 2001; 27: 6.

Cohen RD, Woods HF, eds. Clinical and Biochemical Aspects of Lactic Acidosis. Oxford: Blackwell. 1976.

Cooper DJ, Walley KR, Wiggs BR, et al. Bicarbonate does not improve hemodynamics in critically ill patients who have lactic acidosis. *Ann Intern Med* 1990; 112: 492.

De Backer D. Lactic acidosis. *Intens Care Med* 2003; 29: 699.

Dempsey GA, Lyall HJ, Corke CF, et al. Pyroglutamic acidemia: a cause of high anion gap metabolic acidosis. *Crit Care Med* 2000; 28: 1803.

Editorial. The colon, rumen, and D-lactic acidosis. *Lancet* 1990; 336: 599.

Emmett M, Narins RG. Clinical use of the anion gap. *Medicine* 1977; 56: 38.

Forsythe SM, Schmidt GA. Sodium bicarbonate for the treatment of lactic acidosis. *Chest* 2000; 117: 260.

Fudickar A, Bein B, Tonner PH. Propofol infusion syndrome in anaesthesia and intensive care medicine. *Curr Opin Anaesthesiol* 2006; 19: 404.

Huckabee WE. Abnormal resting blood lactate: II. Lactic acidosis. *Am J Med* 1961; 30: 840.

Iyer VN, Hoel R, Rabinstein AA. Propofol infusion syndrome in patients with refractory status epilepticus: an 11-year clinical experience. *Crit Care Med* 2009; 37: 3024.

Jaber S, Paugam C, Futier E, et al. Sodium bicarbonate therapy for patients with severe metabolic acidaemia in the intensive care unit (BICAR-ICU): a multicentre, open-label, randomised, controlled, phase 3 trial. *Lancet* 2018; 392: 31.

James JH, Luchette FA, McCarter FD, et al. Lactate is an unreliable indicator of tissue hypoxia in injury and sepsis. *Lancet* 1999; 354: 505.

Kraut JA, Madias NE. Lactic acidosis. *N Engl J Med* 2014; 371: 2309.

Kruse JA. Clinical utility and limitations of the anion gap. *Int J Intens Care* 1997; 4: 51.

Linas SL. Disorders of acid-base and potassium balance. In: *Scientific American Medicine*. Nephrology. Hamilton: Dekker Medicine. 2020.

Malhotra D, Shapiro JI. Pathogenesis and management of lactic acidosis. *Curr Opin Crit Care* 1996; 2: 439.

Mizock BA. Lactic acidosis. *Dis Mon* 1989; 35: 233.

Mizock BA, Belyaev S, Mecher C. Unexplained metabolic acidosis in critically ill patients: the role of pyroglutamic acid. *Intens Care Med* 2004; 30: 502.

Mizock BA, Falk JL. Lactic acidosis in critical illness. *Crit Care Med* 1992; 20: 80.

Mo L, Lliang DL, Madden A, et al. A case of delayed onset pyroglutamic acidosis in the sub-acute setting. *Intern Med J* 2016; 46: 747.

Nasraway S, Black R, Sottile F. The anion gap in patients admitted to the medical intensive care unit. *Chest* 1989; 96: 287S.

Riker RR, Glisic EK, Fraser GL. Propofol infusion syndrome: difficult to recognize, difficult to study. *Crit Care Med* 2009; 37: 3169.

Schelling JR, Howard RL, Winter SD, et al. Increased osmol gap in alcoholic ketoacidosis and lactic acidosis. *Ann Intern Med* 1990; 113: 580.

Stacpoole PW. Lactic acidosis: the case against bicarbonate therapy. *Ann Intern Med* 1986; 105: 276.

Suetrong B, Walley KR. Lactic acidosis in sepsis: it's not all anaerobic. *Chest* 2016; 149: 252.

Various. The Janus face of bicarbonate therapy in ICU. *Intens Care Med* 2020; 46: 516, 519, 522.

Vasile B, Rasulo F, Candiani A, et al. The pathophysiology of propofol infusion syndrome: a simple name for a complex syndrome. *Intens Care Med* 2003; 29: 1417.

Langerhans cell histiocytosis See

- Histiocytosis.

Lassa fever

Lassa fever is one of the four forms of **viral haemorrhagic fever** (q.v.) transmitted from person to person. It was first recognized in 1970 in Nigeria and is known to have a rodent reservoir, with person-to-person spread following initial human infection from ingestion of contaminated food. The pathogenesis involves viral interaction with and damage to endothelial cells and platelets, giving rise to a generalized capillary leak.

The incubation period is 6–21 days, which provides sufficient time nowadays for travel anywhere in the world.

The infection is often asymptomatic, but significant illness is apparent initially as influenza-like, with a sore throat, rash and gastrointestinal symptoms. In the second week, encephalopathy (q.v.), hepatitis (q.v.) and pleurisy are seen. Haemorrhage, renal failure and shock may occur in some patients.

The diagnosis is made by viral culture and serology.

The differential diagnosis includes many other infective diseases, including

- malaria (q.v.),
- Ebola haemorrhagic fever (q.v.),
- pneumonia,
- gastroenteritis (q.v.),
- influenza (q.v.),
- typhoid (q.v.).

*Treatment is with **ribavirin** (2 g loading dose, then 1 g qid for 4 days and then 0.5 g tds for 6 days), together with resuscitation and supportive care. Local rodent control with a domestic cat has been recommended.*

When first described, the mortality was 50%, but it is nowadays 1–2%. Prolonged weakness is experienced by survivors, and 25% have permanent deafness. There is no current vaccine.

Bibliography
Howard CR. Viral hemorrhagic fevers: properties and prospects for treatment and prevention. *Antiviral Res* 1984; 4: 169.
McCormick JB, Webb PA, Krebs JW, et al. A prospective study of the epidemiology and ecology of Lassa fever. *J Infect Dis* 1987; 155: 437.

Lateral medullary syndrome See
- Horner's syndrome.

Latex allergy See
- Urticaria.

Lead

Lead (Pb, atomic number 82, atomic weight 207, melting point 328°C) is a soft, dense, malleable, durable and corrosion-resistant grey metal. It is probably the oldest known metal, and although not found free in nature it is readily produced from its major source, namely, lead sulphide (galena). There are many industrial applications for lead or lead-containing compounds, including plumbing, solder, batteries, ammunition, insulation, shielding, glass and formerly in petrol (as the additive tetraethyl lead).

> Lead poisoning may thus occur in a wide variety of circumstances, including the home, industry and agriculture.

Much of the risk of lead poisoning has disappeared since lead salts are no longer used as pigments in white exterior paint, in insecticides or as a fuel additive. Nevertheless, lead may readily accumulate in the body and produce toxicity (referred to as **plumbism**), which takes the form in children particularly of cognitive and behavioural effects and in adults of renal disease. There has been a recent resurgence of lead poisoning in some places due to contamination of illicit narcotics. Moreover, increased lead levels are found in populations who consume either illicitly distilled liquor (moonshine) or game meat shot by hunters using lead shot.

The maximum recommended exposure is not greater than 50 mcg/m^3/8 hr and a whole blood level of <40 mcg/dL. Levels >80 mcg/dL are clearly toxic. However, there may be no safe lower level, as even levels of 5 mcg/dL or lower are associated with decreased intellectual and physical abilities in children and possibly adults. A free RBC protoporphyrin level >35 mcg/dL may be used as a screening test, since lead blocks haemosynthesis and thus produces an acquired porphyrin disease.

Although the toxic effects are widespread throughout the body and especially involve the central nervous system, kidneys, bone marrow and gut, there is very variable individual susceptibility.

Acute toxicity in adults classically gives rise to abdominal colic, haemolytic anaemia (a benign variant of sideroblastic anaemia (q.v.) with coarse basophilic stippling of erythrocytes) and encephalopathy (q.v.) (similar to that seen in hypertension). There may be pallor, irritability, a metallic taste in the mouth, a black line at the base of the gums, anorexia and constipation.

Acute toxicity in children causes neurological damage, which may lead to intellectual impairment and if more severe to deafness, blindness and seizures.

Chronic toxicity is manifest by renal failure, hypertension and saturnine gout (q.v.). Lead nephropathy is a tubulointerstitial nephritis (q.v.), with an unremarkable urinary sediment, and impaired uric acid excretion and increased serum uric acid out of proportion to the degree of renal impairment. Neurological changes of headache, confusion, visual disturbance and peripheral motor neuropathy (q.v.) (e.g. wrist drop) are seen. Permanent mental loss occurs in about one third of patients. Cardiomyopathy (q.v.) with potentially fatal arrhythmias used to be a potential complication of repeated petrol sniffing.

Treatment of lead poisoning requires the **chelating agents**, calcium edetate and/or penicillamine (q.v.). A prolonged course is required, but complete recovery is usual, provided there is no neurological damage.

See also
- Heavy metal poisoning.

Bibliography
Alperstein G, Reznik RB, Duggin GG. Lead: subtle forms and new modes of poisoning. *Med J Aust* 1991; 155: 407.
Balestra DJ. Adult chronic lead intoxication: a clinical review. *Arch Intern Med* 1991; 151: 1718.
Buenz EJ. Lead exposure through eating wild game. *Am J Med* 2016; 129: 457.
Dalvi SR, Pillinger MH. Saturnine gout, redux: a review. *Am J Med* 2013; 126: 450.
Carton JA, Maradona JA, Arribas JM. Acute-subacute lead poisoning: clinical findings and comparative study of diagnostic tests. *Arch Intern Med* 1987; 147: 697.
Flegal AR, Smith DR. Lead levels in preindustrial humans. *N Engl J Med* 1992; 326: 1293.
White JM, Selhi HS. Lead and the red cell. *Br J Haematol* 1975; 30: 133.

Leflunomide

Leflunomide is an immunomodulatory agent which inhibits pyrimidine synthesis and thus T-cell proliferation. It is used as a disease-modifying agent in rheumatoid arthritis, where its efficacy is comparable with that of methotrexate, though the two agents are often used in combination for increased effect.

Pneumonitis (interstitial lung disease) has been reported as an uncommon but important complication of either monotherapy or combined therapy with leflunomide (see Drugs and the lung). It presents as an acute respiratory illness without infection. There are diffuse pulmonary infiltrates, and the associated respiratory failure can be life-threatening.

Treatment involves immediate cessation of the drug. **Colestyramine** administration is recommended to remove the accumulated drug, as its active metabolite has a half-life of up to 4 weeks. Infection with Pneumocystis jirovecii (P. carinii) should be excluded.

A number of other serious side-effects have been reported, including dermatological, haematological, hepatic, neurological and infective complications.

See
- Immunomodulation.

Bibliography

Anon. Leflunomide and interstitial lung disease. *Aust Adv Drug Reactions Bull.* 2009; 28: 15.

Savage RL, Highton J, Boyd IW, et al. Pneumonitis associated with leflunomide: a profile of New Zealand and Australian reports. *Intern Med J* 2006; 36: 162.

Shankaranarayana S, Barrett C, Kubler P. The safety of leflunomide. *Aust Prescriber* 2013; 36: 28.

Lemierre's syndrome

Lemierre's syndrome was described in 1936 as a deep pharyngeal infection associated with septic thrombophlebitis of the internal jugular vein.

It is generally caused by the oral commensal *Fusobacterium necrophorum*, a spindle-shaped anaerobic Gram-negative bacillus. Its most serious complications are septic emboli giving metastatic abscesses, particularly in the lung. It is related to **Vincent's angina**, an erosive tonsillitis with associated soft tissue invasion, caused by similar organisms (see Mouth diseases – 1. Gingivitis).

It occurs in about 20% of cases of **cervical necrotizing fasciitis** (CNF), which is an uncommon but severe complication of ear, nose or throat infections.

In Intensive Care practice, it is one of the rare causes of infections in multiple sites with associated sepsis or septic shock, especially in young and otherwise healthy patients. A recent sore throat may provide a diagnostic clue, but CT scanning is essential for confirmation. Further serious complications may include airway compromise and mediastinitis.

Treatment is with **antibiotics**, *either penicillin (+/– metronidazole) or preferably a β-lactamase-resistant preparation (such as ticarcillin-clavulanate or piperacillin-tazobactam). The course should be prolonged, probably up to 6 weeks, and abscess drainage may be necessary.* **Anticoagulation** *is controversial, as it may entail a risk of spreading the infection.*

Bibliography

Hoehn S, Dominguez TE. Lemierre's syndrome: an unusual cause of sepsis and abdominal pain. *Crit Care Med* 2002; 30: 1644.

Johannesen KM, Bodtger U. Lemierre's syndrome: current perspectives on diagnosis and management. *Infect Drug Resist* 2016; 9: 221.

Lemierre A. On certain septicaemias due to anaerobic organisms. *Lancet* 1936; I; 701.

Nougue H, Le Maho A-L, Boudiaf M, et al. Clinical and imaging factors associated with severe complications of cervical necrotizing fasciitis. *Intens Care Med* 2015; 41: 1256.

Sinave CP, Hardy GL, Fardy PW. The Lemierre syndrome: suppurative thrombophlebitis of the internal jugular vein secondary to oropharyngeal infection. *Medicine* 1989; 68: 85.

Leprosy

Leprosy is a chronic granulomatous disease caused by infection with the organism *Mycobacterium leprae*. It typically presents with
- **anaesthetic skin lesions** which are erythematous or hypopigmented (see Pigmentation disorders – 1. Hypopigmentation (hypomelanosis)), or
- **thickened peripheral nerves** (see Neuropathy – 3. Inflammatory neuropathies).

Given its characteristic features, leprosy and its social consequences were well described in antiquity, as it was associated with severe and obvious deformities and chronic disability. The disease is curable with antibiotics, and it has become rare in developed countries.

Apart from humans, the only animal liable to infection with leprosy is the armadillo.

See
- Infections – Public health reporting.

See also
- Angiotensin-converting enzyme,
- *Mycobacterium ulcerans.*

Leptin

Leptin is a gut hormone which has sometimes been referred to as the 'satiety hormone'. It is also produced in adipose tissue, where it may regulate fat storage. Its presence in lungs and other organs indicates that leptin is both a pleiotropic hormone and a cytokine with multiple but as yet incompletely defined physiological functions.

See
- Ghrelin,
- Non-alcoholic steatohepatitis.

Bibliography
Ahima RS, Flier JS. Leptin. *Annu Rev Physiol* 2000; 62: 413.
Jutant E-M, Tu L, Humbert M, et al. The thousand faces of leptin in the lung. *Chest* 2021; 159: 239.

Leptospirosis

Leptospirosis is due to infection with the small spirochaete *Leptospira interrogans*. It is a zoonosis (q.v.), as the organism is endemic in animals worldwide, both domestic and wild, in which the infection is often asymptomatic and the organism is shed in the urine. Human infection is incidental and occurs after contact of abraded skin or mucous membranes with infected material. In warm and moist conditions, the organism can survive for weeks outside the body. There is an obvious occupational risk for abattoir workers, farmers and veterinarians and a less apparent one from a number of outdoor recreational activities, especially water sports. Although most prevalent in tropical regions in the rainy season, it is now recognized as a re-emerging disease in temperate climates.

Following an incubation period of 7–12 days, there is an acute non-specific febrile illness, which is often severe and lasts for 4–7 days. However, the clinical manifestations are variable, and infection may also be subclinical. Typically, there is bradycardia, rash, conjunctivitis, stiff neck and muscle tenderness. There is occasional hepatosplenomegaly and lymphadenopathy (q.v.). Leptospirae are present in the blood during this phase.

After improvement lasting 1–3 days, recurrent fever and meningitis occur which then last up to some weeks. Specific syndromes at this stage include the following.
- **Weil's disease**
  This is the most severe form of the illness. It is seen in 5–10% of patients and presents with multiorgan failure (q.v.), manifest by jaundice, uraemia, pneumonitis, encephalopathy (q.v.), anaemia (q.v.) and disseminated intravascular coagulation (q.v.). Sometimes there is rhabdomyolysis (q.v.) and vasculitis (q.v.).
- **Aseptic meningitis**
  Initially this mimics viral meningitis, but eventually the CSF shows a lymphocytosis (q.v.), markedly increased protein level and normal glucose.
- **Pretibial fever** (Fort Bragg fever)
  There is splenomegaly (q.v.) and raised, red, painful lesions on the shins.

The diagnosis is made from positive culture or serology. The differential diagnosis is an acute viral illness.

Treatment is primarily with **supportive** *measures, but* **antibiotics** *(doxycycline for 7 days or possibly penicillin) probably shorten the duration of disease and decrease its severity.*

There is no satisfactory prevention. The mortality is 3–6%, and survivors recover completely.

See
- Jarisch–Herxheimer reaction.

Bibliography
Abidi K, Dendane T, Madani N, et al. The clinical picture of severe leptospirosis in critically ill patients. *Intens Care Med* 2017; 43: 1740.
Bharti AR, Nally JE, Ricaldi JN, et al. Leptospirosis: a zoonotic disease of global importance. *Lancet Infect Dis* 2003; 3: 757.
Levett PN. Leptospirosis. *Clin Microbial Rev* 2001; 4: 296.
McBride AJ, Athanazio DA, Reis MG, et al. Leptospirosis. *Curr Opin Infect Dis* 2005; 18: 376.
Meites E, Jay MT, Deresinski S, et al. Reemerging leptospirosis. *Emerg Infect Dis* 2004; 10: 106.
Pappas G, Papadimitriou P, Siozopoulou V, et al. The globalization of leptospirosis: worldwide incidence trends. *Int J Infect Dis* 2008; 12: 351.
Taniguchi LU, Povoa P. Leptospirosis: one of the forgotten diseases. *Intens Care Med* 2019; 45: 1816.
Turner LH. Leptospirosis. *BMJ* 1973; 1: 537.

Leukocytoclastic vasculitis *See*
- Urticaria.

Leukoencephalopathy

Leukoencephalopathy may be encountered in a number of forms, including
- **progressive multifocal leukoencephalopathy** (PML)
  - see Demyelinating diseases,
- **toxic leukoencephalopathy**
  - this may occur either acutely or subacutely following drug overdose, chronic opiate abuse, acute hypoxia,

- **reversible posterior leukoencephalopathy** (q.v.).
  See also
- Encephalopathy,
- Paraneoplastic syndromes – Neurological changes.

Lewisite *See*
- Chelating agents,
- Warfare agents.

Lice

Lice are insects (q.v.) which are common human ectoparasites (see Parasitic infections). They can transmit significant disease under some circumstances.

See
- Arthropods,
- Bites and stings – Insects,
- Cat-scratch disease – Bacillary peliosis hepatis,
- Pediculosis,
- Phthiriasis,
- Relapsing fever,
- Rickettsial diseases – Endemic typhus.

Bibliography
Elston D. Infestations. In: *Scientific American Medicine. Dermatology*. Hamilton: Dekker Medicine. 2020.

Lichenoid skin reaction *See*
- Mercury.

Light chains *See*
- Multiple myeloma.

Lightning

The electrical discharge in **lightning** which strikes the ground has an estimated 10–100 million volts DC with a current of up to 30,000 amperes, although the total duration is <100 msec. Very high temperatures of up to 30,000°C may be produced locally, causing a shock wave which is heard as thunder.

> **Lightning** may strike an individual in several different ways, namely
> - directly,
> - as a splash or flash from a nearby object of high resistance,
> - via contact with a primary object,
> - from the adjacent ground via the legs as a stride potential,
> - via telephone lines.

Burns, electrical injury or blast injury may be produced. The burn is a flash burn over the outside of the body and may even rip clothing apart, the electrical injury is usually minor, and the blast injury is equivalent to blunt trauma.

The injuries are thus neurological, musculoskeletal, cardiovascular, cutaneous and ophthalmological. Direct strike may of course cause immediate death, though an electrically induced respiratory arrest may be reversible for up to 24 hr.

- **Neurologically**, there may be confusion and paralysis. Most patients suffer at least some loss of consciousness. Fixed dilated pupils can be due to local eye damage and not necessarily to brainstem death. From telephone contact, there may be headache, deafness and tinnitus (q.v.).
- **Cardiovascular effects** include any arrhythmia and particularly asystole. Vasoconstriction can be marked, even to the point of tissue ischaemia.
- The **skin** may show a Lichtenberg flower, a delicate branching lesion which is not a burn and disappears within 24 hr. Localized deep burns may also be seen.
- **Eye** damage most commonly results in later development of cataract.

The mortality is 20–30% in humans struck by lightning. There is thus one death per year from this cause per 10 million population. Importantly, long-term sequelae independent of the direct consequences of the injury, including psychiatric illness and cataracts, occur in about two thirds of survivors.

Bibliography
Browne B, Gaasch W. Electrical injuries and lightning. *Emerg Med Clin North Am* 1992; 2: 211.
Hiestant D, Colice G. Lightning-strike injury. *J Intens Care Med* 1988; 3: 303.
Koumbourlis AC. Electrical injuries. *Crit Care Med* 2002; 30: S424.
Makdissi M, Brukner P. Recommendations for lightning protection in sport. *Med J Aust* 2002; 177: 35.

Lipoid pneumonia

Lipoid pneumonia refers to pulmonary inflammation associated with lipid accumulation in the alveoli. Although originally described in the 1920s, it remains an uncommon and poorly understood condition.

Endogenous forms can occur with distal bronchial obstruction from lipid elements, for example in lipid **storage diseases** (q.v.).

Exogenous forms (ELP) are those more usually seen as causing clinical illness.

- **Acute lipoid pneumonia** can follow the inhalation of a variety of lipid materials, either in industry or in recreation (e.g. from vaping – q.v.). Full recovery generally occurs.

- **Chronic lipoid pneumonia** is typically produced by the recurrent inhalation or aspiration of oily substances, such as oil-based laxatives or nose drops, complementary medicines, fish oils, cooking oils, facial cosmetics or commercial oils (see Aspiration).

Clinical features vary greatly in severity and persistence, and indeed many patients remain asymptomatic. Typically, the chest X-ray shows lower lobe opacities, and the CT shows fatty attenuation. Definitive diagnosis can also be made with brochoalveolar lavage (BAL) or lung biopsy.

There is no specific treatment.

Bibliography
Baron SE, Haramati LB, Rivera VT. Radiological and clinical findings in acute and chronic exogenous lipoid pneumonia. *J Thorac Imaging* 2003; 18: 217.
Hu X, Lee JS, Pianosi PT, et al. Aspiration-related pulmonary syndromes. *Chest* 2015; 147: 815.
Samhouri BF, Tandon YK, Hartman TE, et al. Presenting clinicoradiologic features, causes, and clinical course of exogenous lipoid pneumonia in adults. *Chest* 2021; 160: 624.
Sood N, Murin S. Lipoid pneumonia: fat chance of making the diagnosis. *Chest* 2021; 160: 407.
Wright BA, Jeffrey PH. Lipoid pneumonia. *Semin Respir Infect* 1990; 5: 314.

Liquorice

Liquorice is derived from the perennial herb *Glycyrrhiza glabra*, and comprises glycyrrhizic acid (etymologically meaning sweet root). It is obtained from the roots of the plant and is similar to anise.

It has long been used for flavouring and in medicines to disguise unpleasant components. It is also a popular confection and has been used in chewing tobacco. Medically, liquorice has been prescribed in peptic ulcer disease and in Addison's disease (q.v.).

Since liquorice is **salt-retaining**, its excessive use (e.g. >0.45 kg/week) can give rise to oedema or to pseudo-primary aldosteronism and thus secondary hypertension (see Conn's syndrome).

It can also give rise to **hypokalaemic periodic paralysis** (q.v.), although more commonly this condition occurs due to
- potassium loss from the kidney or gut,
- diuretic or corticosteroid use,
- thyrotoxicosis (q.v.).

Bibliography
Blachley JD, Knochel JP. Tobacco chewer's hypokalemia: licorice revisited. *N Engl J Med* 1980; 302: 784.
de Klerk GJ, Nieuwenhuis MG, Beutler JJ. Hypokalaemia and hypertension associated with use of liquorice flavoured chewing gum. *BMJ* 1997; 314: 751.
Farese RV, Biglieri EG, Shackleton CHL, et al. Licorice-induced hypermineralocorticoidism. *N Engl J Med* 1991; 325: 1224.

Listeriosis

Listeriosis is caused by the aerobic Gram-positive bacillus *Listeria monocytogenes*, a saprophyte found widely in soil, plants and animals. It is relatively resistant to heat, including pasteurization, and it can grow even in refrigerated food. It is thus often food-borne, and ready-to-eat foods are a particularly important source of infection.

Despite its ubiquitous nature, human disease is in fact uncommon. However, it is an important cause of neonatal sepsis and of adult meningitis.

> **Meningitis** particularly occurs in the elderly or in compromised hosts.
> It is clinically similar to other forms of meningitis, except that
> - tremor and ataxia are more common,
> - encephalitis (q.v.) especially of the pons may sometimes be seen.

Other less common forms of infection include
- isolated bacteraemia,
- occasional focal lesions,
- an influenza-like illness in pregnancy, with associated amnionitis and fetal damage (see Pregnancy).

The diagnosis is made from bacterial identification, as there is no routine serological test (though an anti-listeriolysin-O test has been developed). The organism may sometimes be difficult to identify, as it can have coccoid forms and may therefore sometimes be confused with streptococci.

Since listeriosis presents to Intensive Care as meningitis, specific diagnosis is important because the third-generation cephalosporins which are commonly used in most forms of meningitis are not appropriate for the treatment of this organism.

*Treatment is with **ampicillin** 2 g IV 4 hrly for 10 days beyond the subsidence of fever. This is longer than is usual for bacterial meningitis and is required because of the frequency of relapse following shorter courses.*
- *Penicillin, erythromycin, tetracycline, cotrimoxazole and vancomycin are also effective.*

- *Gentamicin is synergistic with ampicillin in vitro but probably not in vivo, whereas cotrimoxazole is synergistic with ampicillin in vivo and thus provides a clinically effective combination.*

Bibliography

Calder JAM. Listeria meningitis in adults. *Lancet* 1997; 350: 307.

Crum NF. Update on Listeria monocytogenes infection. *Curr Gastroenterol Rep* 2002; 4: 287.

Durand ML, Calderwood SB, Weber DJ, et al. Acute bacterial meningitis in adults. *N Engl J Med* 1993; 328: 21.

Gellin BG, Broome CV. Listeriosis. *JAMA* 1989; 261: 1313.

Goulet V. What can we do to prevent listeriosis in 2006? *Clin Infect Dis* 2007; 44: 521.

Hearmon CJ, Ghosh SK. Listeria monocytogenes meningitis in previously healthy adults. *Postgrad Med J* 1989; 65: 74.

Nieman RE, Lorber B. Listeriosis in adults: a changing pattern. *Rev Infect Dis* 1980; 2: 207.

Schlech WF. Foodborne listeriosis. *Clin Infect Dis* 2000; 31: 770.

Southwick PS, Purich DL. Intracellular pathogenesis of listeriosis. *N Engl J Med* 1996; 334: 770.

Lithium

Lithium (Li, atomic number 3, atomic weight 7, melting point 179°C) is the lightest solid element. It was discovered in 1817 and is a soft, white substance which floats on water (SG 0.53). Lithium was one of the three elements (together with hydrogen and helium) created during the Big Bang.

Although it has a variety of industrial uses, it is best known medically for its use as lithium carbonate in the treatment of manic-depressive illness, first described in 1949 in Australia. It is still the gold standard medication for mood stabilization, and it remains the most useful drug both for acute treatment of mania and for prevention of relapse in bipolar disorder. In this condition, it is used in a dose of 900–2400 mg per day in divided doses to give a trough therapeutic plasma level of 0.6–1.0 mmol/L. Its volume of distribution equates to the extracellular fluid volume, its half-life is about 18 hr, and it is almost entirely excreted in the urine.

Lithium is a reactive element with a large variety of biological effects. Of particular relevance to its psychopharmacological effects is its inhibition at therapeutic plasma levels of a second messenger system in the central nervous system. At higher levels, it decreases adenyl cyclase and thus cAMP. It is distributed in the total body water and excreted solely by the kidney, where like sodium it undergoes glomerular filtration though not distal tubular reabsorption (hence its excretion is not enhanced by diuretics like thiazides). However, like sodium, with which it competes, it is reabsorbed from the proximal tubule, so that its plasma level is increased in states of sodium depletion and also with NSAIDs.

Lithium has a low therapeutic index, and acute toxicity may be seen with plasma levels >2 mmol/L. Moreover, side-effects are common at any level.

Adverse experiences of lithium are manifest as
- **renal**
  - nephrogenic diabetes insipidus, seen to some degree in about 20% of patients and treated with a thiazide or preferably amiloride,
  - interstitial nephritis (q.v.) or nephrotic syndrome (q.v.), both uncommon but requiring permanent cessation of lithium,
- **neurological**
  - intention tremor, drowsiness, confusion, fits, coma, hyperreflexia, ataxia, dysarthria, blurred vision, tinnitus (q.v.), focal neurological signs,
- **neuropsychiatric**
  - impaired memory, cognition and creativity, though these complaints may be no more than cessation of hypomania,
- **thyroid**
  - non-toxic goitre or hypothyroidism (q.v.), these abnormalities being seen in 5% of patients, particularly women with thyroid antibodies, and requiring thyroid replacement therapy though not cessation of lithium,
- **cardiovascular**
  - arrhythmias, especially conduction defects,
  - hypotension,
  - T-wave inversion on ECG, a benign change,
  - vasculitis (q.v.),
- **dermatological**
  - acne,
  - precipitation or exacerbation of psoriasis (q.v.),
  - stress alopecia (q.v.),
- **haematological**
  - raised white cell count, due to increased neutrophil turnover and mass,
- **gastrointestinal**
  - nausea, vomiting and diarrhoea (q.v.),
- **metabolic**
  - mild hypercalcaemia (q.v.) related to primary hyperparathyroidism (q.v.),

- **general**
  - oedema and weight gain,
- **teratogenic**
  - congenital heart disease (as with rubella).

*The treatment of lithium toxicity is an **emergency**, since high plasma levels may cause permanent neurological damage or death. Therapy is supportive, with sodium and water replacement and enhancement of urinary lithium excretion by alkalinization and osmotic diuresis, though this method of enhancing elimination is not very effective. It is not adsorbed by activated charcoal. Renal replacement therapy is required if toxicity is severe (e.g. plasma level >3.5 mmol/L), though recovery is delayed despite the return to normal of plasma lithium levels, since the intracellular effects themselves are slow to reverse.*

Lithium chloride has been found to be as a suitable marker for the indicator dilution measurement of cardiac output.

Bibliography

Beckmann U, Oakley PW, Dawson AH, et al. Efficacy of continuous venovenous hemodialysis in the treatment of severe lithium toxicity. *J Toxicol Clin Toxicol* 2001; 39: 393.

Brown WA. *Lithium: A Doctor, A Drug, and A Breakthrough.* New York: Liveright. 2019.

Cade JFJ. Lithium salts in the treatment of psychotic excitement. *Med J Aust* 1949; 2: 349.

Jaeger A, Sauder P, Kopferschmitt T, et al. When should dialysis be performed in lithium poisoning. *Clin Toxicol* 1993; 31: 429.

Kulig K. All lithium overdoses deserve respect. *J Emerg Med* 1992;10: 757.

Linton RA, Band DM, Haire KM. A new method of measuring cardiac output using lithium dilution. *Br J Anaesth* 1993; 71: 262.

Malhi GS, Tanious M, Bargh D, et al. Safe and effective use of lithium. *Aust Prescriber* 2013; 36: 18.

Mitchel JE, MacKenzie TB. Cardiac effects of lithium therapy in man: a review. *J Clin Psychiatry* 1982; 43: 47.

Mokhlesi B, Leikin JB, Murray P, et al. Adult toxicology in critical care: part II: specific poisonings. *Chest* 2003; 123: 897.

Nagappan R, Parkin WG, Holdsworth SR. Acute lithium intoxication. *Anaesth Intens Care* 2002; 30: 90.

Oakley PW, Whyte IM, Carter GL. Lithium toxicity: an iatrogenic problem in susceptible individuals. *Aust N Z J Psychiatry* 2001; 35: 833.

Okusa MD, Crystal LJT. Clinical manifestations and management of acute lithium intoxication. *Am J Med* 1994; 97: 383.

Ott M, Stegmayr B, Salander Renberg E, et al. Lithium intoxication: incidence, clinical course and renal function – a population-based retrospective cohort study. *J Psychopharmacol* 2016; 30: 1008.

Salata R, Klein I. Effect of lithium on the endocrine system: a review. *J Lab Clin Med* 1987; 110: 130.

Scharman EJ. Methods used to decrease lithium absorption or enhance elimination. *J Toxicol Clin Toxicol* 1997; 35: 601.

Walker RG. Lithium nephrotoxicity. *Kidney Int* 1993; 42 (suppl.): S93.

Zimmerman JL. Poisonings and overdoses in the intensive care unit: general and specific management issues. *Crit Care Med* 2003; 31: 2794.

Livedo reticularis

Livedo reticularis refers to blue-red mottling of the skin which characteristically takes a fishnet pattern reflecting the underlying vascular anatomy. It is thus a vascular disorder, though its cause is in practice usually unknown.

Idiopathic livedo reticularis occurs chiefly in young to middle-aged women and is typically precipitated by cold or stasis. Symptoms are minimal but may include numbness or tingling.

Treatment is not required.

Secondary livedo reticularis occurs in a number of conditions, including

- antiphospholipid syndrome (q.v.),
- immune vasculitis (q.v.),
- endocarditis (q.v.),
- thrombocythaemia (q.v.),
- hyperviscosity syndromes (see Multiple myeloma),
- cholesterol embolization,
- calciphylaxis (q.v.).

Livedo vasculitis is a related but more serious condition, with a course which is either chronic or relapsing (see Vasculitis).

There is microvascular occlusion with pain and ulceration, especially affecting the lower limbs. The cerebral circulation may be involved with resultant cerebrovascular ischaemia.

Antithrombotic therapy *is recommended.*

Bibliography

Burton JL. Livedo reticularis, porcelain-white scars, and cerebral thromboses. *Lancet* 1988; 1: 1263.

Copeman PW. Livedo reticularis: signs in the skin of disturbance of blood viscosity and of blood flow. *Br J Dermatol* 1975; 93: 519.

Klein K, Pittelkow M. Tissue plasminogen activator for the treatment of livedoid vasculitis. *Mayo Clin Proc* 1992; 67: 923.

Schroeter AL, Diaz-Perez JL, Winkelmann RK, et al. Livedo vasculitis (the vasculitis of atrophie blanche): immunohistopathologic study. *Arch Dermatol* 1975; 111: 188.

Liver abscess

Liver abscess is the most common intra-abdominal visceral abscess. It may arise from either local or systemic infection.

Local causes of liver abscess include
- cholangitis (q.v.),
- direct extension from an adjacent focus,
- portal venous transmission following abdominal surgery or percutaneous transluminal coronary angioplasty (PTCA).

Systemic causes of liver abscess are bacteraemias. In turn, liver abscess may give rise to bacteraemia or metastatic infection elsewhere.

The clinical features of liver abscess may be subtle and include only fever and leukocytosis. Sometimes, there may be abnormal local signs or liver dysfunction.

Although the plain X-ray may show an associated right pleural effusion or even an air-fluid level within the liver, imaging with ultrasound or CT is usually required. Sometimes, there may be difficulty in distinguishing a liver abscess from other types of intrahepatic mass, such as cyst or neoplasm.

> The microorganisms involved in liver abscess are usually Gram-negative enteric bacilli, as for peritonitis or other intra-abdominal abscesses.
> Often the condition is polymicrobial.
> Blood cultures may assist the microbiological diagnosis.
> An amoebic aetiology should be suspected if the abscess is a single right-sided lesion in a traveller.

Treatment is by **percutaneous drainage**, *together with appropriate* **antibiotics**.

The progress and prognosis depend on the underlying cause.

Bibliography

Branum GD, Tyson GS, Branum MA, et al. Hepatic abscess: changes in etiology, diagnosis and management. *Ann Surg* 1990; 212: 655.

Rustgi AK, Richter JM. Pyogenic and amebic abscess. *Med Clin North Am* 1989; 73: 847.

Loeffler's syndrome *See*
- Eosinophilia and lung infiltration.

Ludwig's angina *See*
- Mouth diseases – 1. Gingivitis.

Lung tumours

Primary malignant tumours of the lung are
- (predominantly) bronchogenic carcinoma, i.e. lung cancer,
- (less commonly) mesothelioma, pulmonary lymphoma, melanoma, sarcoma,
- (less malignantly) bronchoadenoma, i.e. carcinoid tumour, cylindroma, others,
- (rarely) papilloma, neurofibroma, haemangiopericytoma, teratoma, plasmacytoma.

Primary benign tumours of the lung include chiefly hamartoma and angioma. Many rare tumours (e.g. chemodectoma) have also been reported.

Secondary (malignant) tumours of the lung are probably more common than in other sites. The most frequent sources of the primary tumour are
- breast,
- gastrointestinal tract,
- urogenital system,
- thyroid,
- connective tissue sarcoma,
- lymphoma.

Primary benign and malignant tumours as well as metastases may also occur in intrathoracic structures other than the lung, such as the mediastinum, chest wall and spine.

> The thoracic signs of lung cancer comprise
> - local wheeze,
> - unresolving pneumonia,
> - pleural effusion,
> - recurrent laryngeal or phrenic nerve involvement,
> - thoracic inlet (Pancoast) syndrome
>   - with shoulder pain, Horner's syndrome (q.v.) and brachial plexus damage,
> - supraclavicular lymph node involvement,
> - superior vena cava obstruction.

Lung cancer is particularly prone to give systemic, non-metastatic manifestations or paraneoplastic phenomena (q.v.). These include
- **general disability**
  - tiredness, weakness, anorexia and weight loss,

- **connective tissue disorders**
  - clubbing, hypertrophic pulmonary osteoarthropathy, acanthosis nigricans (q.v.), dermatomyositis (q.v.),
- **neuromuscular disorders**
  - myasthenia (q.v.), cerebellar degeneration (q.v.), motor and/or sensory neuropathy (q.v.), dementia (q.v.),
- **endocrine disorders**
  - hypercalcaemia (q.v.), Cushing's syndrome (q.v.), syndrome of inappropriate antidiuretic hormone (q.v.), carcinoid syndrome (q.v.), hyperthyroidism (q.v.), hypoglycaemia (q.v.),
- **haematological disorders**
  - thrombophlebitis, venous thromboembolism, non-bacterial thrombotic endocarditis (q.v.), haemolytic anaemia (q.v.), red cell aplasia, thrombocytopenia (q.v.).

Bibliography

Alberts WM, chair. Diagnosis and management of lung cancer: ACCP evidence-based clinical practice guidelines (2nd edition). *Chest* 2007; 132: 2 (suppl.): 1S.

Bains MS. Surgical treatment of lung cancer. *Chest* 1991; 100: 826.

Belani CP, ed. International symposium on thoracic malignancies. *Chest* 1998; 113 (suppl.): 1S.

Clamon GH, Evans WK, Shepherd FA, et al. Myasthenic syndrome and small cell cancer of the lung: variable response to antineoplastic therapy. *Arch Intern Med* 1984; 144: 999.

Crawford J, Strickler J. Lung cancer. In: *Scientific American Medicine. Oncology.* Hamilton: Dekker Medicine. 2020.

Hall TC, ed. Paraneoplastic syndromes. *Ann NY Acad Sci* 1974; 230: 1.

McCaughan BC, Martini N, Bains MS. Bronchial carcinoids. *J Thorac Cardiovsc Surg* 1985; 89: 8.

Menkes MS, Comstock GW, Vuilleumier JP, et al. Serum beta-carotene, vitamins A and E, selenium, and the risk of lung cancer. *N Engl J Med* 1986; 315: 1250.

Miller YE, Keith RL, eds. Lung cancer: early events, early interventions. *Chest* 2004; 125: No. 5 (suppl.).

Minna J, Ihde D, Glatstein E. Lung cancer: scalpels, beams, drugs, and probes. *N Engl J Med* 1986; 315: 1411.

Pass HI, Carbone DP, Johnson DH, et al., eds. *Principles and Practice of Lung Cancer.* 4th edition. Philadelphia: Lippincott Williams & Wilkins. 2010.

Sugarbaker DJ, ed. Multimodality therapy of chest malignancies – update '96. *Chest* 1997; 112: 181S.

The Cancer Council Australia. *Clinical Practice Guidelines for the Prevention, diagnosis and Management of Lung Cancer.* Sydney: NH&MRC. 2004.

Yellin A, Rosenman Y, Lieberman Y. Review of smooth muscle tumours of the lower respiratory tract. *Br J Dis Chest* 1984; 78: 337.

Yesner R, Careter D. Pathology of carcinoma of the lung: changing patterns. *Clin Chest Med* 1982; 3: 257.

Lupus anticoagulant *See*
- Antiphospholipid syndrome.

Lyme disease

Lyme disease is caused by the tick-borne spirochaete, *Borrelia burgdorferi*, and it is the most common vector-borne disease in non-tropical developed countries. It was first observed in the town of Lyme in Connecticut in 1975, its causative agent was confirmed in 1983 and its genome was sequenced in 1997. It is now widely observed around the world, except in Australia, where a Lyme-like disease (referred to as Australian multisystem disorder) has been described. Animal reservoirs include numerous wild and domestic animals and birds, from which a variety of tick species (q.v.) and perhaps other insect vectors become infected.

Humans are inoculated through the skin giving rise to **erythema migrans**, in which the organism can be identified in nearly 90% of cases. The organism then disseminates to the joints, heart and CNS. The disease has protean manifestations, and probably many cases are unrecognized. Infection occurring during pregnancy may cause fetal damage or fetal death at any stage.

The disease has early and late phases.
- **Stage one**

A distinctive skin lesion is noted 3–20 days after the tick bite, which is itself remembered only by about 20% of patients.

The lesion consists of a maculopapule which enlarges to 6–16 cm in diameter and fades after 3–4 weeks.

There may be associated systemic systems including myalgia and a stiff neck.
- **Stage two**

This is a disseminated condition seen in some patients and occurring 1 day to 8 weeks after the skin lesion.

In this condition,
- 80% have arthritis (q.v.), usually involving large joints,
- 15% have neurological abnormalities, including aseptic meningitis, encephalitis (q.v.), cranial and peripheral neuropathy (q.v.), sometimes resembling Guillain–Barré syndrome (q.v.),

- 16% have cardiac dysfunction, with varying degrees of AV block and myocardial but not valvular dysfunction),
- occasional patients have hepatitis (q.v.), pneumonitis resembling ARDS (q.v.), or ocular involvement.

• **Stage three**

This represents late disease, with persistent infection more than 1 year later.

> The diagnosis is primarily a clinical one, supported if in doubt by positive serology, microscopy and culture.
> The differential diagnosis includes
> - erythema marginatum (q.v.),
> - rheumatic fever,
> - reactive arthritis (q.v.), probably due to molecular mimicry,
> - rheumatoid arthritis.
>
> False-positive diagnoses are probably frequent, especially in patients with atypical arthritis and fatigue. In addition, false-positive serology can be produced by unrelated conditions, including autoimmune diseases (q.v.) and bacterial infections.

Treatment is with **tetracycline** *(e.g. doxycycline 100 mg bd for 10–30 days) or amoxicillin, penicillin or ceftriaxone.*

Prophylactic antibiotics have been shown not to be warranted. Antibiotics for the **post-Lyme disease syndrome** *of prolonged asthenia (e.g. >6 months) have also been shown to be ineffective, suggesting that this condition is a postinfectious phenomenon rather than an actual chronic infection.*

Prevention is with protective clothing and removal of ticks from the skin. A vaccine for inhabitants of high-risk areas was subsequently withdrawn, but an ecological approach using an oral vaccine for wildlife carriers of infected ticks has been successfully trialled.

Controversy surrounds the difficult diagnosis of non-specific chronic debilitating symptoms seen in many patients and the temptation to label these symptoms as due to chronic Lyme disease, even in the absence of formal laboratory confirmation (see Chronic fatigue syndrome).

Bibliography

Barbour AG, Fish D. The biological and social phenomenon of Lyme disease. *Science* 1993; 260: 1610.

Beaman MH. Lyme disease: why the controversy? *Intern Med J* 2016; 46: 1370.

Benoist C, Mathis D. Autoimmunity provoked by infection. *Nat Immunol* 2001; 2: 797.

Burgdorfer W, Barbour AG, Benach JL, et al. Lyme disease – a tick-borne spirochetosis? *Science* 1982; 216: 1317.

Collignon PJ, Lum GD, Robson JMB. Does Lyme disease exist in Australia? *Med J Aust* 2016; 205: 413.

Fraser CM, Casjens S, Huang WM, et al. Genomic sequence of a Lyme disease spirochaete, *Borrelia burgdorferi*. *Nature* 1997; 390: 580.

Halperin J, Luft BJ, Volkman DJ, et al. Lyme neuroborreliosis: peripheral nervous system manifestations. *Brain* 1990; 113: 1207.

Nadelman RB, Wormser GP. Lyme borreliosis. *Lancet* 1998; 352: 557.

Shadick NA, Philips CB, Logigian EL, et al. The long-term clinical outcomes of Lyme disease. *Ann Intern Med* 1994; 121: 560.

Spach D, Liles W, Campbell G, et al. Tick-borne diseases in the United States. *N Engl J Med* 1993; 329: 936.

Steere AC. Lyme disease. *N Engl J Med* 2001; 345: 115.

Steere AC, McHugh G, Damle N, et al. Prospective study of serologic tests for lyme disease. *Clin Infect Dis* 2008; 47: 188.

Steere AC, Sikand VJ, Meurice F, et al. Vaccination against Lyme disease with recombinant *Borrelia burgdorferi* outer surface protein A with adjuvant. *N Engl J Med* 1998; 339: 209.

Steere AC, Taylor E, McHugh GL, et al. The overdiagnosis of Lyme disease. *JAMA* 1993; 269: 1812.

Tompkins DC, Luft B. Lyme disease and other spirochetal zoonoses. In: *Scientific American Medicine. Infectious Disease 2*. Hamilton: Dekker Medicine. 2020.

Lymphadenopathy

Lymphadenopathy of a generalized nature may be due to
- infectious diseases
  - viral, bacterial, parasitic, fungal,
- haematological malignancies
  - when it is commonly associated with splenomegaly (q.v.),
- immune disorders,
- miscellaneous conditions, such as
  - Felty's syndrome (q.v.),
  - sarcoidosis (q.v.),
  - systemic lupus erythematosus (SLE) (q.v.),
  - drugs (e.g. phenytoin).

Lymphangioleiomyomatosis

Lymphangioleiomyomatosis (LAM) is a rare cystic lung disease occurring in young women. It is one of the rare causes of **interstitial lung disease** (q.v.).

Many cases are associated with **tuberous sclerosis** (q.v.), which shares a common gene mutation in the control of cell growth, leading to the development of chaotic lymphatic channels. LAM is a chronic progressive condition which is effectively a low-grade neoplasm, sometimes with associated chylothorax or renal angiomyolipomas.

Patients present with progressive dyspnoea, recurrent pneumothorax and chylous pleural effusion. Abdominal symptoms may be caused by lymphadenopathy or angiomyolipomas, which may mimic the features of ovarian cancer, lymphoma or benign renal tumour.

Lung function tests typically show obstruction and impaired gas transfer. The diagnosis is confirmed either by high-resolution CT scanning (HRCT), which shows cystic changes, or by lung biopsy. An elevated serum level of vascular endothelial growth factor-D (VEGF-D) has been shown to be diagnostically specific in patients with typical cystic changes on HRCT. The differential diagnosis is usually emphysema or histiocytosis (q.v.).

Treatment is of limited efficacy, though progesterone and luteinizing-hormone-releasing hormone analogs have been used empirically.

Sirolimus *has been shown to shrink LAMs and improve lung function. There have also been reports of the successful use off-label of* **sunitinib***, an inhibitor of tyrosine kinase and of vascular endothelial growth factor (VEGF) and more typically used for renal cell carcinoma, gastrointestinal stromal tumours (q.v.) and perhaps thyroid cancer. Other more complex opportunities for immunotherapy are under investigation.*

Inhaled bronchodilators can improve airflow obstruction in about 30% of patients. Pleurodesis should be performed in cases of pneumothorax. Lung transplantation has been successful in advanced cases.

Mortality averages 10% at 10 years after diagnosis, which is typically up to 5 years after the onset of symptoms, though the outlook may be better in those presenting with pneumothorax rather than dyspnoea. The median survival is nowadays over 20 years.

Bibliography

Chu SC, Horiba K, Usuki J, et al. Comprehensive evaluation of 35 patients with lymphangioleiomyomatosis. *Chest* 1999; 115: 1041.

Crino PB, Nathanson KL, Henske EP. The tuberous sclerosis complex. *N Engl J Med* 2006; 355: 1345.

Henske EP, McCormack FX. Lymphangioleiomyomatosis – a wolf in sheep's clothing. *J Clin Invest* 2012; 122; 3807.

Johnson SR. Lymphangioleiomyomatosis. *Eur Respir J* 2006; 27: 1056.

Kitaichi M, Nishimura K, Itoh H, et al. Pulmonary lymphangioleiomyomatosis. *Am J Respir Crit Care Med* 1995; 151: 527.

Liu H-J, Krymskaya VP, Henske EP. Immunotherapy for lymphangioleiomyomatosis and tuberous sclerosis: progress and future directions. *Chest* 2019; 156: 1062.

McCormack FX. Lymphangioleiomyomatosis: a clinical update. *Chest* 2008; 133: 507.

McCormack FX, Inoue Y, Moss J, et al. Efficacy and safety of sirolimus in lymphangioleiomyomatosis. *N Engl J Med* 2011; 364: 1595.

Moss J, ed. *LAM (lymphangioleiomyomatosis) and Other Diseases Characterized by Smooth Muscle Proliferation*. New York: Marcel Dekker. 1999.

Taylor JR, Ryu J, Colby TV, et al. Lymphangioleiomyomatosis. *N Engl J Med* 1990; 323: 1254.

Lymphocytosis

Lymphocytosis refers to an increased peripheral blood lymphocyte count of $>4.5 \times 10^9$/L.

It is uncommon, but it is occasionally seen in some infections, such as
- brucellosis (q.v.),
- chicken pox (see Varicella),
- measles,
- tuberculosis (q.v.).

Persistent lymphocytosis suggests the possibility of underlying chronic lymphatic leukaemia.

Atypical lymphocytosis refers to an absolute lymphocytosis with a significant proportion of cells (often about one third) being atypical, i.e. enlarged cells with increased cytoplasm.

This most commonly occurs following viral infection, especially infectious mononucleosis (see Epstein–Barr virus).

It is also seen with
- cytomegalovirus (q.v.),
- toxoplasmosis (q.v.),
- allergic reactions (e.g. serum sickness – q.v.),
- some malignancies (e.g. lymphoma).

It is associated with
- lymphadenopathy (q.v.), usually,
- splenomegaly (q.v.), often,
- hepatomegaly, sometimes,
- signs of meningeal irritation, occasionally.

Lymphomatoid granulomatosis See
- Wegener's granulomatosis.

Lymphopenia

Lymphopenia (lymphocytopenia) refers to an absolute lymphocyte count in peripheral blood of $<1.5 \times 10^9$/L.

It is seen with
- severe infections,
- major surgery or trauma,
- uraemia,
- nutritional deficiency,
- lymphoma,
- immune suppression
  - thus it is an important finding in HIV infection (see Acquired immunodeficiency syndrome).

Bibliography
Castelino DJ, McNair P, Kay TWH. Lymphocytopenia in a hospital population – what does it signify? *Aust NZ J Med* 1997; 27: 170.

Lyssavirus

Lyssavirus is of fruit bat origin and is closely related to classic rabies virus (q.v.). It was first described in 1996 in Australia and has been called Australian bat lyssavirus (ABL). It can cause encephalitis (q.v.), and its management is as for rabies.

See also
- Bites and stings – Bats,
- Zoonoses.

Bibliography
Francis JR, McCall BJ, Hutchinson P, et al. Australian bat lyssavirus: implications for public health. *Med J Aust* 2014; 201: 647.
Warrell MJ, Warrell DA. Rabies and other lyssavirus disease. *Lancet* 2004; 363: 959.

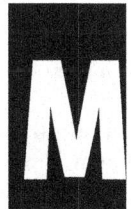

Macrophage activation syndrome (MAS) *See*

- Haemophagocytic syndrome.

'Mad Hatter' syndrome *See*

- Anticholinergic agents,
- Mercury.

Magnesium

Magnesium (Mg, atomic number 12, atomic weight 24) is the lightest structural metal and was first isolated in 1808, though it had long been known in compounds. It is widely distributed in nature and is responsible for much of the bitter taste of sea water, which contains 0.13% magnesium chloride. In biology, it is an important cofactor or catalyst for many enzyme reactions in carbohydrate and other substrate metabolism, particularly intracellular phosphorylation. It is also essential for chlorophyll, upon which plant photosynthesis depends.

The normal plasma level is 0.8–1 mmol/L, of which about 70% is free or ionized and the rest bound to albumin. The total body magnesium is about 1000 mmol (about 25 g), of which the majority is in bone. Magnesium is thus primarily (about 99%) an intracellular cation, being the second most common after potassium. The recommended daily intake is 125–500 mg (5–20 mmol), of which about 40% is absorbed.

Magnesium causes an osmotic diarrhoea (q.v.), and this is seen following the administration of magnesium-containing antacids or magnesium salts which are popular cathartics. Parenterally, it causes systemic and coronary vasodilatation (thus reducing perfusion injury), it is a bronchodilator, and it inhibits platelet function. These effects are due to prostacyclin-mediated smooth muscle relaxation.

Magnesium is useful in a number of **tachyarrhythmias**, especially in torsade de pointes but also in digitalis toxicity and after cardiac surgery, when a dose of 10 mmol (2.5 g of $MgSO_4$ or 5 mL of 50% solution) may be given over 1–2 min. This dose raises the plasma level by about 0.8 mmol/L. A continuous IV infusion of about 5 mmol/hr for 24 hr may then be used.

In acute myocardial infarction, early reports that magnesium decreased mortality (from 10.3% to 7.8%) were not confirmed in the large subsequent ISIS-4 trial. A similar lack of benefit was also found in the later MAGIC trial in patients with STEMI who had received early reperfusion therapy.

Magnesium is effective in a number of other conditions.
- In **pre-eclampsia (q.v.)**, it is the agent of choice to prevent convulsions.
- In **asthma (q.v.)**, it has been shown to be an effective adjunct to treatment when given either intravenously or by nebulization.

- In aneurysmal **subarachnoid haemorrhage**, it is potentially effective in preventing vasospasm and delayed cerebral ischaemia, though the known haemostatic effect of magnesium could also have contributed to the favourable result reported in this condition.

Hypermagnesaemia is uncommon. It is usually seen in patients with renal failure who have been taking magnesium-containing antacids or laxatives. It may give rise to an acquired hypoparathyroidism (q.v.) and thus hypocalcaemia (q.v.).

> Increased plasma magnesium levels are potentially toxic, though the relation between the plasma level and specific abnormalities is only approximate.

- **2–4 mmol/L**
  This is a 'therapeutically increased level', as in pre-eclampsia.
- **>3.0 mmol/L**
  There may be drowsiness, headache, lethargy, sweating, flushing and nausea;
  there may also be diplopia, dysarthria and decreased deep tendon reflexes.
- **>5 mmol/L**
  Toxicity becomes important and is manifest by hyporeflexia and sometimes abnormal cardiac conduction (i.e. prolonged PR interval, widened QRS complex).
- **>7.5 mmol/L**
  There is areflexia, muscle paralysis, narcosis, respiratory failure due to hypoventilation, hypotension and complete heart block.
- **>12.5 mmol/L**
  Asystole occurs.

Treatment is with **hydration** *and* **calcium** *(10–20 mL IV of 10% calcium gluconate over 10 min). The reversal of magnesium toxicity by calcium is temporary, and its persistence may require dialysis.*

Hypomagnesaemia, on the other hand, is common. It occurs in about 10% of hospital patients and in about 40% of seriously ill patients. However, when ionized magnesium instead of the usual total plasma magnesium is measured, hypomagnesaemia is much less frequent, occurring in perhaps only 15% of seriously ill patients. The relationships between measurements of intracellular, ionized plasma and total plasma magnesium are somewhat loose and of uncertain clinical significance. When daily intake is omitted, the magnesium 'stores' become depleted in about a week and hypomagnesaemia occurs.

Decreased intake is compounded by increased loss. This usually arises from

- losses via the gut, especially from GI fistulae,
- losses via the kidney (a fractional magnesium excretion in the urine of >2.5% indicates renal magnesium wasting),
- drugs giving increased urinary loss (aminoglycosides, amphotericin B, cisplatin, ciclosporin, pamidronate, pentamidine, thiazides),
- proton pump inhibitors (PPIs) after prolonged use (the mechanism is unclear, but it appears to be gastrointestinal rather than renal),
- diabetic ketoacidosis,
- alcoholism,
- hypothermia (q.v.),
- burns.

The hypokalaemia associated with diuretic use has concomitant hypomagnesaemia in 40% of cases. Treatment of both is required to correct the hypokalaemia and associated arrhythmias. It is of interest that the potassium-sparing diuretics also conserve magnesium.

> Since magnesium is important in cardiovascular, neurological and endocrine function, its deficiency can give rise to widespread effects and especially tachyarrhythmias, cardiac failure, seizures, tetany and even sudden death.
>
> Hypomagnesaemia is one of the causes of a prolonged QT interval and thus torsade de pointes.

Like hypermagnesaemia, hypomagnesaemia can also give rise to an acquired hypoparathyroidism (q.v.).

Treatment depends on severity.

- *If severe (<0.5 mmol/L), 10–20 mmol should be given, as 5–10 mL IV of 50%* **magnesium** *sulphate in 100 mL of 5% dextrose or 0.9% saline over 10–20 min.*
- *If very severe (<0.4 mmol/L), up to 40–80 mmol may be given in a similar way.*
- *In chronic mild/moderate deficiency, 25–50 mmol should be given daily. Up to a week of treatment may be required to replenish the body's stores, even if continuing losses have ceased.*
- *To prevent deficiency, 5–20 mmol should be given daily, unless there are continuing losses when these too must be taken into account.*

Magnesium is a component in 15% of **renal calculi** in the form of struvite, i.e. magnesium ammonium phosphate (see Nephrolithiasis).

Bibliography
Arsenian MA. Magnesium and cardiovascular disease.
    Progr Cardiovasc Dis 1993; 35: 271.
Casscells W. Magnesium and myocardial infarction.
    Lancet 1994; 343: 807.

Chernow B, Bamberger S, Stoiko M, et al. Hypomagnesemia in patients in postoperative intensive care. *Chest* 1989; 95: 391.

Cholst IN, Steinberg SF, Tropper PJ, et al. The influence of hypermagnesemia on serum calcium and parathyroid hormone levels in human subjects. *N Engl J Med* 1984; 310: 1221.

Connolly E, Worthley LIG. Intravenous magnesium. *Crit Care Resusc* 1999; 1: 162.

Hughes R, Goldkorn A, Masoli M, et al. Use of isotonic nebulised magnesium sulphate as an adjuvant to salbutamol in treatment of severe asthma in adults: randomised placebo-controlled trial. *Lancet* 2003; 361: 2114.

ISIS-4 (Fourth International Study of Infarct Survival) Collaborative Group. ISIS-4: A randomised factorial trial assessing early oral captopril, oral mononitrate, and intravenous magnesium sulphate in 58 050 patients with suspected acute myocardial infarction. *Lancet* 1995; 345: 669.

Lucas MJ, Leveno KJ, Cunningham FG. A comparison of magnesium sulfate with phenytoin for the prevention of eclampsia. *N Engl J Med* 1995; 333: 201.

Mackay JD, Bladon PT. Hypomagnesaemia due to proton-pump inhibitor therapy: a clinical case series. *Q J Med* 2010; 103: 387.

Magnesium in Coronaries (MAGIC) Trial Investigators. Early administration of intravenous magnesium to high-risk patients in the Magnesium in Coronaries (MAGIC) trial: a randomized controlled trial. *Lancet* 2002; 360: 1189.

Magpie Trial Collaborative Group. Do women with pre-eclampsia, and their babies, benefit from magnesium sulphate? The Magpie Trial: a randomized placebo controlled trial. *Lancet* 2002; 359: 1877.

McLean RM. Magnesium and its therapeutic uses. *Am J Med* 1994; 96: 63.

Nadler JL, Rude RK. Disorders of magnesium metabolism. *Endocrinol Metab Clin North Am* 1995; 24: 623.

Noronha JL, Matuschak GM. Magnesium in critical illness: metabolism, assessment, and treatment. *Intens Care Med* 2002; 28: 667.

Silverman RA, Osborn H, Runge J, et al. IV magnesium sulfate in the treatment of acute severe asthma: a multicenter randomized controlled trial. *Chest* 2002; 122: 489.

Teo KK, Yusuf S, Collins R, et al. Effects of intravenous magnesium in suspected acute myocardial infarction: overview of randomized trials. *BMJ* 1991; 303: 1499.

Weisinger JR, Bellorin-Font E. Magnesium and phosphorus. *Lancet* 1998; 352: 391.

Westermaier T, Stetter C, Vince GH, et al. Prophylactic intravenous magnesium sulfate for treatment of aneurysmal subarachnoid hemorrhage: a randomized, placebo-controlled, clinical study. *Crit Care Med* 2010; 38: 1284.

Whang R, Whang D, Ryan M. Refractory potassium depletion: a consequence of magnesium deficiency. *Arch Intern Med* 1992; 152: 40.

Woods KL, Fletcher S, Roffe C, et al. Intravenous magnesium sulphate in suspected acute myocardial infarction: results of the second Leicester Magnesium Intervention Trial (LIMIT-2). *Lancet* 1992; 339: 1553.

Wu J, Carter A. Magnesium: the forgotten electrolyte. *Aust Prescriber* 2007; 30: 102.

Malabsorption

Malabsorption is a commonly used global term encompassing

- **true malabsorption**
  - i.e. failure to absorb nutrients due to damage of the small intestinal mucosa,
- **maldigestion**
  - i.e. due to either deficiency of digestive secretions, especially biliary and/or pancreatic, or to a number of miscellaneous causes.

The causes of **true malabsorption** are

- coeliac disease (q.v.), i.e. a gluten-sensitive enteropathy (GSE),
- tropical sprue,
- miscellaneous conditions, including
  - ischaemia,
  - extensive bowel resection,
  - stasis syndrome, due to bacterial overgrowth, in turn caused by an afferent loop of a gastrojejunostomy, intestinal stricture or diverticulosis, diabetes or scleroderma, and typically aggravated by recent administration of a proton pump inhibitor (PPI) or an opiate,
  - lymphoma,
  - amyloid (q.v.),
  - Crohn's disease (q.v.),
  - Whipple's disease (q.v.),
  - parasitic infection,
  - AIDS (q.v.),
  - irradiation,
  - high altitude (q.v.),
  - hypogammaglobulinaemia,
  - abetalipoproteinaemia,
  - enteropathy caused by the selective angiotensin II receptor antagonists, especially olmesartan (see Coeliac disease, see Renin–angiotensin–aldosterone).

The causes of **maldigestion** include
- chronic pancreatitis or biliary obstruction,
- post-gastrectomy,
- diabetic dysautonomia,
- scleroderma (q.v.),
- drugs, particularly alcohol, colchicine, laxatives.

The clinical features of malabsorption in general comprise
- steatorrhoea, as the presence of fat causes the passage of light and bulky stools, most marked in pancreatic exocrine failure,
- weight loss despite an adequate food intake,
- fatigue,
- the consequences of single or multiple vitamin deficiency (q.v.).

Investigations show anaemia (q.v.), hypoalbuminaemia, hypocalcaemia (q.v.) and hypomagnesaemia (see Magnesium). In true malabsorption, there is impaired xylose absorption, though this test has fallen into disuse. Confirmatory investigations include faecal fat analysis, barium follow-through and small bowel biopsy.

Bibliography

Anderson RP. Coeliac disease: current approach and future prospects. *Intern Med J* 2008; 38: 790.

Campbell CB, Roberts RK, Cowen AE. The changing clinical presentation of coeliac disease in adults. *Med J Aust* 1977; 1: 89.

Corsini G, Gandolfi E, Bonechi I, et al. Postgastrectomy malabsorption. *Gastroenterology* 1966; 50: 358.

Duggan JM. Recent developments in our understanding of adult coeliac disease. *Med J Aust* 1997; 166: 312.

Duggan JM. Coeliac disease: the great imitator. *Med J Aust* 2004; 180: 524.

Feighery C. Coeliac disease. *BMJ* 1999; 319: 236.

Fisher RL, ed. Malabsorption and nutritional status and support. *Gastrenterol Clin North Am* 1989; 18: 467.

Go VLW, et al., eds. *The Pancreas: Biology, Pathobiology and Diseases*. New York: Raven Press. 1993.

Gosh SK, Littlewood JM, Goddard D, et al. Stool microscopy in screening for steatorrhoea. *J Clin Pathol* 1977; 30: 749.

Green PHR, Tall AR. Drugs, alcohol and malabsorption. *Am J Med* 1979; 67: 1066.

Marshak RL, Lindner AE. Malabsorption syndrome. *Semin Roentgenol* 1966; 1: 138.

Matysiak-Budnik T, Candalh C, Dugave C, et al. Alteration of the intestinal transport and processing of gliadin peptides in celiac disease. *Gastroenterolgy* 2003; 125: 696.

Mukherjee R, Kelly CO. Diseases producing malabsorption and maldigestion. In: *Scientific American Medicine. Gastroenterology*. Hamilton: Dekker Medicine. 2020.

Reeves GEM. Coeliac disease: against the grain. *Intern Med J* 2004; 34: 521.

Rubio-Tapia A, Herman ML, Ludviggson JF, et al. Severe sprue-like enteropathy associated with olmesartan. *Mayo Clin Proc* 2012; 87: 732.

Toouli J, Biankin AV, Oliver MR, et al. Management of pancreatic exocrine insufficiency: Australasian Pancreatic Club recommendations. *Med J Aust* 2010; 193: 461.

Malaria

Malaria is a parasitic vector-borne disease, still uncontrolled and causing at least 200 million cases and 1 million deaths per year worldwide, mainly in tropical countries. It is also seen in temperate climates in travellers. The geographic range of disease is expected to extend as future climate change enlarges the range of its main vector, the female *Anopheles* mosquito. Currently, nearly half the world's population lives in areas at risk of malaria transmission.

Occasionally, malaria (particularly due to *Plasmodium falciparum*) has been seen in people who have never been in an endemic area, and presumably this is either
- so-called **airport malaria** (from an infected mosquito which has hitchhiked aboard a plane from a malarious country), or
- **autochthonous malaria** (from a local *Anopheles* mosquito which has fed on a case of imported disease).

Malaria is an ancient disease, and recent genetic evidence suggests that *P. falciparum* may have made a species switch from gorillas at about the time of the first appearance of homo sapiens. Subsequently, relative malarial resistance may have been responsible for the persistence in humans of a number of otherwise adverse conditions, including glucose 6-phosphate dehydrogenase deficiency (q.v.), sickle cell anaemia (q.v.) and thalassaemia (q.v.). The separation of malaria from other causes of fever was greatly assisted by the introduction into Europe in the 1630s of *Cinchona* bark ('Jesuits' bark') from Peru. The plant genus was named *Cinchona* by Linnaeus after the Spanish Countess of Chinchona, who developed tertian ague in Peru and was cured by what was then a local folk medicine. This bark provided a source of quinine and thus specific therapy, and indeed quinine and its derivatives (chloroquine, quinidine, mefloquine, primaquine, tafenoquine, amodiaquine) have remained the front-line treatment for malaria over the succeeding centuries.

Malaria is caused by protozoa of the *Plasmodium* genus, of which several species can cause disease in humans, with most cases caused by *P. falciparum* (46%) and *P. vivax* (43%) and most deaths caused by *P. falciparum*. The parasite has a complex but well documented life-cycle in humans, following the injection of the sporozoite by a mosquito of the anopheline type which is the definitive host. Malaria can also be transmitted by blood transfusion in countries where the disease is prevalent.

> The incubation period is typically 10 days to 4 weeks, but sometimes it is much longer, particularly in those who have been on suppressive antimalarial drugs or who are semi-immune, in whom clinical disease may occur months or years after leaving an endemic area.
>
> The clinical picture is one of high fever (up to 41°C or more), chills, sweating and prostration. Anaemia (q.v.), jaundice and hepatosplenomegaly are observed. Sometimes, there is renal failure, diarrhoea and coma. A rash is not usually present.
>
> *P. falciparum* gives a continuous or intermittent fever, with obstruction of the microcirculation and capillary leakage, especially in the brain (causing cerebral malaria), gut and lung (giving an ARDS-like picture). There is hypoglycaemia, intravascular haemolysis and lactic acidosis (q.v.).
>
> *P. vivax* gives a tertian or second daily fever.

The diagnosis is made by detection of the parasites on blood film, though the parasites may be scanty or absent at the time of severe illness and a repeat smear may be needed. Microscopy includes examination of both thick and thin blood smears. A rapid diagnostic test is available to detect parasite protein in finger-prick samples, and this technique can be used as an inexpensive self-diagnosis kit for travellers. Molecular tests using PCR are available in research laboratories.

Other typical laboratory findings, especially in severe cases, include anaemia (q.v.), thrombocytopenia (q.v.), hypoglycaemia, hypoalbuminaemia, hyperbilirubinaemia, renal impairment and metabolic acidosis (q.v.).

Treatment options have been reduced because drug resistance, most importantly to chloroquine, is now widespread. Normally, acute treatment has been with **chloroquine** 0.6 g then 0.3 g in 6 hr and 0.3 g per day for 2 days, and this remains the preferred treatment in areas where the organism has remained sensitive.

If the parasites are resistant, alternative agents are **quinine** 0.6 g orally tds for three days or **quinidine gluconate** 600 mg IV over 1–2 hr then 1 mg/min IV for 2–3 days. **Pyrimethamine** with a sulphonamide, tetracycline or clindamycin, or **mefloquine** should be added. However, **mefloquine** can cause neuropsychiatric toxicity. The tissue phase of P. vivax infection requires **primaquine** (15 mg per day for two weeks) to eradicate extra-erythrocytic or hepatic infection. Alternatively, the newer analog, **tafenoquine**, may be used in single dosage (300 mg) for eradication. **Proguanil/atovaquone** combination is perhaps the most effective but is expensive. **Halofantrine** is effective, but it is not recommended because it may cause fatal cardiac arrhythmias.

Artesunate (an artemisinin which was originally derived from wormwood) is a relatively new agent which is highly effective in severe cases, though it needs to be followed by another antimalarial, such as proguanil/atovaquone.

In acute malaria, **corticosteroids** have sometimes been given, but they are unhelpful and may even be deleterious in cerebral malaria. **Exchange transfusion** has also been used in severe cases, but its benefit is doubtful.

Fluid resuscitation in severe cases should be conservative, because there is an unpredictable risk of acute pulmonary oedema and an adverse outcome has been associated with liberal fluid regimens in such cases.

Prevention requires avoidance of mosquitoes, prophylactic medication and awareness of its possibility for up to a year after potential exposure. Prophylactic agents in chloroquine-resistant areas comprise chiefly doxycycline (100 mg per day), depending on the region. Mefloquine (250 mg per week) is effective though no longer generally recommended for this purpose (see above), but tafenoquine (a primaquine analog, given as 200 mg per week) has been shown to be effective. There are now malaria vaccines available following extensive research in recent decades, but current formulations show only moderate efficacy.

Bibliography

Brown GV, Good MF. Prospects for a vaccine against malaria. *Intern Med J* 2002; 32: 129.

Iqbal KM, Ahmed N, Aziz L. Malaria: its severe form and its management. *Crit Care Shock* 2000; 3: 69.

Kain KC, Shanks GD, Keystone JS. Malaria chemoprophylaxis in the age of drug resistance. *Clin Infect Dis* 2001; 33: 226.

Knope K, Doggett SL, Jansen CC, et al. Arboviral diseases and malaria: Annual report of the National Arbovirus and Malaria Advisory Committee. *Communicable Diseases Intelligence.* 2019; vol. 43.

Mai NTH, Day NPJ, Chuong LV, et al. Post-malaria neurological syndrome. *Lancet* 1996; 348: 917.

Marks M, Gupta-Wright A, Doherty JF, et al. Managing malaria in the intensive care unit. *Br J Anaesth* 2014; 113: 910.

Martens P, Hall L. Malaria on the move. *Emerg Infect Dis* 2000; 6: 2.

McCarthy JS. Malaria prophylaxis: in war and peace. *Med J Aust* 2005; 182: 148.

Mer M, Dunser MW, Giera R, et al. Severe malaria: current concepts and practical overview: what every intensivist should know. *Intens Care Med* 2020; 46: 907.

Miller LH, Baruch DI, Marsh K, et al. The pathogenic basis of malaria. *Nature* 2002; 415: 673.

Trampuz A, Jereb M, Muzlovic I, et al. Clinical review: severe malaria. *Crit Care* 2003; 7: 315.

White NJ, Pukrittayakamee S, Hien TT, et al. *Malaria. Lancet* 2014; 383: 723.

Wyler DJ. Malaria – resurgence, resistance, and research. *N Engl J Med* 1983; 308: 875.

Zucker JR. Changing patterns of autochthonous malaria transmission in the United States. *Emerg Infect Dis* 1996; 2: 37.

Malignant hyperthermia

Malignant hyperthermia (MH) is a rare and striking complication of general anaesthesia, in which it occurs in about 1 in 50,000 adult cases and more commonly in children. It was first recognized in 1960 in Melbourne. It is usually associated with the use of suxamethonium and volatile agents and mostly occurs during induction, though occasionally it may appear as late as the post-anaesthetic recovery period. Previous anaesthetics may not have caused the syndrome. It can even sometimes occur in the non-anaesthetic situation, such as in stress or exercise.

The aetiology is a genetically determined biochemical defect of muscle metabolism, seen in families who are otherwise normal. Although the condition is inherited as an autosomal dominant in severe cases, there is genetic heterogeneity with recessive inheritance in milder forms of the disease. The regulation of intracellular calcium ions in muscle is abnormal, so that neuronal stimulation and muscle depolarization lead to excessive calcium egress into the cytoplasm, dysregulation of the many calcium-mediated cell processes and thus muscle hypermetabolism. This defect in calcium homeostasis has been attributed in many cases to mutations in the *RYR1* gene which codes for the skeletal muscle ryanodine receptor.

It sometimes occurs in patients with various forms of muscle disease, such as myopathy (q.v.), muscular dystrophy (q.v.) or the neuroleptic malignant syndrome (q.v.).

Clinical features comprise the acute onset of
- rapidly increased core temperature,
- tachyarrhythmias,
- hypercapnia despite tachypnoea,
- metabolic acidosis (q.v.),
- muscular rigidity,
- mottled skin and cyanosis,
- excessive bleeding,
- shock,
- coma.

MH is a hypermetabolic crisis. There is hyperkalaemia, myoglobinuria (q.v.), increased lactate, increased creatine kinase, and the hypercapnia is out of proportion to a seemingly adequate ventilation. Definitive diagnosis in patients or relatives is made by in vitro contracture testing of muscle obtained by biopsy.

Treatment involves cooling, hyperventilation, oxygenation, and therapy for abnormalities of electrolytes (e.g. hyperkalaemia) and acid-base (e.g. metabolic acidosis) or for cardiac arrhythmias or hypotension. If surgery is incomplete, anaesthesia should be maintained with propofol.

*Most importantly, specific therapy is available with **dantrolene**, which decreases calcium ion release from the sarcoplasmic reticulum and thus decreases muscle contractility. It is given in a dose of 2.5 mg/kg IV (formerly 1–2 mg/kg IV) and repeated every 10–15 min until resolution of the hypermetabolic state (pyrexia, acidosis and muscle rigidity). This dosage is usually very effective, but it may need to be repeated 4 hrly and occasionally a total dosage up to 10 mg/kg over 48–72 hr may be required.*

An important but uncommon side-effect of dantrolene is severe hepatitis (q.v.). Severe hypotension can occur if a calcium channel blocker is administered concomitantly.

The untreated mortality used to be 30%, but this has been greatly reduced with prompt and appropriate treatment. After recovery, patient and family counselling should be undertaken, including advice about any future anaesthesia.

Bibliography

Denborough MA, Lovell RR. Anaesthetic deaths in a family. *Lancet* 1960; 2: 45.

Hopkins PM. Malignant hyperthermia: advances in clinical management and diagnosis. *Br J Anaesth* 2000; 85: 118.

Kolb ME, Horne ML, Martz R. Dantrolene in human malignant hyperthermia: a multicenter study. *Anesthesiology* 1982; 56: 254.

MacLennon DH, Phillips MS. Malignant hyperthermia. *Science* 1992; 256: 789.

Nelson TE, Flewellen EH. The malignant hyperthermia syndrome. *N Engl J Med* 1983; 309: 416.

O'Keefe S, Nelson P, Davis M. Malignant hyperthermia. In: Riley R, ed. *Australasian Anaesthesia*. Melbourne: ANZCA. 2017; p 263.

Rosenberg H, Antognini JF, Muldoon S. Testing for malignant hyperthermia. *Anesthesiology* 2002; 96: 232.

Urwyler A, Deufel T, McCarthy T, et al. European Malignant Hyperthermia Group: guidelines for molecular genetic detection of susceptibility to malignant hyperthermia. *Br J Anaesth* 2001; 86: 283.

Waddingham M. Malignant hyperthermia: investigation for the uninitiated. In: Keneally J, ed. *Australian Anaesthesia*. Melbourne: ANZCA. 2005; p 41.

Mallory–Weiss syndrome

Mallory–Weiss syndrome refers to a mucosal or submucosal tear of the lower oesophagus, usually associated with retching or vomiting, particularly if vomiting has been held back. The classical clinical triad consists of vomiting, chest pain and subcutaneous emphysema.

Boerhaave's syndrome refers to a complete oesophageal rupture under similar circumstances.

A Mallory–Weiss tear is reported to be responsible for 5–10% of cases of upper gastrointestinal bleeding.

> In Intensive Care, it is an important cause of acute mediastinitis (q.v.).

Bibliography
Bhatia P, Portin D, Inculet RI, et al. Current concepts in the management of esophageal perforations. *Ann Thorac Surg* 2011; 92: 209.

Manganese

Manganese (Mn, atomic number 25, atomic weight 55) is a hard white brittle metal, first recognized in 1774 and mainly used as an alloy in steel.

It is an essential trace element in animals and plants, but it is toxic in excess causing 'manganese madness'. It is a required cofactor in many enzyme systems and is also required for the action of vitamin K. The most obvious effect of its lack is thus vitamin K deficiency (q.v.). Manganese deficiency has also been associated with osteoarthritis.

It is present in many fruits, nuts and cereals. It is normally excreted in the bile and therefore can accumulate in the body in the presence of cholestasis (q.v.).

The required daily intake is 150–2000 mcg orally, and the recommended IV dose is 5 µmol per day. These doses should be decreased if there is biliary obstruction.

Bibliography
Barceloux DG. Manganese. *J Toxicol Clin Toxicol* 1999; 37: 293.

Marfan's syndrome

Marfan's syndrome (Marfan syndrome) is a generalized disorder of connective tissue which causes extensive physical abnormalities. It has an autosomal dominant inheritance, and its prevalence is about 1 in 5000 of the population. The basic defect is in the gene for fibrillin, a glycoprotein of 350 kDa, which is a structural component of the microfibrils associated with elastin. There is thus disruption of collagen and elastic fibres in many structures, most importantly in the cardiovascular system, but also in the eye and musculoskeletal system.

> The four groups of clinical features of Marfan's syndrome are
> 1. abnormally long limbs (dolichostenomelia) and fingers (arachnodactyly), chest wall abnormalities (kyphoscoliosis – q.v., pectus excavatum – q.v.), increased risk of spontaneous pneumothorax (q.v.) and high arched palate,
> 2. aortic dilatation, with proneness to aortic regurgitation and aortic dissection (q.v.),
> 3. mitral valve prolapse,
> 4. ectopia lentis, which is an upward displacement of the lens, usually bilateral and occurring in up to 80% of subjects. It is due to disrupted ciliary zonular fibres and may be associated with myopia and an increased risk of retinal detachment.

The diagnosis is based on the presence of at least two of the groups of clinical features and is strong if three or four groups and a positive family history are present. Clinical examination and even chest X-ray may be normal, and echocardiography is required to detect significant cardiovascular lesions. Annual echocardiographic screening is often recommended in confirmed cases. The pathogenic *FBN1* mutation may be demonstrated, but in general genetic testing is complex, expensive and often diagnostically unhelpful.

*Prophylactic **beta blockers** are indicated if there is aortic root dilatation.*
- *There should be rigorous control of any hypertension.*
- *Surgical replacement of the ascending aorta and aortic valve is indicated for marked aortic regurgitation.*

Pregnancy in Marfan's syndrome predisposes to aortic dissection.

Bibliography
De Paepe A, Devereux RB, Dietz HC, et al. Revised diagnostic criteria for the Marfan syndrome. *Am J Med Genet* 1996; 62: 417.

Summers KM, West JA, Hattam A, et al. Recent developments in the diagnosis of Marfan syndrome and related disorders. *Med J Aust* 2012; 197: 494.

Summers KM, West JA, Peterson MM, et al. Challenges in the diagnosis of Marfan syndrome. *Med J Aust* 2006; 184: 627.

Marine vertebrate and invertebrate stings See

- Bites and stings.

Mast cells See

- Basophilia
- Drug allergy,
- Eosinophils,
- Immune complex disease,
- Mastocytosis.

Mastocytosis

Systemic mastocytosis produces a similar clinical picture to carcinoid syndrome (q.v.), but the main mediator is histamine rather than serotonin. There is mast cell accumulation not only in skin (in virtually all cases) but also in non-cutaneous sites, such as visceral and bony lesions (in 10–20% of cases). It is probably a clonal proliferative condition related to lymphoproliferative disorders or polycythaemia (q.v.). There may be associated eosinophilia (q.v.). It is an uncommon condition with an estimated prevalence of about 10 per 100,000 of the population.

In addition to urticaria (q.v.), there is flushing (q.v.), headache, fatigue, abdominal pain and diarrhoea (q.v.), all due to histamine release. In severe cases, hypotension may be produced, and ultimately anaphylactoid (i.e. non-Ig-mediated) shock may result. These symptoms are due to acute mast cell degranulation and may be precipitated by alcohol, analgesics or insect stings especially from Hymenoptera, such as ants, bees and wasps.

Even when well, patients may have an elevated serum tryptase level, and this level becomes markedly increased when symptoms are present. There may be coagulopathy due to mast cell release of heparin (q.v.), as mast cell granules contain heparin as well as histamine.

Treatment is with H_1 *and* H_2 **antihistamines**, **anticholinergics** *for gastrointestinal symptoms and oral* **cromoglycate**. *There have been reports of the successful use of* **montelukast** *and of* **interferon alpha** *in this condition. Clearly, histamine-releasing drugs (e.g. opioids) should be avoided.*

See

- Aspirin,
- Flushing,
- Urticaria.

Bibliography

Arthur G, Bradding P. New developments in mast cell biology. *Chest* 2016; 150: 680.

Denburg JA. Basophil and mast cell lineage in vitro and in vivo. *Blood* 1992; 79: 846.

Fine J. Mastocytosis. *Int J Dermatol* 1980; 19: 117.

Lewis RA. Mastocytosis. *J Allergy Clin Immunol* 1984; 74: 755.

Pardanini A. Systemic mastocytosis in adult: 2012 update on diagnosis, risk stratification, and management. *Am J Hematol* 2012; 87: 402.

van der Weide HY, van Westerloo DJ, van den Bergh WM. Critical care management of systemic mastocytosis. *Crit Care* 2015; 19: 238.

May–Thurner syndrome See

- Thrombophilia.

Mediastinal diseases

Acute mediastinitis usually follows oesophageal perforation or rupture. Vomiting may damage the lower oesophagus with either a Mallory–Weiss tear and haemorrhage (q.v.) or a complete perforation, giving rise to Boerhaave's syndrome with pneumomediastinum and left pleural effusion and/or pneumothorax (see Pleural disorders). Oesophageal perforation may also be caused by a procedure, foreign body or carcinoma. Occasionally, mediastinitis may be due to spread of infection from adjacent chest structures, to infection of a mediastinal cyst, or to descending infection from a retropharyngeal abscess. Anterior mediastinitis can be a manifestation of deep sternal wound infection, which is an occasional complication of cardiac surgery.

The clinical features include fever, dysphagia and chest pain. Typically, the patient appears well initially (i.e. up to 48 hr) but then becomes seriously ill.

Treatment comprises appropriate **antibiotic** *therapy (with anaerobic cover) and surgical* **drainage** *of any abscess.*

Chronic mediastinitis is usually associated with a progressive fibrotic process. The cause is unknown, but it may be related to other fibrosing diseases, especially retroperitoneal fibrosis, but also Riedel's thyroiditis, Dupuytren's contracture, Peyronie's disease and sclerosing cholangitis (q.v.). Methysergide therapy for migraine has been implicated in some cases (see Ergot). Tuberculosis (q.v.) and histoplasmosis (q.v.) are sometimes responsible.

Sometimes the disease is localized (e.g. to the hilar region).

There is no effective therapy.

> **Other mediastinal diseases** include chiefly cysts and tumours.
>   The most common, in order, are
> 1. neurogenic tumours, especially neurofibroma,
> 2. cysts, especially bronchogenic or pericardial,
> 3. thymoma, more often benign than malignant,
> 4. teratoma, also more often benign than malignant,
> 5. lymphoma,
> 6. retrosternal thyroid.

However, many different types of lesions may occur in the mediastinum, and their nature depends greatly on their site.
- **Superior mediastinum**
  - thymoma (q.v.),
  - teratoma,
  - lymphoma,
  - retrosternal thyroid or parathyroid mass,
  - cystic hygroma,
  - aortic aneurysm,
  - haemangioma (q.v.),
  - abscess,
  - lymphadenopathy (q.v.),
  - oesophageal lesion.
- **Anterior mediastinum**
  - thymoma (q.v.), or other rarer thymic lesions, such as carcinoma, carcinoid or cyst,
  - teratoma,
  - lymphoma,
  - retrosternal thyroid or parathyroid mass,
  - pericardial or pleuropericardial cyst,
  - cystic hygroma,
  - hernia through the sternocostal or retrosternal hiatus (foramen of Morgagni),
  - neoplasm, especially germ cell or mesenchymal.
- **Middle mediastinum**
  - aortic aneurysm or other great vessel abnormality,
  - bronchogenic or pleuropericardial cyst,
  - lymphoma,
  - lipoma,
  - mediastinitis (see above),
  - tumour related to trachea, lymph nodes, heart,
  - hernia through the sternocostal or retrosternal hiatus (foramen of Morgagni).
- **Posterior mediastinum**
  - neurogenic tumour, i.e. neurofibroma (q.v.),
  - gastro-oesophageal or bronchogenic cyst,
  - oesophageal lesion, such as tumour or diverticulum,
  - meningocoele,
  - aortic aneurysm,
  - hernia through the vertebrocostal or posterolateral hiatus (foramen of Bochdalek),
  - thoracic spine disease,
  - pseudotumour, e.g. due to extramedullary haematopoiesis.

> The clinical features of mediastinal disease may include pain, dysphagia, hoarseness, stridor, cough, haemoptysis (q.v.) and dyspnoea.
>   Physical examination may reveal Horner's syndrome (q.v.), superior vena cava obstruction, enlarged cervical lymph nodes or pleural effusion (q.v.).

Investigations include chest X-ray and particularly CT scanning, and sometimes angiography, bronchoscopy and mediastinoscopy.

Bibliography
Abolnik I, Lossos IS, Breuer R. Spontaneous pneumomediastinum. *Chest* 1991; 100: 93.
Azarow KS, Pearl RH, Zurcher R, et al. Primary mediastinal masses. *J Thorac Cardiovasc Surg* 1993; 106: 67.
Duwe BV, Sterman DH, Musani AI. Tumors of the mediastinum. *Chest* 2005; 128: 2893.
Estrera AS, Landay MJ, Grisham JM, et al. Descending necrotizing mediastinitis. *Surg Gynecol Obstet* 1983; 157: 545.
Freeman RK, Vallieres E, Verrier ED, et al. Descending necrotizing mediastinitis: an analysis of the effects of serial surgical debridement on patient mortality. *J Thorac Cardiovasc Surg* 2000; 119: 260.
Lerner AD, Feller-Kopman D. Disorders of the pleura, mediastinum, and hilum. In: *Scientific American Medicine. Pulmonary & Critical Care Medicine.* Hamilton: Dekker Medicine. 2020.
Schowengerdt CG, Suyemoto R, Main FB. Granulomatous and fibrous mediastinitis. *J Thorac Cardiovasc Surg* 1969; 57: 365.
Strollo DC, de Christenson MLR, Jett JR. Primary mediastinal tumors. *Chest* 1997; 112: 511 & 1344.
Takeda S, Miyoshi S, Minami M, et al. Clinical spectrum of mediastinal cysts. *Chest* 2003; 124: 125.
Whooley BP, Urschel JD, Antkowiak JG, et al. Primary tumors of the mediastinum. *J Surg Oncol* 1999; 70: 95.

Mediastinitis See
- Mediastinal diseases.
  See also
- Anthrax,

- Mallory–Weiss syndrome,
- Pleural effusion.

Mediterranean fever *See*

- Familial Mediterranean fever,
- Pyrexia.

Medullary sponge kidney *See*

- Renal cystic disease.

Medullary thyroid cancer *See*

- Calcitonin,
- Multiple endocrine neoplasia.

Megaloblastic anaemia

Megaloblastic anaemia refers to anaemia (q.v.) characterized by macrocytes seen on the peripheral blood film and megaloblastic erythroid hyperplasia in the bone marrow. There is a defect of DNA synthesis and thus cell division, so that larger cells are produced.

This defect is due most commonly to folic acid or vitamin B_{12} deficiency (see below), but it may also be produced by drugs (e.g. nitrous oxide for >6 hr). It may sometimes be a genetic disorder.

The morphological changes are not confined to the bone marrow and are seen at other sites of rapid cell turnover, such as the gut mucosa. Both folic acid and vitamin B_{12} are required for the metabolism of single carbon units, and both are thus required dietary nutrients.

The diagnosis is suggested from the clinical features and the presence of macrocytosis. It is most readily confirmed by electronic cell counters which provide a sensitive index of macrocytosis (i.e. MCV > 98 fL).

However, macrocytosis is not specific, in that it also occurs in non-megaloblastic disorders, such as

- alcoholism,
- liver disease,
- anti-metabolite therapy.

It can also be masked by concomitant iron deficiency (q.v.) or thalassaemia (q.v.).

The peripheral blood film typically also shows hypersegmented neutrophils (5 or more lobes), occasional nucleated red blood cells and sometimes neutropenia (q.v.) or thrombocytopenia (q.v.). The levels of both folic acid and B_{12} should always be measured, because the administration of folic acid alone to patients with undiagnosed vitamin B_{12} deficiency may mask the anaemia of the latter condition and exacerbate its neurological complications. The reasons for the occurrence of neurological problems in vitamin B_{12} deficiency but not in folic acid deficiency are unclear.

Folic acid deficiency is seen with
- inadequate intake
  - alcoholism, malnutrition, pregnancy,
- impaired absorption
  - intestinal disease,
- certain drugs
  - methotrexate, phenytoin, pyrimethamine, trimethoprim.

Folic acid deficiency can occur rapidly, since the body contains stores for only 2 weeks.

*Treatment is with **folic acid** 1 mg per day or with folinic acid if the deficiency is secondary to specific blocking drugs.*

Vitamin B_{12} deficiency is seen
- classically in pernicious anaemia (q.v.),
- in other causes of impaired absorption, such as
  - post-gastrectomy,
  - pancreatic disease,
  - ileal disease,
  - infection with the fish tapeworm, *Diphyllobothrium latum*, from raw fish,
  - drugs, such as alcohol, colchicine, neomycin,
- also in extreme and prolonged malnutrition,
- following loss of coenzymes
  - e.g. after nitrous oxide,
- in rare congenital disorders.

See
- Folic acid deficiency,
- Pernicious anaemia,
- Vitamin B_{12} deficiency.

Bibliography

Editorial. Nitrous oxide and acute marrow failure. *Lancet* 1982; 2: 856.

Pruthi RK, Tefferi A. Pernicious anemia revisited. *Mayo Clin Proc* 1994; 69: 144.

Romain M, Sviri S, Linton DM, et al. The role of vitamin B12 in the critically ill – a review. *Anaesth Intens Care* 2016; 44: 447.

Melatonin

Melatonin is a serotonin derivative, secreted by the pineal gland when the retina fails to perceive light. It is thus an endogenous hormone, for which there are specific melatonin receptors (MT1, MT2 and MT3). Its name derives from the fact that it lightens amphibian skin by aggregating melanophores, i.e. the opposite effect to that of melanocyte-stimulating hormone, MSH (see Adrenocorticotropic hormone), though such an effect has not been shown in humans.

It was not discovered until 1958, but it has been widely studied since. Its secretion is circadian (diurnal) and thus provides the body with an internal clock in synchrony with the natural day and night. It may therefore influence the function of the brain, psyche, thyroid and gonads. Its circadian rhythm is opposite in direction to that of cortisol. Its effects on the body's **circadian rhythm** (q.v.) and on sleep are mediated via the melatonin receptors, MT1 and MT2. In addition to its effect on circadian rhythm, melatonin has pleiotropic actions, in particular with anti-inflammatory effects.

The circadian rhythm of melatonin secretion has been reported to be lost in patients with sepsis. This is due to failure of daytime suppression, though its mechanism and significance remain uncertain. In general, the plasma level of melatonin is low in critically ill patients, and it does not respond to such darkness as may be practicable in safe Intensive Care practice, but it is increased during catecholamine infusions. Variation in melatonin excretion over time may be assessed by measuring the urinary concentration of its metabolite, 6-sulfatoxymelatonin (aMT6s).

Melatonin is available as a cheap over-the counter drug in many countries and it has become popular in people with a variety of sleep disorders (including 'jet lag'), since unlike sedatives it induces normal REM sleep. However, studies in volunteers and in patients, using 2 mg prolonged-release tablets, have shown it to be only moderately effective. Side-effects reported by some patients have included headache, asthenia and pharyngitis.

Two small studies showed it to be effective in doses of 3 mg and 10 mg in improving sleep quality and preventing sleep deprivation in patients in the traditionally difficult Intensive Care environment. However, a subsequent systematic review showed no clear evidence for efficacy in ICU patients.

The melatonin receptor agonist, **ramelteon**, is more potent, more specific for MT1, longer-lasting and much more expensive than exogenous melatonin. When given in a typical dose of 8 mg, it has been used to treat insomnia, but in ICU patients it has failed to improve either sedation or delirium (q.v.).

The recognition of the **antioxidant properties** of melatonin has led to the study of its use in the treatment of patients with burns and with other forms of skin injury.

Bibliography

Bourne RS, Mills GH. Melatonin: possible implications for the postoperative and critically ill patient. *Intens Care Med* 2006; 32: 371.

Bourne RS, Mills GH, Minelli C. Melatonin therapy to improve nocturnal sleep in critically ill patients: encouraging results from a small randomised controlled trial. *Crit Care* 2008; 12: R52.

Brzezinski A. Melatonin in humans. *N Engl J Med* 1997; 336: 186.

Buscemi N, Vandermeer B, Hooten N, et al. Efficacy and safety of exogenous melatonin for secondary sleep disorders and sleep disorders accompanying sleep restriction: meta-analysis. *BMJ* 2006; 332: 385.

Garfinkel D, Laudon M, Zisapel N. Improvement in sleep quality in elderly people by controlled-release melatonin. *Lancet* 1995; 346: 541.

Hamblin SE, Burka AT. Ramelteon for ICU delirium prevention: is it time to melt away? *Crit Care Med* 2019; 47: 1813.

Jarratt J. Perioperative melatonin use. *Anaesth Intens Care* 2011; 39: 171.

Lewis KS, McCarthy RJ, Rothenberg DM. Does melatonin decrease sedative use and time to extubation in patients requiring prolonged mechanical ventilation? *Anesth Analg* 1999; 88: S123.

Lewis SR, Pritchard MW, Schofield-Robinson OJ, et al. Melatonin for the promotion of sleep in adults in the intensive care unit. *Cochrane Database Syst Rev* 2018; 5: CD012455.

Maas MB, Lizza BD, Abbott SM, et al. Factors disrupting melatonin secretion rhythms during critical illness. *Crit Care Med* 2020; 48: 854.

Maldonado M-D, Murillo-Cabezas F, Calvo J-R, et al. Melatonin as a pharmacologic support in burns patients: a proposed solution to thermal injury-related lymphocytopenia and oxidative damage. *Crit Care Med* 2007; 35: 1177.

Mundigler G, Delle-Karth G, Koreny M, et al. Impaired circadian rhythm of melatonin secretion in sedated critically ill patients with severe sepsis. *Crit Care Med* 2002; 30: 536.

Perras B, Meier M, Dodt C. Light and darkness fail to regulate melatonin release in critically ill humans. *Intens Care Med* 2007; 33: 1954.

Riutta A, Ylitalo P, Kaukinen S. Diurnal variation of melatonin and cortisol is maintained in non-septic intensive care patients. *Intens Care Med* 2009; 35: 1720.

Shilo L, Dagan Y, Smorjik Y, et al. Effect of melatonin on sleep quality of COPD Intensive Care patients. *Chronobiol Int* 2000; 17: 71.

Webb SM, Puig-Domingo M. Role of melatonin in health and disease. *Clin Endocrinol* 1995; 42: 221.

Wurtman RJ, Moskowitz MA. The pineal organ. *N Engl J Med* 1977; 1329: 1383.

Meleney's progressive synergistic gangrene See
- Gangrene.

Melioidosis

Melioidosis is caused by an unusual pseudomonas-like organism, *Burkolderia pseudomallei* (formerly called *Pseudomonas pseudomallei*), a Gram-negative aerobic bacillus found in water and soil in tropical areas up to 20° of latitude either side of the Equator and in particular in South-East Asia and Northern Australia. The organism is enzootic in animals, but these are not a source of direct transmission to humans, nor does person-to-person transmission occur. The organism enters the skin via an abrasion or the lungs via aerosol.

Infection is also seen in travellers, even those who have long left an endemic area.

There are three patterns of infection, namely subclinical, acute and chronic.
- **Subclinical infection**
  This is presumably common, because positive serology is found in up to 30% of populations at risk.
  There may be an asymptomatic pulmonary infiltrate in some patients.
- **Acute infection**
  This comprises a local pustule, pneumonia or systemic sepsis.
  The pustule appears after an incubation period of 2 days and is usually self-limited, though it may lead to sepsis.
  Pneumonia is the most common clinical form and ranges from mild to fulminating. The most severe form is associated with necrosis, cavitation and systemic sepsis.
  Sepsis is similar to that caused by other Gram-negative organisms and can lead to septic shock or metastatic abscess formation.
- **Chronic infection**
  This comprises suppuration, particularly in the lungs and typically with upper lobe cavities.
  It may thus resemble tuberculosis (q.v.).

Recrudescent disease of any form may appear many years later and is usually precipitated by
- diabetes,
- immune suppression,
- infection,
- liver disease,
- trauma.

The diagnosis is made by specific culture, though identification may be difficult and thus delayed. Positive serology in a traveller may assist.

Optimal treatment is not established because of variable susceptibility of the organism.
- *It is commonly **aminoglycoside-resistant**, and treatment was traditionally with chloramphenicol, tetracycline or cotrimoxazole.*
- *Later antipseudomonal agents (e.g. ceftazidime and especially **meropenem**) are of greater value, depending to some extent on their sensitivity merits. High doses and combination therapy are commonly recommended.*
- *The duration of treatment is at least a month and in chronic cases up to 6 months.*

Mortality used to be over 50%, particularly if sepsis was present, but it is nowadays much less, at least in the developed world.

The severity of its illness, together with its difficulty in diagnosis and treatment, make melioidosis a potential agent for germ warfare (q.v.).

Bibliography
Koponen M, Zlock D, Palmer D, et al. Melioidosis: forgotten, but not gone! *Arch Intern Med* 1991; 151: 605.
MacLaren G, Lye DC, Lee VJ. Increasing experience with melioidosis and critical care: medical and military implications. *Crit Care Med* 2016; 44: 1608.
Wiersinga WJ, Currie BJ, Peacock SJ. Melioidosis. *N Engl J Med* 2012; 367: 1035.

Mendelson's syndrome See
- Aspiration.

Meningococcaemia See
- Waterhouse–Friderichsen syndrome.
  See also
- Anorectal infections – Proctitis,
- Conjunctivitis,
- Epididymitis,
- Microangiopathic haemolysis,
- Toxic shock syndrome,
- Vasculitis.

Meningoencephalitis See
- Encephalitis.

Mercury

Mercury (Hg, atomic number 80, atomic weight 201, melting point −39°C, SG 13.5) is a metal of the zinc group. It is the only metal which is liquid at room temperature, and it was well known to the ancients.

Although native mercury occurs in nature, most is readily obtained from the red sulphide (cinnabar), which though rarer than copper or zinc is more abundant than many other common metals, such as tin.

Mercury is a reactive substance which forms metal alloys readily to produce an amalgam. Its uses in thermometers, barometers, sealed electrical switches, vapour lamps and dentistry are well known. It has also been used in fungicides and pharmaceuticals. Mercury is also widely used in industrial processes, the effluent from which can result in biological concentrations via the chain of bacteria to fish to man. The maximum recommended exposure is not greater than 0.1 mg/m^3 or 0.05 mg/m^3/8 hr.

Mercurous chloride (calomel) and mercuric chloride (corrosive sublimate) have antiseptic properties, but mercury-containing therapeutic agents, such as these, diuretics and ointments, are not nowadays used. Mercury poisoning thus usually arises from industrial accidents. Industrial exposure may be indirect, as in the Minamata accident in Japan in the early 1950s when factory effluent into a local bay affected fishermen and their families together with their household cats and the nearby seabirds. Toxicity has also occurred in farmers eating instead of planting grain seed treated with mercury-containing fungicide.

Acrodynia (pink disease) occurs in children from eating house paint containing mercury-based, antimould preparations. For the first half of the twentieth century, it occurred in children given worm cures or teething powders containing mercury in the form of calomel. Its name derived from the bright pink colour of the child's extremities, which were also painful. The patient was also miserable, lethargic and photophobic.

Acute toxicity arises from soluble mercury compounds, which are generally also corrosive. There is nausea, abdominal pain, bloody diarrhoea and renal failure.

Chronic toxicity usually arises from a mercury salt which has been inhaled or absorbed through the skin, the latter for example as mercury nitrate used in felt hat manufacture, giving the '**mad hatter**' syndrome.

- Oral manifestations include salivation, a metallic taste, stomatitis (see Mouth diseases), a blue line on the gums and loose teeth. Anorexia and weight loss may occur.
- Mental effects may include personality change. Weakness, blindness, peripheral neuropathy (q.v.), paralysis, coma and death may result.
- Acute tubulointerstitial disease (q.v.) may be produced.
- A lichenoid skin reaction with purple, flat, irregular papules resembling idiopathic lichen planus may be caused by mercury and indeed by a number of drugs (including beta blockers, methyldopa, NSAIDs, penicillamine, quinidine, quinine).

For treatment modalities, see Chelating agents.

See also
- Acute lung irritation – Toxic gases and fumes,
- Glomerular diseases,
- Heavy metal poisoning,
- Renal tubular acidosis,
- Zinc.

Bibliography

Bernhoft RA, Mercury toxicity and treatment: a review of the literature. *J Environ Public Health* 2012; 2012: 460508.

Black J. The puzzle of pink disease. *J R Soc Med* 1999; 92: 478.

MERS *See*

- Middle East respiratory syndrome.

Mesothelioma *See*

- Asbestos.

See also
- Islet cell tumour,
- Lung tumours,
- Occupational lung diseases,
- Pleural disorders.

Metabolic acidosis *See*

- Lactic acidosis.

See also
- Aspirin,
- Carbon monoxide,
- Carbonic anhydrase inhibitors,
- Drowning,
- Ethylene glycol,
- Heat stroke,
- Hypothermia,
- Malignant hyperthermia,
- Methanol,
- Renal tubular acidosis,
- Syndrome of inappropriate antidiuretic hormone,
- Tubulointerstitial diseases – Chronic interstitial nephritis.

Metabolism and nutrition

Many disorders of **metabolism**, such as the major acid–base and electrolyte abnormalities, and many aspects of **nutrition**, such as enteral and parenteral nutrition, are part of the 'bread and butter' of Intensive Care practice. Numerous other metabolic or nutritional issues and conditions which are less frequently encountered are considered in this book, including

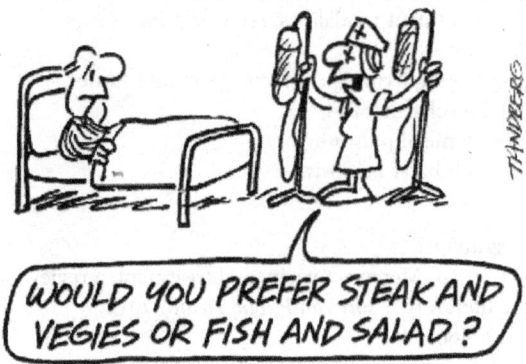

- Beriberi,
- Bicarbonate therapy,
- Caeruloplasmin,
- Calcium,
- Chromium,
- Cobalt,
- Copper,
- Eating disorders,
- Energy expenditure,
- Fabry's disease,
- Fanconi's syndrome,
- Favism,
- Folic acid deficiency,
- Gaucher's disease,
- Glucose-6-phosphate dehydrogenase deficiency,
- Glycogen storage diseases,
- Haemochromatosis,
- Hepcidin,
- Hyperammonaemia,
- Hypercalcaemia,
- Hyperhomocystinaemia,
- Hyperphosphataemia,
- Hyperuricaemia,
- Hypocalcaemia,
- Hypoglycaemia,
- Hypokalaemia,
- Hyponatraemia,
- Hypophosphataemia,
- Inborn errors of metabolism,
- Iron,
- Iron overload disease,
- Lactase deficiency,
- Lactic acidosis,
- Magnesium,
- Manganese,
- Metabolic acidosis,
- Periodic paralysis,
- Porphyria,
- Pseudohyperkalaemia,
- Pseudohyponatraemia,
- Pseudoporphyria,
- Pyroglutamic acid,
- Refeeding syndrome,
- Scurvy,
- Selenium,
- Storage disorders,
- Strontium,
- Thiamine deficiency,
- Trace elements,
- Urea cycle disorders,
- Vitamin deficiency,
- Vitamin B_{12} deficiency,
- Vitamin C deficiency,
- Vitamin D deficiency,
- Vitamin K deficiency,
- Zinc.

Bibliography

Anderson JJB, Toverud SU. Diet and vitamin D: a review with an emphasis on human function. *J Nutr Biochem* 1994; 5: 58.

Biolo G, Grimble G, Preiser J-C, et al. Position paper of the ESICM working group on nutrition and metabolism: metabolic basis of nutrition in intensive care unit patients: ten critical questions. *Intens Care Med* 2002; 11: 1512.

Casaer MP, Van den Berghe G. Nutrition in the acute phase of critical illness. *N Engl J Med* 2014; 370: 1227.

Chandra RK. Effect of vitamin and trace-element supplementation on immune responses and infection in elderly patients. *Lancet* 1992; 340: 1124.

Crowe AV, Griffiths RD. Nutritional failure and drugs. *Curr Opin Crit Care* 1997; 3: 268.

Cynober L, Moore FA, eds. *Nutrition and Critical Care.* Basel: Karger. 2003

DeLuca HF. Vitamin D metabolism and function. *Arch Intern Med* 1978; 138: 836.

Dent CE, Smith R. Nutritional osteomalacia. *Q J Med* 1969; 38: 195.

Editorial. Hepatic osteomalacia and vitamin D. *Lancet* 1982; 1: 943.

Faber P, Siervo M, eds. *Nutrition in Critical Care.* Cambridge: Cambridge University Press. 2014.

Fetterplace K, Holt D, Udy A, et al. Parenteral nutrition in adults during acute illness: a clinical perspective for clinicians. *Intern Med J* 2020; 50: 403.

Fisher RL, ed. Malabsorption and nutritional status and support. *Gastroenterol Clin North Am* 1989; 18: 467.

Herndon DN, Wernerman J, eds. Metabolic support in sepsis and multiple organ failure. *Crit Care Med* 2007; 35: (suppl.) S435.

Kellum JA. Recent advances in acid-base physiology applied to critical care. In: Vincent J-L, ed. *Yearbook of Intensive Care and Emergency Medicine 1998*. Berlin: Springer. 1998; p. 577.

Marik P, Varon J. The obese patient in the ICU. *Chest* 1998; 113: 492.

Mogensen KM, Robinson MK. Enteral and parenteral nutrition. In: *Scientific American Medicine. Gastroenterology.* Hamilton: Dekker Medicine. 2020.

Nasraway S, Black R, Sottile F. The anion gap in patients admitted to the medical intensive care unit. *Chest* 1989; 96: 287S.

Preiser J-C, Chiolero R, Wernerman J. Nutritional papers in ICU patients: what lies between the lines? *Intens Care Med* 2003; 29: 156.

Rose BD, Post TW, Stokes J, eds. *Clinical Physiology of Acid-Base and Electrolyte Disorders*. 6th edition. New York: McGraw-Hill. 2021.

Schelling JR, Howard RL, Winter SD, et al. Increased osmol gap in alcoholic ketoacidosis and lactic acidosis. *Ann Intern Med* 1990; 113: 580.

Taylor BE, McClave SA, Martindale RG, et al. Guidelines for the provision and assessment of nutrition support therapy in the adult critically ill patient: Society of Critical Care Medicine (SCCM) and American Society for Parenteral and Enteral Nutrition (ASPEN). *Crit Care Med* 2016; 44: 390.

Metastatic calcification See

- Calciphylaxis.
  See also
- Hypercalcaemia,
- Hyperphosphataemia.

Methaemoglobinaemia

Methaemoglobinaemia can be either inherited or acquired. The diagnosis of methaemoglobinaemia may be readily confirmed using modern blood gas analyzers which include dyshaemoglobins among their measured parameters.

In methaemoglobin, the iron in haemoglobin is in the ferric (oxidized) form rather than in the normal ferrous (reduced) form. Oxygen binding and thus oxygen carriage are thereby impaired. The oxygen dissociation curve is also shifted to the left, so that oxygen unloading in the tissues is impaired. There is central cyanosis (refractory to oxygen therapy) at levels of 10% or more, in contrast to the requirement of about 30% of deoxyhaemoglobin before cyanosis is apparent. The SaO_2 is usually about 85% by pulse oximetry and is paradoxically low in relation to the PaO_2. Normally, <3% of haemoglobin is present as methaemoglobin.

The relation between blood levels of methaemoglobin and clinical features is shown in the Table.

Blood level (%)	Clinical features
>3	asymptomatic
>10	central cyanosis
>15	hypoxaemia, brown blood
>25	as for anaemia
>40	tissue ischaemia
>50	CNS dysfunction, CVS instability, death

Inherited methaemoglobinaemia is a haemoglobinopathy due to a deficiency of the enzymes required to maintain iron in its reduced or ferrous state. Though worldwide, these disorders are rare.

Acquired methaemoglobinaemia is seen following exposure to many agents,

- classically with nitrites or nitrates (often used in food preservation),
- nowadays, most commonly after the therapeutic use of nitric oxide, particularly in relation to cardiopulmonary bypass,
- also with drugs such as dapsone, glyceryl trinitrate, topical local anaesthetics, primaquine, sulphasalazine and vitamin K analogs.

Treatment of symptomatic disease is with **methylene blue** *(q.v.). Methylene blue is not effective in patients with glucose-6-phosphate dehydrogenase deficiency (q.v.). In severe cases, exchange transfusion and hyperbaric oxygen have sometimes been used.*

Bibliography

Ajayi T, Gropper MA. Methemoglobinemia. *Pulmonary Perspectives* 2001; 18(4): 4.

Barker SJ, Tremper KK, Hyatt J. Effects of methemoglobinemia on pulse oximetry and mixed venous oximetry. *Anesthesiology* 1989; 70: 112.

Charache S. Methemoglobinemia – sleuthing for a new cause. *N Engl J Med* 1986; 314: 776.

Dotsch J, Demirakca S, Hamm R, et al. Extracorporeal circulation increases nitric oxide induced methemoglobinemia in vivo and in vitro. *Crit Care Med* 1997; 25: 1153.

Hall AH, Kulig KW, Rumack BH. Drug- and chemical-induced methemoglobinemia: clinical features and management. *Med Toxicol* 1986; 1: 253.

Mansouri A, Lurie AA. Concise review: methemoglobinemia. *Am J Hematol* 1993; 42: 7.

Mokhlesi B, Leikin JB, Murray P, et al. Adult toxicology in critical care: part II: specific poisonings. *Chest* 2003; 123: 897.

Schweitzer SA. Spurious pulse oximeter desaturation due to methemoglobinemia. *Anesth Intens Care* 1991; 19: 988.

Warren JB, Higenbottam T. Caution with the use of inhaled nitric oxide. *Lancet* 1996; 348: 629.

Methanol

Methanol (methyl alcohol, CH_3OH, 'wood alcohol') is the simplest aliphatic alcohol, with uses in industry and possibly as a fuel. It is occasionally consumed as a substitute for ethyl alcohol, since it causes mild inebriation. Most cases are sporadic, although mini-epidemics are seen following the consumption of contaminated illicit liquor.

> There is considerable variability in the potentially lethal dose.
> - Usually 70–100 mL is fatal.
> - Death has been reported after as little as 6 mL.
> - Total lack of any symptoms has been reported after as much as 500 mL.
>
> Blindness can occur following the ingestion of as little as 4 mL.
>
> The minimum toxic level of methanol is 50 mg/dL.

It is absorbed, distributed and metabolized similarly to ethyl alcohol. Although methanol itself is excreted in the lungs and kidneys, most is metabolized by alcohol dehydrogenase to formaldehyde (HCOH) and then by aldehyde dehydrogenase to formic acid (HCO.OH). These substances and especially the latter are toxic, since they are very reactive, being able to bind proteins and inhibit oxidative metabolism. The further metabolism of formate to carbon dioxide requires folic acid. The oxidation of methanol is 7-fold slower than that of ethanol, so that complete excretion takes several days.

Although methanol is not toxic in itself, toxicity from its metabolites occurs after a latent period of several hours. Typically, although methanol is rapidly absorbed, there is a lag period of 12–24 hr (range 1–72 hr) before toxicity is apparent. The longer delay is especially seen if there has been concomitant ethanol ingestion.

- **Visual impairment** is the most prominent clinical feature, and indeed it occurs to some degree in all cases. Eye damage includes hyperaemia of the optic disc, papilloedema (q.v.), retinal oedema, even fixed dilated pupils and often total permanent blindness.
- **Neurological signs** include headache, drowsiness, vertigo (q.v.), and if severe, fits and coma. There is CT evidence of cerebral oedema and patchy infarction, particularly of the putamen. Permanent motor dysfunction of a Parkinsonian type may be seen.
- **Gastrointestinal symptoms** are common and include nausea, vomiting, severe abdominal pain (possibly pancreatic in origin), actual pancreatitis (q.v.) and haemorrhagic gastritis.
- **Metabolic acidosis** is typically present and can be severe. It is partly due to lactic acidosis (q.v.) associated with circulatory impairment, but mostly it is due to the production of formic acid. The metabolic acidosis is usually uncompensated because of respiratory depression, manifest typically by slow 'fish-like' gasping. There is an increased anion gap (due to the presence of formate) and an increased osmolar gap.

> Treatment priorities are 2-fold, namely,
> - *correction of acidosis,*
> - *alteration of metabolism.*
>
> Other modalities such as gastric lavage (unless very early) and charcoal administration are not effective.

1. **Treatment of the acidosis is urgent.** The metabolic acidosis in this setting is relatively refractory to bicarbonate. Thus, dialysis is indicated if the acidosis is persistently severe and/or if the serum methanol concentration is >0.5 g/L. Dialysis increases the removal of methanol 3-fold. While haemodialysis is very effective, peritoneal dialysis or haemoperfusion are not.
2. **The metabolism of methanol should be decreased** (by ethanol) and **the metabolism of formate increased** (by folic acid).
    - The value of **ethanol** (ethyl alcohol) derives from its competition for the enzyme, alcohol dehydrogenase, so that the degradation of methanol and the accumulation of toxic metabolites are slowed. Ethanol has a greater affinity than methanol for this enzyme and saturates it at a concentration of 1–1.5 g/L (22–33 mmol/L). This blood alcohol level is 2–3 times the maximum legal level permitted for driving and causes marked intoxication in at least a third of subjects.

The required blood level of ethanol is achieved with a loading dose of 0.7 g/kg, equivalent to about 500 mL of 10% alcohol IV over 1 hr or 125 mL of 43% alcohol orally (i.e. 4 'standard drinks'). This level is maintained by about 10–15% of the loading dose given hrly until the osmolar gap becomes (and stays) normal.

In patients who are heavy drinkers or if dialysis is used, this maintenance requirement needs to be increased 2- to 3-fold. The administration of ethanol in this way may need to be modified in patients with pre-existing neurological, cardiac or liver damage. During dialysis, maintenance may also be achieved by adding 1 g/L of alcohol to the dialysate.

*The administration of **fomepizole** (4-methylpyrazole), an expensive agent shown to inhibit alcohol dehydrogenase and thus prevent the production of toxic metabolites, has been used successfully in ethylene glycol poisoning (q.v.), and it was subsequently shown to be similarly useful in methanol poisoning.*

- *The administration of **folate** (e.g. 50–100 mg IV 4 hrly) may be helpful in increasing the metabolism of formate.*

The prognosis of methanol poisoning is related to the degree of metabolic acidosis, with a 50% mortality in patients who have a serum bicarbonate <10 mmol/L.

Bibliography

Barceloux DG, Bond GR, Krenzelok EP, et al. American Academy of Chemical Toxicology practice guidelines on the treatment of methanol poisoning. *J Toxicol Clin Toxicol* 2002; 40: 415.

Brent J, McMartin K, Phillips S, et al. Fomepizole for the treatment of methanol poisoning. *N Engl J Med* 2001; 344: 424.

Burns MJ, Graudins A, Aaron CK, et al. Treatment of methanol with intravenous 4-methylpyrazole. *Ann Emerg Med* 1997; 30: 829.

Jacobsen D, McMartin KE. Methanol and ethylene glycol poisoning: mechanism of toxicity, clinical course, diagnosis and treatment. *Med Toxicol* 1986; 1: 309.

Jacobsen D, McMartin KE. Antidotes for methanol and ethylene glycol poisoning. *J Toxicol Clin Toxicol* 1997; 35: 127.

Kruse JA. Methanol poisoning. *Intens Care Med* 1992; 18: 391.

Kulig K, Duffy JP, Lenden CH, et al. Toxic effects of methanol, ethylene glycol and isopropyl alcohol. *Topics in Emerg Med* 1984; 6: 14.

McCoy HG, Cipolle RJ, Ehlers SM, et al. Severe methanol poisoning: application of a pharmacokinetic model for ethanol therapy and hemodialysis. *Am J Med* 1979; 67: 804.

Megarbane B, Borron, SW, Baud FJ. Current recommendations for treatment of severe toxic alcohol poisonings. *Intens Care Med* 2005; 31: 189.

Mokhlesi B, Leikin JB, Murray P, et al. Adult toxicology in critical care: part II: specific poisonings. *Chest* 2003; 123: 897.

Palatnick W, Redman LW, Sitar DS, et al. Methanol half-life during ethanol administration: implications for management of methanol poisoning. *Ann Emerg Med* 1995; 26: 202.

Zimmerman JL. Poisonings and overdoses in the intensive care unit: general and specific management issues. *Crit Care Med* 2003; 31: 2794.

Methylene blue

Methylene blue is a bright, blue-green organic dye of the phenothiazine family. It was discovered in 1876 and is manufactured from aniline material, most commonly from an organic diazo group. Methylene is a carbene, a class of reactive molecules with divalent carbon atoms (i.e. only two of four potential bonds are formed with other atoms). The generic formula of a carbene is R1-C-R2. Methylene is the most reactive of the carbenes and can attack almost every organic compound.

Methylene blue is used as a dye, a biological stain and a chemical indicator.

> Clinically, methylene blue is used as a reducing agent in the treatment of **methaemoglobinaemia** (q.v.). As a dramatic side-effect, it commonly causes blue-green urine.

Methaemoglobinaemia (q.v.) occurs when the iron in haemoglobin is in the oxidized or ferric form and thus (like carboxyhaemoglobin) cannot bind oxygen. This occurs following exposure to many agents, particularly nitrites and nitrates, but also drugs such as dapsone, glyceryl trinitrate, topical local anaesthetics, primaquine, sulphasalazine and vitamin K analogs.

Methylene blue is given as an IV infusion of 1000 mg in 100 mL from which 1–2 mg/kg is administered over 5 min. Extravasation should be avoided because of the risk of local tissue necrosis. Cyanosis is immediately reversed, though relapse may occur some hours later due to the release from tissues of more oxidizing agent, so that the further administration of methylene blue may be needed, usually the same dose hrly, up to a total dose of 7 mg/kg if needed. A continuous IV infusion of 1 mg/kg/hr may be used but is not generally recommended. If the concentration of methaemoglobin is very high (e.g. 60%), exchange transfusion with or without dialysis is recommended.

Methylene blue is not effective in glucose-6-phosphate dehydrogenase (G6PD) deficiency (q.v.), because it must first be reduced to leuko-methylene blue in red blood cells by NADPH, and NADPH requires G6PD for its formation.

The potential value of methylene blue in **septic shock** has been explored, on the basis that the free radical, nitric oxide (NO), may be an important mediator of the refractory vasodilatation in that condition and methylene blue is of value in nitrate toxicity. Haemodynamic improvement has been observed, though at the expense of hypoxaemia, so that survival data must be awaited before any clinically useful conclusion can be made about the utility of this innovative pharmacological approach.

For similar reasons, methylene blue has been proposed as an appropriate treatment for adverse reactions to **protamine**.

Cases of **serotonin syndrome** (q.v.) after methylene blue localization in parathyroidectomy were found to be associated with previous SSRI use, and it has since been confirmed that this interaction is because methylene blue has some monoamine oxidase inhibitor (MAOI) activity.

Bibliography
Ajayi T, Gropper MA. Methemoglobinemia. *Pulmonary Perspectives* 2001; 18(4): 4.
Blass N, Fung D. Dyed but not dead: methylene blue overdose. *Anesthesiology* 1976; 45: 458.
Gachot B, Bedos JP, Veber B, et al. Short-term effects of methylene blue on hemodynamics and gas exchange in humans with septic shock. *Intens Care Med* 1995; 21: 1027.
Hall HA, Kulig KW, Rumack BH. Drug and chemical-induced methaemoglobinaemia; clinical features and management. *Med Toxicol* 1986; 1: 253.
Kartha SS, Chacko CE, Bumpous JM, et al. Toxic metabolic encephalopathy after parathyroidectomy with methylene blue localization. *Otolaryngol Head Neck Surg* 2006; 135: 765.
Mokhlesi B, Leikin JB, Murray P, et al. Adult toxicology in critical care: part II: specific poisonings. *Chest* 2003; 123: 897.
Pasin L, Umbrello M, Greco T, et al. Methylene blue as a vasopressor: a meta-analysis of randomized trials. *Crit Care Resusc* 2013; 15: 42.
Viaro F, Dalio MB, Evora PRB. Catastrophic cardiovascular adverse reactions to protamine are nitric oxide/cyclic guanosine monophosphate dependent and endothelium mediated: should methylene blue be the treatment of choice? *Chest* 2002; 122: 1061.

Methysergide See
- Ergot.

Microangiopathic haemolysis

Microangiopathic haemolysis refers to the finding on peripheral blood film of fragmented and bizarre-shaped red blood cells with associated haemolysis.

The abnormal red blood cell morphology is caused by shear stress from intravascular obstruction, such as
- local fibrin deposits,
- arteriovenous shunt,
- angiosarcoma,
- intracardiac shunt,
- classically cardiac valve disease or mechanical prostheses, especially the older Starr–Edwards models.

Microangiopathic haemolysis may also be associated with
- vasculitis (q.v.),
- metastatic cancer,
- thrombotic thrombocytopenic purpura (q.v.),
- haemolytic–uraemic syndrome (q.v.),
- meningococcaemia (q.v.),
- rickettsial diseases (q.v.),
- cytomegalovirus infection (q.v.),
- human immunodeficiency virus infection (q.v.),
- bone marrow transplantation,
- abnormal haemodynamic jets,
- ciclosporin.

If it is severe, it may be associated with thrombocytopenia (q.v.) and even disseminated intravascular coagulation (q.v.).

When accompanied by thrombosis, it is referred to as **thrombotic microangiopathy** (TMA) (q.v.). This can be seen in pre-eclampsia (q.v.), severe antiphospholipid syndrome (q.v.) and heparin-induced thrombocytopenia (q.v.), as well as in the conditions listed above.

Treatment is primarily of that of the underlying disease. In TMA, **plasmapheresis** *(q.v.) is the treatment of choice.*

Bibliography
Darmon M, Azoulay E, Thiery G, et al. Time course of organ dysfunction in thrombotic microangiopathy patients receiving either plasma perfusion or plasma exchange. *Crit Care Med* 2006; 34: 2127.
Moake JL. Thrombotic microangiopathies. *N Engl J Med* 2002; 347: 589.
Nand S, Bansal VK, Kozeny G, et al. Red cell fragmentation syndrome with the use of subclavian hemodialysis catheters. *Arch Intern Med* 1985; 145: 1421.
Scully M, Cataland S, Coppo P, et al. Consensus on the standardization of terminology in thrombotic thrombocytopenic purpura and related thrombotic microangiopathies. *J Thromb Haemost* 2017; 15: 312.

Microbiome

The human **microbiome** refers to the constellation of microorganisms which live on or in the body, especially within the gastrointestinal tract. For convenience, the terms microbiome and microbiota are generally used interchangeably.

The **microbiota** are the large and diverse family of microbes familiarly called commensals or normal flora. They have been calculated to number about 4 trillion, which is similar to the number of human cells in the body, though they comprise only about 2% of the body's weight. Since these mostly anaerobic organisms can be hard to culture in the laboratory, they have been more accurately identified by cataloguing their genetic material, collectively called the **microbiome**. This large research program, the Human Microbiome Project, was launched by the NIH in 2007 and has only recently been completed. Even so, a complete census is not possible, given variations between societies, individuals, times, diets, climates and other circumstances. Nevertheless, a core set of some 160 or more species in 20 genera with over a million genes has been identified.

The microbiome is a complex ecosystem of mostly friendly microbes (mainly bacteria, but also viruses, fungi and archaea) which have accompanied humans in a symbiotic way during our evolution, with evidence of greater microbial diversity identified as humans went from hunter-gathering to farming to modern communities. These organisms are important for many aspects of human health, and their disturbance (referred to as **dysbioisis**) can lead to a variety of adverse health outcomes. They may also become directly pathogenic themselves when they sometimes get translocated to a vulnerable area (e.g. the bloodstream) during a disease process.

The gut microbiome is metabolically a very active microbial community, which is responsible for enhancing digestion (especially of fibre and complex carbohydrates), regulating local and systemic immune function, preserving the integrity of the gut barrier, producing vitamins B_{12} and K, clearing ingested toxins, providing resistance to pathogens, and influencing the brain signals related to dietary preference, hunger and satiety. The gut–brain axis involves neuronal, endocrine and immune pathways.

Systemically, gut dysbioisis contributes to many of modern life's chronic illnesses, including the metabolic syndrome (obesity, diabetes, hypertension and hyperlipiaemia), bowel disease, allergy, autoimmunity, cancer and cancer therapy response, bone and joint disease, and many neuropsychiatric conditions (such as mood, anxiety, depression, cognitive function, autism). The consequent immune state in dysbiosis is hyperactive, with an associated chronic inflammatory state. Dysbiosis can be caused by lifestyle changes (particularly a Western diet of highly processed foods), antibiotics, other drugs (e.g. proton pump inhibitors, PPIs), heavy alcohol intake and perhaps the modern obsession with germs (reflecting the 'hygiene hypothesis' of disease).

In ICU, dysbiosis can be an obvious consequence of critical illness due to associated factors including drugs (e.g. antibiotics, protein pump inhibitors, opioids), dietary changes, immobility, and the stress of trauma, surgery or severe illness. In turn, dysbiosis can contribute to multiorgan failure, immune dysfunction and infection.

Restoration of a healthy microbiome may be assisted by a diet richer in fibre, fish and antioxidants, by probiotics (q.v.) and prebiotics and by faecal microbiota transplantation (FMT) (q.v.). FMT has been shown to be effective in some severe gastrointestinal conditions, such as refractory *C. difficile* infection (q.v.). FMT has also been studied in other conditions of known or putative dysbiosis, including inflammatory bowel disease (q.v.), irritable bowel syndrome (q.v.), hepatic encephalopathy, metabolic syndrome and autism, although without convincing efficacy to date.

Bibliography
Almeida A, Mitchell AL, Boland M, et al. A new genomic blueprint of the human gut microbiota. *Nature* 2019; 568: 499.
Bassetti M, Bandera A, Gori A. Therapeutic potential of gut microbiota in the management of sepsis critical care. *Crit Care* 2020; 24: 105.
Dickson RP. The microbiome and critical illness. *Lancet Respir Med* 2016; 4: 59.
Fehily SR, Basnayake C, Wright EK, et al. The gut microbiota and gut disease. *Intern Med J* 2021; 51: 1594.
Gilbert JA, Blaser MJ, Caporaso JG, et al. Current understanding of the human microbiome. *Nat Med* 2018; 24: 392.
Gilbert JA, Quinn RA, Debelius J, et al. Microbiome-wide association studies link dynamic microbial consortia to disease. *Nature* 2016; 535: 94.
Ho KM, Kalgudi S, Corbett J-M, et al. Gut microbiota in surgical and critically ill patients. *Anaesth Intens Care* 2020; 48: 179.
Johnson AL, Backhed F. Role of gut microbiota in atherosclerosis. *Nat Rev Cardiol* 2017; 14: 79.
Relman DA. The human microbiome and the future practice of medicine. *JAMA* 2015; 314: 1127.
Rusting R, ed. *The Microbiome: Your Inner Ecosystem*. New York: Scientific American. 2020.
Sharma A, Das P, Buschmann M, et al. The future of microbiome-based therapeutics in clinical applications. *Clin Pharmacol Ther* 2020; 107: 123.
Soo WT, Bryant RV, Costello SP. Faecal microbiota transplantation: indications, evidence and safety. *Aust Prescriber* 2020 43: 36.

Microcirculation See
- Microvascular dysfunction.

Microscopic polyangiitis See
- Vasculitis,
- Wegener's granulomatosis.

Microvascular dysfunction

Microvascular (or **microcirculatory**) **dysfunction** occurs when there is generalized damage to the small vessels of the circulation, i.e. arterioles, capillaries and venules. Structurally, there is disruption of the **glycocalyx** (q.v.), with endothelial cell damage, microthrombosis and capillary leak, leading to interruption of the normal metabolic support provided at the cellular level to the body's organs and tissues.

Microvascular dysfunction is the end-result or final mechanism of action of a number of adverse clinical states, most typically shock. It may be identified by several techniques, including non-invasive methods such as examination of the sublingual microvasculature by sidestream dark field (SDF) imaging. However, it is most reliably confirmed by evidence of target damage, either systemic (e.g. raised lactate, acidosis) or local (e.g. renal or other organ dysfunction) in situations in which microvascular damage is a relevant mechanism based on known clinicopathological correlates. Tests for shed components of the glycocalyx in plasma or urine may become useful laboratory markers of microcirculatory dysfunction in future Intensive Care practice.

Treatment is primarily that of the underlying condition, but new modalities such as recombinant thrombomodulin (q.v.) may offer therapeutic potential.

The specific conditions in which microvascular dysfunction is a prominent pathogenetic mechanism include
- disseminated intravascular coagulation (q.v.),
- heparin-induced thrombocytopenia (q.v.),
- thrombotic microangiopathy (q.v.),
- vasculitis affecting primarily small vessels (see Vasculitis).

Other conditions in which microvascular dysfunction may also be relevant include
- cryoglobulinaemia (see Multiple myeloma),
- erythromelalgia (see Thrombocytosis/thrombocythaemia),
- livedo vasculitis (see Livedo, see Vasculitis),
- malaria (q.v.),
- petechiae (q.v.),
- pulmonary hypertension (q.v.),
- purpura (q.v.),
- scurvy (q.v.),
- sickle cell anaemia (see Haemoglobin disorders).

Bibliography
De Backer D, Hollenberg S, Boerma C, et al. How to evaluate the microcirculation: report of a round table conference. *Crit Care* 2007; 11: R101.
Den Uil CA, Klijn E, Lagrand WK, et al. The microcirculation in health and clinical disease. *Prog Cardiovasc Dis* 2008; 51: 161.
Edul VS, Enrico C, Lavoille B, et al. Quantitative assessment of the microcirculation in healthy volunteers and in patients with septic shock. *Crit Care Med* 2012; 40: 1443.

Middle East respiratory syndrome

Middle East respiratory syndrome (MERS) is the name which was given by international consensus in 2013 to a new infection that had appeared in the previous year. It was caused by a novel **coronavirus** (q.v.), referred to as MERS-CoV, with a reservoir thought to be originally in bats and later in camels, so that it is a zoonosis (q.v.). While it has primarily been seen in patients who have visited or lived in the Arabian Peninsula, cases have been reported in 20 countries around the world.

Clinically, it can present as a rapidly progressive respiratory illness, with fever, dyspnoea and multiorgan failure (q.v.). Gastrointestinal and neurological symptoms are common.

The case-fatality rate has averaged 35% in the 2000 patients reported to have been infected during the first three years. Specific diagnosis involves PCR testing of respiratory secretions.

There is no specific treatment, but infection control measures are important to prevent further transmission.
See also
- Coronavirus,
- Severe acute respiratory syndrome (SARS).

Bibliography
Alsolamy S. Middle East Respiratory Syndrome: knowledge to date. *Crit Care Med* 2015; 43:1283.
Arabi YM, Mandourah Y, Sindi AA, et al. Critically ill patients with the Middle East respiratory syndrome: a multicenter retrospective cohort study. *Crit Care Med* 2017; 45: 1683.

Mifepristone See
- Cushing's syndrome,
- Pregnancy – 1. Miscarriage.

Miller Fisher syndrome *See*
- Neuropathy – Guillain–Barré syndrome.

Mites

Mites are arachnids (see Arthropods) which are common human ectoparasites. Like lice, they can transmit significant disease under some circumstances.

Non-parasitic mites are also well recognized aetiological factors in other diseases, most notably in asthma due to allergy from house-dust mite.

See
- Parasitic infections,
- Pediculosis.

Mitochondrial diseases

Mitochondrial diseases comprise a heterogeneous group of over 350 genetic disorders due to mutations within the mitochondrial genome (mtDNA). They were first described in 1988. The prevalence of these disorders may be up to 1 in 250 of the population. As mitochondria are derived from ancient aerobic bacteria, they have their own genetic and transcription machinery.

Clearly, a mitochondrial mechanism of disease can cause severe consequences because of the central role of mitochondria in energy (ATP) production. It has been calculated that the body's energy needs of about 100 kCal/hr requires the production of about 65 kg of ATP per day. Thus, skeletal muscles are especially vulnerable, and also cardiac muscle, neurones and retinal cells, i.e. energy-hungry cells and organs.

A severe variant is infantile-onset mitochondrial DNA depletion syndrome, which gives rise to rapidly fatal neurological failure during early childhood. A much publicized case in 2017 at Great Ormond Street Hospital in London was the subject of international controversy regarding terminal care in critically ill children.

The nature of mitochondrial diseases is that they are typically inherited via the mother, but several other modes of inheritance (especially autosomal recessive) are commonly seen. Multiple versions of mtDNA can be present in individual cells (i.e. heteroplasmy), and the threshold for clinical disease can vary between tissues. The variable cell genotypes give rise to variable expressions of disease, and thus there is much clinical as well as genetic heterogeneity, such that mitochondrial diseases can mimic many other conditions.

Mutations can also be acquired from adverse exposure, usually to drugs (e.g. propofol) or the environment. Moreover, mtDNA mutations tend to accumulate with ageing, to which in turn they may contribute. Thus, about 70% of cases are seen in adults.

There are many specific syndromes among the mitochondrial diseases, but the most important manifestations from the Intensive Care perspective are as follows:
- respiratory failure
  - including failure to wean from the ventilator despite exclusion of the usually recognized causes,
- hypertrophic cardiomyopathy
  - often with conduction defects (see Cardiomyopathy),
- lactic acidosis
  - with an anion gap but no hypoxia, shock or sepsis (see Lactic acidosis),
- stroke in young people,
- muscle weakness
  - see Myopathy,
- central sleep apnoea
  - see Sleep apnoea,
- pseudo-obstruction of the colon (q.v.),
- exercise intolerance.

Investigations traditionally involved muscle biopsy, together with specialized metabolic and genetic testing, but high-throughput genetic sequencing is now available for primary assessment in specialized centres. However, the diagnosis can remain elusive, and some cases are referred to as 'possible' when mitochondrial disease is suspected but not proven.

International guidelines for diagnosis and treatment have been published by the Mitochondrial Medicine Society.

Treatment options are limited, non-specific and supportive. Carbohydrate feeding and careful aerobic exercise training are helpful. Clearly, precipitants should be avoided. Novel agents and gene therapies are being investigated.

Genetic prevention may include reproductive biology techniques such as the creation of 'three-person embryos', where the mother's nuclear DNA is transferred to a donor egg that has healthy mitochondria and has been emptied of its own nucleus, after which it is fertilized by the father's sperm.

Mitochondrial DNA (mtDNA) may be released from damaged or dying cells in conditions of severe systemic insult. Under these circumstances, the mtDNA is part of the release of 'damage-associated molecular patterns' (DAMPs), which may then amplify the innate component of the inflammatory process. The measurement of circulating mtDNA may become a biomarker (q.v.) representing a relevant pathogenetic mechanism in critical illness, for example in ARDS (q.v.).

Bibliography
Chinnery PF, Turnbull DM. Mitochondrial DNA and disease. *Lancet* 1999; 354: S117.

Clay AS, Behnia M, Brown KK. Mitochondrial disease: a pulmonary and critical-care perspective. *Chest* 2001; 120: 634.
DiMauro S, Bonilla E, Zeviani M, et al. Mitochondrial myopathies. *Ann Neurol* 1985; 17: 521.
Dziadek MA, Sue CM. Mitochondrial donation. *Med J Aust* 2022; 216: 118.
Howell N. Human mitochondrial diseases: answering questions and questioning answers. *Int Rev Cytol* 1999; 186: 49.
Hutchin T, Cortopassi G. A mitochondrial DNA clone is associated with increased risk of Alzheimer's disease. *Proc Natl Acad Sci* 1995; 92: 6892.
Neupert W. Mitochondrial gene expression: a playground of evolutionary thinking. *Annu Rev Biochem* 2016; 85: 65.
Ng YS, Bindoff LA, Gorman GS, et al. Mitochondrial disease in adults: recent advances and future promise. *Lancet Neurol* 2021; 20: 573.
Ng YS, Turnbull DM. Mitochondrial disease: genetics and management. *J Neurol* 2016; 263: 179.
Shoffner JM. Maternal inheritance and the evaluation of oxidative phosphorylation diseases. *Lancet* 1996; 348: 1283.
Sue CM. Mitocochondrial disease: recognizing more than just the tip of the iceberg. *Med J Aust* 2010; 193: 195.
Sue CM, Balasubramaniam S, Bratkovic D, et al. Patient care standards for primary mitochondrial disease in Australia. *Intern Med J* 2022; 52: 110.
Thorburn DR. Mitochondrial diseases: not so rare after all. *Intern Med J* 2004; 34: 3.
Zhang Q, Raoof M, Chen Y, et al. Circulating mitcochondrial DAMPs cause inflammatory responses to injury. *Nature* 2010; 464: 104.

Mixed connective tissue disease

Mixed connective tissue disease (MCTD) is a clinical syndrome with features common to a number of rheumatic diseases and not specific for any single diagnostic category. It may or may not be a separate disease entity, and some cases have been regarded as a variant of systemic lupus erythematosus (SLE) (q.v.), though without the typical serology.

Clinical features are very variable and are seen mainly in women, though with an age range from 5 to 80 yr. All patients have arthralgia (q.v.), most with an arthritis resembling rheumatoid arthritis but non-deforming, with swollen fingers as in scleroderma (q.v.) and with a rash as in SLE (q.v.). Asymptomatic pulmonary involvement is common, but renal involvement is uncommon. Proximal myopathy resembling polymyositis (q.v.) may be seen. Many patients have neuropsychiatric symptoms.

Investigations typically show leukopenia, raised ESR, increased IgG, positive rheumatoid factor and high titre of antinuclear antibodies. The most typical antibody is to an RNP antigen. Unlike in SLE, LE cells and DNA antibodies are not usually seen and complement levels are usually normal.

*Treatment is with **NSAIDs** in mild disease but otherwise with **corticosteroids**.*

Bibliography
Prockop DJ. Mutations in collagen genes as a cause of connective-tissue diseases. *N Engl J Med* 1992; 326: 540.

Monkey bites *See*
- Bites and stings.

Monosodium glutamate

Monosodium glutamate (MSG) is added to some foods to enhance flavour and in particular to impart a savoury (or umami) taste. The relevant taste buds are normally stimulated by the glutamines present in many natural foods, and added MSG takes advantage of this process.

However, an adverse reaction has been reported in some subjects after excess ingestion of MSG. Symptoms may appear within 20 min and last up to 2 hr. They may comprise a generalized burning feeling, with pressure sensations, sweating and occasionally headache, palpitations and even syncope.

The syndrome is self-limited and harmless, though it can produce consternation, particularly in cardiac patients.

See also
- Food poisoning.

Bibliography
Schaumburg HH, Byck R, Gerstl R, et al. Monosodium L-glutamate. *Science* 1969; 163: 826.

Mosquitoes

Mosquitoes are insects (see Arthropods), and they are important vectors for the transmission of disease to humans from another host. As a blood-sucking flying insect, it can feed on a diseased animal (including humans) and then transmit that disease when it subsequently feeds on a previously uninfected animal (including humans). Disease transmission is thus a two-bite process, though only the females bite. However, of the 35,000 species of mosquitoes identified worldwide, human disease can be carried by only a few species, including *Aedes*, *Anopheles* and *Culex*.

Of passing interest, it has been calculated that
- mosquitoes are the deadliest of all predators of humans, causing over 2 million deaths per year,
- there are over 10,000 mosquitoes for every human on Earth, with particularly high densities in some places in certain seasons, and
- a large and ravenous mosquito swarm covering a human could theoretically drain that person's entire blood volume in about 4 hr, though such a scenario would be extraordinarily rare in practice.

Since disease transmission is generally specific to particular mosquito species, individual diseases are endemic only in areas where that species is found. Exceptions arise of course in travellers from endemic areas. Occasionally, infected mosquitoes can hitchhike on a plane to a non-endemic area or a local mosquito of a suitable species may bite an infected person in a non-endemic area (see Malaria). As predicted, the epidemiology of mosquito-borne infections is being affected by climate change (q.v.), and mosquito control is a complex challenge.

The most important mosquito-borne infections worldwide are
- malaria (q.v.),
- dengue (q.v.),
- yellow fever (q.v.),
- Zika virus infections (q.v.),
- West Nile viral encephalitis (q.v.),
- filiariasis (see Eosinophilia and lung infiltration – Tropical pulmonary eosinophilia),
- chikungunya (q.v.).
See also
- Ross River virus infection.

Bibliography
Strickman D. Buzz kill. *Sci Am* 2018; 319: 59.
Winegard TC. *The Mosquito: A Human History of Our Deadliest Predator.* New York: Dutton (Penguin Random House). 2019.

Motor neuron disease

Motor neuron(e) disease (MND), also called **amyotrophic lateral sclerosis** (ALS, particularly in the USA), or occasionally Charcot's or Lou Gehrig's disease, is a condition of degeneration of the pyramidal motor neurones from the cortex as far as the anterior horn cells of the spinal cord. It thus affects both upper and lower motor neurones. It is a progressive, incurable and eventually fatal neurodegenerative disorder.

It was first described in 1869 by Charcot, the famous French neurologist, and one of its high-profile victims was Lou Gehrig, a baseball champion nicknamed 'Iron Horse', who died in 1941 only two years after being diagnosed with the condition.

It is an uncommon condition of unknown aetiology, most commonly affecting middle-aged men. Although typically a sporadic disorder, a number of genetic defects have been identified. As the condition displays considerable clinical as well as genetic heterogeneity, it may represent an end-result of a number of more primary causes. A number of different phenotypes have been described, including isolated bulbar palsy or predominant upper motor neurone or lower motor neurone involvement.

Clinical features comprise a slowly progressive weakness and wasting, associated with fasciculation, hyper-reflexia and muscle cramps.

The process can be distal or proximal early, but progressive proximal involvement then occurs.

There are no sensory or autonomic features and no eye involvement, but there may be bulbar or pseudobulbar palsy. There may also be associated behavioural disturbances or dementia, typically frontotemporal dementia (FTD).

The EMG shows denervation, but there are no specific diagnostic tests. Genetic testing may be offered.

The differential diagnosis includes
- cervical cord compression,
- polymyositis (q.v.),
- **multifocal motor neuropathy** (MMN). This more recently described condition is similar to motor neuron disease, but it is due to a slowly progressive nerve conduction defect of asymmetric distribution, particularly involving the upper limbs. It responds to immune globulin,
- **lower motor neuron disease** (LMND), an uncommon and more localized member of the overall family of disorders of motor neuron diseases.

*There is no effective treatment for motor neuron disease, though the glutamate inhibitor **riluzole** may increase survival by a few months in some patients. It is perhaps of interest that a large clinical trial of riluzole failed to show efficacy in Parkinson's disease. More recently, the antioxidant **ederavone** has been reported to slow the progress of disease in some patients.*

***Noninvasive ventilation** may prolong survival when respiratory failure ensues. A programme of symptomatic management of nutrition, mobility and emotional needs should be implemented by a multidisciplinary team to maintain quality of life.*

A number of new treatment modalities (including stem cell therapy and antisense oligonucleotide agents) are being investigated, but 'alternative' therapies should be avoided as they provide added cost and unfounded hope but no realistic benefit.

Survival is about 3 yr from diagnosis, though about 10% of patients survive for 10 yr or more. Indeed, the physicist Stephen Hawking lived with the condition for over 50 yr. Eventually, death usually occurs from respiratory failure.

Kennedy's disease is a late-onset variant affecting only men and with a slowly progressive course.

Bibliography
Bach JR. Amyotrophic lateral sclerosis: prolongation of life by noninvasive respiratory aids. *Chest* 2002; 122: 92.
Baumer D, Talbot K, Turner MR. Advances in motor neurone disease. *J R Soc Med* 2014; 107: 14.
Boman K, Meurman T. Prognosis of amyotrophic lateral sclerosis. *Acta Neurol Scand* 1967; 43: 489.
Brown RH, Al-Chalabi A. Amyotrophic lateral sclerosis. *N Engl J Med* 2017; 377: 162.
Dharmadasa T, Henderson RD, Talman PS, et al. Motor neurone disease: progress and challenges. *Med J Aust* 2017; 206: 357.
Greenland KJ, Zajac JD. Kennedy's disease: pathogenesis and clinical approaches. *Intern Med J* 2004; 34: 279.
Kiernan MC. Motor neurone disease: a Pandora's box. *Med J Aust* 2003; 178: 311.
Kiernan MC. Riluzole: a glimmer of hope in the treatment of motor neurone disease. *Med J Aust* 2005; 182: 319.
Kiernan MC, ed. *Motor Neurone Disease.* Sydney: MJA Books. 2007.
Kiernan MC, Vucic S, Cheah BC, et al. Amyotrophic lateral sclerosis. *Lancet* 2011; 377: 942.
Pestronk A. Motor neuropathies, motor neuron disorders, and antiglycolipid antibodies. *Muscle Nerve* 1991; 14: 927.
Petrucelli L, Gitler AD. Unlocking the mystery of ALS. *Sci Am* 2017; 316: 40.
Simmons Z. Management strategies for patients with amyotrophic lateral sclerosis from diagnosis to death. *Neurologist* 2005; 11: 257.
Simon NG, Huynh W, Vucic S, et al. Motor neuron disease: current management and future prospects. *Intern Med J* 2015; 45: 1005.
The ALS/Riluzole Study Group. A controlled trial of riluzole in amyotrophic lateral sclerosis. *N Engl J Med* 1994; 330: 585.

Mouth diseases

Mouth diseases include
- gingivitis,
- glossitis,
- stomatitis,
- parotitis.

1. Gingivitis

Gingivitis (disease of the gums) is commonly of dental origin. The organisms involved are usually anaerobic upper respiratory tract flora, typically peptostreptococci, fusobacteria and bacteroides. In hospital patients, Gram-negative bacilli and staphylococci may also be involved. Uncommon causes include viruses or actinomyces.

Gingivitis may also be associated with
- stomatitis (see below),
- sinusitis,
- Vincent's angina
  - i.e. trench mouth, an erosive tonsillitis with associated local soft tissue invasion,
- Ludwig's angina
  - i.e. sublingual cellulitis,
- peritonsillar abscess
  - sometimes called quinsy,
- haemorrhage
  - seen in bleeding disorders or scurvy,
- hyperplasia
  - classically occurring with phenytoin or more recently with ciclosporin and calcium channel blockers (of the dihydropyridine group, such as nifedipine, amlodipine, felodipine), and generally slowly reversible following cessation of the drug.

> Persistent gingivitis should be remembered as a risk factor for subacute bacterial endocarditis (q.v.).

2. Glossitis

Glossitis (disease of the tongue) occurs in a number of forms.

A. Atrophic glossitis

This is seen in vitamin deficiency, particularly of niacin, riboflavin, B_{12} or folate.

It is commonly associated with
- angular cheilitis, namely, fissuring at the corners of the mouth

This is also and more commonly associated with dribbling of saliva. It may become secondarily infected.
- cheilosis, namely, vertical fissuring of the lips

This also is commonly due to other causes, such as local irritation, solar damage and drugs, such as isotretinoin.

B. Black hairy tongue

This is a benign hyperplasia of the filiform papillae of the tongue.

It is associated with bacterial overgrowth of chromogenic bacteria due to prolonged antibiotic therapy. It may also be caused by tobacco and certain foods.

It is offensive both in appearance and odour.

C. **Xerostomia**

This refers to a dry mouth due to decreased saliva.

This is seen typically in Sjogren's syndrome (q.v.), but it may also be seen following irradiation for head and neck cancer, in chronic sialadenitis, and with some drugs, such as anticholinergics, antidepressants and antihistamines.

D. **Benign migratory glossitis ('geographic tongue')**

This is caused by an irregular loss of papillae of the tongue and is manifest as raised white areas containing red patches.

E. **Strawberry tongue**

This is seen in scarlet fever (q.v.).

F. **Leukoplakia**

This is a pre-malignant condition, manifest as white patches on the tongue.

It is traditionally caused by tobacco, but it is also seen in AIDS (q.v.).

G. **Macroglossia**

This refers to enlargement of the tongue and is seen in acromegaly (q.v.), amyloidosis (q.v.), lymphangioma and myxoedema (q.v.).

H. **Miscellaneous disorders of the tongue include**
- candidiasis due to inhaled corticosteroids,
- herpetic and other ulceration,
- malignancy,
- XII nerve paralysis (see Neuropathy).

3. **Stomatitis**

Although stomatitis (disease of the mouth generally) may be due to local disease, it can more importantly be a manifestation of systemic disease, particularly a generalized dermatosis. In this setting, the mucous membrane is clearly different from skin, in that it has no stratum corneum or appendages and has salivary glands instead of sweat glands.

Important forms of stomatitis associated with systemic disease of this type include
- erythema multiforme and Stevens-Johnson syndrome (q.v.),
- pemphigus (q.v.),
- generalized candidiasis,
- graft-versus-host disease (q.v.),
- Reiter's syndrome (q.v.),
- systemic lupus erythematosus (SLE) (q.v.).
  Other forms of stomatitis include
- aphthous ulceration,
- Behcet's syndrome (q.v.),
- hereditary haemorrhagic telangiectasia (Osler–Weber–Rendu syndrome) (q.v.),
- herpesvirus infection (q.v.)
  - usually HSV type 1, but sometimes HSV type 2 in sexually active young adults,
- other viruses
  - coxsachie virus, which gives herpangina, and VZV and EBV, which have additional clinical features (see Varicella-zoster, see Epstein–Barr virus),
- drugs (e.g. bleomycin – q.v.) and toxins (e.g. mercury – q.v.),
- **Peutz–Jeghers** syndrome

This is an autosomal dominant condition manifest by macules in and around the mouth and often associated with gastrointestinal polyps. These lesions are hamartomas, but they can bleed or obstruct. There may be an associated ovarian tumour.

4. **Parotitis**

Parotitis (inflammation of the parotid gland) is the prominent clinical feature of mumps.

In hospital patients, it is more commonly bacterial (especially staphylococcal), but it may be caused by other infections, e.g. parainfluenza virus.

It may also be seen in
- sarcoidosis (q.v.),
- tumour,
- Sjogren's syndrome (q.v.),
- cat-scratch disease (q.v.),
- anorexia nervosa (q.v.),
- drug usage with anticholinergic agents (q.v.).

Bibliography

Moreland LW, Corey J, McKenzie R. Ludwig's angina. *Arch Intern Med* 1988; 148: 463.

Pruett TL, Simmons RL. Nosocomial gram-negative bacillary parotitis. *JAMA* 1984; 251: 252.

Utsunomiya J, Gocho H, Miyanaga T, et al. Peutz-Jeghers syndrome: its natural course and management. *Johns Hopkins Med J* 1975; 136: 71.

Multidisciplinary topics

Many topics of interest and relevance to Intensive Care practice are necessarily multidisciplinary, in that they cannot be classified by traditional organ/system headings or else they overlap a number of these headings. Examples discussed in this book include
- Abdominal compartment syndrome,
- Arachnids,
- Arthropods,
- Autoinflammatory disease,
- Bathing,
- Bed rest,

- Behcet's syndrome,
- Biomarkers,
- Bradykinin,
- Bromhidrosis,
- Chronic fatigue syndrome,
- Circadian rhythm,
- Conjunctivitis,
- Crustaceans,
- Eating disorders,
- Echinacea,
- Factitious disorders,
- Familial Mediterranean fever,
- Fever,
- Fever of unknown origin,
- Fleas,
- Frailty,
- Gas in soft tissues,
- Genomics,
- Germ warfare,
- Glycocalyx,
- Graft-versus-host disease,
- Haemolacria,
- Haemolytic–uraemic syndromes,
- Haemophagocytic lymphohistiocytosis (HLH),
- Helminths,
- Henoch-Schonlein purpura,
- Hereditary haemorrhagic telangiectasia,
- Histiocytosis,
- Hot flushes,
- Hyperbaric oxygen,
- Hyperdynamic state,
- Hyperhidrosis,
- Hypersplenism,
- Hyperthermia,
- Hyperviscosity,
- Hyposplenism,
- Hypothermia,
- ICU-acquired weakness,
- Immotile cilia syndrome,
- Inflammatory myeloid neoplasia,
- Insects,
- Intensive Care Unit–acquired weakness,
- Intra-abdominal hypertension,
- Isolation,
- Kartagener's syndrome,
- Lactic acidosis,
- Langerhans cell histiocytosis,
- Lice,
- Mastocytosis,
- Melatonin,
- Microbiome,
- Mites,
- Mitochondrial diseases,
- Mosquitoes,
- Multiorgan failure,
- Munchausen syndrome,
- Myalgic encephalomyelitis,
- PADIS,
- Periodic fever,
- Persistent critical illness,
- Pleiotropic effects,
- Post–Intensive Care syndrome,
- Priapism,
- Primary ciliary dyskinesia,
- Protozoa,
- Pyrexia,
- Quarantine,
- Radiation injury,
- Retroperitoneal fibrosis,
- Reye's syndrome,
- Sarcoidosis,
- Serositis,
- Sicca syndrome,
- Situs inversus,
- Sjogren's syndrome,
- Sleep,
- Splenomegaly,
- Sturge–Weber syndrome,
- Sweating,
- Thermoregulation,
- Ticks,
- Tuberous sclerosis,
- Uveoparotid fever,
- Vaping,
- X-linked disorders.

Multifocal motor neuropathy *See*

- Motor neuron disease.

Multiorgan failure

Multiorgan failure (MOF, multiple organ dysfunction syndrome, MODS) is a frequent and major problem in Intensive Care patients. It most commonly complicates sepsis, when it is part of the continuum of the systemic inflammatory response syndrome (SIRS) → sepsis → severe sepsis (with MOF) → septic shock (with MOF). It may also complicate any form of serious circulatory, inflammatory or toxic insult, especially if the insult is prolonged.

Multiorgan dysfunction or failure is best recognized as involvement of some or all of the six main target organs/systems, namely,

- lungs, with acute respiratory distress syndrome (q.v.),
- kidneys, with acute renal failure,

- circulation, with shock,
- liver,
- central nervous system,
- blood, with disseminated intravascular coagulation (q.v.).

However, all of the body's other organs and systems are also affected by such systemic insults, though identification of their dysfunction may be less easy to identify, e.g. gastrointestinal failure. The consequences of systemic insults vary greatly between individuals, presumably because of host factors, underlying diseases and concomitant treatment.

The cause of the systemic insult is usually apparent when it is an infection, other inflammatory process (e.g. pancreatitis) or toxicity (e.g. hypothermia).

In Intensive Care practice, if the cause of multiorgan failure is not readily apparent, there are a number of uncommon causes which should be considered. These include
- catastrophic **antiphospholipid syndrome** (q.v.),
- **Behcet's syndrome** (q.v.),
- **haemophagocytic syndrome** (q.v.),
- **ovarian hyperstimulation syndrome** (q.v.),
- **sickle cell crisis** (see Haemoglobin disorders – 2. Sickle cell anaemia),
- **thyroid storm** (see Hyperthyroidism),
- **toxic shock syndrome** (q.v.),
- unusual **poisoning** (e.g. Colchicine – q.v., Ethylene glycol – q.v., Mushrooms – q.v.),
- **Waterhouse–Friderichsen syndrome** (q.v.).

Bibliography
Marshall JC, Deutschman CS. The multiple organ dysfunction syndrome: syndrome, metaphor, and unsolved clinical challenge. *Crit Care Med* 2021; 49: 1402.

Multiple endocrine neoplasia

The **multiple endocrine neoplasia** (MEN) (or multiple endocrine adenomatosis, MEA) syndromes refer to several patterns of multiple endocrine abnormalities inherited as autosomal dominant conditions. These heterogeneous disorders comprise four phenotypic patterns (MEN1–4). They are relatively rare, with an overall prevalence of about 1 in 20–25,000 of the population.

MEN type I (MEN1) comprises the triad of anterior pituitary, parathyroid and pancreatic islet cell adenomas (or hyperplasia). Pancreatic tumours may sometimes be malignant, although typically they are **neuroendocrine tumours** (NETs), which secrete gastrin, insulin, glucagon, vasoactive intestinal peptide or somatostatin. Carcinoid tumours (q.v.) and rarely other tumours (e.g. meningioma or connective tissue tumour) may also occur.

Although typically a triad, MEN1 may sometimes present as one of these tumours alone. However, in any single tumour presentation in general there is less than a 10% chance of that patient in fact having MEN1. Hyperparathyroidism (q.v.) is the commonest individual clinical manifestation.

The mutation is of the tumour suppressor gene, *MEN1*, located on the long arm of chromosome 11. It was identified in 1988 and cloned in 1997. Its penetrance is high, with virtually all carriers of the mutation developing clinical disease before the age of 40 years. However, over 200 different mutations of this large gene have been described, so that genetic screening is complicated.

*Effective management requires early diagnosis of the component tumours and their surgical **resection**, especially for parathyroid and pancreatic tumours.*

MEN type II (MEN2) comprises
- thyroid medullary carcinoma
  - a rare type of thyroid cancer, which arises in the parafollicular cells and which secretes thyrocalcitonin (see Calcitonin),
- phaeochromocytoma (q.v.)
  - which is often bilateral and may be malignant,
- parathyroid hyperplasia.

MEN2 is subdivided into two groups, namely,
1. MEN2A (referred to recently as **MEN2**), which comprises thyroid medullary cancer, plus phaeochromocytoma in half the cases, plus hyperparathyroidism in 15% of cases,
2. MEN2B (referred to recently as **MEN3**), which comprises thyroid medullary cancer (typically early and aggressive) and phaeochromocytoma, plus other unusual bodily features, including mucosal neuromas and gastrointestinal ganglioneuromatosis.

The mutation is of the *RET* proto-oncogene. Its penetrance is moderate, with about half the carriers of the mutation developing clinical disease before the age of 60 years. Genetic screening is relatively straightforward, since the responsible mutations are tightly clustered.

*Treatment of identified carriers is with prophylactic **thyroidectomy** in childhood or otherwise as soon as possible.*

MEN type IV (MEN4) is a rare and recently described variant, with phenotypic features of MEN1 together with adrenal and ovarian tumours.

Bibliography

Brandi ML. Multiple endocrine neoplasia type 1: general features and new insights into etiology. *J Endocrinol Invest* 1991; 14: 61.

Burgess JR. Multiple endocrine neoplasia type 1: current concepts in diagnosis and management. *Med J Aust* 1999; 170: 605.

Chandrasekharappa SC, Guru SC, Manickam P, et al. Positional cloning of the gene for multiple endocrine neoplasia-type 1. *Science* 1997; 276: 404.

Eng C. RET proto-oncogene in the development of human cancer. *J Clin Oncol* 1999; 17: 380.

Learoyd DL, Delbridge LW, Robinson BG. Multiple endocrine neoplasia. *Aust NZ J Med* 2000; 30: 675.

Mallette LE. The parathyroid polyhormones: new concepts in the spectrum of peptide hormone action. *Endocr Rev* 1991; 12: 110.

McDonnell JE, Gild ML, Clifton-Bligh RJ, et al. Multiple endocrine neoplasia: an update. *Intern Med J* 2019; 49: 954.

Robinson BG. Multiple endocrine neoplasia – who should be screened? *Med J Aust* 1994; 160: 739.

Schimke RN. Multiple endocrine neoplasia: how many syndromes? *Am J Med Genet* 1990; 37: 375.

Multiple myeloma

Multiple myeloma (plasma cell myeloma) is a relatively slowly growing malignant tumour arising in a clone of plasma cells. Since normal plasma cells synthesize immunoglobulins as matched heavy and light chains, malignant plasma cells commonly secrete an abnormal monoclonal immunoglobulin (paraprotein) with a single heavy chain class and a single light chain type giving the classical M protein spike on serum electrophoresis. Commonly, there are excess kappa or lambda light chains (which appear in the urine as Bence Jones proteins – q.v.). Sometimes, there can be no heavy chains at all (with resultant hypogammaglobulinaemia associated with the Bence Jones proteinaemia) or excess heavy chains (either gamma, alpha or mu, giving one of the heavy chain diseases) or neither chain at all (giving panhypogammaglobulinaemia).

An IgG or IgA paraprotein is the result of a clonal disorder of plasma cells (i.e. multiple myeloma), whereas an IgM paraprotein is generally the result of a lymphoproliferative disorder (e.g. Waldenstrom's macroglobulinaemia – see below). Sequencing of the myeloma genome has shown a range of molecular abnormalities rather than any specific defects, and the abnormal clones typically have multiple subclones with varying rates of progression and response to therapy.

Normal plasma cell function is depressed in patients with multiple myeloma, resulting in immunocompromise. The bone marrow is infiltrated with resultant pancytopenia, the bone itself can be eroded by plasmacytomas, and extramedullary infiltration is common in liver, spleen, lymph nodes, gut, subcutaneous tissues, pleural cavity, nasopharynx and nasal sinuses.

A variety of other clinical problems may be produced, including

- **hypercalcaemia** (q.v.),
- **renal disease**, since the abnormal immunoglobulin is typically deposited in the kidney,
- **bone disease**, affecting particularly the axial skeleton and due to increased osteoclastic activity and decreased osteoblastic activity, which has been mediated by plasma cells,
- **hyperviscosity**, especially due to IgA and IgM variants. The abnormal protein aggregates red blood cells, and headache, retinopathy and cardiac failure may result. Sometimes, the abnormal proteins are precipitated by cold (i.e. these are cryoglobulins – see below) and Raynaud's phenomenon (q.v.) results.
- **bleeding** may result from interference with platelets and coagulation factors, particularly factors I, II and VIII.

The diagnosis is made biochemically, histologically and radiologically.

- Biochemically, there is typically Bence Jones protein in the urine and/or a monoclonal spike on serum electrophoresis. No M protein is seen in the serum in 20% of patients, but most of these still have Bence Jones proteins in the urine. An identified paraprotein is then classified by immunofixation as IgG (75% of cases), IgA (25%) or IgM (rare in myeloma and indicative of a lymphoproliferative disorder – see Waldenstrom's macroglobulinaemia below).
- Histologically, typical changes are seen in bone marrow or tissue biopsy material.
- Radiologically, lytic bone lesions may be seen.
- The International Staging System has been reported to be the most useful of the several available staging classifications, and its latest revision provides the basis for current risk stratification.

Treatment is with **radiotherapy** *for local lesions and* **cytotoxic therapy** *for systemic disease. Cytotoxic regimens have been based on* **melphalan** *and* **corticosteroids**, *with or without the additional immunomodulatory agents,* **thalidomide** *(or its analog,* **lenalidomide**, *or more recently,* **pomalidomide**). *Several aggressive and complex cytotoxic regimens have improved the response rate, particularly in patients with poor prognostic factors (including chromosomal abnormalities or increased plasma cell* labelling). In relapsed or refractory cases, a response has been reported to treatment with the new proteasome inhibitor, **bortezomib** (or more recently with **carfilzomib**). The further addition of **daratumumab**, a monoclonal antibody to CD38, has been shown in early trials to improve the response rate greatly in these difficult cases.

- Either autologous or allogeneic **bone marrow transplantation** can be effective, but there have been significant problems with both techniques.
- Hyperviscosity is treated with **plasmapheresis** (q.v.).
- Hypercalcaemia is treated on its usual merits (q.v.).
- Skeletal problems, particularly bone pain, may be relieved by the second-generation bisphosphonate, **pamidronate** (APD) (see Hypercalcaemia). *Osteonecrosis of the jaw* (ONJ) is an occasional complication of this therapy, especially if used for more than 2 yr (see Hypercalcaemia).
- Infectious complications may require **immunoglobulin replacement**.
- Dialysis may be indicated for renal failure, but plasmapheresis (q.v.) has been found to be ineffective for this complication.

Multiple myeloma is currently incurable in most cases. If a response is achieved, there is a mean survival of 4 years in good health. Occasionally, very long survival is seen, particularly in cases of indolent or smouldering myeloma. The sophisticated cytological analysis of minimal residual disease (MRD) can be used as a marker of prognosis. In general, the prognosis is worse in the presence of anaemia (q.v.), hypercalcaemia (q.v.), multiple osteolytic bone lesions or paraproteins in large amounts.

There are several variants of multiple myeloma.

1. **Solitary plasmacytoma** may be seen, especially of bone.
2. **Waldenstrom's macroglobulinaemia** is an indolent variant due to an IgM clone of B cells. It is a form of low-grade non-Hodgkin's lymphoma, i.e. a lymphoproliferative disorder.
3. **Heavy chain disease**, with gamma, alpha or mu fragments, tends to behave as a chronic haematological malignancy.
4. **Monoclonal gammopathy of uncertain significance** (MGUS or benign monoclonal gammopathy) may be seen in older patients. It is typically an incidental finding, and the paraprotein levels are much lower than in myeloma. It generally runs a benign and asymptomatic course. However, classical myeloma develops eventually in about 20% of patients within about 10 years if the gammopathy is IgG or IgA, and other lymphoproliferative disorders develop in about 50% of patients if the gammopathy is IgM.
5. **Cryoglobulinaemia** occurs when the abnormal plasma proteins are precipitated by cold.
   There are three types of cryoglobulinaemia.
   - Type 1 is due to a monoclonal immunoglobulin – IgM, IgG, IgA or BJ in descending order of frequency.
   - Type 2 is a mixed condition.
   - Type 3 is associated with polyclonal immunoglobulins.

   Types 2 and 3 probably represent immune complex diseases (q.v.), in which the immune complexes are precipitated by cold. Most cryoglobulins in this setting have rheumatoid factor activity and can produce a large variety of effects, including inflammation, platelet aggregation, clotting factor consumption, microvascular obstruction, hyperviscosity, bleeding, vascular purpura (q.v.), Raynaud's phenomenon (q.v.), renal dysfunction and neurological changes. Commonly, there is an underlying autoimmune disease or chronic hepatitis (HBV or even more frequently HCV infection).

   *Treatment with **plasmapheresis** (q.v.) is effective, but corticosteroids and cytotoxics are not helpful.*

6. **Amyloidosis** comprises a number of disorders characterized by the accumulation in tissues of protein in fibrillar form (i.e. amyloid). The normally soluble protein is laid down in beta-pleated sheets, so that it is now insoluble, resistant to proteolysis and phagocytosis, it typically stains with Congo red, and it is birefringent under polarizing light. Commonly, the proteins deposit with other extracellular components, such as glycosaminoglycans.

   Several different proteins (currently about 25 in total number) can be modified in this way and different secondary structures result, giving distinct pathophysiological and clinical manifestations for each. Definitive diagnosis of amyloidosis requires biopsy of an affected site.

   A. **Primary amyloidosis** (AL amyloid) is produced by light chain Ig fragments (molecular weight 5–25 kDa) similar to Bence Jones proteins. Deposits occur especially in muscle (e.g. tongue and heart), skin (especially of the upper part of the body), liver, spleen, gut, kidneys (with nephrotic syndrome), joints and peripheral nerves.

   The clinical manifestations are related to the type of local involvement. Bleeding occasionally occurs because of either the trapping of factor X or from increased fibrinolysis (q.v.). Median survival has been reported to be 18 months.

   *No therapy is consistently effective, but **corticosteroids** and **melphalan** have been reported to be helpful in some patients and more so than other therapies such as colchicine. Bone marrow transplantation has been successful in selected patients.*

B. **Secondary amyloidosis** (AA amyloid) is a reactive process to chronic inflammation, especially pyogenic infections, tuberculosis (q.v.) and rheumatoid arthritis. It may also occur in familial Mediterranean fever (q.v.). The protein, amyloid A (AA, molecular weight of 8.5 kDa) is derived from a normal acute phase reactant in plasma, called serum amyloid A (SAA, molecular weight 84–200 kDa and cleaved by monocytes). Since deposits of amyloid occur only in some patients with chronic inflammation, different patterns of monocyte degradation of SAA may be responsible for the individual variation.

> Deposits are seen mostly in liver, spleen, kidneys and adrenals, and the main clinical feature is the nephrotic syndrome.
> *Treatment is with* **colchicine**, *which blocks SAA secretion.*

C. **Miscellaneous amyloidosis** occurs in several forms, including
- **dialysis-related amyloid** (AB_2M amyloid) due to the accumulation of $beta_2$-microglobulin (q.v.) in soft tissues,
- **hereditary amyloid**, due to mutations affecting a number of different proteins, e.g. fibrinogen, transthyretin, lysozyme,
- **senile amyloid** (ATTR amyloid), with chiefly cardiac involvement,
- **local amyloid**, where the amyloid deposit (usually AL amyloid) occurs at the site of production, in contrast to most amyloidoses which are systemic.

Bibliography

Almond JB, Cohen GM. The proteasome: a novel target for cancer chemotherapy. *Leukemia* 2002; 16: 433.

Attal M, Harousseau J-L, Stoppa A-M, et al. A prospective, randomized trial of autologous bone marrow transplantation and chemotherapy in multiple myeloma. *N Engl J Med* 1996; 335: 91.

Bataille R. Management of myeloma with bisphosphonates. *N Engl J Med* 1996; 334: 529.

Bjorkstrand B, Ljungman P, Svensson H, et al. Allogeneic bone marrow transplantation versus autologous stem cell transplantation in multiple myeloma. *Blood* 1996; 88: 4711.

Brouet JC, Clouvel JP, Danon F, et al. Biologic and clinical significance of cryoglobulins. *Am J Med* 1974; 57: 775.

Clark WF, Stewart AK, Rock GA, et al. Plasma exchange when myeloma presents as acute renal failure: a randomized, controlled trial. *Ann Intern Med* 2005; 143: 777.

Dauel TF, Dauth J, Mellstedt H, et al. Waldenstrom's macroglobulinaemia. *Lancet* 1985; 2: 311.

Dowd PM. Cold-related disorders. *Prog Dermatol* 1987; 21: 1.

Frankel AH, Singer DRJ, Winearls CG, et al. Type II essential mixed cryoglobulinemia: presentation, treatment and outcome in 13 patients. *Q J Med* 1992; 82: 101.

Gertz MA, Kyle RA, Greipp PR. Response rates and survival in primary systemic amyloidosis. *Blood* 1991; 77: 257.

Gertz MA, Kyle RA. Secondary systemic amyloidosis. *Medicine* 1991; 70: 246.

Grateau G, Kyle RA, Skinner M, eds. *Amyloid and Amyloidosis*. Boca Baton: CRC Press. 2004.

Greipp PR. Advances in the diagnosis and management of myeloma. *Semin Hematol* 1992; 29: 24.

Hamblin TJ. The kidney in myeloma. *BMJ* 1986; 292: 2.

Joshua DE. Multiple myeloma: the present and the future. *Med J Aust* 2005; 183: 344.

Joshua DE, Bryant C, Dix C, et al. Biology and therapy of multiple myeloma. *Med J Aust* 2019; 210: 375.

Joshua DE, Gibson J. Multiple myeloma – evolving concepts of biology and treatment. *Aust NZ J Med* 2000; 30: 311.

Kintzer JS, Rosenow EC, Kyle RA. Thoracic and pulmonary abnormalities in multiple myeloma. *Arch Intern Med* 1978; 138: 727.

Kwaan HC, ed. The hyperviscosity syndromes. *Semin Thromb Hemost* 2003; 29: 433.

Kyle RA. Amyloidosis: review of 236 cases. *Medicine* 1975; 54: 271.

Kyle RA. 'Benign' monoclonal gammopathy. *Mayo Clin Proc* 1993; 68: 26.

Kyle RA, Gertz MA, Greipp PR, et al. A trial of three regimens for primary amyloidosis. *N Engl J Med* 1997; 336: 1202.

Kyle RA, Rajkumar SV. Multiple myeloma. *N Engl J Med* 2004; 351: 1860.

Kyle RA, Remstein ED, Therneau TM, et al. Clinical course and prognosis of smouldering (asymptomatic) multiple myeloma. *N Engl J Med* 2007; 356: 2582.

Kyle RA, Therneau TM, Rajkumar SV, et al. Prevalence of monoclonal gammopathy of undetermined significance. *N Engl J Med* 2006; 354: 1362.

McGrath MA, Penny R. Paraproteinemia: blood hyperviscosity and clinical manifestations. *J Clin Invest* 1976; 58: 1155.

Mollee P, Renaut P, Gottlieb D, et al. How to diagnose amyloidosis. *Intern Med J* 2014; 44: 7.

Norden CW. Infections in patients with multiple myeloma. *Arch Intern Med* 1980; 140:1150.

Pepys MB. Amyloidosis: some recent developments. *Q J Med* 1988; 67: 283.

Picken MM, Herrera GA, Dogan A, eds. *Amyloid and Related Disorders*. 2nd edition. New York: Springer. 2015.

Richardson P, Hideshima T, Anderson KC. An update of novel therapeutic approaches for multiple myeloma. *Curr Treat Options Oncol* 2004; 5: 227.

Smith A, Wisloff F, Samson D. Guidelines on the diagnosis and management of multiple myeloma 2005. *Br J Haematol* 2006; 132: 410.

Solomon A, Weiss DT, Kattine AA. Nephrotoxic potential of Bence Jones proteins. *N Engl J Med* 1991; 324: 1845.

Talaulikar D, Tam, CS, Joshua D, et al. Treatment of patients with Waldenstrom macroglobulinaemia: clinical practice guidelines from the Myeloma Foundation of Australia Medical and Scientific Advisory Group. *Intern Med J* 2017; 47: 35.

Multiple organ dysfunction/failure See

- Multiorgan failure.

Multiple sclerosis

Multiple sclerosis (MS) is a condition of chronic patchy immune-mediated demyelination which occurs in the white matter in zones called plaques. These are of varying site and size within the CNS. The disease mostly occurs in young adults, especially women, who are predisposed because of certain genetic haplotypes (e.g. the DR2 haplotype of the human leukocyte antigen complex), but these influences are only partly characterized. Its overall prevalence is about 50 per 100,000 of the population.

Its aetiology is unknown, but it includes genetic, environmental and immunological factors.

- Genetically, there is a substantially increased familial risk, and more than 100 gene loci have been so far associated with MS susceptibility.
- Environmentally, an excess of cases is seen with smoking, prior Epstein–Barr virus infection, temperate zones, urban areas and possibly affluence.
- Immunologically, there may be an autoimmune response to viral infection, possibly via molecular mimicry with a homologous sequence within the myelin protein. For example, human herpesvirus type 6, responsible for exanthema subitum (roseola infantum) in children, has been causally linked with cases of multiple sclerosis.

  However, the considerable variation in histological types of lesions suggests that its pathogenesis may be heterogeneous. The animal model of experimental autoimmune encephalomyelitis has assisted understanding of multiple sclerosis.

> The clinical features of multiple sclerosis are characterized by fluctuating neurological signs, attributable to multiple sites of involvement, i.e. the lesions are disseminated in both space and time.
>
> Both its initial onset and subsequent relapses typically occur over a few days. Subsequently, there is stable dysfunction for a few weeks, followed by gradual but usually partial recovery.

Initial symptoms particularly comprise
- **motor changes**
  - weakness, clumsiness, stiffness, mobility impairment, spasticity,
- **sensory changes**
  - paraesthesiae, pain,
- **visual disturbances**, particularly
  - **optic neuritis**, which is manifest by impaired visual acuity, with a central scotoma, loss of pupillary reaction to light and sometimes an oedematous disc on ophthalmoscopy; optic neuritis may sometimes occur as an isolated condition, in which case it is probably a forme fruste of MS,
  - **internuclear ophthalmoplegia**, which is caused by demyelination of the medial longitudinal bundle; on lateral conjugate gaze, there is thus impaired adduction of the following eye and nystagmus in the leading or abducting eye.
- **vestibular disturbance**,
- **incontinence** and/or **impotence**,
- **psychiatric disturbances**,
- **systemic symptoms**
  - fatigue, heat intolerance.

The later course of the disease is very variable, with exacerbations at irregular intervals over long periods but eventually with persistent signs of spastic weakness, incoordination and incontinence. Various clinical patterns are recognized, particularly relapsing-remitting MS (RRMS) and chronic progressive patterns. Relapsing-remitting patterns can sometimes show an aggressive frequency. Progressive patterns may be primary or secondary (i.e. superimposed on a relapsing-remitting pattern). Many cases have quite a benign course, and even permanent remission may occasionally be seen. Sometimes, radiologically isolated MS may be found in a patient who has had an MRI for another indication but has no symptoms of MS.

The diagnosis is based on clinical criteria, but it should be substantiated by special tests, particularly MRI, which shows typical demyelination plaques in over 90% of cases. The MRI should be performed with gadolinium contrast if possible. The CSF shows increased IgG, with oligoclonal banding. The responses to evoked potentials are abnormal. A normal MRI and CSF and the absence of eye signs and incontinence should suggest an alternative diagnosis. An international panel has recently recommended a revised set of diagnostic criteria, referred to as the McDonald criteria.

The differential diagnosis includes hereditary demyelinating or degenerative diseases, chronic infections, vascular disease (including vasculitis – q.v.), sarcoid (q.v.), vitamin B_{12} deficiency (q.v.) and structural lesions.

Treatment is not curative, but new modalities have had increasing efficacy in recent decades.

- **Corticosteroids** *(except as pulsed, high-dose, intravenous methylprednisolone for relapse), cytotoxics, plasmapheresis, immune globulin and hyperbaric oxygen have all been shown to be ineffective.*
- *New immunomodulatory drugs, especially the* **beta-interferons** *and* **glatiramer**, *have shown moderate efficacy over more than two decades of clinical use worldwide, and their long-term value has recently been confirmed. These expensive drugs appear to be of most value in reducing relapses, accumulated disability and MRI evidence of damage. The incomplete efficacy of such therapy and the considerable individual variability in response are thought to reflect both the underlying heterogeneity of the condition and the genetic polymorphisms related to the risk of disease in different patients. On the other hand, these issues may point to the opportunity for more personalized neuroimmunological programs for individual patients in the future.*
- *The monoclonal antibody* **natalizumab** *was initially reported to have some efficacy in preventing relapses, but it was later withdrawn in 2005 after only 4 months on the market because of the unfortunate occurrence of some cases of progressive multifocal leukoencephalopathy (PML) (see Demyelinating diseases). However, it was later reintroduced, with the strict caveat of careful monitoring and avoidance of use in combination regimens (e.g. with interferon beta) that may have been responsible for the PML or other opportunistic infections previously reported.*
- *A number of other new agents (e.g.* **alemtuzumab**) *with different molecular targets and some oral agents ported from other areas of medicine (e.g.* **dimethyl fumarate, fingolimod, teriflunomide, mitoxantrone**) *have also shown efficacy in clinical trials in RRMS.*
- *A small trial of autologous haematopoietic* **stem cell transplantation** *(AHSCT) showed dramatic benefit in some cases of RRMS.*
- *Symptoms of spasticity may be improved with* **baclofen** *(q.v.) or* **diazepam** *and symptoms of urinary urgency with* **propantheline**.
- *Elective surgery carries an increased risk of relapse, but pregnancy is normally well tolerated.*
- *Optimal treatment programs are complex and are best delivered in a specialized MS centre with a multidisciplinary team offering a comprehensive range of clinical, educational, research and support services.*

Bibliography

Anderson DW, Ellenberg JH, Leventhal CM, et al. Revised estimate of the prevalence of multiple sclerosis in the United States. *Ann Neurol* 1992; 31: 333.

Broadley SA, Barnett MH, Boggild M, et al. A new era in the treatment of multiple sclerosis. *Med J Aust* 2015; 203: 139.

Dhib-Jalbut S, McFarlin DE. Immunology of multiple sclerosis. *Ann Allergy* 1990; 64: 433.

Ebers GC. Optic neuritis and multiple sclerosis. *Arch Neurol* 1985; 42: 702.

Editorial. Where to hit MS. *Lancet* 1991; 337: 765.

European Study Group on interferon beta-1b in secondary progressive MS. Placebo-controlled multicentre randomised trial of interferon beta-1b in treatment of secondary progressive multiple sclerosis. *Lancet* 1998; 352: 1491.

Hauser SL, Cree BAC. Treatment of multiple sclerosis: a review. *Am J Med* 2020; 133: 1380.

Jacobs LD, Beck RW, Simon JH, et al. Intramuscular interferon beta-1a therapy initiated during the first demyelinating event in multiple sclerosis. *N Engl J Med* 2000; 343: 898.

Kilpatrick TJ, Soilu-Hanninen M. New treatments for multiple sclerosis. *Aust NZ J Med* 1999; 29: 801.

Lucchinetti C, Brueck W, Parisi J, et al. Heterogeneity of multiple sclerosis lesions: implications for the pathogenesis of demyelination. *Ann Neurol* 2000; 47: 707.

McDonald WI. Multiple sclerosis: diagnostic optimism. *BMJ* 1992; 304: 1259.

McDonald WI, Compston DAS, Edan G, et al. Recommended diagnostic criteria for multiple sclerosis: guidelines from the International Panel on the diagnosis of multiple sclerosis. *Ann Neurol* 2001; 50: 121.

Pender MP. Recent advances in the understanding, diagnosis and management of multiple sclerosis. *Aust NZ J Med* 1996; 26:157.

Pender MP. Multiple sclerosis. *Med J Aust* 2000; 172: 556.

Pender MP, Wolfe NP. Prevention of autoimmune attack and disease progression in multiple sclerosis: current therapies and future prospects. *Intern Med J* 2002; 32: 554.

PRISMS Study Group. Randomized double-blind placebo-controlled study of interferon beta-1a in relapsing/remitting multiple sclerosis. *Lancet* 1998; 352: 1498.

Ron MA, Feinstein A. Multiple sclerosis and the mind. *J Neurol Neurosurg Psychiatry* 1992; 55: 1.

Sedal L, Wilson IB, McDonald EA. Current management of relapsing-remitting multiple sclerosis. *Intern Med J* 2014; 44: 950.

Shaw C, Chapman C, Butzkueven H. How to diagnose multiple sclerosis and what are the pitfalls. *Intern Med J* 2009; 30: 792.

Thompson AJ, Banwell BL, Barkhof F, et al. Diagnosis of multiple sclerosis: 2017 revisions of the McDonald criteria. *Lancet Neurol* 2018; 17: 162.

Thompson AJ, Baranzini SE, Geurts J, et al. Multiple sclerosis. *Lancet* 2018; 391: 1622.

Tyler KL. Human herpesvirus 6 and multiple sclerosis: the continuing conundrum. *J Infect Dis.* 2003; 187: 1360.

Multiple system atrophy *See*

- Shy–Drager disease.

Multisystem inflammatory syndrome in children *See*

- Vasculitis – 2. Vasculitis affecting primarily medium-sized vessels – Kawasaki disease.

Munchausen syndrome *See*

- Factitious disorders.

Murray Valley encephalitis *See*

- Encephalitis.

Muscular dystrophies

Muscular dystrophies comprise a group of hereditary disorders of muscle, characterized by progressive weakness and wasting. The many types of muscular dystrophy can now be classified in some detail according to the genes involved and thus the protein affected. The defective protein may be a component of various muscle structures (the sarcolemma, the sarcomere, the nucleus, the extracellular matrix) or it may be an enzyme. Gene therapy offers promise in many of these conditions.

The three major types of muscular dystrophy are Duchenne's dystrophy, facioscapulohumeral dystrophy and myotonic dystrophy

1. **Duchenne's (pseudohypertrophic) dystrophy (DMD)**
This is an X-linked recessive disorder and is therefore seen in boys of mothers who are carriers. Genetic screening is available, but it has been complicated by the allelic heterogeneity of the condition.

It particularly involves the muscles of the pelvic girdle, resulting in a waddling gait. Most patients have succumbed by their mid-20s to either respiratory failure and/or associated cardiomyopathy.

*No treatment has generally been effective, though **corticosteroids** have been shown to be helpful. Trials to generate full-length muscle protein by gentamicin failed to confirm in humans the promise initially found in experimental animals with a similar condition.*

***Non-invasive nocturnal ventilation** may be useful in advanced disease.*

***Gene therapy** is likely to be the effective treatment of the future, though to date a modified form of such therapy using injected human myoblasts has been ineffective. However, a new gene therapy agent (Exondys 51) has been shown to be effective in those 13% of cases with a particular RNA mutation.*

2. **Facioscapulohumeral dystrophy**
This is an autosomal dominant condition which is very slowly progressive from adolescence onwards.

It primarily involves the muscles of the face and shoulder girdle. There is no associated cardiomyopathy, so that a normal lifespan is common.

3. **Myotonic dystrophy (DM, dystrophia myotonia)**
This is also an autosomal dominant condition, with an onset usually in adolescence. The genetic defect has been identified as mutation which causes an expansion of a trinucleotide repeat sequence. It is the most common muscular dystrophy in adults, with a prevalence of 1 in 10,000 of the population.

While it primarily involves atrophy of the muscles of the face (including eyelids), pharynx and neck, and the small muscles of the hands and feet, there is in fact weakness of all skeletal muscles.

> As its name implies, myotonic dystrophy is associated with myotonia, i.e. delayed muscular relaxation.
> Myotonia is also seen in
> - **myotonia congenita** (a benign myopathy),
> - periodic paralysis (due to hyperkalaemia) (q.v.).

Pathophysiologically, the muscle membrane has decreased permeability to chloride ion, and there is a characteristic EMG.

Myotonic dystrophy is associated with frontal baldness, cardiomyopathy (q.v.) with conduction defects, mental dysfunction, cataracts, glucose intolerance, dysphagia (q.v.) and gonadal atrophy. Hypercalcaemia is common, with features of familial hypocalciuric hypercalcaemia (see Hyperparathyroidism). Often, the condition is mild and the course slow.

Treatment with **phenytoin** or **procainamide** can help the myotonia but not the weakness.

Bibliography

Dent KM, Dunn DM, Niederhausern AC, et al. Improved molecular diagnosis of dystrophinophies in an unselected clinical cohort. *Am J Med* 2005; 134: 295.

Gregorevic P, Chamberlain JS. Gene therapy for muscular dystrophy: a review of promising progress. *Expert Opin Biol Ther* 2003; 3: 803.

Griggs RC, Moxley RT, Mendell JR, et al. Duchenne dystrophy: randomized, controlled trial of prednisone (18 months) and azathioprine (12 months). *Neurology* 1993; 43: 520.

Harper PS. *Myotonic Dystrophy*. 3rd edition. London: WB Saunders. 2001.

Hlaing PM, Scott IA, Jackson RV. Dysregulation of calcium metabolism in type 1 myotonic dystrophy. *Intern Med J* 2019; 49: 1412.

Mankodi A, Thornton CA. Myotonic syndromes. *Curr Opin Neurol* 2002; 15: 545.

Moser H. Duchenne muscular dystrophy: pathogenetic aspects and genetic prevention. *Hum Genet* 1984; 66: 17.

Mushroom poisoning

Mushroom poisoning is a worldwide problem because of the difficulty in identifying the many species which grow in the wild. Commercially available mushrooms, however, are cultured. Poisoning also occurs because of the 'recreational' use of mushrooms for their hallucinogenic properties. In fact, only about 1% of mushrooms are poisonous.

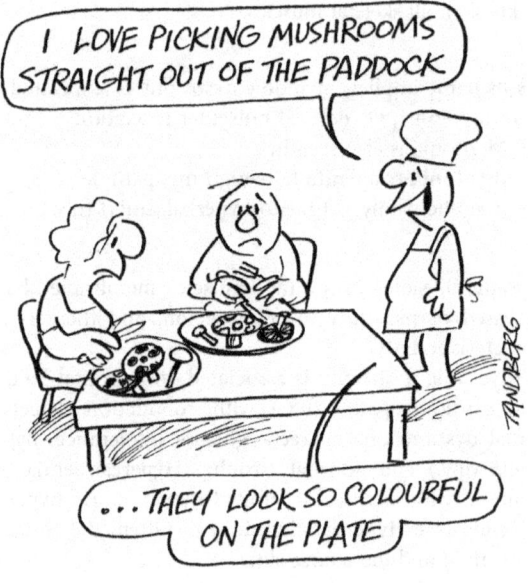

The term 'mushroom' is non-scientific and refers to the edible type of fungus, whereas the equally lay term 'toadstool' refers to any poisonous variety. Mushrooms are the umbrella-shaped, fleshy, fruiting body of fungi of the order Agaricales in the class Basidiomycetes. In the ground, the fungal mycelia may live for hundreds of years as an underground mat of threads, from which a new crop of fruiting sporophores arises each season.

Within the order Agaricales are both
- the family Agaricaceae, which includes *Agaricus campestris* (the common field mushroom) and *Agaricus bisporus* (the common commercial variety),
- the family Amanitaceae, which includes many poisonous varieties and in particular the genus *Amanita* which has about 100 species within it. The most common poisonous mushroom is *Amanita phalloides*, called the death cap, which is responsible for 90% of fatal mushroom poisonings worldwide. It is mostly associated in a symbiotic relationship with older oak and other deciduous trees.

Mushroom poisoning usually occurs in the autumn. There have been many famous deaths of this nature in history, including the Euripides family, the Roman Emperor Claudius, Pope Clement II, Charles VI of France, and of course Babar the elephant's royal predecessor.

> Several syndromes may be produced by mushroom poisoning.
>
> The most common syndromes are
> - **cytotoxic**,
> - **neurotoxic**.

Cytotoxins are primarily amatoxins, cyclic octapeptides from the *Amanita* genus. They are very potent, with as little as 50 g (or one mushroom), containing about 5 mg of toxin, possibly being fatal. They inhibit protein synthesis, giving rise to cell membrane destruction.

Symptoms arise after a latent period of 6–24 hr, by which time the patient may have forgotten having eating a mushroom. There is abdominal pain, nausea and vomiting, but these symptoms usually subside by 24 hr or so. Despite clinical improvement, liver enzymes become abnormal by 48 hr. Between 2 and 4 days, hepatic and renal failure occur.

Optimal treatment is uncertain.
- **Gastric lavage** and **charcoal** are recommended if the diagnosis is made early.
- The administration of high-dose **penicillin** for 3 days inhibits hepatocyte uptake of the toxin.
- **Thioctic acid** has been reported to be helpful.

- *Dialysis* is indicated on its normal merits for renal support, but it does not remove toxin.
- *Liver transplantation* has been used in some severely affected patients.
- *Silibinin* has been reported to be a possible antidote to Amanita poison, but its availability has been limited.
- If alcohol is taken during the first 3 days, a disulfiram-like reaction may be seen.

The mortality is about 20%.

Neurotoxins are varied in type and less commonly fatal.

Symptoms appear within 2 hr, last for 6–12 hr and resolve spontaneously. They comprise chiefly muscarinic effects (with anticholinergic features of sweating, salivation and gastrointestinal upset), hallucinations (which may be LSD-like) or disulfiram-like reactions (with flushing, tachycardia and tachypnoea, following alcohol).

*Atropine may be given for muscarinic effects, but not if there are associated hallucinations as it may worsen these. Hallucinations are best treated with **diazepam**.*

The presence of the rapid and brief neurotoxic reaction does not exclude the possibility of associated amatoxin ingestion and thus later cytotoxic damage.

Mushrooms may cause **flagellate dermatitis** in susceptible subjects who have eaten undercooked shiitake mushrooms (see Dermatitis).

Mushrooms may also cause respiratory illness, since mushroom compost like many organic dusts and mould may cause **hypersensitivity pneumonitis** (q.v.) in people who work with it.

Bibliography

Barbato MP. Poisoning from accidental ingestion of mushrooms. *Med J Aust* 1993; 158: 842.

Diaz JH. Evolving global epidemiology, syndromic classification, general management, and prevention of unknown mushroom poisonings. *Crit Care Med* 2005; 33: 419.

Klein AS, Hart J, Brems JJ, et al. Amanita poisoning: treatment and the role of liver transplantation. *Am J Med* 1989; 86: 187.

Mitchell DH. Amanita mushroom poisoning. *Annu Rev Med* 1980; 31: 51.

Mount P, Harris G, Sinclair R, et al. Acute renal failure following ingestion of wild mushrooms. *Intern Med J* 2002; 32: 187.

Nicholson FB, Korman MG. Death from Amanita poisoning. *Aust NZ J Med* 1997; 27: 448.

Rumack BH, Spoerke DG, eds. *Handbook of Mushroom Poisoning: Diagnosis and Treatment*. 2nd edition. Boca Raton: CRC Press. 1994.

Mustards See
- Warfare agents.

Myalgic encephalomyelitis See
- Chronic fatigue syndrome.

Myasthenia gravis

Myasthenia gravis is a condition of muscle weakness due to impaired neuromuscular transmission.

It is caused by autoantibodies to a subunit of the acetylcholine receptor on the post-junctional muscle membrane, resulting in functional disconnection between the motor neurone and the muscle fibres it relates to. It has a prevalence of about 1 in 10,000 of the population, and it occurs primarily in younger women or older men.

In about 10% of cases, there is an associated thymic tumour (thymoma). Conversely, about 30% of patients with a thymoma have myasthenia gravis. Most thymomas are benign, though they may have the potential to cause paraneoplastic syndromes (q.v.). Occasionally, a microscopic thymoma is found histologically in resected thymic specimens when no thymoma has been apparent macroscopically or on CT scan.

> There is typically a gradual onset of muscle fatigue, characteristically with increasing weakness with repetitive use.
>
> It may range in severity from mild and local to severe and generalized.
>
> It particularly involves the muscles innervated by the cranial nerves (eyes, face, jaw, pharynx and voice). Typically, there is diplopia and ptosis.

The course of the disease is chronic but variable. After the first 5 years, about 20% of patients have undergone spontaneous remission, though later relapse may occur. On the other hand, mild and localized disease often progresses. The response to treatment is also variable, though even effective treatment probably does not alter the natural history of the disease.

The diagnosis is made on the basis of the EMG and confirmed with edrophonium, a short-acting anticholinesterase (q.v.). After edrophonium 10 mg IV, dramatic improvement in muscle power occurs within 60 sec and lasts for a few minutes. Acetylcholine antibodies are present in about 90% of cases, and there may be other associated autoimmune diseases (q.v.), in particular thyroid disease. A CT scan is required to assess the presence of an associated thymoma.

Treatment modalities include
- **anticholinesterase** therapy (in particular pyridostigmine)(q.v.). Dosage requirements vary considerably and range from 15 mg 8 hrly to 120 mg 4 hrly orally (60 mg orally being equivalent to 2 mg IV). The response occurs within minutes but is generally limited and lasts only for a few hours. However, excess dosage (e.g. >480 mg per day) can give a cholinergic crisis (q.v.), which is associated with muscarinic side-effects. It can sometimes be difficult to distinguish this reaction (i.e. drug overdose) clinically from deteriorating disease (i.e. drug underdose), and the response to edrophonium can assist in clarifying this situation.
- **corticosteroids**. These are of value if the response to anticholinesterase is unsatisfactory or the patient is very sick. Usually, prednisolone 1 mg/kg per day is given until there is satisfactory control, when it may be gradually tapered to a maintenance dose. While there may be a response within 2 weeks, more typically it is quite slow, with a median time of 6 months and late plateau of up to 2 years.
- **cytotoxic agents** (usually azathioprine, sometimes cyclophosphamide or more recently mycophenolate). These may enhance the steroid response or be steroid-sparing, but the response to them is very slow. More complex immunosuppression with rituximab (q.v.) or bone marrow ablation and transplantation can be used in desperate situations.
- **plasmapheresis** (q.v.) or **immune globulin**. These are used for an acute crisis and for perioperative support. Both are similarly effective, but there is limited head-to-head comparison, although intravenous immunoglobulin (IVIG) is more convenient. The response occurs within days but lasts only a few weeks.
- **thymectomy**. Even in the absence of a thymoma, this gives a 70% eventual response rate. It is best considered early in the course of the disease.

Two variants of myasthenia gravis may be seen.

1. **Drug-induced myasthenia**

This may be caused by aminoglycosides. Weakness of this type may be caused even in normal subjects, as well as increased weakness in myasthenics.

Penicillamine therapy for rheumatoid arthritis may also be associated with myasthenia.

Needless to say, prolonged neuromuscular junction abnormalities are common after long infusions of neuromuscular blocking drugs, particularly in patients with liver and kidney dysfunction. While this phenomenon is usually due to the persistence of long-acting metabolites (e.g. of vecuronium), a myasthenia-like syndrome has also been reported and is probably due to damage to the neuromuscular junction.

2. **Myasthenic syndrome** (Eaton Lambert syndrome)

This is a paraneoplastic phenomenon (q.v.). It is caused by the binding of antibodies to the presynaptic membrane of the neuromuscular junction.

Although there is typical muscular weakness and fatigue, there is paradoxical improvement with repeated use. It is exacerbated by muscle relaxants and may be improved with successful treatment of the underlying carcinoma (usually of the lung).

It sometimes responds to **pyridostigmine** (perhaps in association with guanidine), **corticosteroids** and/or **plasmapheresis**. Recently, **3,4-diaminopyridine** (3,4-DAP), which is the best tolerated of the aminopyridines, has been shown to be of benefit.

Bibliography

Berrouschot J, Baumann I, Kalischewski P, et al. Therapy of myasthenic crisis. *Crit Care Med* 1997; 25: 1228.

Clamon GH, Evans WK, Shepherd FA, et al. Myasthenic syndrome and small cell cancer of the lung: variable response to antineoplastic therapy. *Arch Intern Med* 1984; 144: 999.

Drachman DB. Myasthenia gravis. *N Engl J Med* 1994; 330: 1797.

Gilhus NE. Myasthenia gravis. *N Engl J Med* 2016; 375: 2570.

Gilhus NE, Verschuuren JJ. Myasthenia gravis: subgroup classification and therapeutic strategies. *Lancet Neurol* 2015; 14: 1023.

Gracey DR, Divertie MB, Howard FM. Mechanical ventilation for respiratory failure in myasthenia gravis. *Mayo Clin Proc* 1983; 58: 597.

Gronseth GS, Bahron RJ. Practice parameter; thymectomy for auto-immune myasthenia gravis (an evidence-based review). *Neurology* 2000; 55: 7.

O'Neill JH, Murray NM, Newsom-Davis J. The Lambert-Eaton myasthenic syndrome. *Brain* 1988; 111: 577.

Segredo V, Caldwell J, Matthay M, et al. Persistent paralysis in critically ill patients after long-term administration of vecuronium. *N Engl J Med* 1992; 327: 524.

Seybold ME. Myasthenia gravis: a clinical and basic science review. *JAMA* 1983; 250: 2516.

Sokoll M, Gergis S. Antibiotics and neuromuscular function. *Anesthesiology* 1981; 55: 148.

Swift TR. Disorders of neuromuscular transmission other than myasthenia gravis. *Muscle Nerve* 1981; 4: 334.

Tonner DR, Schlechte JA. Neurologic complications of thyroid and parathyroid disease. *Med Clin North Am* 1993; 77: 251.

Varelas PN, Chua HC, Natterman J, et al. Ventilatory care in myasthenia crisis: assessing the baseline adverse event rate. *Crit Care Med* 2002; 30: 2663.

Vincent A, Palace J, Hilton-Jones D. Myasthenia gravis. *Lancet* 2001; 357: 2122.

Wolfe GI, Kaminski HJ, Aban IB, et al. Randomized trial of thymectomy in myasthenia gravis. *N Engl J Med* 2016; 375: 511.

Wright EA, McQuillen MP. Antibiotic-induced neuromuscular blockade. *Ann NY Acad Sci* 1971; 183: 358.

Mycetism See

- Mushroom poisoning.

Mycetoma See

- Aspergillosis.

Mycobacterium ulcerans

Mycobacterium ulcerans is an indolent pathogen widely distributed in the environment and responsible for cases of troublesome cutaneous ulceration. It is the third most common mycobaterial infection worldwide, after tuberculosis (q.v.) and leprosy (q.v.). It is found mainly in the Americas, Africa and the Western Pacific (including Australia, where specific endemic areas include coastal Victoria and the tropical north). It is the specific cause of Buruli ulcer (named after the Buruli region in Uganda), also called Bairnsdale or Daintree ulcer in Australia.

Although the environmental reservoir is uncertain (but might involve possums in Australia), the mode of transmission is considered probably via a mosquito vector. There is no human-to-human transmission. The incubation period is prolonged, with a median of 4.5 months and a range of 3 weeks to 1 year.

The initial clinical presentation is with a painless nodule, usually on an exposed limb area. Over the next weeks and months, the lesion shows progressive ulceration with undermined edges. There are no systemic symptoms.

Diagnosis is confirmed either by swab for culture and PCR or by biopsy for identification of acid-fast bacilli.

*Treatment comprises **rifampicin-based oral antibiotic therapy** for 8 weeks. If treatment is delayed and extensive ulceration has occurred, **surgical excision** may be required.*

Bibliography

Boyd SC, Athan E, Friedman MD, et al. Epidemiology, clinical features and diagnosis of *Mycobacterium ulcerans* in an Australian population. *Med J Aust* 2012; 196: 341.

O'Brien DP, Athan E, Blasdell K, et al. Tackling the worsening epidemic of Buruli ulcer in Australia in an information void: time for an urgent scientific response. *Med J Aust* 2018; 208: 287.

WHO. *Treatment of Mycobacterium ulcerans Disease (Buruli Ulcer): Guidance for Health Workers*. Geneva: WHO. 2012.

Mycoplasma hominis See

- Pregnancy.

Mycoplasma pneumoniae See

- Cold agglutinin disease.

Mycotic aneurysms

Mycotic aneurysms arise from destruction of the arterial wall following infection.

This process may be produced by
- direct bacterial invasion of the arterial wall,
- deposition of immune complexes in the arterial wall,
- embolic occlusion of vasa vasorum.

Although the arterial wall damage is an acute process, it may not become clinically evident until long after the original infection has subsided.

A mycotic aneurysm is thus the sterile end-result of a previous infection.
- It may occur in any artery, including the sinus of Valsalva and the pulmonary artery (e.g. following IV heroin use).
- The antecedent infection is a bacteraemia, especially if associated with acute or subacute bacterial endocarditis. The most common organism involved is *Staphylococcus aureus*.

Clinical features can include
- a pulsatile mass (which may be tender and which usually is noted only in a palpable artery, e.g. brachial, femoral or popliteal),
- local pressure problems,
- an abdominal bruit,
- a sudden haemorrhage,

- rupture of a sinus of Valsalva into the right heart giving a left-to-right shunt and a continuous murmur.

*Treatment is **surgical**, if the aneurysm is accessible. Prophylactic surgical excision is recommended, because rupture is a major complication which can be fatal.*

Myelitis See
- Demyelinating diseases,
- Poliomyelitis.

Myelopathy

Myelopathy (spinal cord damage) may be either
- local, or
- associated with encephalopathy (q.v.), as an encephalomyelopathy.

Isolated myelopathy is due to local spinal cord damage, such as that due to
- disc protrusion,
- infection, including rarely human T-cell lymphotropic virus type I or HTLV-I,
- nutritional deficiency, particularly of vitamin B_{12} (q.v.) or sometimes of copper (q.v.),
- radiation.

Myoglobinuria See
- Rhabdomyolysis.
  See also
- Glycogen storage diseases,
- Haematuria,
- Malignant hyperthermia,
- Neuroleptic malignant syndrome.

Myopathy

Myopathy is a general term indicating a muscle disorder. It may be either primary or secondary.

Primary myopathies include
- genetic disorders
  - glycogen storage diseases (q.v.),
  - lipid storage myopathy (see Storage disorders),
  - mitochondrial diseases (q.v.),
- malignant hyperthermia (q.v.),
- muscular dystrophy (q.v.),
- myasthenia gravis (q.v.)
  - in fact a neuromuscular disease,
- periodic paralysis (q.v.),
- poliomyelitis (q.v.)
  - in fact a denervating disease.

Secondary myopathy may be caused by
- inflammation (myositis)
  - **idiopathic inflammatory myopathy** (IIM) refers to a heterogeneous group of systemic autoimmune conditions (see Myositis).
- toxic/metabolic disorders
  - alcoholism,
  - drugs, including antimalarials, colchicine, statins, zidovudine, and especially fluorinated corticosteroids, even in standard doses,
- endocrine disorders, such as adrenal, parathyroid and thyroid disorders of either excess or deficiency,
- metabolic disturbances, such as hypophophataemia, hypokalaemia, hypocalcaemia, hypomagnesaemia (see these separate conditions),
- trauma
  - rhabdomyolysis (q.v.),
  - severe exertion.

Acute necrotizing myopathy is one of the less common forms of critical illness neuromuscular abnormality (q.v.). It may be seen in Intensive Care patients who have received prolonged neuromuscular blockade with any of the non-depolarizing agents, usually with concomitant corticosteroids. It was thus first recognized as a complication of severe asthma, and those paralyzed for more than 24 hr may be at particular risk. Experimental evidence suggests that it may be due to marked enhancement of steroid-induced myopathy by pharmacological denervation. It may be a cause of prolonged ventilator dependence. This condition may be difficult to distinguish from critical illness polyneuropathy (with which it may also coexist).

Critical illness myopathy is a less well understood variant of **critical illness neuromuscular abnormality** (q.v.). It is seen in patients with sepsis and/or multiorgan failure and may have a similar pathogenesis to **critical illness polyneuropathy** (see Neuropathy).

Myopathy due to disuse atrophy may of course occur following any serious illness, particularly if it is prolonged.

Electrophysiological studies and histology may be required to clarify these conditions in an individual patient.

There is evidence in experimental animals that the continuous infusion of pyridostigmine may improve muscle weakness due to prolonged immobilization.

Bibliography
Baer AN. Advances in the therapy of idiopathic inflammatory myopathies. *Curr Opin Rheumatol* 2006; 18: 236.
Batchelor PM, Taylor LP, Thaler HT, et al. Steroid myopathy in cancer patients. *Neurology* 1997; 48: 1234.

Bolton CF. Critical illness polyneuropathy and myopathy. *Crit Care Med* 2001; 29: 2388.

Chad DA, Lacomis D. Critically ill patients with newly acquired weakness: the clinicopathological spectrum. *Ann Neurol* 1994; 35: 257.

De Jonghe B, Cook D, Sharshar T, et al. Acquired neuromuscular disorders in critically ill patients: a systematic review. *Intens Care Med* 1998; 24: 1242.

de Letter M-ACJ, Schmitz PIM, Visser LH, et al. Risk factors for the development of polyneuropathy and myopathy in critically ill patients. *Crit Care Med* 2001; 29: 2281.

Douglass JA, Tuxen DV, Horne M, et al. Myopathy in severe asthma. *Am Rev Respir Dis* 1992; 146: 157.

Hall JB, Griffiths RD, eds. ICU-acquired weakness: proceedings of a round table conference in Brussels, Belgium, March 2009. *Crit Care Med* 2009; 37: S295.

Hamilton-Craig I. Statin-associated myopathy. *Med J Aust* 2001; 175: 486.

Hansen-Flaschen J. Neuromuscular complications of critical illness. *Pulm Perspect* 1997; 14(4): 1.

Hund E. Myopathy in critically ill patients. *Chest* 1999; 27: 2544.

Joffe MM, Love LA, Leff RL, et al. Drug therapy of idiopathic inflammatory myopathies: predictors of response to prednisone, azathioprine, and methotrexate and a comparison of their efficacy. *Am J Med* 1993; 94: 379.

Latronico N. Neuromuscular alterations in the critically ill patient: critical illness myopathy, critical illness neuropathy, or both? *Intens Care Med* 2003; 29: 1411.

Latronico N, Fenzi F, Recupero D, et al. Critical illness myopathy and neuropathy. *Lancet* 1996; 347: 1579.

Layzer RB. McArdle's disease in the 1980s. *N Engl J Med* 1985; 312: 370.

Limaye VS, Blumbergs P, Roberts-Thomson PJ. Idiopathic inflammatory myopathies. *Intern Med J* 2009; 39: 179.

Maramattom BV, Wijdicks EFM. Acute neuromuscular weakness in the intensive care unit. *Crit Care Med* 2006; 34: 2835.

Mastaglia, Phillips BA. Idiopathic inflammatory myopathies: epidemiology, classification and diagnostic criteria. *Rheum Dis Clin North Am* 2002; 28: 723.

Miller FW, Schiffenbauer A. Idiopathic inflammatory myopathies. In: *Scientific American Medicine. Rheumatology.* Hamilton: Dekker Medicine. 2020.

Nates JL, Cooper DJ, Day B, et al. Acute weakness syndromes in critically ill patients – a reappraisal. *Anaesth Intens Care* 1997; 25: 502.

Polkey MI, Moxham J. Clinical aspects of respiratory muscle dysfunction in the critically ill. *Chest* 2001; 119: 926.

Rosenson RS. Current overview of statin-induced myopathy. *Am J Med* 2004; 116: 408.

Schweickert WD, Hall J. ICU-acquired weakness. *Chest* 2007; 131: 1541.

Segredo V, Caldwell JE, Matthay MA, et al. Persistent paralysis in critically ill patients after long-term administration of vecuronium. *N Engl J Med* 1992; 327: 524.

Sieb JP, Gillensen T. Iatrogenic and toxic myopathies. *Muscle Nerve* 2003; 27: 142.

Tonner DR, Schlechte JA. Neurologic complications of thyroid and parathyroid disease. *Med Clin North Am* 1993; 77: 251.

Myositis

Myositis, or inflammation of muscle, may be seen in several settings.

1. **Autoimmune diseases**

A heterogeneous group of systemic autoimmune diseases (q.v.) can be associated with myositis-specific autoantibodies (MSA), particularly to cytoplasmic ribonucleoprotein. The condition is referred to as **idiopathic inflammatory myopathy** (IIM) (see Myopathy).

It includes polymyositis (q.v.), dermatomyositis (q.v.), inclusion body myositis (see Polymyositis), paraneoplastic myopathy/myositis (see Paraneoplastic syndromes), myositis associated with connective tissue disease (q.v.) and Sjogren's syndrome (q.v.).

Clinical features comprise proximal muscle weakness which is symmetrical and subacute. There may be associated myalgia, dysphagia (q.v.) or dyspnoea.

The electromyograph is abnormal, and the diagnosis is confirmed by the presence of myositis-specific antibodies on serological testing. Imaging by MRI can clarify any patchy involvement. Muscle biopsy enables differentiation between the different subtypes of IIM.

Treatment comprises **corticosteroids** *and/or* **immunosuppressive therapy** *(azathioprine, methotrexate, ciclosporin, tacrolimus, mycophenolate, anti-TNF agents, anti-B-cell agents). A multidisciplinary team can assist with non-drug treatment and functional maintenance.*

2. **Infections**

Streptococcal infections with group A streptococci may sometimes cause a potentially fatal gangrenous myositis and/or necrotizing fasciitis (see Gangrene). This is the severe end of the spectrum which ranges from superficial skin infection (impetigo) to deeper infections (such as cellulitis or erysipelas). *Treatment requires surgical drainage and/or debridement, as well as antibiotics.*

Tropical myositis comprises a pyomyositis which is common in the tropics and in AIDS (q.v.). It is usually due to *Staphylococcus aureus*. The muscle abscess is best diagnosed with CT scanning.

Viral myositis is most widely known with influenza virus, but it can also occur with adenovirus, coxsackievirus, echovirus, HIV (q.v.).

Clostridial infections (q.v.) may also cause myositis as part of the condition of gas gangrene.

3. **Myositis ossificans**

This is post-traumatic.

4. **Polymyositis (PM)/dermatomyositis (DM) (q.v.)**

See IIM above.

5. **Inclusion body myositis (IBM)**

See Polymyositis, see IIM above.

6. **Myositis associated with vasculitis**

About 50% of cases of vasculitis (q.v.) have histological evidence of associated myositis, though mostly such muscle involvement is asymptomatic.

Bibliography

Ashton C, Paramalingam S, Stevenson B, et al. Idiopathic inflammatory myopathies: a review. *Intern Med J* 2021; 51: 845.

Hirschmann JV. Fungal, bacterial, and viral infections of the skin. In: *Scientific American Medicine. Dermatology.* Hamilton: Dekker Medicine. 2020.

Limaye VS, Blumbergs P, Roberts-Thomson PJ. Idiopathic inflammatory myopathies. *Intern Med J* 2009; 39: 179.

Mastaglia FL, Phillips BA. Idiopathic inflammatory myopathies: epidemiology, classification and diagnostic criteria. *Rheum Dis Clin North Am* 2002; 28: 723.

Miller FW. Classification and prognosis of inflammatory muscle disease. *Rheum Dis Clin North Am* 1994; 20: 811.

Myotonia See

- Muscular dystrophy.

Myxoedema See

- Hypothyroidism.

Myxoma See

- Cardiac tumours.

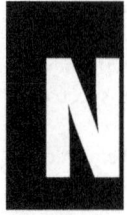

Nails

Nails, especially fingernails, can show a large variety of physical abnormalities, many of which are associated with systemic diseases.

- **Onychomycosis** is usually associated with paronychia and is commonly fungal in origin, though it may also be caused by staphylococci or pseudomonas (in which latter case green nails are sometimes seen). It especially occurs in the immunocompromised. *Both oral and topical antifungal therapy are effective in most cases.*
- **Onycholysis** refers to separation of the nail plate from the nail bed. It may follow drugs (tetracycline, quinolones especially when associated with ultraviolet light), dermatoses (e.g. psoriasis – q.v.), peripheral vascular disease, thyroid disease and trauma.
- **Koilonychia** refers to spoon-shaped nails and is seen typically in iron deficiency anaemia (q.v.) but also in haemochromatosis (q.v.).
- **Clubbing** of the nails may be inherited or may be idiopathic. Most commonly, it arises from malignancy or chronic inflammation in the lungs or mediastinum. Clubbing of a single digit may follow a local vascular abnormality, such as an AV fistula.
- **Leukonychia** indicates white streaking of the nails and is seen in psoriasis (q.v.), systemic infections, and poisoning (arsenic – q.v., thallium – q.v.).
- **Yellow discolouration** of the nails is seen in jaundice, chronic respiratory infections, amyloid (q.v.), thyroid disease and AIDS (q.v.). A discrete **yellow nail syndrome** (YNS) associated with chronic respiratory features (especially pleural effusion) and lymphoedema (especially of the legs) has been described as a rare and usually acquired lymphatic dysfunction.
- **Brown discolouration** of the nails is seen following the use of some antimalarial or cytotoxic drugs, and of course with nicotine staining.
- **Splinter haemorrhages**, while purportedly typical of subacute bacterial endocarditis (q.v.), are usually in fact traumatic in origin.

- **Onychodystrophies** refer to a large variety of alterations of nail shape, surface or colour. They are especially seen in the elderly, in whom for example, brittle or longitudinally ridged nails may be seen.
- **Transverse lines** (Beau lines) may be seen after chemotherapy, heavy metal poisoning (q.v.) or severe systemic illness. The width of the lines and their number depend on the timing and duration of the insult. The lines grow out with time if the insult has subsided.
- **Pitting** of the nails is typical in psoriasis (q.v.) though not pathognomonic. Sometimes, the entire nail plate may be rough, when it is referred to as **trachyonychia (trachonychia)**.
- **Atrophy** or **hypertrophy** of the nails may occasionally be seen as congenital conditions.

Bibliography

Maldonado F, Tazelaar HD, Wang C-W, et al. Yellow nail syndrome. *Chest* 2008; 134: 375.

Myers KA, Farquhar DR. The rational clinical examination: does this patient have clubbing? *JAMA* 2001; 286: 341.

Nguyen J, Cotserelis G. Diseases of the nail unit. In: *Scientific American Medicine. Dermatology*. Hamilton: Dekker Medicine. 2020.

Wolff K, Goldsmith L, Katz S, et al., eds. *Fitzpatrick's Dermatology in General Medicine*. 7th edition. New York: McGraw-Hill. 2007.

Necrolytic migratory erythema See
- Glucagonoma,
- Paraneoplastic syndromes – Dermatoses.

Necrotizing cutaneous mucormycosis See
- Gangrene.

Necrotizing fasciitis See
- Gangrene.

Necrotizing granulomatous vasculitis See
- Wegener's granulomatosis.

Necrotizing pneumonia See
- Cavitation
  See also
- Aspergillosis,
- Pneumothorax.

Necrotizing soft-tissue infection See
- Gangrene.

Nephrogenic fibrosing dermopathy See
- Scleroderma.

Nephrogenic systemic fibrosis See
- Scleroderma

Nephrolithiasis

Nephrolithiasis (renal calculous disease) occurs in about 5% of the population. The calculi may be composed of a variety of substances.

1. **Calcium oxalate**, an octahedron, occurs with or without calcium apatite (70% of calculi).

Such stones form when
- the urine volume is small,
- there is increased urinary calcium or oxalate
  - increased oxalate intake with ingestion of some foods, such as chocolate, peanuts, leafy vegetables, strong tea, star fruit (q.v.),
  - increased oxalate absorption in inflammatory bowel disease (q.v.), the short bowel syndrome (q.v.) or after bariatric surgery,
  - increased oxalate turnover in pyridoxine deficiency or following high IV doses of vitamin C (q.v.),
- there are decreased urinary inhibitors
  - such as citrate, glycoprotein, magnesium (q.v.).

2. **Struvite**, magnesium ammonium phosphate, is typically in the shape of a coffin lid and sometimes forms a staghorn (15% of calculi).

   Such stones form particularly in urinary tract infections when ammonia production is increased from urease secreted by bacteria. These are typically *Proteus*, though other Gram-negative bacilli and staphylococci may also be involved.

3. **Uric acid** calculi occur in the shape of radiolucent diamonds (10% of calculi).
4. **Calcium phosphate** produces an amorphous stone (2% of calculi).
5. **Cystine** produces hexagons (1% of calculi). These occur in cystinuria, which is an autosomal recessive condition.

Clinical consequences of renal calculi include
- pain,
- urinary tract obstruction,
- urinary tract infection,
- haematuria (q.v.).

> Sometimes, the patient may present with
> - renal impairment,
> - ileus,
> - hypovolaemia.

The differential diagnosis of calculi, particularly if radiolucent, includes sloughed renal papilla, clot, tumour or uric acid stone. A diagnosis of renal tubular acidosis (q.v.) is supported by the presence of diffuse tiny nephrocalcinosis and metabolic acidosis with a normal anion gap and high urinary pH. Definitive diagnosis usually requires imaging, either by ultrasound or CT scanning.

Treatment requires **removal of the stone**, unless it is passed spontaneously. Removal options include retrograde **basket extraction** or **lithotripsy**, though in severe cases a **nephrostomy** may be required first.

Antibiotics are commonly required for concomitant infection.

The **high fluid intake** traditionally recommended to decrease stone formation has been confirmed to be effective, though some fluids (e.g. beer) are more effective than others (e.g. grapefruit juice).

Bibliography

Borghi I, Schianchi T, Meschi T, et al. Comparison of two diets for the prevention of recurrent stones in idiopathic hypercalciuria. *N Engl J Med* 2002; 346: 77.

Coe FL, Parks JH, Asplin JR. The pathogenesis and treatment of kidney stones. *N Engl J Med* 1992; 327: 1141.

Curhan GC, Willett WC, Rimm EB, et al. Family history and risk of kidney stones. *J Am Soc Nephrol* 1997; 8: 1568.

Hirvonen T, Pietinen P, Virtanen M, et al. Nutrient intake and use of beverages and the risk of kidney stones among male smokers. *Am J Epidemiol* 1999; 150: 187.

Jackman SV, Potter SR, Regan F, et al. Plain abdominal x-ray versus computerized tomography screening: sensitivity for stone localization after nonenhanced spiral computerized tomography. *J Urol* 2000; 164: 308.

NIH Consensus Development Panel. Prevention and treatment of kidney stones. *JAMA* 1988; 260: 977.

Nishiura JL, Heilberg IP. Nephrolithiasis. In: *Scientific American Medicine. Nephrology.* Hamilton: Dekker Medicine. 2020.

Singer A, Das S. Cystinuria: a review of the pathophysiology and management. *J Urol* 1989; 142: 669.

Stewart C. Nephrolithiasis. *Emerg Med Clin North Am* 1988; 6: 617.

Wilson DM. Clinical and laboratory evaluation of renal stone patients. *Endocrinol Metab Clin North Am* 1990; 19: 773.

Nephrology

Most renal disorders encountered in Intensive Care are very well known, especially the various conditions associated with acute renal failure (acute kidney injury, AKI), chronic renal failure (chronic kidney disease, CKD), dialysis and renal replacement therapy (RRT), transplantation, trauma, and acid–base, fluid and electrolyte disturbances. Nevertheless, a variety of other, less common aspects of renal disease can be relevant to Intensive Care practice and are considered in this book. They include

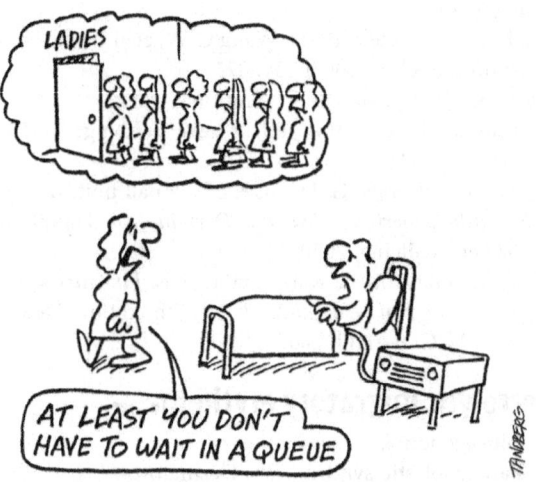

- Aminoaciduria,
- Beta$_2$-microglobulin,
- Calciphylaxis,
- Drugs and the kidney,
- Fanconi's syndrome,
- Glomerular diseases,
- Haematuria,
- Haemoglobinuria,
- Hepatorenal syndrome,
- Interstitial nephritis,
- Medullary sponge kidney,
- Metastatic calcification,
- Myoglobinuria,
- Nephrolithiasis,
- Nephrotic syndrome,
- Pink urine,

- Polycystic kidney disease,
- Proteinuria,
- Renal artery occlusion,
- Renal cortical necrosis,
- Renal cystic disease,
- Renal tubular acidosis,
- Renal vein thrombosis,
- Tubulointerstitial diseases.

Bibliography

Arieff AI, Guisado R, Massry SG, et al. Central nervous system pH in uremia and the effects of hemodialysis. *J Clin Invest* 1976; 58: 306.

Arieff AI, Massry SG, Barrientos A, et al. Brain water and electrolyte metabolism in uremia: effects of slow and rapid hemodialysis. *Kidney Int* 1973; 4: 177.

Aronoff GR, Bennett WM, Berns JS, eds. *Drug Prescribing in Renal Failure: Dosing Guidelines for Adults.* 5th edition. Philadelphia: American College of Physicians. 2007.

Bellomo R, Kellum JA, Ronco C. Defining acute renal failure: physiological principles. *Intens Care Med* 2004; 30: 33.

Berg KJ. Nephrotoxicity related to contrast media. *Scand J Urol Nephrol* 2000; 34: 317.

Caruana RJ. Heparin free dialysis: comparative data and results in high risk patients. *Kidney Int* 1987; 31: 1351.

Chandraker A, ed. Nephrology. In: *Scientific American Medicine.* Hamilton: Dekker Medicine. 2020.

Cronin RE, Kaehny WD, Miller, PD, et al. Renal cell carcinoma: unusual systemic manifestations. *Medicine* 1976; 55: 291.

Dossetor JB. Creatininemia versus uremia: the relative significance of blood urea nitrogen and serum creatinine in azotemia. *Ann Intern Med* 1966; 65: 1287.

Fraser CL, Arieff AI. Nervous system complications of uremia. *Ann Intern Med* 1988; 109: 143.

Hoitsma AJ, Wetzels JFM, Koene RAP. Drug-induced nephrotoxicity: aetiology, clinical features and management. *Drug Safety* 1991; 6: 131.

Hruska KA, Teitelbaum SL. Renal osteodystrophy. *N Engl J Med* 1995; 333: 166.

Keshaviah P, Shapiro FL. A critical examination of dialysis-induced hypotension. *Am J Kidney Dis* 1982; 2: 290.

Kincaid-Smith P. Analgesic abuse and the kidney. *Kidney Int* 1980; 17: 250.

Koyner JL. Assessment and diagnosis of renal dysfunction in the ICU. *Chest* 2012; 141: 1584.

Levey AS, Bosch JP, Lewis JB, et al. A more accurate method to estimate glomerular filtration rate from serum creatinine: a new prediction equation. *Ann Intern Med* 1999; 130: 461.

Li PKT, Burdmann EA, Mehta RL. Acute kidney injury: global health alert. *Intern Med J* 2013; 43: 223.

Massry SG, Glassock RJ, eds. *Textbook of Nephrology.* 4th edition. Baltimore: Williams & Wilkins. 2001.

Mathew T. Recurrence of disease after renal transplantation. *Am J Kidney Dis* 1988; 12: 85.

Morgan DB, Dillon S, Payne RB. The assessment of glomerular function: creatinine clearance or plasma creatinine? *Postgrad Med J* 1978; 54: 302.

Raskin NH, Fishman RA. Neurologic disorders in renal failure. *N Engl J Med* 1976; 294: 143.

Ronco PM, Flahault A. Drug-induced end-stage renal disease. *N Engl J Med* 1994; 331: 1711.

Schrier RW. An odyssey into the milieu interieur: pondering the enigmas. *J Am Soc Nephrol* 1992; 2: 1549.

Schwartz WB, Relman AS. Effects of electrolyte disorders on renal structure and function. *N Engl J Med* 1967; 276: 383 & 452.

Sherman RA, Eisinger RP. The use (and misuse) of urinary sodium and chloride measurements. *JAMA* 1982; 247: 3121.

Stamm WE, Hooton TM. Management of urinary tract infections in adults. *N Engl J Med* 1993; 329: 1328.

Turner NN, Lameire N, Goldsmith DJ, et al. eds. *Oxford Textbook of Clinical Nephrology.* 4th edition. Oxford: Oxford University Press. 2015.

Various. Issue number 6 dedicated to acute kidney injury. *Intens Care Med* 2017; 43: 727.

Nephrotic syndrome *See*

- Glomerular diseases.
  See also
- Antithrombin III,
- Chelating agents – Penicillamine,
- Drugs and the kidney,
- Familial Mediterranean fever,
- Lithium,
- Multiple myeloma – Amyloidosis,
- Pleural effusion,
- Protein S,
- Renal vein thrombosis,
- Systemic lupus erythematosus,
- Thrombophilia.

Neural tube defects *See*

- Alpha-fetoprotein,
- Arnold–Chiari malformation,
- Bathing,
- Folic acid deficiency,
- Syringomyelia.

Neurofibromatosis

Neurofibromatosis arises from dysplasia of the neural and cutaneous ectoderm. It is inherited as an autosomal dominant condition. The genes (*NF-1* and *NF-2*) are on separate chromosomes, *NF-1* being responsible for 90% of cases and *NF-2* for 10%.

It is the most common neurocutaneous disorder, with a prevalence of 1 in 3000 of the population.

The most common form of neurofibromatosis (NF-1) is referred to as **von Recklinghausen's disease**.

This comprises cafe au lait spots (which may be present from birth), freckles in skin folds, neurofibromas, plexiform neuromas, bilateral hamartomas of the iris, neurological impairment and bone involvement.

The neurofibromas are derived from all the nerve elements, including the nerve cells, sheath cells and connective tissue. Histologically, they are therefore multicellular and while not encapsulated they are well circumscribed.

They appear as soft pedunculated lesions from puberty onwards. They are skin-coloured or purplish and may be pruritic. Commonly, they may eventually compress surrounding structures. Sometimes, they may become malignant, with a lifetime risk of 7–10% of sarcomatous change, chiefly in non-cutaneous sites. In the gut, a neurofibroma may be one of the causes of polyp formation.

The less common form of neurofibromatosis (NF-2) is associated with bilateral **acoustic neuromas**. There may also be meningioma or spinal cord neurofibroma, which is usually subdural and found in the thoracic region. Sometimes, there may be associated glioma, cataracts or skin lesions.

Neurofibromatosis may sometimes present with skin lesions in a single dermatome or with an associated **phaeochromocytoma** (q.v.) and thus hypertension.

*Treatment is with **excision** of symptomatic lesions. **Ketotifen** may be useful both for symptoms and to decrease tumour growth.*

Genetic counselling should be undertaken.

See also
- Lung tumours,
- Mediastinal diseases,
- Neuropathy – 7. Guillain–Barré syndrome,
- Pigmentation disorders.

Bibliography

Martuza RL, Eldridge R. Neurofibromatosis 2 (bilateral acoustic neurofibromatosis). *N Engl J Med* 1988; 318: 684.

Reynolds RM, Browning GG, Nawroz I, et al. Von Recklinghausen's neurofibromatosis: neurofibromatosis type 1. *Lancet* 2003; 361: 1552.

Riccardi VM. Von Recklinghausen's neurofibromatosis. *N Engl J Med* 1981; 305: 1617.

Neuroleptic malignant syndrome

The **neuroleptic malignant syndrome** (NMS) is a rare, non-dose-related, idiosyncratic reaction which may occur potentially to any antipsychotic agent, though usually to phenothiazines. Less commonly, it may be caused by the atypical (or 'second-generation') antipsychotics, particularly clozapine, olanzapine, quetiapine and risperidone, though given the great chemical heterogeneity among this group of agents, this complication cannot represent a true class effect. Occasionally, it may be caused by a dopamine antagonist given for non-psychiatric indications, e.g. metoclopramide for nausea.

Its pathogenesis is unclear, but it probably represents dysfunction of the hypothalamus and basal ganglia due to dopamine antagonism.

It may be more common in patients who are already dehydrated or who receive large initial doses of neuroleptic medication. On the other hand, the culprit medication(s) may have been unchanged over many months prior to the onset of this acute complication.

It is associated with fever (q.v.), sweating (q.v.), rigidity, fluctuating consciousness and autonomic instability. These clinical features generally evolve over a few days.

Laboratory investigations usually show elevated CK levels, renal impairment due to myoglobinuria (q.v.) and dehydration and abnormal liver function tests.

The mortality has been reported to be possibly as high as 20%, but the condition is too rare to calculate a true mortality.

> Diagnostic differentiation of NMS both from **agitated delirium** (q.v.) and from the **serotonin syndrome** (q.v.) is clinically important, because
> - treatment of a mistaken diagnosis of agitated delirium with an antipsychotic could exacerbate NMS if the latter instead was present, and
> - treatment of a mistaken diagnosis of NMS with bromocriptine could exacerbate the serotonin syndrome if the latter instead was present.

Treatment comprises drug cessation and general supportive measures.
- ***Bromocriptine**, a dopamine agonist, and **dantrolene**, a direct-acting muscle relaxant (see Malignant hyperthermia), are probably helpful. **Benzodiazepines** may be of symptomatic benefit.*

There is a high incidence of recurrence if the culprit drug is resumed, so that alternative psychiatric therapy is required.

See also
- Baclofen,
- Pyrexia,
- Rhabdomyolysis.

Bibliography

Bienvenu OJ, Neufeld KJ, Needham DM. Treatment of four psychiatric emergencies in the intensive care unit. *Crit Care Med* 2012; 40: 2662.

Caroff SN, Mann SC. Neuroleptic malignant syndrome. *Med Clin North Am* 1993; 77: 185.

Guze BH, Baxter LR. Neuroleptic malignant syndrome. *N Engl J Med* 1985; 313: 163.

Harradine PG, Williams SE, Doherty SR. Neuroleptic malignant syndrome: an underdiagnosed condition. *Med J Aust* 2001; 174: 593.

Kornhuber J, Weller M. Neuroleptic malignant syndrome. *Curr Opin Neurol Neurosurg* 1994; 7: 353.

Rosenberg MR, Green M. Neuroleptic malignant syndrome: review of response to therapy. *Ach Intern Med* 1989; 149: 1927.

Shaw A, Mathews EE. Postoperative neuroleptic malignant syndrome. *Anesthesiology* 1995; 50: 246.

Neurology

Many neurological disorders are commonly seen in Intensive Care, such as those related to cerebrovascular disease, trauma, headache, epilepsy or meningitis. On the other hand, there is a large number of less frequently encountered neurological conditions, many of which raise important issues of diagnosis or management, and these are considered in this book. These conditions include

- Acute flaccid myelitis,
- Amnesia,
- Amyotrophic lateral sclerosis,
- Anorexia nervosa,
- Arnold–Chiari malformation,
- Autonomic dysreflexia,
- Bell's palsy,
- Benign intracranial hypertension,
- Central pontine myelinolysis,
- Cerebellar degeneration,
- Charcot–Marie–Tooth disease,
- CINMA,
- Critical illness myopathy,
- Critical illness neuromuscular abnormality,
- Critical illness polyneuropathy,
- Delirium,
- Dementia,
- Demyelinating disease,
- Eaton Lambert syndrome,
- Encephalitis,
- Encephalopathy,
- Epidural abscess,
- Friedreich's ataxia,
- Guillain–Barré syndrome,
- Hemianopia,
- Horner's syndrome,
- Hydrocephalus,
- Idiopathic inflammatory myopathy,
- Intensive Care Unit-acquired weakness,
- Kennedy's disease,
- Korsakoff syndrome,
- Lateral medullary syndrome,
- Leukoencephalopathy,
- Meningoencephalitis,
- Miller Fisher syndrome,
- Motor neuron disease,
- Multifocal motor neuropathy,

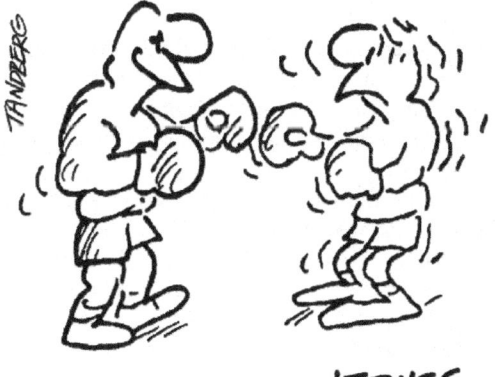

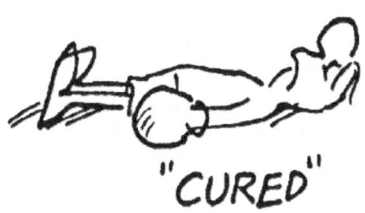

- Multiple sclerosis,
- Muscular dystrophies,
- Myasthenia gravis,
- Myelitis,
- Myelopathy,
- Myopathy,
- Myotonia,
- Neuropathy,
- Neurofibromatosis,
- Neuromyelitis optica,
- Ophthalmoplegia,
- Optic neuritis,
- Osmotic demyelination syndrome,
- Papilloedema,
- Periodic paralysis,
- Peroneal muscular atrophy.
- Polyneuritis,
- Polyneuropathy,
- Posterior reversible encephalopathy,
- PRES,
- Progressive multifocal leukoencephalopathy,
- Ptosis,
- Ramsay Hunt syndrome,
- Restless legs,
- Retinal haemorrhage,
- Retrobulbar neuritis,
- Reversible posterior leukoencephalopathy,
- Shy–Drager disease,
- Subacute sclerosing panencephalitis,
- Syringomyelia,
- Tardive dyskinesia,
- Tinnitus,
- Transverse myelitis,
- Uveitis,
- Vertigo,
- Wernicke–Korsakoff syndrome.

Bibliography

Arieff AI, Guisado R, Massry SG, et al. Central nervous system pH in uremia and the effects of hemodialysis. *J Clin Invest* 1976; 58: 306.

Arieff AI, Massry SG, Barrientos A, et al. Brain water and electrolyte metabolism in uremia: effects of slow and rapid hemodialysis. *Kidney Int* 1973; 4: 177.

Bhardwaj A, Williams MA, Hanley DF, eds. Critical Care of Stroke. In: *New Horizons*. Baltimore: Williams & Wilkins and SCCM. 1997; 5: no. 4.

Bolton CF. Sepsis and the systemic inflammatory response syndrome: Neuromuscular manifestations. *Crit Care Med* 1996; 24: 1408.

Bolton CF. Neuromuscular conditions in the intensive care unit. *Intens Care Med* 1996; 22: 841.

Caplan LR, Brass LM, DeWitt LD, et al. Transcranial Doppler ultrasound: present status. *Neurology* 1990; 40: 696.

Chang CWJ. Neurologic complications of critical illness and transplantation. *Curr Opin Crit Care* 1999; 5: 112.

Charness ME, Simon RP, Greenberg DA. Ethanol and the nervous system. *N Engl J Med* 1989; 321: 442.

Chiappa KH, Ropper AH. Evoked potentials in clinical medicine. *N Engl J Med* 1982; 306: 1140 & 1205.

Ciavarella D, Wuest D, Strauss RG, et al. Management of neurologic disorders. *J Clin Apheresis* 1993; 8: 242.

Fraser CL, Arieff AI. Nervous system complications of uremia. *Ann Intern Med* 1988; 109: 143.

Ghaoui R, Clarke N, Hollingworth P, et al. Muscle disorders: the latest investigations. *Intern Med J* 2013; 43: 970.

Hansen-Flaschen J. Neuromuscular complications of critical illness. *Pulm Perspect* 1997; 14(4): 1.

Hughes AJ, Biggs BA. Parasitic worms of the central nervous system. *Intern Med J* 2002; 32: 541.

Kelly BJ, Luce JM. The diagnosis and management of neuromuscular diseases causing respiratory failure. *Chest* 1991; 99: 1485.

Kirkman MA, Citerio G, Smith M. The intensive care management of acute ischemic stroke: an overview. *Intens Care Med* 2014; 40: 640.

Klebanoff LM, ed. Neurology. In: *Scientific American Medicine*. Hamilton: Dekker Medicine. 2020.

Knochel J. Neuromuscular manifestations of electrolyte disorders. *Am J Med* 1982; 72: 521.

Lansberg MG, O'Donnell MJ, Khatri P, et al. Antithrombotic and thrombolytic therapy for ischemic stroke. *Chest* 2012; 141: S601.

Le Roux P, Menon DK, Vespa G, et al. Consensus summary statement of the International Multidisciplinary Consensus Conference on Multimodality Monitoring in Neurocritical Care. *Intens Care Med* 2014; 40: 1189.

Lyons MK, Meyer FB. Cerebrospinal fluid physiology and the management of increased intracranial pressure. *Mayo Clin Proc* 1990; 65: 684.

Mandel JL. Dystrophin: the gene and its product. *Nature* 1989; 339: 584.

Marton KI, Gean AD. The spinal tap: a new look at an old test. *Ann Intern Med* 1986; 104: 840.

McMahon SB, Kolzenburg M, Tracey I, et al. *Wall and Melzack's Textbook of Pain*. 6th edition. Edinburgh: Elsevier. 2013.

Mirski MA, Varelas PN. Diagnosis and treatment of seizures in the adult intensive care unit. *Contemporary Critical Care* 2003; 1: 1.

Miller DH, Raps EC, eds. *Critical Care Neurology.* Woburn: Butterworth-Heinemann. 1999.

Moore PM. Diagnosis and management of isolated angiitis of the central nervous system. *Neurology* 1989; 39: 167.

Morantz RA, Walsh JW, eds. *Brain Tumors.* New York: Marcel Dekker. 1994.

Moskowitz MA. The visceral organ brain. *Neurology* 1991; 41: 182.

Polkey MI, Moxham J. Clinical aspects of respiratory muscle dysfunction in the critically ill. *Chest* 2001; 119: 926.

Raskin NH, Fishman RA. Neurologic disorders in renal failure. *N Engl J Med* 1976; 294: 143.

Rosenberg RN. Biochemical genetics of neurologic disease. *N Engl J Med* 1981; 305: 1181.

Rosenberg RN, ed. *Atlas of Clinical Neurology.* 4th edition. New York: Springer. 2019.

Schwartzman RJ, McLellan TL. Reflex sympathetic dystrophy: a review. *Arch Neurol* 1987; 44: 555.

Sharshar T, Citerio G, Andrews PJD, et al. Neurological examination of critically ill patients. *Intens Care Med* 2014; 40: 484.

Strandgaard S, Paulson OB. Cerebral autoregulation. *Stroke* 1984; 15: 413.

Strange K. Regulation of solute and water balance and cell volume in the central nervous system. *J Am Soc Nephrol* 1992; 3: 12.

Suarez JI, Bershad EM, Rao CPV, eds. *Critical Care Neurology and Neurosurgery.* 2nd edition. New York: Springer. 2020.

Swift TR. Disorders of neuromuscular transmission other than myasthenia gravis. *Muscle Nerve* 1981; 4: 334.

Tonner DR, Schlechte JA. Neurologic complications of thyroid and parathyroid disease. *Med Clin North Am* 1993; 77: 251.

Torbey MT, ed. *Neurocritical Care.* 2nd edition. Cambridge: Cambridge University Press. 2019.

Wijdicks EFM. *Neurologic Complications of Critical Illness.* 3nd edition. Oxford: Oxford University Press. 2009.

Zweiman B, Levinson AI. Immunologic aspects of neurological and neuromuscular diseases. *JAMA* 1992; 268: 2918.

Neuromyelitis optica See
- Demyelinating diseases – 4. Transverse myelitis.

Neuropathy

Neuropathy is usually a polyneuropathy. Sometimes, it may be a mononeuropathy or an asymmetrical mononeuropathy multiplex. It may be either motor or sensory or more commonly both motor and sensory. Mononeuropathy is commonly due to a local cause.

The types of **polyneuropathy** include
1. genetic neuropathies,
2. toxic neuropathies,
3. inflammatory neuropathies,
4. systemic disease-induced neuropathies,
5. critical illness neuropathy,
6. diabetic neuropathy,
7. Guillain–Barré syndrome (GBS) and its variants,
8. multifocal motor neuropathy.

1. **Genetic neuropathies** include
   - Charcot–Marie–Tooth (CMT) disease (q.v.).
2. **Toxic neuropathies** may be produced by
   - drugs
     - such as amiodarone, antimicrobials (chloramphenicol, dapsone, isoniazid, nitrofurantoin), antiretrovirals, colchicine, cytotoxics, gold, hydralazine, phenytoin, statins,
     - while cessation of the culprit drug leads to recovery, this may take some months and there may even be worsening in the meantime,
   - heavy metals (q.v.)
     - such as arsenic and lead, in particular,
   - poisons, mainly industrial chemical agents
     - such as acrylamide, hexacarbons, organophosphates, rapeseed oil, trichloroethylene.
3. **Inflammatory neuropathies** may occur in
   - AIDS (q.v.),
   - diphtheria (q.v.),
   - leprosy (q.v.).
4. **Systemic disease-induced neuropathies** can be produced by
   - malignancy
     - as a paraneoplastic phenomenon (q.v.),
     - especially in carcinoma of the breast, lung or ovary, or in multiple myeloma (q.v.),
   - collagen-vascular diseases (q.v.),
   - alcoholism,
   - nutritional deficiency,
   - sarcoidosis (q.v.),
   - Lyme disease (q.v.),
   - porphyria (q.v.),
   - uraemia,
   - vitamin B_{12} deficiency (q.v.).

5. **Critical illness neuropathy**
Critical illness neuropathy/polyneuropathy (CIP) is the most common and best recognized **critical illness neuromuscular abnormality** (CINMA)(q.v.). It comprises axonal degeneration of peripheral nerves seen in patients with sepsis and/or multiorgan failure (MOF) of prolonged duration. It may therefore represent the neurological manifestation of MOF (q.v.). It is not generally apparent until after at least a week of critical illness.

This condition was first described in the early 1980s, but no specific aetiology has yet been demonstrated. In patients with multiorgan failure prospectively examined electrophysiologically, the prevalence has been found to be as high as 70%. However, the overall incidence in Intensive Care patients appears to vary greatly, and even mild clinical features are found in only about half of those suspected on EMG of having CIP.

Motor features are generally more prominent than sensory or autonomic, with generalized weakness and wasting due to muscle denervation. There is symmetrical flaccid paresis, particularly of the lower limbs, with reduced deep tendon reflexes. In severe cases, breathing and swallowing can be affected. There is relative preservation of cranial nerve function. If the phrenic nerve is involved, prolonged ventilator dependence may result, and this has been reported to be particularly problematic in some patients with acute respiratory distress syndrome (ARDS)(q.v.).

The diagnosis can of course be difficult, because of the limitations of neurological examination in Intensive Care patients receiving sedation and possibly muscle relaxants and because of the many other causes of neurological dysfunction seen in such patients. The EMG shows an axonal polyneuropathy, and there is abnormal spontaneous muscle activity typical of denervation. Conduction velocities are normal, whereas they are reduced in demyelination (as in Guillain–Barré syndrome – q.v.).

Originally, CIP was distinguished in particular from an acute myopathy, such as that typically seen in Intensive Care patients who have had prolonged neuromuscular blockade and/or corticosteroids (see Myopathy), but more recently it has been recognized that in most patients axonal lesions probably coexist with myopathy. Thus, the better term is **CINMA** or neuromyopathy, which encompasses impairments of nerve, neuromuscular junction and muscle. While it has also been referred to as **critical illness polyneuromyopathy** (CIPNM), the more general term of **intensive care unit–acquired weakness (ICU-AW)** (q.v.) may be more appropriate.

The mortality is reported to be about 60%, but clearly this is also the mortality of the severe underlying conditions. The motor disturbances of CIP are not always reversible, even with prolonged rehabilitation.

Despite extensive study, no specific therapies have been found effective.

6. **Diabetic neuropathy**
A neuropathy may be found in about 60% of patients with either insulin-dependent or non-insulin-dependent diabetes mellitus. The precise mechanism of production of this neuropathy is unclear.

Polyneuropathy is seen in about half of these cases. There is symmetrical distal mainly sensory involvement.

It is often subclinical, but mild symptoms are sometimes seen. These are especially paraesthesiae of the lower limbs, occasionally with sensory loss and even weakness and decreased reflexes. The condition is worse at night and can be very painful.

In some patients, it eventually becomes severe, with associated autonomic involvement, including urinary retention, faecal incontinence, impotence and postural hypotension.

Mononeuropathy is seen in about a third of cases.

Like diabetic polyneuropathy, it is also often subclinical. Symptoms when seen relate usually to the carpal tunnel syndrome. Occasionally, other nerves are involved, either singly or combined, such as
- cranial (especially VII, III and VI),
- ulnar,
- femoral,
- sciatic,
- peroneal,
- lateral femoral cutaneous,
- thoracic roots.

Sometimes, diabetic amyotrophy may be produced, with painful wasting and weakness of the proximal muscles of the lower limbs.

The EMG in diabetic neuropathy typically shows the abnormal nerve conduction of denervation. CSF examination shows a moderately increased protein.

The neuropathy may be improved with good diabetic control. Pain may be alleviated in some cases by **carbamazepine** *or* **tricyclic antidepressants**.

7. **Guillain–Barré syndrome** (GBS) and its variants
See Guillain–Barré syndrome.
8. **Multifocal motor neuropathy**
See Motor neuron disease.

The types of **mononeuropathy** include the following.

- **Carpal tunnel syndrome** (the most common entrapment neuropathy)
- **Brachial plexus neuropathy**
- **Isolated palsies**

These are usually due to a local disease (or sometimes diabetes, see above) and involve the radial, ulnar, peroneal or lateral femoral cutaneous nerves. Peripheral nerve entrapment can occur due to local compression, and about 50 such neuropathies have been described.

- **Cranial neuropathies**

If multiple, they are usually paraneoplastic, though sometimes they may be diabetic.

Individual cranial neuropathies (I–XII) may be caused as follows.

I
- meningioma,
- meningitis,
- post-viral,
- trauma,

II
- optic atrophy, which is often nutritional,
- optic neuritis (q.v.),
- tumour, such as craniopharyngioma, glioma, pituitary adenoma,

III, IV, VI
- see Ophthalmoplegia,

V
- trigeminal neuralgia (tic douloureux),
- disorders of the posterior cranial fossa or base of skull,

VII
- Bell's palsy (q.v.),
- lesions of the pons or cerebellopontine angle,
- sarcoidosis (q.v.),
- Guillain–Barré syndrome (q.v.),
- hemifacial spasm (this and related dystonic disorders are now being usefully treated with botulinum toxin),

VIII
- acoustic neuroma,
- aminoglycoside toxicity,
- brainstem lesions,
- Meniere's disease,
- meningitis,
- vestibular neuronitis,

IX, X, XI
- brainstem lesions,
- cervical infection, trauma or tumour,
- jugular foramen syndrome,
- motor neuron disease (q.v.),

XII
- cervical infection, trauma or tumour,
- motor neuron disease (q.v.).

Bibliography

Ashbury AK. Understanding diabetic neuropathy. *N Engl J Med* 1988; 319: 577.

Bercker S, Weber-Carstens S, Deja M, et al. Critical illness polyneuropathy and myopathy in patients with acute respiratory distress syndrome. *Crit Care Med* 2005; 33: 711.

Berek K, Margreiter J, Willeit J, et al. Polyneuropathies in critically ill patients: a prospective evaluation. *Intens Care Med* 1996; 22: 849.

Bleck TP. The expanding spectrum of critical illness polyneuropathy. *Crit Care Med* 1996; 24: 1282.

Bolton CF. Sepsis and the systemic inflammatory response syndrome: neuromuscular manifestations. *Crit Care Med* 1996; 24: 1408.

Bolton CF. Critical illness polyneuropathy and myopathy. *Crit Care Med* 2001; 29: 2388.

Bolton CF, Gilbert JJ, Hahn AF, et al. Polyneuropathy in critically ill patients. *J Neurol Neurosurg Psychiatry* 1984; 47: 1223.

Bromberg MB, Feldman EL, Albers JW. Chronic inflammatory demyelinating polyradiculoneuropathy. *Neurology* 1992; 42: 1157.

Chad DA, Lacomis D. Critically ill patients with newly acquired weakness: the clinicopathological spectrum. *Ann Neurol* 1994; 35: 257.

Dalakas MC, Engel WK. Chronic relapsing (dysimmune) polyneuropathy: pathogenesis and treatment. *Ann Neurol* 1981; 9 (suppl.): 134.

Davis GA, Day TJ. Peripheral nerve entrapment: how to diagnose and when to refer. *Med J Aust* 2022; 216: 126.

De Jonghe B, Cook D, Sharshar T, et al. Acquired neuromuscular disorders in critically ill patients: a systematic review. *Intens Care Med* 1998; 24: 1242.

De Jonghe B, Sharshar T, Hopkinson N, et al. Paresis following mechanical ventilation. *Curr Opin Crit Care* 2004; 10: 47.

de Letter M-ACJ, Schmitz PIM, Visser LH, et al. Risk factors for the development of polyneuropathy and myopathy in critically ill patients. *Crit Care Med* 2001; 29: 2281.

Dyck PJ, Kratz KM, Karnes JL, et al. The prevalence by staged severity of various types of diabetic neuropathy, retinopathy, and nephropathy in a population-based cohort: the Rochester Diabetic Neuropathy Study. *Neurology* 1993; 43: 817.

Fuller GN, Jacobs JM, Guiloff RJ. Nature and incidence of peripheral neuropathy syndromes in HIV infection. *J Neurol Neurosurg Psychiatry* 1993; 56: 372.

Garnacho-Montero J, Mandrazo-Osuna J, Garcia-Garmendia JL, et al. Critical illness polyneuropathy: risk factors and clinical consequences. *Intens Care Med* 2001; 27: 1288.

Hall JB, Griffiths RD, eds. ICU-acquired weakness: proceedings of a round table conference in Brussels, Belgium, March 2009. *Crit Care Med* 2009; 37: S295.

Halperin J, Luft BJ, Volkman DJ, et al. Lyme neuroborreliosis: peripheral nervous system manifestations. *Brain* 1990; 113: 1207.

Hansen-Flaschen J. Neuromuscular complications of critical illness. *Pulmonary Perspectives* 1997; 14(4): 1.

Harrison MS. 'Epidemic vertigo' – 'vestibular neuronitis': a clinical study. *Brain* 1962; 85: 613.

Hillbom M, Wennberg A. Prognosis of alcoholic peripheral neuropathy. *J Neurol Neurosurg Psychiatry* 1984; 47: 699.

Hund EF, Fogel W, Krieger D, et al. Critical illness polyneuropathy: clinical findings and outcomes of a frequent cause of neuromuscular weaning failure. *Crit Care Med* 1996; 24: 1328.

Latronico N. Neuromuscular alterations in the critically ill patient: critical illness myopathy, critical illness neuropathy, or both? *Intens Care Med* 2003; 29: 1411.

Latronico N, Fenzi F, Recupero D, et al. Critical illness myopathy and neuropathy. *Lancet* 1996; 347: 1579.

Leijten FSS, De Weerd AW, Poortvliet DCJ, et al. Critical illness polyneuropathy in multiple organ dysfunction syndrome and weaning from the ventilator. *Intens Care Med* 1996; 22: 856.

Maramattom BV, Wijdicks EFM. Acute neuromuscular weakness in the intensive care unit. *Crit Care Med* 2006; 34: 2835.

Morantz RA, Walsh JW, eds. *Brain Tumors*. New York: Marcel Dekker. 1994.

Nakamo KK. The entrapment neuropathies. *Muscle Nerve* 1978; 1: 264.

Nates JL, Cooper DJ, Day B, et al. Acute weakness syndromes in critically ill patients – a reappraisal. *Anaesth Intens Care* 1997; 25: 502.

Pestronk A. Motor neuropathies, motor neuron disorders, and antiglycolipid antibodies. *Muscle Nerve* 1991; 14: 927.

Polkey MI, Moxham J. Clinical aspects of respiratory muscle dysfunction in the critically ill. *Chest* 2001; 119: 926.

Schweickert WD, Hall J. ICU-acquired weakness. *Chest* 2007; 131: 1541.

Segredo V, Caldwell JE, Matthay MA, et al. Persistent paralysis in critically ill patients after long-term administration of vecuronium. *N Engl J Med* 1992; 327: 524.

Spies JM. Cranial and peripheral neuropathies. *Med J Aust* 2001; 174: 598.

Sweet WH. The treatment of trigeminal neuralgia (tic douloureux). *N Engl J Med* 1986; 315: 174.

Tonner DR, Schlechte JA. Neurologic complications of thyroid and parathyroid disease. *Med Clin North Am* 1993; 77: 251.

van Mook WNKA, Hulsewe-Evers RPMG. Critical illness polyneuropathy. *Curr Opin Crit Care* 2002; 8: 302.

Walsh TS. Pharmacologic therapies for ICU-acquired weakness: a long road ahead. *Crit Care Med* 2016; 44: 1245.

Williams AC, Sturman S, Kelsey S, et al. The neuropathy of the critically ill. *BMJ* 1986; 293: 790.

Windebank AJ, Blexrud MD, Dyck PJ, et al. The syndrome of acute sensory neuropathy: clinical features and electrophysiologic and pathologic changes. *Neurology* 1990; 40: 584.

Zochodne DW, Bolton CF, Wells GA, et al. Critical illness polyneuropathy: A complication of sepsis and multiple organ failure. *Brain* 1987; 110: 819.

Neutropenia

Neutropenia refers to an absolute neutrophil count in peripheral blood of $<2 \times 10^9/L$. Often it is $<1 \times 10^9/L$; in severe cases, it is $<0.5 \times 10^9/L$. However, in some ethnic populations, neutrophil counts as low as $1 \times 10^9/L$ may in fact be normal.

Since neutrophils have a circulating half-life of only 6–8 hr, the bone marrow must produce and release up to 10^{10} neutrophils daily in healthy individuals, with a much higher production capacity in inflammatory illness. The disappearance of neutrophils from the circulation appears to be a random process, unlike that of red blood cells and platelets which is related to senescence.

The causes of neutropenia are
- decreased production,
- increased removal,
- sequestration.

Decreased production is due usually to
- drugs, the most common cause (see below),
- viral infection,

- bone marrow hypoplasia or infiltration, or less commonly to
- folic acid or vitamin B_{12} deficiency (q.v.),
- Felty's syndrome (q.v.),
- cachexia.

Genetic, cyclic and chronic benign forms of neutropenia due to decreased production sometimes occur.

Increased removal from the circulation occurs
- in immunological disease
  - especially Felty's syndrome (q.v.),
- with drugs (see below).

Sequestration of neutrophils occurs
- in splenomegaly (q.v.),
- with toxic margination
  - best known in Gram-negative sepsis.

Drugs which impair granulopoiesis may do so via cytotoxic, immunological or idiosyncratic mechanisms. Most cases recover within 2 days to 2 weeks.
- **Cytotoxic effects** are produced by a wide variety of agents. These include
  - cancer chemotherapeutic agents (most commonly),
  - benzene and related compounds.
- **Immunological mechanisms** are invoked by
  - beta-lactam antibiotics,
  - hydralazine,
  - procainamide,
  - quinidine.
- **Idiosyncratic mechanisms** are involved with
  - analgesics, especially NSAIDs (classically phenylbutazone but also indomethacin),
  - antibiotics, including ampicillin and chloramphenicol,
  - antihistamines,
  - antithyroid drugs,
  - cimetidine,
  - phenytoin,
  - procainamide,
  - quinidine,
  - ranitidine,
  - sulphonamides,
  - tranquillizers, especially phenothiazines and more recently clozapine.

Clinically, the neutropenia may be found coincidentally or because of an infection. Conversely, infection must be presumed in a patient with known neutropenia who becomes febrile (>38.3°C).

Such infections may produce diminished signs because of the absence of pus, and they typically respond poorly to antibiotics. They particularly involve the skin, respiratory tract and urinary tract, and they are due to an increased risk of infection by those pathogens which normally colonize the body's surfaces. However, in about 40% of patients with fever and neutropenia, no organisms can be identified despite a careful search and antibiotic therapy must therefore be empirical.

*Treatment is primarily of the underlying problem, but occasional cases respond to **corticosteroids** or even **lithium**.*
- ***Granulocyte-colony stimulating factor** (G-CSF) is effective in many types of neutropenia.*
- ***Antibiotics** in this setting need to be bactericidal. Antibiotic regimens need to be carefully considered, because prolonged use of broad-spectrum agents can lead to colonization and infection by resistant organisms, including fungi.*

Recurrent or unusual infections in patients with a normal neutrophil count should raise the possibility of a disorder of neutrophil function.

Bibliography

Bain BJ. Ethnic and sex differences in the total and differential white cell count and platelet count. *J Clin Pathol* 1996; 49: 664.

Cowburn AS, Condliffe AM, Farahi N, et al. Advances in neutrophil biology: clinical implications. *Chest* 2008; 134: 606.

Dale D, Guerry D, Wewerka J, et al. *Chronic neutropenia. Medicine* 1979; 58: 128.

Jones RN. Contemporary antimicrobial susceptibility patterns of bacterial pathogens commonly associated with febrile patients with neutropenia. *Clin Infect Dis* 1999; 29: 495.

Klastersky JA, Meert A-P. Understanding the risk for infection in patients with neutropenia. *Intens Care Med* 2016; 42: 268.

Lingaratnam S, Slavin MA, Koczwara B, et al. Introduction to the Australian consensus guidelines for the management of neutropenic fever in adult cancer patients, 2010/2011. *Intern Med J* 2011; 41 (suppl. 1): 75.

Palmblad JE, von dem Borne AE. Idiopathic, immune, infectious, and idiosyncratic neutropenias. *Semin Hematol* 2002; 39: 113.

Schram AM, Berliner N. Nonmalignant disorders of leukocytes. In: *Scientific American Medicine.* Hamilton: Dekker Medicine. 2020.

van der Klauw MM, Wilson JH, Stricker BH. Drug-associated agranulocytosis. *Am J Haematol* 1998; 57: 206.

Vincent PC. Drug-induced aplastic anemia and agranulocytosis. *Drugs* 1986; 31: 52.

Neutrophilia

Neutrophilia refers to an increased peripheral blood neutrophil count of $>7.5 \times 10^9$/L. A count of $>50 \times 10^9$/L is referred to as a leukemoid reaction.

Neutrophilia is a very common finding and may be produced by several mechanisms, namely
1. **increased production and/or release**, due to
   - inflammatory diseases,
   - malignancy,
   - lithium (q.v.),
   - cytokine administration, e.g. G-CSF or GM-CSF,
2. **decreased exit from the circulation**, due to
   - physical activity,
   - corticosteroids,
3. **decreased sequestration and/or margination**, due to
   - physical activity,
   - corticosteroids,
   - adrenergic influences.

   This third mechanism causes a pseudo-neutrophilia, because the blood pool of neutrophils is not in fact increased.

Spurious or artefactual neutrophilia may occur in the presence of platelet clumping or cryoglobulinaemia (q.v.).
Any treatment is of the underlying disorder.

Newcastle disease *See*
- Conjunctivitis.

Nitric oxide *See*
- Acute pulmonary oedema,
- Heat stroke,
- High altitude – Pulmonary oedema,
- Immune complex disease,
- Methaemoglobinaemia,
- Methylene blue,
- Pulmonary hypertension – Primary pulmonary hypertension.

Nitrous oxide *See*
- Haematology,
- Megaloblastic anaemia,
- Pregnancy,
- Vitamin B_{12} deficiency.

Bibliography
Myles PS, Leslie K, Silbert B, et al. A review of the risks and benefits of nitrous oxide in current anaesthetic practice. *Anaesth Intens Care* 2004; 32: 165.

Nocardiosis

Nocardiosis is an uncommon infection caused by one of the species of the genus *Nocardia*. Like other actinomycetes, *Nocardia* was originally thought to be a fungus because of its filamentous hyphae-like appearance. In fact, it is an unusual Gram-positive bacillus, but unlike *Actinomyces* (see Actinomycosis) it is aerobic and acid-fast on staining.

Many species of *Nocardia* can cause human disease, but the most important is *N. asteroides*, itself now recognized to include several subtypes, so that it is now referred to as the *N. asteroides* complex. *Nocardia* are found in the environment worldwide, particularly in soil, rotting vegetation and water. Inhalation is the usual route of entry into humans.

As the major host defence mechanism is cell-mediated immunity, most infections are found in immunocompromised patients. *Nocardia* infections are suppurative, with the potential to disseminate systemically (particularly to the central nervous system).
- The lungs are the usual site of primary infection, with variable consequences including nodules (q.v.), cavitation (q.v.), lobar consolidation, interstitial infiltrates (q.v.) and pleural effusion (q.v.).
- Because of the particular tropism of *Nocardia* for neural tissue, brain abscess is a common complication. Meningitis may sometimes be seen. A CT scan of the brain should thus be performed in all patients with suspected or confirmed *Nocardia* infection, whatever the original clinical presentation.
- Cutaneous infections are sometimes seen, either as a primary lesion or as a manifestation of disseminated infection.
- Most sites in the body, including prostheses, have been reported as susceptible to *Nocardia* infection when it is disseminated.

Diagnosis requires microbiological identification of the organism in a suitable clinical sample. However, laboratory confirmation can be difficult and delayed, and speciation can be technically challenging. Specialized susceptibility testing is important to guide antibiotic selection.

*Treatment with **cotrimoxazole** is the usual first-line recommendation, but several other agents are also usually* effective, including third-generation cephalosporins, carbapenems, amikacin (but not tobramycin), doxycycline, tigecycline and linezolid. **Combination therapy** given intravenously for up to 6 weeks is required for serious infections. Ongoing oral treatment needs to be continued for at least 1 year in such cases because of the high risk of relapse.

Cerebral or pulmonary abscesses may require **surgical drainage**.

Bibliography
Brown-Elliott BA, Brown JM, Conville PS, et al. Clinical and laboratory features of *Nocardia* spp. based on current molecular taxonomy. *Clin Microbiol Rev* 2006; 19: 259.
Lederman ER, Crum NF. A case series and focused review of nocardiosis: clinical and microbiologic aspects. *Medicine (Baltimore)* 2004; 83: 300.
Lerner PL. Nocardiosis *Clin Infect Dis* 1996; 22: 891.
Threlkeld SC, Hooper DC. Update on management of patients with *Nocardia* infection. *Curr Clin Top Infect Dis* 1997; 17: 1.
Wilson JW. Nocardiosis: updates and clinical overview. *Mayo Clin Proc* 2012; 87: 403.

Non-alcoholic fatty liver disease

Non-alcoholic fatty liver disease (NAFLD) refers to the range of liver injury involving fat accumulation which resembles that seen from alcohol damage but which occurs without alcohol exposure (or at least with <20 g of alcohol consumption per week). The histological spectrum of this clinicopathological entity ranges from simple fat excess in hepatocytes without inflammation (**hepatic steatosis**) to fat accumulation with necrosis and inflammation (**steatohepatitis**, see below).

The cause of the excessive accumulation of triglycerides in the liver remains uncertain, but it theoretically involves excess delivery to the liver of free fatty acids (as in obesity or overfeeding), impaired excretion by the liver of free fatty acids as very-low-density lipoprotein (VLDL), or impaired oxidation of free fatty acids. Insulin resistance is a key association (and perhaps aetiological factor), and there is typically associated obesity, type 2 diabetes, hypertension, dyslipidaemia and metabolic syndrome. Not surprisingly therefore, NAFLD is very common, with a prevalence of 20% or more of the population in developed countries, where it has become the most frequent cause of chronic liver disease.

The diagnosis of NAFLD can be reliably made using a score ('fatty liver index') based on clinical parameters and laboratory tests. The later development of fibrosis in high-risk patients can be assessed using scan evidence (elastography) of liver stiffness.

The majority of patients have no clinically significant consequences of NAFLD, but some patients (up to 10%) eventually develop hepatic fibrosis, end-stage liver disease or hepatocellular carcinoma (q.v.). Thus, given the high prevalence of NAFLD, the absolute numbers of patients with chronic liver disease are greater for NASH than for any other cause of liver disease.

Bibliography
Donnelly KL, Smith CI, Schwarzenberg SJ, et al. Sources of fatty acids stored in liver and secreted via lipoproteins in patients with nonalcoholic fatty liver disease. *J Clin Invest* 2005; 115: 1343.
Huang TD, Behary J, Zekry A. Non-alcoholic fatty liver disease: a review of epidemiology, risk factors, diagnosis and management. *Intern Med J* 2020; 50: 1038.
Matteoni CA, Younossi ZM, Gramlich T, et al. Nonalcoholic fatty liver disease: a spectrum of clinical pathological severity. *Gastroenterology* 1999; 116: 1413.
Younossi Z, Anstee QM, Marietti M, et al. Global burden of NAFLD and NASH: trends, predictions, risk factors and prevention. *Nat Rev Gastroenterol Hepatol* 2018; 15: 11.
Younossi ZM, Koenig AB, Abdelatif D, et al. Global epidemiology of non-alcoholic fatty liver disease: meta-analytic assessment of prevalence, incidence, and outcomes. *Hepatology* 2016; 64: 73.

Non-alcoholic steatohepatitis

Non-alcoholic steatohepatitis (NASH) refers to the severe end of the spectrum of non-alcoholic fatty liver disease (NAFLD, see above). Unlike NAFLD, the prevalence of NASH is uncertain because non-invasive diagnostic methods have poor sensitivity.

Histologically, in addition to steatosis, there are inflammatory changes and hepatocyte degeneration. Pericellular and portal fibrosis commonly occur, and Mallory nuclei may be seen. These changes are indistinguishable from those seen in alcoholic steatohepatitis. Progression to cirrhosis occurs in about 20% of patients with NASH, which is now the most common cause of cryptogenic cirrhosis and its complications (including hepatocellular carcinoma – q.v.).

NASH can also occur after excessive total parenteral nutrition, bariatric surgery and some drugs (e.g. amiodarone, synthetic oestrogens, tetracyclines). Potential roles have been suggested for mitochondrial dysfunction, intestinal microflora, antioxidants, iron and leptin (a peptide produced in adipose tissue as well as in the gut) (q.v.) in providing a putative necessary second hit to cause hepatic damage in this setting.

Clinical features include malaise, upper abdominal discomfort and hepatomegaly.

The liver function tests are abnormal. Ultrasound examination can show the presence of fat in the liver, but it cannot differentiate among the different causes of this finding. Definitive diagnosis requires liver biopsy.

Bibliography
Brunt EM. Nonalcoholic steatohepatitis. *Semin Liver Dis* 2001; 21: 3.
Sheth SG, Gordon FD, Chopra S. Nonalcoholic steatohepatitis. *Ann Intern Med* 1997; 126: 137.
Younossi Z, Anstee QM, Marietti M, et al. Global burden of NAFLD and NASH: trends, predictions, risk factors and prevention. *Nat Rev Gastroenterol Hepatol* 2018; 15: 11.

Non-respiratory thoracic disorders

Non-respiratory thoracic disorders considered in this book are those related to abnormalities of the
- chest wall (q.v.),
- diaphragm (q.v.),
- mediastinum (q.v.),
- pleural cavity (q.v.).

Norovirus

Norovirus (formerly called **Norwalk virus**) is the commonest cause (40%) of non-bacterial gastroenteritis worldwide. It is a calcivirus and was originally named following an outbreak in Norwalk, Ohio, in 1968. There are several members of the norovirus family, and all produce a similar illness.

The virus is faecally transmitted and is thus acquired from food, especially seafood, from water, from other persons or from the environment, with a variable transmission rate reported between 4% and 43%. Outbreaks therefore occur in institutions, at restaurants or on cruise ships. The virus is highly transmissible, and viral shedding can persist for many weeks after symptoms have resolved. There is a year-round risk.

Following an incubation period of 24–48 hr during which time the proximal small bowel becomes infected, there is abdominal cramping, nausea, vomiting, watery diarrhoea (q.v.) and often systemic symptoms of fever (q.v.), myalgia and headache, which generally last for about 48 hr. The patient is rarely seriously ill but is significantly uncomfortable and frequently disabled (as with military personnel, health care workers and travellers).

The specific diagnosis can be made (if required) by electron microscopy or radioimmunoassay of antigen in faeces. Polymerase chain reaction (PCR) techniques have also been developed.

The differential diagnosis includes other calciviruses, enteroviruses, hepatitis, and in children rotavirus.

*Treatment is with **fluid replacement**.*

Infection control measures are important, including careful environmental cleaning after an outbreak. Complete recovery within 2–3 days is expected. A vaccine is under development, but it will need to be polyvalent as there are multiple strains of the virus.

Bibliography
Dolin R, Treanor JJ, Madore HP. Novel agents of viral enteritis in humans. *J Infect Dis* 1987; 155: 365.
Frankhauser RL, Monroe SS, Noel JS, et al. Epidemiologic and molecular trends of Norwalk-like viruses associated with outbreaks of gastroenteritis in the United States. *J Infect Dis* 2002; 186: 1.
Kapikian AZ. Overview of viral gastroenteritis. *Arch Virol* 1996; 12: 7 (suppl.).

See
- Diarrhoea,
- Food poisoning.

Norwalk virus *See*
- Norovirus.

Nutrition *See*
- Metabolism and nutrition.

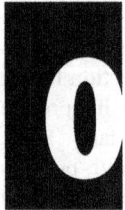

Obstetrics and gynaecology

Several aspects of women's health are of relevance to Intensive Care, particularly obstetric disasters and gynaecological illnesses of a septic or multiorgan nature. Those topics considered in this book include
- Abortion,
- Abruptio placentae (placental abruption),

- Acute fatty liver of pregnancy,
- Amenorrhoea,
- Amniotic fluid embolism,
- Catamenial pneumothorax (see Pneumothorax),
- Fetomaternal haemorrhage,
- HELLP syndrome,
- Oral contraceptives,
- Ovarian hyperstimulation syndrome,
- Pelvic inflammatory disease,
- Pneumonia in pregnancy,
- Polycystic ovary syndrome,
- Pre-eclampsia,
- Pregnancy,
- Salpingitis,
- Trauma in pregnancy.

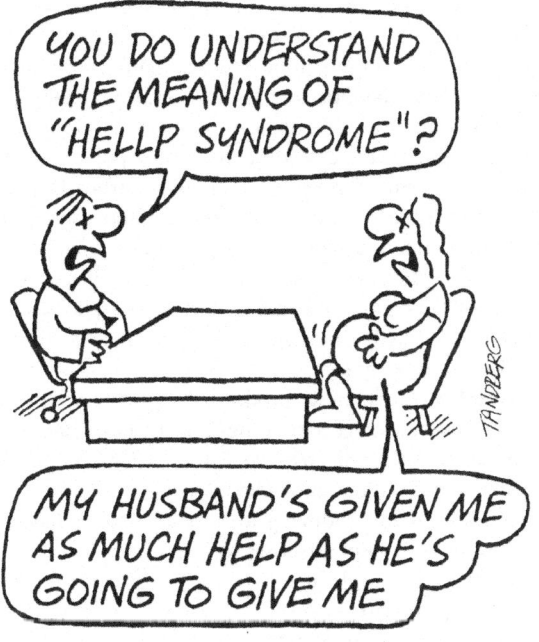

Bibliography

Australian Society for the Study of Hypertension in Pregnancy. Management of hypertension in pregnancy: consensus statement. *Med J Aust* 1993; 158: 700.

Briggs GG, Freeman RL, Towers CV, et al., eds. *Drugs in Pregnancy and Lactation*. 11th edition. Philadelphia: Lippincott Williams & Wilkins. 2017.

Brooks DC, Sznyter LA. Pregnancy. In: *Scientific American Surgery, Section VII Special Problems in Perioperative Care, Chapter 11*. New York: Scientific American. 1998.

Chestnut DH. Critical care in obstetric practice. In: Fuhrman BP, Shoemaker WC, eds. *Critical Care: State of the Art, Chapter 7*. Fullerton: Society of Critical Care Medicine. 1989; 121.

Council on Scientific Affairs, American Medical Association. Fetal effects of maternal alcohol use. *JAMA* 1983; 249: 2517.

Emmerich J, Thomassin C, Zureik M. Contraceptive pills and thrombosis: effects of the French crisis on prescriptions and consequences for medical agencies. *J Thromb Haemost* 2014; 12: 1388.

Guntupalli KK, Hall N, Karnad DR, et al. Critical illness in pregnancy. *Chest* 2015; 148: 1093 & 1333.

Henrich JB, ed. Women's Health. In: *Scientific American Medicine*. Hamilton: Dekker Medicine. 2020.

Hotham N, Hotham E. Drugs in breastfeeding. *Aust Prescriber* 2015; 38: 156.

Jamal S, Maurer JR. Pulmonary disease and the menstrual cycle. *Pulmonary Perspectives* 1994; 11: 3.

Kadir RA, Davies J. Hemostatic disorders in women. *J Thromb Haemost* 2013; 11 (suppl.1): 170.

Kennedy D. Classifying drugs in pregnancy. *Aust Prescriber* 2014; 37: 38.

Lim V, Katz A, Lindheimer M. Acid-base regulation in pregnancy. *Am J Physiol* 1976; 231: 1764.

McLintock C, James AH. Obstetric hemorrhage. *J Thromb Haemost* 2011; 9: 1441.

Middeldorp S. Thrombosis in women. *J Thromb Haemost* 2013; 11 (suppl.1): 180.

Newmark ME, Penry JK. Catamenial epilepsy: a review. *Epilepsia* 1980; 21: 281.

Phelan JP, Pacheco LD, Foley MR, et al., eds. *Critical Care Obstetrics*. 6th edition. Oxford: Wiley. 2018.

Rizk NW, Kalassian KG, Gilligan T, et al. Obstetric complications in pulmonary and critical care medicine. *Chest* 1996; 110: 791.

Sanson B-J, Lensing AWA, Prins MH, et al. Safety of low-molecular-weight heparin in pregnancy: a systematic review. *Thromb Haemost* 1999; 81: 668.

Therapeutic Goods administration. Prescribing medicines in pregnancy database. www.tga.gov.au/mode/4012. 2019.

Wood CE. Menorrhagia: a clinical update. *Med J Aust* 1996; 165: 510.

Occupational lung diseases

Lung damage from inhalation of dusts, fumes or other injurious substances may occur in many occupations in most societies. There is a vast number of such substances which affect air quality in the workplace, and the consequences of their inhalation range from minor to severe with effects possible throughout the entire respiratory tract from the nose to the alveoli. Fortunately, most substances to which the population is exposed are not harmful, and those that are injurious are probably well recognized nowadays. Thus, appropriate preventive measures can generally be taken, with the caveat that there needs to be awareness of new types of exposure as industries continually evolve.

It is worth noting that as a rule occupational diseases are not pathologically unique. They are the same as their counterparts due to other causes and are distinguished primarily by their history. In principle, adverse environmental exposure can exacerbate any pre-existing respiratory disease, and conversely pre-existing respiratory disease renders the patient more susceptible to any adverse environmental exposure.

The major **occupational lung diseases** comprise the following:
- pneumoconiosis,
- occupational asthma,
- hypersensitivity pneumonitis,
- acute lung irritation,
- occupational pulmonary infections,
- occupational pulmonary neoplasms,
- miscellaneous occupational lung diseases.

1. **Pneumoconiosis** refers to the permanent accumulation of inhaled dust in the lungs, together with the tissue reaction to its presence.

   A **dust** is an aerosol of solid, inanimate particles, and their size should be less than 10 μm to be retained in the lung. This size is somewhat unusual, especially in nature, and requires the disruptive forces of industrial processes. Moreover, only a few specific dusts among the many produced give rise to clinical disease. In addition, associated damage due to smoking is very common and may outweigh any effect of inhaled dust.

The chief pneumoconioses are due to
- coal dust,
- silica,
- asbestos.

Less commonly, pneumoconioses can be produced by a number of other dusts.

Coal dust and **silica** give rise to simple pneumoconiosis with few or no symptoms or lung function abnormalities, but the chest X-ray shows diffuse, multiple, rounded opacities, often primarily affecting the upper lobes. If the silica is inhaled as very fine particles, a diffuse interstitial fibrosis rather than a nodular pathology may result.

Coal workers' pneumoconiosis (CWP) is popularly known as 'black lung', and there may be a resurgence of cases, even in developed countries. About 10% of cases continue eventually to **progressive massive fibrosis** (see below).

Silicosis has also undergone a resurgence of cases related to the use of artificial stone (i.e. reconstituted, engineered or manufactured stone) for household benchtops. This phenomenon has been observed since 2010, primarily in developed countries, and it is similar to that previously reported in denim sandblasters. In the manufacture of artificial stone, the main quartz conglomerate is mixed with resins and pigments, then heat cured to produce slabs, which are cut to size. The final step of grinding and polishing with high-powered tools results in high concentration of respirable silica dust. Of those workers who develop pneumoconiosis, many continue to **progressive massive fibrosis**, despite no further exposure.

For reasons that are unclear but may be immunological, some patients develop complicated pneumoconiosis in the form of **progressive massive fibrosis** with large fibrotic lesions, often with cavities and usually in the upper lobes. Symptoms of dyspnoea and cough now appear. The progressive massive fibrosis of silicosis and of coal workers' pneumoconiosis may be complicated by tuberculosis (q.v.) or rheumatoid arthritis (Caplan's syndrome), respectively.

Asbestos (q.v.) may produce progressive, diffuse fibrosis, at which stage symptoms appear. Lung function changes, particularly decreased gas transfer, precede both symptoms and radiographic changes.

In addition to producing a pneumoconiosis (asbestosis), asbestos also predisposes to
- calcified pleural plaques,
- diffuse pleural fibrosis,
- bronchogenic carcinoma,
- pleural and peritoneal mesothelioma.

Other dusts which can produce pneumoconiosis include
- other silicates (e.g. talc and kaolin, but not cement or fibreglass),
- aluminium (q.v.),
- barium sulphate,
- iron oxide,
- tin oxide,
- tungsten carbide,
- beryllium (q.v.), which can also give rise to diffuse granuloma formation.

Pneumoconiosis is irreversible and untreatable, but it is preventable by appropriate public health measures,

including exposure protection, surveillance, screening, reporting and enforcement of international standards.
2. **Occupational asthma** (OA) may be caused by exposure to substances in the workplace which are allergenic, pharmacologically active or directly irritant to the bronchial tree. Up to 10–15% of asthma sufferers may have an occupational contribution to the initiation of their condition. Work-exacerbated asthma (WEA) is less well defined, but it may contribute to illness in a further 10% of all asthma sufferers. Together, OA and WEA comprise the broader entity of work-related asthma (WRA).

Animal danders, vegetable, flower and grain dusts, wood dusts, cotton dusts, isocyanates, latex, soldering flux, insecticides, gases (e.g. sulphur dioxide), and various chemicals and proteolytic enzymes may be incriminated.

Many patients have no past history or family history of asthma or atopy, and symptoms may sometimes be atypical in that wheeze is not always prominent. Typically, the symptoms are worse at work ('Monday morning asthma') and subside at weekends and on holidays, but eventually they may become chronic.

3. **Hypersensitivity pneumonitis** (q.v.).
4. **Acute lung irritation** (q.v.).
5. **Occupational pulmonary infections** include
   - tuberculosis (q.v.)
     - in health workers and in miners with silicosis,
   - Q fever (q.v.)
     - in farmers, veterinarians and abattoir workers,
   - hydatid disease (q.v.)
     - in sheep farmers.
6. **Occupational pulmonary neoplasms** include
   - carcinoma of the lung
     - following exposure to asbestos, uranium mining, arsenic, nickel, chromate, beryllium, mustard gas (see these separate agents),
   - mesothelioma
     - following exposure to asbestos (q.v.).
7. **Miscellaneous occupational lung diseases** include
   - byssinosis
     - a condition found in textile workers inhaling cotton, flax or hemp dust,
     - with cough, chest tightness, dyspnoea and wheeze, especially on Mondays,
     - with an obstructive pattern on spirometry but a normal chest X-ray,
   - pulmonary infiltration due to hair sprays
     - sometimes picturesquely called thesaurosis,
   - paraquat lung
     - a lethal, proliferative and destructive reaction following ingestion of this toxic weed killer (q.v.).

Bibliography

Beach J, Russell K, Blitz S, et al. A systematic review of the diagnosis of occupational asthma. *Chest* 1997; 131: 569.

Bernardo J, Center DM. Hypersensitivity pneumonia. *Dis Mon* 1981; 27: 1.

Berry G. Environmental mesothelioma incidence, time since exposure to asbestos and level of exposure. *Environmetrics* 1995; 6: 221.

Chan-Yeung M, Malo J-L. Occupational asthma. *N Engl J Med* 1995; 333: 107.

Cohen RA, Go LHT. Artificial stone silicosis: removal from exposure is not enough. *Chest* 2020; 158: 862.

Davidoff F. New disease, old story. *Ann Intern Med* 1998; 129: 327.

Hendrick D, Beckett W, Burge SP, et al., eds. *Occupational Disorders of the Lung.* Philadelphia: WB Saunders. 2002.

Ho A, Chan H, Tse KS, et al. Occupational asthma due to latex in health care workers. *Thorax* 1996; 51: 1280.

Hoy RF, Brims F. Occupational lung diseases in Australia. *Med J Aust* 2017; 207: 443.

Malo JL, Chan-Yeung M. Occupational asthma. *J Allergy Clin Immunol* 2001; 108: 317.

Mitchell CA. Occupational lung disease. *Med J Aust* 1997; 167: 498.

Nemery B. Metal toxicity and the respiratory tract. *Eur Respir J* 1990; 3: 202.

Sack CS, Vedal S, Kaufman JD. Occupational and environmental lung diseases. In: *Scientific American Medicine. Pulmonary & Critical Care Medicine.* Hamilton: Dekker Medicine. 2020.

Schwartz DA. Acute inhalational injury. *Occup Med* 1987; 2: 297.

Tarlo SM, Balmes J, Balkissoon R, et al. Diagnosis and management of work-related asthma: American College of Chest Physicians Consensus Statement. *Chest* 2008; 134: suppl.

Taylor AN, Cullinan P, Blanc P, et al., eds. Parkes' *Occupational Lung Disorders.* 4th edition. Oxford: Oxford University Press. 2016.

van Kempen V, Merget R, Baur X. Occupational airway sensitizers. *Am J Ind Med* 2000; 38: 164.

Octreotide See

- Acromegaly,
- Carcinoid syndrome,
- Diarrhoea,
- Glucagonoma,
- Hepatopulmonary syndrome,
- Somatostatin.

Olmesartan *See*

- Coeliac disease,
- Malabsorption,
- Renin–angiotensin–aldosterone.

Oncofetal antigen *See*

- Alpha-fetoprotein,
- Carcinoembryonic antigen.

Ophthalmoplegia

Ophthalmoplegia refers to weakness of the ocular muscles due to damage to the III, IV and/or VI cranial nerves.

- If **unilateral**, it is commonly due to an orbital lesion.
  It may also be associated with
  - an intracavernous carotid artery aneurysm,
  - diabetes,
  - recent viral infection.
- If **bilateral**, it may be caused by
  - cavernous sinus thrombosis,
  - a midbrain lesion, which is usually ischaemic,
  - multiple sclerosis (q.v.),
  - myasthenia gravis (q.v.),
  - Wernicke's encephalopathy (q.v.).

Clinical features are manifest as follows.
- III nerve damage causes weakness of upward, downward and inward eye movement, associated with ptosis and a dilated pupil,
- IV nerve damage causes weakness of downward and inward eye movement,
- VI nerve damage causes weakness of outward eye movement.

Optic neuritis *See*

- Behcet's syndrome,
- Demyelinating diseases – 4. Transverse myelitis,
- Multiple sclerosis,
- Neuropathy – Cranial neuropathies,
- Papilloedema.

Oral contraceptives

Oral contraceptives (OCs) are usually a combination of low-dose oestrogen (ethinylestradiol) and a progoestogen.

Since their introduction in the 1960s, it has been recognized that OCs are associated with a substantially increased relative risk of venous and other thromboembolic complications, although the absolute risk remained small (e.g. 1 case per 1000 years of OC use). Importantly, the progoestogens in the more recently introduced 'third-generation' and 'fourth-generation' OCs have been found to be associated with a doubling of the risk of venous thromboembolism, compared with the safest 'second-generation' OCs (containing levonorgestrel as the progoestogen).

OCs are also associated with problems and complications in many other clinical settings, such as those listed below.

See
- Alopecia,
- Benign intracranial hypertension,
- Cholestasis,
- Drugs and the lung,
- Erythema nodosum,
- Haemoglobin disorders – 2. Sickle cell disease,
- Hepatocellular carcinoma,
- Hirsutism,
- Pigmentation disorders – 2. Hyperpigmentation,
- Porphyria,
- Protein C.

Bibliography
Emmerich J, Thomassin C, Zureik M. Contraceptive pills and thrombosis: effects of the French crisis on prescriptions and consequences for medical agencies. *J Thromb Haemost* 2014; 12: 1388.

Orchitis

The major causes of **orchitis** are
- mumps,
- varicella (q.v.),
- typhoid (q.v.),
- Coxsackie virus B infection,
- filariasis (see Helminths).

In post-pubertal males, mumps causes orchitis in about 10% of patients and is then followed in half by infertility and testicular atrophy.

Orchitis should be distinguished from
- epididymitis (q.v.),
- testicular torsion,
- testicular tumour.

Organophosphates *See*

- Warfare agents.
  See also
- Neuropathy – 2. Toxic neuropathies.

Orthodeoxia *See*

- Platypnoea–orthodeoxia syndrome.

Osler–Weber–Rendu disease *See*
- Arteriovenous malformations.

Osmotic demyelination syndrome *See*
- Central pontine myelinolysis,
- Hyponatraemia.

Osteomalacia *See*
- Aluminium.

Ovarian hyperstimulation syndrome

Ovarian hyperstimulation syndrome (OHSS) is a serious multisystem complication of ovulation induction, first described in 1984. Ovarian stimulation by exogenous hormone administration is used to produce the oocytes needed in IVF and GIFT programs, and OHSS is thus an inadvertent iatrogenic condition.

The pathogenesis of OHSS is presumably an exaggeration of the normal ovulation process, with mediator release, increased capillary permeability, and fluid shift from the intravascular space into the serous cavities. There is thus hypovolaemia and haemoconcentration. There is associated hypercoagulability.

OHSS originally occurred in about 20% of ovarian inductions, with the majority of cases being mild and only about 1% being severe, but its incidence has declined following the replacement of hCG by GnRH antagonists for stimulation in more recent years. It occurs a few days after the start of the luteal phase and usually lasts only a week or so.

OHSS is classified as
- **mild disease**
  - Grade 1, with abdominal discomfort and distension,
  - Grade 2, with nausea, vomiting and diarrhoea (q.v.),
- **moderate disease**
  - Grade 3, with ascites,
- **severe disease**
  - Grade 4, with ascites, pleural effusion (q.v.) and dyspnoea,
  - Grade 5, with hypovolaemia, hypotension, oliguria, coagulopathy.

In the full-blown picture, there is thus
- shock,
- multiorgan failure (acute respiratory distress syndrome, renal failure, liver dysfunction) (q.v.),
- thrombosis and/or haemorrhage.

Treatment is required for all except mild cases, which are self-limiting within about 2 weeks. Appropriate treatment comprises urgent Intensive Care management, with fluid resuscitation, circulatory monitoring, albumin administration, and abdominal and pleural paracenteses. Management principles for intra-abdominal hypertension (q.v.) should be adopted.

No specific pharmacological treatment is established, with antihistamines and prostaglandin inhibitors being disappointing, though ACE inhibitors have shown promise.

Bibliography

Brinsden PR, Wada I, Tan SL, et al. Diagnosis, prevention and management of ovarian hyperstimulation syndrome. *Br J Obstet Gynaecol* 1995; 102: 767.

Budev MM, Arroliga AC, Falcone T. Ovarian hyperstimulation syndrome. *Crit Care Med* 2005; 33 (suppl.): S301.

Golan A, Ron-El R, Herman A, et al. Ovarian hyperstimulation syndrome: an update review. *Obstet Gynecol Surv* 1989; 44: 430.

Myrianthefs P, Ladakis C, Lappas V, et al. Ovarian hyperstimulation syndrome (OHSS): diagnosis and management. *Intens Care Med* 2000; 26: 631.

Nelson SM. Prevention and management of ovarian hyperstimulation syndrome. *Thromb Res* 2017; 151: S61.

Tassone M, Kuhn R, Talbot JM. Ovarian hyperstimulation syndrome. *Aust NZ J Obstet Gynaecol* 1997; 37: 5.

Williamson K, Mushambi MC. Ovarian hyperstimulation syndrome. *Br J Anaesth* 1994; 3: 731.

Oxytocin *See*
- Desmopressin.
  See also
- Syndrome of inappropriate antidiuretic hormone.

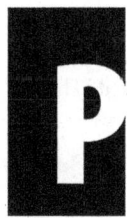

PADIS

PADIS is an acronym for the related conditions of **pain**, **agitation**, **delirium**, **immobility** and **sleep deprivation**.

These adverse experiences are commonly suffered by critically ill patients. Much effort is currently spent improving where possible those aspects of the ICU environment which contribute to these distressful and interrelated symptoms.

See
- Delirium.

Bibliography
Honarmand K, Rafay H, Le J, et al. A systematic review of risk factors for sleep disruption in critically ill adults. *Crit Care Med* 2020; 48: 1066.

Paget's disease

Paget's disease of bone is a local disorder with considerable histological complexity. Although its aetiology is uncertain, there is some familial clustering and variable ethnic prevalence; for example, it is found in up to 3% of older patients in North America and Western Europe but not in Asia. This epidemiology, together with the finding of intranuclear inclusion bodies resembling paramyxovirus nucleocapsids and reacting against measles, respiratory syncytial virus (RSV) or other related viruses, suggests that the disease may be due to an infectious agent acquired some years before.

Histologically, there is a mixed osteolytic/osteoblastic process, the latter becoming predominant later in the disease. In addition to increased bone reabsorption with abnormal osteoclasts, there is osteoblastic activity with new bone formation, typically a mosaic of both lamellar and woven bone. A loose fibrous stroma with prominent vessels replaces the bone marrow. The entire process may be different in different bones at the same time.

The clinical features of a focal bone disorder of this type clearly depend on its site and extent.
- Although commonly asymptomatic, there may be local deformity, local pain, local hyperaemia or pathological fracture. Specific local symptoms include deafness, neural compression or renal calculi (if there has been hypercalcuria).

- Systemically, there may be a hyperdynamic state, if more than 30% of the skeleton is involved. These features are usually seen in middle-aged or elderly patients.

- Occasionally, there may be neoplastic change, either benign giant cell tumour (which is locally destructive) or osteosarcoma (of the osteolytic type). Most osteosarcomas in adults arise in patients with Paget's disease.

Investigations include abnormal X-ray findings, especially in the skull, with lytic lesions surrounded by a somewhat irregular margin. Even if the X-ray is normal, there may be increased uptake on isotope bone scans. There is increased urinary hydroxyproline (reflecting collagen reabsorption) and increased plasma type I procollagen fragments (reflecting collagen synthesis). Although the serum alkaline phosphatase is increased, the urinary calcium is generally normal, unless the patient is confined to bed. Hypercalcaemia (q.v.) is also uncommon despite an increased calcium and phosphate flux which may rise up to 20-fold without changes in plasma levels, and usually this complication occurs only with immobilization such as with bed rest.

*Treatment is often not required. Symptoms respond to **NSAIDs** for clinically significant disease. Specific inhibition of osteoclast formation and function may be obtained with calcitonin, bisphosphonates or plicamycin (mithramycin).*

- ***Calcitonin*** *(q.v.) has been available for several decades and improves most clinical features except deafness. It is given as 50–100 U SC per day or every second day on a long-term basis, since relapse follows its cessation. Although its onset of action is prompt, the fall in alkaline phosphatase, sometimes even to normal values, may take some weeks. Occasional side-effects include nausea, flushing, abnormal taste and local bone pain. More importantly, antibodies develop in some patients, who thus become resistant unless the synthetic human form of calcitonin is then used.*
- ***Bisphosphonates*** *include alendronate, pamidronate and etidronate (see Hypercalcaemia). These too may exacerbate local pain, but improvement tends to be sustained for many months after cessation of therapy.*
- ***Plicamycin*** *(mithramycin) is given in a dose of 15 mcg/kg per day for 10 days. These are much lower doses than are used for cancer chemotherapy, so that although nausea or thrombocytopenia (q.v.) may occur, bone marrow, liver and renal toxicity do not occur. Again, prolonged remissions may be produced.*

Paget's disease of nipple comprises a reddish scaly and often ulcerated plaque, involving the nipple and areola and associated with an underlying carcinoma.

It is unilateral and mostly seen in women. However, extramammary lesions of a similar nature can be seen in either sex, involving apocrine gland sites, especially in the perineum or axilla. These too usually reflect an underlying carcinoma.

Bibliography
Becker C. Diseases of calcium metabolism and metabolic bone disease. In: *Scientific American Medicine*.

Endocrinology & Metabolism. Hamilton: Dekker Medicine. 2020.

Singer FR. Clinical efficacy of salmon calcitonin in Paget's disease of bone. *Calcif Tissue Int* 1991; 49 (suppl. 2): S7.

Singer FR. Paget's disease of bone. In: De Groot LJ, ed. *Endocrinology.* Philadelphia. 1995; p 1259.

Singer FR, Minoofar PN. Bisphosphonates in the treatment of disorders of mineral metabolism. *Adv Endocrinol Metab* 1995; 6: 259.

Walsh JP. Paget's disease of bone. *Med J Aust* 2004; 181: 262.

Palmar erythema

Palmar erythema describes a dark reddish-purple area on the palm of the hand, usually over the hypothenar eminence.

> It is typically associated with **hepatic cirrhosis**, but it is also seen in chronic active hepatitis, thyrotoxicosis (q.v.) and rheumatoid arthritis.

Pancreatic stone protein

Pancreatic stone protein (PSP) was identified in pancreatic calculi several decades ago. Subsequently, it was cloned and sequenced from islet cells, though it appears to be also expressed in a variety of other gastrointestinal cell types and circulating levels are detectable.

As PSP is upregulated in inflammation, its serum level has joined the list of **biomarkers** (q.v.), such as procalcitonin (q.v.) and C-reactive protein (q.v.), which are of potential value in the assessment of intra-abdominal and other sepsis.

Bibliography

Boeck L, Graf R, Eggimann P, et al. Pancreatic stone protein: a marker of organ failure and outcome in ventilator-associated pneumonia. *Chest* 2011; 140: 925.

De Waele JJ. Pancreatic stone protein for predicting outcome in peritonitis: limitations and challenges. *Crit Care Med* 2013; 41: 1150.

Graf R, Schiesser M, Reding T, et al. Exocrine meets endocrine: pancreatic stone protein and regenerating protein – two sides of the same coin. *J Surg Res* 2006; 133: 113.

Pancreatitis

Acute pancreatitis is well known to be precipitated by alcohol or biliary disease in about 80% of cases. Its incidence appears to be rising in developed countries. It has a prevalence of 5–75 per 100,000 of the population, with the highest occurrence in developed countries. Its overall mortality is 2–4%, and severe acute pancreatitis is an important cause of admission to an Intensive Care Unit.

> Less common causes of acute pancreatitis include
> - hypercalcaemia (q.v.),
> - hyperlipoproteinaemia,
> - abdominal trauma
>   - including surgery,
> - infections
>   - particularly mumps, salmonella,
> - drugs
>   - especially azathioprine, cytosine arabinoside, furosemide, oestrogens, sulphonamides, tetracycline, thiazides,
>   - organophosphate poisoning (see Insecticides),
> - genetic abnormalities
>   - multiple mutations of the gene for trypsinogen have been described, giving rise to an autosomal dominant condition of recurrent acute pancreatitis in young people, associated with pancreatic calcification, diabetes and steatorrhoea and eventually with chronic pancreatitis (see below) and sometimes pancreatic carcinoma.

Diagnosis is based on the presence of at least two of the three following criteria – typical abdominal pain, raised serum amylase or lipase, or radiological evidence. Serum lipase is nowadays preferred to amylase, as it is more sensitive and has a more prolonged elevation. Neither enzyme level is useful in assessing the severity or progress of pancreatitis. Levels rise within 3–6 hr of the onset of symptoms, and become diagnostic when elevated at 2–4 times the upper limit of normal. While an elevated amylase may become normal within 24 hr, an elevated lipase may persist for 1–2 wk.

The treatment of severe acute pancreatitis is well known in Intensive Care practice and its elements have recently been critically reviewed (see Bibliography below). International guidelines for its management have been widely promulgated. Newer principles relate to abdominal imaging techniques and early endoscopic retrograde cholangiopancreatography (ERCP).

Chronic pancreatitis is also well known to be associated with
- alcoholism,
- biliary disease,
- hereditary pancreatitis (see above).

It can also be associated with

- abdominal trauma (sometimes),
- autoimmune pancreatic disease, with ductal narrowing and parenchymal swelling, infiltration and fibrosis, causing pancreatic head swelling and obstructive jaundice, and thus potentially mimicking carcinoma.

Bibliography

Baker S. Diagnosis and management of acute pancreatitis. *Crit Care Resusc* 2004; 6: 17.

Baron TH, Morgan DE. Acute necrotizing pancreatitis. *N Engl J Med* 1999; 340: 1412.

Basnayake C, Ratnam D. Blood tests for acute pancreatitis. *Aust Prescriber* 2015; 38: 128.

Berger HG, Matsuno S, Cameron JL, eds. *Diseases of the Pancreas*. Berlin: Springer. 2008.

Chowdhury RS, Forsmark CE. Review article: pancreatic function testing. *Aliment Pharmacol Ther* 2003; 17: 733.

Dellinger EP, Tellado JM, Soto NE, et al. Early antibiotic treatment for severe acute necrotizing pancreatitis. *Ann Surg* 2007; 245: 674.

Dervenis C, Bassi C. Evidence-based assessment of severity and management of acute pancreatitis. *Br J Surg* 2000; 87: 257.

Entock FC, Chong P, Menezes N, et al. A randomized study of early nasogastric versus nasojejunal feeding in severe acute pancreatitis. *Am J Gastroenterol* 2005; 100: 432.

Go VLW, et al., eds. *The Pancreas: Biology, Pathobiology and Diseases*. New York: Raven Press. 1993.

Green PHR, Tall AR. Drugs, alcohol and malabsorption. *Am J Med* 1979; 67: 1066.

Hasibeder WR, Torgersen C, Rieger M, et al. Critical care of the patient with acute pancreatitis. *Anaesth Intens Care* 2009; 37: 190.

Howes N, Greenhall W, Stocken DD, et al. Cationic trypsinogen mutations and pancreatitis. *Gastroenterol Clin North Am* 2004; 33: 767.

Layer P, Yamamoto H, Kalthoff L, et al. The different courses of early- and late-onset idiopathic and alcoholic chronic pancreatitis. *Gastroenterology* 1994; 107: 1481.

Malledant Y, Malbrain MLNG, Reuter DA. What's new in the management of severe acute pancreatitis. *Intens Care Med* 2015; 41: 1957.

Marshall JB. Acute pancreatitis: a review with an emphasis on new developments. *Arch Intern Med* 1993; 153: 1185.

Marshall JC. Surgical approaches to the management of acute severe necrotizing pancreatitis. *Curr Opin Crit Care* 1999; 5: 159.

Mitchell RM, Byrne M, Baillie J. Pancreatitis. *Lancet* 2003; 361: 1447.

Nathens AB, Curtis JR, Beale RJ, et al. Management of the critically ill patient with severe acute pancreatitis. *Crit Care Med* 2004; 32: 2524.

Nesvaderani M, Eslick GD, Cox MR. Acute pancreatitis: update on management. *Med J Aust* 2016; 202: 420.

Pastor CM, Matthay MA, Frossard L-L. Pancreatitis-associated acute lung injury: new insights. *Chest* 2003; 124: 2341.

Rotstein OD. Surgical approach #1 to severe necrotizing pancreatitis. *Curr Opin Crit Care* 1999; 5: 160.

Sheth S, Ketwaroo G, Freedman S. Diseases of the pancreas. In: *Scientific American Medicine. Gastroenterology*. Hamilton: Dekker Medicine. 2020.

Shields CJ, Winter DC, Redmond HP. Lung injury in acute pancreatitis: mechanisms, prevention, and therapy. *Curr Opin Crit Care* 2002; 8: 158.

Starr MG. Surgical approach #2 to severe necrotizing pancreatitis. *Curr Opin Crit Care* 1999; 5: 162.

Steer ML, Meldolesi J. The cell biology of experimental pancreatitis. *N Engl J Med* 1987; 316: 144.

Steer ML, Waxman I, Freedman S. Chronic pancreatitis. *N Engl J Med* 1995; 332: 1482.

Tattersall SJN, Apte MV, Wilson JS. A fire inside: current concepts in chronic pancreatitis. *Intern Med J* 2008; 38: 592.

Wyncoll DL. The management of severe acute necrotizing pancreatitis: an evidence-based review of the literature. *Intens Care Med* 1999; 25: 146.

Yousaf M, McCallion K, Diamond T. Management of severe acute pancreatitis. *Br J Surg* 2003; 90: 407.

Pancytopenia

Pancytopenia refers to the presence of combined anaemia, neutropenia and thrombocytopenia (see Anaemia). Sometimes, the causative process may affect only one or two cell lines.

If the bone marrow has been infiltrated, viable stem cells may circulate and relocate in sites of fetal haemopoiesis. This is referred to as **extramedullary haemopoiesis** and is associated with a **leukoerythroblastic** blood film.

Any cytopenia (affecting one, two or all three cell lines) or a leukoerythroblastic blood film provides an indication for bone marrow examination.

Pandemics

Pandemics are defined as the widespread occurrence of a severe infectious disease. A pandemic occurs when an epidemic crosses international borders and may even become global. An **epidemic** is a large and rapid spread of an infectious disease confined to a localized region, and an **outbreak** is a similar occurrence but of an even more limited extent. By contrast, an **endemic** infectious disease is one where its transmission threshold remains limited and in equilibrium, so that it persists in the relevant population at a low or background level.

The terms *epidemic* or *pandemic* are sometimes applied to non-infectious diseases, such as cardiovascular disease or obesity, but properly these terms should refer to an infectious disease and one which is of some severity.

Epidemic and pandemic spread requires the exposure of a susceptible host population to a new or altered pathogen which is both infectious and pathogenic.

- **Infectivity** is reflected in the disease's basic reproduction number (R_0), i.e. the average number of expected cases caused by a single index case within a susceptible population. For example, the R_0 is generally 1–2 for influenza, 15 for measles and 2–3 for COVID-19.
- **Pathogenicity** is reflected in the disease's case fatality rate (CFR). For example, the CFR has been <0.02% for influenza in recent decades, whereas it was 3% in the Spanish flu pandemic of 1918–19 and is over 50% for Ebola. The CFR for COVID-19 has varied from 1–10%, depending particularly on the extent of testing in the population reported.

An epidemic or pandemic dies out when the R_0 falls below 1, which can occur spontaneously or due to quarantine measures or when herd immunity is achieved (i.e. when $1-1/R_0$ of the population has been infected and is now immune). Mathematical modelling of an epidemic or pandemic takes into account not only the R_0 but also the latent period of the particular disease and other factors reflecting both patient susceptibility to that disease and any public health measures in place.

Epidemics and pandemics have repeatedly devastated humankind over the centuries, with diseases such as smallpox, tuberculosis, measles, cholera and typhus killing tens of millions of people in communities worldwide. Among the best-known pandemic diseases was bubonic plague, which as the 'Black Death' halved the population of fourteenth-century Europe. Recent pandemics have included influenza (1957, 1968, 2009), HIV/AIDS (from the 1970s) and COVID-19 (from 2020). See the separate entries for these conditions.

Papilloedema

Papilloedema or swelling of the optic disc is seen classically in conditions of increased intracranial pressure.

Papilloedema also occurs in
- malignant hypertension,
- hypercapnia,
- optic neuritis (q.v.).

Bibliography
Lyons MK, Meyer FB. Cerebrospinal fluid physiology and the management of increased intracranial pressure. *Mayo Clin Proc* 1990; 65: 684.

Paraganglioma See
- Phaeochromocytoma.

Paragonimiasis

Paragonimiasis occurs following the ingestion of fresh water crustaceans infected with lung flukes (trematodes) from the genus *Paragonimus*. It occurs predominantly in tropical Asia, Africa and Central America.

The flukes migrate from the duodenum via the peritoneal cavity and diaphragm to the lung, where they form a nodule with a necrotic centre surrounded by an inflammatory capsule. After 5–6 weeks, the fluke lays eggs and the capsule ruptures into the bronchial tree, giving sputum containing blood, inflammatory cells and eggs.

The patient often appears well, but sometimes there may be night sweats (q.v.), chronic cough, haemoptysis (q.v.) and pleuritic pain. The effects of a space-occupying lesion are noted if the parasite migrates to other sites, especially the brain.

Chest X-ray shows a transient pulmonary infiltrate as in Loeffler's syndrome (q.v.), and cavities (q.v.) or pleural effusion (q.v.) may subsequently appear. There is an eosinophilia (q.v.).

The diagnosis is made following identification of typical eggs in sputum or faeces (since sputum is often swallowed). Serological confirmation is available.

The differential diagnosis is primarily tuberculosis (q.v.). The illness can thus present as AFB-negative presumed tuberculosis.

*Treatment is with **praziquantel**, which results in a cure rate of 90% within 2 days. However, the lung lesions may take many months to resolve completely.*

Bibliography
Im JG, Chang KH, Reeder MM. Current diagnostic imaging of pulmonary and cerebral paragonimiasis, with pathological correlation. *Semin Roentgenol* 1997; 32:301.
Pachucki CT, Levandowski RA, Brown VA, et al. American paragonimiasis treated with praziquantel. *N Engl J Med* 1984; 311: 582.

Parahaemophilia See
- Haemophilia.

Paralytic shellfish poisoning

Paralytic shellfish poisoning (PSP) results from the ingestion of shellfish which have been filter-feeding on toxic algae or phytoplankton. Under certain conditions, such algae may multiply enormously into toxic blooms called red tides.

PSP is a worldwide public health problem, without simple solutions, since the toxin is very persistent once ingested by the shellfish and is not cleared even after weeks or more of their purging with clean water. Prevention depends on public health monitoring of biotoxin levels in areas of commercial harvesting of shellfish.

The relevant toxin, **saxitoxin**, is a potent water-soluble neurotoxin which is resistant to cooking. Although doses 10-fold lower have also sometimes caused death, the potentially lethal dose in humans is typically about 10 mg, which may be contained is as little as 100 mg of contaminated shellfish meat.

The clinical features of PSP usually occur within about 2 hr of ingestion. They comprise
- in mild cases, paraesthesiae and nausea,
- in moderate cases, weakness, dyspnoea and sweating,
- in severe cases, paralysis and respiratory failure.

The differential diagnosis includes the more common condition of ciguatera (q.v.), botulism (q.v.) and pesticide poisoning.

Treatment is supportive, including respiratory support if necessary, until the toxin is renally excreted over the next few hours.

Mortality is very low (<1%) in developed countries, but it is up to 10% worldwide and up to 50% in younger children.

See also
- Food poisoning.

Bibliography
Lehane L. Paralytic shellfish poisoning. *Med J Aust* 2001; 175: 29.

Paraneoplastic syndromes

Paraneoplastic syndromes occur in malignancies and comprise a variety of local and systemic features not associated with any direct effect of the original cancer, either its primary tumour or its metastases.

They may occur before the cancer itself has been identified and may thus be an early marker of an undetected cancer. They disappear after successful treatment of the underlying cancer, and any reappearance thus signifies a relapse or recurrence.

The most important paraneoplastic syndromes comprise
- **dermatoses**,
- **ectopic hormone production**,
- **neurological changes**.

A variety of other conditions, such as cachexia, disseminated intravascular coagulation (q.v.) and thromboembolism are commonly associated with malignancies, but these are not usually included among the paraneoplastic syndromes.

1. Dermatoses

There are a number of dermatoses specifically suggestive of underlying malignancy. These include
- **hyperpigmentation**
  - due to ACTH production (q.v.),
- **flushing**
  - due to carcinoid syndrome (q.v.),
- **proliferative skin lesions**
  - as in multiple seborrhoeic keratosis due to secretion of growth factors,
- **necrolytic migratory erythema**
  - due to glucagonoma (q.v.).

Other, non-specific, dermatoses are also commonly associated with malignancy.
- **Psoriasis-like lesions** can be associated with metastatic squamous cell carcinoma.
- **Hypertrichosis lanuginosa** can be associated with disseminated carcinoma and consists of fine downy hair in a previously hairless region. It may also be associated with ichthyosis or acanthosis nigricans (q.v.).
- **Pyoderma gangrenosum** (q.v.) may be associated with myeloproliferative disorders, as well as with chronic inflammatory disease.
- **Generalized pruritus** may be associated with polycythaemia vera (q.v.) or lymphoma. Although commonly associated with drugs or scabies, it may also reflect serious non-malignant disease, such as thyrotoxicosis (q.v.), cholestasis (q.v.) or chronic renal disease.
- **Painful red skin plaques with fever and neutrophilia** (Sweet's syndrome) may be associated with myeloproliferative disorders. More often, it is associated with arthritis, and it is also seen after bowel bypass surgery. *Treatment is with corticosteroids.*
- Extramammary lesions resembling **Paget's disease of nipple** (q.v.) can be seen in either sex, involving apocrine gland sites, especially in the perineum or axilla. These lesions comprise reddish scaly and often ulcerated plaques, and they are associated with an underlying carcinoma.
- The skin and internal organs may suffer **concomitant insult** from a potentially cancerous agent, such as arsenic (q.v.).

2. **Ectopic hormone production (q.v.)**
A large variety of biologically active substances may be produced by neoplastic cells. These include particularly a variety of polypeptide hormones, such as ACTH, ADH, calcitonin, glucagon, growth hormone, hCG, LH, MSH, PTH and somatostatin (see the separate entries for these hormones). Corticosteroids, prostaglandins and renin may also be secreted.

> The most frequently encountered clinical feature from ectopic hormone production is the **syndrome of inappropriate antidiuretic hormone** (SIADH) (q.v.).
>
> Cushing's syndrome (q.v.), erythrocytosis (q.v.), hypercalcaemia (q.v.), hyperpigmentation (q.v.), hypoglycaemia (q.v.) may also be produced.
>
> The haematological findings of eosinophilia (q.v.) and raised ESR may be sometimes related to ectopic hormone production.

3. **Neurological changes**
Neurological abnormalities are common and can precede any symptoms directly due to the cancer itself. The mechanisms are uncertain, and there can be a variety of overlapping syndromes. The cancers most commonly involved are lung and ovary but also gastrointestinal tract and breast.

> The neurological abnormalities encountered involve
> - **brain**
>   - progressive multifocal leukoencephalopathy (q.v.),
>   - subacute cerebellar degeneration (q.v.),
>   - brainstem or limbic encephalitis (q.v.),
> - **spinal cord**
>   - degeneration of anterior horn cells,
>   - subacute necrotizing myelopathy (q.v.),
> - **peripheral nerve**
>   - sensory or mixed neuropathy (q.v.),
> - **neuromuscular junction**
>   - myasthenia gravis or related conditions (e.g. Eaton Lambert syndrome) (q.v.),
> - **muscle**
>   - polymyositis (q.v.),
>   - myopathy (q.v.),
>   - neuromyopathy.

Bibliography
Cascino TL. Neurologic complications of systemic cancer. *Med Clin North Am* 1993; 77: 265.
Clamon GH, Evans WK, Shepherd FA, et al. Myasthenic syndrome and small cell cancer of the lung: variable response to antineoplastic therapy. *Arch Intern Med* 1984; 144: 999.
Cohen PR, Kurzrock R. Sweet's syndrome and malignancy. *Am J Med* 1987; 82: 1220.
Cohen PR, Talpaz M, Kurzrock R. Malignancy-associated Sweet's syndrome: review of the world literature. *J Clin Oncol* 1988; 6: 1887.
Cronin RE, Kaehny WD, Miller, PD, et al. Renal cell carcinoma: unusual systemic manifestations. *Medicine* 1976; 55: 291.
Hall TC, ed. Paraneoplastic syndromes. *Ann NY Acad Sci* 1974; 230: 1.
Jemec GBE. Hypertrichosis lanuginosa acquisita. *Arch Dermatol* 1986; 122: 805.
Mallette LE. The parathyroid polyhormones: new concepts in the spectrum of peptide hormone action. *Endocr Rev* 1991; 12: 110.
McLean DI. Cutaneous paraneoplastic syndromes. *Arch Dermatol* 1986; 122: 765.
O'Neill JH, Murray NM, Newsom-Davis J. The Lambert-Eaton myasthenic syndrome. *Brain* 1988; 111: 577.
Peterson K, Rosenblum MK, Kotanides H, et al. Paraneoplastic cerebellar degeneration. *Neurology* 1992; 42: 1931.
Ruther U, Nunnensiek C, Bokemeyer C, eds. Paraneoplastic Syndromes. Basel: Karger. 1998.
Wolff K, Goldsmith L, Katz S, et al., eds. *Fitzpatrick's Dermatology in General Medicine.* 7th edition. New York: McGraw-Hill. 2007.

Paraquat

Paraquat (1,1-dimethyl-4,4-bipyridylium) is a potent phytotoxic herbicide, used worldwide in agriculture since the early 1960s, though banned in recent years in developed countries. It has a low molecular weight of 186 Da and a high volume of distribution of 1.4 L/kg. Most cases of human poisoning have occurred from accidental or deliberate ingestion rather than from inhalation or skin absorption, with as little as 10 mL of the 20% concentrate being potentially lethal. The granular form is considered less toxic.

Although paraquat causes marked local irritation (e.g. of skin, eyes or gastrointestinal tract), its most dramatic effects are systemic, with renal failure, liver damage and in particular pulmonary oedema. Although these complications may be rapidly fatal, more typically death occurs in a few weeks from severe pulmonary fibrosis (q.v.).

Rapid diagnosis is dependent on an accurate history, and confirmation is by a qualitative urine test or plasma radioimmunoassay. Plasma levels >2 mg/L after 4 hr or 0.2 mg/L after 12 hr indicate a poor prognosis. Several nomograms have been published relating plasma levels and time of ingestion to clinical outcome, although they predict death better than survival.

Urgent treatment is with **gastric lavage** and **prevention of further absorption** using Fuller's Earth (30% solution 250 mL 4 hrly), with magnesium sulphate as a purgative to hasten the faecal removal of the paraquat–Fuller's Earth complex. Fuller's Earth is a clay-like material with a high magnesium content able to purify, filter, decolorize or generally degrade oily materials, and it was thus used in the past by 'fullers' in the finishing of woollen cloth.

- Various measures to enhance removal of absorbed paraquat, such as diuresis, dialysis and haemoperfusion, have shown limited efficacy, but possible antidotes, such as corticosteroids and free radical scavengers, have been reported to be helpful in small case series.
- **Propofol** has been found to be protective in experimental animals.
- **Lung transplantation** has been reported, though recurrence of 'paraquat lung' has also been observed in such cases.
- Since the pulmonary effects of paraquat (like those of bleomycin – q.v.) are exacerbated by high concentrations of inspired oxygen, the minimum concentration to provide an arterial oxygen tension of no more than 60 mmHg should be used.

Bibliography
Ariyama J, Shimada H, Aono M, et al. Propofol improves recovery from paraquat acute toxicity in vitro and in vivo. *Intens Care Med* 2000; 26: 981.
Gawarammana IB, Buckley NA. Medical management of paraquat ingestion. *Br J Clin Pharmacol* 2011; 72: 745.
Lin JL, Lin-Tan DT, Chen KH, et al. Repeated pulse of methylprednisolone and cyclophosphamide with continuous dexamethasone therapy for patients with severe paraquat poisoning. *Crit Care Med* 2006; 34: 368.
Ng LL, Naik RB, Polak A. Paraquat ingestion with methaemoglobinaemia treated with methylene blue. *BMJ* 1982; 284: 1445.
Proudfoot AT, Stewart MS, Levitt T, et al. Paraquat poisoning: significance of plasma paraquat concentrations. *Lancet* 1979; 2: 330.
Senarathna L, Eddleston M, Wilks MF, et al. Prediction of outcome after paraquat poisoning by measurement of paraquat concentration. *QJM* 2009; 102: 251.
Suzuki K, Takasu N, Arita S, et al. Evaluation of severity indexes of patients with paraquat poisoning. *Hum Exp Toxicol* 1991; 10: 21.
Vale JA, Meredith TJ, Buckley BM. Paraquat poisoning: clinical features and immediate general management. *Hum Toxicol* 1987; 6: 41.

Parasitic infections

A parasite is an organism that lives on another organism (the host), which provides it with food or shelter. This relationship may be beneficial, harmful or neutral as far as the host is concerned. Humans harbour a large number of commensal organisms, particularly bacteria and viruses (see Microbiome). However, the term 'parasite' usually applies to less ubiquitous organisms harboured by humans and generally refers to **arthropods**, **helminths** and **protozoa** (see below).

These parasites may give rise to significant human disease, particularly infections. However, the parasites which cause human infection are not necessarily human parasites in the first place, as humans can become incidentally infected by parasites of another creature (as also with viral zoonoses – q.v.). The mode of such infections is either direct contact or via a vector.

The chief parasitic infections in humans are due to
- **arthropods** (q.v.)
  - These parasites in humans are necessarily ectoparasites.
  - Some are insects (fleas, lice) and some are arachnids (mites).
  - Primary human ectoparasites include lice (q.v.) and mites (q.v.).
  - Secondary human ectoparasites include animal fleas (q.v.).
- **helminths** (q.v.)
  - These comprise cestodes, nematodes and trematodes (i.e. worms).
  - They are transmitted to humans by ingestion or other close contact.
- **protozoa** (q.v.)
  - These unicellular organisms commonly require a vector for transmission to humans.
  - The vector is typically a mosquito (q.v.).
  - Protozoa cause amoebiasis (q.v.), malaria (q.v.), toxoplasmosis (q.v.).

Bibliography
Elston D. Infestations. In: *Scientific American Medicine. Dermatology*. Hamilton: Dekker Medicine. 2020.
Khemasuwan D, Farver CF, Mehta AC. Parasites of the airways. *Chest* 2014; 145: 883.

Parathyromatosis *See*

- Hyperparathyroidism.

Parotitis *See*

- Mouth diseases.

Paroxysmal nocturnal haemoglobinuria

Paroxysmal nocturnal haemoglobinuria (PNH) is a rare clonal disorder of haematopoietic stem cells, resulting in red cells which cannot bind complement inhibitory protein and are thus prone to complement-induced haemolysis. Its prevalence is about 15 per million of the population.

In addition to anaemia, it is also associated with neutropenia (q.v.), thrombocytopenia (q.v.), uncommon forms of venous thromboembolism (the most frequent cause of death) and occasionally aplastic anaemia (q.v.) or even leukaemia.

Clinical features include systemic symptoms of fatigue, dyspnoea, headache, abdominal pain and erectile dysfunction.

The full blood examination shows anaemia which may resemble that from blood loss (see Anaemia – 1. Anaemia due to blood loss), but diagnostic confirmation is made using flow cytometry studies.

Treatment options currently include erythropoietin (q.v.) and especially the complement inhibitor, **eculizumab** *(q.v.) or its newer analog,* **ravulizumab**. *Although bone marrow transplantation can be curative, it is no longer recommended because of its serious ill effects.*

The natural history of PNH is variable, and the 10-year mortality is nowadays about 30%.

See
- Anaemia – 2. Anaemia due to haemolysis (intracorpuscular defects).

Bibliography
Editorial. Paroxysmal nocturnal haemoglobinuria. *Lancet* 1992; 339: 395.
Henry DH, Spivak JL. Clinical use of erythropoietin. *Curr Opinion Hematol* 1995; 2: 118.
Hillmen P, Lewis SM, Bessler M, et al. Natural history of paroxysmal nocturnal hemoglobinuria. *N Engl J Med* 1995; 333: 1253.
Krantz SB. Erythropoietin. *Blood* 1991; 77: 419.
Young NS, Meyers G, Schrezenmeier H, et al. The management of paroxysmal nocturnal hemoglobinuria: recent advances in diagnosis and treatment and new hope for patients. *Semin Hematol* 2009; 46: S1.

Pectus excavatum

Pectus excavatum ('sunken chest') is one of the congenital **chest wall disorders** (q.v.). It is usually apparent from childhood, and it has an overall prevalence of 1 in 400 of the population.

Its clinical consequences include respiratory, cardiac and cosmetic symptoms. Its severity may be quantified by the Haller index, which is the lateral chest width divided by the minimum sternal to vertebral distance.

Surgical repair is indicated in symptomatic patients.

Bibliography
Eisinger RS, Islam S. Caring for people with untreated pectus excavatum. *Chest* 2020; 157: 590.
Fonkalsrud EW, Dunn JC, Atkinson JB. Repair of pectus excavatum deformities: 30 years of experience in 375 patients. *Ann Surg* 2000; 231: 443.

Pediculosis

Pediculosis is produced by one of two ectoparasites (see Parasitic infestations) which infect the skin and cause a marked itch. Both are arthropods (q.v.). They are
- *Sarcoptes scabiei*, a burrowing **mite** (an arachnid), and
- *Pediculus humanus*, a blood-sucking **louse** (an insect).

Pediculosis is the most prevalent parasitic skin disease in most countries. Infection occurs in one of three body sites, referred to as capitis, corporis and pubis.

Scabies is the more common infestation, except in overcrowding or wartime when lice become more common. Infection occurs from person-to-person transmission or from fomites. The eggs hatch in about 1 week, and the parasites have a lifespan of about 1 month.

Phthiriasis, the 'lousy disease' of antiquity in which lice ate away the flesh of the unfortunate victim as a fatal punishment from the gods, has not been reported for more than a century and may never in fact have existed as such.

Many local treatments are available, including **lindane** *and over-the-counter* **pyrethrins**. *Topical* **permethrin** *has been found to be more effective than oral* **ivermectin**.

The human body louse is also the vector for transmission of *Bartonella quintana*, the aetiological agent in **trench fever** (see Rickettsial diseases). This presents as acute periodic fever with headache and painful shins. Trench fever has recently been noted to have returned to industrialized societies, particularly in homeless people.

Bibliography
Bondeson J. Phthiriasis: the riddle of the lousy disease. *J R Soc Med* 1998; 91: 328.
Elston D. Infestations. In: *Scientific American Medicine. Dermatology.* Hamilton: Dekker Medicine. 2020.
Usha V, Gopalakrishnan Nair TV. A comparative study of oral ivermectin and topical permethrin cream in the treatment of scabies. *J Am Acad Dermatol* 2000: 42: 236.

Pelvic inflammatory disease See
- Salpingitis.

Pemphigus

Pemphigus vulgaris is a vesiculobullous disease, presumably of autoimmune origin (q.v.), since antibodies may be found to the epidermal desmosome adhesion protein, plakoglobulin.

From a local lesion usually in the mouth, it may progress to involve extensive areas of skin and mucous membrane. The affected epidermis can be dislodged by lateral digital pressure, a phenomenon referred to as Nikolsky's sign (which is also seen in the staphylococcal scalded skin syndrome – see Exfoliative dermatitis). The bullae ulcerate and then heal slowly with hyperpigmentation (q.v.). Histologically, there is loss of epidermal cell cohesion (acantholysis).

The differential diagnosis includes the other vesiculobullous diseases (q.v.).

*Treatment is with **corticosteroids**, which may be lifesaving if the disease is extensive, in which case fluid and protein loss also need to be repaired.*

- **Plasmapheresis** *(q.v.), **immune globulin** or pulsed megadoses of **methylprednisolone** are recommended for severe cases with an inadequate steroid response.*
- **Adjuvant therapy** *with cytotoxic, immunosuppressive or anti-inflammatory drugs may be steroid-sparing.*
- **Rituximab** *(q.v.) has been reported to be of benefit in severe, refractory disease.*

Variants of pemphigus include

- **Pemphigus vegetans**, which consists of raised wart-like plaques, which respond to dapsone,
- **Pemphigus foliaceus**, seen in sun-exposed areas and sometimes merging with systemic lupus erythematosus (q.v.),
- **Paraneoplastic pemphigus**, associated with malignancy (see Paraneoplastic syndromes),
- **Bullous pemphigoid**, in which recurrent crops of subepidermal bullae, often with secondary infection, occur in older patients. The condition often begins with urticaria (q.v.) and pruritus (q.v.). Mucosal involvement can sometimes occur. If this includes the conjunctiva, blindness may result. *Treatment with the TNF-α antagonist, **etanercept** (see Tumour necrosis factor), has been reported to be successful in a small case series.*

Drug-related pemphigus can sometimes occur. It may be either induced or triggered. Induced disease recedes after the drug has been ceased, whereas triggered disease continues.

Drugs such as captopril, cephalosporins, penicillamine and penicillin may cause pemphigus foliaceus, which generally regresses when the drug is ceased. Drugs such as enalapril may cause pemphigus vulgaris, which tends to persist when the drug is ceased.

Bibliography

Ahmed AR, Spiegelman Z, Cavacini LA, et al. Treatment of pemphigus vulgaris with rituximab and intravenous immune globulin. *New Engl J Med* 2006; 355: 1772.

Bystryn JC, Jiao D, Natow S. Treatment of pemphigus with intravenous immunoglobulin. *J Am Acad Dermatol* 2002; 47: 358.

Canizares MJ, Smith DI, Conners MS, et al. Successful treatment of mucous membrane pemphigoid with etanercept in 3 patients. *Arch Dermatol* 2006; 142: 1457.

Jolles S, Hughes J, Whittaker S. Dermatological uses of high-dose intravenous immunoglobulin. *Arch Dermatol* 1998; 134: 80.

Korman N. Bullous pemphigoid. *J Am Acad Dermatol.* 1987; 21: 1089.

Provost TT. Pemphigus. *N Engl J Med* 1982; 306: 1224.

Stanley JR, Amagai M. Pemphigus, bullous impetigo and staphylococcal scalded skin syndrome. *N Engl J Med* 2006; 355: 1800.

Turner MS, Sutton D, Sauder DN. The use of plasmapheresis and immunosuppression in the treatment of pemphigus vulgaris. *J Am Acad Dermatol* 2000; 43: 1058.

Wolff K, Goldsmith L, Katz S, et al., eds. *Fitzpatrick's Dermatology in General Medicine.* 7th edition. New York: McGraw-Hill. 2007.

Penicillamine See

- Chelating agents.

Pericarditis

Pericarditis is either post-viral or idiopathic in most cases. However, it can also be a common complication of a number of other primary illnesses, including acute myocardial infarction, endocarditis (q.v.), post-cardiotomy syndrome, radiation injury (q.v.), Still's disease (q.v.) and systemic lupus erythematosus (q.v.).

Although most cases are benign and self-limited, nearly one third of patients develop serious complications, including cardiac tamponade, recurrent disease or constrictive pericarditis.

*Acute pericarditis is treated with **NSAIDs** until symptoms resolve, usually within 2 weeks. The addition of low-dose **colchicine** (0.5–1.0 mg per day) (q.v.) given for 3 months greatly reduces the risk of recurrence. **Corticosteroids** are now given only in refractory cases. **Surgical pericardiectomy** may be required in constrictive pericarditis.*

Bibliography

Adler Y, Charron P, Imazio M, et al. Guidelines for the diagnosis and management of pericardial disease. *Eur heart J* 2015; 36: 2921.

Chiabrando JG, Bonaventura A, Vecchie A, et al. Management of acute and recurrent pericarditis. JACC State-of-the-Art Review. *J Am Coll Cardiol* 2020; 75: 76.

Imazio M, Gaita F, LeWinter M. Evaluation and treatment of pericarditis: a systematic review. *JAMA* 2015; 314: 1498.

Lazaros G, Vlachopoulos C. Acute pericarditis clinical features and outcome: an update on the latest evidence. *Chest* 2020; 158: 2262.

Periodic breathing *See*

- Sleep disorders of breathing.

Periodic fever *See*

- Familial Mediterranean fever,
- Trench fever.

Periodic paralysis

Periodic paralysis is due to an abnormal potassium flux across muscle cell membranes. The serum potassium may be either increased, decreased or normal, thus classifying the condition into three types. All are autosomal dominant conditions.

Muscle weakness, usually generalized, occurs rapidly and lasts for hours to days. Typically, there are recurrent attacks, but they vary greatly in frequency and severity.

A similar condition also occurs in **chronic hypokalaemia** from any other cause (e.g. gut loss).

*All types of periodic paralysis usually respond to **acetazolamide**, 250 mg 6 hrly.*

See also
- Liquorice.

Bibliography

Griggs R, Ptacek L. The periodic paralysis. *Hosp Pract* 1992; 27: 123.

Knochel J. Neuromuscular manifestations of electrolyte disorders. *Am J Med* 1982; 72: 521.

Pernicious anaemia

Pernicious anaemia is an autoimmune-induced vitamin B_{12} deficiency. Normally, vitamin B_{12} binds to intrinsic factor, a 45 kDa glycoprotein secreted by the gastric parietal cells. This complex then binds to specific sites in the distal ileum from where it is absorbed.

In pernicious anaemia, there is an autoimmune antibody to intrinsic factor, and thus vitamin B_{12} deficiency occurs due to impaired absorption. Commonly, the condition is associated with other autoimmune phenomena (q.v.), especially thyroid disease.

Clinical features in addition to anaemia include glossitis (q.v.) and neurological disease. The neurological disease is referred to as **subacute combined degeneration** and comprises peripheral neuropathy (q.v.) as well as spinal cord involvement. It is manifest by paraesthesiae and initially loss of sensations passing through the posterior columns, i.e. loss of vibration sense and proprioception, but the sensations of touch and temperature are preserved until the disease is advanced. There is thus ataxia and spastic weakness. Optic neuropathy may occur. Patients can also suffer from neuropsychiatric impairment, especially memory loss and depression. Neither the presence nor severity of these neurological complications are correlated with the extent of the associated anaemia, but they may be related to impairment of methionine synthase.

*Treatment is with **vitamin B_{12}** 1000 mcg parenterally weekly for 6 weeks, then monthly for life. Even though vitamin B_{12} is poorly absorbed orally in the absence of intrinsic factor, large doses (e.g. 2000 mcg) orally per day may be sufficient to free the patient from monthly injections, since the daily nutritional requirement is only about 1 mcg.*

If the anaemia is severe, transfusion may be considered, but this needs to be administered with great care as volume overload is easily produced in these patients.

Bibliography

Pruthi RK, Tefferi A. Pernicious anemia revisited. *Mayo Clin Proc* 1994; 69: 144.

Romain M, Sviri S, Linton DM, et al. The role of vitamin B12 in the critically ill – a review. *Anaesth Intens Care* 2016; 44: 447.

Wald NJ, Bower C. Folic acid, pernicious anaemia, and prevention of neural tube defects. *Lancet* 1994; 343: 307.

Peroneal muscular atrophy *See*

- Charcot–Marie–Tooth disease.

Persistent critical illness

Persistent critical illness (or **chronic critical illness**) are terms which have been coined to describe the situation of critically ill patients who have survived the acute phase of their illness but who have now entered a more prolonged course of organ failure support and delayed recovery. The time of transition to persistent critical illness is generally about 10 days.

This situation is considered primarily attributable to complications (especially new-onset sepsis) or to prior comorbidities rather than to the condition which initiated the ICU stay in the first place. However, persistent critical illness could also be contributed to by the standard of care in a particular ICU. Theoretically, a more prolonged period of care could result either from excellent care which has led to survival in otherwise fatal settings or from suboptimal care which led to additional complications. Studies suggest that the latter situation is in fact more likely to be relevant.

Persistent critical illness is an important concept, because it represents a clinical situation of worse outcome and of increased ICU resources. For example, it has been calculated that up to 50% of ICU bed-days may be occupied by patients who either have (or will develop) persistent critical illness and who then have a 4-fold increase in ICU mortality.

Bibliography
Bagshaw SM, Stelfox HT, Iwashyna TJ, et al. Timing of onset of persistent critical illness: a multi-centre retrospective cohort study. *Intens Care Med* 2019; 44: 2134.
Darvall JN, Boonstra T, Norman J, et al. Persistent critical illness: baseline characteristics, intensive care course, and cause of death. *Crit Care Resusc* 2019; 21: 110.
Iwashyna TJ, Hodgson CL, Pilcher D, et al. Towards defining persistent critical illness and other varieties of chronic critical illness. *Crit Care Resusc* 2015; 17: 215.
Nelson JE, Cox CE, Hope AA, et al. Chronic critical illness. *Am J Respir Crit Care Med* 2010; 182: 446.
Sakusic A, Gajic O. Chronic critical illness: unintended consequence of intensive care medicine. *Lancet Respir Med* 2016; 4: 531.
Viglianti EM, Bagshaw SM, Bellomo R, et al. Hospital-level variation in the development of persistent critical illness. *Intens Care Med* 2020; 46: 1567.

Pesticides

Pesticides are common causes of chemical poisoning (q.v.), either accidental or suicidal, and some may be used as warfare agents (q.v.). They are responsible for about 10% of all deaths due to poisoning in general.

The most common pesticides are **herbicides** (q.v.) and **insecticides** (q.v.).

Petechiae

Petechiae are the smallest haemorrhagic lesions on the skin and mucous membranes, with echymoses being the largest. Petechiae are manifest as non-blanching red-purple dots.

Petechiae have three mechanisms of causation, namely,
- thrombocytopenia (q.v.),
- platelet function disorders (q.v.),
- microvascular damage (i.e. vascular purpura).

Vascular purpura is especially associated with serious infections, such as sepsis (see Purpura).

Peutz–Jeghers syndrome *See*
- Mouth diseases.

Phaeochromocytoma

Phaeochromocytoma is the only lesion of the adrenal medulla. Similar tumours may sometimes arise elsewhere in the sympathetic nervous system and are referred to as **paragangliomas**.

It is a vascular and secretory tumour associated with the production of hypertension and thus detected mainly in such patients, though given its rarity it is found in less than 1% of patients with hypertension.
- Traditionally, there is paroxysmal hypertension, but this is seen in only 40% of patients and the majority in fact have sustained hypertension.
- An occasional patient may even present with paradoxical hypotension, especially of a postural nature, from excess beta stimulation and hypovolaemia.
- There is associated headache, sweating (q.v.) and tachycardia, with a hypermetabolic state, including glucose intolerance, weight loss and leukocytosis.

Phaeochromocytoma may sometimes be associated with the MEN syndrome type 2 (q.v.), in which case it is often bilateral. Such cases have been found to be associated with genetic mutations. Occasionally, the tumours are found extra-abdominally, e.g. in the thoracic paraaortic region (i.e. a paraganglioma). Most phaeochromocytomas (90%) are benign. Some are clinically undiagnosed during life or are detected incidentally during abdominal imaging for other conditions.

The diagnosis should be considered in young patients with hypertension, in paroxysmal hypertension or if there are associated symptoms.

The differential diagnosis particularly includes
- hypertension with associated anxiety,
- posterior fossa lesions, which can stimulate the medullary sympathetic-adrenal axis.

The diagnosis is confirmed by the demonstration of increased metabolites in the plasma or urine. The most convenient test has been 24-hr urinary secretion of VMA (vanillylmandelic acid) and catecholamines, but the 24-hr urinary excretion of metanephrine is more reliable and elevated plasma catecholamine levels are the most sensitive. Specific provocative or inhibitory tests of catecholamine secretion can be hazardous. Direct imagining of the tumour with CT scanning is required to demonstrate the actual site of lesions >5 mm in diameter. Genetic testing for susceptibility genes is recommended.

Treatment requires careful pre-operative preparation with **alpha blockade** (using phenoxybenzamine) for blood pressure control, followed if necessary by **beta blockade** for heart rate control. Following normalization of blood pressure, heart rate and blood volume, **surgery** is undertaken, preferably laparoscopically. Great care needs to be taken with sudden hypertension during surgical handling of the tumour, followed by hypotension after its removal. Thus, vasodilator and vasopressor infusions need to be prepared for use, as well as parenteral beta blocker and intravenous fluids.

> Rarely, a **phaeochromocytoma crisis** may occur, which produces features similar to those of a number of other conditions, including cerebral trauma, monoamine oxidase inhibitor crisis or abrupt cessation of clonidine.
> It is treated with **blood pressure control**, followed by beta blockade.

Bibliography
Alderazi Y, Yeh MW, Robinson BG, et al. Phaeochromocytoma: current concepts. *Med J Aust* 2005; 183: 201.
Bravo EL, Gifford RW. Pheochromocytoma: diagnosis, localization and management. *N Engl J Med* 1984; 311: 1298.
Bravo EL, Tagle R. Pheochromocytoma: state-of-the-art and future prospects. *Endocr Rev* 2003; 24: 539.
Daly PA, Landsberg L. Phaeochromocytoma: diagnosis and management. *Bailliere's Clin Endocrinol Metab* 1992; 6: 143.
Editorial. The function of adrenaline. *Lancet* 1985; 1: 561.
Golub MS, Tuck ML. Diagnostic and therapeutic strategies in pheochromocytoma. *Endocrinologist* 1992; 2: 101.
Lenders JW, Pacak K, Walther MM, et al. Biochemical diagnosis of pheochromocytoma: which test is best? *JAMA* 2002; 287: 1427.
Naranjo J, Dodd S, Martin YN. Perioperative management of pheochromocytoma. *J Cardiothorac Vasc Anesth* 2017; 31: 1427.
Sutton MG, Sheps SG, Lie JT. Prevalence of clinically unsuspected pheochromocytoma. *Mayo Clin Proc* 1981; 56: 354.
Whalen RK, Althausen AF, Daniels GH. Extra-adrenal pheochromocytoma. *J Urol* 1992; 147: 1.

Phosgene See
- Warfare agents.

Phrenic nerve See
- Diaphragm,
- Neuropathy.

Phthiriasis See
- Pediculosis.

Physical exposures

A large variety of **physical exposures** may be caused by environmental hazards (see Environment, see also Climate change). Some of these can be serious enough to require the attention of Intensive Care clinicians. The physical exposures considered in this book are those related to
- Cold
  - frostbite,
  - hypothermia.
- Heat
  - heat cramps,
  - heat exhaustion/stress,
  - heat stroke,
  - heat rash,
  - heat shock proteins,
  - hot tubs,
  - hyperthermia.
- High altitude.
- Water-related accidents
  - bathing,
  - diving,
  - drowning.

Pigmentation disorders

1. **Hypopigmentation**
- **Albinism**

This is an uncommon condition, in which several types of genetic defect of melanin production may be inherited as an autosomal dominant.
- **Hypomelanosis**

This refers to decreased pigmentation following recent skin trauma or inflammation, including eczema, leprosy (q.v.), psoriasis (q.v.), syphilis (q.v.).

- **Vitiligo**

This refers to patchy depigmentation following loss of melanin and/or melanocytes, especially on the face or limbs. These lesions may coalesce so as to become extensive, but this process is very variable. The same process may also destroy pigment cells in the retina.

It is a common condition with probable multiple aetiologies, including autoimmune, genetic and environmental factors, all leading to an adverse immune response. The condition can be psychologically distressing, especially in darker skinned subjects.

Vitiligo is particularly associated with endocrine disorders, such Addison's disease (q.v.), diabetes, pernicious anaemia (q.v.) and thyroid disease (see Hyperthyroidism, see Hypothyroidism).

Repigmentation of vitiliginous areas has been attempted by psoralen photochemotherapy (PUVA), but later techniques including narrow-band ultraviolet light (UVB phototherapy) and excimer laser therapy (as used for psoriasis – q.v.) have been more successful. Topical calcineurin inhibition (e.g. with tacrolimus or pimecrolimus) have shown both efficacy and safety. Cosmetic surgery may be appropriate in some cases of localized disease.

2. **Hyperpigmentation**

   A. Local hyperpigmentation
   - **Acanthosis nigricans**

   This refers to pigmented papillomatous lesions resembling dirt lines and especially seen in skin folds.

   It may be associated with
   - obesity,
   - autoimmune disease (q.v.),
   - endocrine disease
     - flexural brown thickening of the skin suggests hyperinsulinaemia, typical of the most severe form of insulin-resistant polycystic ovary syndrome (q.v.),
   - malignancy (see Paraneoplastic syndromes)
     - especially abdominal adenocarcinoma,
     - occasionally squamous cell carcinoma of the cervix.

   It may also be seen as a familial trait.
   - **Freckles**, or solar lentigines

   These may be seen after local trauma or inflammation, or in neurofibromatosis (q.v.).
   - **Melasma** (chloasma)

   This occurs on the face and is seen with oral contraceptives (q.v.), pregnancy or liver disease.

   Skin lightening therapies for melasma have been commonly based on combination preparations containing hydroquinone, steroid and tretinoin, but the former agent has been withdrawn in some countries because of concerns about possible ochronosis (extensive skin pigmentation). Laser therapy may be of benefit in difficult cases.

   B. Diffuse hyperpigmentation
   - **Systemic diseases**

   These include
   - Addison's disease (q.v.),
   - haemochromatosis (q.v.),
   - drugs, including amiodarone, antimalarials, cytotoxic agents, oral tanning agents, phenothiazines, tetracycline.
   - **Non-melanin** hyperpigmentation

   This may be due to deposition of
   - carotene,
   - haemoglobin,
   - foreign substances, such as heavy metals (arsenic, silver) (q.v.).

Bibliography

Grimes PE. Melasma: etiologic and therapeutic considerations. *Arch Dermatol* 1995; 131: 1453.

Grimes PE. Disorders of pigmentation. In: *Scientific American Medicine. Dermatology.* Hamilton: Dekker Medicine. 2020.

Hendrix JD, Greer KE. Cutaneous hyperpigmentation caused by systemic drugs. *Int J Dermatol* 1992; 31: 458.

Orlow SJ. Albinism: an update. *Semin Cutan Med Surg* 1997; 16: 24.

Wolff K, Goldsmith L, Katz S, et al., eds. *Fitzpatrick's Dermatology in General Medicine.* 7th edition. New York: McGraw-Hill. 2007.

Pink urine

Pink urine is occasionally seen after the administration of propofol (q.v.). It is related to the deposition of uric acid crystals in acid urine, which dissolve when the urinary pH is raised. It is a benign condition.

Bibliography

Masuda A, Hirota K, Satone T, et al. Pink urine during propofol anesthesia. *Anesth Analg* 1996; 83: 666.

Pituitary

The **hypothalamic–pituitary axis** is the major junction between the body's two chief pathways for integrated systemic responses, namely, the nervous and endocrine systems.

The richly innervated hypothalamus provides the link with the CNS. Since it is outside the blood–brain barrier, it can also sense circulating substances, such as cortisol, glucose and sodium. In addition, it has amine, opioid and peptide receptors. It is thus well placed to house the major homeostatic centres for control of osmolality, temperature, thirst and appetite.

It provides the link with the endocrine system via secretion of stimulatory or inhibitory peptides into the hypophyseal–portal venous system and thus into the anterior pituitary. These peptides include AVP/ADP, CRH, dopamine, GHRH, GnRH, somatostatin, TRH.

The **hypothalamic–pituitary–adrenal** (HPA) axis is also a key player in the human stress response (as described originally by Hans Selye), in which it can mediate and modify the biology involved. Thus, stress-induced effects on the HPA axis are involved in post-traumatic stress disorder (PTSD), anxiety disorders, adjustment disorders and depression.

The **anterior pituitary** secretions, if abnormally increased or decreased, are usually manifest via abnormalities of the target gland. If the pituitary abnormality is caused by a tumour, there may also be local symptoms, particularly of a visual nature. Pituitary tumours may be either microadenomas (<1 cm) or macroadenomas. They arise from cells secreting adrenocorticotropic hormone, follicle stimulating hormone, growth hormone, luteinising hormone, prolactin or thyroid stimulating hormone. Most such tumours are in fact prolactinomas (60%) or growth hormone secreting tumours (20%) which cause acromegaly (q.v.).

Pituitary apoplexy is an emergency condition which can complicate any pituitary tumour (see Acromegaly).

The most common deficiency of anterior pituitary secretion is global, i.e. panhypopituitarism. This is usually due to a tumour, particularly a chromophobe adenoma. Other tumours, such as craniopharyngioma or occasionally metastases, or sometimes other space-occupying lesions, such as granulomas, may be responsible for global pituitary deficiency. In the critically ill, dopamine infusion used to be an important cause of anterior pituitary suppression.

Sheehan's syndrome refers to the rare entity of pituitary deficiency following post-partum shock, though hypophysitis may be a more common cause of pituitary deficiency in the post-partum period.

Pituitary reserve is best tested currently via the response of the pituitary hormones and target hormones to releasing hormones.

*Treatment of pituitary deficiency is traditionally with **target gland hormone replacement** (adrenal, gonadal, thyroid), since pituitary hormones themselves are generally inconvenient to administer clinically.*

*The exception is **human growth hormone**, which is easily given by daily subcutaneous injection. Its indication in adults is controversial, though it is licensed in several countries for use in growth hormone deficiency. It is currently made by recombinant technology and is thus safe, though it is very expensive.*

See Adrenal insufficiency, see Hypothyroidism.

The **posterior pituitary** comprises the terminal parts of the hypothalamic neurones. It is here that vasopressin (AVP or ADH) (q.v.) is secreted, having migrated along the axons from the hypothalamus where it was synthesized.

Vasopressin secretion responds to small changes (e.g. 1%) in osmolality and to larger changes (e.g. 10%) in blood pressure or blood volume. As little as 1% increase in plasma osmolality causes sufficient vasopressin secretion to increase the urine osmolality by 200 mOsm/kg. This response is sensitive in either direction in normal subjects, but it becomes substantially impaired in older patients and in cardiac failure.

Impaired vasopressin secretion due to depleted neurohypophyseal stores may lead to an inappropriately low plasma level of vasopressin in septic shock. Exogenous arginine **vasopressin** in low doses (e.g. 0.03 IU/min) may usefully supplement catecholamine infusion in some cases of poorly responding vasodilatory shock.

The chief disorders of vasopressin (q.v.) are
- diabetes insipidus (q.v.)
  - i.e. ADH deficiency,
- the syndrome of inappropriate antidiuretic hormone (q.v.)
  - i.e. ADH excess.
  See also
- Desmopressin.

Bibliography
Baylis PH. Posterior pituitary function in health and disease. *Clin Endocrinol Metab* 1983; 12: 747.
Bills DC, Meyer FB, Laws ER, et al. A retrospective analysis of pituitary apoplexy. *Neurosurgery* 1993; 33: 602.
Boonen E, Van den Berghe G. Understanding the HPA response to critical illness: novel insights with clinical implications. *Intens Care Med* 2015; 41: 131.
Burke CW. The pituitary megatest: outdated? *Clin Endocrinol* 1992; 36: 133.
Chrousos GP. The hypothalamic-pituitary-adrenal axis and immune-mediated inflammation. *N Engl J Med* 1995; 332: 1351.

Dash RJ, Gupta V, Suri S. Sheehan's syndrome. *Aust NZ J Med* 1993; 23: 26.

Editorial. Corticosteroids and hypothalamic-pituitary-adrenocortical function. *BMJ* 1980; 280: 813.

Elster AD. Modern imaging of the pituitary. *Radiology* 1993; 187: 1.

Hoffman DM, Ho KKY. Growth hormone deficiency in adults: to treat or not to treat. *Aust NZ J Med* 1999; 29: 342.

Holland J, Bakker J, Feelders RA. What's new on the HPA axis? *Intens Care Med* 2015; 41: 1477.

Hurley DM, Ho KKY. Pituitary disease in adults. *Med J Aust* 2004; 180: 419.

Loriaux DL. The polyendocrine deficiency syndromes. *N Engl J Med* 1985; 312: 1568.

Magner JA. Thyroid-stimulating hormone: biosynthesis, cell biology, and bioactivity. *Endocrinol Rev* 1990; 11: 354.

Melmed S. Pituitary. In: *Scientific American Medicine.* Endocrinology & Metabolism. Hamilton: Dekker Medicine. 2020.

Molitch ME, Russell EJ. The pituitary 'incidentaloma'. *Ann Intern Med* 1990; 112: 925.

Robertson GL. Physiology of ADH secretion. *Kidney Int* 1987; 32 (suppl. 21): S20.

Russell JA, Walley KR, Singer J, et al. Vasopressin versus norepinephrine infusion in patients with septic shock. *N Engl J Med* 2008; 358: 877.

Sharshar T, Carlier R, Blanchard A, et al. Depletion of neurohypophyseal content of vasopressin in septic shock. *Crit Care Med* 2002; 30: 497.

Shupnik MA, Ridgway EC, Chin WW. Molecular biology of thyrotropin. *Endocr Rev* 1989; 10: 459.

Vance ML. Hypopituitarism. *N Engl J Med* 1994; 330: 1651.

Van den Berghe G, de Zegher F. Anterior pituitary function during critical illness and dopamine treatment. *Crit Care Med* 1996; 24: 1580.

Vokes TJ, Robertson GL. Disorders of antidiuretic hormone. *Endocrinol Metab Clin North Am* 1988; 17: 281.

Pituitary apoplexy See

- Acromegaly.

Placental abruption (abruptio placentae) See

- Amniotic fluid embolism,
- HELLP syndrome,
- Haemolytic–uraemic syndromes,
- Pre-eclampsia,
- Trauma in pregnancy.

Plague

Plague, more formally called bubonic plague, is caused by the non-motile Gram-negative bacillus *Yersinia* (formerly *Pasteurella*) *pestis*. It is primarily a disease of rodents and of carnivores that prey on them, and it is incidentally transmitted to humans via infected fleas (i.e. insects) or by direct contact. It is thus a zoonosis (q.v.).

The organism can be particularly virulent, with as few as one organism able to cause a lethal infection. Plague is a classic infection model for blood-borne bacterial transmission, because fulminant bacteraemia must be rapidly established in the host mammal for the next wave of feeding fleas to be successfully infected. To achieve this, the organism has developed virulence factors (e.g. T3SS) which can suppress the host's innate immune system.

Of historical interest, the famous plague of Athens in 430 BC was probably not caused by bubonic plague itself but another major contagion, such as epidemic typhus (see Rickettsial diseases), Ebola fever (q.v.) or even post-influenzal toxic shock syndrome (q.v.). However, bubonic plague (which probably originated in Central Asia) was undoubtedly one of the great scourges of humankind over the centuries (see Pandemics). The first pandemic was the Plague of Justinian which devastated much of Europe, Asia and Africa in the sixth century, but it is perhaps best known as the Black Death, which ravaged fourteenth-century Europe. On both occasions, up to half of the population was killed, with disastrous societal consequences which lasted for centuries thereafter. Fortunately, plague is now uncommon worldwide, even in enzootic rural areas of developing countries. On the other hand, interest in plague has recently been stimulated by its potential for use in germ warfare (q.v.) and thus bioterrorism (q.v.).

Plague remains the archetypal pestilence, and it has given its name generically to any infectious disease which is both widespread and virulent or indeed to any other overwhelmingly troublesome condition.

Following an incubation period of 2–6 days after the culprit flea bite, there is painful regional lymphadenopathy, particularly in the axillary and inguinal regions. There is intense local lymph node inflammation with necrosis, producing the buboes characteristic of the disease. After a few further days, bacteraemia and severe sepsis typically ensue, with systemic invasion and haemorrhagic necrotic inflammation, especially of the lungs, liver and spleen. The resultant severe acute pneumonia is commonly associated with septic shock, it can be fatal within a few hours and it is highly infectious to others via droplet spread (in which case the incubation period is much shorter).

Diagnosis is by antibody identification or the finding of typical plump Gram-negative bacilli on lymph node material or in sputum, since culture is too dangerous for routine laboratories.

Treatment is with **antibiotics**, originally streptomycin but subsequently tetracycline or even chloramphenicol. Isolation procedures are required.

A killed vaccine is available for those at high personal risk, but its efficacy is uncertain.

Bibliography

Butler T. A clinical study of bubonic plague: observations of the 1970 Vietnam epidemic with emphasis on coagulation studies, skin histology and electrocardiograms. *Am J Med* 1972; 53: 268.

Inglesby TV, Dennis DT, Henderson DA, et al. Plague as a biological weapon: medical and public health management. *JAMA* 2000; 283: 2281.

Liles WC. Infections due to brucella, francisella, yersinia pestis, and bartonella. In: *Scientific American Medicine. Infectious Disease.* Hamilton: Dekker Medicine. 2020.

Von Reyn CF, Weber NS, Tempest B, et al. Epidemiologic and clinical features of an outbreak of bubonic plague in New Mexico. *J Infect Dis* 1977; 136: 489.

Whitby M, Ruff TA, Street AC, et al. Biological agents as weapons 2: anthrax and plague. *Med J Aust* 2002; 176: 605.

PLAID syndrome *See*
- Urticaria – 4. Physical (Cold urticaria).

Plasmacytoma *See*
- Multiple myeloma.

Plasmapheresis

Plasmapheresis, sometimes referred to as plasma exchange (PEX) or therapeutic plasma exchange (TPE), is a major technique for **immunomodulation** (q.v.).

Although originally using centrifugation, its bedside operation in Intensive Care practice typically involves an extracorporeal circuit (as for renal replacement therapy) with an in-line cartridge containing a membrane filter with a pore size that permits the passage of proteins but not blood cells. The goal is to remove pathological circulating factors (typically culprit antibodies) in systemic conditions which may have an autoimmune pathogenesis, so that the disease process is rapidly controlled while longer-term therapy is established. However, the benefit of plasmapheresis is not fully explained by the removal of pathological factors alone and may involve more complex immunomodulation.

The effective use of plasmapheresis has also been reported in small case-series of poisonings due to protein-bound drugs or toxins. Its possible value in sepsis and septic shock remains controversial.

The chief conditions for which plasmapheresis is indicated include
- antiphospholipid syndrome (q.v.),
- demyelinating diseases (q.v.),
- exfoliative dermatitis (q.v.),
- Goodpasture's syndrome (q.v.),
- Guillain–Barré syndrome (q.v.),
- haemolytic–uraemic syndromes (q.v.),
- HELLP syndrome (q.v.),
- hyperthyroidism (q.v.),
- idiopathic thrombocytopenic purpura (q.v.),
- immune complex disease (q.v.),
- microangiopathic haemolysis (q.v.),
- multiple myeloma (q.v.),
- myasthenia gravis (q.v.),
- pemphigus (q.v.),
- polymyositis (q.v.),
- scleroderma (q.v.),
- systemic lupus erythematosus (q.v.),
- thrombocytopenia – Post-transfusion purpura, Drug-induced thrombocytopenia (q.v.),
- thrombotic thrombocytopenic purpura (q.v.),
- Waterhouse–Friderichsen syndrome (q.v.).

Bibliography

Couriel D, Weinstein R. Complications of therapeutic plasma exchange: a recent assessment. *J Clin Apheresis* 1994; 9: 1.

Madore F. Plasmapheresis. In: *Scientific American Medicine. Nephrology.* Hamilton: Dekker Medicine. 2020.

Reeves HM, Winters JL. The mechanisms of action of plasma exchange. *Br J Haematol* 2014; 164: 342.

Reimann PM, Mason PD. Plasmapheresis: technique and complications. *Intens Care Med* 1990; 16: 3.

Rimmer E, Houston BL, Kumar A, et al. The efficacy and safety of plasma exchange in patients with sepsis and septic shock: a systematic review and meta-analysis. *Crit Care* 2014; 18: 699.

Plasminogen

Plasminogen is the inactive circulating precursor of the fibrinolytic system. Its molecular weight is 92 kDa, its plasma concentration is 220 mcg/mL (2.0 µM) and its half-life is 50 hr.

Its role is described in Fibrinolysis (q.v.).

Platelet function disorders

Platelet function disorders or defects refer to qualitative platelet abnormalities, as opposed to the quantitative platelet abnormality of thrombocytopenia (q.v.).

> They present as a bleeding disorder with prolonged bleeding time but normal platelet count.

Platelet function disorders may be congenital or acquired.
1. **Congenital**
   - absence of platelet membrane receptors, due to the rare conditions involving
     - glycoprotein IIb–IIIa, i.e. Glanzmann's thrombasthenia (see also Antiplatelet agents), in which bleeding episodes have been successfully treated with factor VIIa,
     - glycoprotein Ib–Ix, i.e. Bernard–Soulier disease,
   - platelet granule deficiency, i.e. α- and δ-storage pool disease, which are also rare,
   - von Willebrand's disease (q.v.).
2. **Acquired**
   - storage pool defect
     - in myeloproliferative disorders,
   - miscellaneous abnormalities, as
     - in alcoholism,
     - after cardiopulmonary bypass (q.v.),
     - in sepsis,
     - in uraemia,
     - due to drugs.

> Many **drugs** adversely affect platelet function. However, few do so in a manner quantitative enough to cause clinical bleeding, unless there is some other concomitant haemostatic impairment. On the other hand, antiplatelet drugs have become major modalities in the prevention and treatment of thrombotic disorders, particularly of the arterial system (see Antiplatelet agents).

Of the drugs causing quantitatively significant platelet dysfunction, **aspirin** is the archetypal agent. Like all NSAIDs, it impairs platelet aggregation by inhibiting cyclo-oxygenase and decreasing thromboxane A_2 (TXA_2). Other drugs which cause clinically significant defects include
- beta-lactam antibiotics
  - originally carbenicillin, but also later members of this family to a lesser extent, as well as high doses of penicillin,
- dextran 70,
- selective serotonin reuptake inhibitors (SSRIs).

Many agents can impair platelet function in a minor way, including especially
- anaesthetic agents,
- antihistamines,
- beta blockers,
- calcium channel blockers,
- clofibrate,
- nitrates,
- psychotropic agents,
- radiographic contrast media.

Certain foods can produce similar effects, including
- garlic,
- ginger,
- onions,
- several spices.

Treatment of clinical bleeding due to a platelet function defect is with **platelet concentrates** *and/or* **DDAVP** *(see Desmopressin).*

Bibliography
Cattaneo M. Inherited platelet-based bleeding disorders. *J Thromb Haemost* 2003; 1: 1628.
Desborough MJR, Oakland KA, Landon G, et al. Desmopressin for treatment of platelet dysfunction and reversal of antiplatelet agents: a systematic review and meta-analysis of randomized controlled trials. *J Thromb Haemost* 2017; 15: 263.
Deykin D. Uremic bleeding. *Kidney Int* 1983; 24: 698.
Ferrara JLM. The febrile platelet transfusion reaction: a cytokine shower. *Transfusion* 1995; 35: 89.
George JN, Shattil SJ. The clinical importance of acquired abnormalities of platelet function. *N Engl J Med* 1991; 324: 27.
Hankey GJ, Eikelboom JW. Antiplatelet drugs. *Med J Aust* 2003; 178: 568.
Lacoste L, Hung J, Lam JY. Acute and delayed antithrombotic effects of alcohol in humans. *Am J Cardiol* 2001; 87: 82.
Leung LLK, Zehnder JL. Platelet disorders. In: *Scientific American Medicine. Hematology.* Hamilton: Dekker Medicine. 2020.
Marder VJ, Aird WC, Bennett JS, et al., eds. *Hemostasis and Thrombosis: Basic Principles and Clinical Practice.* 6th edition. Philadelphia: Lippincott Williams & Wilkins. 2012.
Nurden AT, Nurden P. Inherited disorders of platelet function: selected updates. *J Thromb Haemost* 2015; 13: S2.
Pigozzi L, Aron JP, Ball, J, et al. Understanding platelet dysfunction in sepsis. *Intens Care Med* 2016; 42: 583.

Rice TW, Wheeler AP. Coagulopathy in critically ill patient. Part 1: platelet disorders. *Chest* 2009; 136: 1622.

Sattler FR, Weitekamp MR, Ballard JO. Potential for bleeding with the new beta-lactam antibiotics. *Ann Intern Med* 1986; 105: 924.

Schafer AI. Bleeding and thrombosis in the myeloproliferative disorders. *Blood* 1984; 64: 1.

Yang Z, Stulz P, von Segesser L, et al. Different interactions of platelets with arterial and venous coronary bypass vessels. *Lancet* 1991; 337: 939.

Platelets

Platelets are known for their central role physiologically in haemostasis and pathologically in thrombosis. They are the smallest circulating cells in the blood.

However, as with many biological processes, platelets have been increasingly recognized to have diverse functions beyond those originally attributed to them. For example, it has been shown that they may contribute to inflammatory responses by recruiting leukocytes to sites of injury, and they can release both proinflammatory and anti-inflammatory mediators. Thus, platelets may play additional roles in conditions as diverse as sepsis, organ damage, atherosclerosis, cancer progression, wound healing and transplant rejection. Since current antiplatelet drugs (q.v.) target the initial (global) processes of platelet activation and aggregation, therapeutic targeting of other platelet functions would presumably require the development of new and more specific drugs.

Importantly, platelets are more than just anucleate cell fragments. Clearly, they have adhesive properties with numerous receptors which permit interaction both with cells (e.g. endothelial cells, leukocytes and other platelets) and with non-cellular structures (e.g. fibrinogen). The resultant platelet activation leads to the release of a variety of cytokines and mediators, only some of which are involved in coagulation. Many of the secreted mediators are stored in microvesicles. Platelets also contain both relevant RNA (which can then translate into protein) and metabolically competent mitochondria. Thus, platelets retain many of the multifunctional properties of their parent cells in the bone marrow. They also retain some of the functional properties of their evolutionary predecessors, namely the **haemocytes**, which had a combined immunological and haemostatic function in arthropods (q.v.) before more specialized immune and haemostatic cells evolved in later species.

The contribution of platelets to host defence by protection against invading bacteria may explain some of the mechanistic difficulty in understanding the clinical problem of heparin-induced thrombocytopenia (HIT) (q.v.).

Although the normal platelet count has a range from $150-450 \times 10^9$/L, it tends to be higher in women and in youth and to vary considerably between ethnic populations. Variations in the size of platelets are relevant to their functioning (see Thrombocytopenia). About 100 billion platelets are produced in the body each day, but this number may increase up to 20-fold during situations of severe stress. About a trillion platelets are circulating at any one time. Their lifespan is 7–10 days (average half-life 4 days), but as with red blood cells (see Anaemia) the lifespan of transfused platelets is only about 50% of normal, with an initial clearance of about 40% in the spleen due to storage lesions in the donor platelets. The usual half-life of transfused platelets of about 24 hr is greatly reduced (to as low as 1 hr) in severe platelet consumptive disorders.

Dramatic new opportunities for ex vivo platelet production for clinical transfusion may occur with the future use of induced pluripotent stem cells. These can produce megakaryocytes which can be cryopreserved and act as a master source for transfusion services, giving an almost limitless on-demand supply of platelets which can be HLA-deleted (and thus non-alloimmune) and free from blood-borne infections.

Platelet deficiencies result from either

- reduced numbers (i.e. **thrombocytopenia** – q.v.), or
- impaired function (i.e. **platelet function disorders** – q.v.).

Platelet excess occurs when there are

- increased numbers (i.e. **thrombocytosis/ thrombocythaemia** – q.v.).

Bibliography

Bain BJ. Ethnic and sex differences in the total and differential white cell count and platelet count. *J Clin Pathol* 1996; 49: 664.

Bombace NM, Holmes CE. The platelet contribution to cancer progression. *J Thromb Haemost* 2011; 9: 237.

Cognasse F, Garraud O, Pozzetto B, et al. How can nonnucleated platelets be so smart? *J Thromb Haemost* 2016; 14: 794.

Handtke S, Thiele T. Large and small platelets — (when) do they differ? *J Thromb Haemost* 20020; 18: 1256.

Hoylaerts MF, Vanassche T, Verhamme P. Bacterial killing by platelets; making sense of (H)IT. *J Thromb Haemost* 2018; 16: 1182.

Izzi B, Bonaccio M, De Gaetano G, et al. Learning by counting blood platelets in population studies: survey and perspective a long way after Bizzozero. *J Thromb Haemost* 2018; 16: 1711.

Jurk K, Kehrel BE. Platelets: physiology and biochemistry. *Semin Thromb Hemost* 2005; 31: 381.

Koenen RR. The prowess of platelets in immunity and inflammation. *Thromb Haemost* 2016; 116: 605.

Koupenova M, Freedman JE. Platelets: the unsung hero in the immune response. *J Thromb Haemost* 2015; 13: 268.

Pigozzi L, Aron JP, Ball, J, et al. Understanding platelet dysfunction in sepsis. *Intens Care Med* 2016; 42: 583.

Smyth SS, McEver RP, Weyrich AS, et al. Platelet functions beyond hemostasis. *J Thromb Haemost* 2009; 7: 1759.

Platypnoea–orthodeoxia syndrome

Platypnoea–orthodeoxia syndrome (POS) is an uncommon clinical condition of dyspnoea (platypnoea) and oxygen desaturation (orthodeoxia) when upright. It is relieved by lying down.

It is an unusual clinical feature which is occasionally seen in conditions of left-right shunting, either intracardiac or extracardiac. The former conditions most commonly include patent foramen ovale or atrial septal defect, and paradoxical embolism is a recognized complication. The latter conditions are typically pulmonary arteriovenous malformations (see Arteriovenous malformations – Pulmonary AVMs), but they can also include patients with hepatopulmonary syndrome (q.v.), after pneumonectomy or with recurrent pulmonary embolism.

Bibliography
Agrawal A, Palkar A, Talwar A. The multiple dimensions of platypnea-orthodeoxia syndrome: a review. *Respir Med* 2017; 129: 31.

Pleiotropic effects

Pleiotropy (literally 'more ways') refers to the influence of a single gene on multiple, seemingly unrelated phenotypes. In a more familiar pharmacological context, pleiotropy describes the additional actions of a drug separate from those for which it is primarily known. Some of these additional actions may have potential benefit, but in general these have been studied to a limited degree, as they were unexpectedly different from the drug's original marketing indication. This principle does not in general apply to known adverse effects.

Perhaps the most dramatic example of drug pleiotropy in modern medicine is the antiplatelet effect of aspirin (q.v.), which was discovered many decades after its original introduction as an analgesic.

In Intensive Care practice, a number of drugs have interesting pleiotropic effects, which may broaden their appeal in important ways. Examples include ACE inhibitors (see Angiotensin-converting enzyme), heparin (q.v.), melatonin (q.v.), statins (q.v.) and vitamin D (q.v.).

Similar principles of multiple and unexpected actions can also apply to other biological elements, such as hormones (e.g. leptin – q.v.), cytokines, enzymes, proteins (e.g. protein S – q.v., somatostatin – q.v.) and cells (e.g. platelets – q.v.).

Bibliography
Davignon J. Beneficial cardiovascular pleiotropic effects of statins. *Circulation* 2004; 109: 39.

Pleural disorders

Pleural disorders include
1. pneumothorax (q.v.),
2. pleurisy (q.v.),
3. pleural effusion (q.v.),
4. plaques, with pleural thickening and calcification
   - following prior pleural disease,
   - see also Asbestos,
5. tumours
   - mesothelioma (see Asbestos),
   - either localized (i.e. fibroma) or diffuse (i.e. malignant).

The definitive diagnosis of pleural disorders commonly requires **pleural biopsy**. This may be performed with a biopsy needle using a closed technique (with or without ultrasound guidance) or with a biopsy forceps using a visual technique (with pleuroscopy or video-assisted thoracoscopy). The visual technique can also permit cryobiopsy instead of forceps biopsy.

Bibliography
Belani CP, ed. International symposium on thoracic malignancies. *Chest* 1998; 113 (suppl.): 1S.

Cagle PT, Allen TC. Pathology of the pleura: what the pulmonologists need to know. *Respirolory* 2011; 16: 430.

Feller-Kopman D, Light R. Pleural disease. *N Engl J Med* 2018; 378: 1754.

Lerner AD, Feller-Kopman D. Disorders of the pleura, mediastinum, and hilum. In: *Scientific American Medicine. Pulmonary & Critical Care Medicine.* Hamilton: Dekker Medicine. 2020.

Matin TN, Gleeson FV. Interventional radiology of pleural diseases. *Respirology* 2011; 16: 419.

Muller NL. Imaging of the pleura. *Radiology* 1993; 186: 297.

Porcel JM. Pearls and myths in pleural fluid analysis. *Respirology* 2011; 16: 44.

Sahn SA. The pleura. *Am Rev Respir Dis* 1988; 138: 184.

Pleural effusion

Pleural effusion may be either a transudate or exudate, i.e. with less than or greater than 30 g/L protein, respectively. Either may be called a hydrothorax.

A pleural effusion may also contain
- blood (i.e. a haemothorax, see below),
- pus (i.e. an empyema, see below; see Cavitation),
- chyle (i.e. a chylothorax, see below).

An effusion contains at least 500 mL before it can be detected clinically and 100–300 mL before it is apparent on plain X-ray. Ultrasound examination is routinely used to assess the presence and size of a pleural effusion, but it is unable to support a specific diagnosis. The pleural effusion may lie free in the pleural space or be loculated either in the general space or into lobular or subpulmonary spaces.

The chief investigation of pleural effusion is pleural aspiration (with or without pleural biopsy – see Pleural disorders). The fluid is examined for

1. **Macroscopic appearance**
   - straw-coloured
     - transudate, exudate,
   - purulent
     - empyema or pyothorax,
     - >50,000 WBCs/mL gives macroscopic appearance of purulence,
   - blood-stained
     - haemothorax, defined as haematocrit >50% that of peripheral blood,
     - blood-stained exudate, if haematocrit <25% that of peripheral blood,
     - >1 mL of blood/L gives RBC count >5000/mL and a serous appearance,
     - haematocrit >5% gives a red appearance indistinguishable from blood,
     - haematocrit >50% that of peripheral blood indicates frank bleeding,
     - haematocrit <50% but >25% that of peripheral blood does not exclude haemothorax because dilution can occur within a few days
   - milky
     - chylothorax,
     - chyliform (cholesterol-containing), sometimes called a pseudochylothorax, seen occasionally in chronic inflammatory exudates.
2. **Biochemistry**
   - protein
     - <30 g/L indicates transudate,
     - >30 g/L indicates exudate,
   - glucose
     - N > 50% plasma level,
     - decreased in tuberculosis (q.v.), malignancy, rheumatoid disease,
     - postpneumonic empyema,
   - lactate dehydrogenase (LDH)
     - increased in inflammation, i.e. in exudates,
   - cholesterol
     - increased in exudates or lymphatic obstruction,
   - amylase
     - increased in pancreatic disease,
   - pH
     - low (<7.20) in complicated parapneumonic effusions,
     - chest tube drainage is recommended for parapneumonic effusions with pH <7.20, even if they are culture-negative,
   - BNP or NT-proBNP (see Atrial natriuretic factor)
     - increased in serum and pleural fluid in heart failure.
3. **Cytology**
4. **Microbiology**

The chief causes of the different types of pleural effusion are

1. **Transudate**

- congestive cardiac failure
  - bilateral (70%), right-sided (20%) or left-sided (10%),
- constrictive pericarditis (q.v.),
- hypoproteinaemia
  - cirrhosis,
  - nephrotic syndrome,
  - critical illness,
- Meig's syndrome
  - from ovarian carcinoma,
- polyserositis,
- peritoneal dialysis,
- superior vena cava obstruction,
- myxoedema (q.v.).

2. **Exudate**

- bacterial pneumonia
  - parapneumonic sympathetic effusion,
- pulmonary infarction,
- malignancy
  - metastases, especially from cancers of lung, breast, stomach, ovary,
  - primary lung cancer,
  - mesothelioma (q.v.),
- tuberculosis (q.v.),

- subphrenic abscess,
- pancreatitis (q.v.),
- oesophageal perforation (see Mallory-Weiss syndrome),
- collagen-vascular disease (q.v.),
- lymphoma,
- uraemia,
- ascites
  - mostly gives right-sided effusions.

3. **Empyema**

- bacterial pneumonia,
- subphrenic abscess,
- penetrating injury,
- septic embolism,
- haematogenous spread.

4. **Haemothorax**

- trauma
  - including invasive procedures,
- malignancy,
- pulmonary infarction,
- leukaemia,
- tuberculosis (q.v.),
- pancreatitis (q.v.),
- oesophageal perforation (see Mallory-Weiss syndrome),
- pulmonary arteriovenous malformation (q.v.) or fistula,
- 'bloody tap'.

5. **Chylothorax**

- malignancy
  - especially lymphoma,
- trauma,
- surgery,
- left subclavian vein thrombosis,
- lymphangioleiomyomatosis (q.v.),
- lymphangiectasia,
- mediastinitis (q.v.).

Bibliography

Alexandrakis MG, Passam FH, Kyriakou DS, et al. Pleural effusions in hematologic malignancies. *Chest* 2004; 125: 1546.

Alfageme I, Munoz F, Pena N, et al. Empyema of the thorax in adults: etiology, microbiologic findings, and management. *Chest* 1993; 103: 839.

Bartter T, Santarelli R, Akers SM, et al. The evaluation of pleural effusion. *Chest* 1994; 106: 1209.

Bates D, Yang N, Bailey M, et al. Prevalence, characteristics, drainage and outcome of radiologically diagnosed pleural effusions in critically ill patients. *Crit Care Resusc* 2020; 22: 45.

Brogi E, Gargani L, Bignami E, et al. Thoracic ultrasound for pleural effusion in the intensive care unit: a narrative review from diagnosis to treatment. *Crit Care* 2017; 21: 325.

Cagle PT, Allen TC. Pathology of the pleura: what the pulmonologists need to know. *Respirolory* 2011; 16: 430.

Cerfolio RJ, Allen MS, Deschamps C, et al. Postoperative chylothorax. *J Thor Cardiovasc Surg* 1996; 112: 1361.

Gunnels J. Perplexing pleural effusions. *Chest* 1978; 74: 390.

Jamal S, Maurer JR. Pulmonary disease and the menstrual cycle. *Pulmonary Perspectives* 1994; 11(3): 3.

Joseph J, Sahn SA. Thoracic endometriosis syndrome: new observations from an analysis of 110 cases. *Am J Med* 1996; 100: 164.

Lerner AD, Feller-Kopman D. Disorders of the pleura, mediastinum, and hilum. In: *Scientific American Medicine. Pulmonary & Critical Care Medicine.* Hamilton: Dekker Medicine. 2020.

Light RW. Pleural effusions. *Med Clin North Am* 2011; 95: 1055.

Light RW, MacGregor MI, Luchsinger PC, et al. Pleural effusions: the diagnostic separation of transudates and exudates. *Ann Intern Med* 1972; 77: 507.

Lynch TJ. Management of malignant pleural effusions. *Chest* 1993; 103 (suppl.): S385.

Martinez FJ, Villanueva AG, Pickering R, et al. Spontaneous hemothorax. *Medicine* 1992; 71: 354.

Matin TN, Gleeson FV. Interventional radiology of pleural diseases. *Respirology* 2011; 16: 419.

Muller NL. Imaging of the pleura. *Radiology* 1993; 186: 297.

Porcel JM. Pearls and myths in pleural fluid analysis. *Respirology* 2011; 16: 44.

Romero S, Candela A, Martin C, et al. Evaluation of different criteria for the separation of pleural transudates from exudates. *Chest* 1993; 104: 399.

Ryu JH, Tomassetti S, Maldonado F. Update on uncommon pleural effusions. *Respirology* 2011; 16: 238.

Sahn SA. The pleura. *Am Rev Respir Dis* 1988; 138: 184.

Sahn SA. Management of complicated parapneumonic effusions. *Am Rev Respir Dis* 1993; 148: 813.
Shiel WC, Prete PE. Pleuropulmonary manifestations of rheumatoid arthritis. *Semin Arthritis Rheum* 1984; 13: 235.
Taylor JR, Ryu J, Colby TV, et al. Lymphangioleiomyomatosis. *N Engl J Med* 1990; 323: 1254.
Valentine VG, Raffin TA. The management of chylothorax. *Chest* 1992; 102: 586.
Vaz MA, Marchi E, Vargas FS. Cholesterol in the separation of transudates and exudates. *Curr Opin Pulm Med* 2001; 7: 183.
Walker-Renard PB, Vaughan LM, Sahn SA. Chemical pleurodesis for malignant pleural effusions. *Ann Intern Med* 1994; 120: 56.

Pleurisy

Pleurisy or inflammation of the parietal pleura is always due to underlying pulmonary disease, such as infection, inflammation, pulmonary embolism, neoplasm or trauma.

It is associated with chest pain, which is often severe, and with a pleural friction rub on auscultation. Dry or fibrinous pleurisy may be followed later by pleural effusion (q.v.), in which case the friction rub disappears because of separation of the parietal and visceral pleura.

If there is an associated pleural effusion, the causes of the pleurisy may be found among those conditions causing pleural effusions (q.v.). If there is no associated pleural effusion, the pleurisy is likely to be due to
- viral infection
  - especially with enteroviruses, such as Coxsackie B, which is sometimes in the form of epidemic pleurodynia, i.e. Bornholm disease,
- pulmonary embolism,
- serositis
  - usually associated with a collagen-vascular disease (q.v.),
- uraemia,
- pleuropericarditis
  - after myocardial infarction or postcardiotomy.

Bibliography
Cagle PT, Allen TC. Pathology of the pleura: what the pulmonologists need to know. *Respirolory* 2011; 16: 430.
Lerner AD, Feller-Kopman D. Disorders of the pleura, mediastinum, and hilum. In: *Scientific American Medicine. Pulmonary & Critical Care Medicine.* Hamilton: Dekker Medicine. 2020.
Matin TN, Gleeson FV. Interventional radiology of pleural diseases. *Respirology* 2011; 16: 419.
Muller NL. Imaging of the pleura. *Radiology* 1993; 186: 297.
Sahn SA. The pleura. *Am Rev Respir Dis* 1988; 138: 184.

Plumbism *See*
- Lead.

Plummer–Vinson syndrome *See*
- Anaemia,
- Dysphagia.

Pneumatosis coli

Pneumatosis coli describes the uncommon condition of gas-filled cysts within the bowel wall. The cysts can occupy the submucosa and subserosa, and they may affect both the small and large intestine.

Although the aetiology is unknown, there is an association with chronic airways obstruction.

The condition is usually asymptomatic and discovered only incidentally on abdominal X-ray. Occasionally, it may be considered responsible for either diarrhoea (q.v.) or obstruction.

Treatment with **hyperbaric oxygen** *causes the cysts and any associated symptoms to disappear.*

Pneumoconiosis *See*
- Occupational lung diseases.

Pneumomediastinum *See*
- Barotrauma.

Pneumonia, exotic *See*
- Exotic pneumonia.

Pneumonia in pregnancy

Pneumonia in pregnancy presents a special problem, because it is the commonest serious non-obstetric infection in the pregnant patient and because it is the third most frequent cause of indirect maternal death. It can also have a significant effect on fetal well-being.

Although the relative incidence of specific pathogens responsible for pneumonia in pregnancy is the same as in the non-pregnant patient, the decreased immune status of pregnancy renders such infections generally more serious. This particularly applies to viral, fungal and mycobacterial infections, because the chief alteration in maternal defence is in cell-mediated immunity due to the changed hormonal environment. These changes are compounded by secondary anatomical disadvantages in the respiratory system, especially a raised diaphragm, decreased functional residual capacity and reduced ability to clear tracheobronchial secretions.

Pneumonia in pregnancy may be
- community-acquired bacterial or atypical,
- complicating influenza, typically with superinfection (especially due to *Staphylococcus aureus*),
- nosocomial, which is usually Gram-negative,
- aspiration, which is typically polymicrobial with anaerobic and Gram-negative organisms.

The antibiotics which are indicated in pneumonia and which are safe in pregnancy comprise chiefly the **penicillins** *and* **cephalosporins**.
- *A* **macrolide** *(but not erythromycin estolate) is indicated for atypical pathogens.*
- **Aminoglycosides** *and* **vancomycin** *should be used only in very severe infections, because of the risk they pose of fetal ototoxicity and nephrotoxicity.*
  See
- Influenza.

Bibliography
Garland SM, O'Reilly MA. The risks and benefits of antimicrobial therapy in pregnancy. *Drug Safety* 1995; 13: 188.
Goodrum LA. Pneumonia in pregnancy. *Semin Perinatol* 1997; 21: 276.
Rigby FB, Pastorek JG. Pneumonia during pregnancy. *Clin Obstet Gynecol* 1996; 39: 107.
Riley L. Pneumonia and tuberculosis in pregnancy. *Infect Dis Clin North Am* 1997; 11: 119.

Pneumothorax

Pneumothorax refers to the presence of air within the pleural cavity.

This process may be
- spontaneous, or
- traumatic (including iatrogenic).
  Either type may be under 'tension'.

Spontaneous pneumothorax can
- arise in otherwise healthy subjects, i.e. primary pneumothorax, or
- occur as a complication of another lung disorder, i.e. secondary pneumothorax.

Spontaneous pneumothorax is an occasional but well-recognized complication of air travel, particularly in patients with various forms of bullous or cavitating lung disease. This is because a non-communicating air space expands up to 30% during ascent from sea level to the altitude represented by the typical cabin pressures at the cruising altitude of modern aircraft (i.e. 2440 m or 8000 ft), thus exposing thin-walled spaces to potentially disruptive forces.

Primary pneumothorax occurs most commonly in young tall thin males who are otherwise healthy, though they are usually smokers.

This is thought to be due to the greater apical distending forces operating in association with elastic recoil (which declines with age) and the pleural pressure gradient which is proportional to vertical lung height. There is probably an inherent weakness in the subpleural apical tissue, such as a small bleb, presumably due to a congenital bronchial tree anomaly.

Rarely, primary pneumothorax may be **catamenial** (i.e. menses-related), in which case it may be related to thoracic endometriosis. Circulating endometrial cells with particular gene expression profiles may be identified in such patients.

The overall incidence of primary pneumothorax in the population generally is low (about 4 per 10,000 patient-years).

Secondary pneumothorax occurs with
- diffuse disease processes
  - such as airways obstruction, bullae (q.v.), interstitial lung disease (q.v.), Marfan's syndrome (q.v.),
- focal disease processes,
  - such as carcinoma, infarction, necrotizing pneumonia (q.v.), rheumatoid nodule, endometriosis, tuberculosis (commonly in the past) (q.v.), *Pneumocystis jirovecii* pneumonia (PCP) (more commonly nowadays), and acute lobar collapse (causing pneumothorax ex vacuo).

Traumatic pneumothorax may be
- **open**
  - as after a penetrating chest wall injury,
- **closed**
  - as after closed chest wall injury, pulmonary barotrauma (q.v.), transbronchial lung biopsy or central venous catheterization.

The physical signs of pneumothorax may be quite subtle, unless the pneumothorax is large or under tension, when there may be
- compression of the ipsilateral lung,
- displacement of the mediastinum,
- distortion of the contralateral lung,
- circulatory embarrassment.

A chest X-ray is essential to confirm the presence of a pneumothorax and to assess its size and likely cause.

Treatment of a pneumothorax depends on its size and cause.

- *A small spontaneous pneumothorax (up to 25% reduction of lung volume) may be managed conservatively, unless the patient is on mechanical ventilation, in which case as for larger pneumothoraces an intercostal catheter (chest tube) is required. Resolution of a small pneumothorax normally requires 5–7 days, but this can be substantially hastened by administering oxygen which promotes reabsorption by exaggerating the diffusion gradient for nitrogen between the blood and intrathoracic gas.*
- *A moderate spontaneous pneumothorax may be successfully treated by simple aspiration in many cases (again unless the patient is on mechanical ventilation), but conservative management has been shown to be similarly effective, provided the pneumothorax is primary and there is suitable follow-up.*
- *Traumatic pneumothorax is best treated with insertion of an intercostal catheter and underwater seal, since in addition there is often blood in the pleural cavity (haemopneumothorax).*
- *Intercostal (intrapleural) catheter management in patients on mechanical ventilation requires careful attention to the negative intrapleural pressure in order to minimize air leak.*
- *Pleurodesis is usually performed for recurrent pneumothorax, and thoracotomy may be required for a persisting bronchopleural fistula. A number of specialized endobronchial and lung isolation procedures may be considered in selected cases.*

There is a risk of ipsilateral recurrence of spontaneous pneumothorax of about 25% within 2 yr. Review of patients with apparently primary spontaneous pneumothorax is essential to exclude underlying pathology which may require treatment.

See also

- Acute pulmonary oedema,
- Amniotic fluid embolism,
- Barotrauma,
- Cystic fibrosis,
- Gas in soft tissues,
- Histiocytosis,
- Marfan's syndrome,
- Mediastinal diseases.

Bibliography

Alifano M, Roth T, Broet SC, et al. Catamenial pneumothorax: a prospective study. *Chest* 2003; 124: 1004.

Andrivet P, Djedaini K, Teboul JL, et al. Spontaneous pneumothorax: comparison of thoracic drainage vs immediate or delayed needle aspiration. *Chest* 1995; 108: 335.

Baumann MH. Pneumothorax and air travel – editorial. *Chest* 2009; 136: 655.

Baumann MH, Strange C. Treatment of spontaneous pneumothorax. A more aggressive approach? *Chest* 1997; 112: 789.

Baumann MH, Strange C. The clinician's perspective on pneumothorax management. *Chest* 1997; 112: 822.

Baumann MH, Strange C, Heffner JE, et al. Management of spontaneous pneumothorax: an American College of Chest Physicians Delphi Consensus Statement. *Chest* 2001; 119: 590.

Chen K-Y, Jerng J-S, Liao W-Y, et al. Pneumothorax in the ICU: patient outcomes and prognostic factors. *Chest* 2002; 122: 678.

Dugan KC, Laxmanan B, Murgu S, et al. Management of persistent air leaks. *Chest* 2017; 152: 417.

Grotberg JC, Hyzy RC, De Cardenas J, et al. Bronchopleural fistula in the mechanically ventilated patient: a concise review. *Crit Care Med* 2021; 49: 292.

Haynes D, Baumann MH. Pleural controversy: aetiology of pneumothorax. *Respirology* 2011; 16: 604.

Hazelrigg SR. Secondary spontaneous pneumothorax: catamenial pneumothorax. *Chest* 2003; 124: 781.

Henry M, Arnold T, Harvey J, et al. BTS guidelines for the management of spontaneous pneumothorax. *Thorax* 2003; 58 (suppl.): ii39.

Legras A, Mansuet-Lupo A, Rousset-Jablonski C, et al. Pneumothorax in women of child-bearing age. *Chest* 2014; 145: 354.

Lerner AD, Feller-Kopman D. Disorders of the pleura, mediastinum, and hilum. In: *Scientific American Medicine. Pulmonary & Critical Care Medicine*. Hamilton: Dekker Medicine. 2020.

Light RW. Management of spontaneous pneumothorax. *Am Rev Respir Dis* 1993; 148: 245.

Light RW. Pleural controversy: optimal chest tube size for drainage. *Respirology* 2011; 16: 244.

Manaker S. Circulating endometrial cells: a diagnostic test for distinguishing catamenial from spontaneous pneumothorax. *Chest* 2020; 157: 245.

Watt AG. Spontaneous pneumothorax. *Med J Aust* 1978; 1: 186.

Woodring JH, Baker MD, Stark P. Pneumothorax ex vacuo. *Chest* 1996; 110: 1102.

Yarmus L, Feller-Kopman D. Pneumothorax in the critically ill patient. *Chest* 2012; 141: 1098.

Poisoning

Chemical **poisoning** due to drug overdosage is a very commonly encountered problem in Intensive Care and its management principles are well known. Some uncommon drug poisonings (e.g. amphetamines) are considered in this book (see Drugs).

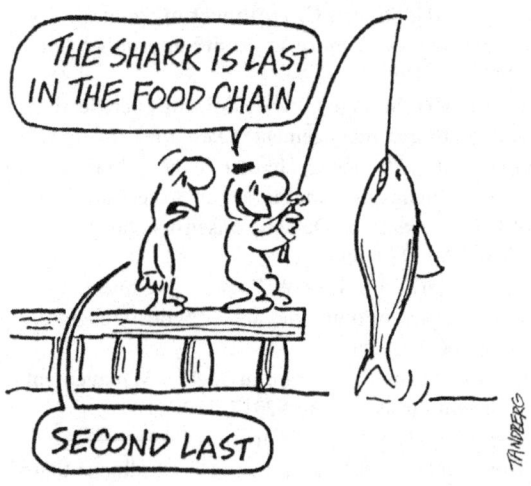

Many other chemical agents, generally of a non-therapeutic nature, may cause uncommon forms of poisoning following ingestion or other exposure (e.g. cyanide, warfare agents), and these are also discussed (see Chemical poisoning).

Food poisoning (q.v.) is considered separately.

Bibliography
Alapat PM, Zimmerman JL. Toxicology in the critical care unit. *Chest* 2008; 133: 1006.
Camporesi EM. Use of hyperbaric oxygen in critical care. In: Lumb PD, Shoemaker WC, eds. *Critical Care: State of the Art*, Chapter 10. Fullerton: Society of Critical Care Medicine. 1990; p 219.
Chiew AL, Reith D, Pomerleau A, et al. Updated guidelines for the management of paracetamol poisoning in Australia and New Zealand. *Med J Aust* 2020; 212: 175.
Kales SN, Christiani DC. Current concepts: acute chemical emergencies. *N Engl J Med* 2004; 350: 800.
Levine M, Brooks DE, Truitt CA, et al. Toxicology in the ICU: part I, II & III. *Chest* 2011; 140: 795, 1072 & 1357.
Ling L, Clark RF, Erickson T, et al., eds. *Toxicology Secrets*. Philadelphia; Hanley & Belfus. 2001.
Mokhlesi B, Garinella, PS, Joffe A, et al. Street drug abuse leading to critical illness. *Intens Care Med* 2004; 30: 1526.
Mokhlesi B, Leiken JB, Murray P, et al. Adult toxicology in critical care: part I: general approach to the intoxicated patient. *Chest* 2003; 123: 577.

Mokhlesi B, Leikin JB, Murray P, et al. Adult toxicology in critical care: part II: specific poisonings. *Chest* 2003; 123: 897.
Olson KR, ed. *Poisoning & Drug Overdose*. 7th edition. New York: McGraw-Hill (Appleton & Lange). 2017.
Rosenstock L, Cullen M, Brodkin C, et al., eds. *Textbook of Clinical Occupational and Environmental Medicine*. 2nd edition. Philadelphia: Saunders. 2004.
Rossoff IS, ed. *Encyclopedia of Clinical Toxicology*. Boca Raton: CRC Press. 2002.
Shannon MW, Borron SW, Burns MJ, eds. *Haddad and Winchester's Clinical Management of Poisoning and Drug Overdose*. 4th edition. Philadelphia: WB Saunders. 2007.
True B-L, Dreisbach RH, eds. Dreisbach's Handbook of Poisoning. Boca Raton: CRC Press. 2002.
Trujillo MH, Guerrero J, Fragachan C, et al. Pharmacologic antidotes in critical care medicine: a practical guide for drug administration. *Crit Care Med* 1998; 26: 377.
Wiegand TJ, Patel MM, Olson KR. Management of poisoning and drug overdose. In: *Scientific American Medicine. Interdisciplinary Medicine*. Hamilton: Dekker Medicine. 2020.
Zimmerman JL. Poisonings and overdoses in the intensive care unit: general and specific management issues. *Crit Care Med* 2003; 31: 2794.

Poliomyelitis

Poliomyelitis has become rare in developed countries since the development of a successful vaccine in 1955. In developed countries, the occasional reported illness was most likely caused by mutation towards a virulent strain of the polio virus (an enterovirus) in a vaccine recipient prior to replacement some years ago of the live attenuated vaccine with the former type of inactivated vaccine (see below).

Poliomyelitis is asymptomatic in 95% of cases. In the remainder, the features are usually similar to mild influenza and gastroenteritis.

It occasionally produces aseptic meningitis and most importantly paralysis from destruction of motor neurones in the spinal cord and brainstem. Paralysis thus occurs of the lower limbs and if severe of the respiratory muscles, with inadequate airway protection and respiratory failure. Residual muscle weakness and wasting are usual, sometimes with resultant skeletal deformity or respiratory impairment.

Over subsequent decades, a number of post-polio sequelae may develop, including increased sensitivity both to cold and to many drugs used in ICU and anaesthesia (e.g. opiates, sedatives, muscle relaxants). Even in developed countries with no acute cases for many decades, patients with these long-term sequelae can currently present management challenges.

An important differential diagnosis has been recognized in **enterovirus type 71** (EV71) infection, which has pathogenic effects and clinical consequences similar to those of poliovirus. Thus, aseptic meningitis, encephalitis (q.v.), acute flaccid paralysis (AFM) and acute pulmonary oedema may occur. Episodes of EV71 infection have been reported worldwide.

Treatment is supportive.

Since 1988, there has been an ambitious WHO plan for the global eradication of poliomyelitis, which was causing over 350,000 cases of paralysis worldwide. This program has had about 99% overall success (with complete eradication of type 2 strains by 2015 and type 3 strains by 2019), and there is now a massive push to eradicate the difficult residual tail. Although the disease has already been controlled throughout most of the world, it is still endemic in Pakistan and Afghanistan. However, vaccination programs in these countries had a major setback in community acceptance following the use of a sham vaccination program by the American CIA in Pakistan in 2011 as part of its hunt for terrorism suspects.

One of the next dilemmas will be when to cease using the live vaccine as the final strain (i.e. type 1) of the wild virus disappears, because this milestone can then be replaced by the potential risk of virulent mutation of one of the attenuated strains used in the vaccine. This unfortunate complication is referred to as vaccine-derived poliovirus (VDPV). Indeed, the phenomenon of VDPV is already emerging in some developing countries in Africa and South-East Asia. Thus, only inactivated strains will likely be used in available vaccines in these countries in due course, as they have been for many years in developed countries.

Even after the eradication of the three wild strains of poliovirus, it would also be theoretically possible for the disease to re-emerge by mutation of one of the eleven closely related Coxsackie A viruses. Indeed, as indicated above, a polio-like illness referred to as enterovirus-associated **acute flaccid myelitis** (AFM) has recently been reported in young people in the USA.

Bibliography
Fine PE, Griffiths UK. Global poliomyelitis eradication: status and implications. *Lancet* 2007; 369: 1321.
Jiang P, Faase JA, Toyoda H, et al. Evidence for emergence of diverse polioviruses from C-cluster coxsackie A viruses and implications for global poliovirus eradication. *Proc Natl Acad Sci USA* 2007; 104: 9204.
May M, Durrheim D, Roberts JA, et al. The risks of medical complacency towards poliomyelitis. *Med J Aust* 2020; 213: 61.
Satcher D. Polio eradication by the year 2000. *JAMA* 1999; 281: 221.

Polyarteritis nodosa

Polyarteritis nodosa (PAN) is a multisystem disease with inflammation and necrosis of small and medium arteries (see Vasculitis).

The cause is unknown, but it can sometimes be associated with
- hepatitis B antigenaemia (q.v.),
- HIV infection (see Acquired immunodeficiency syndrome),
- rheumatoid arthritis,
- amphetamine abuse (q.v.),
- familial Mediterranean fever (q.v.).

The condition is rare, with a prevalence of 1 in 100,000 of the population.

> Clinical manifestations are seen most commonly in middle-aged men.
> - There is fever (q.v.), malaise, anorexia, weight loss, weakness, myalgia, arthralgia (q.v.) and subcutaneous nodules.
> - There may also be hypertension, acute myocardial infarction, asthma, rash, fits, glomerulonephritis (q.v.) and asymmetrical mononeuritis multiplex (see Neuropathy).
> - Renal involvement occurs in 75% of patients and may comprise either glomerulonephritis (q.v.) or vasculitis (q.v.), with haematuria (q.v.), proteinuria (q.v.) and uraemia.
> - Mesenteric arteritis may cause bowel ischaemia and an abdominal crisis.
> - Complications may include aneurysm formation.

Investigations show anaemia (q.v.), leukocytosis, eosinophilia (q.v.) and raised ESR. Definitive diagnosis is made from histological examination of biopsy material from an involved site, especially muscle, though histology while specific is not very sensitive. Visceral angiography may show microaneurysms and segmental arterial narrowing.

*Treatment is that of any underlying disease, together with removal of any identifiable antigen. Otherwise, **corticosteroids** and sometimes **cyclophosphamide** are used.*

Bibliography
Albert DA, Rimon D, Silverstein MD. The diagnosis of poyarteritis nodosa. *Arthritis Rheum* 1988; 31: 1117.

Polycystic kidney disease *See*
- Renal cystic disease.

Polycystic ovary syndrome

Polycystic ovary syndrome (PCOS) has become increasingly recognized as a complex, important and enduring condition, with a prevalence of about 15% in younger women.

It is a metabolic and endocrine disorder exacerbated by obesity, with hormonal changes of insulin resistance (and thus diabetes and the metabolic syndrome) and of increased androgen levels (and thus hirsutism – q.v.). The reproductive consequences can include anovulation and infertility. Psychological health can be impaired, and depression is common.

The diagnosis is confirmed when typical clinical features are supported by the finding of multiple ovarian cysts on ultrasound examination, but it is important first to exclude other endocrine disorders, e.g. thyroid or adrenal dysfunction.

Treatment is primarily supportive, with particular attention to dietary, lifestyle and psychological factors. Metformin may be useful for endocrine management.

See also
- Amenorrhoea,
- Hirsutism,
- Pigmentation disorders – Acanthosis nigricans.

Bibliography
Kidson W. Polycystic ovary syndrome: a new direction in treatment. *Med J Aust* 1998; 169: 537.
Lobo RA, Carmina E. The importance of diagnosing the polycystic ovary syndrome. *Ann Intern Med* 2000; 132:989.
Norman RJ, Wu R, Stankiewixz MT. Polycystic ovary syndrome. *Med J Aust* 2004; 180: 132.
Pal L, Keefe K. Polycystic ovary syndrome. In: *Scientific American Medicine. Women's Health*. Hamilton: Dekker Medicine. 2020.
Shorakae S, Boyle J, Teede H. Polycystic ovary syndrome: a common hormonal condition with major metabolic sequelae that physicians should know about. *Intern Med J* 2014; 44: 720.
Teede HJ, Misso ML, Deeks AA, et al. Assessment and management of polycystic ovary syndrome: summary of an evidence-based guideline. *Med J Aust* 2011; 195 (suppl.): S65.

Polycythaemia

Polycythaemia refers to an increased circulating red cell mass, as opposed to **erythrocytosis** (q.v.), which is an increased red blood cell count without an increased mass.

Relative polycythaemia occurs when there is a decreased plasma volume, as in dehydration, but also in phaeochromocytoma (q.v.) and perhaps in stress.

This group also includes **pseudopolycythaemia** (Gaisbock's syndrome), although its mechanism is unknown.

> **Absolute polycythaemia** may be due to
> 1. hypoxia, i.e. secondary to an appropriate increase in erythropoietin,
> 2. increased erythropoietin without hypoxia, i.e. an inappropriate increase in erythropoietin,
> 3. polycythaemia vera.
>   See
> - Erythropoietin.

1. **Hypoxia** occurs in
   - cardiopulmonary disease,
   - haemoglobinopathy (q.v.),
   - altitude (q.v.),
   - sleep apnoea syndromes (see Sleep disorders of breathing).

   In these settings, if the PaO_2 is <60 mmHg (SaO_2 <90%), erythropoietin is appropriately stimulated.

   An interesting genetic mutation causing excess stability of the factor which regulates erythropoietin has been reported in some Russian families. The resultant Chuvash polycythaemia causes headache, fatigue, dizziness, dyspnoea and thromboembolism, often commencing in adolescence.

2. **Increased erythropoietin without hypoxia** occurs in erythropoietin-secreting tumours. These tumours are usually
   - renal,
   - adrenal,
   - hepatic,
   - ovarian,
   - cerebellar.

   Polycythaemia occurs either transiently or persistently in up to 20% of patients after renal transplantation and may require venesection to prevent thromboembolism.

   Polycythaemia may also be produced illegally in athletes following blood doping or erythropoietin injections. Deaths in these cases have been reported after supervening dehydration due to exercise.

3. **Polycythaemia vera** is an autonomous increase in red cell mass associated with decreased erythropoietin. It is a myeloproliferative disorder, in which the initial clonal change arises in a pluripotent stem cell, so that

there are abnormal markers in granulocytic as well as erythroid precursors. However, the red cell series predominates, probably because of inhibition of apoptosis rather than increased sensitivity to erythropoietin.

Clinical features are usually seen in older patients, in whom there is hepatosplenomegaly, ischaemic disease, and typically pruritus (q.v.), especially after bathing (i.e. aquagenic pruritus).

Increased viscosity gives rise to thromboembolism, which may be unusual or multiple, and may include the Budd–Chiari syndrome (q.v.).

Investigations show an increased red blood cell mass of >36 mL/kg (unless there is concomitant bleeding) in the absence of hypoxia, and leukocytosis and thrombocytosis. Cytogenetic abnormalities may be found in some patients, but the demonstration of the JAK2 V617F point mutation on PCR testing is found in virtually all patients.

Treatment is with **hydroxyurea**, *with* **venesection** *to a haematocrit of 0.40–0.45 or with* **radiotherapy**.
- *Radiophosphorous is used if the patient is refractory to venesection.*
- *Cytotoxic therapy causes a significantly increased risk of the development of leukaemia.*

The prognosis without treatment is a 50% mortality within 1.5 years. This is increased to 3.5 years with successful venesections and 12.5 years following radiotherapy. About 20% of patients develop myeloid metaplasia, considered the burnt-out phase of the myeloproliferative disorders.

The laboratory findings of polycythaemia vera in the absence of clinical features is sometimes referred to as **primary erythrocytosis** and is probably a forme fruste of polycythaemia vera.

Bibliography
Berlin NI. Polycythemia vera: an update. *Semin Hematol* 1986; 23: 131.
Broudy VC. The polycythemias. In: *Scientific American Medicine. Hematology.* Hamilton: Dekker Medicine. 2020.
Campbell PJ, Green AR. The myeloproliferative disorders. *N Engl J Med* 2006; 355: 2452.
Challoner T, Briggs C, Rampling MW, et al. A study of the haematological and haemorrheological consequences of venesection. *Br J Haematol* 1986; 62: 671.
Editorial. Pseudopolycythaemia. *Lancet* 1987; 2: 603.
Gareau R, Audran M, Barnes R, et al. Erythropoietin abuse in athletes. *Nature* 1996; 380: 113.
Golde DW, Hocking WG, Koeffler HP, et al. Polycythemia: mechanisms and management. *Ann Intern Med* 1981; 95: 71.
Gordeuk VR, Sergueeva AI, Miasnikova GY, et al. Congenital disorder of oxygen sensing: association of the homozygous Chuvash polycythemia VHL mutation with thrombosis and vascular abnormalities but not tumors. *Blood* 2004; 103: 3924.
Gruppo Italiano Studio Policitemia. Polycythaemia vera. *Ann Intern Med* 1995; 123: 656.
Hinshelwood S, Bench AJ, Green AR. Pathogenesis of polycythaemia vera. *Blood Rev* 1997; 11: 224.
Krantz SB. Erythropoietin. *Blood* 1991; 77: 419.
Kwaan HC, ed. The hyperviscosity syndromes. *Semin Thromb Hemost* 2003; 29: 433.
Noakes TD. Tainted glory: doping and athletic performance. *N Engl J Med* 2004; 351: 847.
Schafer AI. Bleeding and thrombosis in myeloproliferative disorders. *Blood* 1984; 64: 1.
Tefferi A. Myelofibrosis with myeloid metaplasia. *N Engl J Med* 2000; 342: 1255.
Watts EJ, Lewis SM. Spurious polycythaemia. *Scand J Haematol* 1983; 31: 241.

Polymyalgia rheumatica

Polymyalgia rheumatica (PMR) is a clinical syndrome of profound proximal limb girdle pain and stiffness, usually seen in older patients.

Polymyalgia rheumatica is at one end of a spectrum, with giant cell arteritis, most commonly temporal arteritis (q.v.) at the other, and with overlap in some patients.

Not uncommonly, rheumatoid arthritis may present with a clinical picture of PMR, with overt peripheral synovitis becoming apparent only subsequently.

Clinical manifestations may include fever (q.v.), fatigue, weight loss and depression, as well as the proximal muscle symptoms. The onset is usually acute but may sometimes be insidious.

Investigations show a markedly increased ESR or CRP, often with anaemia (q.v.), increased alkaline phosphatase, normal CK and increased fibrinogen. Imaging confirms peri-articular inflammation.

Treatment with **corticosteroids** *(usually 15 mg per day of prednisolone) gives a dramatic response within days. Higher doses are needed initially for temporal arteritis. The dose should usually be tapered to a low dose for up to 2 yr before attempting withdrawal.*

See
- Arteritis.

Bibliography

Hamilton CR, Shelley WM, Tumulty PA. Giant cell arteritis: including temporal arteritis and polymyalgia rheumatica. *Medicine* 1971; 50: 1.

Hunder GG, Bloch DA, Michel BA, et al. The American College of Rheumatology 1990 criteria for the classification of giant cell arteritis. *Arthritis Rheum* 1990; 33: 1122.

Owen CE, Buchanan RRC, Hoi A. Recent advances in polymyalgia rheumatica. *Intern Med J* 2015; 45: 1102.

Zilko PJ. Polymyalgia rheumatica and giant cell arteritis. *Med J Aust* 1996; 165: 438.

Polymyositis/dermatomyositis

Polymyositis (PM) is an uncommon but often serious condition affecting skeletal muscles. When associated with skin eruptions, it is referred to as **dermatomyositis** (DM). It is a member of the group of conditions referred to as **idiopathic inflammatory myopathies** (see Myopathy, see Myositis).

Although its cause is unknown, it may sometimes be associated with

- malignancy, as a paraneoplastic phenomenon (q.v.),
- other rheumatic diseases, especially systemic lupus erythematosus (q.v.) and scleroderma (q.v.).

The pathogenesis is presumably immunological, and autoantibodies of various types may be identified in most patients. However, such antibodies are probably markers rather than causes of disease, since they are not usually directed to muscle components, and the muscle injury is more likely to be cell-mediated, since lymphocytes may produce muscle cell cytotoxin.

Clinical features are dominated by proximal muscle weakness, i.e. shoulder and pelvic girdles.
In severe cases, distal muscles and even the pharynx and diaphragm may be involved, with dysphagia, aspiration and respiratory failure.

Multiorgan involvement may be seen.
- **Skin**
  - A dark-red eruption is typical, particularly on the face, neck, chest and hands.
  - Extensor surface rash may include either palpable papules (Gottron papules) or plaques (Gottron sign).
  - The eyelids may be discoloured and oedematous (heliotrope rash).
  - There may be generalized cutaneous vasculitis (q.v.).
  - Some patients may have the typical rash without apparent muscle involvement or with only subclinical myositis, a condition referred to as amyopathic DM' or 'DM sine myositis'.
- **Lungs**
  - In about 50% of cases, there is either interstitial fibrosis (q.v.) or associated pneumonia.
  - Pulmonary involvement carries a high mortality.
- **Heart**
  - Arrhythmias and conduction defects may be seen.
  - Myocarditis is now recognized to be present in most patients.
- **Carcinoma**
  - This may be apparent if the polymyositis is a paraneoplastic phenomenon (q.v.).

Investigations show increased muscle enzymes, especially CK, the most specific muscle enzyme, and particularly the CK-MM isoenzyme. An elevated CK-MB is not necessarily indicative of acute myocardial infarction in this setting, as this isoenzyme is also produced in regenerating skeletal muscle. The AST and LDH are also elevated. The EMG shows characteristic changes of asynchronous muscle fibre contraction. Biopsy shows degeneration and fragmentation of muscle fibres with patchy inflammation. Older patients with dermatomyositis should be screened for an underlying malignancy.

Diagnosis is made on the basis of the clinical features, together with the elevated muscle enzymes and typical biopsy and perhaps EMG. Imaging with MRI may be useful. Other causes of myopathy (q.v.) and of myalgia (e.g. polymyalgia rheumatica – q.v., or fibromyalgia) should be excluded.

A particularly difficult differential diagnosis is **inclusion body myositis (IBM)** (see Myositis), suggested by a poor therapeutic response and confirmed by biopsy.

Treatment is with **corticosteroids**, *the dose depending on the severity of the disease. Although most patients improve with corticosteroids, the response is often partial. Following a satisfactory clinical response and normalization of muscle enzymes, the dosage may be tapered. If the response to corticosteroids is inadequate or the dose required for maintenance is unacceptably high, other modalities may be required, including cytotoxic agents (azathioprine or methotrexate), ciclosporin, tacrolimus, high-dose immune globulin or plasmapheresis (q.v.).*

The rash is photosensitive, so that protection from the sun is important. Beta-carotene, antimalarials and tacrolimus have also been reported to relieve the rash.

The course of the disease is very variable, ranging from fulminant over a few days to indolent over many years. Typically, there is gradual progression over weeks to months. The mortality is 15–20% at 5 yr and is worse in older patients or with associated cardiac, pulmonary or malignant processes. Occasionally there is spontaneous improvement, and sometimes complete and permanent remission may occur with therapy.

Bibliography

Dalakas MC. Polymyositis, dermatomyositis, and inclusion-body myositis. *N Engl J Med* 1991; 325: 1487.

Fathi M, Lundberg IE. Interstitial lung disease in polymyositis and dermatomyositis. *Curr Opin Rheumatol* 2005; 17: 701.

Gerami P, Schope JM, McDonald L, et al. A systematic review of adult-onset clinically amyopathic dermatomyositis (dermatomyositis sine myositis): a missing link within the spectrum of the idiopathic inflammatory myopathies. *J Am Acad Dermatol* 2006; 54: 597.

Jorizzo JL. Dermatomyositis; practical aspects. *Arch Dermatol* 2002; 138: 114.

Limaye VS, Blumbergs P, Roberts-Thomson PJ. Idiopathic inflammatory myopathies. *Intern Med J* 2009; 39: 179.

Marie I, Hatron PY, Levesque H, et al. Influence of age on characteristics of polymyositis and dermatomyositis in adults. *Medicine* 1999; 78: 139.

Miller FW. Classification and prognosis of inflammatory muscle disease. *Rheum Dis Clin North Am* 1994; 20: 811.

Schwarz MI. The lung in polymyositis. *Clin Chest Med* 1998; 19: 701.

Sigurgeirsson B, Lindelof B, Edhag O, et al. Risk of cancer in patients with dermatomyositis or polymyositis. *N Engl J Med* 1992; 326: 363.

Tazelaar HD, Viggiano RW, Pickersgill J, et al. Interstitial lung disease in polymyositis and dermatomyositis: clinical features and prognosis as correlated with histologic findings. *Am Rev Resp Dis* 1990; 141: 727.

Polyneuritis *See*

- Neuropathy.

Polyneuropathy *See*

- Neuropathy.

Porphyria

The **porphyrias** comprise a group of six diseases of abnormal porphyrin metabolism. Porphyrin synthesis produces the iron-containing moiety, **haeme**, which is the chief component in haemoglobin, cytochromes and other oxidative enzymes. It is thus responsible for the red colour of blood.

The enzymic steps from the initial components, glycine and succinyl-CoA, to the eventual production of haeme give rise to ring structures via progressive deamination, decarboxylation, oxidation and finally iron chelation. These steps clearly provide multiple sites for enzymic defects, and indeed an abnormality at each of the **six steps** after the initial production of porphobilinogen causes a distinct disease, as described below.

The major sites of haeme production are the liver and bone marrow, and thus the sites of the defects in porphyrias are either hepatic (the four most common forms) or erythropoietic (one rare form) or both (one form). Most porphyrias are inherited disorders.

Porphyrias were among the first inborn errors of metabolism to be described, because of their familial pattern, their characteristic clinical features (either neurovisceral or cutaneous photosensitivity) and their obvious chemical markers in the urine (since porphyrins fluoresce under ultraviolet light).

The typical clinical course is one of acute attacks separated by long latent periods. This fluctuating course is explained by the fact that the enzyme defects affect non-rate-limiting steps, whereas the chief endogenous or exogenous stimuli for acute attacks induce the normally rate-limiting initial step controlled by the enzyme, δ-amino laevulinic acid (ALA) synthetase. Thus, precursor production now overwhelms the defective step, and intermediate products spill into the circulation and then into the urine.

Other diseases are also associated with acquired abnormalities of porphyrin metabolism, namely, chronic liver disease, haemolysis, malignancy and especially lead poisoning (q.v.).

1. **Acute intermittent porphyria** (AIP) is an autosomal dominant disease due to deficiency of porphobilinogen (PBG) deaminase to about 50% of normal levels. It is thus due to an abnormality at the first of the six steps from porphobilinogen to haeme.

More than 100 different mutations have been described as affecting PBG deaminase in this way. However, 80–90% of those with genetic abnormalities have only latent disease, since many mutations are expressed mildly, and nearly half of those with overt biochemical defects are asymptomatic.

AIP comprises about 5% of porphyrias. Most patients are female.

> Like the other hepatic porphyrias, AIP is characterized by the five 'Ps', namely,
> i. onset after Puberty,
> ii. Pain, especially abdominal,
> iii. Polyneuropathy,
> iv. Photosensitivity,
> v. Psychiatric features.

In over 90% of symptomatic patients, attacks have occurred before the age of 40 years. They are precipitated by the four 'Ms', namely
i. Medicines

> - especially alcohol, barbiturates, carbamazepine, chloramphenicol, chlordiazepoxide, ergot, griseofulvin, methyldopa, oestrogens, phenytoin, sulphonamides, tolbutamide.
> - Fortunately, many drugs are safe, including analgesics, beta blockers, benzodiazepines, chlorpromazine, corticosteroids, penicillin and warfarin.

ii. Medical illnesses
   - especially infections.
iii. Malnutrition
   - especially carbohydrate deprivation.
iv. Menstruation.

The clinical features are very diverse.
- More than half the attacks are precipitated by drugs (usually barbiturates, oral contraceptives – q.v., phenytoin, sulphonamides, though many others have varying degrees of reported porphyrinogenicity), followed by menstruation or pregnancy (13%), infections (10%), alcohol (3%), starvation (3%), while in about 15% no clear precipitating factor can be defined.
- Abdominal pain and tenderness are universal.
- The urine is dark (since PBG in urine polymerizes to form porphobilin, so that the urine becomes dark red on standing).
- Peripheral neuropathy (q.v.), more motor than sensory, is found in 75% of patients, of whom 15% develop respiratory paralysis.
- About half the patients show neuropsychiatric changes of behaviour and/or mood, often with cranial nerve involvement and sometimes with fits.
- Fever, tachycardia and labile hypertension are common.

Investigations show increased urinary δ-ALA and PBG in all patients, even in remission. Urinary uroporphyrin (>40 nmol per day) and faecal coproporphyrin are increased in all cases acutely. Other investigations show leukocytosis, hyponatraemia, hypochloraemia, hypovolaemia, abnormal EEG and EMG, sometimes an abnormal CSF, and dilated bowel loops on abdominal X-ray.

The differential diagnosis includes in particular any cause of acute abdominal pain.

*Treatment is **symptomatic** with analgesics.*

- **Glucose** in the form of 10% dextrose 200 mL/hr is recommended, though added insulin may be required.
- Tachycardia and hypotension respond to **beta blockers**.
- Fits may be controlled with **gabapentin**.
- If respiratory paralysis occurs, ventilatory support is required, but even then the reported mortality is up to 50%.
- Fluids, electrolytes and nutritional support are required, together with avoidance of known precipitating drugs and treatment of any concurrent diseases.
- Specific treatment in the form of **haematin**, the ferric form of haeme (200 mg IV over 20 min bd), provides improvement within a few days but can give rise to disseminated intravascular coagulation (q.v.) This complication is primarily due to degradation of haematin after its reconstitution in water.
- **Liver transplantation** has been successful in patients with severe, recurrent and refractory disease.

The prognosis is probably better than traditionally reported, since modern screening now shows that many patients are asymptomatic, and prophylactic avoidance of precipitating factors is effective. Family screening is recommended.

2. **Variegate porphyria** (VP, or porphyria variegata, PV) is due to a decreased protoporphyrinogen oxidase. It is thus due to an abnormality at the fifth of the six steps from porphobilinogen to haeme. It is inherited and comprises about 5% of porphyrias.

It is associated with solar skin lesions, as there is photosensitivity, even indoors or under transparent sunscreens, because long wavelength ultraviolet light penetrates transparent media. There is associated skin fragility and also neuropathic lesions, and blisters, ulcers and scars of various stages are seen.

Acute, systemic attacks can occur, similar to those in acute intermittent porphyria. The two conditions are distinguished by the demonstration of the appropriate porphyrins, usually in faeces, since the defective enzyme itself is not readily assayed.

Treatment is the same as for acute intermittent porphyria.

3. **Hereditary coproporphyria** (HC or HCP) is the least common hepatic porphyria (2% of porphyrias) and is due to a deficiency of coproporphyrinogen oxidase. It is thus due to an abnormality at the fourth of the six steps from porphobilinogen to haeme. A number of culprit gene mutations as been described.

It is clinically indistinguishable from variegate porphyria and thus overlaps acute intermittent porphyria.

Treatment principles are therefore similar.

4. **Porphyria cutanea tarda** (PCT) is the most common porphyria (80% of porphyrias) and is due to a deficiency of uroporphyrinogen decarboxylase. It is thus due to an abnormality at the third of the six steps from porphobilinogen to haeme. Unlike the other porphyrias, most cases (up to 90%) are not familial.

   The majority (75%) of affected cases are men, and the peak age of onset is in the 50s. More than half the cases are precipitated by alcohol and the rest by either oestrogens or liver disease, in which case there are abnormal liver function tests and histology. The condition can thus be associated with hepatitis (q.v.), biliary disease or hepatocellular carcinoma (q.v.).

   All patients show photosensitivity, with vesiculation, hyperpigmentation (q.v.), hypertrichosis (q.v.) and skin fragility. In 50% of cases, the urine becomes dark on standing.

   Investigations show an increased urinary uroporphyrin (>40 nmol per day) and increased total porphyrins in urine and in plasma. Iron overload is seen in 75% of cases and may require venesection or even desferrioxamine (see Haemochromatosis).

   *Treatment measures include **avoidance** of sun, alcohol, iron and oestrogens.*
   - **Beta-carotene** may be useful.
   - **Iron depletion therapy** is required in most patients (see Haemochromatosis).
   - Low doses of **chloroquine** or **hydroychloroquine** can be effective if repeated venesection (phlebotomy) is poorly tolerated.

5. **(Erythropoietic) Protoporphyria** (EPP) is due to a deficiency of ferrochelatase. It is thus due to an abnormality at the last of the six steps from porphobilinogen to haeme. The deficient enzyme occurs in erythrocytes, as well as in liver cells. It is inherited and comprises about 8% of porphyrias.

   The chief clinical feature is photosensitivity. Cholelithiasis and hepatopathy are recognized complications.

   *It may be treated with **beta-carotene**.*

6. **Congenital erythropoietic porphyria** is a very rare autosomal recessive condition with a deficiency of uroporphyrinogen cosynthetase. It is thus due to an abnormality at the second of the six steps from porphobilinogen to haeme. The deficient enzyme occurs only in the erythrocyte series.

   It is associated with photosensitivity, haemolysis, dark urine and red teeth.

   *It has been successfully treated with **bone marrow transplantation**.*

7. **Pseudoporphyria** is a phototoxic skin eruption which occurs as soon as 1 day or as long as 1 year after the commencement of any of a number of drugs, particularly furosemide, naproxen, tetracycline, voriconazole. There are blisters and scarring in exposed areas, resembling the lesions seen in PCT or EPP (see above), but porphyrin metabolism is normal.

Bibliography

Anderson KE, Bloomer JR, Bonkovsky H, et al. Recommendations for the diagnosis and treatment of the acute porphyrias. *Ann Intern Med* 2005; 142: 439.

Anderson KE, Kappas A. The porphyrias. In: *Scientific American Medicine. Endocrinology & Metabolism.* Hamilton: Dekker Medicine. 2020.

Brodie MJ, Moore MR, Thompson GG, et al. Pregnancy and the acute porphyrias. *Br J Obstet Gynaec* 1977; 84: 726.

Grandchamp B. Acute intermittent porphyria. *Semin Liver Dis* 1998; 18: 17.

Kauppinen R, Mustajoki P. Prognosis of acute porphyria: occurrence of acute attacks, precipitating factors, and associated diseases. *Medicine* 1992; 71: 1.

Lamon JM, Bennett M, Frykholm BC, et al. Prevention of acute porphyric attacks by intravenous haematin. *Lancet* 1978; 2: 492.

Moore MR. Biochemistry of porphyria. *Int J Biochem* 1993; 25: 1353.

Mustajoki P, Heinonen J. General anesthesia in 'inducible' porphyrias. *Anesthesiology* 1980; 53: 15.

Mustajoki P, Nordman Y. Early administration of heme arginate for acute porphyric attacks. *Arch Intern Med* 1993; 153: 2004.

Puy H, Gouya L, Deybach JC. Porphyrias. *Lancet* 2010; 375: 924.

Ratnaike S, Blake D, Campbell D, et al. Plasma ferritin levels as a guide to the treatment of porphyria cutanea tarda by venesection. *Aust J Dermatol* 1988; 29: 3.

Yeung Laiwah AC, Moore MR, Goldberg A. Pathogenesis of acute porphyria. *Quart J Med* 1987; 63: 377.

Portopulmonary hypertension *See*

- Pulmonary hypertension.

Posterior reversible encephalopathy *See*

- Reversible posterior leukoencephalopathy.

Post–Intensive Care syndrome

Post–Intensive Care syndrome is a term used to describe the combination of persistent cognitive, mental and physical disabilities that may follow critical illness in some patients and may therefore impair their recovery process.

A similar mental disability may also be seen in family members of critically ill patients and resembles the post-traumatic stress disorder (PTSD) seen after other circumstances of severe psychological stress.

See also
- Critical illness neuromuscular abnormality.

Post-transfusion purpura *See*
- Thrombocytopenia.

Pre-eclampsia

Pre-eclampsia (toxaemia of pregnancy, gestosis in Eastern Europe) occurs in 5–10% of all pregnancies, most commonly in the third trimester of the first pregnancy. It occurs earlier, even in the first trimester, in the presence of hydatidiform mole or underlying renal disease. Severe pre-eclampsia occurring before 34 weeks of gestation is associated with increased fetal mortality and maternal morbidity and mortality.

The aetiology remains unknown but clearly requires the presence of the trophoblast, as the condition is unique to pregnancy. It is associated with uteroplacental ischaemia, which in turn is associated with structural abnormalities of the spiral arteries, abnormalities of prostaglandin metabolism, increased platelet responsiveness, generalized increase in pressor responsiveness and endothelial cell swelling in the glomeruli. It thus becomes a multisystem disorder with widespread endothelial dysfunction. Its pathogenesis may be immunological and perhaps an abnormal response to feto-placental tissue, or there may be mediator release from placental ischaemia.

Pre-eclampsia consists of the gradual onset of
- **hypertension** (to >140/90 mmHg), and
- **proteinuria** (q.v.).

Proteinuria may be assessed by urine dipstick (> trace), 24-hour urine collection (>0.3 g per day) or protein/creatinine ratio (>30 mg/mmol). There is a normal renal sediment, and the renal function is normal. Important causes of proteinuria also present in the non-pregnant patient should be excluded, particularly renal disease, urinary tract disease, diabetes and systemic lupus erythematosus (q.v.).

As about 10% of patients with otherwise documented pre-eclampsia do not have proteinuria, other criteria are required to support its diagnosis in a pregnant patient with new-onset hypertension and no proteinuria. These additional criteria include thrombocytopenia (q.v.), abnormal liver enzymes (transaminitis), marked oedema or neurological symptoms (see below).

The plasma uric acid level is typically increased above 300 µmol/L.

The progression from pre-eclampsia to eclampsia is indicated by convulsions and occurs in about 1 in 200 cases. Even in the absence of convulsions (eclampsia), severe pre-eclampsia is associated with neurological features of headache, visual disturbance and increased reflexes. The disparity in the responses of eclamptic and epileptic seizures to benzodiazepines and phenytoin suggests that their mechanism of production is different.

There may be upper abdominal tenderness due to liver distension, which may herald the onset of **acute fatty liver of pregnancy** (q.v.) or the **HELLP syndrome** (q.v.). Acute fatty liver of pregnancy is a rare complication, but about 10% of more severe cases of pre-eclampsia may experience the HELLP syndrome.

> In 20–30% of cases of eclampsia, the onset is post-partum and any ante-partum pre-eclampsia may have been mild.
> Eclampsia may thus be an unpredictable complication for up to 7 days after delivery.

Since pre-eclampsia does not cause renal impairment, the presence of renal failure indicates another associated complication, such as
- sepsis,
- placental abruption (abruptio placentae) (q.v.),
- urinary tract obstruction,
- haemolytic–uraemic syndrome (q.v.), especially postpartum,
- hypovolaemia, due either to hyperemesis or to diabetes insipidus (q.v.), the latter occasionally seen from excess placental metabolism of vasopressin by vasopressinase).

The differential diagnosis is underlying hypertension or renal disease. Pre-existing hypertension tends to be manifest before the 20th week and to cause minimal proteinuria.

*Treatment is by **delivery** if the mother is stable and fetal maturity is satisfactory (e.g. >34 weeks' gestation).*
- ***Hypertension** may be treated effectively with beta blockers (including labetalol), methyldopa, hydralazine or calcium channel inhibitors (usually nifedipine), but ACE inhibitors should be avoided because of increased fetal morbidity and because of possible hypovolaemia.*
- ***Hypovolaemia** should be treated, and cardiac filling pressures may need to be monitored.*
- ***Magnesium** sulphate is the agent of choice for the prevention and treatment of convulsions (i.e. eclampsia). To achieve a 'therapeutic serum magnesium level' of 2–4 mmol/L, 20 mmol (0.5 g) of magnesium (i. e. 5 g of magnesium sulphate) should be*

given, as 10 mL IV of 50% magnesium sulphate in 100 mL of 5% dextrose over 20 min. This should be followed by a continuous IV infusion of 5–10 mmol/hr for 24 hr to maintain a magnesium level which is effective but not toxic. If seizures recur, 50% of the initial loading dose is repeated. Toxicity is monitored by assessment of tendon reflexes for hyporeflexia and by measurement of the serum magnesium level. See Magnesium.

- Effective prophylaxis in high-risk patients may be achieved with low-dose **aspirin**.
- Management based on international evidence-based guidelines has been associated with improved maternal outcome.

The maternal prognosis is good in developed countries. There is probably little increased incidence of subsequent hypertension or renal disease, though there is an increased risk of cardiovascular disease and the metabolic syndrome in later life. If the disease has progressed to frank eclampsia, there is a risk of maternal mortality from cerebral haemorrhage. There is an increased fetal risk.

There is a low likelihood of recurrence, unless

- the condition is severe,
- it has had an early onset,
- it has occurred in a multigravida,
- there is a different partner for a subsequent pregnancy,
- there is underlying renal disease.

Bibliography

Arbogast BW, Taylor RN. *Molecular Mechanisms of Pre-eclampsia.* Berlin: Springer-Verlag. 1997.

Brown MA, Lowe SA. Current management of pre-eclampsia. *Med J Aust* 2009; 190: 3.

Bucher HC, Guyatt GH, Cook RJ, et al. Effect of calcium supplementation on pregnancy-induced hypertension and preeclampsia. A meta-analysis of randomised controlled trials. *JAMA* 1996; 275: 1113.

Chua S, Redman CWG. Are prophylactic anticonvulsants required in severe pre-eclampsia? *Lancet* 1991; 337: 250.

CLASP (Collaborative Low-dose Aspirin Study in Pregnancy) Collaborative Group. CLASP: a randomised trial of low-dose aspirin for the prevention and treatment of pre-eclampsia among 9364 pregnant women. *Lancet* 1994; 343: 619.

Cunningham FG, Grant NF. Prevention of preeclampsia – a reality? *N Engl J Med* 1989; 321: 606.

Davison JM, Shiells EA, Barron WM, et al. Changes in the metabolic clearance of vasopressin and plasma vasopressinase throughout human pregnancy. *J Clin Invest* 1989; 83: 1313.

Dekker GA, Sibai B. Primary, secondary, and tertiary prevention of pre-eclampsia. *Lancet* 2001; 357: 209.

Douglas KA, Redman CWG. Eclampsia in the United Kingdom. *BMJ* 1994; 309: 1395.

Durr JA, Hoggard JG, Hunt JM, et al. Diabetes insipidus in pregnancy associated with abnormally high circulating vasopressinase activity. *N Engl J Med* 1987; 316: 1070.

Editorial. Are ACE inhibitors safe in pregnancy? *Lancet* 1989; 2: 482.

Gant NF, Worley RJ, Everett RB, et al. Control of vascular responsiveness during human pregnancy. *Kidney Int* 1980; 18: 253.

Higby, Suiter CR, Phelps JY, et al. Normal values of urinary albumin and total protein excretion during pregnancy. *Am J Obstet Gynecol* 1994; 171: 984.

Hod T, Cerdeira AS, Karumanchi SA. Molecular mechanisms of preeclampsia. *Cold Spring Harb Perspect Med* 2015; 5: a023473.

Ihle BU, Long P, Oats J. Early onset pre-eclampsia: recognition of underlying renal disease. *BMJ* 1987; 294: 79.

Leone M, Einav S. Severe preeclampsia: what's new in intensive care? *Intens Care Med* 2015; 41: 1343.

Lucas MJ, Leveno KJ, Cunningham FG. A comparison of magnesium sulfate with phenytoin for the prevention of eclampsia. *N Engl J Med* 1995; 333: 201.

Magpie Trial Collaborative Group. Do women with pre-eclampsia, and their babies, benefit from magnesium sulphate? The Magpie Trial: a randomized placebo controlled trial. *Lancet* 2002; 359: 1877.

Martin JN, Files FC, Blake PG. Plasma exchange for preeclampsia: I. Postpartum use for persistently severe preeclampsia with HELLP syndrome. *Am J Obstet Gynecol* 1990; 162: 126.

Myatt L, Webster RP. Vascular biology of preeclampsia. *J Thromb Haemost* 2009; 7: 375.

Need JA. Pre-eclampsia in pregnancies by different fathers: immunological studies. *BMJ* 1975; 1: 548.

Perry KG, Martin JN. Abnormal hemostasis and coagulopathy in preeclampsia and eclampsia. *Clin Obstet Gynecol* 1992; 35: 338.

Redman C. Platelets and the beginnings of preeclampsia. *N Engl J Med* 1990; 323: 478.

Redman CWG, Roberts JM. Management of pre-eclampsia. *Lancet* 1993; 341: 1451.

Roberts J, Taylor R, Goldfen A. Clinical and biochemical evidence of endothelial cell dysfunction in pregnancy syndrome eclampsia. *Am J Hypertens* 1991; 4: 700.

Sibai BM, El-Nazer A, Gonzalez-Ruiz A. Severe preeclampsia in young primigravid women: subsequent pregnancy outcome and remote prognosis. *Am J Obstet Gynecol* 1986; 155: 1011.

The Eclampsia Trial Collaborative Group. Which anticonvulsant for women with eclampsia? Evidence from the Collaborative Eclampsia Trial. *Lancet* 1995; 345: 1455.

Williams D. Pre-eclampsia and long-term maternal health. *Obstet Med* 2012; 5: 98.

Williams DJ, de Swiet M. The pathophysiology of pre-eclampsia. *Intens Care Med* 1997; 23: 620.

Pregnancy

Pregnancy problems account for about 2% of admissions to ICU, and thus a number of either general or specific maternal problems have relevance for Intensive Care clinicians.

The **general problems** are discussed below and include
1. miscarriage (abortion),
2. drugs,
3. systemic disorders,
4. teratogenicity,
5. trophoblastic neoplasia,
6. post-partum problems.

The **specific problems** of importance are discussed separately, namely,
- acute fatty liver of pregnancy (q.v.),
- amniotic fluid embolism (q.v.),
- aspiration (q.v.),
- HELLP syndrome (q.v.),
- ovarian hyperstimulation syndrome (OHSS)(q.v.),
- pneumonia in pregnancy (q.v.),
- pre-eclampsia (q.v.),
- trauma in pregnancy (q.v.).

The most common direct complications of pregnancy comprise pre-eclampsia (q.v.), intrauterine growth retardation (IUGR), fetal death in utero (FDIU) and placental abruption (q.v.), and these together occur in 1–5% of pregnancies.

Maternal deaths are defined by the WHO as deaths 'during pregnancy, childbirth or in the 42 days of the puerperium, irrespective of the duration and site of the pregnancy, from any cause related to or aggravated by the pregnancy or its management'.

Maternal deaths may be
- **direct**, i.e. due to a complication of the pregnancy itself,
- **indirect**, i.e. due to some other disease but possibly aggravated by pregnancy, or
- **incidental** to the pregnancy, e.g. from trauma, suicide, cancer.

> The most common direct causes of maternal mortality in developed countries are
> - thromboembolism,
> - hypertensive disorders,
> - peripartum haemorrhage,
> - amniotic fluid embolism (q.v.).

Total maternal mortality in Australia is recorded from all three groups of causes (i.e. direct, indirect and incidental), and over the past decade it has averaged only about 1 per 10,000 births. However, 99% of maternal deaths worldwide occur in developing countries.

By contrast, the total perinatal mortality in Australia has been 6.9 per 1000 births (or 4.3 per 1000 births using the more restricted WHO recommendations for international comparison), of which about two thirds of the deaths are stillbirths (i.e. at least 500 g or over 22 weeks' gestation) and one third neonatal (i.e. at least 500 g or over 22 weeks' gestation, and within 28 days of birth). The infant death rate (i.e. total mortality of liveborn babies up to 1 year) was 3.8 per 1000 live births. This low figure has been particularly contributed to by the progressive decline in sudden infant death syndrome (SIDS, cot death) over the past decade from about 30% to 10% of infant deaths.

1. The **risk of miscarriage (abortion)** is increased
   - in the antiphospholipid syndrome (APS) (q.v.),
   - in systemic infection, especially brucellosis (q.v.), toxoplasmosis (q.v.), typhoid (q.v.),
   - with misoprostol, a synthetic PGE_1 analog used for NSAID-induced peptic ulceration,
   - after mifepristone (RU486), a progestogen antagonist which is available for medical abortion (see also Cushing's syndrome).

About 15% of pregnancies result in fetal loss. However, even after recurrent fetal loss (i.e. 3 times), successful pregnancy still occurs in about 50% of cases. Chromosomal abnormalities are the cause of most cases of fetal loss, although maternal thrombophilia (q.v.) is particularly related to recurrent fetal loss.

More than half of all cases of recurrent miscarriage can be related to a procoagulant abnormality (i.e. thrombophilia – q.v.), which then leads to placental vascular occlusion via thrombosis and infarction. The antiphospholipid syndrome is responsible for two thirds of these abnormalities. Virtually all patients with a procoagulant abnormality can subsequently proceed to term with treatment, usually with aspirin before conception and with aspirin and heparin from conception to delivery.

While thrombophilia is associated with fetal loss, in fact most cases of fetal loss are not due to the thrombophilia itself but to associated chromosomal abnormalities

The **complications of miscarriage** are numerous, the most important acute ones being infective, namely,
- acute pelvic inflammatory disease (q.v.),
- clostridial or Gram-negative anaerobic infections,
- *Mycoplasma hominis* infection (which may also occur post-partum) giving a mild, self-limited, febrile illness.

2. **Drugs** may cause fetal and sometimes maternal problems.
    - Antibiotics
        - erythromycin estolate, quinolones, tetracycline and trimethoprim are contraindicated in pregnancy,
        - aminoglycosides, chloramphenicol, metronidazole and sulphonamides are also best avoided,
        - penicillin and cephalosporins are safe.
    - Analgesics and sedatives
        - codeine and paracetamol are safe,
        - narcotics are safe except near term,
        - benzodiazepines and barbiturates are not recommended for long-term use,
        - aspirin should be used only for specifically defined indications, e.g. pre-eclampsia.
    - Anaesthetics
        - muscle relaxants are safe,
        - nitrous oxide is safe in late pregnancy,
        - local anaesthetics should be used with caution in late pregnancy.
    - Angiotensin-converting enzyme (ACE) inhibitors and angiotensin receptor blockers (ARBs)
        - early fetal exposure (in the first trimester) may be associated with congenital abnormalities,
        - later fetal exposure (in the second and third trimesters) may be related to neonatal renal dysfunction.

3. Common **systemic disorders**, such as the antiphospholipid syndrome (q.v.), carbon monoxide exposure (q.v.), cardiac disease, cholestasis (q.v.), collagen-vascular diseases (q.v.), diabetes, epilepsy, folic acid deficiency (q.v.), hypertension, immune thrombocytopenic purpura (q.v.), infectious diseases (e.g. listeriosis – q.v., toxoplasmosis – q.v.), inflammatory bowel disease (q.v.), obesity, renal disease, thromboembolism and thyroid disease, all present additional problems during pregnancy.

Pulmonary oedema in pregnancy may be
- cardiogenic,
- associated with pre-eclampsia (q.v.),
- tocolytic-induced (i.e. a complication of β-agonist therapy).

Pneumonia in pregnancy (q.v.) and trauma in pregnancy (q.v.) present particular problems and are discussed separately.

4. Some occupational and environmental exposures are **teratogenic**.
5. **Neoplasia** may arise in the gestational trophoblast. Such neoplasia includes
    - hydatidiform mole, which can be partial, complete or invasive,
    - choriocarcinoma, the most invasive form. Choriocarcinoma usually arises from a molar pregnancy, but it can also occur after spontaneous abortion (1 in 5000 cases), ectopic pregnancy (1 in 15,000 cases) or full-term pregnancy (1 in 150,000 cases).

A molar pregnancy should be considered if there is excessive uterine enlargement, pre-eclampsia (q.v.), hyperemesis or abnormal vaginal bleeding. The hCG level is markedly elevated, associated hyperthyroidism (q.v.) is sometimes seen, and occasionally trophoblastic lung emboli may occur. In choriocarcinoma, metastases occur particularly to the lung and later to the brain and liver.

Treatment with combination **chemotherapy** *carries a very high cure rate, even for advanced metastatic disease (85% in such cases).*

6. **Post-partum problems** are similar to the systemic problems encountered during pregnancy and listed above, but they can especially include thromboembolism, hypertension and haemorrhage.

Post-partum haemorrhage (PPH) is most commonly caused by uterine atony, surgical trauma or placenta praevia. PPH is a major cause of maternal mortality in developing countries, but it can be reduced by one third with the early IV administration of tranexamic acid (TXA) (q.v.). Pre-emptive measures include optimization of haemoglobin during pregnancy, identification of high-risk cases antenatally, careful management of the third stage of labour, the use of uterotonics, and the availability of blood products.

In developed countries, PPH may develop without an obvious bleeding source, in which case it is generally associated with disseminated intravascular coagulation (q.v.) due to placental abruption (q.v.), amniotic fluid embolism (q.v.) or fetal death in utero.

Additional post-partum problems may sometimes be seen, and they include

- endocrine abnormalities, e.g. pituitary infarction,
- cardiomyopathy (q.v.),
- streptococcal infection,
- depression.

Bibliography

Al-Kalbani M, Lapinsky SE. Prgenancy and risk. *Crit Care Med* 2020; 48: 765.

Arnout J, Spitz B, Wittevrongel C, et al. High-dose intravenous immunoglobulin treatment of a pregnant patient with an antiphospholipid syndrome. *Thromb Haemost* 1994; 71: 741.

Australian Society for the Study of Hypertension in Pregnancy. Management of hypertension in pregnancy: consensus statement. *Med J Aust* 1993; 158: 700.

Barron WM. The pregnant surgical patient: medical evaluation and management. *Ann Intern Med* 1984; 101: 683.

Bates SM, Greer IA, Pabinger I, et al. Venous thromboembolism, thrombophilia, antithrombotic therapy, and pregnancy. *Chest* 2008; 133 (suppl.): 844S.

Battino D, Granata T, Binelli S, et al. Intrauterine growth in the offspring of epileptic mothers. *Acta Neurol Scand* 1992; 86: 555.

Beeley L. Adverse effects of drugs in later pregnancy. *Clin Obstet Gynaecol* 1981; 24: 275.

Bick RL. Recurrent miscarriage syndrome due to blood coagulation protein/platelet defects: prevalence, treatment and outcome results. *Clin Appl Thromb Hemost* 2000; 6: 115.

Branch DW, Scott JR, Kochenour NK, et al. Obstetric complications associated with the lupus anticoagulant. *N Engl J Med* 1985; 313: 1322.

Brenner B, Conard J, eds. Women's issues in thrombophilia. *Semin Thromb Hemost* 2003; 29: 1.

Briggs GG, Freeman RL, Towers CV, et al., eds. *Drugs in Pregnancy and Lactation*. 11th edition. Philadelphia: Lippincott Williams & Wilkins. 2017.

Brodie MJ, Moore MR, Thompson GG, et al. Pregnancy and the acute porphyrias. *Br J Obstet Gynaec* 1977; 84: 726.

Brooks DC, Sznyter LA. Pregnancy. In: *Scientific American Surgery, Section VII Special Problems in Perioperative Care*, Chapter 11. New York: Scientific American. 1998.

Brown M, Whitworth J. The kidney in hypertensive pregnancies – victim and villain. *Am J Kidney Dis* 1992; 20: 427.

Brown MA, Buddle ML. Hypertension in pregnancy: maternal and foetal outcomes according to laboratory and clinical features. *Med J Aust* 1996; 165: 360.

Burrow GN. The management of thyrotoxicosis in pregnancy. *N Engl J Med* 1985; 313: 562.

Cheah S, Gao Y, Mo S, et al. Fertility, pregnancy and post partum management after bariatric surgery: a narrative review. *Med J Aust* 2022; 216: 96.

Chestnut DH. Critical care in obstetric practice. In: Fuhrman BP, Shoemaker WC, eds. *Critical Care: State of the Art*, Chapter 7. Fullerton: Society of Critical Care Medicine. 1989; 121.

Cope I. Medicines in pregnancy. *Med J Aust* 1991; 155: 214.

Council on Scientific Affairs, American Medical Association. Fetal effects of maternal alcohol use. *JAMA* 1983; 249: 2517.

Cowchock FS, Reece EA, Balaban D, et al. Repeated fetal losses associated with antiphospholipid antibodies. *Am J Obstet Gynecol* 1992; 166: 1318.

Dansky LV, Rosenblatt DS, Andermann E. Mechanisms of teratogenesis: folic acid and antiepileptic therapy. *Neurology* 1992; 42 (suppl. 5): 32.

Editorial. Are ACE inhibitors safe in pregnancy? *Lancet* 1989; 2: 482.

Farmer JC, ed. Critical illness of pregnancy. *Crit Care Med* 2005; 33 (suppl.): S248.

Fildes J, Reed L, Jones N, et al. Trauma: the leading cause of maternal death. *J Trauma* 1992; 32: 643.

Gilbert GL. Infections in pregnant women. *Med J Aust* 2002; 176: 229.

Ginsberg JS, Bates SM. Management of venous thromboembolism during pregnancy. *J Thromb Haemost* 2003; 1: 1435.

Ginsberg JS, Brill-Edwards P, Johnston M, et al. Relationship of antiphospholipid antibodies to pregnancy loss in patients with systemic lupus erythematosus. *Blood* 1992; 80: 975.

Ginsberg JS, Hirsh J. Use of antithrombotic agents during pregnancy. *Chest* 1992; 102 (suppl. 4): 385S.

Greer IA. Thrombosis in pregnancy: maternal and foetal issues. *Lancet* 1999; 353: 1258.

Grunfeld J-P, Pertuiset N. Acute renal failure in pregnancy. *Am J Kidney Dis* 1987; 9: 359.

Guntupalli KK, Hall N, Karnad DR, et al. Critical illness in pregnancy. *Chest* 2015; 148: 1093 & 1333.

Hanly JG, Gladman DD, Rose TH, et al. Lupus pregnancy: a prospective study of placental changes. *Arthritis Rheum* 1988; 31: 358.

Hayslett JP. Postpartum renal failure. *N Engl J Med* 1985; 312: 1556.

Hazelgrove JF, Price C, Pappachan VJ, et al. Multicenter study of obstetric admissions to

14 intensive care units in southern England. *Crit Care Med* 2001; 29: 770.

Henriquez DDCA, Bloemenkamp KWM, Van Der Bom JG. Management of postpartum haemorrhage: how to improve maternal outcomes? *Thromb Haemost* 2018; 16: 1523.

Hiilesmaa VK. Pregnancy and birth in women with epilepsy. *Neurology* 1992; 42 (suppl. 5): 8.

Homans DC. Peripartum cardiomyopathy. *N Engl J Med* 1985; 312: 1432.

Horowitz MD, Gomez GA, Santiesteban R, et al. Acute appendicitis during pregnancy. *Arch Surg* 1985; 120: 1362.

Hotham N, Hotham E. Drugs in breastfeeding. *Aust Prescriber* 2015; 38: 156.

Imperiale TF, Petrulis AS. A meta-analysis of low-dose aspirin for the prevention of pregnancy-induced hypertensive disease. *JAMA* 1991; 266: 237.

Johns KR, Morand EF, Littlejohn GO. Pregnancy outcome in systemic lupus erythematosus. *Aust NZ J Med* 1998; 28: 18.

Johnson MJ. Obstetric complications and rheumatic disease. *Rheum Dis Clin North Am* 1997; 23: 169.

Jones WB, Lewis JL. Integration of surgery and other techniques in the management of trophoblastic malignancy. *Obstet Gynecol Clin North Am* 1988; 15: 565.

Kaaja E, Kaaja R, Hiilesmaa V. Major malformations in offspring of women with epilepsy. *Neurology* 2003; 50: 575.

Kennedy D. Classifying drugs in pregnancy. *Aust Prescriber* 2014; 37: 38.

Kjellberg U, Andersson N-E, Rosen S, et al. APC resistance and other haemostatic variables during pregnancy and puerperium. *Thromb Haemost* 1999; 81: 527.

Koch S, Losche G, Jager-Roman E, et al. Major and minor birth malformations and antiepileptic drugs. *Neurol* 1992; 42 (suppl. 5): 83.

Koshy M, Burd L. Management of pregnancy in sickle cell anemia. *Hematol Oncol Clin North Am* 1991; 5: 585.

Lapinsky SE. Respiratory care of the critically ill pregnant patient. *Curr Opin Crit Care* 1996; 3: 1.

Lapinsky SE. Cardiopulmonary complications of pregnancy. *Crit Care Med* 2005; 33: 1616.

Laskin CA, Bombardier C, Hannah ME. Prednisolone and aspirin in women with autoantibodies and unexplained recurrent fetal loss. *N Engl J Med* 1997; 337: 148.

Ledger WJ. Antibiotics in pregnancy. *Clin Obstet Gynaecol* 1977; 20: 411.

Lemire RJ. Neural tube defects. *JAMA* 1988; 259: 558.

Leung AS, Millar LK, Koonings PP, et al. Perinatal outcome in hypothyroid pregnancies. *Obstet Gynecol* 1993; 81: 349.

Lim V, Katz A, Lindheimer M. Acid-base regulation in pregnancy. *Am J Physiol* 1976; 231: 1764.

Lindheimer MD, Katz AI. Hypertension in pregnancy. *N Engl J Med* 1985; 313: 675.

Lockshin MD. Lupus pregnancy. *Clin Rheum Dis* 1985; 11: 611.

Loverro G, Pansini V, Greco P, et al. Indications and outcome for intensive care unit admission during puerperium. *Arch Gynecol Obstet* 2002; 265: 195.

McDonald CF, Burdon JGW. Asthma in pregnancy and lactation: a position paper for the Thoracic Society of Australia and New Zealand. *Med J Aust* 1996; 165: 485.

McLintock C, James AH. Obstetric hemorrhage. *J Thromb Haemost* 2011; 9: 1441.

McPartin J, Halligan A, Scott JM, et al. Accelerated folate breakdown in pregnancy. *Lancet* 1993; 341: 148.

Oakley CM. Anticoagulants in pregnancy. *Br Heart J* 1995; 74: 107.

Oats JJN (chairman). *Annual Report for the Year 2007.* Melbourne: Consultative Council on Obstetric and Paediatric Mortality and Morbidity. 2008.

Persellin RH. The effect of pregnancy on rheumatoid arthritis. *Bull Rheum Dis* 1977; 27: 922.

Phelan JP, Pacheco LD, Foley MR, et al., eds. *Critical Care Obstetrics.* 6th edition. Oxford: Wiley. 2018.

Pisani RJ, Rosenow EC. Pulmonary edema associated with tocolytic therapy. *Ann Intern Med* 1989; 110: 714.

Pollock W, Rose L, Dennis C-L. Pregnant and postpartum admissions to the intensive care unit: a systematic review. *Intens Care Med* 2010; 36: 1465.

Rabinovich A, Abdul-Kadir R, Thachil J, et al. DIC in obstetrics: Diagnostic score, highlights in management, and international registry – communication from the DIC and Women's Health SSCs of the International Society of Thrombosis and Haemostasis. *J Thromb Haemost* 2019; 17: 1562.

Rand JH, Wu X-X, Andree HAM, et al. Pregnancy loss in the antiphospholipid-antibody-syndrome – a possible thrombogenic mechanism. *N Engl J Med* 1997; 337: 154.

Rizk NW, Kalassian KG, Gilligan T, et al. Obstetric complications in pulmonary and critical care medicine. *Chest* 1996; 110: 791.

Rubin PC. Beta-blockers in pregnancy. *N Engl J Med* 1981; 305: 1323.

Sanson B-J, Lensing AWA, Prins MH, et al. Safety of low-molecular-weight heparin in pregnancy: a systematic review. *Thromb Haemost* 1999; 81: 668.

Schrier RW. Pathogenesis of sodium and water retention in high-output and low-output cardiac failure, nephrotic syndrome, cirrhosis, and pregnancy. *N Engl J Med* 1988; 319: 1065 & 1127.

Seely EW, Ecker J. Medical complications in pregnancy. In: *Scientific American Medicine. Women's Health.* Hamilton: Dekker Medicine. 2020.

Smith A, Eccles-Smith J, D'Emden M, et al. Thyroid disorders in pregnancy and postpartum. *Aust Prescriber* 2017; 40: 214.

Stirrat GM. Recurrent miscarriage. *Lancet* 1990; 336: 673.

Therapeutic Goods administration. Prescribing medicines in pregnancy database. www.tga.gov.au/mode/4012. 2019.

Vasquez DN, Estenssoro E, Canales HS, et al. Clinical characteristics and outcomes of obstetric patients requiring ICU admission. *Chest* 2007; 131: 718.

Wald NJ, Bower C. Folic acid, pernicious anaemia, and prevention of neural tube defects. *Lancet* 1994; 343: 307.

Yerby M, Koepsell T, Darling J. Pregnancy complications and outcomes in a cohort of women with epilepsy. *Epilepsia* 1985; 26: 631.

Yerby MS. Pregnancy and epilepsy. *Epilepsia* 1991; 32 (suppl. 6): S51.

Yerby MS, Friel PN, McCormick K. Antiepileptic drug disposition during pregnancy. *Neurology* 1992; 42 (suppl. 5): 12.

Yerby MS, Leavitt A, Erickson DM, et al. Antiepileptics and the development of congenital anomalies. *Neurology* 1992; 42 (suppl. 5): 132.

Zeeman GG. Obstetric critical care: a blueprint for improved outcomes. *Crit Care Med* 2006; 34 (suppl.): S208.

Zwart JJ, Dupuis JRO, Richters A, et al. Obstetric intensive care unit admission: a 2-year nationwide population-based cohort study. *Intens Care Med* 2010; 36: 256.

PRES *See*

- Reversible posterior leukoencephalopathy.

Priapism

Priapism refers to prolonged (>4 hr) erection of the penis, without sexual stimulation. It is generally painful after about 6 hr, especially in the low-flow or ischaemic form.

It is an uncommon complication of
- sickle cell anaemia (q.v.),
- spinal cord lesions,
- polycythaemia vera (q.v.),
- rarely other thrombotic disorders,
- trauma.

It is sometimes seen as a complication of local therapy for impotence, especially intracavernosal papaverine, while priapism itself may in turn lead to impotence.

It has occasionally been reported as a side-effect of the non-tricyclic antidepressant agent trazodone, though it can in fact occur after any antipsychotic medication as most have some antiadrenergic properties.

Treatment of the low-flow form of priapism is a urological emergency. A variety of surgical and antithrombotic measures have been employed. Alpha-adrenergic agonists may be helpful.

Bibliography

Hodgson D. Of gods and leeches: treatment of priapism in the nineteenth century. *J R Soc Med* 2003; 96: 562.

Melman A, Serels S. Priapism. *Int J Impot Res* 2000; 12: S133.

Pautler SE, Brock GB. Priapism: from Priapus to the present time. *Urol Clin North Am* 2001; 28: 391.

Primary alveolar hypoventilation *See*

- Sleep disorders of breathing.

Primary ciliary dyskinesia

Primary ciliary dyskinesia (PCD) is the umbrella term referring to conditions of abnormalities of cilial motility. Abnormal cilial motility is a cardinal feature of **Kartagener's syndrome** (immotile cilia syndrome) (q.v.). More recently, other abnormalities of disturbed microtubular configurations have also been described, with consequent motility disturbances including incoordination instead of immotility.

Investigations include examination of the cilia in vitro or their clearance ability in vivo, e.g. by using radioaerosols. Low nasal nitric oxide measurements are typically found. Specific diagnosis of ciliary dyskinesia may be made in specialist centres by high-speed video microscopy analysis.

See
- Bronchiectasis,
- Situs inversus.

Bibliography

Afzelius BA. A human syndrome caused by immotile cilia. *Science* 1976; 193: 317.

Corbelli R, Bringolf-Isler B, Amacher A, et al. Nasal nitric oxide measurements to screen for primary ciliary dyskinesia. *Chest* 2004; 126: 1054.

Horani A, Ferkol TW. Advances in the genetics of primary ciliary dyskinesia: clinical implications. *Chest* 2018; 154: 645.

Kennedy MP, Noone PG, Cardon J, et al. Calcium stone lithoptysis in primary ciliary dyskinesia. *Respir Med* 2007; 101: 76.

Marthin JK, Mortensen J, Pressler T, et al. Pulmonary radioaerosol mucociliary clearance in diagnosis of primary ciliary dyskinesia. *Chest* 2007; 132: 966.

Mygind N, Nielsen MH, Pedersen M. Kartagener's syndrome and abnormal cilia. *Eur J Respir Dis* 1983; 64 (suppl. 127): 1.

Noone PG, Leigh MW, Sannuti A, et al. Primary ciliary dyskinesia: diagnostic and phenotypic features. *Am J Respir Crit Care Med* 2004; 169: 459.

Probiotics

Probiotics are living micro-organisms which are purported to provide a variety of health benefits when ingested. This concept particularly derives from the food industry, where yoghurts containing live bacterial cultures have been traditionally regarded as healthy, and it was first given scientific credence by Metchnikoff in the early twentieth century as part of his theory related to immunity and gut health.

Probiotics are widely marketed as nutritional supplements rather than as therapeutic agents, though they may be referred to as nutraceuticals when specific health benefits are claimed. The possible enhancement of mucosal immunity by probiotics could be relevant in a number of clinical situations, including some in critically ill patients, such as antibiotic-associated colitis, ventilator-associated pneumonia, hospital-acquired infections, pancreatitis and hepatic encephalopathy. Probiotics may also be of value in traveller's diarrhoea and atopic dermatitis.

There are many commercial preparations of probiotics available, and a number of different micro-organisms may be included. While the trial evidence to support the therapeutic use of probiotics has been tantalizing, the overall results are conflicting and a major recent study in prevention of ventilator-associated pneumonia has been negative. Clearly, more research data are required before definitive recommendations can be made.

See
- Colitis – Antibiotic-associated colitis.
- Dermatitis – Atopic dermatitis.
- Inflammatory bowel disease – Crohn's disease.
- Microbiome.

Bibliography

Hempel S, Newberry SJ, Maher AR, et al. Probiotics for the prevention and treatment of antibiotic-associated diarrhea: a systematic review and meta-analysis. *JAMA* 2012; 307: 1959.

Ho KM, Kalgudi S, Corbett J-M, et al. Gut microbiota in surgical and critically ill patients. *Anaesth Intens Care* 2020; 48: 179.

Johnstone J, Meade M, Lauzier F, et al. Effect of probiotics on incident ventilator-associated pneumonia in critically ill patients: a randomized clinical trial. *JAMA* 2021; 326: 1024.

Manzanares W, Lemieux M, Langlois PL, et al. Probiotic and synbiotic therapy in critical illness: a systematic review and meta-analysis. *Crit Care* 2016; 19: 262.

Morrow LE, Wischmeyer P. Blurred lines: dysbiosis and probiotics in the ICU. *Chest* 2017; 151: 492.

Procalcitonin *See*
- Calcitonin.

Proctitis *See*
- Anorectal infections.

Progressive multifocal leukoencephalopathy *See*
- Demyelinating diseases.

Propofol

Propofol is a widely used sedative drug in Anaesthesia and Intensive Care. Its particular value lies in its rapid onset and short duration of action. In common with most parenteral sedative drugs, propofol can produce some circulatory and respiratory depression, but in general it has a wide margin of safety.

However, it can cause an unusual but serious metabolic complication, referred to as the **propofol infusion syndrome** (PRIS). This has been observed as an uncommon but potentially fatal metabolic acidosis complicating propofol infusion, particularly in patients with an acute neurological condition, such as traumatic brain injury. It was first described in 1992 in children and was given its present name in 1999. It has been reported in up to 4% of Intensive Care patients receiving propofol.

The syndrome comprises lactic acidosis (q.v.), rhabdomyolysis (q.v.), acute renal failure, hyperkalaemia, refractory bradycardia or tachyarrhythmia (with wide QRS complexes), myocardial failure, fever (q.v.), hyperlipidaemia and green urine. Clearly, many of these clinical features are frequent in critically ill patients for a variety of common reasons, and the recognition of an iatrogenic cause can be difficult or delayed.

It has generally followed prolonged infusions at high dose, often with associated catecholamine and/or corticosteroid administration. Thus, the dosage should be limited to 3 mg/kg/hr (maximum 300 mg/hr) and the duration at this dose to 48 hr. However, there have been some reports of its occurrence even following short courses at low doses, prompting the suggestion that patients with a specific genetic susceptibility causing mitochondrial dysfunction may be at particular risk.

Treatment requires awareness of the complication, limitation of dosage, and alertness to an early warning finding of a rising blood lactate. Cardiovascular collapse can be treated with venoarterial extracorporeal membrane oxygenation (VA-ECMO) as it is potentially reversible. Fatality can be avoided only if the condition is identified promptly or preferably prevented in the first place by care with dosage (see above).

See also
- Lactic acidosis,
- Malignant hyperthermia,
- Mitochondrial diseases,
- Paraquat,
- Pink urine.

Bibliography

Chukwuemeka A, Ko R, Ralph-Edwards A. Short-term low-dose propofol anaesthesia associated with severe metabolic acidosis. *Anaesth Intens Care* 2006; 34: 651.

De Waele JJ, Hoste E. Propofol infusion syndrome in a patient with sepsis. *Anaesth Intens Care* 2006; 34: 676.

Ernest D, French C. Propofol infusion syndrome – report of an adult fatality. *Anaesth Intens Care* 2003; 31: 316.

Fudickar A, Bein B, Tonner PH. Propofol infusion syndrome in anaesthesia and intensive care medicine. *Curr Opin Anaesthesiol* 2006; 19: 404.

Hempill S, McMenamin L, Bellamy MC, et al. Propofol infusion syndrome: a structured literature review and analysis of published case reports. *Br J Anaesth* 2019; 122: 448.

Iyer VN, Hoel R, Rabinstein AA. Propofol infusion syndrome in patients with refractory status epilepticus: an 11-year clinical experience. *Crit Care Med* 2009; 37: 3024.

Krajcova A, Waldauf P, Andel M, et al. Propofol infusion syndrome: a structured review of experimental studies and 153 published case reports. *Crit Care* 2015; 19: 398.

Masuda A, Hirota K, Satone T, et al. Pink urine during propofol anesthesia. *Anesth Analg* 1996; 83: 666.

Mizock BA, Falk JL. Lactic acidosis in critical illness. *Crit Care Med* 1992; 20: 80.

Riker RR, Glisic EK, Fraser GL. Propofol infusion syndrome: difficult to recognize, difficult to study. *Crit Care Med* 2009; 37: 3169.

Vasile B, Rasulo F, Candiani A, et al. The pathophysiology of propofol infusion syndrome: a simple name for a complex syndrome. *Intens Care Med* 2003; 29: 1417.

Prostacyclin *See*
- Antiplatelet agents,
- Pulmonary hypertension.

Protein C

Protein C is an important natural inhibitor of coagulation, first described in 1979 (see Anticoagulants). It is a vitamin K-dependent factor (q.v.), and it is a serine protease, like most coagulation factors.

Protein C is activated when thrombin couples with thrombomodulin on the endothelial cell surface. This reaction is greatly amplified by the endothelial protein C receptor (EPCR), which binds protein C and aligns it with the nearby thrombin/thrombomodulin complex. Activated protein C then combines with membrane-bound protein S to form an active complex. This complex antagonizes the large activated cofactors, Va and VIIIa, as they assist the activation of II to IIa and X to Xa, respectively (see Haemophilia).

Protein C has a molecular weight of 62 kDa, plasma concentration of 4 mcg/mL (0.065 μM) and half-life of about 6 hr. Laboratory testing for protein C levels can be complex, with the usual chromogenic assay subject to occasional false-positive and false-negative results.

Protein C deficiency is implicated in the rare **warfarin-induced skin necrosis** (q.v.). This is because protein C has a shorter half-life than the four vitamin K–dependent coagulation factors (factors II, VII, IX and X) and the initial effect of warfarin, especially in higher dose, must therefore be transiently thrombotic, i.e. the anticoagulant factors are decreased before the coagulation factors. Similarly, in vitamin K deficiency, the administration of vitamin K must result in a transiently haemorrhagic state, i.e. the anticoagulant factors are increased before the coagulation factors.

Protein C deficiency may be either congenital or acquired and leads to a hypercoagulable state.

Congenital protein C deficiency is inherited as an autosomal dominant condition, with over 200 gene mutations having been found to cause either a quantitative or more rarely a qualitative deficiency. The condition is lethal (with purpura fulminans) in early life if it is homozygous, but heterozygotes are common, with a prevalence of 1 in 250 of the population. In these subjects, protein C levels overlap the low normal range, and thromboses can occur even with levels of about 50% of normal. Venous and arterial thromboses may occur, and these are sometimes unusual in affecting e.g. cerebral or splenic vessels.

*Treatment is normally with lifelong **warfarin**, though acute episodes can be treated with **protein C concentrates**.*

Acquired protein C deficiency occurs in
- vitamin K deficiency (q.v.),
- liver disease,
- disseminated intravascular coagulation (q.v.).

Activated protein C resistance is a familial thrombophilia (q.v.), with a relatively high Caucasian population prevalence of about 5–15%. It is inherited as an autosomal dominant condition. It has been found to be the major risk factor for venous thrombosis, being demonstrated in 20–50% of such patients, the higher prevalence being found in patients with a family history of thromboembolism.

The phenomenon was first described in 1993 and is most commonly due to a point mutation with a single-base substitution of adenine for guanine in the Factor V gene. In the resultant factor V molecule (**Factor V Leiden**), an arg at amino acid 506 is replaced by a glu at the cleavage site for protein C, thus rendering factor Va resistant to inactivation by activated protein C (APC) and consequently with a 10-fold longer half-life. This procoagulant or 'gain-of-function' mutation arose in Caucasians about 30,000 years ago, and it has been postulated to have conferred in the past some evolutionary benefit, i.e. a higher survival and/or fertility to compensate for the loss of the gene pool due to thrombosis. Indeed, favourable phenotypes related to haemostasis, inflammation and fertility have been reported among carriers. Several other genetic conditions can also lead to APC resistance.

Heterozygous subjects have a thrombotic risk which is similar to that seen in heterozygous protein C or protein S deficiency and which increases with age, malignancy and oral contraceptives (q.v.). APC resistance may also predispose to arterial thrombosis.

Paradoxically, the risk of pulmonary embolism is not increased in patients with the Factor V Leiden variant. It is believed that the venous thrombi in these patients while more frequent are also more stable and that for reasons as yet unresolved they are therefore less liable to embolize.

APC resistance may also be an acquired phenotype in certain circumstances, such as pregnancy, oral contraceptive use (q.v.), antiphospholipid syndrome (q.v.). An increased risk of stroke and venous thrombosis also accompanies acquired APC resistance.

Treatment principles are the same as those previously established for protein C or S deficiency (q.v.).

Protein C levels have been found to be low in sepsis and to be correlated with outcome. Protein C replacement was reported to be of benefit in the treatment of small numbers of patients with this condition, and the results of a subsequent large multicentre randomized controlled study using **recombinant human activated protein C** (drotrecogin alfa) were positive. However, these results were later criticized, and importantly they were not replicated in later studies, so that this agent has been withdrawn from the market.

Bibliography

Bernard GR, Vincent J-L, Laterre P-F, et al. Efficacy and safety of recombinant human activated protein C for severe sepsis. *N Engl J Med* 2001; 344: 699.

Bertina RM, Koeleman RPC, Koster T, et al. Mutation in blood coagulation factor V associated with resistance to activated protein C. *Nature* 1994; 369: 64.

Castoldi E, Rosing J. APC resistance: biological basis and acquired influences. *J Thromb Haemost* 2009; 8: 445.

Dhainaut J-F, Aird WC, Esmon CT, eds. Protein C pathways: bedside to bench. *Crit Care Med* 2004; 32; suppl.

Dowd P, Ham S-W, Naganathan S, et al. The mechanism of action of vitamin K. *Annu Rev Nutr* 1995; 15: 419.

Esmon C. The protein C pathway. *Crit Care Med* 2000; 28: 556.

Esmon CT, Johnson AE, Esmon NL, et al. Initiation of the protein C pathway. *Ann NY Acad Sci* 1991; 614: 30.

Hillarp A, Dahlback B. Activated protein C resistance. *Vessels* 1997; 3: 4.

Kisiel W. Human plasma protein C: isolation, characterization and mechanism of activation by alpha-thrombin. *J Clin Invest* 1979; 64: 761.

Kjellberg U, Andersson N-E, Rosen S, et al. APC resistance and other haemostatic variables during pregnancy and puerperium. *Thromb Haemost* 1999; 81: 527.

Koster T, Rosendaal FR, de Ronde H, et al. Venous thrombosis due to poor anticoagulant response to activated protein C. *Lancet* 1993; 342: 1503.

Mannucci PM, Franchini M. Classic thrombophilic gene variants. *Thromb Haemost* 2015; 114: 885.

Matsuzaka T, Tanaka H, Fukuda M, et al. Relationship between vitamin K dependent coagulation factors and anticoagulants (protein C and protein S) in neonatal vitamin K deficiency. *Arch Dis Child* 1993; 68: 297.

Papinger I, Kyrle PA, Heistinger M, et al. The risk of thromboembolism in asymptomatic patients with protein C and protein S deficiency. *Thromb Haemost* 1994; 71: 441.

Rodeghiero F, Tosetto A. Activated protein C resistance and factor V Leiden mutation are independent risk factors for venous thromboembolism. *Ann Intern Med* 1999; 130: 643.

Rose VL, Kwaan HC, Williamson K, et al. Protein C antigen deficiency and warfarin necrosis. *Am J Clin Pathol* 1986; 86: 653.

Shearer MJ. Vitamin K. *Lancet* 1995; 345: 229.

Smith OP, White B, Vaughan D, et al. Use of protein C concentrate, heparin, and haemodiafiltration in meningococcus-induced purpura fulminans. *Lancet* 1997; 350: 1590.

Svensson PJ, Dahlback B. Resistance to activated protein C as a basis for venous thrombosis. *N Engl J Med* 1994; 330: 517.

Yan SB, Helterbrand JD, Hartman DL, et al. Low levels of protein C are associated with poor outcome in severe sepsis. *Chest* 2001; 120: 915.

Zoller B, Hillarp A, Dahlback B. Activated protein C resistance: Clinical implications. *Clin Appl Thromb Hemost* 1997; 3: 25.

Protein S

Protein S is, like protein C, vitamin K–dependent (q.v.). It was first described in 1984 in Seattle (hence its name). It is a cofactor for protein C in the inactivation of factors Va and VIIIa. It can also act as a cofactor for another of the body's natural anticoagulants, tissue factor pathway inhibitor (TFPI), which inactivates factor Xa (see Anticoagulants).

It has a molecular weight of 69 kDa (comprising 635 AAs). Its average plasma concentration is 25 mcg/mL (0.35 μM), with about 40% free and 60% protein-bound, and a further small moiety circulating in the α-granules of platelets. Its half-life is possibly 40 hr, though calculation of a circulating half-life is to some extent unrealistic, because it functions as a membrane-bound cofactor. Its laboratory assay is based on its activated protein C (APC) effect only, which may limit appreciation of its other physiological potential.

Protein S is a pleiotropic protein, which provides one of the links between the processes of inflammation and thrombosis (see Pleiotropic effects). Thus, in addition to its well recognized role in coagulation, it is also involved in the regulation of inflammation, vasculogenesis and cell proliferation. Physiologically, circulating protein S is bound to the C4b component of complement (q.v., an acute phase reactant) and is thereby inhibited. In addition, interleukin 1 (IL-1) decreases thrombomodulin on endothelial cells by two thirds, so that the protein C–protein S complex functions at only about 10% of its normal capacity in this setting.

Protein S deficiency may be either congenital or acquired. Like protein C deficiency, congenital protein S deficiency is inherited as an autosomal dominant condition, and nearly 200 gene mutations having been found to cause either a quantitative or more rarely a qualitative deficiency. Acquired protein S deficiency may be seen in pregnancy and in the nephrotic syndrome.

Protein S deficiency is a cause of a thrombotic tendency with clinical features similar to those for protein C deficiency. Such thromboses can affect cerebral, mesenteric, renal and other veins, as well as causing typical venous thromboembolism. Compared with protein C deficiency, its prevalence is about 50% and its thrombotic risk about 25%.

Treatment is with lifelong **warfarin**.

Bibliography

Borgel D, Gandrille S, Aiach M. Protein S deficiency. *Thromb Haemost* 1997; 78: 351.

Comp PC. Laboratory evaluation of protein S status. *Semin Thromb Haemost* 1990; 16: 177.

Comp PC, Esmon CT. Recurrent venous thromboembolism in patients with a partial deficiency of protein S. *N Engl J Med* 1984; 311: 1525.

Dahlback B. Vitamin K-dependent protein S: beyond the protein C pathway. *Semin Thromb Haemost* 2018; 44: 176.

Dowd P, Ham S-W, Naganathan S, et al. The mechanism of action of vitamin K. *Annu Rev Nutr* 1995; 15: 419.

Engesser L, Broekmans AW, Briet E, et al. Hereditary protein S deficiency: clinical manifestations. *Ann Intern Med* 1987; 106: 677.

Gierula M, Ahnstrom J. Anticoagulant protein S – new insights on interactions and functions. *J Thromb Haemost* 2020; 18: 2801.

Mannucci PM, Franchini M. Classic thrombophilic gene variants. *Thromb Haemost* 2015; 114: 885.

Matsuzaka T, Tanaka H, Fukuda M, et al. Relationship between vitamin K dependent coagulation factors and anticoagulants (protein C and protein S) in neonatal vitamin K deficiency. *Arch Dis Child* 1993; 68: 297.

Papinger I, Kyrle PA, Heistinger M, et al. The risk of thromboembolism in asymptomatic patients with protein C and protein S deficiency. *Thromb Haemost* 1994; 71: 441.

Shearer MJ. Vitamin K. *Lancet* 1995; 345: 229.

Protein Z

Protein Z is, like proteins C and S, vitamin K–dependent (q.v.). Although it was first identified in humans in 1984, it still has not been found to have a defined physiological role.

It is structurally related to other serine proteases, specifically the vitamin K–dependent factors VII, IX, X and protein C. It has a molecular weight of 62 kDa, but its plasma levels are unusually wide.

While protein Z does not itself possess enzymatic activity, it forms a complex with protein Z–dependent protease inhibitor (ZPI), thereby enhancing the normal effect of PZI as a cofactor in reducing the activation of factor V and consequently in leading to the inhibition of factor X. Thus, its deficiency should theoretically predispose to thrombosis, and there is some variable literature to support this possibility. On the other hand, some studies have linked protein Z deficiency to bleeding and protein Z excess to thrombosis (particularly stroke).

Bibliography
Vasse M. Protein Z, a protein seeking a pathology.
  Thromb Haemost 2008; 100: 548.

Proteinuria

Proteinuria, like haematuria (q.v.), is a common abnormality detected on urinalysis.

> Proteinuria is defined as total urinary protein >150 mg per day (or total urinary albumin >20 mg per day). In pregnancy, the threshold is considered to be 300 mg per day (see Pre-eclampsia).
> Proteinuria is considered
> - mild if total urinary protein is <1 g per day,
> - severe if total urinary protein is >3 g per day and this is referred to as the nephrotic range.

The gold standard for the measurement of proteinuria requires a 24-hr urine collection. Because of its limitations and inconvenience, this test is commonly replaced by a spot urine protein–creatinine ratio (PCR) or albumin–creatinine ratio (ACR), their upper limits of normal in the non-pregnant patient being 17 and 3.5 mg/mmol, respectively.

For screening, the usual test for proteinuria is the dipstick test, but it should be remembered that this test
- does not detect non-albumin protein,
- has a threshold of detection of albumin of about 20 mg/dL (thus about 300 mg per day of protein),
- is only semiquantitative and is dependent on urine concentration,
- may sometimes be falsely positive, e.g. with high urine pH or specific gravity (SG), marked haematuria, radiocontrast agents, antiseptics, some drugs,
- may sometimes be falsely negative, e.g. with dilute urine, non-albumin proteinuria.

Microalbuminuria is a term formerly used to describe urinary albumin excretion greater than normal but less than the threshold of detection by dipstick test (i.e. 20–300 mg per day). It may be an early marker of kidney disease and is associated with an increased cardiovascular risk. **Macroalbuminuria** refers to urinary albumin excretion >300 mg per day.

Proteinuria is considered benign and not to require complex investigation, if it is
- transient,
- solely orthostatic,
- isolated and mild.

Transient proteinuria is common in young patients, in whom a routine dipstick test is positive on a single occasion. The patients are typically asymptomatic, but there may have been associated fever or exercise. As there may also be haematuria (q.v.), it is probably due to transiently increased glomerular permeability. The proteinuria is mild and comprises chiefly albumin.

Orthostatic proteinuria is also common in young asymptomatic patients. This condition comprises persistent proteinuria in the upright position (during the day) and normal protein excretion in the supine position (during the night). Its mechanism is uncertain but is presumed to be glomerular. The proteinuria is usually mild and comprises albumin. After this diagnosis, the patient should be periodically re-evaluated.

Isolated proteinuria refers to persistent proteinuria in the absence of abnormal urinary sediment, decreased glomerular filtration rate (GFR) or evidence of systemic disease. It is typically mild in degree and benign in outlook.

Proteinuria of clinical importance and requiring more complex investigation may be classified as due to one or more of the following four conditions.

1. **Glomerular disease** (q.v.)

  In this case, the protein is chiefly albumin. There may be an orthostatic element in some cases. This form of proteinuria is variable in severity.

2. **Tubulointerstitial disease** (including reflux nephropathy) (q.v.)

  In this case, the protein is chiefly the low molecular weight material, beta$_2$-microglobulin (q.v.). This form of proteinuria is not usually severe.

3. **'Overflow'**

  Increased production of some low molecular weight proteins may lead to their increased renal excretion and thus overflow proteinuria, such as with light chains in multiple myeloma (q.v.), lysozyme in acute leukaemia, myoglobin in rhabdomyolysis (q.v.) or haemoglobin in intravascular haemolysis (see Anaemia). This form of proteinuria is variable in severity.

4. **Post-renal disease**

  Typically, this is seen in urinary tract inflammation, in which small amounts of non-albumin protein are commonly excreted. This form of proteinuria is usually mild.

Appropriate investigations of proteinuria include examination of urine, ultrasound examination and renal biopsy. Specialist referral is important for detailed diagnosis and ongoing management.

Since there is a documented association between proteinuria and declining renal function, it is recommended that proteinuria be decreased if possible below 0.5 g per day in patients with chronic renal disease.

*Treatment with an **ACE inhibitor** and/or an **ARB agent** can be effective in this setting.*

Bibliography
Gosling P, Czyz J, Nightingale P, et al. Microalbuminuria in the intensive care unit: clinical correlates and association with outcomes in 431 patients. *Crit Care Med* 2006; 34: 2158.
Robinson RR. Isolated proteinuria in asymptomatic patients. *Kidney Int* 1980; 18: 395.
Turner NN, Lameire N, Goldsmith DJ, et al. eds. *Oxford Textbook of Clinical Nephrology*. 4th edition. Oxford: Oxford University Press. 2015.

Prothrombin G20210A abnormality

The **prothrombin G20210A abnormality** refers to a prothrombin variant caused by a mutation at nucleotide 20210, where there has been a guanine to adenine substitution. It was first described in Leiden in 1996. It is inherited as an autosomal dominant condition.

As this abnormality causes a 30% increase in prothrombin levels, it is referred to as a 'gain-of-function' abnormality. It is the second most common cause of **thrombophilia** (q.v.) after Factor V Leiden (see Protein C), with a population prevalence of 2–3% rising 2-fold in patients with venous thromboembolism. The risk of thrombosis is similar to that seen in activated protein C resistance (see Protein C).

In the past, a 'gain-of-function' defect (like prothrombin G20210A abnormality) with thrombotic potential may have conferred a survival benefit by the offset of a reduced bleeding potential, resulting in the persistence in the population of the relevant polymorphisms.

Bibliography
Poort SR, Rosendaal FR, Reitsma PH, et al. A common genetic variation in the 3'-untranslated region of the prothrombin gene is associated with elevated plasma prothrombin levels and an increase in venous thrombosis. *Blood* 1996; 88: 3698.

Prothrombin complex concentrate

Prothrombin complex concentrate (PCC) contains the vitamin K–dependent clotting factors. Three-factor PCC contains factors II, IX and X, and four-factor PCC also contains factor VII. Small amounts of proteins C and S are also present, and heparin has been added to prevent activation, as activated PCCs may cause thrombotic overshoot.

PCCs are used to treat vitamin K deficiency when it is severe enough to be associated with bleeding. This is usually in the context of excess warfarin dosage. In practice, there is little clinical difference in effect between the two PCCs, although resultant laboratory tests necessarily differ; for example, four-factor PCC must affect the PT/INR more because it contains factor VII. PCC is also helpful in reducing bleeding in non-anticoagulated patients, such as after trauma or cardiac surgery. Activated PCC (aPCC) is used for the treatment of haemophilia with inhibitors.

PCC is standardized by factor IX concentration (typically 250 IU per vial), but the concentrations of the other coagulation factors are similar. Vial contents are reconstituted, such that (for example) 2500 IU is contained in 100 mL for IV administration. An average therapeutic dose is 50 IU per kg.

Protozoa

Protozoa are unicellular organisms which may be transmitted incidentally to humans (see Parasitic infections). This transmission commonly requires a vector, typically a mosquito (q.v.).
See
- Amoebiasis,
- Diarrhoea – 3. Exudative diarrhoea (giardia),
- Malaria,
- Toxoplasmosis.

Bibliography
Van Voorhis WC. Protozoan infections. In: *Scientific American Medicine. Infectious Disease*. Hamilton: Dekker Medicine. 2020.

Pruritus

Pruritus refers to the troublesome symptom of skin itching. It can provide a diagnostic challenge, especially if chronic and generalized, as it can have numerous dermatological, neurological, psychogenic and systemic causes.
See
- Biliary cirrhosis,
- Bleomycin,
- Dermatology,
- Drug allergy,
- Paraneoplastic syndromes – 1. Dermatoses,
- Pemphigus,
- Polycythaemia – Polycythaemia vera,
- Psoriasis,
- Scombroid.

Bibliography
Champion RH. Generalised pruritus. *BMJ* 1984; 289: 751.
Denman ST. A review of pruritus. *J Am Acad Dermatol* 1986; 14: 375.

Prussian blue

Prussian blue, also called Parisian blue, was the first artificial paint pigment and was developed in the early 1700s. It was the original blue in blueprints. It has a complex structure with the idealized generic formula of a hydrated ferrocyanide ion. Thus, due to its ion exchange properties, it can be used as an antidote in certain heavy metal poisonings (q.v.).

See
- Prussic acid,
- Thallium.

Prussic acid

Prussic acid (hydrogen cyanide) was originally derived from the artificial pigment Prussian blue (q.v.), hence its name.

See
- Cyanide.

Pseudogout See
- Gout.

Pseudohyperkalaemia

Pseudohyperkalaemia is not a clinical problem but solely an in vitro phenomenon.

It is best known as a consequence of in vitro haemolysis, but it also occurs in the presence of marked leukocytosis ($>100 \times 10^9$/L) or thrombocytosis ($>1000 \times 10^9$/L) (q.v.).

Hyperkalaemia in these circumstances should always raise some suspicion as to its correctness. Sometimes, of course, the hyperkalaemia is correct, though unexpected and transient.

Bibliography
Greenberg S, Reiser IW, Chou SY, et al. Trimethoprim-sulfamethoxazole induces reversible hyperkalemia. *Ann Intern Med* 1993; 119: 291.

Pseudohyponatraemia

Pseudohyponatraemia refers to a decreased plasma sodium in the presence of a normal or increased plasma osmolality. It may be referred to as isotonic hyponatraemia.

True hyponatraemia (q.v.) is always associated with hypo-osmolality, i.e. <275 mOsm/kg. It is thus referred to as hypotonic hyponatraemia.

Pseudohyponatraemia is due to the presence of other active osmols in plasma, which therefore cause water to move from the intracellular space to the extracellular space and thus dilute the plasma sodium. It thus occurs in the presence of high concentrations of glucose or mannitol. As a rule of thumb, an increased plasma glucose of 5 mmol/L decreases the plasma sodium by 2 mmol/L. The presence of mannitol sufficient to cause hyponatraemia may be confirmed by the finding of an osmolar gap, i.e. a difference between the measured and calculated plasma osmolality.

Increased concentrations of lipids and proteins can cause up to one third decrease in plasma sodium, because there is less water per litre of plasma, and the phenomenon is thus a measurement artefact. An interesting example is the hyponatraemia seen following the administration of IV immune globulin. Diagnostic difficulty can then arise of course if the IVIG is being given for a condition which may itself be independently accompanied by hyponatraemia, e.g. Guillain–Barré syndrome with its associated syndrome of inappropriate antidiuretic hormone (SIADH) (q.v.).

Glycine irrigation solution as sometimes used in urology gives isosmotic dilution of plasma sodium, which can fall as low as 100 mmol/L. Consequent symptoms such as fits are due to glycine toxicity as well as to hyponatraemia.

The diagnosis of pseudohyponatraemia is important, because it is the underlying disease and not the low plasma sodium which requires treatment. When the plasma osmolality is measured in such circumstances, it is important to subtract any contribution from a raised urea, as in renal failure, to provide an estimate of the true osmolality.

See
- Central pontine myelinolysis,
- Hyponatraemia,
- Syndrome of inappropriate antidiuretic hormone.

Bibliography
Bonventre JV, Leaf A. Sodium homeostasis: steady states without a set point. *Kidney Int* 1982; 21: 880.
Colls BM. Guillain–Barré syndrome and hyponatraemia. *Intern Med J* 2003; 33: 5.
Dixon B, Ernest D. Hyponatraemia in the transurethral resection of prostate syndrome. *Anaesth Intens Care* 1996; 24: 102.

Spasovski G, Vanholder R, Allolio B, et al. Clinical practice guideline on diagnosis and treatment of hyponatraemia. *Intens Care Med* 2014; 40: 320.

Weinberg LS. Pseudohyponatremia: a reappraisal. *Am J Med* 1989; 86: 315.

Pseudohypoparathyroidism See

- Hypoparathyroidism.

Pseudolymphoma See

- Sjogren's syndrome.

Pseudomembranous colitis See

- Colitis,
- Diarrhoea.

Pseudomyxoma peritonei

Pseudomyxoma peritonei is a rare intra-abdominal malignancy which mostly arises from a perforated mucus-secreting tumour of the appendix. Peritoneal spread then occurs, and although there are generally no systemic metastases, the malignant process is eventually fatal because of the progressive abdominal infiltrate.

Current treatment modalities include **cytoreductive surgery** followed by **chemotherapy**. The surgery itself involves multiple lengthy procedures to remove all macroscopic disease. The chemotherapy then involves hyperthermic intraperitoneal instillation to remove microscopic disease.

The procedure is relevant to Intensive Care clinicians, because the surgery results in significant blood loss and complex coagulopathy associated with hypofibrinogenaemia.

Bibliography

Hinson FL, Ambrose NS. Pseudomyxoma peritonei. *Br J Surg* 1998; 85: 1332.

Moran BJ, Cecil TD. The etiology, clinical presentation, and management of pseudomyxoma peritonei. *Surg Oncol Clin N Am* 2003; 12: 585.

Pseudo-obstruction of the colon

Pseudo-obstruction of the colon (Ogilvie syndrome) is a relatively common acute complication of a number of conditions in sick hospitalized patients, including surgery, trauma, sepsis, diabetes, neurological disorders, scleroderma (q.v.), amyloid (q.v.), and of course drugs which inhibit gastrointestinal motility. As its name suggests, there is no mechanical obstruction, though the pathogenesis is uncertain.

Colonic dilatation is evidenced by a caecal diameter at least 10 cm shown radiologically. Although the condition tends to resolve with conservative treatment, it is a serious condition, because it can sometimes cause perforation and thus peritonitis and even death.

Its clinical features are abdominal pain, tenderness and distension, and its differential diagnoses include ileus and mechanical obstruction.

Treatment is chiefly of the underlying condition. If this fails, early **colonoscopic decompression** *is recommended, though this procedure can be both difficult and hazardous in some patients.*

The anticholinesterase **neostigmine***, given in a dose of 2 mg IV over 3–5 min, has been shown to be rapidly effective, with decompression in less than 30 min. This agent should be given only in the Intensive Care Unit, because significant muscarinic effects including bradycardia (requiring atropine) may occur, as well as abdominal pain. Needless to say, subtle as well as overt mechanical bowel obstruction (e.g. volvulus) must be excluded before this cholinergic agent can be safely given. Urgent laparotomy is required if perforation or mechanical obstruction is suspected.*

Bibliography

Ponec RJ, Saunders MD, Kimmey MB. Neostigmine for the treatment of acute colonic pseudo-obstruction. *N Engl J Med* 1999; 341: 137.

Pseudoporphyria See

- Porphyria.

Pseudo primary aldosteronism See

- Conn's syndrome.

Psittacosis

Psittacosis is caused by infection with the bacterium *Chlamydia psittaci*. As this organism may be transmitted to humans from birds, both wild and domestic, psittacosis is thus a zoonosis (q.v.). The route of transmission is the inhalation of avian excreta.

The clinical features vary in severity from a subclinical infection to a fulminating state. Typically, there is fever and flu-like symptoms. An atypical pneumonia of variable duration may result.

The diagnosis is confirmed serologically.

Treatment with **tetracycline** *(e.g. doxycycline 100 mg bd) for 10–14 days is rapidly effective.*

Bibliography

Kaplan RM. Budgies and bugs: our homegrown contribution to pandemics. *Med J Aust* 2021; 214: 509.

Stewardson AJ, Grayson ML. Psittacosis. *Infect Dis Clin North Am* 2010; 24: 7.

Psoriasis

Psoriasis is a chronic papulosquamous disease, with a population prevalence of 1–6%. Although it is most obviously an inflammatory skin condition, other organs can also be affected, most notably the joints. There is an increased incidence of important comorbidities, including metabolic syndrome, cardiovascular disease, psychosocial disorders and malignancy.

Its aetiology has been recognized as autoimmune, but both hereditary and environmental factors are also involved, as a number of susceptibility genes have been identified and there is a markedly increased incidence in smokers and in alcoholics. There is an association with other autoimmune conditions, especially inflammatory bowel disease (q.v.).

Although an uncommon cause of a major clinical problem in its own right in Intensive Care practice, psoriasis is of particular interest as it has been a model for many new biological therapies (see below), some of which have also found use in other less common autoimmune conditions (q.v.).

The Auspitz sign refers to small bleeding points following scraping of the lesion's scales and is diagnostically helpful. The Kobner response refers to the production of a new lesion following local trauma at an uninvolved site, though this phenomenon is not specific for psoriasis. Scratching thus can aggravate the condition.

The individual lesions tend to coalesce to form plaques which can become extensive, especially on the elbows, knees, lower back and scalp. Even the palms, soles and genitals may be involved, and the nails can become pitted. The lesions can last for many years unless treated. Discomfort and pruritus occur in 60% of cases.

Local treatment includes dithranol, phototherapy (including excimer laser therapy), steroids and tar. New combinations and vehicles have greatly improved topical therapy. Narrow band ultraviolet B has reduced the risk of subsequent squamous cell carcinoma of the skin compared with older forms of phototherapy.

- *Systemic therapy* chiefly includes methotrexate, acitretin or its prodrug etretinate (retinoids related to isotretinoin) and ciclosporin, though many other agents have also been used with some benefit. Liver biopsy should be considered in patients who have received a cumulative dose of methotrexate of more than 1 g, though hepatotoxicity may be reduced by the concomitant administration of folic acid in patients given this drug for non-malignant conditions. Since these agents, while effective, are potentially toxic, they have been referred to as 'blunt instruments' in this setting.
- More targeted **biological therapies** have considerable attraction because of their greater safety, but all to date are very expensive. Moreover, since they are immune modifiers, there is the potential for opportunistic infection and tumour formation. Examples of effective biological agents include inhibitors of tumour necrosis factor (TNF), such as infliximab, etanercept and adalimumab, which have been shown to offer rapid and long-term benefit. Alefacept and efalizumab (since withdrawn) are biological agents which have also been of benefit in some patients. Monoclonal antibodies to IL-17 (ixekizumab, secukinumab) and to IL-23 (guselkumab, tildrakizumab, ustekinumab) have recently been introduced, based on the finding that increases in interleukin 17 and 23 (IL-17 and IL-23) can lead to the proliferation of keratinocytes in psoriasis. Clinical trials of fumaric acid esters (fumarates) showed promising results in moderate to severe cases.
- Drugs including antimalarials, beta blockers, indometacin and lithium may adversely affect psoriasis and should be avoided if possible.

The prognosis is very variable and the condition can greatly fluctuate spontaneously.

> Variants of psoriasis include
> - **Erythroderma** (see Exfoliative dermatitis),
> - **Guttate psoriasis**, occurring especially after upper respiratory tract infection, because infecting organisms can act as superantigens and boost the immune response, causing guttate flares,
> - **Seborrhoeic psoriasis**, also included in the spectrum of seborrhoeic dermatitis (see Dermatitis),
> - **Psoriasis associated with arthritis** and overlapping with Reiter's syndrome (q.v.), There is often considerable disparity between the extent of joint and skin involvement and between the symptoms and signs of the arthritis.
> - **Pustular psoriasis**, either generalized (in 8% of cases and associated with hypocalcaemia – q.v.) or localized (usually to the palms and soles). The lesions appear infected but in fact are not.

Bibliography

Abel EA, Lebwohl M. Psoriasis. In: *Scientific American Medicine. Dermatology*. Hamilton: Dekker Medicine. 2020.

Calvert HT, Smith MA, Wells RS. Psoriasis and the nails. *Br J Dermatol* 1963; 75: 415.

Dawe RS, Cameron H, Yule S, et al. UV-B phototherapy clears psoriasis through local effects. *Arch Dermatol* 2002; 138: 1071.
Farber EM, Nall ML. The natural history of psoriasis in 5,600 patients. *Dermatologica* 1974; 148: 1.
Farber EM, Nall ML. An appraisal of measures to prevent and control psoriasis. *J Am Acad Dermatol* 1992; 26: 736.
Fox BJ, Odom RB. Papulosquamous diseases: a review. *J Am Acad Dermatol* 1985; 12: 597.
Ingram JT. Pustular psoriasis. *Arch Dermatol* 1958; 77: 314.
Kovitwanichkanont T, Chong AH, Foley P. Beyond skin deep: addressing comorbidities in psoriasis. *Med J Aust* 2020; 212: 528.
Lebwohl M. Advances in psoriasis therapy. *Dermatol Clin* 2000; 18: 13.
Smith D. Fumaric acid esters for psoriasis: a systematic review. *Ir J Med Sci* 2017; 186: 161.
Whyte HJ, Baughman RD. Acute guttate psoriasis and streptococcal infection. *Arch Dermatol* 1964; 89: 350.
Wolff K, Goldsmith L, Katz S, et al., eds. *Fitzpatrick's Dermatology in General Medicine*. 7th edition. New York: McGraw-Hill. 2007.

Psychiatric issues

Psychiatric issues permeate much of Intensive Care practice, as they do of medicine generally. Clearly, the major psychoses can present as primary conditions to the ICU with drug overdose (see Poisoning, see Chemical poisoning) or with other self-inflicted harm. Moreover, people with a psychiatric disorder of any type can be incidentally affected by any of the range of acute illnesses that result in critical illness generally. Finally, critically ill patients and their families can suffer a variety of long-term adverse outcomes after discharge from ICU and some of these outcomes are psychiatric in nature (see Post–Intensive Care syndrome).

More frequently in Intensive Care practice, psychiatric or neuropsychiatric features may be displayed in a number of serious conditions which are not primarily psychiatric in themselves. Relevant conditions and issues include

- carbon monoxide poisoning (q.v.),
- delirium (q.v.),
- dementia (q.v.),
- eating disorders (see Anorexia nervosa),
- factitious disorders,
- hepatitis type C (see Hepatitis),
- hyperparathyroidism (q.v.),
- lightning (q.v.),
- mefloquine administration (see Malaria),
- microbiome (q.v.),
- mixed connective tissue disease (q.v.),
- multiple sclerosis (q.v.),
- Munchausen syndrome (q.v.),
- N-acetyl-D-aspartate receptor encephalitis (see Encephalitis),
- pernicious anaemia (q.v.),
- porphyria (q.v.),
- Sjogren's syndrome (q.v.),
- stress alopecia (see Alopecia),
- systemic lupus erythematosus (q.v.),
- Wernicke–Korsakoff syndrome (q.v.).

Finally, antipsychotic drugs (e.g. lithium, monoamine oxidase inhibitors, phenothiazines, selective serotonin reuptake inhibitors (SSRIs), tricyclic antidepressants) can cause a number of problems of relevance to the care of the critically ill. These drug issues include

- amnesia (q.v.),
- anticholinergic agents (q.v.),
- carcinoid syndrome (q.v.),
- cholestasis (q.v.),
- drug-induced SLE (see Systemic lupus erythematosus),
- haematuria (q.v.),
- heat stroke (q.v.),
- hyperpigmentation (see Pigmentation disorders),
- lithium (q.v.),
- neuroleptic malignant syndrome (q.v.),
- neutropenia (q.v.),
- platelet function disorders (q.v.),
- pseudotetanus (see Tetanus),
- serotonin syndrome (q.v.),
- syndrome of inappropriate antidiuretic hormone (q.v.),
- tardive dyskinesia (q.v.),
- valproate (q.v.)

Bibliography
Bienvenu OJ, Neufeld KJ, Needham DM. Treatment of four psychiatric emergencies in the intensive care unit. *Crit Care Med* 2012; 40: 2662.
Black DW, ed. Psychiatry. In: *Scientific American Medicine*. Hamilton: Dekker Medicine. 2020.
Cucci MD, Chester KW, Hamilton LA. Concise definitive review for reinitiation of antidepressants, antipsychotics, and gabapentinoids in ICU patients. *Crit Care Med* 2022; 50: 665.

Ptosis

Ptosis, or drooping eyelid, may be unilateral or bilateral.
- If **unilateral**, it is due to
    - III nerve lesion,
    - Horner's syndrome (q.v.).

- If **bilateral**, it is associated with
  - ophthalmoplegia (q.v.),
  - generalized muscle disorder (see Myopathy).

Pulmonary alveolar proteinosis

Pulmonary alveolar proteinosis (PAP) is a disease of unknown cause and indeed with no known precipitating factor, first described in 1958. It is probably an autoimmune disorder (q.v.), though occasional cases may be secondary to inhaled insults.

There is an accumulation in the alveoli of glycoprotein and lipid material resembling surfactant. It was found to be associated with deficient surfactant clearance by alveolar macrophages. It is of interest that granulocyte-macrophage colony-stimulating factor (GM-CSF) 'knockout' mice develop a strikingly similar condition.

Microscopically, this material is amorphous and eosinophilic, with a characteristic positive reaction to periodic acid–Schiff (PAS) reagent. On electron microscopy, there are lamellar bodies similar to those seen in alveolar type II cells. Inflammation is usually minimal, and the lung structure remains intact.

Clinical features comprise cough and dyspnoea, through some patients are asymptomatic. Chest signs are minimal. While occasionally it may cause respiratory failure, most patients are not seriously ill.

The chest X-ray shows a bilateral, butterfly-shaped, pulmonary infiltrate resembling pulmonary oedema (q.v.) but without cardiomegaly, pulmonary vascular congestion, Kerley B lines or pleural effusion (q.v.). The disease is thus one of the uncommon causes of this common X-ray picture in seriously ill patients.

> The diagnosis is made by the demonstration in turbid fluid obtained by bronchoalveolar lavage of abundant PAS-positive material.
> - Since secondary infection may occur, particularly with *Mycobacteria*, *Nocardia* or fungi, the lavage fluid should always be cultured for these microorganisms.
> - PAS-positive material and a somewhat similar chest X-ray may be found in pneumonia due to *Pneumocystis jirovecii* (*P. carinii*). Thus, the presence of this microorganism should always be sought in such cases.

Treatment is indicated only if dyspnoea is significant or if the disease fails to remit spontaneously as it does in most cases within a few months.

- *Therapy consists of unilateral **lung lavage**, using a double-lumen endotracheal tube to isolate the contralateral lung from the procedure. The other lung is similarly treated on a subsequent occasion. Corticosteroids are contraindicated.*
- **GM-CSF** therapy has been reported to be dramatically helpful in some patients, particularly when administered by inhalation.
- ***Rituximab*** *(q.v.) and **plasmapheresis** (q.v.) have been reported to have some effect.*

Bibliography

Claypool WD, Rogers RM, Matuschak GM. Update on the clinical diagnosis, management, and pathogenesis of pulmonary alveolar proteinosis (phospholipidosis). *Chest* 1984; 85: 550.

Goldstein LS, Kavuru MS, Curtis-McCarthy P, et al. Pulmonary alveolar proteinosis: clinical features and outcome. *Chest* 1998; 114: 1357.

Greenhill SR, Kotton DN. Pulmonary alveolar proteinosis: a bench-to-bedside story of granulocyte-macrophage colony-stimulating factor dysfunction. *Chest* 2009; 136: 571.

Jouneau S, Menard C, Lederlin M. Pulmonary alveolar proteinosis. *Respirology* 2020; 10: 1111.

Michaud G, Reddy C, Ernst A. Whole-lung lavage for pulmonary alveolar proteinosis. *Chest* 2009; 136: 1678.

Rosen SH, Castleman B, Liebow AA. Pulmonary alveolar proteinosis. *N Engl J Med* 1958: 258: 1123.

Seymour JF, Presneill JJ. Pulmonary alveolar proteinosis: progress in the first 44 years. *Am J Respir Crit Care Med* 2002; 166: 215.

Seymour JF, Presneill JJ, Schoch OD, et al. Therapeutic efficacy of granulocyte-macrophage colony-stimulating factor in patients with idiopathic acquired alveolar proteinosis. *Am J Respir Crit Care Med* 2001; 163: 531.

Trapnell BC, Whitsett JA, Nakata K. Pulmonary alveolar proteinosis. *N Engl J Med* 2003; 349: 2527.

Pulmonary hypertension

Pulmonary hypertension is a common association of many lung diseases. It also follows a number of non-pulmonary disorders, especially those of a cardiac nature.

> Pulmonary hypertension is defined as an increase in the pulmonary artery pressure (PAP) above 30/15 mmHg or preferably a mean PAP > 20–25 mmHg.

Cor pulmonale refers to right ventricular hypertrophy and/or dilatation secondary to pulmonary disease and in response to pulmonary hypertension. There may or may not be overt right ventricular failure. The development of right ventricular hypertrophy implies that the process is chronic. Right ventricular dilatation, however, may be acute.

> Traditionally, three groups of causes of pulmonary hypertension were identified, as initially described by Paul Wood in 1956.
> 1. **Increased left atrial pressure**
> This is due to left heart failure and causes passive pulmonary hypertension. Since the pulmonary venous pressure is increased, pulmonary oedema eventually occurs.
> 2. **Increased pulmonary blood flow**
> This is due to left-to-right shunt and causes hyperkinetic pulmonary hypertension.
> 3. **Increased pulmonary vascular resistance**
> This may be due to
> - vascular constriction, usually caused by hypoxia,
> - vascular obliteration, usually caused by diffuse parenchymal damage, sometimes by vasculitis (q.v.) or rarely by pulmonary veno-occlusive disease (q.v.),
> - vascular obstruction, usually caused by pulmonary embolism.
>
> More recently, pulmonary hypertension (PH) has been classified into five broad clinical categories. These are associated with
> 1. **pulmonary arterial disease**
>   - leading to pulmonary arterial hypertension (**PAH**) and thus to increased pulmonary vascular resistance (>3 Wood units),
>   - e.g. primary pulmonary hypertension (idiopathic or familial), collagen-vascular diseases (q.v.), HIV (q.v.), drugs, toxins,
> 2. **pulmonary venous hypertension**
>   - e.g. left heart disease, pulmonary veno-occlusive disease (q.v.),
> 3. **intrinsic lung disease**
>   - e.g. chronic airways obstruction, interstitial lung disease (q.v.), sleep disorders of breathing (q.v.), chronic high altitude (q.v.),
> 4. **thromboembolism**
>   - i.e. chronic thromboembolic pulmonary hypertension (CTEPH),
> 5. **other pulmonary vasculopathy**
>   - e.g. pulmonary capillary haemangiomatosis, extrinsic compression.

Regardless of the initial cause, secondary structural changes eventually occur in the pulmonary arteries. In addition, plexiform (or microaneurysmal) lesions, microvascular thromboses or reactive vasoconstriction occur in some patients. These complications further exacerbate the hypertension.

Chronic airways obstruction, particularly chronic bronchitis, is the main cause of pulmonary hypertension due to parenchymal lung disease. Other causes include diffuse interstitial lung disease (q.v.), bronchiectasis (q.v.), kyphoscoliosis (q.v.), vasculitis (q.v.), primary pulmonary hypertension (see below) and pulmonary veno-occlusive disease (q.v.).

However, any lung disease if sufficiently severe and widespread can cause pulmonary hypertension. Rare causes include tumour or talc embolization, HIV infection (q.v.), amyloidosis (q.v.), and familial capillary haemangiomatosis.

> There may also be an association with portal hypertension and chronic liver disease in some patients, when the condition is called **portopulmonary hypertension** (PPHT or PoPH). Like the **hepatopulmonary syndrome** (q.v.), this rare condition is one of the pulmonary complications of liver disease, especially cirrhosis. The impaired clearance of vasoactive mediators is thought to give rise to prolonged vasostimulation with consequent hyperplasia of terminal pulmonary arterioles. The presence of PPHT is a contraindication to liver transplantation unless successfully treated first (as for PPH – see below).

Clusters of cases of pulmonary hypertension have been reported following the ingestion of denatured rapeseed oil or appetite suppressants (initially aminorex and subsequently fenfluramines, which were therefore later withdrawn from the market). Indeed, later surveillance has suggested that anorexigens may not only cause primary pulmonary hypertension but also contribute to the secondary pulmonary hypertension associated with other underlying diseases.

Chronic thromboembolic pulmonary hypertension (CTEPH) may seem to be an obvious potential consequence of acute pulmonary embolism, but in fact CTEPH occurs in only about 2% of patients following acute venous thromboembolism. CTEPH is more common with recurrent pulmonary embolism and also in the presence of malignancy, inflammatory bowel disease (q.v.) and antiphospholipid syndrome (q.v.), but not thrombophilia (q.v.). About 50% of patients with CTEPH have no clinical history of prior venous thromboembolism. Thus, the relationship between CTEPH and previous pulmonary embolism is not clear-cut and suggests the presence of additional mechanisms, such as the inflammatory processes involved in thrombus resolution. Inflammation is thought to promote fibrous transformation of thrombus and thus impair vascular remodelling.

> The clinical features of pulmonary hypertension include symptoms due to low cardiac output, such as fatigue, dyspnoea and angina.
>
> Physical examination shows a prominent 'a' wave of the jugular venous pulse, right ventricular hypertrophy, loud pulmonary component with narrowed split of the second sound, and right heart gallop. In advanced cases, systolic ejection click and pulmonary diastolic and tricuspid pansystolic murmurs may be heard.
>
> There may be evidence of overt right ventricular failure, with increased jugular venous pressure, hepatomegaly and peripheral oedema.

The investigation of patients with pulmonary hypertension requires chest X-ray, ECG, echocardiography and appropriate lung function tests. In addition, right heart catheterization will confirm the presence and degree of pulmonary hypertension, indicate the left atrial pressure (indirectly by the pulmonary artery wedge pressure), demonstrate the presence of left-to-right shunt by right heart blood gas sampling, permit calculation of pulmonary vascular resistance, allow pulmonary angiography and test for vasoreactivity. The possibility of associated obstructive sleep apnoea (q.v.) should be investigated. The possibility of CTEPH is assessed by ventilation/perfusion scanning or CTPA.

The treatment of pulmonary hypertension and cor pulmonale is that of the underlying condition.
- *Diuretics and especially digitalis should be used with considerable caution.*
- *In cases with significant arterial hypoxaemia, long-term **oxygen** therapy is helpful.*
- *CTEPH may be treated effectively by **thrombendarterectomy** in specialized surgical centres. **Balloon angioplasty** may be considered in patients who are not suitable for surgery. Long-term **anticoagulation** is indicated.*

Primary pulmonary hypertension (PPH), more recently called idiopathic pulmonary arterial hypertension (IPAH or more simply PAH), is an uncommon condition of unknown aetiology primarily affecting young women. Some cases are familial and may be associated with abnormalities of the bone morphogenetic protein receptor type II (*BMPR2*) gene.

Its prevalence is about 15 per million of the population and its incidence about 1 per million of the population per year. Its distinction from chronic, recurrent, pulmonary thromboembolism (i.e. CTEPH) is not always possible. A greatly increased risk of developing this condition has been reported among patients who have previously used the stimulant drugs amphetamine, methamphetamine and cocaine.

The chief symptoms are fatigue, dyspnoea (of unknown mechanism) and syncope on exertion, and sometimes chest pain. Physical signs of cor pulmonale are usually marked. Often there is peripheral vasoconstriction, including Raynaud's phenomenon (q.v.) and cyanosis.

The median age of diagnosis is 36 years, which is usually at least 2 yr after the onset of symptoms. The condition is incurable and the previously reported average survival of about 3 yr from diagnosis has increased only modestly to 5–6 yr with the more recently introduced target-specific agents. It thus remains a cause of substantial morbidity and mortality.

Treatment includes avoidance of systemic vasodilators, of pregnancy and of high altitude (q.v.) >2000 m (including air travel) without supplemental oxygen.

Specific treatment modalities should be assessed and supervised in a multidisciplinary environment in a specialist centre. Treatment guidelines are based primarily on expert consensus rather than on high-level evidence. Recently updated guidelines include a visual algorithm to assist understanding of the place of the now 14 medications which have been approved in past years.

- *Long-term **anticoagulation** is commonly prescribed, because the distinction from CTEPH in which anticoagulation is indicated is not always possible and because supervening pulmonary artery thrombosis may occur. However, no clear recommendation can be made either way based on available clinical trial evidence.*
- *Pulmonary **vasodilator** therapy is tempting, but in fact most available pulmonary vasodilators are also systemic vasodilators. Thus, even if the pulmonary vascular resistance is decreased by medication, cardiac output may be increased, so that the pulmonary artery pressure may be unchanged or even increased, while there may be associated systemic hypotension. Assessment of such agents therefore requires complex haemodynamic monitoring in an Intensive Care setting. Vasoreactivity is defined for this purpose as a fall in mean PAP of >10 mmHg without a fall in cardiac output. If a favourable acute vasodilator response is obtained, high-dose calcium channel blockers (e.g. nifedipine 240 mg per day, amlodipine*

30 mg per day or diltiazem 720 mg per day, but not verapamil) may be used. A suitable pulmonary vascular response may perhaps be best assessed following prostacyclin (epoprostenol) infusion or aerosol. Inhaled nitric oxide gives a similar though transient effect.

- Symptomatic patients who are not suitable for calcium channel blocker treatment should be given either an **endothelin receptor antagonist** (see below) or a **phosphodiesterase inhibitor** (see below) or both in combination.
- Endothelin receptor antagonists (ERA, ETRA) include **bosentan**, ambrisentan and macitentan. A more highly selective ERA (to ET-1 or ET-A), **sitaxsentan**, was withdrawn from marketing due to its association with occasional cases of severe liver injury.
- Phosphodiesterase inhibitors include **sildenafil** and **tadalafil**. These agents were originally introduced for the treatment of male erectile dysfunction.
- More recently, the guanyl cyclase stimulant, **riociguat**, has been shown to be a useful pulmonary vasodilator, with a mechanism of action similat to that of nitric oxide and a clinical effect similar to that of the endothelin receptor antagonists and phosphodiesterase inhibitors.
- Severely symptomatic patients should be considered for additional treatment with a prostanoid. **Epoprostenol** (prostacyclin) may be given by continuous IV infusion. **Iloprost** (a stable analog of prostacyclin) may be given by inhalation. Other prostacyclin analogs include **treprostinil** which may be given parenterally or orally and **selexipag** which may be given orally.
- **Nesiritide**, synthetic human brain natruiretic peptide (BNP), has been reported to be useful in refractory cases (see Atrial natriuretic peptide).
- It has been reported that the **selective serotonin reuptake inhibitors** (SSRIs) may have a favourable effect both on the outcome of pulmonary hypertension and on its initial development, but this potential benefit has not been subsequently confirmed.
- Single (or preferably bilateral) lung or heart–lung **transplantation** has been reported to be relatively effective.

Unfortunately, the chief index of efficacy in treatment trials has been limited to exercise tolerance, so that there is little documentation of the effects of the various treatment modalities on other important aspects of the condition, ranging from pathophysiology to survival.

Bibliography

Auger WR, Channick RN, Kerr KM, et al. Evaluation of patients with suspected chronic thromboembolic pulmonary hypertension. *Semin Thorac Cardiovasc Surg* 1999; 11: 179.

Badesch DB, Abman SH, Simonneau G, et al. Medical therapy for pulmonary arterial hypertension: updated ACCP evidence-based clinical practice guidelines. *Chest* 2007; 131: 1917.

Barst RJ, Rubin LJ, Long WA, et al. A comparison of continuous intravenous epoprostenol (prostacyclin) with conventional therapy for primary pulmonary hypertension. *N Engl J Med* 1996; 334: 296.

Bauer M, Fuhrmann V, Wendon J. Pulmonary complications of liver disease. *Intens Care Med* 2019; 45: 1433.

Budhiraja R, Hassoun PM. Portopulmonary hypertension: a tale of two circulations. *Chest* 2003; 123: 562.

Chin KM, Channick RN, Rubin LJ. Is methamphetamine use associated with idiopathic pulmonary arterial hypertension? *Chest* 2006; 130: 1657.

Dantzker DR, Grant BJB. Pulmonary hypertension. In: Shoemaker WC, Thompson WL, eds. *Critical Care: State of the Art*. Fullerton: Society of Critical Care Medicine. 1983; p F1.

Dartrevelle P, Fadel E, Mussor S, et al. Chronic thromboembolic pulmonary hypertension. *Eur Respir J* 2004; 23: 637.

Ewert R, ed. *Iloprost in Intensive Care Medicine*. Bremen: Uni-Med Verlag. 2006.

Farber HW, Loscalzo J. Pulmonary arterial hypertension *N Engl J Med* 2004; 351: 1655.

Fedullo PF, Auger WR, Kerr KM, et al. Chronic thromboembolic pulmonary hypertension. *N Engl J Med* 2001; 345: 1465.

Fishman AP. Aminorex to fen/phen: an epidemic foretold. *Circulation* 1999; 99: 156.

Fishman AP. Clinical classification of pulmonary hypertension. *Clin Chest Med* 2001; 22: 385.

Gabbay E, Reed A, Williams TJ. Assessment and treatment of pulmonary arterial hypertension. *Intern Med J* 2007; 37: 38.

Gaine SP, Rubin LJ. Primary pulmonary hypertension. *Lancet* 1998; 352: 719.

Gaine S. Pulmonary hypertension. *JAMA* 2000; 284: 3160.

Hemnes AR, Opotowsky AR, Assad TR, et al. Features associated with discordance between pulmonary arterial wedge pressure and left ventricular end diastolic pressure in clinical practice: implications for pulmonary hypertension classification. *Chest* 2019; 154: 1099.

Humbert M, Sitbon O, Simonneau G. Treatment of pulmonary arterial hypertension. *N Engl J Med* 2004; 351: 1425.

Keogh AM, McNeil KD, Williams T, et al. Pulmonary arterial hypertension: a new era in management. *Med J Aust* 2003; 178: 564.

Klinger JR, Elliott CG, Levine DJ, et al. Therapy for pulmonary arterial hypertension in adults: update of the CHEST guideline and expert panel report. *Chest* 2019; 155: 565.

Klok FA, Delcroix M, Bogaard HJ. Chronic thromboembolic pulmonary hypertension from the perspective of the patient with pulmonary embolism. *J Thromb Haemost* 2018; 16: 1040.

Langleben, D. Endothelin receptor antagonists in the treatment of pulmonary arterial hypertension. *Clin Chest Med* 2007; 28: 117.

Libby DM, Briscoe WA, Boyce B, et al. Acute respiratory failure in scoliosis or kyphosis: prolonged survival and treatment. *Am J Med* 1982; 73: 532.

Martin KB, Klinger JR, Rounds SIS. Pulmonary arterial hypertension: new insights and new hope. *Respirology* 2006; 11: 6.

McGregor M, Sniderman A. On pulmonary vascular resistance: the need for more precise definition. *Am J Cardiol* 1985; 55: 217.

Moll M, Sardana M, Farber HW. Pulmonary hypertension, cor pulmonale, and other pulmonary vascular conditions. In: *Scientific American Medicine. Pulmonary & Critical Care Medicine.* Hamilton: Dekker Medicine. 2020.

Naeije R. Pulmonary vascular resistance: a meaningless variable? *Crit Care Med* 2003; 29: 526.

Newman JH. Treatment of primary pulmonary hypertension – the next generation. *N Engl J Med* 2002; 346: 933.

Newman JH. Pulmonary hypertension by the method of Paul Wood. *Chest* 2020; 158: 1164.

Niemann CU, Mandell SM. Pulmonary hypertension and liver transplantation. *Pulmonary Perspectives* 2003; 20(1): 4.

Palevsky HI, Fishman AP. The management of primary pulmonary hypertension. *JAMA* 1991; 265: 1014.

Pengo V, Lensing AW, Prins MH, et al. Incidence of chronic thromboembolic pulmonary hypertension after pulmonary embolism. *N Engl J Med* 2004; 350: 2257.

Pepke-Zaba J, Higenbottam TW, Dinh-Xuan AT, et al. Inhaled nitric oxide as a cause of selective pulmonary vasodilatation in pulmonary hypertension. *Lancet* 1991; 338: 1173.

Prasad S, Wilkinson J, Gatzoulis MA. Sildenafil in primary pulmonary hypertension. *N Engl J Med* 2000; 343: 1342.

Prior DL, Adamas H, Williams TJ. Update on pharmacotherapy for pulmonary hypertension. *Med J Aust* 2016; 205: 271.

Rich S. Primary pulmonary hypertension. *Prog Cardiovasc Dis* 1988; 31: 205.

Rich S. The current treatment of pulmonary arterial hypertension: time to redefine success. *Chest* 2006; 130: 1198.

Rich S, Herskowitz A, eds. Pulmonary vascular disease: the global perspective. *Chest* 2010; 6 (suppl.): 1S.

Rich S, Rubin L, Walker AM, et al. Anorexigens and pulmonary hypertension in the United States. *Chest* 2000; 117: 870.

Robalino BD, Moodie DS. Association between pulmonary hypertension and portal hypertension: analysis of its pathophysiology and clinical, laboratory and hemodynamic manifestations. *J Am Coll Cardiol* 1991; 17: 492.

Roberts WC. A simple histologic classification of pulmonary arterial hypertension. *Am J Cardiol* 1986; 58: 385.

Rubin LJ. Primary pulmonary hypertension. *N Engl J Med* 1997; 336: 111.

Rubin LJ, ed. Brenot memorial symposium on the pathogenesis of primary pulmonary hypertension. *Chest* 1998; 114: no.3 (suppl.).

Rubin LJ. Therapy of pulmonary hypertension: targeting pathogenic mechanisms with selective treatment delivery. *Crit Care Med* 2001; 29: 1086.

Rubin LJ, ed. Diagnosis and management of pulmonary arterial hypertension: ACCP evidence-based clinical practice guidelines. *Chest* 2004; 126: no.1 (suppl.).

Rubin LJ, Badesch DB, Barst RJ, et al. Bosentan therapy for pulmonary artery hypertension. *N Engl J Med* 2002; 346: 896.

Runo JR, Loyd JE. Primary pulmonary hypertension. *Lancet* 2003; 361: 1533.

Salvador ML, Loaiza CAQ, Padial LR, et al. Portopulmonary hypertension: prognosis and management in the current treatment era – results from the REHAP registry. *Intern Med J* 2021; 51: 355.

Shah SJ, Gomberg-Maitland M, Thenappan T, et al. Selective serotonin reuptake inhibitors and the incidence and outcome of pulmonary hypertension. *Chest* 2009; 136: 694.

Shure D. Primary pulmonary hypertension – good news and bad. *Pulmonary Perspectives* 1996; 13(3): 6.

Simonneau G, Galie N, Rubin LJ, et al. Clinical classification of pulmonary hypertension. *J Am Coll Cardiol* 2004; 43: 5S.

Smith I. Pulmonary hypertension: an overview for the non-cardiac anaesthetist. In: Riley R, ed. *Australasian Anaesthesia*. Melbourne: ANZCA. 2015; p 75.

Taichman DB, Omelas J, Chung L, et al. Pharmacologic therapy for pulmonary arterial hypertension in adults: CHEST guideline and expert panel report. *Chest* 2014; 146: 449.

Various. 47th annual Thomas L Petty lung conference: cellular and molecular pathobiology of pulmonary hypertension. *Chest* 2005; 128 (suppl.): 547S.

Versprille A. Pulmonary vascular resistance: a meaningless variable. *Intens Care Med* 1984; 10: 51.

Walmrath D, Schneider T, Pilch J, et al. Effects of aerosolized prostacyclin in severe pneumonia. *Am J Respir Crit Care Med* 1995; 151: 724.

Winter M-P, Schernthaner GH, Lang IM. Chronic complications of venous thromboembolism. *J Thromb Haemost* 2017; 15: 1531.

Pulmonary infiltrates

> The chief causes of a diffuse **pulmonary infiltrate** are
> 1. pneumonia,
> 2. pulmonary oedema (q.v.),
> 3. acute respiratory distress syndrome (q.v.),
> 4. aspiration pneumonitis (q.v.),
> 5. interstitial lung disease (q.v.)
>   - idiopathic interstitial pneumonias (q.v.),
>   - sarcoidosis (q.v.),
>   - haemorrhagic infiltrates, e.g. Goodpasture's syndrome (q.v.),
>   - pulmonary infiltration with eosinophilia (q.v.),
>   - angiitis and granulomatosis, e.g. Wegener's granulomatosis (q.v.),
>   - rare pulmonary infiltrative conditions,
> 6. malignancy
>   - lymphoma,
>   - metastases,
>   - lymphangitis carcinomatosa,
>   - alveolar cell carcinoma,
> 7. pneumoconiosis (q.v.),
> 8. hypersensitivity pneumonitis (q.v.),
> 9. drug reaction (see Drugs and the lung),
> 10. lung involvement in systemic disease (see Systemic diseases and the lung),
> 11. miliary tuberculosis (q.v.),
> 12. radiation pneumonitis (q.v.),
> 13. uraemia.

Most of these conditions are separately considered elsewhere in this book.

Bibliography

Crystal RG, Bitterman PB, Rennard SI, et al. Interstitial lung diseases of unknown cause. *N Engl J Med* 1984; 310: 154 & 235.

Muller NL, Miller RR. Computed tomography of chronic diffuse infiltrative lung disease. *Am Rev Respir Dis* 1990; 142: 1440.

Pulmonary infiltration with eosinophilia (PIE) See

- Eosinophilia and lung infiltration.

Pulmonary Langerhans cell histiocytosis See

- Histiocytosis – Eosinophilic granuloma.

Pulmonary nodules

Pulmonary nodules may be
- small and single (i.e. a 'coin' lesion),
- large (>6 cm diameter) and single,
- multiple.

The diagnosis cannot usually be made from the clinical features, since most patients are asymptomatic. However, patient characteristics and nodule features, such as size, density, location and margins, can guide assessment. Nevertheless, diagnosis generally requires comparison with previous X-ray films (if available), CT or PET scanning (with percutaneous needle biopsy/aspiration), bronchoscopy, and sometimes thoracotomy (or video-assisted thoracoscopic surgery, VATS) and resection.

Management guidelines for small incidental pulmonary nodules have been published by the Fleischner Society and others, as these lesions generally cause the most diagnostic difficulty.

> The chief causes of a **small and single pulmonary nodule** are
> 1. carcinoma
>   - usually primary and especially adenocarcinoma,
>   - mostly resectable and thus potentially curable at this stage,
> 2. infection
>   - granuloma, especially tuberculous or fungal, and often calcified,
> 3. hamartoma
>   - typically with 'popcorn' calcification,
> 4. arteriovenous malformation (q.v.),
> 5. bronchogenic cyst
>   - for which there may also be a clue from 'popcorn' calcification.

The chief causes of a **large and single pulmonary nodule** are
1. neoplasm
   - usually primary, and especially large cell carcinoma or alveolar cell carcinoma,
   - sometimes lymphoma,
2. infection
   - bacterial pneumonia, fungal infection,
3. sequestration,
4. bronchogenic cyst.

The chief causes of **multiple pulmonary nodules** are
1. neoplasm
   - usually metastases,
   - sometimes in women 'benign metastasizing' uterine leiomyoma,
2. infection
   - septic emboli, especially in *S. aureus* infection,
   - granulomas, as in fungal or nocardial infection, or in melioidosis (q.v.) or paragonimiasis (q.v.),
3. arteriovenous malformations (q.v.),
4. Wegener's granulomatosis (q.v.),
5. rheumatoid lung,
6. sarcoidosis (q.v.),
7. amyloid (q.v.).

Bibliography
Baldwin DR. Development of guidelines for the management of pulmonary nodules. *Chest* 2015; 148: 1365.
Cruickshank A, Stieler G, Ameer F. Evaluation of the solitary pulmonary nodule. *Intern Med J* 2019; 49: 306.
Dines DE, Arms RA, Bernatz PE, et al. Pulmonary arteriovenous fistulas. *Mayo Clin Proc* 1974; 48: 460.
Faughnan ME, Lui YW, Wirth JA, et al. Diffuse pulmonary arteriovenous malformations: characteristics and prognosis. *Chest* 2000; 117: 31.
Gould MK, Tang T, Liu IL, et al. Recent trends in the identification of incidental pulmonary nodules. *Am J Respir Crit Care Med* 2015; 192: 1208.
Lee P, Minai OA, Mehta AC, et al. Pulmonary nodules in lung transplant recipients: etiology and outcome. *Chest* 2004; 125: 165.
Lillington GA. Management of the solitary pulmonary nodule. *Hosp Pract* 1993; 28: 41.
MacMahon H, Naidich DP, Goo JM, et al. Guidelines for management of incidental pulmonary nodules detected on CT images: from the Fleischner Society 2017. *Radiology* 2017; 284: 228.
Ost D, Fein A. Evaluation and management of the solitary pulmonary nodule. *Am J Respir Crit Care Med* 2000; 162: 782.
Patel VK, Naik SK, Naidich DP, et al. A practical algorithmic approach to the diagnosis and management of solitary pulmonary nodules: Parts 1 & 2. *Chest* 2013; 143: 825 & 840.
Savic B, Birtel FJ, Tholen W, et al. Lung sequestration. *Thorax* 1979; 34: 96.
Steele JD. The solitary pulmonary nodule. *J Thorac Cardiovasc Surg* 1963; 46: 21.
Terry PB, Barth KH, Kaufman SL, et al. Balloon embolization for the treatment of pulmonary arteriovenous fistulas. *N Engl J Med* 1980; 302: 1189.
Wiener DC, Wiener RS. Patient-centred guideline-concordant discussion and management of pulmonary nodules. *Chest* 2020; 158: 416.
White RJ, Lynch-Nyhan A, Terry P, et al. Pulmonary arteriovenous malformation: techniques and long-term outcome of embolotherapy. *Radiology* 1988; 169: 663.

Pulmonary oedema *See*

- Acute pulmonary oedema.

Pulmonary veno-occlusive disease

Pulmonary veno-occlusive disease (PVOD) may be seen in a number of settings. In primary pulmonary hypertension (PPH) (q.v.), about 5% of patients have involvement predominantly affecting the pulmonary veins instead of the arteries, with intimal proliferation, thrombosis, obliteration and fibrosis. In these cases, it appears to be an uncommon variant of PPH. Sometimes, the condition may be seen in association with mediastinal fibrosis (see Mediastinum). It has also been reported in collagen-vascular diseases (q.v.), and after radiation (q.v.), cancer chemotherapy (e.g. mitomycin) and bone marrow transplantation. Genetic mutations may be responsible for some cases.

The chest X-ray shows pulmonary congestion, and the lung scan shows patchy abnormality. Although the pulmonary artery wedge pressure is often increased, it underestimates the true pulmonary capillary or filtration pressure, because in this condition the capillary pressure is much greater than the venous pressure. Lung function tests show marked impairment of gas transfer. Lung biopsy shows intimal fibrosis and eventual arterialization, particularly of the smaller pulmonary veins.

Medical treatment is ineffective. Vasodilator drugs are not usually of value and may paradoxically exacerbate acute pulmonary oedema or even death.

Lung transplantation is the only potentially curative treatment.

Bibliography

Heath D, Segal N, Bishop J. Pulmonary veno-occlusive disease. *Circulation* 1966; 34: 242.

Holcomb BW, Loyd JE, Ely EW, et al. Pulmonary veno-occlusive disease. *Chest* 2000; 118: 1671.

Palevsky HI, Pietra GG, Fishman AP. Pulmonary veno-occlusive disease and its response to vasodilator agents. *Am Rev Respir Dis* 1990; 142: 426.

Palmer SM, Robinson LJ, Wand A, et al. Massive pulmonary edema and death after prostacyclin infusion in a patient with pulmonary veno-occlusive disease. *Chest* 1998; 113: 237.

Purpura

Purpura refers to skin and mucous membrane bleeding, with lesions that can range from as small as petechiae (q.v.) to as large as ecchymoses.

> Purpura is caused by
> - thrombocytopenia (q.v.),
> - platelet function disorders (q.v.),
> - increased microvascular permeability.

Increased **microvascular permeability** (with vascular purpura) may be due to
- endothelial cell damage,
- damage to supporting structures,
- miscellaneous conditions.

These vascular thrombohaemorrhagic conditions may be either hereditary or acquired. They are clinically manifest as bleeding disorders with a normal platelet count and normal platelet function.

Endothelial cell damage may be
- toxic, from
  - infections, especially Gram-negative or rickettsial,
  - snake venom (see Bites and stings),
- embolic, due to
  - sepsis,
  - disseminated intravascular coagulation (q.v.),
  - thrombotic thrombocytopenic purpura (q.v.),
  - subacute bacterial endocarditis (see Endocarditis),
  - cholesterol,
  - fat,
- leukocytoclastic (see Vasculitis), due to immune-mediated neutrophil aggregation, as
  - in Henoch–Schonlein (or Schonlein–Henoch) purpura (q.v.),
  - in collagen-vascular disease (q.v.),
  - in hepatitis B infection (q.v.),
  - with some drugs, e.g. sulphonamides,
- thrombotic (as in purpura fulminans), due to
  - microvascular damage (q.v.), with resultant haemorrhagic skin necrosis,
  - microangiopathy (q.v.),
  - in protein C deficiency (q.v.),
  - in meningococcaemia,
  - in idiopathic cases, but sometimes associated with hyposplenism.

Damage to supporting structures occurs with
- scurvy (q.v.),
- corticosteroids,
- senile purpura,
- hereditary haemorrhagic telangiectasia (q.v.),
- amyloid (see Multiple myeloma),
- hereditary connective tissue disorders (see Connective tissue diseases)
  - Ehlers–Danlos syndrome, Marfan's syndrome (q.v.), pseudoxanthoma elasticum.

Miscellaneous conditions primarily include **auto-erythrocyte purpura**. This is an unusual and uncommon condition in middle-aged women.

It is manifest as large painful subcutaneous haematomas. Its name derives from its reproduction by subcutaneous injection of the patient's own red blood cells.

Treatment is ineffective.

See
- Connective tissue diseases.

Bibliography

Bick R. Vascular thrombohaemorrhagic disorders: hereditary and acquired. *Clin Appl Thromb Hemost* 2001; 7: 178.

Cameron JS. Henoch-Schonlein purpura: clinical presentation. *Contrib Nephrol* 1984; 40: 246.

Connell NT. Microangiopathic and vascular disorders. In: *Scientific American Medicine. Hematology.* Hamilton: Dekker Medicine. 2020.

Stein RH, Sapadin AN. Purpura fulminans. *Int J Dermatol* 2003; 42: 130.

Thachil J. History of the word 'purpura' and its current relevance. *J Thromb Haemost* 2021; 191: 2381.

Pyoderma gangrenosum

Pyoderma gangrenosum (PG) is a rare condition in which purple, non-crepitant, painful nodules develop, usually on the limbs or lower body. The lesions vesiculate, coalesce and ulcerate, leaving a ragged and undermined edge. They can become large and are often multiple. There is no systemic toxicity. The aetiology is non-infective and probably immunological.

The course is very variable from acute to chronic. The condition is most commonly associated with serious underlying systemic disease, such as a myeloproliferative disorder, rheumatoid arthritis, chronic active hepatitis, gastrointestinal malignancy or especially inflammatory bowel disease (q.v.). Sometimes, it occurs at the site of recent skin trauma.

The diagnosis is clinical. Biopsy shows only non-specific inflammation but may be helpful in excluding other conditions.

The chief differential diagnoses are infectious gangrenous cellulitis (see Gangrene), vasculitis (q.v.), malignant ulceration or tissue injury (e.g. spider bite – q.v.).

Treatment is local, though systemic **corticosteroids** *may be required. There is no response to antibiotics, and there may be worsening with debridement.*

- *In resistant cases,* **immunosuppression** *with cyclophosphamide, ciclosporin, thalidomide or tacrolimus (a macrolide antibiotic with an action similar to that of ciclosporin) is indicated.*
- **Dapsone** *and* **hyperbaric oxygen** *have been reported to be helpful in some cases.*

Bibliography

Cooper A, Powell FC. Pyoderma gangrenosum – a frequently misdiagnosed skin condition. *Med J Aust* 2013; 199: 382.

Hecker MS, Lebwohl MG. Recalcitrant pyoderma gangrenosum: treatment with thalidomide. *J Am Acad Dermatol* 1998; 38: 490.

Newell LM, Malkinson FD. Pyoderma gangrenosum. *Arch Dermatol* 1982; 118: 769.

Schwaegerle SM, Bergfeld WF, Senitzer D, et al. Pyoderma gangrenosum: A review. *J Am Acad Dermatol* 1988; 18: 559.

Teagle A, Hargest R. Management of pyoderma gangrenosum. *J R Soc Med* 2014; 107: 228.

Pyrexia

It is well known that normal body temperature is defended within very narrow limits, with an additional circadian range from about 36.1°C in the morning to 37.4°C in the evening. However, circadian rhythms (q.v.) tend to be lost in the seriously ill.

Heat is produced by metabolic processes, particularly by the liver and heart at rest and by skeletal muscles on exercise. Skeletal muscle can generate large amounts of energy and the body is only about 25% efficient in translating metabolic energy to external work, the rest being converted to heat.

Heat is lost from the skin (90%) and lungs (10%), two thirds by radiation and one third by evaporation, though the latter component increases with increased environmental temperature and on exercise, when sweating which may reach up to 2 L/hr becomes the body's main method of achieving external heat loss. Normally, this external heat loss is very efficient, so that even a prolonged increase in metabolic rate of 15-fold or more for 2 hours or more, as in elite marathoners, raises the body temperature to only 38–40°C (whereas without such heat loss, the temperature would increase by 1°C each 5 min).

The temperature control centre resides in the preoptic nucleus in the anterior hypothalamus, from where it stimulates the autonomic nervous system to produce either vasodilatation and sweating to increase heat loss or vasoconstriction and shivering to decrease heat loss.

Increased body temperature is referred to as **pyrexia**. Pyrexia may take one of two forms, namely,
- **hyperthermia**
  - i.e. failure of heat control, so that heat production exceeds heat loss,
- **fever**
  - i.e. an increased set-point of the hypothalamic thermostat, so that heat control achieves an increased temperature.

Hyperthermia can be caused by
- increased heat production,
- decreased heat loss,
- hypothalamic disease.

In practice, hyperthermia is usually associated with exercise (in which heat production can increase 20-fold), particularly in association with dehydration or adverse environmental conditions (see Heat stroke).

However, some disease states also produce hyperthermia rather than fever, often with very high body temperatures (e.g. >41°C).
These diseases include
- alcohol withdrawal, i.e. delirium tremens,
- baclofen withdrawal (q.v.),
- drug abuse, e.g. amphetamines (q.v.,) cocaine (q.v.), anticholinergic agents (q.v.),
- malignant hyperthermia (q.v.),
- neuroleptic malignant syndrome (q.v.),
- salicylate poisoning (see Aspirin),
- serotonin syndrome (q.v.),
- status epilepticus,
- tetanus (q.v.),
- thyroid storm (q.v.),

- phaeochromocytoma (q.v.),
- hypothalamic disease,
  - due to encephalitis (q.v.), cerebrovascular disease, neurotrauma, neoplasia, sarcoidosis (q.v.), drugs.

The clinical distinction between hyperthermia and fever cannot be made on the basis of temperature level and can be particularly difficult in endocrine or hypothalamic disease. Recurrent pyrexia makes fever more likely than hyperthermia.

The treatment for hyperthermia is that of the underlying disease, with specific therapy if possible. In addition, systemic measures are important, including physical cooling and circulatory support (see treatment of Fever below).

Fever, unlike hyperthermia, is always due to disease. It has been known since antiquity to be one of the cardinal signs of significant disease.

Fever arises from the production, especially by mononuclear phagocytes, of cytokines which are acute inflammatory mediators. These include especially interleukin-1 (IL-1) and tumour necrosis factor (TNF) but also IL-6 and interferon-gamma (IFNγ). The cytokine, interleukin-1 receptor antagonist (IL-1ra), opposes the inflammatory response.

IL-1 in particular is a pyrogen, in which role it acts as a hormone rather than a cytokine. Thus, it is distributed by the circulation and acts on receptors remote from the original site of inflammation and cytokine production. Following binding to cell membrane receptors in the hypothalamus, IL-1 activates phospholipase to release from membrane phospholipids the family of arachidonic acid metabolites and in particular prostaglandins (especially of the E series). These substances increase the temperature set-point in the hypothalamus and activate the heat control mechanisms accordingly. It is because of the central role of prostaglandins in this pathway that aspirin is so effective in fever.

Several other cytokines are also pyrogenic, including TNF (see Tumour necrosis factor) (which is indirect and acts via stimulating IL-1) and IL-6 and IFNγ (which are direct). As is well known, the 'pro-inflammatory' cytokines are also immunostimulatory, with a variety of actions incorporated into the **acute phase response**. These include stimulation of T and B cells, activation of macrophages, release of other cytokines, stimulation of neutrophil release from the bone marrow, stimulation of neutrophil chemotaxis (thus causing leukocytosis systemically and inflammatory cell infiltration locally), stimulation of production by the liver of acute phase proteins (thus causing an increased ESR), increased procoagulant activity and platelet adhesion, vasodilatation and increased vascular permeability, and subsequently fibroblast proliferation for repair.

The net effect of the endocrine–immune interactions and the consequent inflammatory and related responses is the 'sick everything' syndrome.

This is a pyrexial, euthyroid, diabetogenic and hypogonadal state, whose details are more apparent as laboratory than as clinical findings.

Apart from being a marker of potentially serious illness, the clinical significance of this state remains uncertain.

Fever of unknown origin (FUO) should perhaps more properly be termed **pyrexia of unknown origin** (PUO). This is because no assumption should be made in advance as to whether the set-point is or is not increased, though in most cases of course the set-point is in fact increased and the condition may rightly be termed fever. FUO was originally described and defined in 1961.

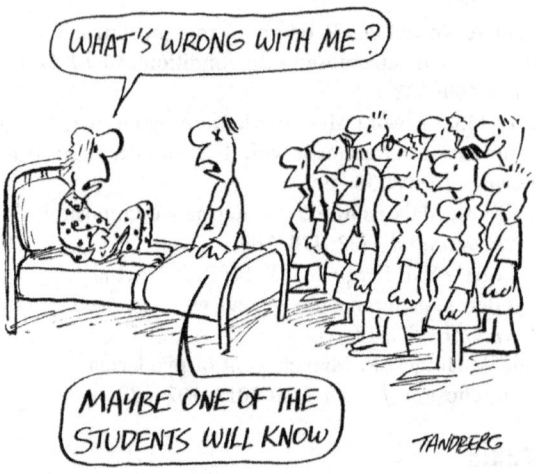

Fever of unknown origin (FUO) has been defined as
- core body temperature >38.3°C,
- of at least 3 weeks' duration,
- excluding major well-known infective and postoperative causes, and
- unclarified despite 1 week of investigations.

This definition immediately excludes the majority of cases of fever, since although one third of hospital patients develop fever (most due to infection), nearly

90% of these have straightforward diagnoses and in most of the rest the fever is short-lived and has no ill effects.

The causes of FUO have been well documented in published series, and it is worth remembering that in this, as in many situations of diagnostic difficulty, the uncommon manifestations of common diseases are more likely to be encountered than the common manifestations of uncommon diseases. It is interesting to note that the main causes of FUO have remained substantially unchanged for over 50 years.

The causes of FUO have thus been found to be
1. infections (20–36%),
2. neoplasms (19–31%),
3. collagen-vascular diseases (9–19%),
4. other less common specific diseases (18–25%),
5. undiagnosed (7–34%).

1. **Infections**

   a) **Systemic**
   - Brucellosis (q.v.), leptospirosis (q.v.), listeriosis (q.v.), mycosis, psittacosis, toxoplasmosis (q.v.) should be considered.
   - Viral infections do not produce fever for >3 weeks, except for cytomegalovirus (CMV, q.v.), which is especially seen in transplant recipients.
   - Endocarditis (q.v.) and tuberculosis (q.v.) should always be specifically excluded.
   - Other infections are rare, except in travellers.

   b) **Local**
   - A localized collection or abscess should always be sought, especially if there has been local injury, particularly to the abdomen. Subphrenic, intrahepatic or other intra-abdominal collections should be considered in such cases.
   - Occult local infection sometimes involves the urinary tract, paranasal sinuses or teeth.

2. **Neoplasms**

   - Lymphoma.
   - Haematological malignancy.
     - In these cases, however, the usual cause of fever is infection rather than the malignancy itself, but if the latter it typically responds to NSAIDs.
   - Carcinoma of the kidney.
   - Phaeochromocytoma (q.v.).
   - Extensive metastatic disease.

3. **Collagen-vascular diseases**

   - Especially systemic lupus erythematosus (q.v.).
   - In the elderly, polymyalgia rheumatica (q.v.) and temporal arteritis (q.v.) should be considered.
   - Associated arthralgia and high ESR are useful clues to this category of illness.

4. **Other less common specific diseases**

   - Alcoholic hepatitis.
   - CNS lesions
     - usually associated with coma and known brain damage.
   - Drugs (see Drug fever)
     - particular culprits are beta-lactam antibiotics, isoniazid, hydralazine, methyldopa, phenytoin, sulphonamides.
     - The presence of a rash and/or eosinophilia (q.v.) may provide a useful clue.
     - In addition, the responsible drug has usually been administered only recently, except that both methyldopa and phenytoin can produce late-presenting fever.
   - Factitious (q.v.).
   - Familial Mediterranean fever (q.v.).
   - Granulomatous diseases, especially sarcoidosis (q.v.).
   - Inflammatory bowel disease (q.v.).
   - Pulmonary thromboembolism
     - though fever prolonged for >1 week is uncommon.
   - Whipple's disease (q.v.).

The height and pattern of fever are not usually diagnostically helpful. Diagnosis requires detailed history and clinical examination, and appropriate investigations (particularly microbiological, imaging and histological) to cover the conditions listed above. Details of travel, occupation, recreation, contacts and drugs need to be specifically explored. Fever in a returned traveller can present a particularly challenging problem, as the diagnostic net may need to be cast wider than usual. Occasionally, diagnosis may be assisted by antibiotics or corticosteroids in a therapeutic trial. Otherwise, specific treatment without a diagnosis should be avoided, unless the suspected condition is life-threatening, e.g. disseminated tuberculosis (q.v.).

Fever in the Intensive Care patient is a very common finding. While in general it may or may not be clinically significant, fever which is high or prolonged is associated with an adverse outcome. However, an exact temperature in an individual patient may be difficult to define with precision, as there are a number of different methods of measuring body temperature in ICU and these can give somewhat differing readings.

It may be considered as a core temperature >38.3°C (Society of Critical Care Medicine definition). For practical purposes, temperature elevations less than this do not usually warrant complex investigation in themselves. Instead, the acute phase reactant, C-reactive protein (q.v.), has been reported to be more useful than traditional indices such as temperature or leukocytosis in diagnosing and monitoring infection in Intensive Care patients. A cut-point of 50 mg/L has been recommended for this purpose.

Most cases of fever in ICU are caused by obvious infections,
- particularly
  - nosocomial pneumonia,
  - line-related sepsis,
  - abdominal sepsis,
  - wound infection,
- sometimes
  - sinusitis,
  - urinary tract infection,
  - C. difficile colitis (q.v.).

Some cases of fever in ICU are due to non-infectious causes and can be frustrating to clarify. While most such causes usually produce only minor elevations of temperature, sometimes they may produce genuine fever. These conditions include
- pancreatitis (q.v.),
- acalculous cholecystitis,
- gut ischaemia,
- gut bleeding,
- thromboembolism,
- drug fever (q.v.),
- transfusion,
- myocardial infarction,
- cerebral haemorrhage or other brain injury,
- haematoma,
- phlebitis.

While the hazards of pyrexia are well known, the possible benefits of fever remain controversial.

The **adverse consequences of pyrexia** include,
- catabolic state,
- hyperdynamic circulation (see Hyperdynamic state),
- delirium (q.v.),
- convulsions (usually in children),
- cellular damage if the temperature is extreme (i.e. >41°C), though usually such damage may be primarily attributable to the underlying disease.

The **beneficial consequences of fever** have not been established in humans, although cytokine release appears to have evolved over hundreds of millions of years, so that in many species it presumably enhances host defence. Certainly, fever benefits some infected poikilotherms and even mammals.

However, fever is not helpful in humans, since although some infecting organisms are heat sensitive the body temperatures achieved during fever are not high enough to take advantage of this potential microbial weakness.

Similarly,
- fever therapy as used in the past was not helpful in infections, though it was not harmful, and
- antipyretic medication is not harmful, though it is not helpful except symptomatically.

Whole body hyperthermia has been used in some oncology centres as part of a range of cancer treatment modalities.

Treatment of fever is that of the underlying disease, together with symptomatic measures (aspirin or paracetamol) and general support. Since the temperature set-point is increased, physical cooling can be distressing, though it may be considered useful (as in hyperthermia) if the temperature is particularly high (i.e. >40–41°C), especially at extremes of age and in cardiovascular disease. To prevent shivering and its associated physiological stress and psychological distress, sedation may be required, sometimes to the point of requiring ventilatory support.

It should be remembered that the active treatment of fever is controversial in most critically ill patients (except particularly in acute brain injury), and while it is the subject of ongoing clinical investigation, neither beneficial nor adverse effects on mortality have been shown to date.

Bibliography

Aduan RP, Fauci AS, Dale DC, et al. Factitious fever and self-induced infection. *Ann Intern Med* 1979; 90: 230.

Aronoff DM, Neilson EC. Antipyretics: mechanisms of action and clinical use in fever suppression. *Am J Med* 2001; 111: 304.

Axelrod P. External cooling in the management of fever. *Clin Infect Dis* 2000; 31: S224.

Ben-Chetrit E, Levy M. Familial Mediterranean fever. *Lancet* 1998; 351: 659.

Beresford RW, Gosbell IB. Pyrexia of unknown origin: causes, investigation and management. *Intern Med J* 2016; 46: 1011.

Bernheim HA, Block LH, Atkins E. Fever: pathogenesis, pathophysiology, and purpose. *Ann Intern Med* 1979; 91: 261.

Blumenthal I. Fever – concepts old and new. *J R Soc Med* 1997; 90: 391.

Cunha BA. Fever in the intensive care unit. *Intens Care Med* 1999; 25: 648.

Dallimore J, Ebmeier S, Thayabaran D, et al. Effect of active temperature management on mortality in intensive care patients. *Crit Care Resusc* 2018; 20: 150.

Dinarello CA, Cannon JG, Wolff SM. New concepts on the pathogenesis of fever. *Rev Infect Dis* 1988; 10: 168.

Drenth JPH, van der Meer JWM. Hereditary periodic fever. *New Engl J Med* 2001; 345: 1748.

Editorial. Familial Mediterranean fever. *BMJ* 1980; 281: 2.

Eliakim M, Levy M, Ehrenfeld M. *Recurrent Polyserositis (Familial Mediterranean Fever, Periodic Disease)*. Amsterdam: Elsevier. 1981.

Gherardin A, Sisson J. Assessing fever in the returned traveller. *Aust Prescriber* 2012; 35; 10.

Hasday JD, Garrison A. Antipyretic therapy in sepsis. *Clin Infect Dis* 2000; 31: S234.

Jacoby GA, Swartz MN. Fever of undetermined origin *N Engl J Med* 1973; 289: 1407.

Kluger MJ, Ringler DH, Anver MR. Fever and survival. *Science* 1975; 188: 166.

Knockaert DC, Vanneste LJ, Vanneste SB, et al. Fever of unknown origin in the 1980s. *Arch Intern Med* 1992; 152: 51.

Laupland KB. Fever in the critically ill patient. *Crit Care Med* 2009; 37 (suppl.): S273.

Laupland KB, Shahpori R, Kirkpatrick AW, et al. Occurrence and outcome of fever in critically ill adults. *Crit Care Med* 2008; 36: 1531.

Lefrant J-Y, Muller L, Coussaye JE, et al. Temperature measurement in intensive care patients: comparison of urinary bladder, oesophageal, rectal, axillary, and inguinal methods versus pulmonary artery core method. *Intens Care Med* 2003; 29: 414.

Mackowiak PA. Fever: blessing or curse? A unifying hypothesis. *Ann Intern Med* 1994; 120: 1037.

Mackowiak PA. Concepts of fever. *Arch Intern Med* 1998; 158: 1870.

Mackowiak PA, LeMaistre CF. Drug fever: a critical appraisal of conventional concepts. *Ann Intern Med* 1987; 106: 728.

Marik PE. Fever in the ICU. *Chest* 2000; 117: 855.

Musher DM, Fainstein V, Young EJ. Fever patterns: their lack of clinical significance. *Arch Intern Med* 1979; 139: 1225.

Netea MG, Kullberg BJ, Van der Meer JW. Circulating cytokines as mediators of fever. *Clin Infect Dis* 2000; 31: S178.

Nimmo SM, Kennedy BW, Tullet WM, et al. Drug-induced hyperthermia. *Anaesthesia* 1993; 48: 892.

O'Grady NP, Barie PS, Bartlett J, et al. Practice guidelines for evaluating new fever in critically ill adult patients. *Crit Care Med* 1998; 26: 392.

Olson KR, Benowitz NL. Environmental and drug-induced hyperthermia: pathophysiology, recognition and management. *Emerg Med Clin North Am* 1984; 2: 459.

Petersdorf RG, Beeson PB. Fever of unexplained origin. *Medicine* 1961; 40: 1.

Plaisance KI, Mackowiak PA. Antipyretic therapy: physiologic rationale, diagnostic implications, and clinical consequences. *Arch Intern Med* 2000; 160: 449.

Point/Counterpoint Editorial. Should antipyretic therapy be given routinely to febrile patients in septic shock? Yes or no. *Chest* 2013; 144: 1096 & 1098.

Rehman T, deBloisblanc BP. Persistent fever in the ICU. *Chest* 2014; 145: 158.

Reny J-L, Vuagnat A, Ract C, et al. Diagnosis and follow-up of infections in intensive care patients: value of C-reactive protein compared with other clinical and biological variables. *Crit Care Med* 2002; 30: 529.

Roberts NJ. Impact of temperature elevation on immunologic defenses. *Rev Infect Dis* 1991; 13: 462.

Robins HI, Longo W. Whole body hyperthermia. *Intens Care Med* 1999; 25: 898.

Rosenberg J, Pentel P, Pond S, et al. Hyperthermia associated with drug intoxication. *Crit Care Med* 1986; 14: 964.

Saper CB, Breeder CD. The neurologic basis of fever. *N Engl J Med* 1994; 330: 1880.

Shafazand S, Weinacker AB. Blood cultures in the critical care unit: improving utilization and yield. *Chest* 2002; 122: 1727.

Shann F. Antipyretics in severe sepsis. *Lancet* 1995; 345: 338.

Simon HB. Hyperthermia. *N Engl J Med* 1993; 329: 483.

Simon HB. Hyperthermia, fever, and fever of undetermined origin. In: *Scientific American Medicine. Infectious Diseases*. Hamilton: Dekker Medicine. 2020.

Simon HB, Daniels GH. Hormonal hyperthermia: endocrinologic causes of fever. *Am J Med* 1979; 66: 257.

Sohar E, Gafni J, Heller H. Familial Mediterranean fever. *Am J Med* 1967; 43: 227.

Young PJ, Nielsen N, Saxena M. Fever control. *Intens Care Med* 2018; 44: 227.

Young PJ, Prescott HC. When less is more in the active management of elevated body temperature of ICU patients. *Intens Care Med* 2019; 45: 1275.

Pyroglutamic acid *See*

- Lactic acidosis.

Bibliography

Dempsey GA, Lyall HJ, Corke CF, et al. Pyroglutamic acidemia: a cause of high anion gap metabolic acidosis. *Crit Care Med* 2000; 28: 1803.

Mo L, Lliang DL, Madden A, et al. A case of delayed onset pyroglutamic acidosis in the sub-acute setting. *Intern Med J* 2016; 46: 747.

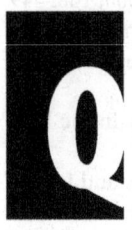

Q fever *See*

- Rickettsial diseases.

Quarantine

Quarantine refers to the isolation of healthy people (or animals) who may be harbouring a communicable disease due to actual or potential exposure. It was so named because of the 40-day period imposed on travellers in the Middle Ages who had come from an area where plague was endemic. The number 40 is 'quaranta' in Italian (derived from the Latin 'quadraginta'), and its choice for this purpose was somewhat arbitrary. Quarantine is a public health measure, and WHO guidelines for its use include a set of regulatory processes which also include surveillance, response procedures and coordination among relevant authorities.

It is a separate concept from the **isolation** process used in Intensive Care, whereby sick patients who are either infectious (and thus at risk of infecting others) or immunocompromised (and thus at risk of becoming infected themselves) are cared for in separated pressure-regulated areas by staff who are themselves properly protected. Isolation is recommended for patients with a number of infectious diseases described in this book, including anthrax, COVID-19, diphtheria, Ebola haemorrhagic fever (and related conditions), influenza, Middle East respiratory syndrome (MERS), plague, rabies, severe acute respiratory syndrome (SARS), tuberculosis, varicella-zoster and yellow fever.

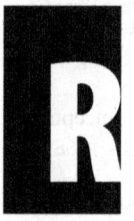

Rabies

Rabies is a dramatic example of one of many viral zoonoses in animals which may be incidentally transmitted to humans, where an entirely different disease is produced from that seen in the original reservoir.

Rabies is found in many carnivores in most countries (except Australia, the United Kingdom and Hawaii). Dogs are the main source of infection in humans, followed by monkeys. The disease is particularly prevalent in Asia, Africa, and Central and South America, where it is responsible for about 60,000 deaths per year.

Usually, direct inoculation occurs from infected saliva following a bite, most commonly to the hand or arm.

- The virus replicates in adjacent muscle cells and then passes via the nerves to the CNS.
- There is an incubation period of about 30 days (though 12 days to >4 yr have been reported).
- Clinical features comprise local pain and numbness and systemic features of irritability, apprehension, dyspnoea, nausea and diarrhoea (q.v.).
- Hydrophobia occurs in some patients and is characteristic.
- Subsequently, excitation occurs with hyperventilation, seizures and disorientation.
- Finally, paralysis occurs, even involving autonomically innervated structures, and death follows from cardiorespiratory failure.

The diagnosis requires a careful history, especially of travel. It is confirmed by viral isolation and positive serology.

Treatment is with local wound cleaning and general supportive measures.

- Although no person-to-person transmission has been reported, **isolation** is usually recommended.
- Post-exposure prophylactic **vaccination** is now very effective, but it is complex and requires consultation with local health authorities. No vaccination, however, is required if a suspected animal remains healthy after 10 days of observation or if the animal is killed and laboratory tests are negative.
- Pre-exposure vaccination may be considered in those about to enter a high-risk area.

The condition is always fatal within 3 weeks of illness in unvaccinated patients.

The ability of the rabies virus to pass from neurone to neurone (and thus avoid immune detection) has been harnessed in the neuroscience laboratory using engineered forms of the virus to study neurotransmission and map complex brain circuits.

See
- Bites and stings – Bats, Dogs,
- Lyssavirus,
- Zoonoses.

Bibliography

Emergency ID Net Study Group. Appropriateness of rabies postexposure prophylaxis treatment for animal exposures. *JAMA* 2000; 284: 1001.

Fishbein DB, Robinson LE. Rabies (review). *N Engl J Med* 1993; 329: 1632.

Krebs JW, Smith JS, Rupprecht CE, et al. Mammalian reservoirs and epidemiology of rabies diagnosed in human beings in the United States, 1981–1998. *Ann NY Acad Sci* 2000; 916: 345.

Warrell MJ, Warrell DA. Rabies and other lyssavirus disease. *Lancet* 2004; 363: 959.

Radiation injury

Radiation has dose-related consequences, both local and systemic. In particular, the patient may become a compromised host with
- loss of integrity of the mucocutaneous surface barrier, especially the gut,
- decreased number and impaired function of circulating neutrophils and lymphocytes,
- impaired function of both circulating and fixed mononuclear phagocytes.

In radiotherapy, either subatomic particle radiation or electromagnetic radiation (megavoltage X-ray or gamma-rays from radioactive isotopes) may be used. Both modalities deliver photons to the tissues where intracellular structures (e.g. DNA) are ionized in both malignant and normal cells. Some malignant tissues (lymphoma, seminoma) are much more sensitive to radiation than are normal tissues, but unfortunately the converse applies for the gut, kidneys, liver, lungs and nervous system. Radiation injury is an important complication of therapeutic radiation, even though appropriate precautions are taken to minimize the exposure of normal tissues.

Acute effects of radiation include damage to proliferating cells with erythema, desquamation, nausea, oesophagitis and bone marrow suppression.

Late effects of radiation are due to vascular occlusion, tissue necrosis or possibly stem cell damage.

Carcinogenic influences in the environment, including radiation, can affect almost all organs by activation of cellular oncogenes. The tumours which may result include especially leukaemia but also carcinoma of the skin, thyroid and breast, bone and soft tissue sarcomas, and brain tumours. Previous radiotherapy for conditions such as Hodgkin's disease or ankylosing spondylitis may give rise to such tumours subsequently (as well as to an excess cardiac mortality).

Local effects of radiation can be prominent.
- In the **pelvis**, proctitis (q.v.) and cystitis may result.
- In the **head and neck**, there may be hoarseness, sore and dry mouth and throat, with loss of taste, mucositis, ulcers, fistulae and cutaneous erythema.
- **Neurological** changes of encephalopathy (q.v.) or myelopathy (q.v.) may be produced from local vascular damage.
- Late **pericarditis** (q.v.) may be produced.
- **Radiation pneumonitis** is an acute, primary, vascular reaction, initially with pulmonary vascular congestion and alveolar oedema, and later with small vessel thrombosis and alveolar epithelial desquamation. It is of variable extent and severity, but it occurs to some degree in all patients having chest irradiation, whether for cure or for palliation. It may resemble *Pneumocystis jirovecii* (*P. carinii*) pneumonia, from which it therefore needs to be distinguished.

Symptoms appear some weeks after radiation and include dry cough and dyspnoea. The overlying skin may show increased pigmentation.

Chest X-ray shows a new pulmonary infiltrate, often typically confined to the area of the radiation port. Bronchoalveolar lavage (BAL) helps exclude infection or malignancy and may show lymphocytes and dysplastic or damaged alveolar type II cells.

*Severe symptoms are probably helped with **corticosteroids**, and concomitant **antibiotics** are usually given because of the likelihood of superinfection.*

- **Radiation fibrosis** is a natural progression of radiation pneumonitis over the succeeding months.

The process is often clinically silent, but dyspnoea can occur and may be progressive and disabling.

Chest X-ray shows infiltration and contraction of the affected part of the lung.

There is no effective treatment.

Bibliography

Gross NJ. Pulmonary effects of radiation injury. *Ann Intern Med* 1977; 86: 81.

Hanania AN, Mainwaring W, Ghebre Y, et al. Radiation-induced lung injury. *Chest* 2019; 156: 150.

Ricks RC, Berger ME, O'Hara FM, eds. *The Medical Basis for Radiation-Accident Preparedness*. Boca Raton: CRC Press. 2002.

Ramsay Hunt syndrome *See*

- Bell's palsy,
- Varicella-zoster.

Rat bites *See*

- Bites and stings.

Raynaud's phenomenon/disease

Raynaud's phenomenon is a peripheral vasospastic disorder, secondary to organic disease, such as systemic lupus erythematosus (SLE) (q.v.) or scleroderma (q.v.), which it often precedes.

Less commonly, it may be associated with
- **vascular disease**, such as vasculitis (q.v.) or thromboangiitis obliterans,
- **haematological disease**, especially myeloproliferative disorders, cryoglobulinaemia (q.v.) and cold agglutinin disease (q.v.),
- **trauma**, including frostbite (q.v.).
- **drugs**, e.g. ergot (q.v.), methysergide (q.v.), beta blockers.

Raynaud's disease is a primary or idiopathic form of the condition, which in its mildest form occurs in about 25% of young women. It may represent an increased sensitivity to $α_2$ agonists due to an increased density of receptors in the digital arteries.

Treatment is primarily symptomatic and physical.
- Low-dose **aspirin** is generally recommended.
- **Calcium channel blockers** are effective, though direct vasodilator agents are ineffective.
- **Captopril, prazosin** and **ketanserin** are reportedly helpful.
- **Topical nitroglycerin gel** can be effective, but associated headache is common.
- **Sildenafil** has been reported to be helpful in resistant cases.
- Novel therapies include **statins** (q.v.) and **selective serotonin reuptake inhibitors (SSRIs)**.
- **Thoracic sympathectomy** may be considered in severe and refractory cases.
- **Smoking cessation** is important.

Bibliography

Coffman JD. Raynaud's phenomenon: an update. *Hypertension* 1991; 17: 593.

Creager MA. Peripheral artery diseases. In: *Scientific American Medicine. Cardiovascular Medicine*. Hamilton: Dekker Medicine. 2020.

Fries R, Shariat K, von Wilmowsky H, et al. Sildenafil in the treatment of Raynaud's phenomenon resistant to vasodilator therapy. *Circulation* 2005; 112: 2980.

Sturgill MG, Seibold JR. Rational use of calcium-channel antagonists in Raynaud's phenomenon. *Curr Opin Rheumatol* 1998; 10: 584.

Thompson AE, Pope JE. Calcium channel blockers for primary Raynaud's phenomenon: a meta-analysis. *Rheumatology* 2005; 44: 145.

Reactive arthritis *See*

- Reiter's syndrome.
  See also
- Histocompatibility complex,
- Lyme disease,
- Spondyloarthritis.

Refeeding syndrome

Refeeding syndrome comprises potentially harmful changes in fluid and electrolyte balance which may occur when previously malnourished patients are acutely and intensively fed. The consequent rapid synthesis of glycogen and protein causes a decreased plasma level of the major intracellular electrolytes, i.e. potassium, magnesium and phosphate. Serious adverse effects may result from these changes, especially from **hypophosphataemia** (q.v.).

See
- Anorexia nervosa.
  See also
- Magnesium.

Bibliography

Mehanna HM, Moledina J, Travis J. Refeeding syndrome: what it is, and how to prevent and treat it. *BMJ* 2008; 336: 1495.

Reiter's syndrome

Reiter's syndrome comprises the triad of arthritis (q.v.), urethritis and conjunctivitis (q.v.). Occasionally, there may be a tetrad, with the additional features of painless ulcers (q.v.) in the mouth or rash on the glans penis (circinate balanitis). The joint involvement is a **reactive arthritis**.

As with Wegener's granulomatosis (q.v.), consideration has been given to renaming this condition without any eponymous recognition because of Dr Reiter's strong Nazi affiliations before and during World War II. The revised name most generally used is simply 'reactive arthritis'.

It occurs particularly in young men, in whom it is the commonest inflammatory monoarthropathy or oligoarthropathy, with a prevalence of 3.5 per 100,000 of the population. There is a 37-fold increased incidence in subjects with the specific genetic HLA antigen B27, and 70–90% of patients with the condition are B27-positive.

Reiter's syndrome usually follows a specific infection, either epidemic or endemic.

- Epidemic causes are usually dysenteric, especially from salmonella, shigella, campylobacter or *Yersinia enterocolitica*.
- Endemic infections are usually venereal, either from chlamydia or mycoplasma.

Although the pathogenetic mechanisms of the illness are uncertain, there may be cross-reactivity between bacterial antigens and self-antigens.

Clinical features prominently include **arthritis**, usually asymmetrical and involving the knees, ankles or feet.
- Achilles tendonitis, plantar fasciitis and tenosynovitis are common.
- There may be associated sacroiliitis or overlap with ankylosing spondylitis (q.v.).
- There may sometimes be associated skin lesions, namely keratoderma blennorrhagicum with hyperkeratotic lesions.
- Conjunctivitis is usual, and there may sometimes be uveitis (q.v.).
- In AIDS (q.v.), the condition is more severe, though probably not more frequent. This is in contrast to other rheumatic disorders, such as rheumatoid arthritis and systemic lupus erythematosus (q.v.), which may improve in the presence of AIDS.

Investigations usually show a raised ESR. Examination of the synovial fluid shows a high complement level, reflecting inflammation (in contrast to rheumatoid arthritis in which the level is low). In chronic disease, there may be IgA antibodies to the trigger organism, consistent with a continuing mucosal infection. The diagnosis is made on the basis of the clinical features and not the laboratory tests.

Treatment is with **NSAIDs**, to which symptoms of arthritis usually respond.
- In occasional severe cases, **salazopyrine** or **methotrexate** and sometimes **corticosteroids** may be required (though some of these agents are contraindicated in HIV-positive cases).
- Any predisposing urethritis or bacterial gastroenteritis is treated on its merits.

The condition is usually self-limited, but sometimes it may progress to produce considerable and prolonged disability.

See also
- Spondyloarthritis.

Bibliography

Amor B. Reiter's syndrome. *Rheum Dis Clin North Am* 1998; 24: 677.

Editorial. Reactive arthritis. *BMJ* 1980; 281: 311.

Gibofsky A, Zabriskie JB. Rheumatic fever and poststreptococcal reactive arthritis. *Curr Opin Rheumatol* 1995; 7: 299.

Keat A. Reactive arthritis. *Adv Exp Med Biol* 1999; 455: 201.

McEwen C, DiTata D, Lingg C, et al. Ankylosing spondylitis and spondylitis accompanying ulcerative colitis, regional enteritis, psoriasis and Reiter's disease. *Arthritis Rheum* 1971; 14: 291.

Panush RS, Paraschiv D, Dorff RE. The tainted legacy of Hans Reiter. *Semin Arthritis Rheumatol* 2003; 32: 231.

Winblad S. Arthritis associated with *Yersinia enterocolitica* infections. *Scand J Infect Dis* 1975; 7: 191.

Relapsing fever

Relapsing fever occurs following infection with one of several species of spirochaete of the genus *Borrelia*, which are transmitted by lice or ticks. These are arthropod vectors (q.v.), lice being insects and ticks being arachnids.
- Louse-borne infection often occurs in epidemics and follows natural or man-made disasters. It has thus been associated with typhus (q.v.) and has occurred mainly in Africa, Asia and South America.
- Tick-borne infection is widely distributed and usually arises from exposure to infected rodents.

Both forms of infection are clinically similar.
- Following an incubation period of about 7 days,
  - symptoms comprise high fever (q.v.) with chills, headache, myalgia, prostration, confusion, cough and gastrointestinal complaints,
  - clinical findings include tachycardia, hyperventilation, rash, splenomegaly (q.v.),
  - sometimes, there is hepatomegaly, lymphadenopathy (q.v.), disseminated intravascular coagulation (q.v.).
- After 3–6 days,
  - the febrile illness comes to an abrupt end in a drenching sweat.
- In another 6–10 days,
  - there is a febrile recurrence, but the illness on this occasion is shorter.
  - Sometimes, there may be only one relapse, but often there are many.
  - However, on each occasion the symptom-free interval is longer and the actual relapse is milder and briefer.
  - Resolution occurs because of the production of antibody, but recurrence occurs because of the process of antigen variation.

Spirochaetes are seen on the blood film, except during symptom-free intervals. *Borrelia* cannot be cultured on artificial media. There is anaemia (q.v.), thrombocytopenia (q.v.) and disseminated intravascular coagulation (q.v.), but the white cell count is normal. Liver function tests are abnormal in severe cases.

The differential diagnosis includes
- bacteraemia,
- infectious mononucleosis (see Epstein–Barr virus),
- malaria (q.v.),
- salmonellosis (see Typhoid fever),
- leptospirosis (q.v.),
- spotted fevers (q.v.).

Treatment is with **tetracycline** for 10 days, though a single dose of doxycycline 100 mg has been used in epidemics.
- *Chloramphenicol, penicillin and ceftriaxone are also effective.*
- Treatment can be associated with the **Jarisch–Herxheimer reaction** (q.v.).

The mortality is usually 2–5%, though it can increase to 40% in epidemics because of concomitant diseases.

Bibliography
Spach D, Liles W, Campbell G, et al. Tick-borne diseases in the United States. *N Engl J Med* 1993; 329: 936.

Renal artery occlusion

Renal artery occlusion may be due to
- emboli
- thrombi,
- vascular disease.

Emboli arise from
- **cardiac thrombi**, due to acute myocardial infarction or atrial arrhythmias

A frequent consequence of embolization of such material is renal artery occlusion, because the kidneys take 20% of the cardiac output.
- **athero-emboli** (cholesterol emboli)

This is usually seen in older patients with extensive atherosclerotic disease who have had a radiological or surgical procedure proximal to the kidneys.

An acute increase in plasma creatinine after such procedures is an important clue to this mechanism, though it requires differentiation from contrast-induced renal damage.

It may be associated with more peripheral embolization and livedo reticularis (q.v.).
- **subacute bacterial endocarditis** (q.v.), **tumour** or **fat**

These are uncommon sources of clinically significant renal artery emboli.

Thrombi are usually associated with underlying arterial damage from atheroma or trauma.

Vascular disease is usually associated with abdominal aortic aneurysm.

Renal artery occlusion causes ischaemic damage to the kidney, with a typically wedge-shaped infarct or more general atrophy. The consequences depend on the speed, extent and duration of the process, with irreversible changes often appearing after 2 hr of occlusion.

Clinical features typically comprise
- loin pain and tenderness,
- systemic symptoms of fever (q.v.) and nausea.

Sometimes, the process may be clinically silent. Often in embolic disease there are emboli apparent elsewhere, and the site of embolization is apparent. Hypertension is common. A skin rash may be seen, in the form of livedo reticularis (q.v.).

Investigations show haematuria (q.v.) in one third of cases. The LDH but not the AST is typically elevated. A renal isotope scan is the preferred technique to show either segmental or generalized decrease in renal perfusion.

> The diagnosis of renal artery occlusion can be difficult, especially if there is no apparent initiating event and the process is persistent or recurrent.

> In severe cases, the differential diagnosis includes acute kidney injury (AKI, acute tubular necrosis).
>
> The urine sediment is sometimes 'active', with haematuria, red blood cell casts and occasionally eosinophils.
>
> Eosinophilia may be noted on peripheral blood examination.

*Treatment is with **anticoagulation**, though local thrombolytic therapy has also been reported to be successful in selected cases.*

Bibliography

Bell SP, Frankel A, Brown EA. Cholesterol emboli syndrome – uncommon or unrecognized? *J R Soc Med* 1997; 90: 543.

Corwin HL, Korbet SM, Schwartz MM. Clinical correlates of eosinophiluria. *Arch Intern Med* 1985; 145: 1097.

Crosby RL, Miller PD, Schrier RW. Traumatic renal artery thrombosis. *Am J Med* 1986; 81: 890.

Lessman RK, Johnson SF, Coburn JW, et al. Renal artery embolism. *Ann Intern Med* 1978; 89: 477.

Peat DS, Mathieson PW. Cholesterol emboli may mimic systemic vasculitis. *BMJ* 1996; 313: 546.

Smith MC, Ghose MK, Henry AR. The clinical spectrum of renal cholesterol embolization. *Am J Med* 1981; 71: 174.

Turner NN, Lameire N, Goldsmith DJ, et al. eds. *Oxford Textbook of Clinical Nephrology*. 4th edition. Oxford: Oxford University Press. 2015.

Renal calculous disease *See*

- Nephrolithiasis.

Renal cortical necrosis

Renal cortical necrosis refers to infarction of the entire renal cortex with consequent acute anuric renal failure. The juxtamedullary glomeruli probably survive and are responsible for the partial recovery seen in some patients.

> Renal cortical necrosis is
> - traditionally associated with prolonged shock or severe hypovolaemia,
> - classically associated with obstetric disasters.

Clinically, there may be loin pain, hypotension and anuria, preceded sometimes by haematuria (q.v.).

Urinalysis shows casts (as in acute kidney injury, AKI), and renal function is non-specifically abnormal.

The differential diagnosis includes
- AKI, acute tubular necrosis,
- post-renal obstruction,
- severe glomerulonephritis (see Glomerular diseases),
- bilateral vascular occlusion (see Renal artery occlusion),
- haemolytic–uraemic syndrome (q.v.), rarely.

An ultrasound examination is required to exclude obstruction, and diagnostic confirmation may require renal biopsy.

*Treatment is **supportive**.*

About one third of patients recover sufficiently to be dialysis-free but with renal function only 15–50% of normal and with proneness to a gradual decline thereafter.

Renal cystic disease

Renal cystic disease comprises a wide variety of conditions.

1. **Simple cysts** are fluid-filled, epithelial-lined structures.

   They are clinically silent and are found in about 50% of older patients.

2. **Acquired cystic disease** refers to the presence of more than five cysts, accompanied by renal impairment and usually with small, scarred kidneys.

   This process arises in the proximal tubules and occurs in about 50% of patients on long-term dialysis.

   These cysts can cause haematuria (q.v.), loin pain and erythrocytosis (q.v.). They may also become infected or malignant.

3. **Polycystic disease** is a common condition inherited as an autosomal dominant. It is often referred to as **autosomal-dominant polycystic kidney disease** (ADPKD) and has a prevalence of at least 1 in 1000 of the population. In 90% of cases, there is an abnormal gene on the short arm of chromosome 16 (ADPKD1 locus).

   Though the cysts commence in utero as outpouchings of the renal tubule and Bowman's capsule, the condition is clinically silent until adult life. There is interstitial scarring and compression of adjacent normal tissue, giving rise to
   - loin pain,
   - hypertension,
   - a palpable abdominal mass,
   - urinary tract infection,
   - renal calculi (q.v.),
   - haematuria (q.v.),
   - renal impairment.

   The most useful diagnostic imaging is with ultrasound.

There may also be
- cysts elsewhere, especially in the liver, pancreas or spleen,
- cerebral arterial berry aneurysms, and thus subarachnoid haemorrhage,
- mitral valve prolapse,
- colonic diverticula.

*Since antidiuretic hormone (ADH) promotes renal tubular cyst growth (via cAMP), the potential utility of the vasopressin-2 (V2) receptor antagonist, **tolvaptan**, has been assessed in ADPKD. Although tolvaptan was shown to reduce kidney growth in ADPKD by about 50%, the associated side-effect of liver injury then prevented its routine use in ADPKD. Subsequently, it was recommended that patients with ADPKD drink at least 2 L of water per day to help suppress ADH production, but the efficacy of this revised regimen has not yet been confirmed.*

See Vasopressin.

4. **Medullary cystic disease** is an autosomal dominant condition of cystic development in the medulla.

    It presents in young adults with
    - scarred, shrunken kidneys,
    - loss of concentrating ability and thus polyuria,
    - renal failure.

5. **Medullary sponge kidney** is due to cystic outpouching from the collecting ducts, giving rise to the characteristic flower-spray appearance on intravenous pyelogram. Some cases are familial.

    The condition presents with
    - haematuria (q.v.),
    - renal calculi (q.v.),
    - occasional tubular effects, e.g. renal tubular acidosis (q.v.),
    - but not renal failure.

Bibliography

Amis ES, Cronan JJ, Yoder IC, et al. Renal cysts: curios and caveats. *Urol Radiol* 1982; 4: 199.

Gabow PA. Autosomal dominant polycystic disease. *N Engl J Med* 1993; 329: 332.

Harris PC, Torres VE. Polycystic kidney disease. *Annu Rev Med* 2009; 60: 321.

Ishikawa I. Acquired cystic disease: mechanisms and manifestations. *Semin Nephrol* 1991; 11: 671.

Rangan GK, Tchan MC, Tong A, et al. Recent advances in autosomal-dominant polycystic kidney disease. *Intern Med J* 2016; 46: 883.

Turner NN, Lameire N, Goldsmith DJ, et al. eds. *Oxford Textbook of Clinical Nephrology*. 4th edition. Oxford: Oxford University Press. 2015.

Renal tubular acidosis

Renal tubular acidosis (RTA) refers to the inability of the kidney to excrete the acid load required to maintain the body's normal acid–base balance, despite a relatively normal glomerular filtration rate. It is one of the causes of a metabolic acidosis with a normal anion gap. The diagnosis is usually suspected in a patient with metabolic acidosis (q.v.) but an inappropriately raised urinary pH.

RTA has traditionally been classified on clinical grounds as distal (more common) and proximal (less common).

Classical renal tubular acidosis (distal RTA or type 1) is caused by a defect of the distal tubules preventing H^+ excretion.

Thus,
- the urine cannot be fully acidified,
- the urine pH is always >5.3,
- there is a metabolic acidosis with a normal anion gap.

The urinary anion gap is positive.

A similar phenomenon is found in some cases of diarrhoea (q.v.), but this should be apparent clinically. Moreover, the normal negative urinary anion gap is still seen in such patients with diarrhoea.

H^+ is normally secreted as NH_4^+ from the alpha-intercalated cell into the lumen of the collecting tubule under the action of aldosterone via an ATP-ase pump. The urinary anion gap is an approximate index of urinary ammonium, with a negative anion gap suggesting normal acidification. Potassium is excreted from the adjacent principal cell also under aldosterone action to restore electrochemical neutrality following the active reabsorption of Na^+ from the lumen. When H^+ is secreted from the cell, bicarbonate remains and diffuses into the blood in exchange for Cl^-, also to maintain electrical neutrality. In RTA only potassium secretion is available to compensate for sodium reabsorption, so that hypokalaemia results. Since citrate excretion is also impaired, the less soluble phosphate appears in the tubules, and this precipitates with calcium to give nephrocalcinosis. A similar phenomenon may occur in chronically alkaline urine from other causes.

RTA type 1 may be
- genetic
    - sometimes associated with Marfan's syndrome (q.v.),
- idiopathic,
- associated with
    - drugs, e.g. amphotericin B, lithium (q.v.),

- autoimmune disease (q.v.),
- hypocalcaemia (q.v.),
- hypergammaglobulinaemia,
- medullary sponge kidney (see Renal cystic disease).

A rare form of RTA may be hyperkalaemic and associated with
- urinary tract obstruction,
- renal transplant rejection,
- systemic lupus erythematosus (q.v.),
- sickle cell anaemia (q.v.),
- drugs, e.g. amiloride, silver sulfadiazine.

Proximal renal tubular acidosis (proximal RTA or type 2) is associated with a defect of proximal tubular reabsorption of bicarbonate.

Thus,
- there is excess sodium bicarbonate in the urine,
- the urine pH is >5.3 (when the filtered load exceeds the absorptive capacity),
- the plasma bicarbonate is low.

This condition is usually associated with other proximal tubular defects, for example of glucose, amino acids, phosphates and uric acid, so that these substances appear in excess in the urine, a condition called the **Fanconi syndrome** (q.v.).

By contrast, carbonic anhydrase inhibitors (q.v.) which also increase bicarbonate in the urine do not cause any of these additional abnormalities.

RTA type 2 may be
- hereditary
  - as in a variety of metabolic disorders, such as glycogen storage diseases (q.v.), Wilson's disease (q.v.),
- acquired
  - following heavy metals or drugs, e.g. cadmium, copper, lead, mercury, outdated tetracycline,
  - associated with multiple myeloma (q.v.) or hyperparathyroidism (q.v.).

Bibliography
Kamel KS, Briceno LF, Sanchez MI, et al. A new classification for renal defects in net acid secretion. *Am J Kidney Dis* 1997; 29: 136.
Turner NN, Lameire N, Goldsmith DJ, et al. eds. *Oxford Textbook of Clinical Nephrology*. 4th edition. Oxford: Oxford University Press. 2015.
Unwin RJ, Capasso G. The renal tubular acidosis. *J R Soc Med* 2001; 94: 221.

Renal vein thrombosis

Renal vein thrombosis is generally associated with the nephrotic syndrome (q.v.), but it can also occur in renal carcinoma and thus with normal renal function. The nephrotic syndrome occurs with acute occlusion, but if the thrombosis is gradual, there may be appropriate compensation and the process may be silent.

While renal vein thrombosis may cause the nephrotic syndrome in association with a thrombophilic state (q.v.), membranous nephropathy (see Glomerular diseases) may also lead to renal vein thrombosis in its own right in about 50% of patients.

Renal vein thrombosis may be bilateral and may be acute enough to cause infarction. Usually it is more gradual and may even be clinically silent, though it can lead to loin pain and haematuria (q.v.).

Diagnosis is by renal vein Doppler ultrasound examination.

Treatment is with long-term **anticoagulation**.

Bibliography
Cronin RE, Kaehny WD, Miller, PD, et al. Renal cell carcinoma: unusual systemic manifestations. *Medicine* 1976; 55: 291.
Llach F. Hypercoagulability, renal vein thrombosis, and other thrombotic complications of the nephrotic syndrome. *Kidney Int* 1985; 28: 429.
Llach F, Papper S, Massry SG. The clinical spectrum of renal vein thrombosis: acute and chronic. *Am J Med* 1980; 69: 819.

Renin–angiotensin–aldosterone

The **renin–angiotensin–aldosterone** (RAA) system is one of the key mechanisms for salt and water balance and thus for circulatory control.

Renin is a proteolytic enzyme produced (initially as the inactive protein, prorenin) by modified smooth muscle cells in the afferent arteriole of the kidney in the juxtaglomerular cells. Its release is regulated by tubular sodium concentration, sensed in the adjacent epithelial cells of the macula densa in the distal convoluted tubule. Renin release is also influenced by adrenergic stimuli.

The substrate for renin is a circulating α_2-globulin (angiotensinogen) which is produced in the liver. From it, renin cleaves the inactive decapeptide, angiotensin I. Angiotensin I is converted to the octapeptide, angiotensin II, in the lungs by angiotensin-converting enzyme (see Angiotensin-converting enzyme), and angiotensin II is the main stimulus to the production of aldosterone in the adrenal gland (see Aldosterone). Angiotensin II also activates the adrenergic system and is thus a vasopressor and mild inotrope. These well-known effects are mediated via the AT_1 receptors.

Stable formulations of synthetic human **angiotensin II** are now available as clinical vasopressors, and initial studies have confirmed their physiological efficacy. Thus, when selecting vasopressors in vasodilatory (i.e. vasoplegic or distributive) shock (see Hyperdynamic state), angiotensin II may add a further option to the established regimens of catecholamines and subsequently vasopressin (q.v.).

In addition to these effects which have been recognized for many decades, it has been appreciated that angiotensin II has a second subtype of receptors, AT_2, which mediate a variety of other less well-defined actions. Thus, angiotensin II also increases intracellular Ca^{++} release and cell growth (i.e. it affects gene expression by enhancing protein synthesis in smooth muscle and myocardial cells). Angiotensin II is thus an extracellular messenger, and its mechanism of action is via binding to the specific cell surface receptors, which initiates a complex signalling cascade to release intracellular Ca^{++} and to activate protein kinase C.

Angiotensin II receptor antagonists (ARAs) or **blockers** (ARBs) include losartan, followed later by candesartan, eprosartan, irbesartan, telmisartan and valsartan, and finally by olmesartan – a class of agents referred to generically as the '**sartans**'. They target the AT_1 receptor and thus provide more complete angiotensin blockade than do the inhibitors of angiotensin-converting enzyme (ACE, q.v.), because angiotensin can also be formed to some extent via pathways other than renin. Since the angiotensin receptor antagonists do not block the inactivation of bradykinin (BK) like the ACE inhibitors do, they were not expected to produce cough or angioedema, but this early promise has not been entirely borne out in practice. On the other hand, the potentiation of BK may be responsible also for some of the beneficial effects of the ACE inhibitors. In addition, the ARAs have been reported to cause occasional sprue-like enteropathy (see Coeliac disease, see Malabsorption) and hepatotoxicity. They may exacerbate hyperglycaemia in some diabetics. In clinical trials, angiotensin receptor antagonists have been found to be as effective as ACE inhibitors in hypertension and possibly more effective in reducing mortality in heart failure.

Since renin release is influenced by sodium concentration, adrenergic stimuli and renal perfusion pressure, it is ideally attuned to controlling blood volume.

A newer class of drug, **direct renin inhibitors** (DRIs) (e.g. aliskiren) have been introduced for the treatment of hypertension, though long-term clinical results are still awaited. Such successful targeting of the first step in the eventual generation of angiotensin II has long been a therapeutic goal, and DRIs now complement ACE inhibitors and ARAs in completing the therapeutic inhibition of each step in the renin–angiotensin pathway. Hperkalaemia has been a reported complication of DRI therapy.

Abnormalities of renin secretion include both
- **overproduction** in
  - renal artery stenosis,
  - the rare Bartter's syndrome, in which there is an increased renal synthesis of PGE_2 and hypokalaemic metabolic alkalosis,
- **deficiency** in
  - renal disease, especially diabetic nephropathy,
  - Conn's syndrome (q.v.).

Abnormalities of aldosterone production follow the abnormalities of renin secretion, though there are also other causes of **dysaldosteronism**.
- **Hypoaldosteronism** may be
  - hyporeninaemic,
  - idiopathic.
- **Hyperaldosteronism** may be
  - hyperreninaemic,
  - primary,
  - secondary to cardiac, hepatic or renal disease.

Bibliography
Bellomo R, Hilton A. The ATHOS-3 trial, angiotensin II and the three musketeers. *Crit Care Resusc* 2017; 19: 3.
Curry SC, Arnold-Capell P. Nitroprusside, nitroglycerin, and angiotensin-converting enzyme inhibitors. *Crit Care Clin* 1991; 7: 555.
Harel Z, Gilbert C, Wald R, et al. The effect of combination treatment with aliskrein and blockers of the renin-angiotensin system on hyperkalaemia and acute kidney injury: systematic review and meta-analysis. *BMJ* 2012; 344: 42.
Khanna A, English SW, Wang XS, et al. Angiotensin II for the treatment of vasodilatory shock. *New Engl J Med* 2017; 377: 419.
Melby JC. Diagnosis of hyperaldosteronism. *Endocrinol Metab Clin North Am* 1991; 20: 247.
Oparil S, Haber E. The renin-angiotensin system. *N Engl J Med* 1974; 291: 389 & 446.
Pitt B, Segal R, Martinez FA, et al. Randomised trial of losartan versus captopril in patients over 65 with heart

failure (Evaluation of Losartan in the Elderly Study, ELITE). *Lancet* 1997; 349: 747.

Quinn SJ, Williams GH. Regulation of aldosterone secretion. *Ann Rev Physiol* 1988; 50: 409.

Stoll M, Steckelings UM, Paul M, et al. The angiotensin AT2-receptor mediates inhibition of cell proliferation in coronary endothelial cells. *J Clin Invest* 1995; 95: 651.

Williams GH. Hyporeninemic hypoaldosteronism. *N Engl J Med* 1986; 314: 1041.

Respiratory burns *See*

- Inhalation injury.

Respiratory diseases

Issues related to the management of major **respiratory diseases**/problems comprise much of the backbone of Intensive Care, particularly problems concerning mechanical ventilation, acute (adult) respiratory distress syndrome and nosocomial pneumonia. While many other respiratory problems are also common, especially asthma, acute pulmonary oedema, community-acquired pneumonia and pulmonary thromboembolism, some may have uncommon causes or differential diagnoses. These uncommon aspects of common conditions, together with the more clearly uncommon conditions themselves, are therefore considered in this book, and they include

- Acute lung irritation,
- Acute pulmonary oedema,
- Acute respiratory distress syndrome (ARDS),
- Alpha$_1$-antitrypsin deficiency,
- Aspiration,
- Asthma,
- Barotrauma,
- Bornholm disease,
- Bronchiectasis,
- Bronchiolitis obliterans,
- Bronchocentric granulomatosis,
- Broncholithiasis,
- Bullae,
- Burns, respiratory complications,
- Byssinosis,
- Cancer,
- Cavitation,
- Chest X-ray,
- Cheyne–Stokes respiration,
- Churg–Strauss syndrome,
- Chylothorax,
- Cough,
- Cystic fibrosis,
- Diffuse alveolar haemorrhage,
- Diffuse fibrosing alveolitis,
- Diffuse parenchymal lung diseases,
- Drowning,
- Drugs and the lung,
- Emphysema,
- Empyema,
- Eosinophilia and lung infiltration,
- Eosinophilic granuloma.
- Exotic pneumonia,
- Extrinsic allergic alveolitis,
- Goodpasture's syndrome,
- Granulomatosis with polyangiitis,
- Haemoptysis,
- Hepatopulmonary syndrome,
- Histiocytosis,
- Hypersensitivity pneumonitis,
- Idiopathic interstitial pneumonias,
- Idiopathic pulmonary fibrosis,
- Idiopathic pulmonary haemosiderosis,
- Inhalation injury,
- Interstitial lung diseases,
- Interstitial pneumonia,
- Langerhans cell histiocytosis,
- Loeffler's syndrome,
- Lung tumours,
- Lymphangioleiomyomatosis,
- Lymphomatoid granulomatosis,
- Mendelson's syndrome,
- Mesothelioma,
- Necrotizing granulomatous vasculitis,
- Necrotizing pneumonia,
- Occupational lung diseases,
- Orthodeoxia,
- Pectus excavatum,
- Periodic breathing,
- Platypnoea–orthodeoxia syndrome,
- Pneumoconiosis,
- Portopulmonary hypertension,
- Primary alveolar hypoventilation,
- Pulmonary alveolar proteinosis,
- Pulmonary hypertension,
- Pulmonary infiltrates,
- Pulmonary infiltration with eosinophilia (PIE),
- Pulmonary Langerhans cell histiocytosis,
- Pulmonary nodules,
- Pulmonary oedema,
- Pulmonary veno-occlusive disease,
- Radiation injury,
- Respiratory burns,
- Sarcoidosis,
- Silicosis,
- Sleep disorders of breathing,
- Smoke inhalation,

- Stridor,
- Systemic diseases and the lung,
- Thesaurosis,
- Tropical pulmonary eosinophilia,
- Wegener's granulomatosis.

Non-respiratory thoracic disorders are also considered, in relation to the
- Chest wall
  - congenital conditions,
  - kyphoscoliosis,
  - ankylosing spondylitis,
  - old thoracoplasty,
  - obesity,
  - neuromuscular disorders,
  - inflammation (costochondritis),
  - trauma,
  - tumour (primary or secondary).
- Diaphragm
  - congenital conditions,
  - inflammation,
  - paralysis,
  - neuromuscular disorders,
  - postoperative,
  - spasmodic disorders,
  - trauma,
  - tumour.
- Mediastinum
  - acute mediastinitis,
  - chronic mediastinitis,
  - mediastinal cysts and tumours.
- Pleural cavity
  - pneumothorax,
  - pleurisy,
  - pleural effusion,
  - plaques, thickening and calcification,
  - tumours.

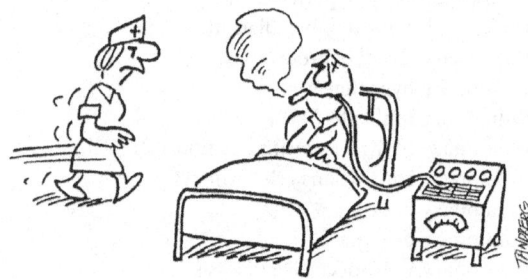

Bibliography

Abraham E, Terada L, eds. Acute lung injury. *Chest* 1999; 116 (suppl. 1).

Albertson TE, Walby WF, Derlet RW. Stimulant-induced pulmonary toxicity. *Chest* 1995; 108: 1140.

Bascom R, Bromberg PA, Costa DL, et al. Health effects of outdoor pollution. *Am J Respir Crit Care Med* 1996; 153: 3 & 477.

Berger AJ, Mitchell RA, Severinghaus JW. Regulation of respiration. *N Engl J Med* 1977; 297: 92, 138 & 194.

Cade JF, Pain MCF. *Essentials of Respiratory Medicine*. Oxford: Blackwell. 1988.

Caruana-Montaldo B, Gleeson K, Zwillich CW. The control of breathing in clinical practice. *Chest* 2000; 117: 205.

Chang DW, White GC, Waugh J, et al. *Respiratory Critical Care*. Sudbury: Jones & Bartlett Learning. 2020.

Craddock PR, Fehr J, Brigham KL, et al. Complement and leukocyte-mediated pulmonary dysfunction in hemodialysis. *N Engl J Med* 1977; 296: 769.

Davidson C, Treacher D, eds. *Respiratory Critical Care*. London: Arnold. 2002.

Editorial. Polycythaemia due to hypoxaemia: advantage or disadvantage? *Lancet* 1989; 2: 20.

Gardner WN. The pathophysiology of hyperventilation disorders. *Chest* 1996; 109: 516.

Goldstein RA, Rohatgi PK, Bergofsky EH, et al. Clinical role of bronchoalveolar lavage in adults with pulmonary disease. *Am Rev Respir Dis* 1990; 142: 481.

Green M. Air pollution and health. *BMJ* 1995; 311: 401.

Heffner JE, Harley RA, Schabel SI. Pulmonary reactions from illicit substance abuse. *Clin Chest Med* 1990; 11: 151.

Hughes M, Black R, eds. *Advanced Respiratory Critical Care*. Oxford: Oxford University Press. 2011.

Irwin RS, ed. Managing cough as a defense mechanism and as a symptom: a consensus panel report of the American College of Chest Physicians. *Chest* 1998; 114: no.2 (suppl.).

Jamal S, Maurer JR. Pulmonary disease and the menstrual cycle. *Pulm Perspect* 1994; 11(3): 3.

Kopec SE, Irwin RS, Umali-Torres CB, et al. The postpneumonectomy state. *Chest* 1998; 114: 1158.

Kryger M, Bode F, Antic R, et al. Diagnosis of obstruction of the upper and central airways. *Am J Med* 1976; 61: 85.

Leatherman JW, Davies SF, Hoidal JR. Alveolar hemorrhage syndromes: diffuse microvascular lung hemorrhage in immune and idiopathic disorders. *Medicine* 1984; 63: 343.

Leatherman JW, Mcdonald FM, Niewohner DE. Fluid-containing bullae in the lung. *South Med J* 1985; 78: 708.

McGregor M, Sniderman A. On pulmonary vascular resistance: the need for more precise definition. *Am J Cardiol* 1985; 55: 217.

Nemery B. Metal toxicity and the respiratory tract. *Eur Respir J* 1990; 3: 202.

Parsons PE. Respiratory failure as a result of drugs, overdoses, and poisonings. *Clin Chest Med* 1994; 15: 93.

Ray CS, Sue DY, Bray G, et al. Effects of obesity on respiratory function. *Am Rev Respir Dis* 1983; 128: 501.

Savic B, Birtel FJ, Tholen W, et al. Lung sequestration. *Thorax* 1979; 34: 96.

Schatz M, Wasserman S, Patterson R. Eosinophils and immunologic lung disease. *Med Clin North Am* 1981; 65: 1055.

Schraufnagel DE, Balmes JR, Cowl CT, et al. Air pollution and noncommunicable diseases. *Chest* 2019; 155: 409.

Sugarbaker DJ, ed. Multimodality therapy of chest malignancies – update '96. *Chest* 1997; 112: 181S.

Terry PB, Barth KH, Kaufman SL, et al. Balloon embolization for the treatment of pulmonary arteriovenous fistulas. *N Engl J Med* 1980; 302: 1189.

Trulock EP. Lung transplantation. *Am J Respir Crit Care Med* 1997; 155: 789.

Versprille A. Pulmonary vascular resistance: a meaningless variable. *Intens Care Med* 1984; 10: 51.

Wahidi MM, Herth FJF, Chen A, et al. State of the art: interventional pulmonology. *Chest* 2020; 157: 724.

Walmrath D, Schneider T, Pilch J, et al. Effects of aerosolized prostacyclin in severe pneumonia. *Am J Respir Crit Care Med* 1995; 151: 724.

Weinhouse GL, ed. Pulmonary & Critical Care Medicine. In: *Scientific American Medicine*. Hamilton: Dekker Medicine. 2020.

White RJ, Lynch-Nyhan A, Terry P, et al. Pulmonary arteriovenous malformation: techniques and long-term outcome of embolotherapy. *Radiology* 1988; 169: 663.

Winterbauer RH, Belic N, Moores KD. Clinical interpretation of bilateral hilar adenopathy. *Ann Intern Med* 1973; 78: 65.

Wohl MEB, Chernick V. Bronchiolitis. *Am Rev Respir Dis* 1978; 118: 759.

Wright BA, Jeffrey PH. Lipoid pneumonia. *Semin Respir Infect* 1990; 5: 314.

Wu T-C, Tashkin DP, Djahed B, et al. Pulmonary hazards of smoking marijuana as compared with tobacco. *N Engl J Med* 1988; 318: 347.

Restless legs syndrome

Restless legs syndrome (akathisia) is a condition of sensory discomfort leading to motor restlessness of the legs in bed at night. It is classically a benign idiopathic disorder, often with an autosomal inheritance. Secondary causes can include iron or vitamin deficiency, diabetes, renal failure, peripheral neuropathy (q.v.), psychotropic drugs and pregnancy, and it may even be a precursor to other clinical manifestations of these disorders, particularly toxic/metabolic neuropathy, such as that due to uraemia.

There is aching of the legs, with crawling sensations, especially at night, and an irresistible urge to move the legs. It is associated with sleep disruption, and it is relieved by voluntary movement or walking about.

It is of variable severity, and its course is often progressive, though symptoms may be present for a long time without any progression. Its prevalence is about 10% of the population.

Investigations include tests for secondary causes and polysomnography if sleep deprivation is marked.

Treatment is not required in mild cases, apart from that of any underlying cause. Sleep optimization techniques should be adopted.

More severe cases are treated with analgesics, benzodiazepines (usually clonazepam), carbamazepine, levodopa or dopaminergic drugs (e.g. bromocriptine or more recently cabergoline and pergolide). The newer non-ergot dopaminergic drugs, ropinirole and pramipexole, have been found to be effective, but subsequent refractoriness and later rebound may be problematic. Cardiac valvulopathy can be caused by ergot-derived drugs, and nausea, dizziness and pathological impulses can occur with any dopamine agonist.

The condition may be exacerbated by anticholinergic drugs.

Bibliography

Allen, RP, Picchieti D, Hening WA, et al. Restless legs syndrome: diagnostic criteria, special considerations, and epidemiology. *Sleep Med* 2003; 4: 101.

Earley CJ. Clinical practice: restless legs syndrome. *N Engl J Med* 2003; 348: 2103.

O'Keefe ST. Restless legs syndrome: a review. *Arch Intern Med* 1996; 156: 243.

Telstad W, Sorensen O, Larsen S, et al. Treatment of the restless legs syndrome with carbamazepine. *BMJ* 1984; 288: 444.

Thyagarajan D. Restless legs syndrome. *Aust Prescriber* 2008; 31: 90.

Reticulocytes

The red blood cell is produced when the late normoblast extrudes its nucleus. For the first 4 days of its lifespan (3 days in the bone marrow and 1 in the peripheral blood), the new red blood cell is termed a **reticulocyte**, because it contains residual ribosomes which are apparent on supravital stain, since the RNA is precipitated by methylene blue. Following the loss of this residual ribosomal material, the red blood cell becomes mature. When nuclei are extruded from even earlier normoblasts, as in severe anaemia (q.v.), 'stress reticulocytes' are produced.

The reticulocyte count reflects the vigour of marrow production.

The absolute reticulocyte count may be calculated as
- the red blood cell count,
- multiplied by the percentage of reticulocytes,
- corrected for the time in the peripheral circulation (normally 1 day).

Maturation time in the peripheral blood is prolonged in anaemia, for example it is 2 days when the packed-cell volume (PCV) has fallen to 0.25. Since the reticulocyte count is normally 0.5–2.5% of the total red blood cell count, the normal corrected reticulocyte count is $50 \pm 25 \times 10^9/L$.

- **An increased reticulocyte count**
  - is seen in increased marrow production.
  - This occurs in many forms of anaemia (q.v.).
- **A decreased reticulocyte count**
  - is seen in decreased marrow production.
  - This occurs in renal disease, aplastic anaemia, megaloblastic anaemia (q.v.), sideroblastic anaemia (q.v.), thalassaemia (q.v.) and myelofibrosis.

Retinal haemorrhage

Retinal haemorrhage is seen most typically
- in uncontrolled hypertension,
- with increased local venous pressure, as in cavernous thrombosis.
  It may also be seen in
- some infections,
  - such as with cytomegalovirus (CMV) (q.v.) or in subacute bacterial endocarditis (see Endocarditis),
- a number of other settings,
  - such as carbon monoxide poisoning (q.v.), fat embolism and high altitude (q.v.).

Retrobulbar neuritis

Retrobulbar neuritis is usually due to demyelination (see Demyelinating diseases).
  It may also be caused by
- cyanide poisoning (q.v.),
- nicotine
  - tobacco amblyopia, traditionally seen in pipe smokers,
- vitamin B_{12} deficiency (q.v.).

Retroperitoneal fibrosis See
- Ergot,
- Mediastinal diseases.

Reversible posterior leukoencephalopathy

Reversible posterior leukoencephalopathy (RPL) or posterior reversible encephalopathy (PRES) is a syndrome first described in 1996 and characterized by headache, visual disturbance and seizures, often with acute hypertension. It typically presents in the setting of hypertensive encephalopathy, eclampsia (q.v.), cancer chemotherapy or renal failure (particularly when associated with haemolytic–uraemic syndrome, q.v.). It is thought to be caused by vasogenic oedema.

Since there may be involvement of areas of the brain other than the posterior parietal and occipital lobes and of grey as well as white matter, and since the condition is not necessarily completely reversible even with early treatment, the label RPL (or PRES) is probably not ideal.

The diagnosis is made most reliably by MRI.
Treatment requires
- prompt **antihypertensive** and **anticonvulsant** medication,
- withdrawal of any cytotoxic and immunosuppressant drugs, and
- specific management of any underlying condition.

Bibliography
Hinchey J, Chaves C, Appignani B, et al. A reversible posterior leukoencephalopathy syndrome. *N Engl J Med* 1996; 334: 494.
Marinella MA, Markert RJ. Reversible posterior leucoencephalopathy syndrome associated with anticancer drugs. *Intern Med J* 2009; 39: 826.
Servillo G, Bifulco F, De Robertis E, et al. Posterior reversible encephalopathy syndrome in intensive care medicine. *Intens Care Med* 2007; 33: 230.
Stott VL, Hurrell MA, Anderson TJ. Reversible posterior leukoencephalopathy syndrome: a misnomer revisited. *Intern Med J* 2005; 35: 83.

Reye's syndrome

Reye's syndrome is a serious systemic disorder, which follows a viral infection and which involves particularly the brain and liver. Although originally described in children, it is now known also to affect young adults and even sometimes older patients.

Epidemiologically, it has been linked to prior influenza (and probably other viral infections, such as varicella), together with the concomitant use of salicylates. However, its pathogenesis remains unknown. Moreover, its incidence appears to have declined significantly since the 1980s, perhaps partly because of greater avoidance of aspirin and partly because many cases became reclassified as due to other, metabolic disorders.

> Clinical features comprise the rapid onset, some days after the viral illness, of
> - refractory vomiting,
> - hepatomegaly,
> - fits,
> - drowsiness,
> - eventually coma.

Investigations show abnormal liver function tests, except that the bilirubin usually remains normal. Liver biopsy shows microvesicular steatosis, with minimal inflammation (a similar fatty infiltration occurring in other viscera). The CSF is normal, except that the pressure may be raised.

The diagnosis is generally made clinically, because liver biopsy may be unsafe due to the associated coagulopathy (q.v.).

Treatment is **supportive** *with clotting factor replacement, mechanical ventilation, lactulose, and measures to decrease intracranial hypertension (including mannitol and/or dexamethasone).*

Prevention includes the use of paracetamol rather than aspirin for young people with acute viral infections and influenza vaccine for those few patients who need to have aspirin.

Bibliography

Atkins JN, Haponik EF. Reye's syndrome in the adult patient. *Am J Med* 1979; 67: 672.

Reye RDK, Morgan G, Baral J. Encephalopathy and fatty degeneration of the viscera: a disease entity in children. *Lancet* 1963; 2: 749.

Sarnaik AP. Reye's syndrome: hold the obituary. *Crit Care Med* 1999; 27: 1674.

Rhabdomyolysis

Rhabdomyolysis refers to the necrosis of muscle tissue. There is consequent release of myoglobin and muscle enzymes into the circulation.

The causes of rhabdomyolysis include the following.
- **Idiopathic**
  - paroxysmal, with muscle pain, tenderness and weakness,
  - usually after exertion and lasting for 2–3 days,
  - sometimes familial, in which there may be an enzyme defect indicating an underlying myopathy (q.v.),
  - associated with an increased intracellular Ca^{++} and thus dantrolene (q.v.) may be helpful by inhibiting calcium release from the sarcoplasmic reticulum.
- **Heat stroke** (q.v.)
- **Malignant hyperthermia** (q.v.)
- **Neuroleptic malignant syndrome** (q.v.)
- **Metabolic disorders**
  - hypokalaemia, hypophosphataemia (q.v.), diabetic ketoacidosis, hyperosmolality, hypothyroidism (q.v.).
- **Muscle damage**
  - from ischaemia, severe exertion, status epilepticus, trauma.
- **Polymyositis** (q.v.)
- **Toxic agents**
  - alcohol, cocaine (q.v.), drug overdose, snake venom,
  - statins, particularly when taken with grapefruit juice or star fruit (q.v.),
  - rarely following the eating of migrating quail in Europe, i.e. coturnism (q.v.).
- **Viral (and rarely bacterial) infection**
  - especially influenza (q.v.),
  - also adenovirus, EBV, HSV,
  - occasionally Gram-positive bacteria.

> The most important clinical consequence of rhabdomyolysis is **acute renal failure** from tubular obstruction due to pigment casts. There may also be tubular cell damage and afferent–efferent arterial imbalance, as well as hypovolaemia.

Rhabdomyolysis is thus similar to haemolysis (q.v.), with myoglobinuria causing problems similar to those from haemoglobinuria, but with some clearly distinguishing features, as indicated in the following Table.

Myoglobinuria v. haemoglobinuria

	Myoglobinuria	Haemoglobinuria
Molecular weight	170 kDa	69 kDa
Plasma colour	normal	dark red
Urine colour	dark red	dark red
Urine dipstick test for blood	positive	positive
Urine red blood cells	negative	negative
Renal damage	yes	yes

Other renal investigations show
- pigment casts in the urine sediment,
- raised plasma creatinine and urea,
- hyperkalaemia,
- hyperphosphataemia (q.v.),
- hypercalcaemia (q.v.),
- very low urine sodium concentration, in contrast to the more normal level in typical acute kidney injury (AKI, acute tubular necrosis).

The plasma CK is also high, as are other muscle enzyme levels. The plasma CK level is more convenient than the plasma myoglobin level for clinical monitoring, but it should be remembered that CK has a much slower elimination half-life than myoglobin.

Treatment is with **hydration** *with IV saline to improve renal perfusion and urine flow. A urine output of 300 mL/hr should be obtained, if necessary with mannitol diuresis. The urine pH should be maintained >6.5 until the urine colour has normalized. A positive fluid balance may be expected in the first 6–12 hr, because of fluid sequestration in damaged muscle. Because of the likelihood of renal failure, and difficulties with fluid balance, cardiac filling pressures should be monitored.*

Although **hypocalcaemia** *(q.v.) is usual in the early phases due to calcium transit into ischaemic muscle, and although it may be aggravated by alkalinization, hypercalcaemia (q.v.) occurs in 20–30% of cases during the recovery. This may be an unexpected phenomenon and arises from mobilization of calcium from injured muscle. Calcium administration should thus be avoided, even during the early stages of hypocalcaemia.*

Bibliography
de Meijer AR, Fikkers BG, de Keijzer MH, et al. Serum creatine kinase as predictor of clinical course in rhabdomyolysis. *Intens Care Med* 2003; 29: 1121.
Gabow PA, Kaehny WD, Kelleher SP. The spectrum of rhabdomyolysis. *Medicine* 1982; 61: 141.
Holt SG, Moore KP. Pathogenesis and treatment of renal dysfunction in rhabdomyolysis. *Intens Care Med* 2001; 27: 803.
Knochel JP. Rhabdomyolysis and myoglobinuria. *Semin Nephrol* 1981; 1: 75.
Lappalainen H, Tiula E, Uotila L, et al. Elimination kinetics of myoglobin and creatine kinase in rhabdomyolysis; implications for follow-up. *Crit Care Med* 2002; 30: 2212.
Miller FW. Classification and prognosis of inflammatory muscle disease. *Rheum Dis Clin North Am* 1994; 20: 811.
Warren JD, Blumbergs PC, Thompson PD. Rhabdomyolysis: a review. *Muscle Nerve* 2002; 25: 332.
Zimmerman JL, Shen MC. Rhabdomyolysis. *Chest* 2013; 144: 1058.

Rheumatology

Disorders affecting joints, connective tissue and musculoskeletal structures (i.e. the domain of **rheumatology**) mostly have no currently identifiable specific aetiology. However, as for other conditions, a classification is useful, though it must necessarily be somewhat arbitrary.

Many **rheumatological conditions** are very common in the population, including soft tissue rheumatic syndromes, osteoarthritis, post-traumatic damage, rheumatoid arthritis and vasomotor disorders. Thus, while some connective tissue and musculoskeletal conditions may have manifestations severe enough to require Intensive Care admission, more common reasons for Intensive Care in such patients are either comorbidity, because of the chronicity of many of these conditions, or other illness, with the rheumatic disorder being coincidental.

A large variety of rheumatological conditions may therefore be seen in Intensive Care patients, and while not usually primary problems they can give rise to added difficulties of management of pain, immobility, stiffness and concomitant drug needs. The chief such conditions include
- Ankylosing spondylitis,
- Antinuclear antibodies,
- Arthritis,
- Arthropathies,
- Bone failure,
- Collagen-vascular diseases,
- Connective tissue diseases,
- CREST syndrome,
- Cricoarytenoid arthritis,
- Dermatomyositis,
- Felty's syndrome,
- Gout,
- Hyperuricaemia,
- Kyphoscoliosis,
- Leflunomide,
- Microscopic polyangiitis,
- Mixed connective tissue disease,
- Myositis,
- Osteomalacia,
- Paget's disease,
- Polyarteritis nodosa,
- Polymyalgia rheumatica,

- Polymyositis,
- Pseudogout,
- Reactive arthritis,
- Reiter's syndrome,
- Rhabdomyolysis,
- Scleroderma,
- Sjogren's syndrome,
- Spondyloarthritis,
- Still's disease,
- Systemic lupus erythematosus,
- Systemic sclerosis,
- Temporal arteritis.

Bibliography

Ahern MJ, Smith MD. Rheumatoid arthritis. *Med J Aust* 1997; 166: 156.

Firestein G, Budd R, Gabriel SE, et al. *Firestein & Kelley's Textbook of Rheumatology.* 11th edition. Philadelphia: Elsevier. 2020.

Fox DA, ed. Rheumatology. In: *Scientific American Medicine.* Hamilton: Dekker Medicine. 2020.

Gibofsky A, Zabriskie JB. Rheumatic fever and poststreptococcal reactive arthritis. *Curr Opin Rheumatol* 1995; 7: 299.

Hamerman D. The biology of osteoarthritis. *N Engl J Med* 1989; 320: 1322.

Hruska KA, Teitelbaum SL. Renal osteodystrophy. *N Engl J Med* 1995; 333: 166.

Jowsey J. *Metabolic Disease of Bone.* Philadelphia: WB Saunders. 1977.

Klippel JH, ed. *Primer on the Rheumatic Diseases.* 13th edition. New York: Springer. 2008.

Littlejohn GO. Fibromyalgia syndrome. *Med J Aust* 1996; 165: 387.

Mandell BF, ed. *Acute Rheumatologic and Immunological Diseases: Management of the Critically Ill Patient.* New York: Marcell Dekker. 1994.

Miller FW. Classification and prognosis of inflammatory muscle disease. *Rheum Dis Clin North Am* 1994; 20: 811.

Mills PR, Sturrock RD. Clinical associations between arthritis and liver disease. *Ann Rheum Dis* 1982; 41: 295.

Parniapour M, Nordin M, Skovron ML, et al. Environmentally induced disorders of the musculoskeletal system. *Med Clin North Am* 1990; 74: 347.

Posen S. Paget's disease: current concepts. *Aust NZ J Surg* 1992; 62: 17.

Prockop DJ. Mutations in collagen genes as a cause of connective-tissue diseases. *N Engl J Med* 1992; 326: 540.

Rodan GA. Introduction to bone biology. *Bone* 1992; 13: 53.

Shiel WC, Prete PE. Pleuropulmonary manifestations of rheumatoid arthritis. *Semin Arthritis Rheum* 1984; 13: 235.

Simon LS, Mills JA. Drug therapy: nonsteroidal antiinflammatory drugs. *N Engl J Med* 1980; 302: 1179 & 1237.

Rickettsial diseases

Rickettsial diseases are produced by infection with members of a genus of small pleomorphic obligate intracellular parasites, which contain both DNA and RNA and are coccobacillary in appearance. In general, they have an animal reservoir and an arthropod vector (q.v.), and they are transmitted to humans only incidentally. They are taxonomically related to various proteobacteria, such as legionella. A revised taxonomy of these organisms has been proposed, with new families, genera and species within the overall order of Rickettsiales.

The organisms multiply at the site of entry and then disseminate so as to infect endothelial cells throughout the body. This results in

- capillary leak syndrome (see Microvascular dysfunction),
- hypovolaemia,
- circulatory failure,
- multiorgan failure (q.v.).

> There are three main groups of rickettsial diseases, namely,
> - the spotted fevers,
> - the typhus group,
> - Q fever.
>
> In addition, many new rickettsioses have been identified worldwide in recent years, involving ehrlichiosis and bartonella infection, including.
> - Cat scratch disease (q.v.),
> - Trench fever (q.v.),
> - Bacillary angiomatosis (q.v.).

1. **Spotted fevers** are widely distributed, particularly in the Rocky Mountains of the USA, the Mediterranean, Asia and Northern Australia.

    A generalized maculopapular rash is accompanied by fever and systemic features.

2. The **typhus group** includes
    - endemic (murine) typhus,
    - epidemic (louse-borne) typhus,
    - scrub typhus.

    Endemic typhus occurs worldwide and is transmitted by rodent fleas (insects). The responsible organism is *R. typhi.*

Following an incubation period of 6–14 days, there is fever (q.v.), an eventual rash and systemic symptoms, especially headache. There may be a pulmonary infiltrate (q.v.).

The illness lasts 10–12 days if untreated.

Epidemic typhus is due to *R. prowazekii* and is transmitted by the body louse (an insect), especially in times of war. It has been suggested as a possible cause of the famous plague of Athens in 430 BC (see Plague).

Following an incubation period of 7 days, there is an abrupt onset of high fever (q.v.), an eventual rash, severe headache and diffuse vascular lesions. There is often a pulmonary infiltrate (q.v.) and splenomegaly (q.v.), and if severe, hypotension, confusion, respiratory failure and disseminated intravascular coagulation (q.v.).

Lysis occurs after 2 weeks without treatment, and mortality is 10–50%, especially in the debilitated.

A recrudescence of epidemic typhus may occur many years later and is referred to as **Brill–Zinsser disease**. The organism has presumably persisted dormant in the reticuloendothelial system prior to reactivation. There is an irregular fever and severe headache but no rash. The illness lasts 7–11 days, following which there is complete recovery.

Scrub typhus is produced by the organism *Orientia tsutsugamushi* (formerly called *R. tsutsugamushi*) and is transmitted by an infected mite, an arachnid ectoparasite of small mammals which are the organism's natural reservoir. The condition usually occurs in South-East Asia, the Western Pacific or Northern Australia.

The bite site may show infection with a painless ulcer (q.v.), and there is regional lymphadenopathy (q.v.), a high fever (q.v.), headache, myalgia and a rash. Pneumonitis can occur, with progression to ARDS (q.v.) and multiorgan failure (q.v.) in severe cases.

3. **Q fever** is caused by the organism, *Coxiella burnetii*, following transmission via milk, faeces or products of conception. The animal reservoir in cattle and sheep and related animals is worldwide, and the organism is very infectious, although no person-to-person transmission occurs. It is usually seen in animal workers. The transmission is air-borne.

The incidence of Q fever may be much higher than that based on clinical reports, as seropositivity surveys suggest that many cases must be asymptomatic or misdiagnosed.

Following an incubation period of about 20 days, there are non-specific initial symptoms followed after 4–5 days by fever (q.v.), headache, cough, chest pain and primary atypical pneumonia. There is no rash but there is occasionally hepatosplenomegaly. Spontaneous recovery occurs after 1–2 weeks.

Chronic recurrent illness may occur in up to 10% of patients in the months to years after the acute illness. This can be associated with potentially fatal endocarditis (q.v.). Persistent fatigue (q.v.) is common for up to a year or more after an acute infection.

The differential diagnosis is difficult, as in the early phases it is similar to many acute febrile illnesses. The history of contact with livestock is important. When pneumonitis appears, the differential diagnosis becomes more confined and includes viral, chlamydial, legionella and mycoplasma infections. In endocarditis, it mimics bacterial infection.

Vaccination is available for those at high risk and is recommended for adults with significant animal exposure.

The diagnosis of rickettsial diseases is confirmed serologically.

The organisms are sensitive to **tetracycline** *(0.5 g qid or doxycycline 100 mg bd) or* **chloramphenicol** *(0.5 g qid), to either of which antibiotic group a rapid response is seen.* **Ciprofloxacin** *is also effective.*

Bibliography

Blanton LS. Infections due to rickettsia and related organisms. In: *Scientific American Medicine. Infectious Diseases.* Hamilton: Dekker Medicine. 2020.

Caron F, Meurice JC, Ingrand P, et al. Acute Q fever pneumonia. *Chest* 1998; 114: 808.

Francis JR, Robson JM. Q fever: more common than we think, and what this means for prevention. *Med J Aust* 2019; 210: 305.

Kempschreur LM, Dekker S, Hagenaars JC, et al. Identification of risk factors for chronic Q fever. *Emerg Infect Dis* 2012; 18: 563.

Marmion B. Q fever: the long journey to control by vaccination. *Med J Aust* 2007; 186: 164.

Raoult D, Tissot-Dupont H, Foucault C, et al. Q fever 1985–1998: clinical and epidemiologic features of 1,383 infections. *Medicine (Baltimore)* 2000; 79: 109.

Sloan-Gardner TS, Massey PD, Hutchinson P, et al. Trends and risk factors for human Q fever in Australia, 1991–2014. *Epidemiol Infect* 2017; 145: 787.

Spach D, Liles W, Campbell G, et al. Tick-borne diseases in the United States. *N Engl J Med* 1993; 329: 936.

Watt G, Parola P. Scrub typhus and tropical rickettsioses. *Curr Opin Infect Dis* 2003; 16: 429.

Winkler HH. *Rickettsia* species. *Annu Rev Microbiol* 1990; 44: 131.

Rituximab

Rituximab is a monoclonal antibody to CD20, originally used in non-Hodgkin's lymphoma (NHL) and subsequently in rheumatoid arthritis. It is also used in a variety of other lymphomas, haematological malignancies and autoimmune disorders.

More recently, it has been used effectively as an immunosuppressive agent (see Immunomodulation) in a wide variety of refractory conditions, including autoimmune haemolytic anaemia, antiphospholipid syndrome, Bell's palsy, Churg–Strauss syndrome, cold agglutinin disease, exophthalmos, haemophagocytic syndrome, idiopathic thrombocytopenic purpura, myasthenia gravis, pemphigus, pulmonary alveolar proteinosis, sarcoidosis, Sjogren's disease, systemic lupus erythematosus, thrombotic thrombocytopenic purpura and Wegener's granulomatosis (see these other conditions).

A rare but major complication of rituximab treatment has been the development of **progressive multifocal leukoencephalopathy** (PML) (see Demyelinating diseases – 3. Progressive multifocal leukoencephalopathy).

Ross River virus disease

Ross River virus (RRV) **disease** (epidemic polyarthritis) was originally described in New South Wales in 1928 and later outbreaks occurred among the military in Northern Australia during World War II. The responsible arbovirus was identified in a mosquito from Ross River in Queensland in 1959 and eventually from a patient in 1985. Marsupials appear to be the main natural reservoir. Outbreaks have occurred throughout Australia and the Western Pacific Islands, though particularly in Northern Australia during the rainy season.

The incubation period is about 1 week. While one third of those infected are asymptomatic, in the others the disease is debilitating.

Clinical features comprise an acute polyarthritis (q.v.), commonly with fever (q.v.), headache, myalgia and rash. Occasionally, renal involvement, encephalitis (q.v.) or splenomegaly (q.v.) have been reported. Prolonged arthralgia and asthenia can persist for many months in some patients, with a picture of chronic fatigue (q.v.) similar to that recognized as sometimes occurring after Epstein–Barr infection (q.v.).

Diagnosis is confirmed serologically.

Treatment is symptomatic, with **NSAIDs** being generally the most helpful medication. Corticosteroids are not effective.

Bibliography
Barber B, Denholm JT, Spelman D. Ross River virus. *Aust Family Physician* 2009; 38: 586.
Mylonas A, Brown A, Carthew T, et al. Natural history of Ross River-induced epidemic polyarthritis. *Med J Aust* 2002; 177: 356.

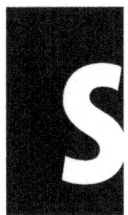

Salicylism *See*

- Aspirin.

Salpingitis

Salpingitis or infection involving the Fallopian tubes commonly also involves the uterus and adjacent structures, and together these infections comprise **acute pelvic inflammatory disease**. Most obviously clinically, there is typically evidence of mucopurulent cervicitis.

Except when the organisms are directly implanted following abortion, pregnancy or surgery, the pathogens usually have ascended from the vagina. Thus, aerobic and anaerobic faecal flora and cervicovaginal flora (especially bacteroides and anaerobic Gram-negative cocci) are responsible for 50% of infections. Other organisms commonly involved include *Neisseria gonorrhoeae*, *Chlamydia trachomatis*, *Mycoplasma hominis*, and *Ureaplasma urealyticum*.

There are both local and systemic features of infection and occasionally extension to produce peritonitis.

Subsequent problems include recurrent abdominal pain, ectopic pregnancy and infertility.

The differential diagnosis can sometimes be difficult and includes

- appendicitis,
- mesenteric adenitis,
- endometriosis,
- ruptured ovarian cyst,
- ovarian tumour,
- ectopic pregnancy.

In 25% of cases presenting with a putative diagnosis of salpingitis, no definitive diagnosis is made even at laparoscopy.

Treatment is with **antibiotics**, *preferably tetracycline (doxycycline) and a cephalosporin (cefoxitin).*

Quinolones have also been shown to be effective. If severe, gentamicin plus metronidazole or even a carbapenem may be indicated. In either event, doxycycline should also be given for up to 2 weeks to cover chlamydia.

If poor compliance with such a regimen is anticipated, a single dose of azithromycin 1 g is a cost-effective alternative.

Failure of antibiotic therapy indicates the likelihood of an abscess, which needs to be identified by imaging (usually CT) and drained.

Bibliography

Peterson HB, Walker CK, Kahn JG, et al. Pelvic inflammatory disease: key treatment issues and options. *JAMA* 1991; 266: 2605.

Rice PA, Schachter J. Pathogenesis of pelvic inflammatory disease: what are the questions? *JAMA* 1991; 265: 2587.

Webster DP, Schneider CN, Cheche S, et al. Differentiating acute appendicitis from pelvic inflammatory disease in women of child-bearing age. *Am J Emerg Med* 1993; 11: 569.

Sarcoidosis

Sarcoidosis is a multisystem disease characterized by non-caseating granulomas. It is found worldwide, but there is great regional variation in incidence. In general, it is more common in temperate than in tropical climates. Occasional familial clustering is seen, perhaps indicating some genetic predisposition.

The aetiology remains unknown, but it is most likely to be an exaggerated immune response to one or more, as yet unidentified, transmissible agents or environmental antigens. Although it has been linked with a number of infections, none of these associations have stood up to close scrutiny, except perhaps for reports of its occurrence after *Yersinia* infections. In turn, sarcoidosis may predispose to listeria (q.v.) or cryptococcal (q.v.) infection. Moreover, many conditions both infectious (e.g. histoplasmosis – q.v., non-caseating tuberculosis – q.v.) and non-infectious (e.g. berylliosis – q.v.) may also produce granulomas similar to those seen in sarcoidosis. The aetiological controversy has been refuelled by the discovery in sarcoidosis tissue specimens of molecular sequences from mycobacterial species and by lymphocyte proliferation tests showing sensitization to inorganic occupational antigens in some patients.

It is a relatively common condition, especially in young adults, with a prevalence generally from 5 to 20 per 100,000 of the population. It is less common in tobacco smokers.

Although the clinical features are protean, the chief manifestations are pulmonary, with over 95% of patients having an abnormal chest X-ray. Physical examination of the chest is frequently normal, but crackles and wheezes are sometimes noted. Respiratory symptoms correlate much better with functional or pathological changes than with radiological changes, the latter often being either considerably greater or less than the symptoms would suggest.

Clinical staging is based on the lung involvement, though there is no necessary progression or retrogression serially through the individual stages.

- **Stage I** (50% of cases)

This consists of bilateral hilar lymphadenopathy which is usually asymptomatic.

There are however systemic features of fever (q.v.), malaise, weight loss, arthralgia (q.v.) and erythema nodosum (q.v.).

About 10% of these patients have extrapulmonary involvement (especially of CNS, eyes, lacrimal glands).

Most cases (75%) resolve after 2 years, and only 10–15% develop progressive pulmonary disease.

An acute onset with erythema nodosum especially heralds a self-limited course and spontaneous resolution.

- **Stage II** (25% of cases)

This involves both bilateral hilar lymphadenopathy and diffuse lung infiltration (q.v.).

In addition to systemic features, there are usually pulmonary symptoms of cough and dyspnoea.

Remission occurs in about 50% of patients within 2 years, but some progress to develop chronic disease.

- **Stage III** (15% of cases)

This refers to diffuse lung infiltration (q.v.) without hilar lymphadenopathy.

Respiratory symptoms are usual, though these are much less striking than the chest X-ray would predict.

Although most patients at this stage have progressed through the previous stages, about 10% of cases in fact present at this stage.

Remission still occurs in about one third of patients by two years, though progression to relentless progressive chronic pulmonary fibrosis (i.e. Stage IV) is common, especially in patients with an insidious onset.

Extrapulmonary involvement is frequent.

- **Stage 0** (the remaining 10% of cases)

This term is sometimes applied to those who have a normal chest X-ray.

Uncommon intrathoracic manifestations include the following.

- **Pleural effusion** or pleural thickening is seen in 1–4% of cases. The effusion is usually small, and there is a high lymphocyte count in the pleural fluid. See Pleural effusion.
- **Lung nodules** can often be large (i.e. 2–10 cm diameter) and need to be distinguished from

tuberculosis (q.v.), mycetoma or carcinoma. See Pulmonary nodules.
- **Airway involvement** affects both the lower and upper tracts, with mucosal inflammation, airway distortion, airflow limitation, bronchiolitis, dysphagia (q.v.) and laryngeal dysfunction.
- **Cavitation** (q.v.) occurs rarely.
- **Calcification of hilar lymph nodes** is seen in 5% of cases as a late phenomenon.
- **Atelectasis** can occur due to endobronchial involvement and may be associated with wheeze.
- **Respiratory failure** may result from extensive consolidation.
- An unusual variant is **necrotizing sarcoid granulomatosis with pulmonary arteritis**.

Extrapulmonary manifestations are numerous and varied, and they may be apparent in virtually any organ system.
- **Skin** involvement comprises erythema nodosum (q.v.) in 90% of patients with stage I disease. Sometimes, there may be skin granulomas, nodules or lupus pernio (usually in stage III disease).
- **Eyes** are involved in 25% of patients. Typically, there is uveitis (q.v.) with painless photophobia and lacrimation. Classically but uncommonly, there may be **uveoparotid fever** (with associated salivary gland enlargement, systemic symptoms, meningitis and cranial nerve palsies) or chorioretinitis (with blurred vision). Keratoconjunctivitis sicca may occur (see also Sicca syndrome).
- **Neurological changes** are seen in <5% of patients. These changes may involve either the central nervous system (encephalopathy – q.v., hypothalamic lesions, granulomas, cranial nerve palsies, fits, chronic meningitis in which the CSF shows increased protein and lymphocytes) or the peripheral nervous system (with peripheral neuropathy of a sensory and/or motor form – q.v.).
- **Liver** and **spleen** may contain granulomas, with occasional overt enlargement or dysfunction, and there may be associated lymphadenopathy (q.v.).
- **Musculoskeletal system** is involved in 1–10% of patients, with arthritis (q.v.), swelling and cystic lesions in the bones of the digits.
- **Endocrine changes** comprise hypercalcaemia (q.v.) and especially hypercalcuria, and occasionally pituitary dysfunction, especially with diabetes insipidus (q.v.).
- **Heart** problems are due to granulomas, which may cause failure, arrhythmias and pericardial disease, though in fact most cardiac involvement is occult.
- **Upper respiratory tract** symptoms are due to either nasal granulomatous involvement simulating rhinitis or supraglottic laryngeal plaque involvement causing hoarseness.
- **Renal** involvement is generally tubulointerstitial nephritis (q.v.), associated with either interstitial infiltration, granulomas or nephrocalcinosis. There is sterile pyuria, mild proteinuria (q.v.) and defects of concentration and acidification and thus tubular function. However, renal involvement is usually asymptomatic, and like any cardiac involvement it is generally found only at autopsy.

The diagnosis is established most securely when clinicoradiographic findings are supported by histological evidence of widespread non-caseating epithelioid-cell granulomas in more than one organ. Although often only lung material obtained by transbronchial lung biopsy is available for examination (with a diagnostic sensitivity of 60–90%), additional biopsy of lymph node, Kveim nodule (formerly) or other tissue greatly assists diagnostic precision. Transbronchial needle aspiration of mediastinal lymph nodes may be made under endobronchial ultrasound guidance. Bronchoalveolar lavage fluid shows lymphocytosis, though this is non-specific.

Chest X-ray shows that the diffuse lung involvement may be miliary, nodular or reticular. Confluent infiltrates may occur and are sometimes massive. Chest radiography is always essential, as clinically silent pulmonary involvement is usual, even if the presentation is extrapulmonary. PET scanning may be used to assess overall inflammatory activity.

Lung function tests may show decreased ventilatory capacity, usually restrictive but occasionally obstructive in pattern, hypoxaemia and hypocapnia, decreased lung volumes, decreased compliance and decreased gas transfer. The latter is probably the most sensitive functional test and the best for serial follow-up. Although these functional changes correlate quite well with pathological changes, they are not helpful prognostically.

There is depressed cell-mediated immunity (i.e. anergy, with a negative Mantoux test) but often enhanced humoral or B lymphocyte activity (with raised or abnormal immunoglobulins).

Historically, a positive Kveim test was obtained in about 80% of cases, though this test is no longer performed.

Microbiological examination of sputum should exclude acid-fast bacilli.

Hypercalcaemia (q.v.) and especially hypercalcuria may be demonstrated. The alkaline phosphatase may be elevated. Full blood examination may show that one or more of the formed elements is decreased, due to either splenic sequestration or bone marrow involvement.

The serum angiotensin-converting enzyme (ACE) (q.v.) level is increased in most patients with acute disease. However, this finding is non-specific, importantly being also seen in miliary tuberculosis (q.v.), as well as in pneumoconiosis (q.v.), biliary cirrhosis (q.v.) and leprosy (q.v.). Clearly, this test is unreliable in patients who are receiving ACE inhibitors, as these agents can substantially reduce serum ACE levels.

The chief differential diagnosis is
- tuberculosis (q.v.),
- lymphoma,
- metastatic carcinoma,
- amyloid (q.v.),
- talc granulomas, e.g. from the filler in illicit IV drugs.

Treatment is not required in many patients, because the disability is mild and remission is usual, but **corticosteroids** are indicated in symptomatic disease. Corticosteroids both relieve symptoms and suppress inflammation and granuloma formation. They thus suppress the manifestations of acute sarcoidosis, but whether they alter the long-term outcome remains unproven. Most clinicians, however, would use corticosteroids in Stage II or III disease with dyspnoea and abnormal lung function and in serious extrapulmonary disease. Low doses are usually effective, and treatment can often be ceased after 1 year.
- The addition of **methotrexate** but not **ciclosporin** to corticosteroids has been shown to be useful.
- There is some trial evidence to suggest that prolonged treatment with **chloroquine** may be helpful in some patients and that **thalidomide** may ameliorate lupus pernio. **Infliximab** and other **TNF-α blockers** (e.g. etanercept) have also been used with success, particularly for skin lesions and arthritis.
- **Rituximab** (q.v.) has been reported to be effective in some cases.
- A cocktail of **levofloxacin, ethambutol, azithromycin** and **rifabutin** (CLEAR) has been found to be useful in cases of cutaneous and pulmonary involvement.

The prognosis is usually good, because about 75% of patients with stage I disease undergo a complete remission within 2 years. In about 10% of patients, progression to fibrosis occurs. In individual patients, the course and prognosis may correlate with the mode of onset, as indicated above. Severe chronic extrapulmonary lesions are usually associated with pulmonary fibrosis. The overall mortality is less than 5% and is most commonly due to respiratory failure secondary to severe pulmonary fibrosis.

Bibliography

Ahmadzai H, Huang S, Steinfort C, et al. Sarcoidosis: a state of the art review from the Thoracic Society of Australia and New Zealand. *Med J Aust* 2018; 208: 499.

Baughman RP, Culver DA, Judson MA. A concise review of pulmonary sarcoidosis. *Am J Respir Crit Care Med* 2011; 183: 573.

Baughman RP, Drent M, Kavuru M, et al. Infliximab therapy in patients with chronic sarcoidosis and pulmonary involvement. *Am J Respir Crit Care Med* 2006; 174: 795.

Baughman RP, Judson MA, Teirstein AS, et al. Thalidomide for chronic sarcoidosis. *Chest* 2002; 1222: 227.

Baughman RP, Scholand MB. Sarcoidosis. In: *Scientific American Medicine. Pulmonary & Critical Care Medicine.* Hamilton: Dekker Medicine. 2020.

Conron M, Young C, Beynon H. Calcium metabolism in sarcoidosis and its clinical implications. *Rheumatology* 2000; 39: 707.

Crouser ED, Maier LA, Wilson KC, et al. Diagnosis and detection of sarcoidosis: an official American Thoracic Society clinical practice guideline. *Am J Respir Crit Care Med* 2020; 201: 26.

Drake WP, Pei Z, Pride DT, et al. Molecular analysis of sarcoidosis tissues for mycobacterium species DNA. *Emerg Infect Dis* 2002; 8: 1334.

Gardner DG. Hypercalcemia and sarcoidosis – another piece of the puzzle falls into place. *Am J Med* 2001; 110: 736.

Gibson GJ, Prescott RJ, Muers MF, et al. British Thoracic Society Sarcoidosis Study: Effects of long term corticosteroid treatment. *Thorax* 1996; 51: 238.

Judson MA. Extrapulmonary sarcoidosis. *Semin Respir Crit Care Med* 2007; 28: 83.

Judson MA. The diagnosis of sarcoidosis. *Clin Chest Med* 2008; 29: 415.

Judson MA, Thompson BW, Rabin DL, et al. The diagnostic pathway to sarcoidosis. *Chest* 2003; 123: 406.

Lodha S, Sanchez M, Prystowsky S. Sarcoidosis of the skin: a review for the pulmonologist. *Chest* 2009; 136: 583.

Morgenthau AS, Ianuzzi MC. Recent advances in sarcoidosis. *Chest* 2011; 139: 174.

Newman LS. Beryllium disease and sarcoidosis: clinical and laboratory links. *Sarcoidosis* 1995; 12: 7.

Newman LS, Rose CS, Maier LA. Sarcoidosis. *N Engl J Med* 1997; 336: 1224.

Patterson KC, Chen ES. The pathogenesis of pulmonary sarcoidosis and implications for treatment. *Chest* 2018; 153: 1432.

Polychronopoulos VS, Prakash UBS. Airway involvement in sarcoidosis. *Chest* 2009; 136: 1371.

Reich JM. What is sarcoidosis? *Chest* 2003; 124: 367.

Selroos O, Astra Draco AB. Glucocorticosteroids and pulmonary sarcoidosis. *Thorax* 1996; 51: 229.

Statement on sarcoidosis. Joint Statement of the American Thoracic Society (ATS), the European Respiratory Society (ERS) and the World Association of Sarcoidosis and Other Granulomatous Disorders (WASOG). *Am J Respir Crit Care Med* 1999; 160: 736.

Thomas PD, Hunninghake GW. Current concepts of the pathogenesis of sarcoidosis. *Am Rev Respir Dis* 1987; 135: 747.

Valevre D, Prasse A, Nunes H, et al. Sarcoidosis. *Lancet* 2014; 383: 1155.

Winterbauer RH, Belic N, Moores KD. Clinical interpretation of bilateral hilar adenopathy. *Ann Intern Med* 1973; 78: 65.

Wyser CP, van Schalkwyk EM, Alheit B, et al. Treatment of progressive pulmonary sarcoidosis with cyclosporin A. *Am J Respir Crit Care Med* 1997; 156: 1371.

SARS *See*

- Severe acute respiratory syndrome.

Scalded skin syndrome *See*

- Exfoliative dermatitis.
  See also
- Pemphigus.

Scarlet fever

Scarlet fever is usually produced by the Group A beta-haemolytic streptococcus, *S. pyogenes*. This organism produces the type A erythrogenic toxin, which causes extensive capillary damage. Although scarlet fever declined in incidence and severity following the introduction of penicillin, there has been a recent re-emergence of the condition.

> The original site of streptococcal infection can be skin and soft tissue, e.g. cellulitis or necrotizing fasciitis (q.v.), rather than an upper respiratory tract infection. Usually, there is associated bacteraemia.

Following a fever and sore throat, there is a fine, red, sandpaper-like rash within 1–5 days. Although the rash includes the oral cavity, it typically tends to spare the perioral region. There is nausea and even severe prostration. When the rash fades, desquamation accompanies the healing process.

Complicating features, often in the absence of a rash, include

- acute respiratory distress syndrome (ARDS) (q.v.),
- renal failure,
- a toxic shock syndrome resembling that caused by staphylococci (see Toxic shock syndrome). In this setting, the mortality is 30% despite treatment with high-dose penicillin and Intensive Care.

Schistosomiasis

Schistosomiasis (bilharzia) arises from infection with a trematode (i.e. fluke), one of the major groups of helminthic parasites (see Helminths).

The three major species of fluke are *Schistosoma mansoni*, *S. japonicum* and *S. haematobium*. They are mostly found in tropical and subtropical regions of Africa, Asia, and Central and South America. Because of the absence of an intermediate host, they are not found in developed countries, though infection may be seen in travellers and of course in refugees from endemic regions.

Following passage of the eggs in human faeces into water, the hatchlings become free-swimming miracidia which enter the fresh water snail, the immediate host. These release free-swimming cercaria, which penetrate human skin and become schistosomula, which in turn circulate in the blood and mature and mate in portal vessels. These then lodge in blood vessels in different parts of the body, where they shed eggs, which are excreted or transported elsewhere. In particular, *S. mansoni* lodges in the colon, *S. japonicum* in the entire intestine and *S. haematobium* in the bladder. Adult worms may survive for over 10 years in a human host.

There are three stages of clinical disease.

- **First stage**

There is dermatitis at the site of penetration of the parasite into the skin.

- **Second stage**

About 4–8 weeks later, if the original infestation has been heavy, acute disease now occurs (**Katayama fever**).

There is fever (q.v.), malaise, myalgia, urticarial rash, cough, abdominal pain, haematuria (q.v.), hepatosplenomegaly and eosinophilia (q.v.).

- **Third stage**

The eggs are now found in the liver, gut and bladder. This gives rise to fever (q.v.), malaise, diarrhoea (q.v.), haematuria (q.v.), hepatosplenomegaly and later portal hypertension. Liver failure does not occur, because the hepatic parenchyma is spared. Renal failure and bladder cancer may occur.

Embolization of eggs to the lungs may cause pulmonary hypertension (q.v.) and to the brain may cause irreversible damage with focal CNS signs.

The diagnosis is made following serological testing or demonstration of the eggs in faeces or urine.

Treatment is with **praziquantel** *(40–60 mg/kg) taken in 2–3 divided doses 4 hr apart. This drug is very effective and has few side-effects, except for transient systemic symptoms thought to be due to an immune response to the dying worms.*

Bibliography
Bierman WF, Wetsteyn JC, van Gool T. Presentation and diagnosis of imported schistosomiasis: relevance of eosinophilia, microscopy for ova, and serology. *J Travel Med* 2005; 12: 9.
Hiatt RA, Sotomayor ZR, Sanchez G, et al. Factors in the pathogenesis of acute schistosomiasis mansoni. *J Infect Dis* 1979; 139: 659.

Schonlein–Henoch purpura See

- Henoch–Schonlein purpura,
- Purpura.

Scleredema See

- Scleroderma.

Scleroderma

Scleroderma (systemic sclerosis) is a generalized disorder of connective tissue of unknown aetiology. It is characterized by degenerative and inflammatory changes that lead to intense fibrosis, particularly in the skin. Possible fetal microchimerism with a consequent form of graft-versus-host disease has been reported as an interesting pathogenetic mechanism in some cases of scleroderma in women. Some familial aggregation and ethnic clustering supports a genetic component, perhaps via the gene for fibrillin. Mathematical modelling of its epidemiology has suggested that its pathogenesis is complex, multifactorial, multi-event-related and unpredictable.

The pathological process may be extensive and involve many other organs, especially lungs and kidneys, but sometimes it may be localized to skin and subcutaneous tissue and even comprise a single linear lesion. Pathogenetically, the fibrous proliferation comprises quantitatively but not qualitatively abnormal collagen. There is an associated vasculopathy involving small arteries (see Vasculitis). It is considered an autoimmune disorder (q.v.).

Clinical manifestations of scleroderma can be widespread, with multiorgan involvement.

- **Skin**
  - There is early thickening and later atrophy.
  - There is loss of pliability, mobility and appendages, especially on the hands (sclerodactyly) and face.
  - There is often associated telangiectasia (q.v.).
  - The involvement of cutaneous vessels may give Raynaud's phenomenon (q.v.).
  - Sometimes, there is subcutaneous calcinosis.
- **Musculoskeletal**
  - There is polyarthralgia and sometimes polyarthritis (q.v.), and tenosynovitis.
  - Acral osteolysis with loss of terminal bone and soft tissue from the digits is seen.
  - There can be flexion contractures and myopathy (q.v.).
- **Gastrointestinal tract**
  - There is dilatation and impaired contractility of the oesophagus.
  - This process may also involve the intestine, and sometimes there may be pneumatosis intestinalis (q.v.).
  - Some patients have associated Sjogren's syndrome (q.v.).
- **Lungs**
  - There may be diffuse interstitial fibrosis (q.v.) and pulmonary hypertension (q.v.).
  - There is a 6-fold increased incidence of lung cancer.
- **Heart**
  - Cardiomyopathy (q.v.), arrhythmias, conduction defects and cardiac failure may occur.
- **Kidneys**
  - Malignant hypertension (renal crisis) can be produced.
- **Nerves**
  - Trigeminal neuralgia and other cranial neuropathies (q.v.) may be seen rarely.

Investigations show a positive ANA test in most patients, and diffuse hypergammaglobinaemia may be present. A specific antibody is demonstrable to the enzyme, topoisomerase I (Scl-70).

Treatment is **symptomatic** *and depends on the extent of involvement and the speed of progression. Symptoms should be managed on their individual merits.*

Corticosteroids *and* **cyclophosphamide** *arrest the progress of pulmonary fibrosis.* **Tacrolimus** *has been reported to delay sclerosis in rapidly progressive cases.* **ACE inhibitors** *are recommended in renal crisis.*

Sildenafil*, *epoprostenol and ***bosentan*** have been useful in cases with pulmonary hypertension or Raynaud's phenomenon. ***Penicillamine*, *methotrexate*** and more recently a ***monoclonal antibody to transforming growth factor β1*** have been found to be ineffective. **Lung transplantation** may be considered in advanced cases, provided there is not significant oesophageal or systemic involvement. Autologous **stem cell transplantation** has been reported to provide long-term remission, and the use of mesenchymal stem cells is under study.

The prognosis depends on the extent and type of involvement. Renal crisis used to be fatal, but patients now generally survive with aggressive antihypertensive therapy, particularly with ACE inhibitors (see Angiotensin-converting enzyme). Pulmonary involvement is now the chief cause of death. The mortality is very variable, though the average is 50% at 5 yr in diffuse disease and 35% at 10 yr overall. At death, the mean duration of disease has been about 15 yr. Although the condition only occasionally remits, its progress is usually slow, especially after the first 2–5 yr. Localized disease itself does not adversely affect life expectancy.

Variants of scleroderma include the following.

- **Overlap syndromes**
  - mixed connective tissue disease (q.v.).
- **Limited cutaneous scleroderma**
  - CREST syndrome, namely, calcinosis, Raynaud's phenomenon, oesophageal immobility, sclerodactyly, telangiectasia. However, it has been suggested that this acronym be abandoned, because it fails to reflect the internal organ involvement which may be seen.
  - This variant of scleroderma is a milder form with limited skin involvement, less organ damage (except for biliary cirrhosis) and less progression.
  - However, some patients develop severe pulmonary hypertension (q.v.) late in the course of this illness.
  - An anti-centromere antibody is usually demonstrable.

The more recently described condition of **nephrogenic systemic fibrosis** (NSF or nephrogenic fibrosing dermopathy) may mimic scleroderma closely.

NSF is a rare but life-threatening condition caused by fibrosis of the skin and connective tissues. It presents as rapidly progressing patches of discolouration, swelling and thickening of the skin, usually on the extremities. Later, there may be joint contractures and organ involvement. It has been reported to follow the use of gadolinium-containing contrast agents for MRI, particularly in patients with existing renal impairment, e.g. if the GFR is <30 mL/min. Pregnancy is a contraindication to the use of these agents, since fetal NSF may occur.

There is no effective treatment, but **plasmapheresis** (q.v.) has been reported to be helpful in some cases, and any measures that might improve renal function would be expected to improve the condition.

Scleredema is a separate condition comprising induration of the neck and back. It occurs in some obese diabetic patients and occasionally briefly after streptococcal pharyngitis.

It may respond to **corticosteroids**.

Bibliography

Cheung PP, Dorai Raj AK. Nephrogenic fibrosing dermopathy: a new clinical entity mimicking scleroderma. *Intern Med J* 2007; 37: 139.

Cowper SE, Robin HS, Steinberg SM, et al. Scleromyxedema-like cutaneous disease in renal-dialysis patients. *Lancet* 2000; 356: 1000.

Donohoe J. Scleroderma and the kidney. *Kidney* 1992; 41: 462.

Englert HJ, Manolios N. Systemic sclerosis: new hope for an unyielding disease. *Med J Aust* 2009; 191: 365.

Evans PC, Lambert N, Maloney S, et al. Long-term fetal microchimerism in peripheral blood mononuclear cell subsets in healthy women and women with scleroderma. *Blood* 1999; 93: 2033.

Hissaria P, Lester S, Hakendorf P, et al. Survival in scleroderma: results from the population-based South Australian register. *Intern Med J* 2011; 41: 381.

Phillips K. Scleroderma and related disorders. In: *Scientific American Medicine. Rheumatology.* Hamilton: Dekker Medicine. 2020.

Rasaratnam I, Ryan PFJ. Systemic sclerosis and the inflammatory myopathies. *Med J Aust* 1997; 166: 322.

Sahhar J, Littlejohn G, Conron M. Fibrosing alveolitis in systemic sclerosis. *Intern Med J* 2004; 34: 626.

Silver RM, Miller KS, Kinsella MB, et al. Evaluation and management of scleroderma lung disease using bronchoalveolar lavage. *Am J Med* 1990; 88: 470.

Sinnathurai P, Schrieber L. Treatment of Raynaud phenomenon in systemic sclerosis. *Intern Med J* 2013; 43: 476.

Steen VD. The lung in systemic sclerosis. *J Clin Rheumatol* 2005; 11: 40.

Steen VD, Medger TA. Long-term outcomes of scleroderma renal crisis *Ann Intern Med* 2000; 133: 600.

Tan FK, Arnett FC. Genetic factors in the etiology of systemic sclerosis and Raynaud phenomenon. *Curr Opin Rheumatol* 2000; 12: 511.

Scombroid

Scombroid poisoning is the commonest seafood poisoning worldwide. It is named after the Scombridae family of fish, which comprises over 50 species, including tuna, mackerel and bonito. These fish contain high concentrations of the amino acid histidine (in the dark meat), which enteric marine flora can degrade to form histamine, the likely toxin in this condition. This process arises when caught fish are not promptly cooled, and it can occur within even a few hours at room temperature. Once formed, the toxin is not destroyed by subsequent freezing, smoking or cooking.

The victim may note that the fish tasted metallic or peppery. The onset of symptoms is rapid with headache, flushing, pruritus (q.v.), gastrointestinal symptoms and occasionally bronchospasm. It generally lasts for no more than about 12 hr. It is a toxic rather than an allergic process.

*The administration of **antihistamines**, including H2 antagonists, are recommended for symptomatic relief. For severe symptoms, IV fluids, adrenaline (epinephrine) and corticosteroids are helpful.*

The condition is non-fatal and self-limited. In recent years, affected batches of canned tuna from South-East Asia, China and West Africa have been identified and confiscated by public health authorities in several countries.

See
- Food poisoning.

Bibliography
Morrow JD, Margolies GR, Rowland J, et al. Evidence that histamine is the causative toxin of scombroid-fish poisoning. *N. Engl J Med* 1991; 324: 716.

Scorpion stings See
- Bites and stings.

Scrotal fire See
- Gangrene.

Scurvy

Scurvy is due to vitamin C deficiency (q.v.) and is the oldest known nutritional disorder of humans. It was well described during the Crusades, and later it afflicted sailors during long voyages. It was recognized in 1753 as dietary in origin. Since vitamin C (ascorbic acid) cannot be synthesized endogenously (in humans), its source must be dietary.

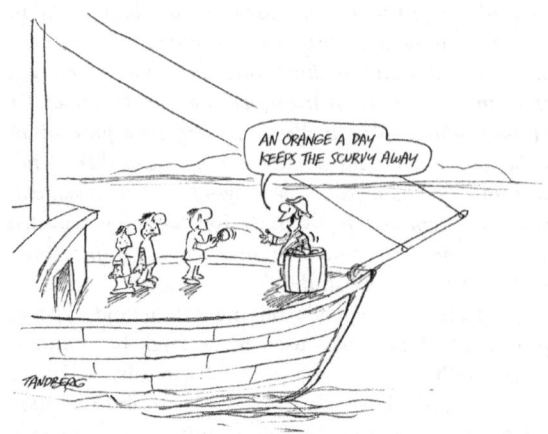

Vitamin C is required for the synthesis of collagen, so patients with scurvy have deficient supporting structures for small vessels. There is thus microvascular bleeding (especially of the gums), commonly with vascular purpura (q.v.) and sometimes with deep haematomas. Poor wound healing is typical. There are also abnormalities of the hair shafts and of keratinization.

Scurvy is commonly associated with other vitamin deficiencies (q.v.) and with malnutrition. It may also be related to some extreme dietary fads, even in a modern society.

The normal vitamin C level in serum is 40–100 μmol/L.

*Treatment is with **vitamin C** 1 g per day, to which there is a prompt response within days.*

Bibliography
Jones AR, Kumareswaran K. The scourge of C. *Med J Aust* 2018; 209: 62.
Levavasseur M, Becquart C, Pape E, et al. Severe scurvy: an underestimated disease. *Eur J Clin Nutr* 2015; 69: 1076.
Wallerstein RO, Wallerstein RO Jr. Scurvy. *Semin Hematol* 1976; 13: 211.

Selenium

Selenium (Se, atomic number 34, atomic weight 79) was discovered in 1818 and is related chemically and physically to sulphur, being intermediate between metals and non-metals. It is widely distributed in nature in small quantities, and it is ingested in grains, meats and seafood.

In the body, where it is present in a total amount of 10–20 mg, it is an essential trace element (q.v.) and acts as an antioxidant. Over the past decade, it has become apparent that, like iodine, selenium is required for normal thyroid metabolism (see Euthyroid sick syndrome).

Selenium deficiency has been reported to be associated with cardiomyopathy (q.v.), myositis (q.v.) and osteoarthropathy. Subsequently, it was appreciated that low selenium levels may occur in sepsis and trauma and that they are then associated with increased morbidity and mortality. Follow-up studies suggested that increased selenium supplementation might reduce mortality in septic patients, perhaps via an antioxidant effect, but this benefit was not confirmed in larger subsequent studies. Selenium supplementation has been found in preliminary studies to reduce substantially the risk of prostate cancer. This finding may explain some of the presumed environmental influence evident with this cancer because of its geographic heterogeneity. Selenium may be helpful in treating exophthalmos (see Hyperthyroidism).

In excess doses, selenium is highly toxic, with refractory vomiting, abdominal pain, salivation, haemolysis (q.v.), liver necrosis, pulmonary oedema (q.v.), coma and even death. In modest excess, it may cause unpleasant body odour in humans and 'blind staggers' in animals.

The normal plasma level is 0.8–1.2 µmol/L, and most is protein-bound. The daily requirement is 30–80 mcg orally, and the recommended IV dose is 0.4–1.5 µmol per day.

Bibliography

Alhazzini W, Jacobi J, Sindi A, et al. The effect of selenium therapy on mortality in patients with sepsis syndrome: a systematic review and meta-analysis of randomized controlled trials. *Crit Care Med* 2013; 41: 1555.

Angstwurm MW, Engelmann L, Zimmermann T, et al. Selenium in intensive care (SIC): results of a prospective randomized placebo-controlled multiple-center study in patients with severe systemic inflammatory response syndrome, sepsis and septic shock. *Crit Care Med* 2007; 35: 118.

Barceloux DG. Selenium. *J Toxicol Clin Toxicol* 1999; 37: 145.

Bar-Or D, Garrett RE. Is low plasma selenium concentration a true reflection of selenium deficiency and redox status in critically ill patients? *Crit Care Med* 2011; 39: 2000.

Berger MM, Cavadini C, Chiolero R, et al. Copper, selenium and zinc status and balances after major trauma. *J Trauma* 1996; 40: 103.

Brawley OW, Barnes S, Parnes H. The future of prostate cancer prevention. *Ann NY Acad Sci* 2001; 952: 145.

Daniels LA. Selenium: does selenium status have health outcomes beyond overt deficiency? *Med J Aust* 2004; 180: 373.

Diplock AT, Chaudhry FA. The relationship of selenium biochemistry to selenium-responsive disease in man. In: Prasad AS, ed. *Essential and Toxic Trace Elements in Human Health and Disease.* New York: Liss. 1988, p 211.

Forceville X. Selenium and the 'free' electron. *Intens Care Med* 2001; 27: 16.

Heyland DK, Dhaliwal R, Suchner U, et al. Antioxidant nutrients: a systematic review of trace elements and vitamins in the critically ill patient. *Intens Care Med* 2005; 31: 327.

Levander OA, Burk RF. ASPEN research workshop on selenium in clinical nutrition. *JPEN* 1986; 10: 545.

Rayman MP. The importance of selenium to human health. *Lancet* 2000; 356: 233.

Valenta J, Brodska H, Drabek T, et al. High-dose selenium substitution in sepsis: a prospective randomized clinical trial. *Intens Care Med* 2011; 37: 808.

Serositis

Serositis refers to inflammation of a serosal surface, i.e. pleura, pericardium or peritoneum. **Polyserositis** refers to inflammation of all the serosal surfaces. As inflammation is accompanied by fluid extravasation, there are typically pleural effusions (q.v.), pericardial effusion (q.v.) and abdominal ascites.

While such fluid accumulation may be associated with generalized oedema, as with cardiac, renal or liver failure, more specific polyserositis can be due to a number of uncommon conditions, including

- collagen-vascular diseases (q.v.), especially systemic lupus erythematosus (q.v.),
- familial Mediterranean fever (q.v.),
- HELLP syndrome (q.v.),
- Meig's syndrome, due to ovarian carcinoma,
- ovarian hyperstimulation syndrome (q.v.).

Serotonin syndrome

The 'serotonin syndrome' was first described in 1982 and comprises the acute onset of the triad of

- **altered mental state**, with agitation, confusion,
- **autonomic dysfunction**, with sweating (q.v.), shivering, fever (q.v.), diarrhoea (q.v.), postural hypotension,
- **increased neuromuscular activity**, with hyperreflexia, tremor, myoclonus.

It thus has some features in common with **carcinoid syndrome** (q.v.).

In severe cases, disseminated intravascular coagulation (q.v.), rhabdomyolysis (q.v.) and seizures may occur. Hyponatraemia due to the syndrome of inappropriate antidiuretic hormone secretion (q.v.) has been described.

Its incidence is uncertain; because the diagnosis can be difficult, mild cases may be overlooked and many of the culprit drugs are prescribed in general practice where familiarity with this complication may be limited. Recently, it has been calculated to occur in as many as 1 in 6 patients taking selective serotonin reuptake inhibitors (SSRIs), though its incidence has also been calculated as only 1 per 200 patient-years of treatment with SSRIs. It generally follows usual therapeutic doses rather than an overdose of the culprit drugs.

> Serotonin syndrome is produced by increased serotonergic neurotransmission due to increased release, decreased reuptake or catabolism, or direct activation. It is thus generally caused by a drug reaction involving one or more usually a combination of serotonergic agents, including
> - amphetamine and related compounds (q.v.),
> - SSRIs, e.g. fluoxetine, paroxetine, sertraline,
> - tricyclic antidepressants,
> - monoamine oxidase inhibitors, including methylene blue (q.v.),
> - anti-migraine agents (ergot-related drugs – q.v., sumatriptan and related 'triptan' drugs),
> - the synthetic opioids, pethidine and tramadol, especially in combination with SSRIs,
> - pseudoephedrine,
> - St John's Wort, a complementary medicine sometimes used to treat depression,
> - miscellaneous drugs, such as linezolid, lithium (q.v.).

Diagnosis is clinical, and there are no laboratory tests routinely available for confirmation. The diagnosis should be suspected in appropriate patients, even if the particular drug or drug combination has been taken for some weeks (average 5 weeks), because the time-course of action of some culprit drugs can be very long.

The differential diagnosis, in addition to the carcinoid syndrome (q.v.) referred to above, includes
- neuroleptic malignant syndrome (q.v.),
- malignant hyperthermia (q.v.),
- sepsis,
- tetanus (q.v.),
- meningoencephalitis (q.v.),
- hyperthyroidism (q.v.),
- anticholinergic overdose (q.v.),
- baclofen withdrawal (q.v.).

It usually responds rapidly to drug cessation and supportive care, and death is thus rare. Occasionally, it may be fulminating and require serotonin antagonist therapy, such as with **cyproheptadine** in particular (e.g. 4–8 mg IV 1–4 hrly). Methysergide, chlorpromazine, olanzapine or especially benzodiazepines may also be useful in this setting. Dantrolene and bromocriptine are contraindicated, and antipyretics and beta blockers are not effective.

Bibliography
Bienvenu OJ, Neufeld KJ, Needham DM. Treatment of four psychiatric emergencies in the intensive care unit. *Crit Care Med* 2012; 40: 2662.
Bodner RA, Lynch T, Lewis L, et al. Serotonin syndrome. *Neurology* 1995; 45: 219.
Boyer EW, Shannon M. The serotonin syndrome. *N Engl J Med* 2005; 352: 1112.
Chan BSH, Graudins A, Whyte IM, et al. Serotonin syndrome resulting from drug interactions. *Med J Aust* 1998; 169: 523.
Gillman PK. Serotonin syndrome: history and risk. *Fundam Clin Pharmacol* 1998; 12: 482.
Gillman PK. The serotonin syndrome and its treatment. *J Psychopharmacol* 1999; 13: 100.
Isbister GK, Buckley NA, Whyte IM. Serotonin toxicity: a practical approach to diagnosis and treatment. *Med J Aust* 2007; 187: 361.
Jones D, Story DA. Serotonin syndrome and the anaesthetist. *Anaesth Intens Care* 2005; 33: 181.
Lappin RI, Auchincloss EL. Treatment of the serotonin syndrome with cyproheptadine. *N Engl J Med* 1994; 331: 1021.
Mills KC. Serotonin syndrome: a clinical update. *Crit Care Clin* 1997; 13: 763.
Mokhlesi B, Leikin JB, Murray P, et al. Adult toxicology in critical care: part II: specific poisonings. *Chest* 2003; 123: 897.
Sternbach H. The serotonin syndrome. *Am J Psych* 1991; 148:705.

Serpins

Serpins (serine protease inhibitors) are a large group of protease inhibitors (i.e. antiproteases), including several of importance in coagulation, e.g. alpha$_1$-antitrypsin (q.v.), antithrombin (q.v.), heparin cofactor II (see Anticoagulants, see Thrombophilia) and protein C (q.v.).

Bibliography
Low RH, Zhang Q, McGowan S, et al. An overview of the serpin superfamily. *Genome Biol* 2006; 7: 216.

Serum sickness *See*
- Immune complex disease.
  See also
- Arthritis,
- Drug allergy,
- Lymphocytosis.

Severe acute respiratory syndrome

Severe acute respiratory syndrome (SARS) was first reported in November 2002 in China, from where it spread rapidly throughout South-East Asia over the next few months, with sporadic cases elsewhere in the world, most notably in Toronto, Canada. By the time the outbreak had subsided in mid-2003, the WHO has calculated that there had been over 8000 cases in 37 countries across 5 continents, with a mortality of about 10%. Subsequently, sporadic cases have been reported in laboratory workers.

It was found to be caused by a novel coronavirus (SARS-CoV), more familiar coronaviruses (q.v.) being the second most frequent cause of the common cold. The newly identified virus probably derived from wild animals (particularly palm civets) sold for meat in markets in Guangdong province in China. The original animal reservoir appears to have been in asymptomatic bats. The incubation period is usually 2–7 days but can be up to 10 days.

Clinical features initially reflect a non-specific febrile illness. After 3–7 days, respiratory symptoms occur, and this phase can progress to respiratory failure due to severe, refractory pneumonia, with bilateral involvement and a peak severity at 8–10 days. Pneumothorax (q.v.) is an important complication. Later, bronchiolitis obliterans and organizing pneumonia (see Interstitial pneumonias) may occur.

Diagnosis requires viral identification in nasopharyngeal aspirates or demonstration of a specific antibody response. Radiologically, the appearances can progress from patchy bronchopneumonia to resemble acute respiratory distress syndrome (ARDS) (q.v.).

Treatment of severe disease requires mechanical ventilation, but other modalities including antiviral agents (e.g. ribavirin), immune globulin and corticosteroids have been of undocumented value.

As the organism is highly infectious (primarily by the air-borne route), meticulous infection control is required to protect clinical staff and others at risk of exposure. The epidemic was controlled in 2003 by concerted public health measures, and detailed guidelines for future outbreaks of this or other potential epidemics have been published. The stimulus to develop a commercial vaccine may have been dampened by the absence of any further outbreaks.

Bibliography
Chan-Yeung M, Yu WC. Outbreak of severe acute respiratory syndrome in Hong Kong Special Administrative Region. *BMJ* 2003; 326: 850.
Christian MD, Poutanen SM, Loutfy MR, et al. Severe acute respiratory distress syndrome. *Clin Infect Dis* 2004; 38: 1420.
Ksiazek TG, Erdman D, Goldsmith CS, et al. A novel coronavirus associated with severe acute respiratory syndrome. *N Engl J Med* 2003; 348: 1953.
Li W, Shi Z, Yu M, et al. Bats are natural reservoirs of SARS-like coronaviruses. *Science* 2005; 310: 676.
Manocha S, Walley KR, Russell JA. Severe acute respiratory distress syndrome (SARS): a critical care perspective. *Crit Care Med* 2003; 31: 2684.
Peiris M, Anderson L, Osterhaus ADME, et al., eds. *Severe Acute Respiratory Syndrome: A Clinical Guide*. Oxford: Blackwell. 2005.
Poutanen SM, Low DE, Henry B, et al. Identification of severe acute respiratory syndrome in Canada. *N Engl J Med* 2003; 348: 1995.
Sprung CL, Cohen R, Adini B, eds. Recommendations and standard operating procedures for intensive care unit and hospital preparations for an influenza epidemic or mass disaster. Summary report of the European Society of Intensive Care Medicine's Task Force for intensive care unit triage during an influenza epidemic or mass disaster. *Intens Care Med* 2010; 36 (suppl. 1): S1.
Tan TK. How severe acute respiratory syndrome (SARS) affected the Department of Anaesthesia at Singapore General Hospital. *Anaesth Intens Care* 2004; 32: 394.
Tomlinson B, Cockram C. SARS: experience at Prince of Wales Hospital, Hong Kong. *Lancet* 2003; 361: 1486.
Tsang K, Zhong NS. SARS: pharmacotherapy. *Respirology* 2003; 8: S25.
Weinstein RA. Planning for epidemics – the lessons of SARS. *New Engl J Med* 2004; 350: 2332.

Sheehan's syndrome See

- Pituitary.

Short bowel syndrome

The **short bowel syndrome** occurs following extensive surgical removal of the small intestine usually for ischaemia or malignancy, though sometimes it may follow irradiation.

Malabsorption (q.v.) results, especially when the ileum is lost, because although the ileum can compensate for the loss of the jejunum, vice versa does not apply, especially for specialized absorption sites within the ileum for vitamin B_{12} (q.v.) and bile salts.

The predominant clinical feature is profuse diarrhoea (q.v.). This occurs because of the increased osmotic load, especially of carbohydrates. Steatorrhoea, weight loss, and vitamin or mineral deficiencies, may occur (see Vitamin deficiency, see Trace elements).

Treatment is with dietary control (i.e. small, frequent and readily absorbed meals), vitamin and mineral supplementation, and anti-diarrhoeal medication.

In severe cases, long-term parenteral nutrition is required. In these cases, dependence on parenteral nutrition may be reduced by the new agent, **teduglitide**, which is an analog of the peptide hormone, glucagon-like peptide-2 (GLP-2). GLP-2 is secreted by the L cells in the distal intestine and causes the release of growth factors which repair intestinal mucosa by enhancing the height of villi and the depth of crypts. Teduglitide is given in a dose of 0.05 mg/kg per day SC, but it may have multiple gastrointestinal side-effects including cancer risk so that routine colonoscopic screening is recommended.

See also
- Lactic acidosis,
- Nephrolithiasis.

Shy–Drager disease

Shy–Drager disease is a neurodegenerative disease of unknown aetiology described in 1960 as a condition with Parkinsonian, cerebellar and autonomic features, particularly with decreased sweating and postural hypotension. It has been recently renamed **multiple system atrophy** (MSA).

There is no specific treatment, and it is generally fatal in 7–8 yr.

See
- Sweating.

Sicca syndrome See
- Conjunctivitis,
- Hepatitis,
- Sarcoidosis,
- Sjogren's syndrome.

Sickle cell anaemia See
- Haemoglobin disorders.

See also
- Anaemia,
- High altitude,
- Priapism,
- Renal tubular acidosis.

Sideroblastic anaemia

Sideroblastic anaemia refers to a diverse group of conditions associated with ineffective erythropoiesis and thus anaemia (q.v.). The name derives from the presence in peripheral blood of normoblasts with iron-encrusted mitochondria, the so-called ringed sideroblasts. The peripheral blood film shows hypochromic, distorted red blood cells, but the iron-binding capacity is saturated.

> The following types may be found.
> 1. **Hereditary benign sideroblastic anaemia**
>   This can occur as either a sex-linked or autosomally inherited condition.
> 2. **Acquired benign sideroblastic anaemia**
>   This is seen in
>   - alcoholism,
>   - lead poisoning (q.v.),
>   - pyridoxine deficiency,
>   - use of anti-tuberculous drugs, such as isoniazid.
> 3. **Acquired malignant sideroblastic anaemia**
>   This is a myelodysplastic disorder, accompanied by neutropenia (q.v.) and thrombocytopenia (q.v.). It may evolve into a myeloproliferative disorder or acute myeloid leukaemia.

See also
- Reticulocytes.

Bibliography
Doll DC, List AF. Myelodysplastic syndromes. *Semin Oncol* 1992; 19: 1.
Jacobs A. Primary acquired sideroblastic anaemia. *Br J Haematol* 1986; 64: 415.

Silicosis See
- Occupational lung diseases – 1. Pneumoconiosis.

Situs inversus

Situs inversus refers to left–right reversal of the normal asymmetrical position of the body's internal organs. If this process involves just the heart, it is called isolated **dextrocardia**. Less complete disorders of laterality ('abnormal sidedness') are referred to as **situs ambiguous** or heterotaxy. These conditions are developmental disorders.

Situs inversus is a characteristic feature of **Kartagener's syndrome** (q.v.).

Sjogren's syndrome

Sjogren's syndrome is a chronic inflammatory condition involving the exocrine glands. It may be associated with other autoimmune diseases (q.v.), especially rheumatoid arthritis, but also systemic lupus erythematosus (q.v.) and scleroderma (q.v.). It is the second most common rheumatic disease of autoimmune cause after rheumatoid arthritis.

Since the changes can be subtle, its total incidence is uncertain, but its prevalence may be up to 1 in 100 of the population.

The pathology comprises an inflammatory cellular infiltrate of glandular tissue with associated acinar atrophy.

> Clinical manifestations are dominated by the **sicca syndrome**.
> - This comprises dry eyes and mouth, because the lacrimal and salivary glands are affected.
> - Sometimes, the respiratory tract is also dry, with hoarseness, bronchitis and pneumonia.
> - The skin and genital mucous membranes may be similarly affected.
>
> There may be associated myositis (q.v.), neuropathy (q.v.) and thyroiditis.
>
> Sometimes, there is concomitant biliary cirrhosis (q.v.), cryoglobulinaemia (q.v.), drug hypersensitivity (q.v.), pancreatitis (q.v.), renal tubular acidosis (q.v.), chronic hepatitis C infection (q.v.) or interstitial lung disease (q.v.).
>
> Neuropsychiatric abnormalities may be seen.

Investigations show decreased tear production, which can be conveniently assessed by the Schirmer filter paper test. There is filamentous keratitis on slit-lamp examination and conjunctival staining with Rose Bengal dye. There is decreased salivary flow, e.g. <0.5 mL/min from the parotid duct after lemon juice. Sialography may be useful, but salivary gland biopsy provides the gold standard for diagnosis if this remains uncertain after less invasive procedures. The ESR and IgG are increased. Rheumatoid factor is positive in most patients, antinuclear antibodies are often present in high titre with a speckled pattern, and antibodies to Ro(SS-A) and La(SS-B) are present in about 60% of patients. There is some genetic predisposition, with primary Sjogren's syndrome associated with HLA B8, DR3.

An unusual complication is lymphoid proliferation to produce either
- **pseudolymphoma**, if the proliferation is pleomorphic, or even
- non-Hodgkin's lymphoma.

Apart from this complication, the outcome in patients with Sjogren's syndrome is similar to that of the general population.

*Treatment is usually **symptomatic** with oral fluids and artificial tears. A multidisciplinary team approach to care is advised in complex cases.*

*Low-dose corticosteroids or hydroxychloroquine are occasionally indicated. Immunosuppression (q.v.), most recently with **rituximab** (q.v.), is a useful adjunct if severe manifestations are present.*

Bibliography

Hansen A, Lipsky PE, Dorner T. New concepts in the pathogenesis of Sjogren's syndrome: many questions, fewer answers. *Curr Opin Rheumatol* 2003; 15: 563.

Kassan SS, Moutsopoulos HM. Clinical manifestations and early diagnosis of Sjogren's syndrome. *Arch Intern Med* 2004; 164: 1275.

Lee AS, Scofield H, Hammitt KM, et al. Consensus guidelines for evaluation and management of pulmonary disease in Sjogren's. *Chest* 2021; 159: 683.

Parambil JG, Myers JL, Lindell RM, et al. Interstitial lung disease in primary Sjogren syndrome. *Chest* 2006; 130: 1489.

Patel R, Shahane A. The epidemiology of Sjogren's syndrome. *Clin Epidemiol* 2014; 6: 247.

Vivino FB. Sjogren's syndrome: clinical aspects. *Clin Immunol* 2017; 182: 48.

Skin necrosis

Warfarin-induced skin necrosis is a rare complication of coumarin therapy (see Warfarin), usually seen within the first 10 days of treatment in protein C deficient patients (q.v.). Red haemorrhagic bullae, which become necrotic and then scar, occur particularly on the breasts, thighs and buttocks of women and on the penis of men.

Heparin-induced skin necrosis is also rare and is similar to that seen after warfarin (see Heparin). It is presumed to be due to immune-mediated platelet aggregation, though the non-necrotic skin lesions seen after heparin administration are due to delayed hypersensitivity and not to HIT.

Skin necrosis is also a feature of a number of other toxic or inflammatory conditions
- see Bites and stings – Marine invertebrates, Marine vertebrates,
- see Calciphylaxis,
- see Gangrene – 1. Necrotizing fasciitis,
- see Purpura – Purpura fulminans.

Bibliography

Schindewolf M, Kroll H, Ackermann H, et al. Heparin-induced non-necrotizing skin lesions: rarely associated with heparin-induced thrombocytopenia. *J Thromb Haemost* 2010; 8: 1486.

Skin signs of internal malignant disease *See*

- Paraneoplastic syndromes.

Bibliography
Lebwohl M. Cutaneous manifestations of systemic diseases. In: *Scientific American Medicine. Dermatology.* Hamilton: Dekker Medicine. 2020.

SLE *See*

- Systemic lupus erythematosus.

Sleep *See*

- Circadian rhythm,
- Delirium,
- Melatonin,
- PADIS,
- Sleep disorders of breathing.

Sleep disorders of breathing

Sleep disorders of some degree have been reported to occur in the majority of people, even if healthy. However, they are especially common in patients with a variety of common medical disorders, including chronic lung or kidney disease, cancer, infectious diseases, neurological disorders, chronic pain syndromes, gastro-oesophageal reflux disease and menopause. Disordered sleep may become even more prominent when patients are hospitalized, and sleep deprivation is a main component in the constellation of distressful symptoms referred to as PADIS (q.v.) in critically ill patients. Properly structured sleep is clinically important, not just for psychological well-being but also for cardiovascular, metabolic and immune health.

> Sleep disorders include
> - insomnia,
> - various hypersomnias (including narcolepsy),
> - parasomnia,
> - sleep-related movement disorders,
> - **sleep-related breathing disorders**, i.e. the **sleep apnoea syndromes** (which are considered here).
>
> In some of these settings, there is the possibility of sleep-related violence, which then has forensic implications.

In addition, disordered breathing syndromes which are not primarily sleep-related become more marked during sleep, including

- **periodic and other abnormalities of breathing pattern**, and
- **primary alveolar hypoventilation**,

1. **Periodic breathing** is best known in the form of **Cheyne–Stokes respiration**, in which cycles occur of gradually increasing tidal volume followed by decreasing tidal volume and then transient apnoea, when the cycle is repeated.

   It is best explained by a lag in the normal control loop of ventilation. It is thus an expected feature of advanced cardiac disease with a prolonged circulation time. It is also seen in patients with central nervous system lesions involving the deep structures in the cerebral hemispheres and basal ganglia, as in ischaemia or encephalopathy (q.v.). For uncertain reasons, it may be seen during haemodialysis, in chronic pulmonary disease and in some normal subjects, e.g. at altitude (q.v.).

   Other related abnormal breathing patterns include
   - random, ataxic or Biot's breathing
     - due to medullary, pontine or cerebellar lesions, usually haemorrhage or trauma,
     - in these cases, apnoea is readily produced by sedatives or narcotics,
   - apneustic breathing
     - due to lower pontine lesions and characterized by an end-inspiratory pause.

2. **Primary alveolar hypoventilation** is usually due to a brainstem lesion, commonly vascular or inflammatory, though it may sometimes be congenital. However, even autopsy is usually unable to identify a specific structural abnormality.
   There is
   - hypoxaemia,
   - hypercapnia,
   - grossly impaired ventilatory response to carbon dioxide, hypoxia and exercise,
   - normal pulmonary function,
   - normal neuromuscular function,
   - normal chest wall,
   - normal blood gases on voluntary hyperventilation.

   Clinical features include headache, lethargy and somnolence but not dyspnoea. There is cyanosis, polycythaemia (q.v.) and cor pulmonale.

   > The extreme of the condition has been picturesquely **Ondine's curse**. When associated with obesity and often also obstructive sleep apnoea (see below), it is sometimes referred to as the **Pickwickian syndrome** or the **obesity–hypoventilation syndrome (OHS)**. The current worldwide epidemic of obesity has led to an increase in the recognition of this condition.

3. The **sleep apnoea syndromes** comprise those impairments of breathing, either hypoventilation or

frank apnoea, that occur chiefly or solely during sleep. They are classified as either central or obstructive (or both). The sleep-related hypoventilation and hypoxaemia syndromes are nowadays incorporated into the wider International Classification of Sleep Disorders.

- **Central sleep apnoea** (CSA) is due to impaired respiratory drive, which can arise from a number of mechanisms, including narcotic drugs, obesity and high-altitude (q.v.). Decreased respiratory drive during sleep is commonly due to modern polypharmacy.

When hypoventilation occurs in the setting of obesity without obstruction (as in pure OHS), there are often abnormal respiratory mechanics (i.e. 'can't' breathe as well as, or instead of, 'won't' breathe). The changes during sleep which lead to abnormal respiratory mechanics include decreased upper airway patency, position, decreased functional residual capacity (FRC) and muscle hypotonia. These changes are exacerbated in patients with pre-existing chronic airways obstruction, neuromuscular disease or chest wall abnormality.

- **Obstructive sleep apnoea** (OSA) is the severe end (and chronic snoring is the mild end) of the spectrum of conditions referred to as sleep-disordered breathing (SDB) due to increased upper airway resistance. OSA is commonly associated with OHS (see above) or with chronic obstructive airways disease. It probably affects over 5% of the population, though about 90% of cases are calculated to be undiagnosed. On the other hand, the mere presence of OSA does not necessarily imply clinical relevance in any particular patient.

The sleep apnoea syndromes are most commonly due to upper airway obstruction, though the cause may be sometimes either central or a combination of both mechanisms, as described above. Although most patients are overweight middle-aged men, the condition is in fact widespread, as described above.

It may also occur as a new phenomenon in patients discharged from Intensive Care after prolonged mechanical ventilation.

Although the sleep apnoea syndromes are heterogeneous with varying phenotypes, clinical features are dominated by
- somnolence during the daytime (also called excessive daytime sleepiness or EDS)
  - due to nocturnal sleep fragmentation and sleep deprivation,
  - causing fatigue, inattention, irritability, proneness to error (e.g. at work or driving),
  - with impaired cognition, memory, general functioning and quality of life,
  - also commonly associated with depression,
- snoring, restlessness and apnoeic episodes during the night
  - observed by bed partners,
- the longer-term consequences of repeated asphyxia
  - polycythaemia (q.v.), hypercapnia, cor pulmonale, intellectual deterioration, sexual dysfunction, headache,
- cardiovascular consequences
  - arrhythmias, hypertension, an increased incidence of acute myocardial infarction and stroke.

Pathogenetic mechanisms, generally worse during REM-sleep in most patients, include relaxation of the muscles of the upper airway during sleep (a process exacerbated by alcohol or sedative drugs), decreased ventilatory response to carbon dioxide during sleep, or pathological abnormalities of the upper airway, chest wall or neuromuscular function. Sedative drugs impair the arousal response to obstruction, i.e. hypoxaemia and hypercapnia, and they thus prolong the apnoeic episodes.

The diagnosis is suggested by clinical suspicion based on the constellation of features described above, but it should be confirmed by formal polysomnography in a sleep laboratory. Such studies show that sleep disruption with apnoea and arousal may occur up to 60 times or more per hour. Various numeric indices may be used to quantify the respiratory disturbances caused by sleep apnoea, including the number of apnoeas per hour, the number of desaturations per hour, the number of arousals per hour and the proportion of sleep spent snoring.

Treatment options include
- *cessation of alcohol and sedatives,*
- *weight control,*
- *attention to any local pathology, e.g. tonsillar hypertrophy,*
- *exclusion of hypothyroidism (q.v.),*
- *avoidance of androgens,*
- *use of drugs, such as acetazolamide (see Carbonic anhydrase inhibitors), medroxyprogesterone (a respiratory stimulant), protryptyline (to decrease REM-sleep), modafinil (to promote daytime wakefulness), or more recently solriamfetol (a dopamine-noradrenaline*

reuptake inhibitor) and pitolisant (a histamine H3 agonist) to treat the EDS component,
- low-flow oxygen if hypoxaemia is the dominant consequence,
- **nasal continuous positive airway pressure (CPAP)**, the most dramatically effective measure, even in non-obstructive cases,
- other mechanical aids, but those available are generally less effective than CPAP,
- nasal (non-invasive) positive pressure ventilation (NIPPV) or variants (e.g. bilevel positive pressure) in severe cases,
- attention to non-obstructive causes,
- **surgery**, which is occasionally indicated, usually tracheostomy but sometimes uvulopalatopharyngoplasty (UPPP), though the results are often disappointing and there is an absence of good trial data,
- neurostimulatory techniques, a variety of which are currently being explored.

OSA is of particular relevance to Intensive Care practice, because increasing numbers of such patients are having elective surgery and many may need short-term ICU admission postoperatively to optimize their oxygenation, positive pressure therapy and analgesia. While this need may be apparent preoperatively, in many patients OSA has not been previously diagnosed and respiratory problems become apparent only in the post-anaesthetic care area (recovery room), resulting then in an urgent rather than elective ICU admission.

See also
- Melatonin.

Bibliography

Aldrich MS. Narcolepsy. *Neurology* 1992; 42 (suppl.): 34.

Benjafield AV, Ayas NT, Eastwood PR, et al. Estimation of the global prevalence and burden of obstructive sleep apnoea: a literature-based analysis. *Lancet Respir Med* 2019; 7: 687.

Bradley TD, Floras JS. Obstructive sleep apnoea and its cardiovascular consequences. *Lancet* 2009; 373: 82.

Burwell CS, Robin ED, Whaley RD, et al. Extreme obesity associated with alveolar hypoventilation: a Pickwickian syndrome. *Am J Med* 1956; 21: 811.

Canto RG, Zwillich CW. Central sleep apnea. Pulmonary *Perspectives* 1993; 10(3): 4.

Casey KR, Cantillo KO, Brown LK. Sleep-related hypoventilation/hypoxemic syndromes. *Chest* 2007; 131: 1936.

Chan ASL, Phillips CL, Cistulli PA. Obstructive sleep apnoea – an update. *Intern Med J* 2010; 40: 102.

Chan CS, Grunstein RR, Bye PT, et al. Obstructive sleep apnea with severe chronic airflow limitation. *Am Rev Respir Dis* 1989; 140: 1274.

Cherniack NS, Longobardo GS. Cheyne–Stokes breathing: instability in physiologic control. *N Engl J Med* 1973; 288: 952.

Chishti A, Batchelor AM, Bullock RE, et al. Sleep-related breathing disorders following discharge from intensive care. *Intens Care Med* 2000; 26: 426.

Chokroverty S. Sleep disorders. In: *Scientific American Medicine*. Neurology, Psychiatry. Hamilton: Dekker Medicine. 2020.

Douglas JA, Chai-Coetzer cl, McEvoy D, et al. Guidelines for sleep studies in adults: a position statement of the Australasian Sleep Association. *Sleep Med* 2017; 36: S2.

Dyken ME, Afifi AK, Lin-Dyken DC. Sleep-related problems in neurologic diseases. *Chest* 2012; 141: 528.

Eastwood PR, Malhotra A, Palmer LJ, et al. Obstructive sleep apnoea: from pathogenesis to treatment: current controversies and future directions. *Respirology* 2010; 15: 587.

Eckert DJ, Jordan AS, Merchia P, et al. Central sleep apnea: pathophysiology and treatment. *Chest* 2007; 131: 595.

Exar EN, Collop NA. The upper airway resistance syndrome. *Chest* 1999; 115: 1127.

Fishman AP, Goldring RM, Turino GM. General alveolar hypoventilation: a syndrome of respiratory and cardiac failure in patients with normal lungs. *Q J Med* 1966; 35: 261.

Flemons WW. Obstructive sleep apnea. *N Engl J Med* 2002; 347: 498.

Hamilton GS, Solin P, Naughton MT. Obstructive sleep apnoea and cardiovascular disease. *Intern Med J* 2004; 34: 420.

Holt NR, Downey G, Naughton MT. Perioperative considerations in the management of obstructive sleep apnoea. *Med J Aust* 2019; 211: 326.

Hudgel DW, Thanakitcharu S. Pharmacologic treatment of sleep-disordered breathing. *Am J Respir Crit Care Med* 1998; 158: 691.

Ingbar DH, Gee JBL. Pathophysiology and treatment of sleep apnea. *Annu Rev Med* 1985; 36: 369.

Javaheri S, Javaheri S. Update on persistent excessive daytime sleepiness in OSA. *Chest* 2020; 158: 776.

Johns MW. A new method for measuring daytime sleepiness: the Epworth sleepiness scale. *Sleep* 1991; 14: 540.

Jordan AS, McSharry DG, Malhotra A. Adult obstructive sleep apnoea. *Lancet* 2014; 383: 736.

Kales A, Vela-Bueno A, Kales JD. Sleep disorders: sleep apnea and narcolepsy. *Ann Intern Med* 1987; 106: 434.

Kessler R, Chaouat A, Schinkewitch P, et al. The obesity-hypoventilation syndrome revisited. *Chest* 2001; 120: 369.

Khan Z, Trotti LM. Central disorders of hypersomnolence. *Chest* 2015; 148: 262.

Krachman SL, D'Alonzo GE, Griner JG. Sleep in the intensive care unit. *Chest* 1995; 107: 1713.

Kushida CA, ed. *Obstructive Sleep Apnea (2 volumes)*. Boca Raton: CRC Press LLC. 2007.

Lang AO, ed. *Sleep Apnea Syndrome Research Focus*. New York: Nova Science. 2007.

Levenson JC, Kay DB, Buysse DJ. The pathophysiology of insomnia. *Chest* 2015; 147: 1179.

Mansfield DR, McEvoy RD, eds. Sleep disorders: a practical guide for Australian health care practitioners. *Med J Aust* 2013; 199 (suppl. 8): S1.

McEvoy RD, Antic NA, Heeley E, et al. CPAP for prevention of cardiovascular events in obstructive sleep apnea. *N Engl J Med* 2016; 375: 919.

McNicholas WT. Sleep apnoea and driving risk. *Eur Respir J* 1999; 13: 1225.

McNicholas WT, Philipson EA. *Breathing Disorders in Sleep*. London: WB Saunders. 2002.

McNicholas WT, Ryan S. Obstructive sleep apnoea syndrome: translating science to clinical practice. *Respirology* 2006; 136: 144.

Mohammadieh A, Sutherland K, Cistulli PA. Sleep disordered breathing: management update. *Intern Med J* 2017; 47: 1241.

Mokhlesi B, Tulaimat A. Recent advances in obesity hypoventilation syndrome. *Chest* 2008; 132: 1322.

Naughton M, Pierce R. *Snoring, Sleep Apnoea and Other Sleep Problems*. 2nd edition. Spring Hill: Australian Lung Foundation. 2000.

Neill AM, McEvoy RD. Obstructive sleep apnoea and other sleep breathing disorders. *Med J Aust* 1997; 167: 376.

O'Keefe ST. Restless legs syndrome: a review. *Arch Intern Med* 1996; 156: 243.

Overeem S, Mignor E, Van Dijk, et al. Narcolepsy: clinical features, new pathophysiologic insights and future prospects. *J Clin Neurophysiol* 2001; 18: 78.

Pack AI. Obstructive sleep apnea. *Adv Intern Med* 1994; 39: 517.

Pack AI. *Sleep Apnea: Pathogenesis, Diagnosis, and Treatment*. Lung Biology in Health & Disease – Volume 166. New York: Marcel Dekker. 2002.

Parish JM. Sleep-related problems in common medical conditions. *Chest* 2009; 135: 563.

Patil SP, Schneider H, Schwartz AR, et al. Adult obstructive sleep apnea: pathophysiology and diagnosis. *Chest* 2007; 132: 325.

Phillips B. Sleep apnea and public health. *Pulmonary Perspectives* 2005; 22 (4): 1.

Phillips B, Naughton MT. *Obstructive Sleep Apnea*. Basel: Health Press. 2004.

Powell NB, Riley RW, Robinson A. Surgical management of obstructive sleep apnea syndrome. *Clin Chest Med* 1998; 19: 77.

Ray CS, Sue DY, Bray G, et al. Effects of obesity on respiratory function. *Am Rev Respir Dis* 1983; 128: 501.

Riley RW, Powell NB. Maxillofacial surgery and obstructive sleep apnea syndrome. *Otolaryngol Clin North Am* 1990; 23: 809.

Saunders NA, Sullivan CE, eds. *Sleep and Breathing. Lung Biology in Health and Disease,* Vol 21. New York: Marcel Dekker. 1984.

Severinghaus JW, Mitchell RA. Ondine's curse – failure of respiratory center automaticity while awake. *Clin Res* 1962; 10: 122.

Schmickl CN, Landry SA, Orr JE, et al. Acetazolamide for OSA and central sleep apnea: a comprehensive systematic review and meta-analysis. *Chest* 2020; 158: 2632.

Strohl KP, Redline S. Nasal CPAP therapy, upper airway muscle activation, and obstructive sleep apnea. *Am Rev Respir Dis* 1986; 134: 555.

Strollo PJ, Rogers RM. Obstructive sleep apnea. *N Engl J Med* 1996; 334: 99.

Strollo PJ, Soose RJ, Maurer JT, et al. Upper-airway stimulation for obstructive sleep apnea. *N Engl J Med* 2014; 370: 139.

Sullivan CE, Issa FG, Berthon-Jones M, et al. Reversal of obstructive sleep apnoea by continuous positive airway pressure applied through the nares. *Lancet* 1981; 1: 862.

Venkateshiah SB, Collop NA. Sleep and sleep disorders in the hospital. *Chest* 2012; 141: 1337.

Young T, Palta M, Dempsey J, et al. The occurrence of sleep-disordered breathing among middle-aged adults. *N Engl J Med* 1993; 328: 1230.

Weingarten JA, Collop NA. Air travel: effects of sleep deprivation and jet lag. *Chest* 2013; 144: 1394.

Worsnop C, Pierce R, McEvoy RD. Obstructive sleep apnoea. *Aust NZ J Med* 1998; 28: 421.

Smallpox See
- Germ warfare.

Smoke inhalation See
- Cyanide,
- Inhalation injury.

Snake bites See
- Bites and stings.
  See also
- Anaemia – 2. Anaemia due to haemolysis,
- Purpura,
- Rhabdomyolysis.

Sodium nitroprusside See
- Cyanide.
  See also
- Amphetamines,
- Aortic dissection,
- Lactic acidosis,
- Phaeochromocytoma.

Somatomedin C See
- Acromegaly.

Somatostatin

Somatostatin (SST) inhibits the release of growth hormone (and also to some extent the release of TSH and LH) by the anterior pituitary (q.v.). It is secreted by the hypothalamus for this purpose.

However, it is also secreted by cells elsewhere in the body, including delta cells in the pancreas (where alpha cells secrete glucagon and beta cells secrete insulin), epithelial cells in the gastrointestinal tract and myenteric neural plexus cells. Thus, it has a broad range of actions related to pancreatic and gastrointestinal function, via the inhibition of the secretion of insulin, glucagon and gastrointestinal hormones (gastrin, cholecystokinin and others), with resultant decrease in gastric acid production, gastrointestinal motility, pancreatic function, biliary flow and nutrient absorption.

Somatostatin exists as 28 and 14 amino acid peptides, and it acts via a specific family of SST receptors. It is impractical as a therapeutic agent, since it has a short half-life of <5 min, so that a number of analogs have been prepared. The best-known analog is **octreotide** (q.v.), an 8 amino acid peptide, which comprises the C-terminal ring of SST and which has a half-life of 1–2 hr. Octreotide is mostly metabolized by the liver, but about one third is excreted unchanged in the urine.

Octreotide offers therapeutic options in a wide variety of conditions, including
- acromegaly (q.v.),
- carcinoid syndrome (q.v.) and other neuroendocrine disorders,
- chylous pleural effusion, by decreasing the production of chyle (see Pleural effusion),
- secretory diarrhoea, such as that due to hormone-producing gastrointestinal tumours (see Diarrhoea),
- glucagonoma (q.v.),
- hepatorenal syndrome (q.v.), in combination with vasopressin (see Desmopressin),
- hypoglycaemia due to sulphonylurea (sulfonylurea) overdose in regions where these drugs are still commonly used for diabetes,
- variceal bleeding, with similar efficacy to vasopressin (see Desmopressin).

Octreotide is generally given in doses of 50–200 mcg SC tds or 50 mcg/hr IV (but see the individual conditions listed above).

The side-effects of octreotide are usually minor, with occasional abdominal symptoms, headache, fatigue or hyperglycaemia. Tolerance may develop with prolonged dosage (e.g. >1 month).
  See also
- Ectopic hormone production,
- Paraneoplastic syndromes – 2. Ectopic hormone production,
- Pituitary.

Bibliography
Chan MM, Chan MM, Mengshol JA, et al. Octreotide. *Chest* 2013; 114: 1937.
Lamberts SW, van der Lely AJ, de Herder WW, et al. Octreotide. *N Engl J Med* 1996; 334: 246.

Spider bites See
- Bites and stings.
  See also
- Gangrene –1. Necrotizing fasciitis,
- Sweating,
- Tetanus.

Splenomegaly

Splenomegaly may be caused by
- **congestion**, due to
  - portal or splenic vein obstruction,
  - hepatic cirrhosis,
  - cardiac failure,

- **infectious diseases**, either
  - generalized, e.g. malaria (q.v.), infectious mononucleosis (see Epstein–Barr virus),
  - local and granulomatous, e.g. tuberculosis (q.v.),
- **connective tissue disorders**, such as
  - collagen-vascular diseases (q.v.),
  - vasculitis (q.v.),
- **infiltrations**, such as
  - sarcoidosis (q.v.),
  - amyloid (q.v.),
  - lipoidosis,
- **neoplasia**, particularly
  - lymphoma, which is often associated with non-tender lymphadenopathy (q.v.),
  - myeloproliferative disorders,
- **haemolytic diseases**.

See also
- Hypersplenism.

Bibliography
Bohnsack JF, Brown EJ. The role of the spleen in resistance to infection. *Annu Rev Med* 1986; 37: 49.
Rose WF. The spleen as a filter. *N Engl J Med* 1987; 317: 704.

Spondyloarthritis

Spondyloarthritis refers to combined sacroiliitis and peripheral arthropathy (q.v.). Although the chief such condition is **ankylosing spondylitis** (q.v.), other diseases may cause a similar condition and indeed there may be considerable overlap between them. Sometimes, the specific type is difficult to characterize and the term 'undifferentiated spondyloarthritis' is used. They are associated with the major histocompatibility complex class I molecule (q.v.), the human leukocyte antigen HLA-B27. They are typically 'seronegative', i.e. there are no IgM autoantibodies to IgG (rheumatoid factor). There is a probable inflammatory pathogenesis, most obviously found in **reactive arthritis** (see below).

The other causes of spondyloarthritis include
- **enteropathic** spondyloarthritis,
  - associated with Crohn's disease (q.v.) or ulcerative colitis (q.v.),
- **psoriatic** spondyloarthritis (see Psoriasis),
- **Reiter's syndrome** (q.v.),
- **reactive arthritis**,
  - occurring after various infections, but without direct microbial joint invasion (see Arthritis),
  - best regarded as a limited form of Reiter's syndrome (q.v.),
- possibly **Behcet's syndrome** (q.v.),
- possibly **Whipple's disease** (q.v.).

Bibliography
Kahn MA, ed. Spondyloarthropathies. *Curr Opin Rheumatol* 1994; 6: 351.
Khan MA. Update on spondyloarthropathies. *Ann Intern Med* 2002; 136: 896.
Maksymowych WP. Seronegative spondyloarthritis. In: *Scientific American Medicine. Rheumatology*. Hamilton: Dekker Medicine. 2020.
McEwen C, DiTata D, Lingg C, et al. Ankylosing spondylitis and spondylitis accompanying ulcerative colitis, regional enteritis, psoriasis and Reiter's disease. *Arthritis Rheum* 1971; 14: 291.
Reveille JD. HLA-B27 and the seronegative spondyloarthropathies. *Am J Med Sci* 1998; 316: 239.
Reveille JD, Arnett FC. Spondyloarthritis: update on pathogenesis and management. *Am J Med* 2005; 118: 592.
Robinson PC, Benham H. Advances in classification, basic mechanisms and clinical science in ankylosing spondylitis and axial spondyloarthritis. *Intern Med J* 2015; 45: 127.
Sheehan NJ. The ramifications of HLA-B27. *J R Soc Med* 2004; 97: 10.
Stafford L, Youssef PP. Spondyloarthropathies: a review. *Intern Med J* 2002; 32: 40.

Spotted fevers *See*
- Rickettsial diseases.

Sprue-like enteropathy *See*
- Coeliac disease,
- Renin–angiotensin–aldosterone.

Staphylococcal scalded skin syndrome *See*
- Exfoliative dermatitis.

Star fruit poisoning

Star fruit (carambola) is a tropical fruit from Asia, but it is now readily available in markets worldwide. It has purported health benefits due to its content of vitamin C and antioxidants. In addition, like grapefruit, it can inhibit cytochrome P450 and thus increase the effective dosage of some drugs, including benzodiazepines and statins (q.v.).

Star fruit are rich in oxalic acid and thus predispose to nephrolithiasis (q.v.) due to the formation of calcium oxalate stones. More seriously, **neurotoxicity** from star fruit intoxication can readily occur in patients with even moderate renal impairment, especially when there is concomitant dehydration. This is manifest by confusion, hiccups and seizures, and it carries a serious prognosis.

Treatment with conventional anticonvulsants is poorly effective, and **renal replacement therapy** is required.

Bibliography
Herbland A, El Zein I, Valentino R, et al. Star fruit poisoning is potentially life-threatening in patients with moderate chronic renal failure. *Intens Care Med* 2009; 35: 1459.

Statins

Statins is the generic name for the group of HMG-CoA reductase inhibitors which, as lipid-lowering agents, have become an integral part of the management of cardiovascular disease for the past several decades. These drugs include atorvastatin, fluvastatin, lovastatin, pravastatin, rosuvastatin and simvastatin.

However, despite their undoubted benefits in this setting, a variety of uncommon side-effects have been reported, particularly related to liver dysfunction and muscle damage (see Myopathy, see Neuropathy, see Rhabdomyolysis).

Interestingly, statins have been increasingly recognized to have pleiotropic effects (q.v.), independent of their lipid-lowering properties. Clinically, they have been found to have favourable effects on endothelial and immune function. Thus, they have shown probable benefit in conditions as diverse as antiphospholipid syndrome (q.v.), autoinflammatory diseases (see familial Mediterranean fever), bronchiectasis (q.v.), Raynaud's phenomenon/disease (q.v.), sepsis and vasospasm in subarachnoid haemorrhage.

Stevens–Johnson syndrome *See*

- Erythema multiforme,
- Exfoliative dermatitis.
  See also
- Conjunctivitis,
- Dengue,
- Mouth diseases – 3. Stomatitis,
- Systemic diseases and the lung,
- Toxic shock syndrome,
- Ulcers.

Still's disease

Adult-onset **Still's** (or **Still**) **disease** (AOSD) is a generalized inflammatory condition of unknown aetiology. Formerly regarded as a systemic variant of rheumatoid arthritis, it is now considered to have an autoimmune origin (see Autoimmune disorders). It is more commonly seen in children, in whom it is nowadays referred to as idiopathic juvenile arthritis.

Clinical features include fever, rash, arthritis (q.v.), lymphadenopathy (q.v.), hepatosplenomegaly and pleuropericarditis, as in the **haemophagocytic syndrome** (q.v.).

Treatment is with **NSAIDs** in mild disease and with **corticosteroids** in more severe disease. Biologic **disease-modifying anti-rheumatic drugs** (DMARDs) are recommended in severe or refractory cases (see Immunomodulation).

Stings *See*

- Bites and stings.

Stomatitis *See*

- Mouth diseases.

Storage disorders

Storage disorders (lysosomal storage disorders, LSDs) are one of the groups of inborn errors of metabolism (q.v.). They are inherited disorders with an overall prevalence of about 2 per 10,000 live births. They result in defects of monocyte/macrophage function. These cells normally scavenge cellular debris, a process which involves their lysosomes. Mutations involve lysosomal proteins (particularly enzymes), causing defects of lysosomal constituents (e.g. hydrolases) and thus resulting in storage abnormalities. The accumulated substrates are then responsible for cellular dysfunction and damage.

These rare disorders are classified according to the composition of the retained product, which include glycoproteins, mucopolysaccharides, neutral lipids and sphingolipids. There is thus considerable biochemical heterogeneity among the various LSDs. Of the almost 50 such disorders described to date, the most common are Gaucher's disease (q.v.) and Fabry's disease (q.v.).

Bibliography
Beutler E, Gelbart T. Glucocerebrosidase (Gaucher disease). *Hum Mutat* 1996; 8: 207.
Charrow J, Esplin JA, Gribble TJ, et al. Gaucher disease: recommendations on diagnosis, evaluation and monitoring. *Arch Intern Med* 19 98; 158: 1754.
Meikle PJ, Hopwood JJ, Clague AE, et al. Prevalence of lysosomal storage disorders. *JAMA* 1999; 281: 249.
Various. Treatable lysosomal storage diseases in the advent of disease-specific therapy. *Intern Med J* 2020; 50 (suppl 4).
Wenger DA, Copploa S, Liu SL. Insights into the diagnosis and treatment of lysosomal storage diseases. *Arch Neurol* 2003; 60: 322.

Stridor *See*

- Asthma.

Strontium

Strontium (Sr, atomic number 38, atomic weight 88) is a soft metal like lead with a relatively low melting point. It is an alkaline-earth metal and is chemically related to (and intermediate between) calcium (q.v.) and barium. Its biological properties are closest to those of calcium.

Strontium does not occur free in nature and was first isolated by Davy in 1808. Its compounds have limited commercial value, because the corresponding compounds of calcium or barium are more readily available and serve similar purposes. They are, however, used in pyrotechnics, including red flares.

Strontium isotopes are the main health hazard from the radioactive fallout after nuclear explosions. Their harmful effects are primarily due to their replacement of calcium in bones, where they produce long-lived radiation (e.g. from ^{90}Sr) which is damaging to the bone marrow and is carcinogenic. Therapeutically, controlled isotopes of strontium (e.g. ^{89}Sr) can be used in radiotherapy for bone metastases. Commercially, they are used in the generation of electricity in small lightweight power sources for remote locations.

There is no biological requirement for strontium, and thus there is no defined daily intake or level in the body.

Strontium ranelate is marketed for the treatment of osteoporosis. In postmenopausal women, it reduces the risk of vertebral fractures. It is given in a dose of 2 g per day. It is contraindicated in patients with renal impairment. Serious adverse reactions have been reported, including both venous thromboembolism and acute myocardial infarction, and a syndrome of severe skin rash, eosinophilia (q.v.) and systemic symptoms. The latter complication may be steroid-responsive.

Bibliography
Burlet N, Reginster JY. Strontium ranelate: the first dual acting treatment for postmenopausal osteoporosis. *Clin Orthop Relat Res* 2006; 443: 55.
Friedland J. Local and systemic radiation for palliation of metastatic disease. *Urol Clin North Am* 1999; 26: 391.
O'Donnell S, Cranney A, Wells GA, et al. Strontium ranelate for preventing and treating postmenopausal osteoporosis. *Cochrane Database Syst Rev* 2006; 4: CD005326.

Strychnine

Strychnine is an alkaloid (q.v.) which was discovered in 1818 in the woody vine called St Ignatius' beans, *Strychnos ignatii*, in the Philippines. It also occurs in the seeds of the Indian tree *S. nux-vomica*. It is a very bitter substance and was used until the early 1900s as a tonic or cathartic in medicinals, usually in doses of about 2–5 mg. Its common clinical use at the time was paralleled by its frequency in suicide and homicide. Now, however, it is used only as a rodent poison in agriculture, so that human toxicity is rare. The average lethal dose is 100 mg.

It is rapidly absorbed, and having a low protein-binding it is also rapidly cleared, 80% being metabolized by the liver and 20% excreted unchanged in the urine. The urine thus provides the best sample for clinical measurement.

Neurological toxicity is rapid (within 10–30 min) and dramatic. Since strychnine blocks the inhibitory neurones in the thalamus, brainstem and spinal cord, it produces a hyperexcitable state with powerful spasms and fits and eventually death from brainstem paralysis. There is facial stiffness, trismus and opisthotonos. Tetanic contraction of the respiratory muscles produces apnoea. A series of fits each followed by exhaustion lasts several hours. Since the patient is awake during these episodes, there is considerable somatic and psychic discomfort. Death occurs primarily from respiratory failure. There may be associated lactic acidosis (q.v.), rhabdomyolysis (q.v.) and even fractures.

The differential diagnosis includes epilepsy, tetanus (q.v.) and rabies (q.v.).

*Treatment consists of **sedation**, particularly with a benzodiazepine.*

- *Muscle relaxation and mechanical ventilation are usually required, together with cardiovascular and metabolic support.*
- *Dialysis is not effective.*

If the patient survives for 6 hours, i.e. the usual period of seizures, total recovery is the rule.

Bibliography
Ball CM, Featherstone PJ. Pharmacological treatment of shock – strychnine. *Anaesth Intens Care* 2017; 45: 3.

Sturge–Weber syndrome

Sturge–Weber syndrome (encephalo-trigeminal angiomatosis) is a rare neurocutaneous disorder most obviously manifest by a craniofacial naevus, which is a port-wine stain (naevus flammaeus or capillary angioma) of the face. It involves the skin innervated by the first branch of the trigeminal nerve and is due to dilated capillaries in the dermis. Although it is apparent at birth, after puberty the lesion becomes thicker and more nodular, and little regression occurs.

Neurological features include contralateral fits from ipsilateral leptomeningeal and cortical angiomatosis, usually in the parieto-occipital region. There may also be hemiparesis and hemianopia, as well as mental retardation. There is commonly ipsilateral glaucoma.

*Treatment is **symptomatic**, apart possibly from laser therapy for the skin lesion.*

See also
- Tuberous sclerosis (another rare inherited neurocutaneous disorder).

Subacute sclerosing panencephalitis *See*
- Encephalitis.

Sucralfate *See*
- Aluminium
- Hypothyroidism.

Sweating

Sweating is an important physiological mechanism of temperature control. However, pathological abnormalities are frequent.

Decreased sweating occurs in the following:

- Autonomic nervous system disease.
  - This is usually part of diabetic or alcoholic peripheral neuropathy (q.v.) and is associated with other neurological features, such as hyporeflexia and impotence.
  - Commonly, there is orthostatic hypotension without tachycardia.
- Dehydration.
- Heat stroke (q.v.).
- Shy–Drager disease (q.v.).

Increased sweating occurs in the following:

- Acromegaly (q.v.).
- Acute myocardial infarction.
- Anticholinesterase overdose (q.v.)
  - i.e. cholinergic crisis.
- Carcinoid syndrome (q.v.).
- Cardiac tumours (q.v.).
- Collagen-vascular diseases (q.v.)
  - especially rheumatoid arthritis.
- Drug withdrawal
  - especially from anxiolytic, hypnotic or sedative drugs (colloquially referred to as 'cold turkey').
  - severe or even life-threatening features can occur within 24–36 hr of withdrawal of such drugs, with hyperthermia (q.v.), fits and coma, as well as sweating.
- Dumping syndrome
  - occurring shortly after a meal.
- Dyshidrosis (or pompholyx)
  - a form of eczematous dermatitis, manifest by recurrent vesicles on the sides of the fingers and on the palms and soles.
- Endocarditis (q.v.).
- Exercise
  - sweating being of course the major physiological response to the hyperthermia of exercise.
- Envenomation (see Bites and stings)
  - e.g. spider bite.
- Hot flushes (hot flashes) (see Flushing)
  - which are part of the vasomotor disturbance associated with declining oestrogen levels, particularly at the female menopause.
- Hyperhidrosis (HH)
  - a common and embarrassing condition, affecting (in order) the axillary, palmar and plantar, and facial regions, and with a probable prevalence of 5% of the population,
  - *treatment options include antiperspirants, anticholinergic agents and botulinum toxin injections,*
  - sometimes associated with bromhidrosis (i.e. foul-smelling body odour).
- Hyperthyroidism (q.v.).
- Hypoglycaemia (q.v.).
- Irritable bowel syndrome (q.v.)
  - which is associated with vasomotor instability in many patients.
- Monosodium glutamate ingestion (q.v.).
- Myeloproliferative disorders.
- Phaeochromocytoma (q.v.).
- Pre-syncope
  - in which there is increased cholinergic stimulation, with pallor, nausea and increased intestinal peristalsis, as well as sweating (see Cholinergic crisis).
- Needless to say, increased sweating is one of the accompaniments of fever or hyperthermia (q.v.).

Night sweats are prominent in the following:

- AIDS (q.v.).
- Chronic myeloid leukaemia.
- Cryptococcosis (q.v.).
- Eosinophilic pneumonia (q.v.).
- Fungal infections.
- Hodgkin's disease.
- Melioidosis (q.v.).
- Paragonimiasis (q.v.).
- Pulmonary aspergillosis (q.v.).

- Renal abscess.
- Tuberculosis (q.v.).

Bibliography
Doolittle J, Walker P, Mills T, et al. Hyperhidrosis: an update on prevalence and severity in the United States. *Arch Dermatol Res* 2016; 308: 743.
Nawrocki S, Cha J. The etiology, diagnosis, and management of hyperhidrosis: a comprehensive review. *J Am Acad Dermatol* 2019; 81: 657 & 669.
Quinton P. Physiology of sweat secretion. *Kidney Int* 1987; 2 (suppl. 21): S102.

Sweet's syndrome *See*
- Paraneoplastic syndromes – 1. Dermatoses.

Swimming *See*
- Bathing,
- Diving,
- Drowning.

Swine flu *See*
- Influenza.

Syndrome of inappropriate antidiuretic hormone

The **syndrome of inappropriate antidiuretic hormone** (SIADH) secretion occurs in any of three groups of clinical settings.

1. **Increased ADH**
   Either increased ADH synthesis in the hypothalamus or increased ADH release from the posterior pituitary may be produced by
   - CNS disorders, e.g. infection, neoplasia, vascular disease,
   - the postoperative state,
   - prolonged nausea.
2. **Ectopic ADH**
   This may be produced in a number of tumours (see Ectopic hormone production),
   - particularly carcinoma of the lung,
   - also tumours of the gut or thymus,
   - neuroblastoma.
3. **Increased sensitivity to ADH**
   This may be produced by a number of drugs, such as
   - carbamazepine,
   - chlorpropamide,
   - cyclophosphamide,
   - proton pump inhibitors (PPIs), particularly omeprazole,
   - many psychotropic drugs, especially selective serotonin reuptake inhibitors (SSRIs).

Of course, vasopressin or oxytocin may also have been administered in its own right (see Desmopressin, see Vasopressin).

In SIADH, the osmostat gets reset at a lower level for ADH release, e.g. as low as 275 mOsm/kg instead of the normal threshold of 280 mOsm/kg. The serum sodium is thus stabilized at a new low level (usually 120–130 mmol/L), despite an abnormally increased urinary sodium concentration and osmolality. This is a relatively stable state, since water restriction gives rise to thirst (when the plasma osmolality rises to about 290 mOsm/kg) and thus to further stimulation of ADH, so that the urine becomes more concentrated.

The clinical features are those of hyponatraemia (q.v.). These features are chiefly neurological, with headache, malaise, nausea, fits and eventually coma. The patient is typically euvolaemic.

The differential diagnosis of SIADH is primarily the other causes of hyponatraemia (q.v.), in particular
- volume depletion,
- dilution
  - as in psychogenic polydypsia, exercise-induced (or exercise-associated) hyponatraemia, and with amphetamine abuse (q.v.),
- pseudohyponatraemia (q.v.)
- possibly cerebral salt wasting (q.v.).

Adrenal insufficiency (q.v.), hypothyroidism (q.v.) and recent use of diuretics (especially thiazides) should be specifically excluded.

The diagnosis is confirmed by measurements of the plasma and urine sodium concentration and osmolality, as indicated in the accompanying Table. In addition, the plasma urea and uric acid tend to be low, and the hyponatraemia is not corrected by the administration of 0.9% saline.

Differential diagnosis of hyponatraemia

Condition	Plasma Na^+	Plasma osmolality	Urine Na^+	Urine osmolality
SIADH	⇓	⇓	⇑	⇑
Hypovolaemia	⇓	⇓	⇓	⇑
Dilution	⇓	⇓	⇔	⇓
Pseudohyponatraemia	⇓	⇔	⇔	⇔

Increased urine Na^+ refers to >20 mmol/L and decreased urine Na^+ refers to <15 mmol/L.
Increased urine osmolality refers to >200 mOsm/kg.

> In hyponatraemia due to hypovolaemia, if there is associated
> - **hypokalaemia and metabolic alkalosis**
>   - hypovolaemia is probably due to vomiting, diuretic therapy or perhaps a villous adenoma,
> - **hypokalaemia with metabolic acidosis** (q.v.)
>   - hypovolaemia is probably due to diarrhoea,
> - **hyperkalaemia and metabolic acidosis** (q.v.)
>   - hypovolaemia is probably due to adrenal insufficiency (q.v.).

*Treatment is primarily with **water restriction**.*
- **Saline** may be cautiously administered in severe cases but clearly must be more hypertonic than the urine, so that isotonic saline is generally unsuitable. This is because normal sodium excretion takes less water with it than is administered, so that the plasma sodium falls further.
- In persistent cases, an **ADH antagonist** may be used, such as a loop diuretic (e.g. furosemide), demethyltetracycline, possibly lithium, or one of the new **vaptans** (see Vasopressin).

See also
- Antidiuretic hormone,
- Central pontine myelinolysis (for further discussion of the treatment of hyponatraemia, including speed of correction and complications).

Bibliography
Adrogue HJ, Madias NE. Hyponatremia. *N Engl J Med* 2000; 342: 1581.
Barnes A, Li JYZ, Gleadle JM. Lack of appropriate investigations in making a diagnosis of syndrome of inappropriate antidiuretic syndrome. *Intern Med J* 2017; 47: 336.
Berl T. Treating hyponatremia: damned if we do and damned if we don't. *Kidney Int* 1990; 37: 1006.
Fazekas AS, Funk G-C, Klobassa DS, et al. Evaluation of 36 formulas for calculating plasma osmolality. *Intens Care Med* 2013; 39: 302.
Goudie AM, Tunstall-Pedoe DS, Kerins M, et al. Exercise-induced hyponatraemia after a marathon: case series. *J R Soc Med* 2006; 99: 363.
Madhusoodanan S, Bogunovi OJ, Moise D, et al. Hyponatraemia associated with psychotropic medications: a review of the literature and spontaneous reports. *Adverse Drug React Toxicol Rev* 2002; 21: 17.
Noakes TD. Overconsumption of fluids by athletes. *BMJ* 2003; 327: 113.
Robertson GL. Physiology of ADH secretion. *Kidney Int* 1987; 32 (suppl. 21): S20.
Rose BD. New approach to disturbances in the plasma sodium concentration. *Am J Med* 1986; 81: 1033.
Spasovski G, Vanholder R, Allolio B, et al. Clinical practice guideline on diagnosis and treatment of hyponatraemia. *Intens Care Med* 2014; 40: 320.
Sterns RH. Severe symptomatic hyponatremia: treatment and outcome. *Ann Intern Med* 1987; 107: 656.
Vokes TJ, Robertson GL. Disorders of antidiuretic hormone. *Endocrinol Metab Clin North Am* 1988; 17: 281.

Syphilis

Syphilis is a sexually transmitted disease produced by infection with the thin motile spirochaete *Treponema pallidum*. Humans are its only known host. Because of its many manifestations, it has been referred to as the great mimicker.

The incidence of syphilis declined markedly after the introduction of penicillin in the 1940s, but there has been a recent resurgence, particularly among homosexual men or men who have sex with men (MSM).

Although not culturable in vitro and very labile to heat, cold, drying and soap, a 50% effective inoculum requires only 50–60 organisms. Since most inocula in contacts of even heavily infected cases do not produce the disease, most inocula are therefore presumably very small. Following penetration of mucous membrane or broken skin, there is parasitaemia which lasts 10–60 days.

The **primary lesion** appears as a painless chancre at the site of inoculation after an incubation period of usually 3–4 weeks. It lasts for 1–6 weeks and then heals. A chancre is highly infective.

A **secondary stage** appears 6–12 weeks later, with
- widespread mucocutaneous lesions,
- lymphadenopathy (q.v.),
- systemic illness.

This stage resolves after 2–6 weeks. The disease then becomes latent for a variable period up to 20 years or more, during which time there are no symptoms but positive serology.

The **tertiary stage** eventually appears with destructive lesions in the CNS, aorta, bones, skin and elsewhere.
- Neurosyphilis takes the form of meningovascular disease, general paresis, optic atrophy, tabes dorsalis (a motor ataxia accompanied by ptosis), Argyll–Robertson pupils, Charcot's joints, incontinence, visceral crises and lightning pains in the legs.
- The aortic lesions include aortitis (q.v.) and aortic valve incompetence.
- Elsewhere, necrotic granulomas called gummas appear.

The diagnosis is made by dark-field microscopy of infected lesions, which show the parasite, and by serological demonstration of a non-specific antibody directed against the lipoidal antigen produced by the interaction of the parasite with host tissues. Such tests (e.g. venereal disease research laboratory (VDRL)) have a high sensitivity but numerous false-positives. A specific antitreponemal antibody may be demonstrated for confirmation, but such tests do not necessarily indicate current activity as they remain positive indefinitely even after treatment.

Confirmation of syphilis in a particular patient should prompt a search for other concomitant sexually transmitted infections (STIs), such as gonorrhoea, chlamydia and HIV (q.v.). The patient's sexual partners need to be notified, tested and treated.

*Treatment is with **penicillin** for 7–14 days, though a long-acting preparation such as benzathine penicillin may be given in a single dose of 1.8 g (2.4 million U). An effective alternative is **azithromycin** (2 g given as a single dose).*
- *Erythromycin, tetracycline, chloramphenicol and cephalosporins are also effective.*
- *The **Jarisch–Herxheimer** reaction may occur during treatment (q.v.).*

Bibliography
Augenbraun M. Syphilis and the nonvenereal treponematoses. In: *Scientific American Medicine. Infectious Diseases.* Hamilton: Dekker Medicine. 2020.
Hook EW, Marra CM. Acquired syphilis. *N Engl J Med* 1992; 326: 1060.
Read PJ, Donovan B. Clinical aspects of adult syphilis. *Intern Med J* 2012; 42: 614.

Syringomyelia

Syringomyelia refers to local dilatation of the central canal within the cervical and/or thoracic spinal cord. It is usually associated with the Arnold–Chiari malformation (q.v.), but it can follow local injury or be associated with a spinal glioma.

Clinically it causes a myelopathy (q.v.), with both motor and sensory deficits in one or both arms. The sensory deficit involves especially pain and temperature. There may be neck pain, extending up to the occiput. Occasionally, there is an ipsilateral Horner's syndrome (q.v.). Eventually, the pyramidal tracts also become involved, with spastic weakness of the lower limbs.

Proximal extension to the medulla gives rise to **syringobulbia**, with abnormal signs related to the V, VII, IX, X and XII cranial nerves.

Diagnosis is optimally made by MRI.

*Treatment is with **surgical decompression**.*
See
- Neural tube defects.

Bibliography
Lemire RJ. Neural tube defects. *JAMA* 1988; 259: 558.
Milunsky A, Ulcickas M, Rothman K, et al. Maternal heat exposure and neural tube defects. *JAMA* 1992; 268: 882.
Paul KS, Lye RH, Strang FA, et al. Arnold-Chiari malformation. *J Neurosurg* 1983; 58: 183.
Wald NJ, Bower C. Folic acid, pernicious anaemia, and prevention of neural tube defects. *Lancet* 1994; 343: 307.

Systemic diseases and the lung

Many systemic diseases may have significant pulmonary involvement, either directly or indirectly.

They include
- collagen-vascular diseases (q.v.)
  - systemic lupus erythematosus (q.v.),
  - scleroderma (q.v.),
  - dermatomyositis (q.v.),
- rheumatoid arthritis,
- Sjogren's disease (q.v.),
- polyarteritis nodosa (q.v.),
- ankylosing spondylitis (q.v.),
- Stevens-Johnson syndrome (q.v.),
- obesity,
- neurological disease,
- renal disease
  - uraemia,
  - dialysis problems,
  - disseminated intravascular coagulation (q.v.),
  - acute glomerulonephritis (see Glomerular diseases),
  - collagen-vascular diseases (q.v.),
  - Goodpasture's syndrome (q.v.),
  - Wegener's granulomatosis (q.v.),
  - drug reactions (see Drugs and the lung),
  - transplant complications.

Bibliography
Craddock PR, Fehr J, Brigham KL, et al. Complement and leukocyte-mediated pulmonary dysfunction in hemodialysis. *N Engl J Med* 1977; 296: 769.
Davies D. Ankylosing spondylitis and lung fibrosis. *Q J Med* 1972; 41: 395.
Marik P, Varon J. The obese patient in the ICU. *Chest* 1998; 113: 492.

Matthay RA, Schwarz MI, Petty TL. Pulmonary manifestations of systemic lupus erythematosus. *Medicine* 1975; 54: 397.

Ray CS, Sue DY, Bray G, et al. Effects of obesity on respiratory function. *Am Rev Respir Dis* 1983; 128: 501.

Segal AM, Calabrese LH, Muzaffar A, et al. The pulmonary manifestations of systemic lupus erythematosus. *Semin Arthritis Rheum* 1985; 14: 202.

Shiel WC, Prete PE. Pleuropulmonary manifestations of rheumatoid arthritis. *Semin Arthritis Rheum* 1984; 13: 235.

Systemic lupus erythematosus

Systemic lupus erythematosus (SLE) is a chronic multisystem autoimmune disease (q.v.). It is a complex condition of great clinical heterogeneity. Its cause or causes are as yet unknown.

Pathogenetically, it arises from the loss of immune regulation and tolerance, so that there is an autoimmune reaction to host antigens giving rise to inflammatory damage of vessels and tissues. There is some genetic predisposition, and there may be viral disruption of the suppressor T-cell population. Eventually, there is excess B-cell proliferation and circulating immune complexes, with deposits containing DNA, complement and immunoglobulins. It is of immunological interest that similar antibodies and even overt SLE have been reported in some patients following treatment with the anti-TNF-α agents, infliximab, etanercept and adalimumab, for rheumatoid arthritis, psoriatic arthritis (see Psoriasis), ankylosing spondylitis (q.v.) and Crohn's disease (q.v.).

The clinical features are extremely variable and are seen primarily in young women, in whom there is an incidence of 1 in 15,000 of the population per year. The overall community prevalence is 5–50 per 100,000 of the population.

The most common features are rash, fever (q.v.) and arthritis (q.v.), but there are very many others and indeed the condition can rightly be called protean due to the widespread immunological attack on the body's many organs and structures.

- **Rash** is characteristically manifest as facial erythema, typically of the transient butterfly type, but more commonly it is apparent elsewhere, particularly on the neck and hands. It may be exacerbated by ultraviolet light, and it can be associated with alopecia (q.v.) or mouth ulcers (q.v.).
- **Fever** is present in many patients, and the differential diagnosis from infection can be difficult (see Pyrexia).
- **Arthritis** is usually of the non-deforming type and comprises symmetrical polyarthritis with pain, swelling and morning stiffness. Sometimes, it may be indistinguishable from rheumatoid arthritis. There may be associated tendonitis and sometimes avascular necrosis of bone. Arthralgia is common. See Arthritis.
- **Heart** involvement is especially manifest by pericarditis (q.v.). Sometimes, there may be myocarditis or non-infective endocarditis (q.v.). Accelerated atherosclerosis occurs in long-standing SLE.
- **Kidneys** are commonly involved, as evidenced by haematuria (q.v.), proteinuria (q.v.), pyuria and urinary casts. Minor mesangial changes occur in most patients but are asymptomatic. Focal proliferative changes are also common but are benign and reversible. Membranous glomerulonephritis may sometimes occur with consequent nephrotic syndrome, though this too can remit. Diffuse proliferative glomerulonephritis is the most serious renal complication and may lead to renal failure. Advanced glomerulosclerosis can eventually occur. The renal pathology may vary during the course of the disease. The classification of the various forms of lupus nephritis has recently been revised. See Glomerular diseases.
- **Neurological** involvement occurs in about 50% of patients, although it is often mild. Neuropsychiatric features are common early in the course of the disease. Depression is especially marked, but there may also be organic psychosis or fits. Pyramidal tract or cranial nerve involvement may be seen (especially the latter, with VII nerve and extra-ocular signs). Aseptic meningitis, chorea, peripheral neuropathy (q.v.) may sometimes be seen. Except for cognitive dysfunction, most neurological changes are transient. The CSF is often normal, there are minimal histological changes, and abnormalities noted on MRI in subcortical white matter are reversible.
- **Lungs** are commonly involved, with pleurisy and pleural effusion (see Pleural disorders), diffuse pulmonary infiltrates (q.v.) and propensity to pneumonia. Pulmonary hypertension (q.v.) is sometimes seen. The lungs may also be involved if there is cardiac failure, renal failure or thromboembolism.
- **Liver** involvement may be caused by drugs (especially chemical hepatitis due to NSAIDs), primary biliary cirrhosis (q.v.) or autoimmune hepatitis (q.v.).

- **Antiphospholipid syndrome** (q.v.) is a hypercoagulable state associated with autoantibodies to phospholipid, the so-called lupus anticoagulant, occurring in about 50% of patients with SLE.
- **Myopathy** may be seen (q.v.).
- **Splenomegaly** and sometimes **hepatomegaly** may occur (q.v.).
- **Raynaud's phenomenon** (q.v.) is common.

Pregnancy can be associated with specific problems in SLE, since pregnancy may sometimes be a cause of SLE exacerbation. Pregnancy-related problems also occur if there is hypertension, renal disease or antiphospholipid syndrome, and there is an increased incidence of spontaneous abortion (q.v.), pre-eclampsia (q.v.) and neonatal lupus. See Pregnancy.

Investigations show anaemia (q.v.), sometimes of an acute haemolytic nature. There is typically leukopenia and thrombocytopenia (q.v.). Many autoantibodies can be demonstrated, especially ANA (in >90% of cases), as well as antibodies to dsDNA, RNP, Ro and La. Antiphospholipid antibodies (aPL) are usually found (see Antiphospholipid syndrome). Complement levels (C3, C4) are typically reduced in active disease. The changes of individual organ involvement (especially kidneys) may be demonstrated, and classic inflammatory markers (e.g. CRP and ESR) are raised. The investigations which best reflect disease activity are the levels of anti-dsDNA antibody and complement.

In practice, the diagnosis is based on the combination of clinical features, autoantibodies and organ involvement.

Treatment must be individualized, because of the very variable clinical course and the difficulty in evaluating progress.

- *It is usual to recommend **avoidance of sun exposure**, because 30% of patients are photosensitive and a flare-up involves not just the skin but systemic changes.*
- *Skin manifestations are treated with avoidance of excessive ultraviolet light exposure, topical corticosteroids, and sometimes hydroxychloroquine and low-dose systemic corticosteroids.*
- *Joint manifestations are treated with NSAIDs, hydroxychloroquine and sometimes low-dose corticosteroids.*
- *Problems such as pleurisy or pericarditis may require moderate-dose corticosteroids.*
- *Severe neurological manifestations or diffuse proliferative glomerulonephritis are treated with high-dose **corticosteroids**, e.g. commencing with pulse methylprednisolone (500 mg per day for 3 days) then oral prednisolone (60–75 mg per day for 3–6 months). Plasmapheresis (q.v.) may be useful at this time. End-stage renal disease is treated with chronic haemodialysis or transplantation, after which recurrence of lupus nephritis is fortunately rare.*
- ***Immunosuppressive therapy*** *(cyclophosphamide, azathioprine, mycophenolate, rituximab) may be used for steroid-sparing or for uncontrolled disease, though these drugs have not been shown to enhance the efficacy of steroids in controlled trials (except for cyclophosphamide IV).*
- *Although **corticosteroids** may be strikingly helpful symptomatically in a number of situations as described above, it is doubtful whether they alter survival.*
- ***Plasmapheresis*** *(q.v.) was found not to be effective in a controlled trial, although it may be useful for acute rescue (see above).*
- *The role of novel targeted therapy with biological agents is still to be defined, although early evidence has shown that **belimumab**, a monoclonal antibody which inhibits B-cell cytokines, can be a helpful additional agent, especially in severe disease and in lupus nephritis.*

The prognosis is difficult to assess in an individual patient, but it is often good. An average 5 yr mortality of 20% is sometimes quoted from referral centres, though the actual rate is greatly dependent on the patient sample studied, with much lower rates applying to the overall population of SLE-affected patients. There is no cure, and while there may be complete remission for several years on the one hand, on the other hand there may be recurrences which can range from mild to severe multiorgan disease. Exacerbations may be precipitated by infection, surgery, some drugs and sometimes pregnancy. The prognosis is worse if there is severe neurological or renal involvement. Death is usually from either infection or renal failure.

Variants include the following:

1. **Drug-induced SLE**

This has been mainly seen after hydralazine and procainamide. It may also follow penicillamine, isoniazid, phenytoin, sometimes phenothiazines and occasionally other drugs (see anti-TNF-α agents above).

The risk is about 1% with the high-risk drugs, though about 50% of patients exposed to these drugs develop positive ANA titres and some may have subclinical SLE.

This form of lupus is usually milder and with less renal disease, though sometimes the entire lupus complex may be seen.

Usually, drug-induced SLE follows the continuous administration of the offending drug for some time

> (range 3 weeks to 2 years). It is reversible on stopping the drug, though the abnormal laboratory tests may take many months to resolve, unlike the symptoms which usually subside in a few days.

2. **Discoid lupus**

This comprises skin lesions only and involves the face, scalp, chest and arms. Systemic disease rarely occurs. The serology is negative.

Bibliography

Connelly K, Morand EF. Systemic lupus erythematosus: a clinical update. *Intern Med J* 2021; 51: 1219.

Contreras G, Pardo V, Leclerrcq B, et al. Sequential therapies for proliferative lupus nephritis. *N Engl J Med* 2004; 350: 971.

Doherty NE, Siegel RJ. Cardiovascular manifestations of systemic lupus erythematosus. *Am Heart J* 1985; 110: 1257.

Durcan L, O'Dwyer T, Petri M. Management strategies and future directions for systemic lupus erythematosus in adults. *Lancet* 2019; 393: 2332.

Ginsberg JS, Brill-Edwards P, Johnston M, et al. Relationship of antiphospholipid antibodies to pregnancy loss in patients with systemic lupus erythematosus. *Blood* 1992; 80: 975.

Golder V, Hoi A. Systemic lupus erythematosus: an update. *Med J Aust* 2017; 206: 215.

Hanly JG, Gladman DD, Rose TH, et al. Lupus pregnancy: a prospective study of placental changes. *Arthritis Rheum* 1988; 31: 358.

Johns KR, Morand EF, Littlejohn GO. Pregnancy outcome in systemic lupus erythematosus. *Aust NZ J Med* 1998; 28: 18.

Kirou KA, Lockshin MD. Systemic lupus erythematosus. In: *Scientific American Medicine. Rheumatology.* Hamilton: Dekker Medicine. 2020.

Lee LS, Chase PH. Drug-induced systemic lupus erythematosus. *Semin Arthritis Rheum* 1975; 5: 83.

Lockshin MD. Lupus pregnancy. *Clin Rheum Dis* 1985; 11: 611.

Matthay RA, Schwarz MI, Petty TL. Pulmonary manifestations of systemic lupus erythematosus. *Medicine* 1975; 54: 397.

Rahman A, Isenberg DA. Systemic lupus erythematosus. *N Engl J Med* 2008; 358: 929.

Rasaratnam I, Ryan PFJ. Systemic lupus erythematosus. *Med J Aust* 1997; 166: 266.

Reeves GEM. Update on the immunology, diagnosis and management of systemic lupus erythematosus. *Intern Med J* 2004; 34: 338.

Segal AM, Calabrese LH, Muzaffar A, et al. The pulmonary manifestations of systemic lupus erythematosus. *Semin Arthritis Rheum* 1985; 14: 202.

Steinberg AD. The treatment of lupus nephritis. *Kidney Int* 1986; 30: 769.

Tan EM, Cohen AS, Fries JF, et al. The 1982 revised criteria for the classification of systemic lupus erythematosus. *Arthritis Rheum* 1982; 25: 1271.

Weening JJ, D'Agan VD, Schwartz MM, et al. The classification of glomerlonephritis in systemic lupus erythematosus revisited. *Kidney Int* 2004; 65: 521.

Systemic sclerosis *See*

- Scleroderma.

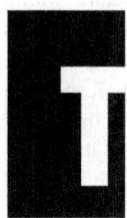

Takayasu's disease *See*

- Aortic coarctation,
- Vasculitis.

Takotsubo cardiomyopathy

Takotsubo cardiomyopathy (Takotsubo syndrome (TTS) or stress-induced cardiomyopathy) is an acute reversible event simulating an acute coronary syndrome but with normal coronary arteries. It was first described in Japan in 1991 and so named because echocardiography showed typical acute systolic ballooning of the apex of the left ventricle which resembled a Japanese octopus trap. Sometimes the mid-ventricular segment is involved, and occasionally both ventricles are affected. The condition has since been reported worldwide. Most patients are middle-aged women.

There is cardiac stunning due to coronary artery spasm, and the condition has been colloquially referred to as the 'broken heart syndrome' due to its association with stress. The aetiology is extreme emotional or sometimes physical stress, and the pathogenetic mechanism is thought be a severe catecholamine surge. A similar condition has long been known to occur after severe neurological injury.

> The condition can thus occur in the setting of critical illness.

Clinically, there is chest pain with associated ECG changes of ST elevation or T-wave inversion and with elevated levels of cardiac enzymes. There may be significant acute but transient cardiac dysfunction, with arrhythmias, left ventricular failure or even cardiogenic shock. However, the condition is reversible, usually within a week or so, and mortality is very low. Complete recovery is usual, and recurrence is uncommon.

It has been estimated that about 2% of patients presenting with the features of an acute coronary syndrome may in fact have Takotsubo cardiomyopathy. The diagnosis in this setting is one of exclusion, but it should be suspected in postmenopausal women with typical clinical and ECG abnormalities after intense stress. Phaeochromocytoma (q.v.) or myocarditis as well as coronary artery disease with acute plaque rupture should be excluded. The diagnosis is confirmed by echocardiography or other imaging, such as cardiac MRI.

Treatment is as for an acute coronary syndrome. Beta blocker or ACE inhibitor treatment is recommended until full recovery.

Bibliography
Boland TA, Lee VH, Bleck TP. Stress-induced cardiomyopathy. *Crit Care Med* 2015; 43: 686.
Connelly KA, MacIsaac AI, Jelinek VM. Stress, myocardial infarction, and the 'tako-tsubo' phenomenon. *Heart* 2004; 90: e52.
Dote K, Sato H, Tateishi H, et al. [Myocardial stunning due to simultaneous multivessel coronary spasms. [Japanese] *J Cardiol* 1991; 21: 203.
Park JH, Kang SJ, Song JK, et al. Left ventricular apical ballooning due to severe physical stress in patients admitted to the medical ICU. *Chest* 2005; 128: 296.
Pernicova I, Garg S, Bourantas CV, et al. Takotsubo cardiomyopathy: a review of the literature. *Angiology* 2010; 61: 166.
Samardhi H, Raffel OC, Savage M, et al. Takotsubo cardiomyopathy: an Australian single centre experience with medium term follow-up. *Intern Med J* 2012; 42: 35.
Samuels MA, The brain-heart connection. *Circulation* 2007; 116: 77.
Sharkey SW, Windenburg DC, Lesser, JR, et al. Natural history and expansive clinical profile of stress (takotsubo) cardiomyopathy. *J Am Coll Cardiol* 2010; 55: 333.

Tardive dyskinesia

Tardive dyskinesia (TD) describes a syndrome of involuntary facial movements and choreoathetotic movements of the limbs.

It is a severe neurological complication, reportedly seen in about 20% of patients on long-term antipsychotic drugs. The best-known drugs in this setting are the phenothiazines, but similar effects may be produced by other unrelated antipsychotics (though not apparently by the atypical antipsychotic agent, clozapine). It is more common in older patients.

> Sometimes there may be impairment of swallowing, airway control and breathing.

The condition may slowly resolve when the drug is stopped. It is otherwise untreatable.

Telangiectasia See
- Arteriovenous malformations.
  See also
- Carcinoid syndrome,
- Haemangioma,
- Immunodeficiency – 2. Cell-mediated immunodeficiency,
- Mouth diseases – 3. Stomatitis,
- Purpura,
- Scleroderma.

Temporal arteritis See
- Arteritis,
- Polymyalgia rheumatica,
- Pyrexia,
- Vasculitis.

Tetanus

Tetanus results from infection with the anaerobic Gram-positive bacillus *Clostridium tetani*, which is widely distributed in soil and animal (and occasionally human) faeces. Since active immunization is so effective, the disease is most commonly seen in developing countries, where an estimated million deaths per year occur from tetanus worldwide due to the fact that the organism is ubiquitous and trauma so frequent. Clinical tetanus does not provide immunity against subsequent episodes.

Inoculated spores germinate at the site of injury and produce a potent neurotoxin, referred to as tetanospasmin. This migrates centrally along motor neurone axons to the spinal cord, where it suppresses the inhibition of the reflex arc by internuncial neurones. The reflex antagonist relaxation normally activated during contraction is thus lost, and muscular spasm occurs with a result which depends on the relative strengths of the agonist and antagonist muscle groups involved. Thus, opisthotonos is typical, with upper limb flexion and lower limb extension.

> Most commonly, the organisms penetrate a site of skin injury following trauma,
>   Sometimes, they follow bites, burns, surgery, parenteral narcotic use, delivery or abortion.
>   In 10–20% of cases, there is no identifiable initial lesion.

There is an incubation period of usually more than 2 weeks, but it may range from 1 to 55 days. The shorter the incubation period, the higher the mortality will be, which is reportedly 100% if the incubation period is only 1–2 days and about 30% if it is greater than 10 days.

> - Trismus (lockjaw) is the first clinical feature noted in over half the patients.
> - There is
>   - restlessness,
>   - generalized muscle spasm and stiffness,
>   - hyperreflexia, with downgoing plantar reflexes,
>   - dysphagia (q.v.).
> - The spasms become progressively violent within 72 hr, though there is no loss of consciousness. Tonic seizures follow even minor stimuli and may involve the respiratory muscles, thus potentially giving respiratory arrest.
> - There is moderate fever (q.v.) and sympathetic overactivity.
> - The illness is severe for the first week, then gradually decreases over several weeks.
> - Complications include
>   - respiratory failure,
>   - pulmonary aspiration (q.v.),
>   - arrhythmias,
>   - fractures of the thoracic vertebrae,
>   - pulmonary embolism.

Laboratory results are generally normal, and the organism can be isolated in only 30% of patients.

The differential diagnosis includes
- strychnine poisoning (q.v.)
  - this is very similar,
- pseudotetanus with trismus
  - this may be caused by phenothiazines and resolves with IV phenytoin,
- spider bite (q.v.),
- trismus from other causes
  - such as jaw infection or encephalopathy (q.v.),
- hysteria.

However, the diagnosis of tetanus in developed countries can be delayed, because most clinicians will have never seen a case.

Treatment principles are 3-fold, namely, to **treat the source**, **neutralize the toxin** and **manage the complications**.
1. **Treat the source**.
   The wound requires debridement and culture.
2. **Neutralize the toxin**.
   Antitoxin, nowadays of human origin, is given in a single dose of 3000–5000 U IM or IV. The wound should be infiltrated with antitoxin also. Antitoxin is not effective for toxin which has already become bound. If human immunoglobulin is not available, equine antitoxin is used in a dose of 100,000 U.
3. **Manage the complications**.
   Intensive Care is required with administration of muscle relaxants, sedation, IV fluids and mechanical ventilation. Sedation should be with diazepam, and beta blockers IV are used for arrhythmias. Dantrolene can usefully reduce muscle tone. Magnesium sulphate has been found to be ineffective in reducing muscle spasms. Penicillin is given IV in large doses for 1 week, but it is of limited value in that it affects only the vegetative cells in the wound, though in this way new toxin production is prevented.
   Interestingly, **botulinum toxin** (which acts peripherally and causes a flaccid paralysis) has been used successfully by local injection into muscles in spasm due to tetanus (whose toxin acts centrally and causes a spastic paralysis).

See also
- Agammaglobulinaemia,
- Bites and stings,
- Clostridial infections,
- Frostbite,
- Ulcers.

Bibliography
Edsall G. Problems in the immunology and control of tetanus. *Med J Aust* 1976; 2: 216.
Gaber T A-Z K, Mannemela S. Botulinum toxin for muscle spasm after tetanus. *J R Soc Med* 2005; 98: 63.

Tidyman M, Prichard JG, Deamer RL, et al. Adjunctive use of dantrolene in severe tetanus. *Anesth Analg* 1985; 64: 538.

Tetrachlorethylene *See*

- Carbon tetrachloride.

Tetrachlormethane *See*

- Carbon tetrachloride.

Tetrahydroaminoacridine (THA) *See*

- Anticholinergic agents.

Tetralogy of Fallot

Tetralogy of Fallot is the commonest cyanotic congenital heart disease.

It comprises
- pulmonary stenosis (more commonly infundibular than valvular),
- ventricular septal defect,
- an overriding dextroposed aorta.
- right ventricular hypertrophy.

There is thus a right-to-left shunt, the degree of which varies with the degree of pulmonary stenosis.

The shunt causes hypoxaemia, cyanosis and secondary polycythaemia (q.v.). Coagulopathy due to reduced vitamin K-dependent clotting factors (q.v.) and platelet dysfunction (q.v.) give rise to a bleeding tendency, which is especially marked after cardiac surgery.

Surgical correction should be performed in childhood (before the age of 5 yr). Such surgery nowadays always involves a complete repair.

In adults who have had an incomplete repair or no surgery, there is an increased risk of
- infective endocarditis (q.v.),
- paradoxical embolism, especially of the brain and thus the production of a brain abscess,
- sudden death from arrhythmias.

Bibliography
Nora JJ. Causes of congenital heart disease: old and new modes, mechanisms, and models. *Am Heart J* 1993; 125: 1409.
Wilson NJ, Neutze JM. Adult congenital heart disease: principles and management guidelines. *Aust NZ J Med* 1993; 23: 498 & 697.

Tetrodotoxin *See*

- Bites and stings – Marine invertebrates, Marine vertebrates.

Thalassaemia *See*

- Haemoglobin disorders.

See also
- Anaemia,
- Chelating agents – Desferrioxamine,
- Fetal haemoglobin,
- Megaloblastic anaemia,
- Reticulocytes.

Thallium

Thallium (Tl, atomic number 81, atomic weight 204, melting point 304°C) is a soft, blue-grey metal, malleable like lead but tarnishing in air. It is present in small amounts in lead and zinc ores and was discovered in them in 1861. Neither the metal nor its compounds have major commercial application, but since it is a poor conductor of electricity it has found limited industrial use in photoelectric cells and in optics.

However, its toxicity made it popular in insecticides and rodenticides until the 1960s. As it was readily available for these purposes, its use as the 'poisoner's poison' naturally followed, especially as it was tasteless, colourless, odourless and hard to detect. Following its accidental or deliberate ingestion in humans, there is a classical picture of initial gastroenteritis (q.v.) followed by peripheral neuropathy (q.v.) and later alopecia (q.v.). The peripheral neuropathy is generally mixed and is manifest particularly by ptosis (q.v.), retrobulbar neuritis (q.v.) and facial paralysis. A Guillain–Barré-like polyneuritis (q.v.) has also been reported.

> Since thallium ions behave like those of potassium, they are secreted into the gut where they may be sequestered by the antidote **Prussian blue** (potassium ferrihexacyanoferrate) (q.v.), via exchange of potassium for thallium in its molecular lattice.

Prussian blue is given in a dose of 10 g bd orally or by nasogastric or nasoduodenal tube, a tube usually being needed because of associated gastrointestinal stasis. For the same reason, a purgative is generally required to treat the severe constipation which typically occurs. The antidote is continued not only until plasma and urinary levels have declined but more importantly until faecal excretion has ceased. Potassium given intravenously enhances thallium excretion into the gut, but oral potassium is contraindicated since it interferes with the thallium-potassium exchange by the antidote in the gut.

Thermoregulation *See*

- Heat,
- Heat stroke,

- Hypothermia,
- Pyrexia.

Thesaurosis *See*

- Occupational lung diseases.

Thiamine deficiency *See*

- Beriberi,
- Dementia,
- Vitamin deficiency,
- Wernicke–Korsakoff syndrome.

Thrombasthenia *See*

- Antiplatelet agents,
- Platelet function disorders.

Thrombocythaemia *See*

- Thrombocytosis.

Thrombocytopenia

Thrombocytopenia refers to a decreased peripheral blood platelet count (see Platelets). A decreased platelet count is common in critically ill patients, especially in the more seriously ill and in non-survivors.

Like deficiencies of the other formed elements, it is due to one or more of the same three mechanisms, namely decreased production, increased removal or sequestration.

The mechanism of platelet production from megakaryocytes has been greatly clarified by the discovery of **thrombopoietin** (TPO) and by its later cloning and characterization. TPO deficiency may occur in liver disease, since the liver is a major site of its production, and TPO excess may be involved in some states of thrombocytosis (q.v.). Exogenous TPO is available for clinical trial use in thrombocytopenic conditions, but more recently developed thrombopoietin receptor agonists have more practical utility (see Idiopathic thrombocytopenic purpura).

The relationship between the platelet count and the risk of bleeding is inexact.
- Thus, there is no single level below which bleeding occurs and above which bleeding does not occur.
- Nevertheless, a platelet count of 20×10^9/L is commonly regarded as the 'magic number' below which the risk of serious haemorrhage becomes significant. In haemato-oncology patients, a lower threshold of 10×10^9/L is generally recommended.
- However, a platelet count of at least double this is required for protection against bleeding from invasive procedures (i.e. 40–50×10^9/L) and double this again (about 100×10^9/L) for haemostatic safety in high-risk procedures, such as neurosurgery.
- In general, one unit of platelet concentrate raises the platelet count by about 10×10^9/L per m^2, so that 5–6 units or packs are generally required for haemostasis.
- However, unlike the normal half-life of 4 days (i.e. lifespan of 7–10 days), the half-life of transfused platelets is usually only about 24 hr and perhaps as short as only 1 hr in severe platelet consumptive disorders.

In addition, a number of other factors both platelet-related and platelet-independent affect bleeding.
- **Platelet-related factors** include platelet size and thus their age and metabolic and functional activity, with larger platelets being younger and generally more active, though the relationship between platelet size and function is inexact. In addition, platelet function abnormalities (q.v.) increase the risk of bleeding for any given platelet count.
- **Platelet-independent factors** affecting bleeding include any concomitant haemostatic defect, particularly those of coagulation, as in liver disease, vitamin K deficiency (q.v.) and disseminated intravascular coagulation (q.v.).

The diagnosis of the cause of thrombocytopenia is assisted by both the associated clinical features and the full blood examination. Platelet kinetics are not feasible as a routine study, though the response to a standard six-unit platelet transfusion gives indirect kinetic information and is thus diagnostically helpful.

The types of thrombocytopenia are (as indicated above)
- decreased production,
- increased removal,
  - either immune or non-immune mediated,
- sequestration.

Decreased production occurs with
- marrow infiltration,
- aplastic anaemia (q.v.),
- dysplastic megakaryopoiesis
  - due to alcoholism, or deficiency of vitamin B$_{12}$ (q.v.) or folic acid (q.v.),
- drugs
  - alcohol, gold, sulphonamides, thiazides.

Increased removal may be either immune or non-immune mediated. The two mechanisms are not always clearly separable.

1. **Immune mechanisms** include
   - autoantibodies (q.v.)
     - immune (idiopathic) thrombocytopenic purpura (ITP) (q.v.),
     - lymphoma, systemic lupus erythematosus (q.v.),
     - occasionally triggered by drugs, including gold, laevodopa, penicillamine, procainamide, sulphonamides,
   - drugs (see also Drug-induced thrombocytopenia below)
     - quinine/quinidine particularly,
     - heparin (q.v.),
     - fluoroquinolones (e.g. ciprofloxacin), presumably because they are structurally similar to quinine,
     - amiodarone, antibiotics (especially beta-lactams, linezolid, rifampicin, vancomycin), anticonvulsants, diuretics, NSAIDs, paracetamol, platinum-containing compounds, sulphonamides,
     - the anti-GPIIb-IIIa antiplatelet drugs (q.v.), including abciximab, tirofiban and eptifibatide, to which naturally occurring antibodies may already be present in some patients,
   - infections
     - infectious mononucleosis (see Epstein–Barr virus), malaria (q.v.), hepatitis C (q.v.), HIV infection (see Acquired immunodeficiency syndrome),
   - **post-transfusion purpura** (PTP).

> **Post-transfusion purpura** is an uncommon condition occurring 2–10 days after the transfusion of any blood products containing platelets.
>
> PTP is considered due to antibody production to the platelet allo-antigen Zwa, a platelet antigen occurring in 90% of the population. Patients with PTP are thus Zwa negative.
>
> The condition is usually seen in middle-aged or elderly women. There tends to be severe thrombocytopenia and clinically significant bleeding.
>
> The chief differential diagnosis is heparin-induced thrombocytopenia (q.v.), disseminated intravascular coagulation (q.v.) and sepsis.
>
> *Treatment with high doses of **corticosteroids** may be effective.*
> - ***Plasmapheresis** (q.v.) may be used in severe and refractory cases.*
> - *The best therapy is **immune globulin** (40 g IV over 40 min), followed by 10 units of platelets which are now effective because of reticuloendothelial blockade. The condition is reversible within 1–4 months.*

2. **Non-immune destruction** occurs because of activation of coagulation, platelet aggregation or endothelial cell damage.
   It is due to
   - disseminated intravascular coagulation (DIC)(q.v.)
     - or related conditions, such as haemolytic-uraemic syndrome (q.v.), thrombotic thrombocytopenic purpura (q.v.), vasculitis (q.v.), pre-eclampsia (q.v.),
   - giant haemangioma (q.v.)
     - possibly via DIC,
   - Gram-negative sepsis
     - typically accompanied by DIC if severe,
     - without DIC in milder cases, e.g. platelet count $>50 \times 10^9$/L,
   - massive transfusion
     - and thus platelet washout.

   Sequestration occurs with
   - splenomegaly (q.v.)
     - when the intrasplenic platelet pool may rise from the normal 25% to 50–80%,
   - coronary artery bypass grafting
     - when a platelet count $<50 \times 10^9$/L may persist for up to one week or more, especially in the elderly,
   - pre-eclampsia (q.v.) and HELLP syndrome (q.v.).

Normal pregnancy (q.v.) is incidentally associated with mild asymptomatic thrombocytopenia in 5–8% of cases.

Thrombocytopenia due to sequestration is usually mild and not clinically significant unless there is concomitant disease. The reason for the failure of the bone marrow to compensate is uncertain.

Drug-induced thrombocytopenia (DITP) may be difficult to distinguish from ITP, though the history may provide a clue (see Immune thrombocytopenic purpura). Its incidence has been estimated as about 10 per million of the population per year. While drugs may of course cause thrombocytopenia by impairing platelet production (see above), increased platelet removal due to an immune pathogenesis is much more common. There are several mechanisms by which drugs may cause an immune thrombocytopenia, but specific laboratory testing based on these is difficult. The diagnosis is therefore made clinically (see drugs listed above).

Thrombocytopenia due to quinine/quinidine is the archetypal form of DITP. It typically develops after about 2 weeks, and it is treated with corticosteroids and platelet transfusion if severe and possibly with immune globulin or plasmapheresis if prolonged.

DITP due to other drugs generally follows a similar course, except after GPIIb-IIIa antiplatelet agents (see

Antiplatelet agents), when thrombocytopenia occurs within a few hours of initial exposure.

Occasionally, there may be systemic symptoms or antibody-induced anaemia (q.v.) or neutropenia (q.v.). The risk of bleeding is inversely related to the platelet count, as discussed above. The thrombocytopenia generally resolves within a week of cessation of the culprit drug, though occasionally it may persist for several weeks, and sometimes the haemolytic–uraemic syndrome (q.v.) may occur (particularly after quinine).

Heparin (q.v.) has nowadays become the most common cause of drug-associated thrombocytopenia (see Heparin-induced thrombocytopenia).

Inherited thrombocytopenia is rare, but it can present first in adult life. It can comprise many different forms, which require sophisticated laboratory investigation to elucidate. Their importance in adult medicine lies in the fact that their genetic component may not be appreciated, that they are then misdiagnosed as immune thrombocytopenia and that they may therefore be treated inappropriately.

Bibliography

Akca S, Haji-Michael P, de Mendonca A, et al. Time course of platelet counts in critically ill patients. *Crit Care Med* 2002; 30: 753.

Aster RH, Bougie DW. Drug-induced immune thrombocytopenia. *N Engl J Med* 2007; 357: 904.

Aster RH, Curtis BR, McFarland JG, et al. Drug-induced immune thrombocytopenia: pathogenesis, diagnosis, and management. *J Thromb Haemost* 2009; 7: 911.

Balduini CL, Savoia A, Seri M. Inherited thrombocytopenias frequently diagnosed in adults. *J Thromb Haemost* 2013; 11: 1006.

Beutler E. Platelet transfusions: the 20,000/μL trigger. *Blood* 1993; 81: 1411.

Chong BH. Heparin-induced thrombocytopenia. *J Thromb Haemost* 2003; 1: 1471.

Cines DB, Blanchette VS. Immune thrombocytopenic purpura. *N Engl J Med* 2002; 346: 995.

Ferrara JLM. The febrile platelet transfusion reaction: a cytokine shower. *Transfusion* 1995; 35: 89.

George JN. Thrombotic thrombocytopenic purpura. *N Engl J Med* 2006; 354: 1927.

George JN, El-Harake M, Raskob GE. Chronic idiopathic thrombocytopenic purpura. *N Engl J Med* 1994; 331: 1207.

Handtke S, Thiele T. Large and small platelets – (when) do they differ? *J Thromb Haemost* 20020; 18: 1256.

Haznedaroglu IC, Goker H, Turgut M, et al. Thrombopoietin as a drug: biologic expectations, clinical realities, and future directions. *Clin Appl Thromb Hemost* 2002; 8: 193.

Hui P, Cook DJ, Lim W, et al. The frequency and clinical significance of thrombocytopenia complicating critical illness. *Chest* 2011; 139: 271.

Italiano JE, Shivdasani A. Megakaryocytes and beyond: the birth of platelets. *J Thromb Haemost* 2003; 1: 1174.

Marder VJ, Aird WC, Bennett JS, et al., eds. *Hemostasis and Thrombosis: Basic Principles and Clinical Practice*. 6th edition. Philadelphia: Lippincott Williams & Wilkins. 2012.

Moake JL. Thrombotic microangiopathies. *N Engl J Med* 2002; 347: 589.

Mueller-Eckhardt C. Post-transfusion purpura. *Br J Haematol* 1986; 64: 419.

Papadopoulos J, Kane-Gill S, Cooper B, eds. Identification and prevention of common adverse drug events in the intensive care unit. *Crit Care Med* 2010; 36: 6 (suppl.).

Payne BA, Pierre RV. Pseudothrombocytopenia: a laboratory artifact with potentially serious consequences. *Mayo Clin Proc* 1984; 59: 123.

Pene F, Benoit DD. Thrombocytopenia in the critically ill: considering pathophysiology rather than looking for a magic threshold. *Intens Care Med* 2013; 39: 1656.

Rice TW, Wheeler AP. Coagulopathy in critically ill patient. Part 1: platelet disorders. *Chest* 2009; 136: 1622.

Selleng K, Warkentin TE, Greinacher A. Heparin-induced thrombocytopenia in intensive care patients. *Crit Care Med* 2007; 35: 1165.

Thiolliere F, Serre-Serpin AF, Reignier J, et al. Epidemiology and outcome of thrombocytopenic patients in the intensive care unit: results of a prospective multicenter study. *Intens Care Med* 2013; 39: 1460.

Various. Drug-induced thrombocytopenia. *Chest* 2005; 127(2): suppl.

Warkentin TE, Greinacher A, eds. *Heparin-Induced Thrombocytopenia*. 5th edition. London: CRC Press. 2012.

Warkentin TE, Greinacher A, Koster A, et al. Treatment and prevention of heparin-induced thrombocytopenia: ACCP evidence-based clinical practice guidelines *Chest* 2008; 133 (suppl.): 340S.

Warkentin TE, Levine MN, Hirsh J, et al. Heparin-induced thrombocytopenia in patients treated with low-molecular-weight heparin or unfractionated heparin. *N Engl J Med* 1995; 332: 1330.

Warkentin TE, Sheppard J-AI, Heels-Ansdell D, et al. Heparin-induced thrombocytopenia in medical surgical critical illness. *Chest* 2013; 144: 848.

Williamson DR, Albert M, Heels-Ansdell D, et al. Thrombocytopenia in critically ill patients receiving thromboprophylaxis. *Chest* 2013; 144: 1207.

Yang Z, Stulz P, von Segesser L, et al. Different interactions of platelets with arterial and venous coronary bypass vessels. *Lancet* 1991; 337: 939.

Thrombocytosis/thrombocythaemia

Thrombocytosis refers to an increased platelet count above 400×10^9/L, and **thrombocythaemia** refers to disease associated with such an increased count.

Thrombocytosis is usually 'reactive' to
- inflammation,
- trauma,
- neoplasia,
- splenectomy.

The platelets themselves are normal. There are no clinical consequences, even in the presence of a very high count.

> Such high platelet counts can however be a cause of pseudohyperkalaemia (q.v.).

Thrombocythaemia is an autonomous increase in the peripheral blood platelet count, with megakaryocyte proliferation in the bone marrow. It is usually due to a clonal chronic myeloproliferative disorder, such as chronic myeloid leukaemia, polycythaemia vera (q.v.), myelofibrosis, and essential thrombocythaemia.

The platelet count is commonly much $>1000 \times 10^9$/L. Platelet function is commonly abnormal as well.

Life expectancy is relatively unimpaired, but there is an increased prevalence of bleeding (about 20%) and/or thromboembolism (about 10%).

It is one of the causes of secondary livedo reticularis (q.v.).

Erythromelalgia may be produced and is due to microvascular dysfunction. It is manifest by cyanotic, ischaemic and burning digits.

*Treatment is generally with **aspirin**, which reduces vascular complications. In this setting, aspirin 100 mg should probably be given twice rather than once daily.*

- *Cytotoxics (alkylating agents), **radiophosphorus** (^{32}P), **hydroxycarbamide (hydroxyurea)** or **interferon** are used in severe cases to reduce the platelet count. However, alkylating agents, radiophosphorus and hydroxycarbamide have been shown to increase the incidence of leukaemic transformation and are therefore best avoided in younger patients, but the newer agent, **anagrelide**, is not mutagenic.*
- ***Plateletpheresis** may be used in emergency cases.*
- *The new agent, **ruxolitinib**, has been found useful in refractory cases.*

Bibliography

Anagrelide Study Group. Anagrelide, a therapy for thrombocythemic states. *Am J Med* 1992; 92: 69.

Bentley MA, Taylor KM, Wright SJ. Essential thrombocythaemia. *Med J Aust* 1999; 171: 210.

Layzer RB. Hot feet: erythromelalgia and related disorders. *J Child Neurol* 2001; 16: 199.

Kurzrock R, Cohen PR. Erythromelalgia: review of clinical characteristics and pathophysiology. *Am J Med* 1991; 91: 416.

Marder VJ, Aird WC, Bennett JS, et al., eds. *Hemostasis and Thrombosis: Basic Principles and Clinical Practice.* 6th edition. Philadelphia: Lippincott Williams & Wilkins. 2012.

Michiels JJ, ed. Platelet-dependent vascular complications and bleeding symptoms in essential thrombocythemia and polycythemia vera. *Semin Thromb Hemost* 1997; 23: 333.

Michiels JJ, Abels J, Steketee J, et al. Erythromelalgia caused by platelet mediated arteriolar inflammation and thrombosis in thrombocythemia. *Ann Intern Med* 1985; 102: 466.

Sroren EC, Tefferi A. Long-term use of anagrelide in young patients with essential thrombocythemia. *Blood* 2001; 97: 863.

Tefferi A, Elliott M, Solberg L, et al. New drugs in essential thrombocythemia and polycythemia vera. *Blood Rev* 1997; 11: 1.

Thromboembolism See

- Thrombophilia.
  See also
- Anaemia – Paroxysmal nocturnal haemoglobinuria,
- Antithrombin III,
- Bed rest,
- Cancer complications,
- Eosinophilia – Hypereosinophilic syndrome,
- Heparin-induced thrombocytopenia,
- High altitude,
- Lung tumours,
- Paraneoplastic syndromes,
- Polycythaemia,
- Pregnancy – 3. Common systemic problems, 6. Post-partum problems,
- Protein C,
- Pulmonary hypertension,
- Pyrexia,

- Systemic lupus erythematosus,
- Thrombocytosis/thrombocythaemia.

Bibliography

Leung LLK. Thrombotic disorders. In: *Scientific American Medicine. Hematology.* Hamilton: Dekker Medicine. 2020.

Marder VJ, Aird WC, Bennett JS, et al., eds. *Hemostasis and Thrombosis: Basic Principles and Clinical Practice.* 6th edition. Philadelphia: Lippincott Williams & Wilkins. 2012.

Winter M-P, Schernthaner GH, Lang IM. Chronic complications of venous thromboembolism. *J Thromb Haemost* 2017; 15: 1531.

Thrombohaemorrhagic disorders See

- Thrombotic microangiopathy.

Thromboinflammation See

- Coagulation disorders.

Thrombolysis

Thrombolysis may be considered for the treatment of both arterial and venous thrombi, if acute and severe, such as acute myocardial infarction, non-haemorrhagic stroke and pulmonary embolism. It carries a significant risk of bleeding, so that it is contraindicated if there is an existing haemorrhagic tendency.

Thrombolytic agents include

- **streptokinase**, the original thrombolytic agent but now used only in developing countries because it is much cheaper than the expensive newer agents,
- **urokinase**, of comparable efficacy to streptokinase and still sometimes used as an adjunct in vascular clearance procedures,
- **tissue plasminogen activator** (tPA, alteplase), a naturally occurring agent but produced commercially by genetic engineering, with greater efficacy than earlier agents,
- **tenecteplase** and **reteplase**, which are tPA variants with longer duration of action and simplified dosing regimens.

Thrombomodulin

Thrombomodulin (TM) is a glycoprotein which is bound to the vascular endothelial cell membrane. It can bind to and neutralize thrombin and accelerate the anticoagulant and anti-inflammatory action of protein C (q.v.).

Some thrombomodulin circulates in a soluble truncated form (sTM) when shed from the endothelium. Both high and low levels of sTM have been associated with a variety of conditions, particularly vascular diseases. The rare disorder of inherited dysfunctional thrombomodulin is associated with bleeding.

Recombinant thrombomodulin (rhTM, ART-123) has been produced to enable this natural anticoagulant to be studied for its concomitant anti-inflammatory potential. However, like the other natural anticoagulants (q.v.), including antithrombin III (AT-III), tissue factor pathway inhibitor (TFPI, tifacogin), and activated protein C (drotrecogin alfa), recombinant thrombomodulin has not been found in controlled trials to have a significant mortality benefit in sepsis. Nevertheless, it has been licensed in Japan since 2008 for use in sepsis-associated coagulopathy and disseminated intravascular coagulation (q.v.), and early studies have suggested potential utility in various other conditions associated with endothelial injury and microvascular thrombosis, such as acute respiratory distress syndrome (ARDS) (q.v.).

See also

- Anticoagulants,
- Antithrombin,
- Protein C,
- Trauma in pregnancy.

Bibliography

Conway EM. Thrombomodulin and its role in inflammation. *Semin Immunopathol* 2012; 34: 107.

Maruyama I. Recombinant thrombomodulin and activated protein C in the treatment of disseminated intravascular coagulation. *Thromb Haemost* 1999; 82: 718.

Saito H, Maruyama I, Shimazaki S, et al. Efficacy and safety of recombinant human soluble thrombomodulin (ART-123) in disseminated intravascular coagulation: results of a phase III randomized double-blind clinical trial. *J Thromb Haemost* 2007; 5: 31.

Valeriani E, Squizzato A, Gallo A, et al. Efficacy and safety of recombinant human soluble thrombomodulin in patients with sepsis-associated coagulopathy: a systematic review and meta-analysis. *J Thromb Haemost* 2020; 18: 1618.

Vincent JL, Francois B, Zabolotskikh I, et al. Effect of recombinant human soluble thrombomodulin on mortality in patients with sepsis-associated coagulopathy: the SCARLET randomized clinical trial. *JAMA* 2019; 321: 1993.

Yamakawa K, Fujimi S, Mohri T, et al. Treatment effects of recombinant human soluble thrombomodulin in patients with severe sepsis: a historical control study. *Crit Care* 2011; 15: R123.

Thrombophilia

Thrombophilia refers to a thrombotic or clotting tendency. It may be inherited or acquired, or perhaps more commonly it can result from an interaction between environmental and genetic factors. The term was coined in 1965 (when hereditary antithrombin deficiency was first reported) and is a broader term than 'hypercoagulability', as it includes abnormalities of platelets and fibrinolysis as well as of coagulation. It does not, however, include the other two components of Virchow's triad for thrombosis, namely, abnormalities of the vessel wall or of blood flow, nor does it include local or anatomical conditions, such as the May–Thurner syndrome of left iliac vein compression by the right common iliac artery.

Thrombophilia is typically associated with the occurrence of venous thrombi which are familial, unusual, recurrent or multiple. Inherited thrombophilias now explain about 40% of hitherto idiopathic episodes of venous thromboembolism. The risk of thromboembolism is highest in the rarer and the homozygotic defects and it is lowest in the more common and the heterozygote defects, where additional trigger factors are usually present. Thus, routine laboratory testing for thrombophilia should be tempered by an appreciation of the variable clinical utility of the many individual biomarkers. Laboratory testing is least likely to be useful in cases of secondary thromboembolism, where acquired risk factors are usually prominent.

Inherited thrombophilia includes
- activated protein C resistance (Factor V Leiden defect) (see Protein C),
- deficiencies (or abnormalities) as follows:
  - antithrombin-III deficiency (q.v.),
  - protein C deficiency (q.v.),
  - protein S deficiency (q.v.),
  - prothrombin G20210A abnormality (q.v.),
  - plasminogen deficiency (see Fibrinolysis),
  - fibrinogen abnormality, specifically dysfibrinogenaemia,
  - low factor XII, with 46 C → T mutation which has been considered paradoxically to be a possible thrombophilic rather than a haemostatic risk (after all, Mr Hageman, whose name was originally given to factor XII, died of pulmonary embolism),
- hyperhomocystinaemia
  - generally due to a mutant variant (called C677T) of the enzyme, 5,10-methylenetetrahydrofolate reductase (MTHFR), which causes a relative deficiency of the enzyme responsible for converting homocysteine to methionine,
  - a fasting plasma homocysteine level >18.5 mmol/L is significantly associated with arterial and probably venous thrombosis, possibly via a direct pathogenetic mechanism,
  - possibly ameliorated with folate supplementation.
- non-O blood groups (i.e. A, B and AB)
  - associated with a 2-fold risk of venous thromboembolism, probably because the half-lives of von Willebrand factor (q.v.) and factor VIII (see Haemophilia) are shorter in patients with blood group O (e.g. 10 hr v 25 hr for vWF) and their levels are therefore lower (by 25–30%).

A number of other abnormalities have been reported to have a probable association with thrombophilia, as follows:
- increased factors VII, VIII, IX or XI,
- increased plasminogen activator inhibitor type 1 (PAI-1),
- heparin cofactor II deficiency,
- thrombomodulin deficiency (q.v.),
- platelet glycoprotein abnormality,
- increased lipoprotein a (Lpa).

Many other, less well defined, genetic variants have been increasingly described, many of which are polymorphic and some of which affect other organ systems as well.

Interestingly, factor XIII mutation (val34leu) has been described as significantly protective against thrombophilia.

Acquired thrombophilia includes
- antiphospholipid syndrome (q.v.),
- asparaginase chemotherapy (see Antithrombin III),
- collagen-vascular diseases (q.v.),
- COVID-19 (q.v.),
- malignancy (including chemotherapy),
- nephrotic syndrome (q.v.),
- myeloproliferative disorders.

Bibliography
Baglin T. Unraveling the thrombophilia paradox: from hypercoagulability to the prothrombotic state. *J Thromb Haemost* 2009; 8: 228.
Bick RL, Kaplan H. Syndromes of thrombosis and hypercoagulability: congenital and acquired thrombophilias. *Clin Appl Thromb Hemost* 1998; 4: 25.
Brenner B, Conard J, eds. Women's issues in thrombophilia. *Semin Thromb Hemost* 2003; 29: 1.
Casini A, Neerman-Arbez M, Ariens RA, et al. Dysfibrinogenemia: from molecular anomalies to clinical manifestations and management. *J Thromb Haemost* 2015; 13: 909.

Cattaneo M. Hyperhomocysteinemia, atherosclerosis and thrombosis. *Thromb Haemost* 1999; 81: 165.
de Moerloose P, Bounameaux HR, Mannucci PM. Screening tests for thrombophilic patients: which tests, for which patient, by whom, when, and why? *Semin Thromb Hemost* 1998; 24: 321.
den Heijer M, Rosendaal FR, Blom HJ, et al. Hyperhomocystinemia and venous thrombosis: a meta-analysis. *Thromb Haemost* 1998; 80: 874.
Franchini M, Mannucci PM. ABO blood group and thrombotic vascular disease. *Thromb Haemost* 2014; 112: 1103.
Franchini M, Martinelli I, Mannucci PM. Uncertain thrombophilia markers. *Thromb Haemost* 2016; 115: 25.
Franco RF, Reitsma PH, Lourenco D, et al. Factor XIII val34leu is a genetic factor involved in the aetiology of venous thrombosis. *Thromb Haemost* 1999; 81: 676.
Harbin MM, Lutsey PL. May-Thurner syndrome: history of understanding and need for defining population prevalence. *J Thromb Haemost* 2020; 18: 534.
Hirsh J, Guyatt G, Albers GW, et al., eds. Antithrombotic and thrombolytic therapy: ACCP evidence-based clinical practice guidelines (8th edition). *Chest* 2008; 133: no. 6 (suppl.).
Iba T, Levy JH, Levi M, et al. Coagulopathy of coronavirus disease 2019. *Crit Care Med* 2020; 48: 1358.
Kearon C, Crowther M, Hirsh J, et al. Management of patients with hereditary hypercoagulable disorders. *Annu Rev Med* 2000; 51: 169.
Khan S, Dickerman JD. Hereditary thrombophilia. *Thromb J* 2006; 4: 15.
Lane DA, Mannucci PM, Bauer KA, et al. Inherited thrombophilia. *Thromb Haemost* 1996; 76: 651.
Leung LLK. Thrombotic disorders. In: *Scientific American Medicine. Hematology.* Hamilton: Dekker Medicine. 2020.
Mannucci PM, Franchini M. Classic thrombophilic gene variants. *Thromb Haemost* 2015; 114: 885.
Marder VJ, Aird WC, Bennett JS, et al., eds. *Hemostasis and Thrombosis: Basic Principles and Clinical Practice.* 6th edition. Philadelphia: Lippincott Williams & Wilkins. 2012.
May R, Thurner J. The cause of predominantly sinistral occurrence of thrombosis in the pelvic veins. *Angiology* 1957; 8: 419.
Miletich JP, Prescott SM, White R, et al. Inherited predisposition to thrombosis. *Cell* 1993; 72: 477.
Oldenburg J, Schwaab R. Molecular biology of blood coagulation. *Semin Thromb Hemost* 2001; 27: 313.
Prins MH, Hirsh J. A critical review of the evidence supporting a relationship between impaired fibrinolytic activity and venous thromboembolism. *Arch Intern Med* 1991; 151: 1721.
Sacher RA, ed. Thrombophilia: a forum on diagnosis and management in obstetrics, gynecology and surgery. *Semin Thromb Hemost* 1998; 24: suppl. 1.
Winter M, Gallimore M, Jones DW. Should factor XII assays be included in thrombophilia screening? *Lancet* 1995; 346: 52.

Thrombopoietin See

- Thrombocytopenia.

Thrombotic microangiopathy

The **thrombotic microangiopathies** (TMAs) are thrombohaemorrhagic disorders characterized by

- microangiopathic haemolysis (q.v.),
- thrombocytopenia (q.v.),
- platelet-fibrin thrombi in small vessels, and
- ischaemic organ damage, especially involving the kidneys, but also affecting the brain, liver, lungs and skin.

Although a disparate group, the TMAs share the common pathogenetic mechanism of complement activation.

The TMA disorders include
- antiphospholipid syndrome (q.v.),
- disseminated intravascular coagulation (q.v.),
- haemolytic–uraemic syndromes (q.v.),
- heparin-induced thrombocytopenia (q.v.),
- pre-eclampsia (including HELLP syndrome)(q.v.),
- purpura (q.v.),
- thrombocytosis/thrombocythaemia (q.v.),
- thrombotic thrombocytopenic purpura (q.v.).

Bibliography
Fox LC, Cohney SJ, Kausman JY, et al. Consensus opinion on diagnosis and management of thrombotic microangiopathy in Australia and New Zealand. *Intern Med J* 2018; 48: 624.

Thrombotic thrombocytopenic purpura

Thrombotic thrombocytopenic purpura (TTP) is an uncommon but life-threatening condition, which has a prevalence of about 10 per million of the population and which causes about one death per million population per year. It occurs at all ages and is twice as common in women.

TTP was originally described in 1924 by Moschowitz, but it was only in 1982 that its relation to platelet adhesion to damaged endothelial cells via unusually large von Willebrand factor multimers was discovered (see Von Willebrand's disease). The mechanism for this damage was finally elucidated in 1996, when it was found that a metalloprotease is normally responsible for cleaving the large vWF multimers after they are secreted into the plasma by endothelial cells. This vWF-cleaving protease (ADAMTS13) is deficient in TTP, being removed by a specific autoantibody in acute TTP and being absent in chronic relapsing TTP. The protease is normal in the seemingly related haemolytic–uraemic syndrome (q.v.). An ADAMTS13 level of activity <10% (10 IU/dL) provides a specific diagnosis, though this assay is not universally available. Autoantibodies to ADAMTS13 may also be found.

Most cases of TTP represent acquired immune-mediated TTP, with about 50% being idiopathic and about 50% being associated with other conditions (see below). Less than 5% of cases of TTP have an underlying genetic deficiency of ADAMTS13, which is inherited as an autosomal recessive condition.

TTP is manifest by
- thrombocytopenia (q.v.),
- microangiopathic haemolysis (q.v.),
- generalized symptoms of fever (q.v.) and damage to the brain and kidneys (and sometimes to the bowel, heart, liver and skin).

It is thus a **thrombotic microangiopathy** (q.v.), and it has many clinical features in common with **haemolytic-uraemic syndrome** (q.v.).

There are a number of variants of TTP as yet unclarified as to mechanism, but their predisposing factors include
- bone marrow transplantation,
- pregnancy (q.v.),
- the drugs ciclosporin and ticlopidine,
- HIV infection (see Acquired immunodeficiency syndrome),
- autoimmune disorders (q.v.).

Treatment has not been subjected to formal trials (given the rarity of TTP), but plasmapheresis (q.v.) has become the favoured therapy, with daily exchanges for 1 week in severe cases. Plasmapheresis may be increased to twice daily in cases which do not respond within 3 days. Plasmapheresis helps restore ADAMTS13 levels and remove the responsible antibodies. Electrolytes, plasma proteins and the platelet count need careful monitoring during plasmapheresis.
- *Corticosteroids in high doses are traditionally given, but the use of former modalities such as aspirin, dipyridamole, vincristine, dextran and prostacyclin is now historic.*
- *The adjunctive use of the immunomodulating agent, **rituximab** (q.v.) can remove anti-ADAMTS13 antibodies, though its effect is delayed for about 2 weeks. Although it may lead to normalization of the ADAMTS13 levels, it does not cure the underlying autoimmune response.*
- *In severe and refractory cases, **splenectomy** may produce a striking remission.*
- *Platelet microthrombi formation may be blocked by a new nanobody product with anti-vWF effect, **caplacizumab**, which has shown efficacy in acquired TTP.*
- **Gene therapy** *appears successful in animal models of hereditary TTP.*

Modern treatment has greatly improved the previously rapidly fatal course of this condition, so that survival is now over 80%. However, while many patients remain in complete and long-term remission, about one third relapse during the following 10 yr, and 10% of patients develop other serious disease. The outcome is worse in patients over 60 yr of age.

Several international guidelines have been published for the diagnosis and management of TTP, initially by a British committee in 2012, later by a Japanese team in 2017, and most recently by the International Society on Thrombosis and Haemostasis (ISTH, 2019). Guidelines providing expert assistance for clinicians are particularly important for rare conditions, such as TTP, where individual experience is usually limited, where research evidence is not robust and where international practice is varied.

See
- Thrombocytopenia.

See also
- Haemolytic–uraemic syndromes,
- Microangiopathic haemolysis,
- Purpura.

Bibliography

Azoulay E, Bauer PR, Mariotte E, et al. Expert statement on the ICU management of patients with thrombotic thrombocytopenic purpura. *Intens Care Med* 2019; 45: 1518.

Bell WR, Braine HG, Ness PM, et al. Improved survival of thrombotic thrombocytopenic purpura-hemolytic uremic syndrome: clinical experience in 108 patients. *N Engl J Med* 1991; 325: 398.

Blombery P, Kivivali L, Pepperell D, et al. Diagnosis and management of thrombotic thrombocytopenic purpura (TTP) in Australia. *Intern Med J* 2016; 46: 71.

Cines DB, Konkle BA, Furlan M. Thrombotic thrombocytopenic purpura: a paradigm shift? *Thromb Haemost* 2000; 84: 528.
Editorial. TTP – desperation, empiricism, progress. *N Engl J Med* 1991; 325: 426.
George JN. Thrombotic thrombocytopenic purpura. *N Engl J Med* 2006; 354: 1927.
Hovinger JAK, Heeb SR, Skowronska M, et al. Pathophysiology of thrombotic thrombocytopenic purpura and hemolytic uremic syndrome. *J Thromb Haemost* 2018; 16: 618.
ISTH guidelines for the diagnosis and treatment of thrombotic thrombocytopenic purpura. *J Thromb Haemost* 2020; 18: 2486 & 2496.
Mannucci PM. Thrombotic thrombocytopenic purpura: a simpler diagnosis at last? *Thromb Haemost* 1999; 82: 1380.
Mannucci PM. Understanding organ dysfunction in thrombotic thrombocytopenic purpura. *Intens Care Med* 2015; 41: 715.
Mariotte E, Blet A, Galicier L, et al. Unresponsive thrombotic thrombocytopenic purpura in critically ill patients. *Intens Care Med* 2013; 39: 1272.
Moake JL, Rudy CK, Troll JH, et al. Unusually large plasma factor VIII: von Willebrand factor multimers in chronic relapsing thrombotic thrombocytopenic purpura. *N Engl J Med* 1982; 307: 1432.
Sadler JE. Von Willebrand factor, ADAMTS-13, and thrombotic thrombocytopenic purpura. *Blood* 2008; 112: 11.
Saha M, McDaniel JK, Zheng XL. Thrombotic thrombocytopenic purpura: pathogenesis, diagnosis and potential novel therapeutics. *J Thromb Haemost* 2017; 15: 1889.
Schleinitz N, Ebbo M, Mazodier K, et al. Rituximab as preventative therapy of a clinical relapse in TTP with ADAMTS 13 inhibitor. *Am J Hematol* 2007; 82: 417.
Scully M, Cataland S, Coppo P, et al. Consensus on the standardization of terminology in thrombotic thrombocytopenic purpura and related thrombotic microangiopathies. *J Thromb Haemost* 2017; 15: 312.
Scully M, Cataland S, Peyvandi F, et al. Caplacizumab for acquired thrombotic thrombocytopenic purpura. *N Engl J Med* 2019; 380: 335.
Tsai HM, Lian ECY. Antibodies to von Willebrand factor-cleaving protease in acute thrombotic thrombocytopenic purpura. *N Engl J Med* 1998; 339: 1585.
VeyradierA, Meyer D. Thrombotic thrombocytopenic purpura and its diagnosis. *J Thromb Haemost* 2005; 3: 2420.
Zheng XL. The standard of care for immune thrombotic thrombocytopenic purpura today. *J Thromb Haemost* 2021; 191: 1864.
Zheng X, Chung D, Takayama TK, et al. Structure of von Willebrand factor-cleaving protease (ADAMTS13), a metalloprotease involved in thrombotic thrombocytopenic purpura. *J Biol Chem* 2001; 276: 41059.

Thymoma *See*

- Anaemia,
- Mediastinal diseases,
- Myasthenia gravis.

Thyroid function

Disorders of **thyroid function** are the most common endocrine disorders seen in clinical practice. They can be a particular diagnostic challenge in critically ill patients.
See
- Euthyroid sick syndrome,
- Hyperthyroidism,
- Hypothyroidism.

Bibliography
Ladenson PW. Hypothyroidism and thyrotoxicosis. In: *Scientific American Medicine. Endocrinology & Metabolism*. Hamilton: Dekker Medicine. 2020.
Mortimer R. Thyroid function tests. *Aust Prescriber* 2011; 34: 12.

Thyroid storm *See*

- Hyperthyroidism.

Ticks

Ticks are arachnids (like spiders). They are common blood-sucking ectoparasites in many species of mammals and birds, and they cause human disease only incidentally when contact occurs following specific exposures. They may contain a variety of microorganisms, including viruses, rickettsiae, bacteria and protozoa, which can cause infection following a bite.

Tick bites can also cause allergic reactions (IgE-related), including reactions at the site of the bite, systemic anaphylaxis and strangely later **mammalian meat allergy** (and gelatin allergy).
See
- Arthropods,
- Bites and stings – Insects, Arachnids,
- Lyme disease,
- Relapsing fever.

Bibliography
Graves SR, Stenos J. Tick-borne infectious diseases in Australia. *Med J Aust* 2017; 206: 320.

Tinnitus

Tinnitus is the distressing symptom of ringing in the ear(s).

It is due to any of the causes of VIII nerve damage (see Neuropathy), provided the nerve has not been actually destroyed.

It is also seen in
- lithium toxicity (q.v.),
- migraine,
- motion sickness,
- salicylism (q.v.),
- in persons struck by lightning (q.v.).
  See also
- Vertigo.

Tirofiban *See*
- Antiplatelet agents.

Tisagenlecleucel *See*
- CAR T-cell therapy (i.e. Chimeric antigen receptor T-cell therapy).

Tocilizumab

Tocilizumab is a monoclonal antibody to interleukin 6 (IL-6) receptors, which has been shown to be effective in a number of conditions associated with a severe cytokine storm, such as CAR T-cell therapy (q.v.) and haemophagocytic syndrome (q.v.). It has also been recommended in giant cell arteritis (see Arteritis). It is given in a dose of 8 mg/kg IV over 1 hr and repeated if necessary every 8 hr to a maximum of 4 doses.

See
- Autoimmune disorders,
- Immunomodulation.

Tongue *See*
- Mouth diseases.

Torulosis *See*
- Cryptococcosis.

Toxic epidermal necrolysis *See*
- Exfoliative dermatitis.

Toxic erythemas *See*
- Erythema multiforme,
- Exfoliative dermatitis.

Toxic gases and fumes *See*
- Acute lung irritation.
  See also
- Asthma – Stridor,
- Interstitial pneumonias – Bronchiolitis obliterans,
- Mercury.

Toxic shock syndrome

Toxic shock syndrome (TSS) consists of hypotension, shock and rash following an acute febrile staphylococcal infection.

It was first described in 1978 in children, and by 1980 there had been reports of about 1000 cases, with 95% in women. Of these, by far the majority had occurred during menstruation and were associated with super-absorbent tampon use. In retrospect, post-influenzal toxic shock syndrome has been postulated to have been the cause of the plague of Athens in 430 BC known as the 'Thucydides syndrome', although other conditions have been more plausibly implicated (see Plague).

The syndrome is due to the effects of staphylococcal toxin, TSST-1, in those few patients who do not already have antibodies to TSST-1. The toxin is secreted following a localized superficial and not necessarily overt staphylococcal infection. One of a considerable variety of local infections (or even just colonizations) may be identified. The cause may also include deep staphylococcal infections, such as wound infection, abscess, pneumonia (especially post-influenzal), empyema or osteomyelitis. Sometimes, no culprit source of the infection can be identified. TSST-1 stimulates interleukin 1 (IL-1) and TNF release, and the entire sequence may be enhanced by impaired host immunity.

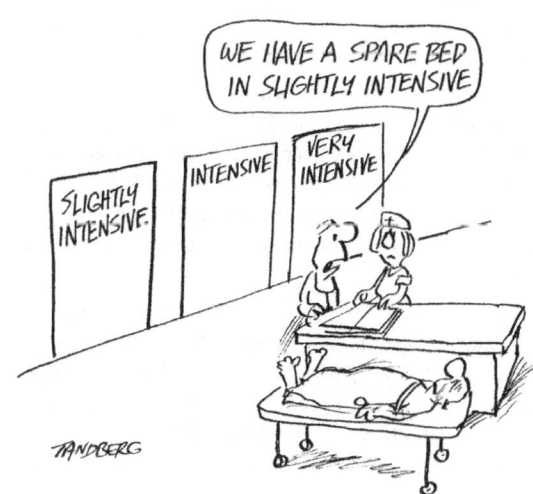

Clinical features include
- high fever (q.v.),
- scarlatiniform rash with subsequent desquamation, especially on the palms,
- strawberry tongue and sore throat, though without a pharyngeal exudate,
- conjunctival injection,
- vomiting and diarrhoea (q.v.),
- hypotension and eventually shock.

Multiorgan involvement is demonstrated by
- myalgia,
- toxic encephalopathy (q.v.),
- liver dysfunction,
- renal failure,
- thrombocytopenia (q.v.),
- hypocalcaemia (q.v.).

The diagnosis is based on the clinical features and the identification of *Staphylococcus aureus* in culture. The condition is rarely caused by *S. epidermidis*.

The differential diagnosis includes
- scarlet fever (q.v.),
- meningococcaemia,
- viral exanthems,
- spotted fevers (q.v.),
- drug toxicity, e.g. the Stevens–Johnson syndrome (q.v.).

*Treatment includes **resuscitation**, **management of the local infection** and **systemic antibiotics**. The antibiotics should be either a beta-lactamase-resistant penicillin or a cephalosporin. If methicillin-resistance is suspected, vancomycin should be given. It is suggested that concomitant clindamycin or linezolid may reduce the possibility of further toxin production when other, bacteriocidal antibiotics are first given.*

- The potential value of **corticosteroids** is uncertain, but **immune globulin** may be helpful.

The prognosis is good, with recovery in 1–2 weeks and a mortality of only 5%. The incidence has declined and the fatality rate has decreased since super-absorbent tampons were withdrawn from the market in 1981. Nowadays, most cases bear no relation to menstruation. The condition can be recurrent given appropriate circumstances.

A similar syndrome is produced by some group-A strains of *S. pyogenes* which secrete erythrogenic toxin type A, i.e. the toxin responsible for scarlet fever, though in the **'toxic strep syndrome'** scarlatiniform eruptions may be paradoxically absent (see Scarlet fever).

Non-group A streptococcal strains have also been reported to cause this condition.

Massive soft tissue destruction (see Gangrene – 1. Necrotizing fasciitis) is usual, but sometimes the preceding streptococcal infection may not be severe.

The diagnosis can be particularly difficult, with only flu-like symptoms in some patients and negative blood cultures in 40% of cases. Comorbidities are common, as many patients are immunocompromised.

*The general principles of the treatment of staphylococcal TSS also apply to streptococcal TSS. A β-lactam antibiotic should be combined with clindamycin, because of the latter's additional antitoxin effect (even if some organisms are resistant to it in vitro). In addition, **immune globulin** is probably useful, and there has been a preliminary report that the administration of high doses of **C1-esterase inhibitor** IV may also be helpful.*

Bibliography
Burnham JP, Kollef MH. Understanding toxic shock syndrome. *Intens Care Med* 2015; 41: 1707.
Cone LA, Woodard DR, Schlievert PM, et al. Clinical and bacteriologic observations of a toxic shock-like syndrome due to *Streptococcus pyogenes*. *N Engl J Med* 1987; 317: 146.
Davis JP, Chesney PJ, Wand PJ, et al. Toxic-shock syndrome: epidemiologic features, recurrence, risk factors, and prevention. *N Engl J Med* 1980; 303: 1429.
Fronhoffs S, Luyken J, Steuer K, et al. The effect of C1-esterase inhibitor in definite and suspected streptococcal toxic shock syndrome. *Intens Care Med* 2000; 26: 1566.
Kain KC, Schulzer M, Chow AW. Clinical spectrum of nonmenstrual toxic shock syndrome (TSS): comparison with menstrual TSS by multivariate discriminant analysis. *Clin Infect Dis* 1993; 16: 100.
Langmuir AD, Worthen TD, Solomon J, et al. The Thucydides syndrome: a new hypothesis for the cause of the plague of Athens. *N Engl J Med* 1985; 313: 1027.
Schlievert PM, MacDonald KL. *Toxic Shock Syndrome*. 2nd ed. Philadelphia: WB Saunders.1998.
Seal DV. Necrotizing fasciitis. *Curr Opin Infect Dis* 2001; 14: 127.
Stevens DL. Streptococcal toxic-shock syndrome: spectrum of disease, pathogenesis, and new concepts in treatment. *Emerg Infect Dis* 1995; 1: 3.
Stevens DL, Tanner MH, Winship J, et al. Severe group A streptococcal infections associated with a toxic shock-like syndrome and scarlet fever toxin. *N Engl J Med* 1989; 321: 1.

Toxoplasmosis

Toxoplasmosis is caused by infection with the obligate intracellular protozoan parasite, *Toxoplasma gondii*, which has a worldwide distribution and can infect all mammalian species.

Human infection usually arises from ingestion of contaminated raw food or cat faeces (the cat being the definitive host), but it can also arise from transplacental passage, organ transplantation or blood transfusion. Following the ingestion of cysts, trophozoites are liberated in the gut giving rise to parasitaemia and tissue invasion with eventual cyst formation. Though quiescent, the cysts remain viable.

- Most infections are clearly asymptomatic, since positive serology is found in up to 50% of populations, even in developed countries.
- In adults, there is fever (q.v.), myalgia, fatigue, rash, lymphadenopathy (q.v.), hepatosplenomegaly, atypical lymphocytosis (q.v.) and sometimes uveitis (q.v.).
- The disease is usually mild and subsides after several weeks.
- In immunocompromised hosts, a severe opportunistic infection may occur with
  - pneumonitis,
  - myocarditis,
  - meningoencephalitis (q.v.),
  - a mass lesion.

The diagnosis is made serologically. The differential diagnosis includes
- infectious mononucleosis (see Epstein–Barr virus),
- cytomegalovirus (CMV) infection (q.v.),
- lymphoma,
- sarcoidosis (q.v.).

Treatment is required if the disease is severe or there is multisystem involvement. **Pyrimethamine** *is used in a dose of 25–50 mg per day for 4–6 weeks. Concomitant folinic acid therapy is recommended.*
- *It is usual to add a* **sulphonamide** *or* **clindamycin** *for cerebral toxoplasmosis in patients with AIDS.*

Bibliography

Joiner KA, Dubremetz JF. Toxoplasma gondii: a protozoan for the nineties. *Infect Immun* 1993; 61: 1169.

McCabe R, Remington JS. Toxoplasmosis. *N Engl J Med* 1988; 318: 313.

Wong S, Remington JS. Toxoplasmosis in pregnancy. *Clin Infect Dis* 1994; 18: 853.

Trace elements

Trace elements are micronutrients, i.e. chemical substances required by living organisms in very small amounts. Each is present in the body in an amount <0.01% of total body weight, and they are usually associated with enzyme function. Confirmation of the essential nature of a particular trace element requires that its deficiency is associated with dysfunction and that its addition prevents or reverses this dysfunction.

The **essential trace elements** (ETEs) include
- boron,
- chromium (q.v.),
- cobalt (q.v.),
- copper (q.v.),
- iodine,
- manganese (q.v.),
- molybdenum,
- selenium (q.v.),
- zinc (q.v.),
- possibly nickel,
- possibly silicon,
- possibly vanadium.

Deficiency of any one of these elements gives rise to clinical disease. The major deficiencies are discussed elsewhere in relation to the individual elements.

In recent decades, there has been new understanding of the requirements for trace elements in critical illness and of their IV dosage in that setting, with particular emphasis on prevention of deficiency. The elements with defined daily dosage for this purpose are listed in the accompanying Table.

Trace element requirements

Element	Dosage
Chromium	0.2–0.4
Copper	5–20
Iodine	1.0
Iron	20
Manganese	5
Molybdenum	0.4
Selenium	0.4–1.5
Zinc	50–100

Doses are in μmol per day for IV administration in patients receiving total parenteral nutrition (TPN).

They may be conveniently obtained by adding a commercial multi-element preparation to the TPN solution. Major minerals such as sodium, potassium, calcium, magnesium and phosphate have to be added separately, as their needs can vary greatly between individual patients.

Bibliography

Barceloux DG. Cobalt. *J Toxicol Clin Toxicol* 1999; 37: 201.

Barceloux DG. Molybdenum. *J Toxicol Clin Toxicol* 1999; 37: 231.

Barceloux DG. Nickel. *J Toxicol Clin Toxicol* 1999; 37: 239.

Barceloux DG. Vanadium. *J Toxicol Clin Toxicol* 1999; 37: 265

Berger MM, Cavadini C, Chiolero R, et al. Influence of large intakes of trace elements on recovery after major burns. *Nutrition* 1994; 10: 327.

Casaer MP, Bellomo R. Micronutrient deficiency in critical illness: an invisible foe? *Intens Care Med* 2019; 45: 1136.

Chandra RK. Effect of vitamin and trace-element supplementation on immune responses and infection in elderly patients. *Lancet* 1992; 340: 1124.

Elia M. Changing concepts of nutrient requirements in disease: implications for artificial nutritional support. *Lancet* 1995; 345: 1279.

Fleming CR. Trace element metabolism in adult patients requiring total parenteral nutrition. *Am J Clin Nutr* 1989; 49: 573.

Heyland DK, Dhaliwal R, Suchner U, et al. Antioxidant nutrients: a systematic review of trace elements and vitamins in the critically ill patient. *Intens Care Med* 2005; 31: 327.

Mertz W. The essential trace elements. *Science* 1981; 213: 1332.

Prasad AS, ed. *Essential and Toxic Trace Elements in Human Health and Disease.* New York: Liss. 1988.

Shenkin A. Vitamin and essential trace element recommendations during intravenous therapy: theory and practice. *Proc Nutr Soc* 1986; 45: 383.

Simmer K, Thompson RPH. Trace elements. In: Cohen RD, Lewis B, Alberti KGMM, Denman AM, eds. *The Metabolic and Molecular Basis of Acquired Disease.* London: Baillere Tindall. 1990, p 670.

Singer P, Manzanares W, Berger MM. What's new in trace elements? *Intens Care Med* 2018; 44: 643.

Supplement. The trace elements: their role and function in nutritional support. *Nutrition* 1995; 2: no.1.

Tranexamic acid

Tranexamic acid (TXA) is currently the antifibrinolytic agent of choice, having superseded epsilon aminocaproic acid (see Aminocaproic acid). Both are low molecular weight drugs (about 150 kDa) and are synthetic analogs of the amino acid lysine. The lysine-binding site on fibrin is the target for fibrinolysis by plasmin.

Its indications include primary or secondary **fibrinolysis** (q.v.), in which it may be given orally or IV in a typical dose of 1 g tds. It may also be administered locally, when focal bleeding has been attributed to local rather than systemic fibrinolysis.

However, good published evidence is required to support its use in specific settings, as its potential efficacy needs to be balanced against its potential adverse (mainly thromboembolic) effects. For example:

- TXA has been shown to reduce both bleeding and mortality after major trauma or post-partum haemorrhage.
- TXA was found to decrease bleeding but increase mortality after major gastrointestinal haemorrhage.
- TXA after traumatic brain injury has been the subject of conflicting reports in the literature, and meta-analyses have suggested reduction in haematoma expansion but no overall effect on mortality or disability.

See
- Angioedema,
- Anticoagulants,
- Arteriovenous malformations,
- Cystic fibrosis,
- Pregnancy – 6. Post-partum problems,
- Von Willebrand's disease.

Transverse myelitis *See*

- Demyelinating diseases.
 See also
- Epidural abscess,
- Guillain–Barré syndrome,
- Optic neuritis.

Trauma

The principles of the management of patients with **trauma**, even those with uncommon aspects of common injuries, are well known in the Intensive Care setting. This book thus considers injuries and complications which themselves are generally less common, including

- Autonomic dysreflexia,
- Barotrauma,
- Bites and stings,
- Envenomation,
- Irukandji syndrome,
- Lightning,
- Respiratory burns,
- Tranexamic acid,
- Trauma in pregnancy,
- Trauma-induced coagulopathy,

- Water-related accidents
    - bathing,
    - diving,
    - drowning.

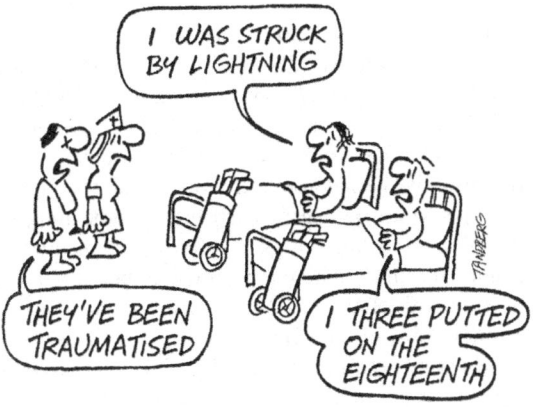

Bibliography

Barton RN. Trauma and its metabolic products. *Br Med Bull* 1985; 41: 3.

Blaisdell FW, Holcroft JW, eds. *Scientific American Surgery Handbook of Trauma.* New York: Scientific American. 1999.

Green DR. Trauma and the immune response. *Immunol Today* 1988; 9: 253.

Frayn KN. Hormonal control of metabolism in trauma and sepsis. *Clin Endocrinol* 1986; 24: 577.

Moore EE, Cogbill TH, Malagoni MA, et al. Scaling systems for organ specific injuries. *Curr Opin Crit Care* 1996; 2: 450.

Nelson LD, ed. New advances in the care of critically injured patients. *New Horizons: The Science and Practice of Acute Medicine* 1999; 7: 1.

Smith RM, Giannoudis PV. Trauma and the immune response. *J R Soc Med* 1998; 91: 417.

Wisner DH. Current priorities in the management of multiple injury. *Curr Opin Crit Care* 1996; 2: 463.

Trauma-induced coagulopathy See

- Coagulation disorders.

Bibliography

Spahn DR, Bouillon B, Duranteau J, et al. The European guideline on management of major bleeding and coagulopathy following trauma: fifth edition. *Crit Care* 2019; 23: 98.

Trauma in pregnancy

Trauma in pregnancy is the commonest cause of maternal death, although only 1 in 20 cases of maternal trauma requires hospitalization. Fetal risk is greater than maternal risk, but in general fetal loss is minimized if maternal health can be maintained.

Trauma during pregnancy may present special problems of assessment and management. This is not just because two patients have to be simultaneously considered, but especially because of the alterations in abdominal anatomy and general physiology at the time.

While **hypotension** in the pregnant trauma patient may be due to hypovolaemia, it may also be positional. This distinction may be especially difficult, because the blood volume is increased by up to 35% in pregnancy (about 1500 mL at term) and the cardiac output is concomitantly increased, thus masking the usual clinical signs of hypovolaemia. However, putting the patient in the left lateral position will help to differentiate these two causes, because in the supine position inferior caval (or even aortocaval) obstruction can occur. This may reduce the cardiac output by up to 30% and the systolic blood pressure by up to 30 mmHg due to diminished preload.

Early **vascular access** for volume resuscitation is important, because the uterine blood flow is not autoregulated and fetal shock may occur early. Vasopressors are best avoided.

Abdominal examination in pregnancy can be misleading, because the normal anatomical relationships are altered due to stretching of the abdominal wall, relocation of viscera and compartmentalization. Diagnostic peritoneal lavage can be safely performed in any trimester provided it is above the uterus.

Placental abruption (abruptio placentae) occurs in 2–4% of patients with minor injuries and in up to 40% of those with major injuries. The maternal mortality is very low (<1%), but the fetal mortality is high (about 25%), and it is thus the major cause of fetal death following maternal trauma. This complication occurs particularly with deceleration forces, and there may therefore be few external signs of injury. It also complicates about 1% of pregnancies in general, particularly when risk factors such as advanced maternal age, smoking or hypertension are present.

Clinical features may include abdominal cramps, uterine tenderness, vaginal bleeding, amniotic fluid leakage (with the resultant vaginal fluid having a pH of 7–7.5), amniotic fluid embolism (q.v.), hypovolaemia (since up to 2 L of blood can accumulate in the

> uterus), a uterine size which is 'larger than dates', and altered fetal heart rate.
>
> The detection of increased plasma levels of thrombomodulin (q.v.), a marker of endothelial cell damage, has been reported to have the highest sensitivity of any test for placental abruption.
>
> Cardiotocographic monitoring should be performed for at least 4 hr and continued for up to 24 hr if any of the clinical features described above are present.

Fetomaternal haemorrhage occurs in 8–30% of cases after trauma. It is detected by the Kleihauer–Betke (KT) acid elution technique on maternal blood. One fetal cell per 1000 maternal cells corresponds to a fetomaternal haemorrhage of 5 mL. All Rh-negative mothers who have a negative indirect Coomb's test and who suffer abdominal trauma during pregnancy should receive Rh immune globulin prophylactically. The dose will depend on the KT test result, but 125 mcg IM is a commonly given dose.

See also
- Pregnancy.

Bibliography

Fildes J, Reed L, Jones N, et al. Trauma: the leading cause of maternal death. *J Trauma* 1992; 32: 643.

Knudson MM. Acute abdominal injuries during pregnancy. *Curr Opin Crit Care* 1996; 2: 469.

Magriples U, Chan DW, Bruzek D, et al. Thrombomodulin: a new marker for placental abruption. *Thromb Haemost* 1999; 81: 32.

Pearlman MD, Tintinalli JE, Lorenz RP. Blunt trauma during pregnancy. *N Engl J Med* 1990; 323: 1609.

Sorensen VJ, Bivins BA, Obeid FN, et al. Management of general surgical emergencies in pregnancy. *Am Surg* 1990; 56: 245.

Trauma Service. *Trauma Guidelines Booklet*. Melbourne: Royal Melbourne Hospital. 2011.

Weinberg L, Steele RG, Pugh R, et al. The pregnant trauma patient. *Anaesth Intens Care* 2005; 33: 167.

Trench fever See
- Pediculosis,
- Rickettsial diseases.

Trichlorethylene See
- Carbon tetrachloride.

Tropical pulmonary eosinophilia See
- Eosinophilia and lung infiltration.

Tuberculosis

Tuberculosis (TB) is one of the best-known chronic infectious diseases. Although in recent decades its incidence has greatly reduced in developed countries (e.g. <5 notifications per 100,000 of the population per year), it has remained one of the major causes of death worldwide, particularly among the poor. It has been calculated that about one third of the world's population has been infected with the tubercle bacillus (*Mycobacterium tuberculosis*, first identified by Koch in 1882), with an annual burden of about 10 million new cases and 1.5 million deaths.

Importantly, TB has also lately had a small resurgence in developed countries, particularly in migrants, indigenous peoples, disadvantaged groups (especially the homeless) and the immunocompromised (especially as a coinfection with HIV – see Acquired immunodeficiency syndrome). A major conference has emphasized its many different visages and thus the need for adaptable control strategies. Issues related to diagnostic difficulties, complex treatment options and effective vaccine development remain challenges both for basic research and for public health. The proposed goal of global eradication of TB by 2035 may be ambitious.

Although treatment principles (standard 6 months chemotherapy with 4-drug combinations) are well established with almost 100% cure rates and at low cost, perhaps one of the main new challenges is the increasing frequency of multidrug-resistant strains, selected because of inappropriate therapy and evident not only in developing countries. The occurrence of multidrug-resistant tuberculosis (MDR-TB) ranges from <1% of cases of TB in Australia (i.e. about 10 cases per year) to over 13% in India (i.e. about 250,000 cases per year). Current agents which may be of use in the treatment of such patients include new fluoroquinolones (e.g. ciprofloxacin), macrolides (e.g. clarithromycin) and rifamycins (e.g. rifabutin), but depressingly no agents are suitable for prophylaxis after contact with isoniazid-resistant strains. Successful therapy requires attention to social (and societal) as well as clinical factors.

> Clinical staff need to be aware of the risks of hospital-acquired tuberculosis and the need for scrupulous preventative measures, including rapid diagnosis, effective treatment, thorough isolation of infected patients, filtered ventilation, proper disposal of medical waste, monitoring of staff and chemoprophylaxis of close contacts. Latent infection in exposed staff (and others) may now be identified most expeditiously with one of the new blood tests based on T-cell interferon-γ release.

Bibliography

Blumberg HM, Leonard MK, Jasmer RM. Update on the treatment of tuberculosis and latent tuberculosis infection. *JAMA* 2005; 293: 2776.

Catanzaro A. How to increase the accuracy of the diagnosis of tuberculosis. *Pulmonary Perspectives* 2004; 21(2): 1.

Darby J, Black J, Buising K. Interferon-gamma release assays and the diagnosis of tuberculosis: have they found their place? *Intern Med J* 2014; 44: 624.

Davies PDO. The challenge of tuberculosis. *J R Soc Med* 2003; 96: 262.

Davies PDO, De Cock KM, Leese J, et al. Tuberculosis 2000. *J R Soc Med* 1996; 89: 431.

Donoghue HD, Spigelman M, Greenblatt CL, et al. Tuberculosis: from prehistory to Robert Koch, as revealed by ancient DNA. *Lancet Infect Dis* 2004; 4: 584.

Fordham von Reyn C. Correcting the record on BCG before we license new vaccines against tuberculosis. *J R Soc Med* 2017; 110: 428.

Frieden TR, Sterling TR, Munsiff SS, et al. Tuberculosis: a review. *Lancet* 2003; 362: 887.

Keal JL, Davies PDO. Tuberculosis: a forgotten plague? *J R Soc Med* 2011; 104: 182.

Lancet Conference. The challenge of tuberculosis: statements on global control and prevention. *Lancet* 1995; 346: 809.

Lawn SD, Zumla AI. Tuberculosis. *Lancet* 2011; 378: 57.

Madkour MM, ed. *Textbook of Tuberculosis*. Berlin: Springer-Verlag. 2003.

Milburn H. Key issues in the diagnosis and management of tuberculosis. *J R Soc Med* 2007; 100: 134.

Millard FJC. The rising incidence of tuberculosis. *J R Soc Med* 1996; 89: 497.

Ormerod P, Campbell J, Novelli V. Chemotherapy and management of tuberculosis in the United Kingdom: recommendations 1998. *Thorax* 1998; 53: 536.

Parr JB, Leonard MK, Blumberg HM. Tuberculosis. In: *Scientific American Medicine. Infectious Diseases*. Hamilton: Dekker Medicine. 2020.

Reichman LB, Tanne JH. *Timebomb: The Global Epidemic of Multi-Drug-Resistant Tuberculosis*. New York: McGraw-Hill. 2002.

Snider DE, La Montagne JR. The neglected global tuberculosis problem. *J Infect Dis* 1994; 169: 1189.

Snider DE, Roper WL. The new tuberculosis. *N Engl J Med* 1992; 326: 703.

Tuberous sclerosis

Tuberous sclerosis (Bourneville's disease) is a rare inherited neurocutaneous disorder or phakomatosis. It has a variable hereditary pattern and a reported prevalence of about 1 in 100,000 of the population, although recent surveys have suggested up to a 10-fold greater frequency.

It is characterized by the triad of facial sebaceous adenoma (i.e. butterfly rash over the nose and cheeks), epilepsy and mental retardation. There may also be cafe-au-lait spots. It is one of the uncommon causes of a diffuse pulmonary infiltrate (q.v.), with an interstitial pattern of extensive fine thin-walled cysts seen on high-resolution CT scanning due to **lymphangioleiomyomatosis** (q.v.). There may be associated cardiac, cerebral or renal tumours, which are typically hamartomatous.

Treatment is **symptomatic**, *but opportunities for immunotherapy are under investigation.*

See also
- Sturge–Weber syndrome (another rare inherited neurocutaneous disorder).

Bibliography

Crino PB, Nathanson KL, Henske EP. The tuberous sclerosis complex. *N Engl J Med* 2006; 355: 1345.

Critchley M, Earle C. Tubero-sclerosis and allied conditions. *Brain* 1932; 55: 311.

Curatolo P, Bombardieri R, Jozwiak S. Tuberous sclerosis. *Lancet* 2008; 372: 657.

Lenoir S, Grenier P, Brauner MW, et al. Pulmonary lymphangiomyomatosis and tuberous sclerosis: comparison of radiographic and thin-section CT findings. *Radiology* 1990; 175: 329.

Liu H-J, Krymskaya VP, Henske EP. Immunotherapy for lymphangioleiomyomatosis and tuberous sclerosis: progress and future directions. *Chest* 2019; 156: 1062.

McCormack FX. Lymphangioleiomyomatosis: a clinical update. *Chest* 2008; 133: 507.

Tubulointerstitial diseases

Tubulointerstitial diseases, glomerular diseases (q.v.) and vascular diseases comprise the three main groups of renal disorders. The tubulointerstitial diseases have a large variety of causes and display a considerable spectrum of severity and reversibility and thus clinical features.

The urine usually shows
- haematuria (q.v.),
- sterile pyuria,
- white blood cell casts,
- proteinuria (q.v.)
  - the protein is of low molecular weight, i.e. beta$_2$-microglobulin (q.v.),
  - rather than albumin as in glomerular diseases.

Renal dysfunction shows tubular defects, including

- impaired concentration with polyuria and possibly hypovolaemia,
- hypokalaemia or hyperkalaemia,
- magnesium loss (q.v.),
- glycosuria,
- aminoaciduria (q.v.),
- renal tubular acidosis (q.v.).

Acute interstitial nephritis (AIN) is usually an allergic response, especially to drugs (q.v.). Many drugs (currently more than 50) can be potential causes, but the most common are
- beta-lactam antibiotics
  - especially with the anti-staphylococcal agents, flucloxacillin and dicloxacillin, and more commonly with the latter (in contrast to hepatic reactions which are more common with the former),
- other antibiotics
  - including ciprofloxacin, cotrimoxazole, erythromycin, rifampicin, vancomycin,
- NSAIDs,
- cimetidine (but not ranitidine), proton pump inhibitors (PPIs),
- diuretics, such as thiazides,
- phenytoin, carbamazepine,
- other drugs
  - allopurinol, methyldopa, propranolol.

AIN is clinically associated with fever (q.v.), rash and eosinophilia (q.v.), which occur on average about 2 weeks (range 3–42 days) after the drug has been commenced. Oliguria is usual. There is a sterile pyuria, often with eosinophiluria and occasionally with haematuria (q.v.).

Definitive diagnosis requires renal biopsy.

AIN is an important cause of renal dysfunction, because
- it is third in frequency after pre-renal uraemia and acute kidney injury (AKI, acute tubular necrosis),
- it is reversible if the drug is stopped,
- it can complicate recovery from sepsis-induced acute kidney injury, in which setting its recognition can sometimes be difficult.

Treatment with **corticosteroids** is probably helpful, but there is currently no satisfactory trial evidence to confirm this. The best results have been with prompt treatment, though in practice corticosteroids are more commonly given if recovery is delayed beyond a few days after withdrawal of the culprit drug.

Dialysis is required in perhaps one third of cases, occasionally for several weeks.

Chronic interstitial nephritis may be caused by a large variety of factors. It is a toxic nephropathy, and some years ago it was commonly called **analgesic nephropathy**, because in most cases it had been associated with excessive oral analgesic consumption (particularly phenacetin), although the mechanism for this type of damage remains unclear.

The many aetiological factors include
- drugs most commonly, especially
  - analgesics, not just phenacetin, which was later withdrawn from the market, but also paracetamol/aspirin combinations as well as other NSAIDs,
  - cisplatin,
  - ciclosporin,
  - lithium (q.v.),
- toxic/metabolic agents
  - cadmium (q.v.),
  - lead (q.v.),
  - hypokalaemia,
  - hypercalcaemia (q.v.),
- physical agents
  - irradiation,
  - obstruction,
  - reflux,
- infection
  - chronic pyelonephritis,
  - systemic infection,
- vascular diseases,
- cystic renal disease (q.v.),
- transplant rejection,
- systemic diseases
  - systemic lupus erythematosus (q.v.),
  - sarcoidosis (q.v.),
  - dysproteinaemias.

Chronic interstitial nephritis is commonly associated with papillary necrosis. It typically presents as two sequential problems, namely,
- renal dysfunction
  - with failure of urinary concentration, acidification and sodium conservation,
  - with consequent metabolic acidosis (q.v.) and hypovolaemia,
- slowly progressive renal failure
  - sometimes with severe hypertension,
  - eventually with dialysis-dependent end-stage renal disease.

Bibliography
Abraham PA, Keane WF. Glomerular and interstitial disease induced by nonsteroidal anti-inflammatory drugs. *Am J Nephrol* 1984; 4: 1.

Appel GB, Bhat P, Canetta P. Tubulointerstitial diseases. In: *Scientific American Medicine*. Nephrology. Hamilton: Dekker Medicine. 2020.

Corwin HL, Korbet SM, Schwartz MM. Clinical correlates of eosinophiluria. *Arch Intern Med* 1985; 145: 1097.

Fored CM, Ejerblad E, Lindblad P, et al. Acetaminophen, aspirin, and chronic renal failure. *N Engl J Med* 2001; 345: 1801.

Hoitsma AJ, Wetzels JFM, Koene RAP. Drug-induced nephrotoxicity: aetiology, clinical features and management. *Drug Safety* 1991; 6: 131.

Kincaid-Smith P. Analgesic abuse and the kidney. *Kidney Int* 1980; 17: 250.

Linton AL, Clark WF, Driedger AA, et al. Acute interstitial nephritis due to drugs. *Ann Intern Med* 1980; 93: 735.

Neilson EG. Pathogenesis and therapy of interstitial nephritis. *Kidney Int* 1989; 35: 1257.

Ronco PM, Flahault A. Drug-induced end-stage renal disease. *N Engl J Med* 1994; 331: 1711.

Rossert J. Drug-induced acute interstitial nephritis. *Kidney Int* 2001; 60: 804.

Turner NN, Lameire N, Goldsmith DJ, et al. eds. *Oxford Textbook of Clinical Nephrology*. 4th edition. Oxford: Oxford University Press. 2015.

Tumour-lysis syndrome

The **tumour-lysis syndrome** (TLS) results from the massive release of intracellular components, especially purines from DNA breakdown as well as potassium and phosphate, following the extensive acute lysis of tumour cells. The syndrome is particularly seen following induction chemotherapy in haematological malignancies and reflects the presence of a large tumour burden. Although acute, transient and to some extent predictable, it can be severe and even life-threatening. It is thus one of the important **cancer complications** (q.v.).

The clinical features of TLS include renal, cardiac and neurological manifestations. The laboratory features of TLS comprise hyperkalaemia, hyperphosphataemia (q.v.), hyperuricaemia (q.v.) and hypocalcaemia (q.v.).

Purine metabolism gives rise to uric acid and phosphate release.

- The former may give rise to oliguric renal failure due to acute uric acid nephropathy.
- The latter leads to hypocalcaemia (q.v.) and thus cardiac arrhythmias and fits.

Prevention is with

- fluid loading, e.g. saline to give a urine output of at least 100 mL/hr,
- bicarbonate to give a urinary pH of at least 6.5, since uric acid is then converted to the more soluble urate, though there is now a recognized risk of crystal nephropathy from this practice,
- allopurinol (a xanthine oxidase inhibitor – see Gout).

Treatment is with

- fluid administration, which should be titrated against cardiac filling pressures,
- loop diuretics,
- management of hyperkalaemia and hypocalcaemia,
- renal replacement therapy if necessary.

Recombinant urate oxidase, rasburicase, is the most effective agent for the prevention and treatment of hyperuricaemia associated with haematological tumour lysis, but it is expensive. It may be given in a single standard dose of 3 mg.

Bibliography

Arrambide K, Toto RD. Tumor lysis syndrome. *Semin Nephrol* 1993; 13: 273.

Barton JC. Tumor lysis syndrome in nonhematopoietic neoplasms. *Cancer* 1989; 64: 738.

Coiffier B, Mounier N, Bologna S, et al. Efficacy and safety of rasburicase (recombinant urate oxidase) for the prevention and treatment of hyperuricemia during induction chemotherapy of aggressive non-Hodgkin's lymphoma. *J Clin Oncol* 2003; 21: 4402.

Howard SC, Jones DP, Pui C-H. The tumor lysis syndrome *N Engl J Med* 2011; 364: 1844.

McCurdy MT, Shanholtz CB. Oncologic emergencies. *Crit Care Med* 2012; 40: 2212.

Zafrani L, Canet E, Darmon M. Understanding tumor lysis syndrome. *Intens Care Med* 2019; 45: 1608.

Tumour markers/biomarkers

Tumour markers (or **biomarkers**) are substances whose bloods levels are elevated in the presence of a specific tumour. In principle, such assays can provide clinical assistance in monitoring treatment and in prognosis generally, but they are not as yet appropriate for routine screening of asymptomatic patients or for diagnosis of non-specific clinical features.

The controversy over their potential role in screening is best exemplified by the recent debate over the utility of **prostate-specific antigen** (PSA) in the early diagnosis of prostate cancer. Moreover, the limitation of using serum tumour (bio)markers in screening is illustrated by calculating that for a tumour with an incidence of (say) 40 per 100,000 of the population per year, a test with 99.6% specificity would still have a positive predictive value of only 10%.

The other commonly used markers include

- **carcinoembryonic antigen** (q.v.)
  - for colorectal cancer,

- **alpha fetoprotein** (q.v.)
  - for hepatocellular carcinoma (q.v.), some hepatic metastases, non-seminoma testicular cancer, germ cell tumours,
- **CA 19.9**
  - for pancreatic cancer,
- **CA 125**
  - for ovarian cancer,
- **CA 15.3**
  - for breast cancer,
- **hCG**
  - for gestational trophoblast tumours (see Pregnancy), germ cell tumours,
- **thyroglobulin**
  - for thyroid cancer,
- **calcitonin** (q.v.)
  - for medullary thyroid cancer,
- **paraproteins**
  - for multiple myeloma (q.v.).

With the exception of paraproteins, all the other tumour biomarkers may also be elevated sometimes in a number of malignant and non-malignant conditions in addition to those for which they are more specifically used.

Immunophenotype markers identified by flow cytometry are extensively used in the diagnosis and classification of haematological malignancies.

In the future, the opportunities for useful tumour (and other) screening are expected to be revolutionized by the new techniques of functional genomics and proteomics and by the development of 'liquid biopsies'. The latter seeks to identify DNA, proteins of cellular fragments specific to multiple types of cancers.

Bibliography
Pezaro C, Woo, HH, Davis ID. Prostate cancer: measuring PSA. *Intern Med J* 2014; 44: 433.
Smith RA, Cokkinides V, Brooks D, et al. Cancer screening in the United States, 2010: a review of current American Cancer Society guidelines and issues in cancer screening. *CA: A Cancer Journal for Clinicians* 2010; 60: 99.
Sturgeon CM, Lai LC, Duffy MJ. Serum tumour markers: how to order and interpret them, *BMJ* 2010; 339: 852.

Tumour necrosis factor

Tumour necrosis factor (TNF) is a small protein of 18 kDa secreted by activated macrophages and other immune cells in response to infection. It is a member of a superfamily of related proteins involved in regulating the body's complex responses to infection and injury. It was originally identified because of its anticancer activity and initially called cachectin (cachexin).

TNF is a cytokine which acts as an endogenous pyrogen, inducing fever, inflammation, apoptosis, cachexia, and tumour inhibition. It is a key mediator in the response to endotoxin and thus in septic shock.

Its dysregulation has been implicated in the pathogenesis of many diseases, most notably inflammatory bowel disease (q.v.), psoriasis (q.v.), some cancers and Alzheimer's disease. It may be produced ectopically by some cancers.

While recombinant TNF may be used as a potential immunostimulant, more importantly **TNF inhibitors** have become front-line tools of **immunomodulation** (q.v.) in a large variety of autoimmune and related conditions. TNF inhibitors are monoclonal antibodies to TNF-α and include infliximab, etanercept and adalimumab. Potential side-effects include atypical infections (particularly with opportunistic intracellular organisms) and tumour formation.

Conditions in which TNF inhibitors have been shown to be effective include
- ankylosing spondylitis (q.v.),
- Behcet's syndrome (q.v.),
- eosinophilia – hypereosinophilic syndrome (q.v.),
- haemophagocytic syndrome, (q.v.)
- inflammatory bowel disease (q.v.),
- Jarisch–Herxheimer reaction (q.v.),
- myopathy – idiopathic inflammatory myopathy (q.v.),
- pemphigus (q.v.),
- psoriasis (q.v.),
- rheumatoid arthritis,
- sarcoidosis (q.v.),
- Wegener's granulomatosis (q.v.)
  See
- Autoimmune disorders.

Bibliography
Chu W-M. Tumor necrosis factor. *Cancer Lett* 2013; 328: 222.
Jani M, Dixon WG, Chinoy H. Drug safety and immunogenicity of tumour necrosis factor inhibitors. *Rheumatology* 2018; 57: 1896.
Kalliolias GD, Ivashkiv LB. TNF biology, pathogenic mechanisms and emerging therapeutic strategies. *Nature Rev Rheum* 2015; 12: 49.
Lundy SK, Gizinski A, Fox DA. Introduction to clinical immunology: overview of immune response, autoimmune conditions, and immunosuppressive therapeutics for rheumatic diseases. In: *Scientific American Medicine. Allergy & Immunology*. Hamilton: Dekker Medicine. 2020.
Monaco C, Nanchahal J, Taylor P, et al. Anti-TNF therapy: past, present and future. *Int Immunol* 2015; 27: 55.

Old LJ. Tumor necrosis factor. *Sci Am* 1988; 258: 59.
Udalova I, Monaco C, Nanchahal J, et al. Anti-TNF therapy. *Microbiol Spectr* 2016; 4: 4.

Typhoid fever

Typhoid fever (enteric fever) is caused by the exclusively human pathogen *Salmonella typhi*. Transmission is via water or food contaminated with human faeces. The disease thus occurs primarily in developing countries, and the rare outbreaks in developed countries usually arise because of food handling by chronic salmonella carriers.

Typhoid was a serious transmissible disease of past centuries with a case fatality rate of 10–20% in pre-antibiotic times. Famous victims included Prince Albert (Queen Victoria's husband), Henry Prince of Wales ('Henry IX'), Franz Schubert (composer), Hakaru Hashimoto (Japanese physician) and Wilbur Wright (early American aviator).

Clinical features comprise
- fever (q.v.),
- paradoxical bradycardia,
- headache,
- cough,
- abdominal pain,
- splenomegaly (q.v.),
- a transient rose-coloured macular rash on the body,
- watery diarrhoea (q.v.), which occurs early with constipation later.

The lymphoid hyperplasia in the terminal ileum may be complicated by haemorrhage or perforation.

Blood cultures are usually positive in the first 2 weeks, and faecal and urinary cultures become positive during the second and third weeks. Positive serology occurs after 2–3 weeks.

Continued excretion of the organism occurs in up to 3% of patients. Biliary disease predisposes to chronic enteric carriage, and schistosomiasis (q.v.) predisposes to chronic urinary carriage. Chronic carriers are asymptomatic but remain a risk to others (e.g. 'Typhoid Mary', the New York cook reported as the first such carrier in *JAMA* 1907).

Treatment traditionally was with **chloramphenicol**, *but* **ciprofloxacin** *is nowadays the antibiotic of choice.* **Ampicillin** *and* **cotrimoxazole** *are also effective.*
- In cases of fluoroquinolone resistance (e.g. in South and South-East Asia), a third-generation cephalosporin or azithromycin is preferred.
- Chronic carriage requires prolonged antibiotic therapy, and **cholecystectomy** is generally curative in carriers with biliary disease who do not respond completely to antibiotics.

Prevention is with public health measures and immunization.

Non-typhoidal salmonellosis is common in developed countries, with the usual sources being inadequately cooked hen's eggs, exotic pets such as turtles and the smoking of contaminated marijuana.

Bibliography
Hornick RB, Greisman SE, Woodward TE, et al. Typhoid fever. *N Engl J Med* 1970; 283: 686 & 739.
Parry CM. Typhoid fever. *Curr Infect Dis Rep* 2004; 6: 27.
Rabsch W, Tschape H, Baumler AJ. Non-typhoidal salmonellosis: emerging problems. *Microbes Infect* 2001; 3: 237.

Typhus *See*
- Rickettsial diseases.

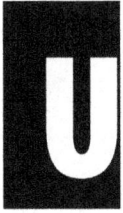

Ulcerative colitis *See*
- Inflammatory bowel disease.

Ulcers

Ulcers refer to breaches in the skin or mucous membranes. Though common, they may have a large list of causes, some of which are unusual.

Skin ulcers are seen with

- Anthrax (q.v.),
- Basal cell carcinoma,
- Blastomycosis,
- Chancroid,
- Chromium poisoning (q.v.),
- Cryptococcosis (q.v.),
- Decubitus (i.e. pressure, a classic ICU risk),
- Diphtheria (q.v.),
- Ecthyma (q.v.),
- Erythema multiforme (q.v.),
- Felty's syndrome (q.v.),
- Graft-versus-host disease (q.v.),
- Granuloma inguinale,
- Histiocytoma (see Histiocytosis),

- Kaposi's sarcoma (see Acquired immunodeficiency syndrome),
- Ischaemia (including diabetes),
- Leishmaniasis,
- Livedo vasculitis (q.v.),
- Lymphogranuloma venereum,
- Mucormycosis,
- Mycobacteria (non-tuberculous),
- Mycosis fungoides (cutaneous T-cell lymphoma),
- Nicorandil (a synthetic nicotine derivative) use in patients with chronic angina,
- Pemphigus vulgaris (q.v.),
- Plague (q.v.),
- Porphyrias (q.v.),
- Progressive bacterial synergistic gangrene (see Gangrene),
- Pseudomonas,
- Pyoderma gangrenosum (q.v.),
- Scleroderma (q.v.),
- Sporotrichosis,
- Squamous cell carcinoma,
- Syphilis (q.v.),
- Tetanus (q.v.),
- Tularaemia,
- Venereal inguinal buboes,
- Venous disease,
- Yaws.

Oral ulcers are seen in

- Aphthous states,
- Behcet's syndrome (q.v.),
- Bejel,
- Erythema multiforme (q.v.),
- Graft-versus-host disease,
- Hand-foot-and-mouth disease (q.v.),
- Herpes simplex virus (q.v.),
- Leishmaniasis,
- Neutropenia (q.v.),
- Nicorandil (a synthetic nicotine derivative) use in patients with chronic angina,
- Pemphigus vulgaris, including bullous mucosal pemphigoid (q.v.),
- Reiter's syndrome (q.v.),
- Stevens–Johnson syndrome (q.v.),
- Systemic lupus erythematosus (q.v.).

See also
- Mouth diseases – 3. stomatitis.

Genital ulcers occur in

- Amoebiasis (q.v.),
- Behcet's syndrome (q.v.),
- Chancroid,
- Epstein–Barr virus infection (q.v.),
- Granuloma inguinale,
- HSV (type 2) infection (see Herpesviruses),
- Lymphogranuloma venereum,
- Reiter's syndrome (q.v.),
- Stevens–Johnson syndrome (q.v.),
- Syphilis (q.v.),
- Trauma.

Bibliography

Antoon JW, Miller RL. Aphthous ulcer – a review of the literature on etiology, pathogenesis, diagnosis, and treatment. *JAMA* 1980; 101: 803.

Wolff K, Goldsmith L, Katz S, et al., eds. *Fitzpatrick's Dermatology in General Medicine*. 7th edition. New York: McGraw-Hill. 2007.

Urea cycle disorders See
- Hyperammonaemia.

Urticaria

There are a number of urticarial conditions, but apart from hives they are uncommon.

1. **Urticaria** thus usually refers to **hives**, which are areas of transient, localized, pruritic oedema, varying in size from 1 to 20 cm and in number from one to more than 100. They are usually caused by food sensitivity (mostly due to the degranulating chemicals used as colouring and flavouring agents) and aspirin (q.v.). There was a flurry of reports of cases associated with the anti-smoking drug bupropion.

Latex allergy has in recent years become the archetypal form of contact urticaria. It is an IgE-mediated hypersensitivity reaction to proteins present in the natural rubber from which latex is derived. Risk factors include an existing allergic diathesis, frequent use of latex gloves, and multiple procedural exposure, especially of mucosal surfaces, to latex. In addition to contact urticaria, there may be generalized urticaria, respiratory allergy, angioedema (q.v.) or even anaphylaxis (q.v.). Fatalities have been reported. Needless to say, latex allergy has important occupational as well as medical implications.

*The main treatment of hives and indeed of urticaria in general is with **antihistamines**, e.g. loratidine or fexofenadine in the morning and cetirizine in the evening. If further treatment is needed, 4–6 days of histamine suppression can be produced by a single nocturnal dose of doxepin. If severe, treatment with adrenaline (epinephrine) and* *corticosteroids may be required. Photochemotherapy has been used. There have been reports of the successful use of cytotoxic agents (e.g. azathioprine, mycophenolate) in severe and refractory cases.*

2. **Angioedema** (q.v.).
3. **Chronic urticaria** can be difficult to treat, and corticosteroid supplementation of routine H1-antihistamine medication is often required for control.

    It has been appreciated that many cases are not allergic but have autoantibodies to IgE or IgE receptors. Thus, the new monoclonal antibody to IgE, **omalizumab** (originally introduced for atopic asthma), and/or molecules which could block the receptor itself, may offer potent future therapy (see Asthma, see Churg–Strauss syndrome).

4. **Physical**, due especially to cold (q.v.), but also to heat (q.v.) or sun.

    Cold urticaria is produced in some patients by IgE autoantibodies to a cold-dependent skin antigen. The gene for the familial form of this condition has been identified.

    Cold urticaria occurs particularly during rewarming and is usually associated with systemic symptoms, such as headache, tachycardia, syncope and wheeze. If severe, it resembles **leukocytoclastic vasculitis** (see below).

    Cold urticaria is a major feature of the **PLAID syndrome** (PLCG2-associated immune dysregulation), in which recurrent bacterial infections and skin granulomas also occur.

5. **Systemic mastocytosis** (q.v.) produces urticaria, as well as flushing (q.v.), headache, fatigue, abdominal pain and diarrhoea (q.v.), all due to histamine release. In severe cases, hypotension may be produced. These symptoms may be precipitated by alcohol or analgesics.

6. **Leukocytoclastic vasculitis** is sometimes considered among the urticarial conditions.
    - It comprises necrosis of the walls of vessels up to arterioles with extravasation of formed blood elements.
    - This usually gives rise to palpable purpura (q.v.), but some lesions begin as urticaria.
    - In addition, chronic lesions tend to become urticarial.

    Although it may be idiopathic, it is more usually associated with
    - systemic disease, especially collagen-vascular disease (q.v.), lymphoma, other malignancy,
    - infections, e.g. infectious mononucleosis (see Epstein–Barr virus,) hepatitis (q.v.), streptococcal,
    - drugs, such as aspirin (q.v.), cephalosporins, penicillin, procainamide, thiazides.

Bibliography

Chen JR, Khan DA. Urticaria and angioedema. In: *Scientific American Medicine. Allergy & Immunology.* Hamilton: Dekker Medicine. 2020.

Denburg JA. Basophil and mast cell lineage in vitro and in vivo. *Blood* 1992; 79: 846.

Dowd PM. Cold-related disorders. *Prog Dermatol* 1987; 21: 1.

Ekenstam E, Callen JP. Cutaneous leukocytoclastic vasculitis. *Arch Dermatol* 1984; 120: 484.

Fine J. Mastocytosis. *Int J Dermatol* 1980; 19: 117.

Gibson LE. Cutaneous vasculitis: approach to diagnosis and systemic associations. *Mayo Clin Proc* 1990; 65: 221.

Greaves M. Chronic urticaria. *J Allergy Clin Immunol* 2000; 105: 664.

Greaves MW. Pathology and classification of urticaria. *Immunol Allergy Clin North Am* 2014; 34: 1.

Hoffman HM, Wright FA, Broide DH, et al. Identification of a locus on chromosome 1q44 for familial cold urticaria. *Am J Hum Genet* 2000; 66: 1693.

Katelaris C. Treatment of urticaria. Aust *Prescriber* 2001; 24: 124.

Lewis RA. Mastocytosis. *J Allergy Clin Immunol* 1984; 74: 755.

Mehregan RD, Hall MJ, Gibson LE. Urticarial vasculitis: a histopathologic and clinical review of 72 cases. *J Am Acad Dermatol* 1992; 26: 441.

Milner JD. PLAID: a syndrome of complex patterns of disease and unique phenotypes. *J Clin Immunol* 2015; 35: 527.

Monroe EW. Urticarial vasculitis: an updated review. *J Am Acad Dermatol* 1981; 5: 88.

Pardanini A. Systemic mastocytosis in adults: 2019 update on diagnosis, risk stratification and management. *Am J Hematol* 2019; 94: 363.

Philpott H, Kette F, Hissaria P, et al. Chronic urticaria: the autoimmune paradigm. *Intern Med J* 2008; 38: 852.

Singleton R, Halverstam CP. Diagnosis and management of cold urticaria. *Cutis* 2016; 97: 59.

Taylor JS, Erkek E. Latex allergy: diagnosis and management. *Dermatol Ther* 2004; 17: 289.

Trevisonno J, Balram B, Netchiporouk E, et al. Physical urticaria: review on classification, triggers and management with special focus on prevalence including a meta-analysis. *Postgrad Med* 2015; 127: 565.

Wolff K, Goldsmith L, Katz S, et al., eds. *Fitzpatrick's Dermatology in General Medicine*. 7th edition. New York: McGraw-Hill. 2007.

Uveitis

Uveitis refers to inflammation of the structures of the eye, including the iris, vitreous and retina, as well as outer structures including the cornea and sclera.

Its importance in acute medicine lies in the fact that many cases are associated with serious underlying systemic diseases, including ankylosing spondylitis, (q.v.), Behcet's disease (q.v.), inflammatory bowel disease (q.v.), Reiter's syndrome (q.v.), sarcoidosis (q.v.) and toxoplasmosis (q.v.). The vulnerability of the eye to such insults relates to its content of immune competent cells.

Treatment has traditionally included **corticosteroids**, but **immunomodulatory agents** (e.g. methotrexate, adalimumab) are now used both for disease control and for steroid-sparing effect.

Bibliography
Trivedi A, Katelaris C. The use of biologic agents in the management of uveitis. *Intern Med J* 2019; 49: 1352.

Uveoparotid fever See

- Sarcoidosis.

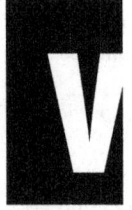

Valerian See

- Hepatitis.

Valproate

Sodium **valproate** is an important anticonvulsant and antipsychotic, unrelated to other such agents. In the brain, it has a GABAergic effect, but it has little effect on other organs and systems.

In epilepsy, it is widely effective in grand mal, petit mal and partial seizures and in myoclonus. In psychiatry, it is effective in mania. Interestingly, it also has some thromboprophylactic action, as it promotes the release of tissue-type plasminogen activator (t-PA) and thus stimulates endogenous fibrinolysis (q.v.).

Although usually given orally, it may be given IV in similar doses. Acutely, 400–800 mg may be given over 3–5 min, followed by up to 2400 mg per day by continuous IV infusion. Orally, the usual daily dose ranges from 600–2500 mg per day. It is highly protein-bound and is metabolized prior to excretion.

> In Intensive Care practice, valproate is important because of its extensive drug interactions, its potential adverse effects and its difficult management in overdose.
> 1. **Drug interactions** of importance include increased benzodiazepine levels when valproate is given and decreased valproate levels when carbapenems are given.
> 2. **Adverse effects** include pancreatitis (q.v.), hepatic dysfunction, hyperammonaemia (q.v.), thrombocytopenia (q.v.) and suicidal behaviour.
> 3. **Overdose** may result in severe and prolonged neurological and respiratory depression, sometimes with cerebral oedema and intracranial hypertension. Intensive Care support may be enhanced with naloxone and renal replacement therapy.

Bibliography
Zawab A, Carmody J. Safe use of sodium valproate. *Aust Prescriber* 2014; 37: 124.

Vaping

Vaping refers to the inhalation of the vapours produced by e-cigarettes (electronic cigarettes). The inhaled toxic substances, especially nicotine, are rapidly absorbed into the bloodstream (within seconds) and can cause cardiovascular disturbances, respiratory abnormalities and seizures. A large number of different substances are present in available products, and chemical analysis has shown that they may differ substantially from those officially listed for that product. Moreover, these substances may change both with time and with the heating involved.

Vaping has also been reported to be associated with the development of severe and life-threatening lung injury, referred to as VARDS, i.e vaping-associated respiratory distress syndrome (see Acute pulmonary oedema), probably due to contaminated product (e.g. with vitamin E and plant oils). This form of lung injury has also been referred to as EVALI, i.e. e-cigarette or vaping use–associated lung injury. The clinical, radiological and pathological features are non-specific. Steroid therapy may be helpful in severe cases. Overall, although recovery is usual, deaths have been reported.

Much controversy surrounds the claim that vaping may assist in the cessation of tobacco smoking or alternatively may be an entry to nicotine and other recreational drug use.

Bibliography

Bozier J, Chivers EK, Chapman DG, et al. The evolving landscape of e-cigarettes: a systematic review of recent evidence. *Chest* 2020; 157: 1362.

Hajek P, Phillips-Waller A, Przulj D, et al. A randomized trial of e-cigarettes versus nicotine-replacement therapy. *N Engl J Med* 2019; 380: 629.

Hartnett KP, Kite-Powell A, Patel MT, et al. Syndromic surveillance for e-cigarette or vaping product use-associated lung injury. *N Engl J Med* 2020; 382: 766.

Jonas AM, Raj R. Vaping-related acute parenchymal lung injury: a systematic review. *Chest* 2020; 158: 1555.

Kiernan E, Click ES, Melstrom P, et al. A brief overview of the national outbreak of e-cigarette, or vaping, product use-associated lung injury and the primary causes. *Chest* 2021; 159: 426.

Kligerman SJ, Kay FU, Raptis CA, et al. CT findings and patterns of e-cigarette or vaping product use-associated lung injury. *Chest* 2021; 160: 1492.

Shao XM, Fang ZT. Severe acute toxicity of inhaled nicotine and e cigarettes: seizures and cardiac arrhythmia. *Chest* 2020; 157: 506.

Werner AK, Koumans EH, Chatham-Stephens K, et al. Hospitalizations and deaths associated with EVALI. *N Engl J Med* 2020; 382: 1589.

Vaptans *See*

- Vasopressin.

Varicella-zoster

The **varicella-zoster** virus (VZV) is a member of the human herpesvirus group (q.v.). It undergoes latency and reactivation as do other herpesviruses. Following an initial episode of varicella, the virus lies relatively dormant in the cytoplasm of the neurones of the sensory ganglia, whence it may be reactivated.

Varicella (chickenpox) is a highly communicable illness, with an incubation period of 11–20 days following droplet or direct contact. The virus is carried by the white blood cells to the skin and viscera.

- A vesiculating rash appears in successive crops, especially on the face and trunk. This resolves over 7–10 days. There is associated fever (q.v.), headache and malaise.
- In adults, a diffuse reticulonodular pneumonitis may occur, which can eventually calcify. There is cough, tachypnoea and prolonged abnormality of gas exchange. It may predispose to fulminating secondary bacterial infection, particularly with invasive group A streptococci (see Gangrene – 1. Necrotizing fasciitis).
- Rarely, arthritis (q.v.), encephalitis (q.v.), myocarditis, nephritis (q.v.), orchitis (q.v.) and thrombocytopenia (q.v.) may occur.
- Disseminated disease occurs chiefly in the presence of associated malignancy.
- Reinfection does not occur, except in immunocompromised hosts when it is usually mild.

Zoster (shingles) arises from reactivation and is thus usually seen in older patients (because of waning immunity with time) and especially in the immunocompromised. Its incidence has increased in recent years, perhaps paradoxically associated with the introduction of varicella vaccination in children, since the lowered viral background in the community has reduced the re-exposure necessary to maintain otherwise waning immunity in adults. On the other hand, the reported lack of an increased occurrence of zoster in French monks who had no exposure to children suggests that this explanation may be overly simplistic.

Complications include
- postherpetic neuralgia, which may be severe, prolonged and refractory, especially in the elderly,
- ocular involvement, i.e. herpes ophthalmicus,
- Ramsay–Hunt syndrome (see Bell's palsy),
- Guillain-Barré syndrome (q.v.),
- encephalitis (q.v.), mainly in the immunocompromised.

Varicella does not lead to zoster in another person, but vice versa applies, though such transmission is probably much less than from a case of chickenpox itself. Recurrent attacks of shingles can occur.

The diagnosis is made clinically, and if necessary it can be confirmed by virus isolation or positive serology.

The chief differential diagnosis is disseminated herpes simplex infection, but contact dermatitis (q.v.), folliculitis (q.v.) or insect bites (q.v.) may be considered.

Treatment is with **acyclovir** (q.v.) or the related compounds famciclovir or valaciclovir, if commenced within 72 hr of the onset of the rash. Although treatment reduces the severity and duration of the acute illness, the incidence of postherpetic neuralgia may not be similarly reduced.

- *Isolation* is recommended to prevent nosocomial transmission to susceptible patients. Patients so exposed should receive prophylactic immune globulin.
- Varicella *vaccine* of live attenuated VZV is recommended for universal use. Unlike immunity from natural infection, immunization from varicella vaccine may require booster doses to maintain optimal immunity. Interestingly, the administration of a much more potent vaccine to older patients has been shown to reduce greatly the incidence of subsequent herpes zoster and postherpetic neuralgia, and this vaccine has now been recommended as a specific zoster vaccine for older people.
- *Postherpetic neuralgia* is treated with a lidocaine 5% patch, gabapentin 300–3600 mg per day or carbamazepine in high doses (e.g. at least 600 mg per day). Local measures, such as transcutaneous electrical nerve stimulation (TENS), may provide short-term benefit.

Bibliography

Chaves SS, Gargiullo P, Zhang JX, et al. Loss of vaccine-induced immunity to varicella over time. *N Engl J Med* 2007; 356: 1121.

Cohen JI. Herpes zoster, *N Engl J Med* 2013; 369: 255.

Cohen JI, Brunell PA, Straus SE, et al. Recent advances in varicella-zoster virus infection. *Ann Intern Med* 1999; 130: 922.

Dwyer DE, Cunningham AL. Herpes simplex and varicella-zoster virus infections. *Med J Aust* 2002; 177: 267.

Gilden DH, Kleinschmidt-DeMasters BK, LaGuardia JJ, et al. Neurologic complications of reactivation of varicella-zoster virus. *N Engl J Med* 2000; 342: 636.

Oxman MN, Levin MJ, Johnson GR, et al. A vaccine to prevent herpes zoster and postherpetic neuralgia in older patients. *N Engl J Med* 2005; 352: 2271.

Straus SE, Ostrove JM, Inchauspe G, et al. Varicella-zoster virus infections: biology, natural history, treatment, and prevention. *Ann Intern Med* 1988; 108: 221.

Strassels, SA, Sullivan SD. Clinical and economic considerations of vaccination against varicella. *Pharmacotherapy* 1997; 17: 133.

Watson CP. A new treatment for postherpetic neuralgia. *N Engl J Med* 2000; 343: 1563.

Vasculitis

Vasculitis refers to inflammation of the blood vessels and comprises a group of conditions of variable aetiology, clinical features and outcome.

Most cases of generalized or systemic vasculitis are of unknown aetiology, but presumably they have an immune pathogenesis.
- Clinical features include fever (q.v.), weight loss, malaise, myalgia, arthropathy (q.v.) and neuropathy (q.v.).
- There is anaemia (q.v.), thrombocytosis (q.v.), raised erythrocyte sedimentation rate (ESR) and hypoalbuminaemia.
- The most specific and sensitive test is biopsy of an affected area.
- In general, serological tests should be used to support a clinical and histological diagnosis rather than to define one. In particular, they are unsuitable for indiscriminate screening.
- The diagnosis can often be difficult.
- **Corticosteroids** *are the mainstay of initial treatment, associated with a* **second immunosuppressant agent**, *usually cyclophosphamide to induce remission and then azathioprine or methotrexate for maintenance.*

Vasculitis may also be
- **secondary** to systemic autoimmune inflammatory conditions, such as
  - rheumatoid arthritis,
  - Sjogren's syndrome (q.v.),
- **organ-specific**, such as
  - primary angiitis or arteritis of the central nervous system (see Arteritis),
  - neutrophilic dermatoses, e.g. Behcet's syndrome (q.v.),
  - chronic lymphocytic vasculitis, e.g. pyoderma gangrenosum (q.v.).

There are a number of specific groups of vasculitis, including those
- affecting mostly large vessels,
- affecting primarily medium-sized vessels,
- affecting primarily small vessels,

- associated with thrombosis,
- associated with spasm,
- associated with vessel wall degeneration.

1. **Vasculitis affecting mostly large vessels**
   - **Takayasu's arteritis** (pulseless disease, occlusive thromboaortopathy)

   This particularly affects the upper extremities of young Asian women. It primarily involves the aorta and its major branches. The intima becomes thickened and inflamed with granulomas, and later there is sclerosis with medial degeneration and adventitial fibrosis. The coronary and pulmonary arteries may sometimes be involved, though they are usually spared. The condition is probably an autoimmune vasculitis with a genetic predisposition.

   Clinically, it may present as a prolonged flu-like illness, but the typical features of ischaemia of the affected areas are usually prominent. It is diagnosed arteriographically, at which time the opportunity should also be taken to measure the central or aortic blood pressure.

   It may respond to corticosteroids.
   - giant cell arteritis or temporal arteritis (q.v.)

   This is often associated with polymyalgia rheumatica (q.v.).
   - aortitis (see Endarteritis)

   This may sometimes be secondary to rheumatoid arthritis, ankylosing spondylitis (q.v.) or syphilis (q.v.).
   - primary angiitis of the central nervous system (see Cerebral arteritis)

2. **Vasculitis affecting primarily medium-sized vessels**
   - polyarteritis nodosa (PAN) (q.v.)
   - **microscopic polyangiitis**

   This was formerly considered a variant of polyarteritis nodosa (q.v.), but it is now recognized to be one of the anti-neutrophil cytoplasmic antibody (ANCA)-associated systemic necrotizing vasculitides (see Wegener's granulomatosis).
   - granulomatous arteritis (Wegener's granulomatosis – q.v.)

   In addition, vessels as small as capillaries may also be involved in this condition.
   - Churg–Strauss syndrome (q.v.)
   - Behcet's disease (q.v.)
   - **Kawasaki disease** (KD, mucocutaneous lymph node syndrome)

   This acute, self-limited vasculitis is seen chiefly in young children, with the highest incidence in East Asia. It appears to be an immune-related inflammatory response to a recent viral infection. During 2020, cases began being reported in children with COVID-19 disease (q.v.), when it has been called **multisystem inflammatory syndrome in children** (MIS-C in the USA or PIMS-TS in the UK). The preceding viral infection may have been mild or even asymptomatic, and it usually occurred several weeks earlier. Its typical features include fever (q.v.), rash, shock and multiorgan failure (q.v.), but its most important complications are coronary artery abnormalities. The cardiac injury can cause left ventricular dysfunction and dilatation. An important differential diagnosis is toxic shock syndrome (q.v.).

   A similar syndrome has recently been reported in young adults, and its distinction from prolonged COVID-19 illness required the presence of specific antibodies but a negative COVID PCR. The condition has been referred to as MIS-A.

   It is treated with immune globulin, corticosteroids and aspirin, and it requires Intensive Care support.
   - vasculitis due to hepatitis B (q.v.)
   - vasculitis due to HIV infection (see Acquired immunodeficiency syndrome)

3. **Vasculitis affecting primarily small vessels**
   - **hypersensitivity angiitis**

   This term, which may now be outdated though it is still commonly used, refers usually to drug-related vasculitis. It can be associated with crops of palpable purpura (q.v.) or even Henoch–Schonlein purpura (q.v.). Although small vessels are primarily involved, all cutaneous vessels may be affected. There may be associated renal, gut, lung or neurological involvement.

   *It responds to **corticosteroids**.*
   - Goodpasture's syndrome (q.v.) and cryoglobulinaemia (q.v.)

   These can be associated with a similar picture.
   - **leukocytoclastic vasculitis**

   This comprises necrosis of the walls of vessels up to arterioles with extravasation of formed blood elements. It is more commonly considered among the urticarias (q.v.).
   - vasculitis due to
     - meningococcaemia,
     - hepatitis B or C infection (sometimes)(q.v.),
     - other bacterial, rickettsial or viral infections (occasionally).
   - drug-induced cutaneous necrotizing vasculitis may be associated with prolonged urticaria, palpable purpura, haemorrhagic bullae, subcutaneous nodules, digital necrosis and multiorgan involvement. It is especially due to
     - antimicrobials, including beta-lactams, cotrimoxazole, quinolones, sulphonamides,

- NSAIDs,
- diuretics,
- granulocyte-colony stimulating factor (G-CSF),
- insulin,
- phenytoin,
- quinine,
- streptokinase.
* cutaneous necrotizing vasculitis due to miscellaneous immunological, inflammatory, connective tissue and neoplastic conditions.
4. **Vasculitis associated with thrombosis**
   * antiphospholipid syndrome with anticardiolipin antibody (q.v.),
   * livedo vasculitis (see Livedo reticularis).
5. **Vasculitis associated with spasm**
   * Raynaud's disease (q.v.),
   * migraine,
   * eclampsia (see Pre-eclampsia),
   * ergotism (see Ergot).
6. **Vasculitis associated with vessel wall degeneration**
   * atherosclerosis,
   * connective tissue diseases (q.v.).

Bibliography

Arend WP, Michel BA, Bloch DA, et al. The American College of Rheumatology 1990 criteria for the classification of Takayasu arteritis. *Arthritis Rheum* 1990; 33: 1129.

Booher AM, Eagle KA. Diseases of the aorta. In: *Scientific American Medicine. Cardiovascular Medicine.* Hamilton: Dekker Medicine. 2020.

Bourrillon A. Kawasaki's disease: multiple and various aspects. *Arch Pediatr* 2008; 15: 825.

Calabrese L, Dune G, Lie J. Vasculitis in the central nervous system. *Arthritis Rheum* 1997; 40: 1189.

Carter MJ, Shankar-Hari M, Tibby SM. Paediatric inflammatory multisystem syndrome temporally-associated with SARS-CoV-2 infection: an overview. *Intens Care Med* 2021; 47: 90.

Coffman JD. Raynaud's phenomenon: an update. *Hypertension* 1991; 17: 593.

Conn DL. Update on systemic necrotizing vasculitis. *Mayo Clin Proc* 1989; 64: 535.

Feldstein LR, Rose EB, Horwitz SM, et al. Multisystem inflammatory syndrome in US children and adolescents. *N Engl J Med* 2020; 383: 334.

Frankel SK, Cosgrove GP, Fischer A, et al. Update in the diagnosis and management of pulmonary vasculitis. *Chest* 2006; 129: 452.

Gatenby PA. Vasculitis - diagnosis and treatment. *Aust NZ J Med* 1999; 29: 662.

Gatenby PA. Anti-neutrophil cytoplasmic antibody-associated systemic vasculitis: nature or nurture? *Intern Med J* 2012; 42: 351.

Gibson LE. Cutaneous vasculitis: approach to diagnosis and systemic associations. *Mayo Clin Proc* 1990; 65: 221.

Hamilton CR, Shelley WM, Tumulty PA. Giant cell arteritis: including temporal arteritis and polymyalgia rheumatica. *Medicine* 1971; 50: 1.

Han RK, Sinclair B, Newman A, et al. Recognition and management of Kawasaki disease. *CMAJ* 2000; 162: 807.

Hunder GG, Bloch DA, Michel BA, et al. The American College of Rheumatology 1990 criteria for the classification of giant cell arteritis. *Arthritis Rheum* 1990; 33: 1122.

Jayne DRW, Davies MJ, Cox CJV, et al. Treatment of systemic vasculitis with pooled intravenous immunoglobulin. *Lancet* 1991; 337: 1137.

Jennette JC, Falk RJ. Small-vessel vasculitis. *N Engl J Med* 1997; 337: 1512.

Jennette JC, Falk RJ, Andrassy K, et al. Nomenclature of systemic vasculitides: proposal of an international consensus conference. *Arthritis Rheum* 1994; 37: 187.

Kerr GS, Hallahan CW, Giordano J, et al. Takayasu arteritis. *Ann Intern Med* 1994; 120: 919.

Lie JT. Classification and immunodiagnosis of vasculitis: a new solution or promises unfulfilled? *J Rheumatol* 1988 15: 728.

Lupi-Herrera E, Sanchez-Torres G, Marcushamer J, et al. Takayasu's arteritis: clinical study of 107 cases. *Am Heart J* 1997; 93: 94.

Mehregan RD, Hall MJ, Gibson LE. Urticarial vasculitis: a histopathologic and clinical review of 72 cases. *J Am Acad Dermatol* 1992; 26: 441.

Moore PM. Diagnosis and management of isolated angiitis of the central nervous system. *Neurology* 1989; 39: 167.

Numano F, Kobayashi Y. Takayasu arteritis: beyond pulselessness. *Intern Med* 1999; 38: 226.

Oz MC, Brener BJ, Buda JA, et al. A ten-year experience with bacterial aortitis. *J Vasc Surg* 1989; 10: 439.

Riphagen S, Gomez X, Gonzales-Martinez C, et al. Hyperinflammatory shock in children during COVID-19 pandemic. *Lancet* 2020; 395: 1607.

Royle J, Williams K, Elliott E, et al. Kawasaki disease in Australia, 1993–95. *Arch Dis Child* 1998; 78: 33.

Savage COS, Harper L, Adu D. Primary systemic vasculitis. *Lancet* 1997; 349: 553.

Sheikhzadeh A, Tettenborn I, Noohi F, et al. Occlusive thromboaortopathy (Takayasu disease): clinical and angiographic features and a brief review of literature. *Angiology* 2002; 53: 29.

Szer I. Henoch–Schonlein purpura: when and how to treat. *J Rheumatol* 1996; 23: 1661.

Villa-Forte A, Mandell BF. Systemic vasculitis syndromes. In: *Scientific American Medicine. Rheumatology.* Hamilton: Dekker Medicine. 2020.

Zilko PJ. Polymyalgia rheumatica and giant cell arteritis. *Med J Aust* 1996; 165: 438.

Vasopressin

Natural (arginine) **vasopressin** (i.e. antidiuretic hormone – q.v.) is an agonist with non-selective effects on both V1a and V2 receptors. Stimulation of V1a receptors is responsible for the vasopressor effect and possible immunomodulatory action, whereas stimulation of V2 receptors causes vasodilatation, antidiuresis and procoagulant activity. **Selepressin** is a selective V1a agonist, and **desmopressin** (q.v.) is a selective V2 agonist.

There has been a resurgence of interest in **vasopressin** (as arginine vasopressin, AVP) as an agent for haemodynamic support in patients with septic shock. The results of a large randomized clinical trial in this area confirmed its efficacy, though the results failed to show superiority over noradrenaline (norepinephrine) in terms of survival. However, vasopressin may usefully supplement catecholamine infusion in poor responders, and it may improve renal outcome in septic shock. It is used in a dose of 0.03 U/min by continuous IV infusion.

By contrast, the new **vasopressin-2 (V2) receptor antagonists** ('vaptans', e.g. tolvaptan) have been shown to be useful in treating the hyponatraemia associated with the syndrome of inappropriate antidiuretic hormone (q.v.), cirrhosis and cardiac failure (i.e. hyponatraemia with either hypervolaemia or euvolaemia). They act by causing a pure water diuresis ('aquaresis'). They are, of course, contraindicated in hypovolaemia.

See
- Antidiuretic hormone,
- Desmopressin,
- Pituitary – Posterior pituitary.

See also
- Adrenocorticotropic hormone,
- Amphetamines,
- Ectopic hormone production,
- Pre-eclampsia,
- Syndrome of inappropriate antidiuretic hormone.

Bibliography

Gordon AC, Russell JA, Walley KR, et al. The effects of vasopressin on acute kidney injury in septic shock. *Intens Care Med* 2010; 36: 83.

Holmes CL, Patel BM, Russell JA, et al. Physiology of vasopressin relevant to management of septic shock. *Chest* 2001; 120: 989.

Russell JA, Walley KR, Singer J, et al. Vasopressin versus norepinephrine infusion in patients with septic shock. *N Engl J Med* 2008; 358: 877.

Vertigo

Vertigo is the distressing symptom of a spinning or revolving sensation, often loosely referred to as dizziness.

While it may be due to the same conditions as cause **tinnitus** (q.v.), the most common causes are
1. Peripheral
   - vestibular neuronitis (*best treated with corticosteroids*),
   - Meniere's disease,
2. Central
   - migraine-associated vestibulopathy,
   - multiple sclerosis (q.v.),
   - posterior circulation stroke,
3. Mixed
   - trauma,
   - a recurrent condition called **benign paroxysmal positional vertigo** (BPPV).

Bibliography

Fetter M. Assessing vestibular function: which test, when? *J Neurol* 2000; 247: 335.

Furman JM, Cass SP. Benign paroxysmal positional vertigo *N Engl J Med* 1999; 341: 1590.

Harrison MS. 'Epidemic vertigo' – 'vestibular neuronitis': a clinical study. *Brain* 1962; 85: 613.

Rivlin W, Habershon C, Tsang BK-T, et al. Practical approach to vertigo: a synthesis of the emerging evidence. *Intern Med J* 2022; 52: 356.

Strupp M, Zingler VC, Arbusow V, et al. Methylprednisolone, valacyclovir, or the combination for vestibular neuritis. *N Engl J Med* 2004; 351: 354.

Tsang BKT, Chen ASK, Paine M. Acute evaluation of the acute vestibular syndrome: differentiating posterior circulation stroke from acute peripheral vestibulopathies. *Intern Med J* 2017; 47: 1352.

Vesiculobullous diseases

Vesiculobullous diseases compromise a large and heterogeneous group of blistering disorders.

They include
- **pemphigus vulgaris** and its variants (q.v.),
- **dermatitis herpetiformis** (see Dermatitis),
- **erythema multiforme** (q.v.),

- **epidermolysis bullosa** (q.v.),
- **other conditions**, such as contact dermatitis (q.v.), drug eruptions (q.v.), heat rash (q.v.), herpes infections (q.v.), scabies (see Pediculosis) and systemic lupus erythematosus (q.v.), which may sometimes produce blistering.

*Corticosteroids are commonly prescribed, but **rituximab** and **immune globulin** can also provide effective first-line therapy and are steroid-sparing in autoimmune cases.*

Bibliography

Katz SI, Hall RP, Lawlwy TJ, et al. Dermatitis herpetiformis: the skin and the gut. *Ann Intern Med* 1980; 93: 857.

Levitt J, Czernik A, Koo B. Vesiculobullous diseases. In: *Scientific American Medicine. Dermatology.* Hamilton: Dekker Medicine. 2020.

Sehgal VN, Gangwani OP. Fixed drug eruption: current concepts. *Int J Dermatol* 1987; 26: 67.

Wolff K, Goldsmith L, Katz S, et al., eds. *Fitzpatrick's Dermatology in General Medicine.* 7th edition. New York: McGraw-Hill. 2007.

Vincent's angina See

- Mouth diseases – 1. Gingivitis.

VIPoma See

- Diarrhoea.

Viral haemorrhagic fever

Viral haemorrhagic fever (VHF) describes a number of types of similar infections, due to Ebola (q.v.), Lassa (q.v.), Marburg and Crimean–Congo viruses. Extensive endothelial cell damage is the common pathogenetic mechanism of all the viral haemorrhagic fevers.

See
- Ebola haemorrhagic fever,
- Lassa fever.

See also
- Dengue.

Bibliography

Howard CR. Viral hemorrhagic fevers: properties and prospects for treatment and prevention. *Antiviral Res* 1984; 4: 169.

Vitamin deficiency

It has long been known that certain foods are required for health. In 1906, Hopkins found that in addition to protein, carbohydrate, fat, minerals and water, there were certain essential 'accessory factors'. In 1912, Frank showed that the anti-beriberi fraction in unpolished rice was an amine, which he therefore called a vital amine or vitamine. This name was then applied to all 'accessory factors', though later the 'e' was dropped, as the substances were found to be chemically very different and not many were in fact amines.

Later in the same year, Hopkins and Frank proposed the theory of diseases due to **vitamin deficiency**, and the individual vitamins were subsequently discovered, being given letters according to their perceived function. As with **trace elements** (q.v.), deficiency of any one of these substances gives rise to clinical disease, and the major deficiencies are discussed elsewhere in relation to the individual vitamins.

As with trace elements also, there have been published guidelines for the appropriate IV dosage of vitamins in critical illness, with particular emphasis on prevention of deficiency. However, unlike those for trace elements, the guidelines for vitamins re-emphasize previous knowledge and practice. The recommended minimum daily IV doses of vitamins for this purpose are listed in the accompanying Table.

Vitamin requirements

Vitamin	Dosage
A	1 mg (3000 IU)
C	100 mg
D	5 µg (200 IU)
E	10 mg (10 IU)
K	–
Thiamine (B_1)	3 mg
Riboflavin (B_2)	3.6 mg
Pyridoxine (B_6)	4 mg
Niacin (B_3)	40 mg
Biotin (B_7)	60 µg
Pantothenic acid (B_5)	15 mg
Folic acid	400 µg
B_{12}	5 µg

Doses are in µg or mg per day for IV administration in patients receiving total parenteral nutrition (TPN).

They may be conveniently obtained by adding a commercial multi-vitamin preparation to the TPN solution. The dose requirements for vitamin K vary greatly between individual patients and may be conveniently assessed by measurement of the prothrombin time, since this test is largely determined by the plasma levels of the vitamin K-dependent coagulation factors (see Vitamin K deficiency).

> Although low levels of vitamins have been found in a number of acute and chronic disease states (apart from those conditions specifically due to vitamin deficiency), the use of vitamin supplements has not generally been followed by identifiable clinical improvement in these conditions.

However, even in the absence of clinical or defined vitamin deficiency, vitamin supplementation in the community has reached epidemic proportions in response to the intensive marketing of complementary medicines by the multibillion-dollar industry in these products. A huge range of health benefits is claimed, but none has any evidence base in otherwise healthy individuals with a normal diet. The disadvantages of this practice include not only the enormous but wasted cost to consumers but also the risk of adverse effects of some vitamins when taken in excess.

See
- Beriberi,
- Folic acid deficiency,
- Hypoparathyroidism,
- Scurvy,
- Vitamin B_{12} deficiency,
- Vitamin C deficiency,
- Vitamin D deficiency,
- Vitamin K deficiency,

Bibliography

Amrein K, Oudemans-van Straaten, Berger MM. Vitamin therapy in critically ill patients: focus on thiamine, vitamin C and vitamin D. *Intens Care Med* 2018; 44: 1940.

Anderson JJB, Toverud SU. Diet and vitamin D: a review with an emphasis on human function. *J Nutr Biochem* 1994; 5: 58.

Casaer MP, Bellomo R. Micronutrient deficiency in critical illness: an invisible foe? *Intens Care Med* 2019; 45: 1136.

Chandra RK. Effect of vitamin and trace-element supplementation on immune responses and infection in elderly patients. *Lancet* 1992; 340: 1124.

DeLuca HF. Vitamin D metabolism and function. *Arch Intern Med* 1978; 138: 836.

Heyland DK, Dhaliwal R, Suchner U, et al. Antioxidant nutrients: a systematic review of trace elements and vitamins in the critically ill patient. *Intens Care Med* 2005; 31: 327.

Kennedy M. The vitamin epidemic: what is the evidence for harm or value? *Intern Med J* 2018; 40: 901.

Ordonez-Moran P, Larriba MJ, Pendas-Franco N, et al. Vitamin D and cancer: an update of in vitro and in vivo data. *Front Biosci* 2005; 10: 2723.

Shearer MJ. Vitamin K. *Lancet* 1995; 345: 229.

Shenkin A. Vitamin and essential trace element recommendations during intravenous therapy: theory and practice. *Proc Nutr Soc* 1986; 45: 383.

Thomas MK, Lloyd-Jones DM, Thadhani RI, et al. Hypovitaminosis D in medical inpatients. *N Engl J Med* 1998; 338: 777.

Vitamin B_{12} deficiency *See*

- Megaloblastic anaemia,
- Pernicious anaemia.

See also
- Dementia,
- Folic acid deficiency,
- Mouth diseases – 2. Glossitis,
- Myelopathy,
- Neuropathy – 4. Systemic disease-induced neuropathies,
- Neutropenia,
- Retrobulbar neuritis,
- Short bowel syndrome,
- Thrombocytopenia.

Bibliography

Romain M, Sviri S, Linton DM, et al. The role of vitamin B12 in the critically ill – a review. *Anaesth Intens Care* 2016; 44: 447.

Vitamin C deficiency

Vitamin C deficiency is known as scurvy (q.v.). However, a relative vitamin C deficiency (like other 'deficiencies') may be seen in critically ill patients, although normalization of its plasma levels has not been shown to confer clinical benefit. In general, vitamin C administration has not been found to confer outcome benefit either in ICU patients overall or in ICU patients after cardiac surgery.

More recently, studies have examined whether high doses of vitamin C might be helpful in the management of sepsis in the critically ill. This concept is based on the fact that vitamin C is a powerful antioxidant and is thus able to prevent reactive oxygen species generation by neutrophils. It can also increase endogenous vasopressor synthesis, provide endothelial barrier protection, enhance cellular host defences and support wound healing. This is a modern extension of the flawed concept promoted by Linus Pauling in the 1970s that mega doses of vitamin C had universal health benefits. While recent small results have suggested that high doses of vitamin C (e.g. 1.5 g IV qid) might improve the outcome of sepsis in critically ill patients, larger subsequent studies have failed to confirm this initial promise. Moreover, such doses can sometimes have adverse effects, including oxalate nephropathy (see Nephrolithiasis), hypernatraemia and haemolysis in glucose-6-phosphate dehydrogenase deficiency (q.v.).

Bibliography

Carr AC, Shaw GM, Fowler AA, et al. Ascorbate-dependent vasopressor synthesis: a rationale for vitamin C administration in severe sepsis and septic shock? *Crit Care* 2015; 19: 418.

Fuji T, Luethi N, Young PJ, et al. Effect of vitamin C, hydrocortisone, and thiamine vs hydrocortisone alone on time alive and vasopressor support among patients with septic shock: the VITAMINS randomized clinical trial. *JAMA* 2020; 323: 423.

Hooper MH, Hager DN. Understanding vitamin C in critical illness: focus on dose, route, and disease. *Crit Care Med* 2019; 47: 867.

Long CL, Maull KI, Krishnan RS, et al. Ascorbic acid dynamics in the seriously ill and injured. *J Surg Res* 2003; 109: 144.

Marik PE. Vitamin C for the treatment of sepsis: the scientific rationale. *Pharmacol Ther* 2018; 189: 63.

Marik P, Khangora V, Rivera R, et al. Hydrocortisone, vitamin C, and thiamine for the treatment of severe sepsis and septic shock: a retrospective before-after study. *Chest* 2017; 151: 1229.

McNamara R, Deane A, Anstey J, et al. Understanding the rationale for parenteral ascorbate (vitamin C) during an acute inflammatory reaction: a biochemical perspective. *Crit Care Resusc* 2018; 20: 174.

Mohammed BM, Fisher BJ, Kraskauskas D, et al. Vitamin C: a novel regulator of neutrophil extracellular trap formation. *Nutrients* 2013; 5: 3131.

Moskowitz A, Huang DT, Hou PC, et al. Effect of ascorbic acid, corticosteroids, and thiamine on organ injury in septic shock: the ACTS randomized clinical trial. *JAMA* 2020; 324: 642.

Oudemans-van Straaten HM, Elbers PW, Spoelstra-de Man AME. How to give vitamin C a cautious but fair chance in severe sepsis. *Chest* 2017; 151: 1199.

Putzu A, Daems A-M, Lopez-Delgado JC, et al. The effect of vitamin C on clinical outcome in critically ill patients: a systematic review with meta-analysis of randomized clinical trials. *Crit Care Med* 2018; 47: 774.

Yanase F, Fujii T, Naorungroj T, et al. Harm of high-dose vitaimin C therapy in adult patients: a scoping review. *Crit Care Med* 2020;

Vitamin D deficiency

Vitamin D is best known for its role in maintaining bone health. However, as a steroid hormone with pleiotropic actions (q.v.), it has been also implicated in various non-skeletal effects, including reducing the risk of cardiovascular disease, cancer, diabetes, tuberculosis (q.v.), asthma (q.v.) and cognitive decline, and in modulating immune function and the inflammatory response.

In Intensive Care practice, vitamin D is of relevance in hypercalcaemia (q.v.), which may sometimes be due to excess vitamin D from either increased dietary intake or from ectopic production by some malignancies. Conversely, vitamin D deficiency has been associated with an increased risk of sepsis and of mortality in seriously ill patients, though routine replacement therapy is not recommended due to lack of identified outcome benefit.

The major source of vitamin D is the conversion by ultraviolet light from sunlight of the precursor 7-dehydrocholesterol to colecalciferol (vitamin D_3) in the skin, provided the skin is not protected from direct sunlight by clothing, sunscreen or glass. For this purpose, an average of 15 min exposure several days a week is considered adequate, though this recommendation needs to be balanced by the need to prevent skin cancer by protection from excessive sun exposure. Detailed consensus guidelines have been recently published to assist in the understanding and management of these conflicting issues under different circumstances.

Vitamin D_3 is also present in some fish and meat, and vitamin D_2 (ergocalciferol) is found in some vegetables. Vitamin D is then converted in the liver to 25-hydroxyvitamin D (25(OH)D), which is the chief circulating form and the one measured in most laboratory assays. Further conversion occurs in the kidney with the production of 1, 25-dihydroxyvitamin D (1, 25 (OH)2D) (calcitriol), which is the active form.

Active vitamin D enhances calcium absorption from the gut, inhibits parathyroid hormone secretion and promotes bone mineralization. Calcium balance is thus co-regulated by vitamin D and parathyroid hormone.

Vitamin D deficiency is generally asymptomatic, though there can be muscle weakness and discomfort. It is confirmed by the finding of a plasma level of 25(OH)D <50 nmol/L (20 ng/mL). Levels <25 nmol/L indicate moderate to severe deficiency. Unfortunately, the substantial variability in current laboratory assays can affect the reliability with which an accurate diagnosis of vitamin D deficiency can be made.

Interestingly, high levels (i.e. >125 nmol/L) have also been associated with adverse health effects. Vitamin

D toxicity does not occur naturally (i.e. from sunlight) and is seen only with excessive doses of supplements or in malignancy (see Hypercalcaemia).

Although the normal dietary requirement of vitamin D is as little as 200 IU, treatment of deficiency requires doses at least 10-fold higher than this, together with supplemental calcium. **Colecalciferol** is available in 1000 IU capsules, which is the usually recommended daily dose for bone benefit in patients with vitamin D deficiency. Higher doses are not generally necessary, though doses up to 4000 IU per day do not cause toxicity. On the other hand, **calcitriol** can readily lead to hypercalcaemia, and it should be used only in patients with renal failure. Replenishment of body stores, in muscle and fat, can take over 3 months to achieve.

See
- Aluminium,
- Calcitonin,
- Fanconi syndrome,
- Hypercalcaemia,
- Hyperparathyroidism,
- Hypoparathyroidism.

Bibliography

Amrein K, Christopher KB, McNally JD. Understanding vitamin D deficiency in intensive care patients. *Intens Care Med* 2015; 41: 1961.

Anderson JJB, Toverud SU. Diet and vitamin D: a review with an emphasis on human function. *J Nutr Biochem* 1994; 5: 58.

Cancer Council of Australia, in conjunction with the Australasian College of Dermatologists, the Australian and New Zealand Bone and Mineral Society, the Endocrine Society of Australia and Osteoporosis Australia. Position statement: sun exposure and vitamin D – risks and benefits. 2016. http://wiki.cancer.org.au/policy/Position_statement_-_Risks_and_benefits_of_sun_exposure

DeLuca HF. Vitamin D metabolism and function. *Arch Intern Med* 1978; 138: 836.

Ginde AA, Brower RG, Caterino JM, et al. Early high-dose vitamin D3 for critically ill, vitamin D-deficient patients. *N Engl J Med* 2019; 381: 2529.

Joshi D, Center JR, Eisman JA. Vitamin D deficiency in adults. *Aust Prescriber* 2010; 33: 103.

Lai JKC, Lucas RM, Banks E, et al. Variability in vitamin D assays impairs clinical assessment of vitamin D status. *Intern Med J* 2012; 42: 43.

Lee P, Eisman JA, Center JR. Vitamin D deficiency in critically ill patients. *N Engl J Med* 2009; 360: 1912.

Moromizato T, Litonjua AA, Braun AB, et al. Association of low serum 25-hydroxyvitamin D levels and sepsis in the critically ill. *Crit Care Med* 2014; 42: 97.

Ordonez-Moran P, Larriba MJ, Pendas-Franco N, et al. Vitamin D and cancer: an update of in vitro and in vivo data. *Front Biosci* 2005; 10: 2723.

Reid IR, Bolland MJ. Controversies in medicine: the role of calcium and vitamin D supplements in adults. *Med J Aust* 2019; 211: 468.

Truswell AS. Vitamin D and tuberculosis. *Med J Aust* 2013; 199: 641.

Vitamin K deficiency

Vitamin K deficiency was initially thought to cause solely decreased plasma levels of four coagulation factors or clotting proteins, namely prothrombin (factor II) and factors VII, IX and X (see Coagulation disorders). This coagulation abnormality is most readily demonstrated by an increased prothrombin time (or INR), as during anticoagulant treatment with a vitamin K antagonist, e.g. **warfarin** (q.v.).

Although vitamin K was discovered in 1929 (and later named K for 'koagulation'), it was not until 1974 that its unique mechanism of action was elucidated, and this in turn has led to the recognition of other vitamin K–dependent proteins. When precursor proteins (PIVKA) bind to vitamin K–dependent γ-carboxylase, several glutamic acid residues (Glu) are converted to γ-carboxyglutamic acid residues (Gla). Gla residues are essential for the vitamin K–dependent proteins to form active complexes able to bind calcium and attach to phospholipids, so that in vitamin K deficiency only inactive proteins are produced.

The other vitamin K–dependent proteins discovered subsequently include
- the anticoagulant factors, **protein C** (q.v.) and **protein S** (q.v.),
- **bone Gla protein** (osteocalcin) and **matrix Gla protein** (MGP)
  - a deficiency of MGP leads to vascular calcification,
  - long-term warfarin therapy in patients with atrial fibrillation has thus been reported to be associated with increased calcification of cardiac valves, of arteriovenous fistulae and of atherosclerotic plaques, even after adjusting for confounding factors (see also Calciphylaxis),
  - these adverse 'off-target' effects are not seen following anticoagulant treatment with non–vitamin K antagonists, such as DOACs (see Anticoagulanta),
- other less well-defined proteins in lung, liver, kidney, pancreas, and placenta.

Anticoagulant-related nephropathy (ARN) has been described as an occasional complication of long-term treatment with a vitamin K antagonist, such as warfarin (q.v.), e.g. in patients with atrial fibrillation.

The action of vitamin K is manganese-dependent, so that **manganese deficiency** is in turn one of the uncommon causes of vitamin K deficiency (see Manganese).

See also
- Brodifacoum.

Bibliography
Berkner KL, Runge KW. The physiology of vitamin K nutriture and vitamin K-dependent protein function in atherosclerosis. *J Thromb Haemost* 2004; 2: 2118.
Dam H. The antihaemorrhagic vitamin of the chick: occurrence and chemical nature. *Nature* 1935; 135: 652.
Dowd P, Ham S-W, Naganathan S, et al. The mechanism of action of vitamin K. *Annu Rev Nutr* 1995; 15: 419.
Hasific S, Ovrehus KA, Gerke O, et al. Extent of arterial calcification by conventional vitamin K antagonist treatment. *PLoS ONE* 2020; 15: e0241450.
Lerner RG, Aronow WS, Sekhri A, et al. Warfarin use and the risk of valvular calcification. *J Thromb Haemost* 2009; 7: 2023.
Presnell SR, Stafford DW. The vitamin K-dependent carboxylase. *Thromb Haemost* 2002; 87: 937.
Shearer MJ. Vitamin K. *Lancet* 1995; 345: 229.
Stafford DW. The vitamin K cycle. *J Thromb Haemost* 2005; 3: 1873.
Stenflo J, Fernlund P, Egan W, et al. Vitamin K dependent modifications of glutamic acid residues in prothrombin. *Proc Natl Acad Sci* 1974; 71: 2730.
Tie J-K, Stafford DW. Structural and functional insights into enzymes of the vitamin K cycle. *J Thromb Haemost* 2016; 14: 236.
Yang Y, Liu T, Zhao J, et al. Warfarin-related nephropathy: prevalence, risk factors and prognosis. *Int J Cardiol* 2014; 176: 1297.

Vitiligo *See*

- Autoimmune disorders,
- Pigmentation disorders –1. Hypopigmentation.

Von Recklinghausen's disease *See*

- Neurofibromatosis.

Von Willebrand's disease

Von Willebrand's disease (vWD) or perhaps preferably disorder (also vWD) or syndrome (vWS) is the most common congenital coagulation abnormality. It has a heterozygous prevalence of about 1% of the population. It was first described in 1926 in Helsinki by Professor Erik von Willebrand. The disease arises because of either deficient or defective von Willebrand's factor (vWF), a plasma protein coded for by a gene on chromosome 12. Like many other coagulation abnormalities, vWD can be either congenital (most commonly) or acquired (occasionally).

Von Willebrand's factor circulates as variable multimers from 0.5–20×10^3 kDa (average 255 kDa), with a plasma concentration of 10 mcg/mL (0.04 µM) and half-life of 12 hr. Its haemostatic function is to carry and protect factor VIII:C and assist platelet adhesion by associating platelet receptors with subendothelial structures, such as collagen. VWF can effect this process because it has specific binding sites for factor VIII:C, platelet glycoprotein receptors and collagen.

Very large multimers of vWF are synthesized and stored in the endothelial cells as organelles called Weibel–Palade bodies, from where they are released both basally and in response to injury. They are also stored in the α-granules of platelets. Proteolytic cleavage of ultra-large multimers produced by the metalloprotease ADAMTS13 is required for normal haemostasis (see also Thrombotic thrombocytopenic purpura).

Recently, vWF has been found to be a multi-purpose protein, with roles beyond haemostasis extending to inflammation, angiogenesis (see Angiodysplasia), vascular permeability, cell proliferation (e.g. smooth muscle cells) and conversely in proapoptosis with limiting of tumour cell survival. Some cancers can acquire vWF expression, which may then increase their metastatic potential, perhaps via the formation of platelet-tumour aggregates.

Elevated vWF levels are associated with an increased risk of ischaemic cardiovascular events. Conversely, the presence of vWD is associated with a decrease in cardiovascular disease (of about 15%), though such protection is unlikely to explain the genetic persistence of a disease causing the adverse condition of bleeding, since the likely clinical benefit from decreased cardiovascular disease occurs after reproductive age.

Von Willebrand's disease may be classified as follows:
- **type I**, the classical type (80% of cases)

This is inherited as an autosomal dominant and is usually seen in its heterozygous form, with mild to moderate disease. It is twice as common in women as in men. There is a quantitative abnormality of vWF.
- **type II** (up to 20% of cases)

This consists of several sub-types of abnormal multimer patterns. There is normal total vWF but a qualitative abnormality. This condition may be inherited as a recessive disorder (with features similar to haemophilia – q.v.). It is also the form that may sometimes be **acquired**, for example in severe aortic stenosis or prolonged extracorporeal life support due to multimer damage from high shear stress (see also Angiodysplasia).

- **type III** (only 1% of cases)
  This is the severe and homozygous form of type I.

> Clinical features often commence only in adult life and comprise bleeding, either spontaneously or in excess after surgery or trauma. Unlike haemophilia (q.v.), the bleeding in vWD is less frequent and is most commonly mucosal.

There is commonly a spontaneous improvement during pregnancy, presumably related to the temporary elevation of the vWF level during that time.

The diagnosis is suspected from screening tests, which show a prolonged APTT, together with a normal platelet count and an increased bleeding time. The vWF quantity is measured immunologically (as vWF:Ag), and vWF function is commonly measured via impaired ristocetin-induced platelet aggregation. VWF multimer analysis is a reference standard, especially for acquired vWD, but this test is complex and time-consuming. Since vWF levels are typically elevated during the inflammatory state, vWF measurements made in Intensive Care patients may be unreliable.

*Treatment is with **cryoprecipitate**, which contains large and functionally active vWF multimers. Typically, 10 bags may be given 12 hrly until bleeding ceases.*

***DDAVP** (desmopressin – q.v.) causes release of vWF from endothelial cells and is usually given in a dose of 20 mcg IV, which may be repeated in 6 hr. DDAVP is most suitable for preoperative prophylaxis, although sometimes tachycardia, headache, flushing and water retention may result. Since DDAVP may stimulate fibrinolysis (q.v.), concomitant **tranexamic acid** (TXA, 1 g 6 hrly) (q.v.) should be used as a fibrinolytic inhibitor in those cases where local fibrinolysis may be enhanced (e.g. dental extraction).*

Aspirin should be avoided.

See also

- Coagulation disorders,
- Thrombotic thrombocytopenic purpura.

Bibliography

Bloom AL. Von Willebrand factor: clinical features of inherited and acquired disorders. *Mayo Clin Proc* 1991; 66: 743.

Lenting PJ, Casari C, Christophe OD, et al. Von Willebrand factor: the old, the new and the unknown. *J Thromb Haemost* 2012; 10: 2428.

Michiels JJ, ed. Diagnosis and management of congenital von Willebrand's disease. *Semin Thromb Hemost* 2002; 28: 109.

Mohri H. Acquired von Willebrand syndrome: features and management. *Am J Hematol* 2006; 81: 616.

Oldenburg J, Schwaab R. Molecular biology of blood coagulation. *Semin Thromb Hemost* 2001; 27: 313.

Patmore S, Dhami SPS, O'Sullivan JM. Von Willebrand factor and cancer: metastasis and coagulopathies. *J Thromb Haemost* 2020; 18: 2444.

Sadler JE, Budde U, Eikenboom JCJ, et al. Update on the pathophysiology and classification of von Willebrand disease. *J Thromb Haemost* 2006; 4: 2103.

Sadler JE, Mannucci PM, Berntorp E, et al. Impact, diagnosis and treatment of von Willebrand disease. *Thromb Haemost* 2000; 84: 160.

Seaman CD, Yabes J, Comer DM, et al. Does deficiency of von Willebrand factor protect against cardiovascular disease? Analysis of a national discharge register. *J Thromb Haemost* 2015; 13: 1999.

Veyradier A, Jenkins CSP, Fressinaud E, et al. Acquired von Willebrand syndrome: from pathophysiology to management. *Thromb Haemost* 2000; 84: 175.

Vincentelli A Susen S, Le Tourneau T, et al. Acquired von Willebrand syndrome in aortic stenosis. *N Engl J Med* 2003; 349: 343.

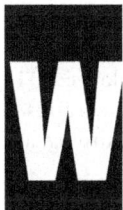

Waldenstrom's macroglobulinaemia *See*

- Multiple myeloma.

Warfare agents

Chemical **warfare agents** are substances which cause military incapacity via nausea, asphyxia, blindness, paralysis or burns. These effects may or may not be fatal. The term usually includes defoliants but not smoke. They were first used in World War I, in the form of chlorine, phosgene and mustard gas. Gas masks containing a mixture of charcoal and soda lime as absorbents were able to provide some protection. Subsequently, because of public outrage and because they usually had minimal military efficacy, these agents became banned, and though available they were not used in World War II. However, some of these agents remain stocked and have even been used in local combat in recent years. They also remain a potential concern in terrorist attacks. Tear gas continues to be widely available for civilian riot control.

The different agents may be classified as follows:

1. **Nerve agents**

These most commonly are organophosphates, related to **insecticides** (q.v.). They are thus easy to manufacture and can be possessed by 'rogue' military regimes or terrorist groups. They are potent and irreversible inhibitors of acetylcholinesterase (see Anticholinesterases), and they are lethal at about 1 mg (G agents). One of the most toxic of such compounds is sarin (isopropyl methylphosphonofluoridate).

> Nerve agents produce a cholinergic crisis (q.v.) with dramatic muscarinic and nicotinic effects.
> - The former effects predominate in milder forms of poisoning. They include 'SLUDGE' (i.e. salivation, lacrimation, urination, diarrhoea, GI cramps, emesis), as well as sweating, bronchospasm, blurred vision and bradycardia.
> - The latter effects predominate in more severe forms of poisoning. They include weakness, fasciculation, paralysis, hypertension and tachycardia.
>
> Coma and fits are seen, and death may occur from acute respiratory failure and arrest within a few minutes.
>
> Uncommon complications include a prolonged QT interval due to cardiac toxicity and acute pancreatitis.
>
> Survivors may suffer permanent neurological defects.

Laboratory investigations include measurement of plasma and especially red cell cholinesterase, as well as the non-specific screening tests of biochemistry and haematology usually undertaken in any seriously ill patient.

Urgent respiratory support is required with intubation and mechanical ventilation to prevent immediate death from respiratory failure.

Specific treatment to reverse the muscarinic effects is with **atropine** *in large doses, i.e. 2–6 mg IV and up to 15 mg in the first 30 min. Dosage should be doubled every 5–10 min until muscarinic symptoms are relieved. A continuous IV infusion of 6 mg/hr may be used for maintenance, since in severe cases prolonged treatment may be required, with hundreds of mg given over days or even weeks.*

The most effective antidote to reverse the nicotinic and central nervous system effects is an oxime, such as **pralidoxime**, *which complexes with the agent and thus removes it from acetylcholinesterase (see Anticholinergic agents). It should be given promptly and is used in a dose of 1–2 g IV in 100 mL saline over 15 min. If there is continued absorption or if muscle weakness persists, the dose may be repeated once or twice hrly or a continuous IV infusion of 0.5 g/hr given for 24 hr or more.*

Diazepam *up to 10 mg IV may be concomitantly useful, especially for fits.*

Pyridostigmine *is paradoxically effective as a prophylactic agent, because it binds reversibly to cholinesterase and thus protects it.*

Contaminated clothing must be removed, the skin and hair cleansed, and staff protected from accidental exposure via the patient.

Intensive Care monitoring is generally required for 1–2 weeks, and it may take some weeks for complete regeneration of the body's cholinesterases. The average mortality of organophosphate poisoning in general is 25%.

2. **Mustards**

These act as vesicants.

They are chiefly treated locally and **symptomatically**, *though IV fluids and possibly sodium thiosulphate (see Cyanide) may be useful.*

3. **Lewisite**

This is a vesicant arsenical.

It requires treatment as for the mustards, with the addition of **BAL** *parenterally (q.v.) and also as an eye ointment.*

4. **Phosgene**

This is carbonyl chloride, a colourless but reactive and toxic gas with a smell of musty hay. It is denser than air and becomes a liquid at 8°C. Carbonyl is a polar chemical unit of carbon and oxygen and is a reactive constituent in many organic compounds, including aldehydes, ketones, esters, amides, quinones and carboxylic acids. Phosgene is thus widely used industrially in chemical processes. It was first prepared in 1811 from carbon monoxide and chlorine, but it dissolves in water to give carbon dioxide and hydrochloric acid. It is thus a potent respiratory irritant with a progressive effect over several hours (see Acute lung irritation).

Its effects are treated **symptomatically** *and with intravenous and inhaled* **corticosteroids**.

5. **Cyanide** (q.v.)

6. **Incapacitating agents**

These are usually anticholinergics (q.v.).

*They are treated with **physostigmine**.*
7. **Local irritants and nauseants**

These include tear gas and pepper (capsicum) spray. They require no specific treatment and spontaneous recovery occurs.

See also
- Germ warfare.

Bibliography

Bardin PG, Van Eeden SF, Moolman JA, et al. Organophosphate and carbamate poisoning. *Ann Intern Med* 1994; 154: 1433.

Dunn MA, Sidell FR. Progress in medical defense against nerve agents. *JAMA* 1989; 262: 649.

Eddleston M, Szinicz L, Eyer P, et al. Oximes in acute organophosphorus pesticide poisoning: a systematic review of clinical trials. *Quart J Med* 2002; 95: 275.

Emad A, Rezaian GR. The diversity of the effects of sulfur mustard gas inhalation on respiratory system 10 years after a single heavy exposure. *Chest* 1997; 112: 734.

Kvetan V, Farmer JC, et al., eds. Critical care medicine for disasters, terrorism, and military conflict. Crit Care Med 2005; 33 (1, suppl.).

Leikin JB, Thomas RG, Walter FG, et al. A review of nerve agents for the critical care physician. *Crit Care Med* 2002; 30: 2346.

Marrs TC. Organophosphate poisoning. *Pharmacol Ther* 1993; 58: 51.

Mokhlesi B, Leikin JB, Murray P, et al. Adult toxicology in critical care: part II: specific poisonings. *Chest* 2003; 123: 897.

Nozaki H, Aikawa N, Shinozawa Y, et al. Sarin poisoning in Tokyo subway. *Lancet* 1995; 345: 980.

Rickett DL, Glenn JF, Houston WE. Medical defense against nerve agents: new directions. *Milit Med* 1987; 152: 35.

Sidell FR, Borak J. Chemical warfare agents. *Ann Emerg Med* 1992; 21: 865.

Smythies J. Nerve gas antidotes. *J R Soc Med* 2004; 97: 32.

Tafuri J, Roberts J. Organophosphate poisoning. *Ann Emerg Med* 1987; 16: 193.

Vedder EB. *The Medical Aspects of Chemical Warfare*. Baltimore: Williams & Wilkins. 1925.

Zimmerman JL. Poisonings and overdoses in the intensive care unit: general and specific management issues. *Crit Care Med* 2003; 31: 2794.

Warfarin

Warfarin, a vitamin K antagonist (VKA), is the classic oral anticoagulant. For decades, it has been an effective and cheap agent for the long-term prevention of arterial and venous thromboembolic disease.

The coumarins were discovered by Link in 1933, and warfarin was found to be the best coumarin for use as a rodenticide in 1944. It was named after the Wisconsin Alumni Research Foundation in 1948 and marketed initially as a rat poison. In 1954, it was commercialized for clinical use, and together with heparin it became part of the standard therapeutic regimen for the anticoagulant management of venous thromboembolism over succeeding decades.

It has a narrow therapeutic window, necessitating close laboratory monitoring, typically using an international normalized ratio (INR) of 2–3. The INR is a version of the classic prothrombin time, which takes account of variation in test reagents in different laboratories.

Because of the need for laboratory monitoring and because of its multiple drug interactions, warfarin is being progressively replaced in many settings by the newer direct-acting oral anticoagulants (DOACs), which are safer, more effective and simpler to manage.

See
- Anticoagulants,
- Brodifacoum,
- Calciphylaxis,
- Protein C,
- Prothrombin complex concentrate,
- Skin necrosis,
- Vitamin K deficiency.

Wasp stings *See*
- Bites and stings.

Water-related accidents *See*
- Bathing,
- Diving,
- Drowning.

Waterhouse–Friderichsen syndrome

The **Waterhouse–Friderichsen syndrome** refers to acute fulminant meningococcaemia with resultant shock.

> This form of severe sepsis is seen in about 10% of cases of meningococcaemia and presents as typical endotoxaemia.
> It is commonly complicated by
> - myocarditis,
> - disseminated intravascular coagulation (q.v.),
> - acute adrenal failure (see Adrenal insufficiency), due to haemorrhage,
> - acute oliguric renal failure,
> - acute respiratory distress syndrome (q.v.).

Although typically caused by meningococcaemia, it is not distinguishable from similar conditions caused by other Gram-negative bacteria (including *Haemophilus influenzae* type b in children) and also by *Streptococcus pneumoniae* in asplenic patients.

Treatment is with **resuscitation** and supportive therapy, high-dose parenteral **antibiotics, corticosteroids** and possibly **heparin** if disseminated intravascular coagulation (DIC) is severe. **Plasmapheresis** (q.v.) has been reported to be helpful.

Recombinant human activated protein C (drotrecogin alfa) was reported to decrease mortality significantly in severe sepsis in general and in this condition in particular (see Protein C), but it was later withdrawn from the market since its early promise was not replicated in later studies. Previously, encouraging initial results from the use of **monoclonal antibodies to endotoxin** also failed to be confirmed in later studies, so that this product too was withdrawn from the market.

Prevention is important for contacts and for patients at risk. Although there is a high mortality, there are usually no long-term sequelae for survivors.

Bibliography

Hamilton D, Harris MD, Foweraker J, et al. Waterhouse–Friderichsen syndrome as a result of non-meningococcal infection. *J Clin Pathol* 2004; 57: 208.

Vella A, Nippoldt TB, Morris JC. Adrenal hemorrhage: a 25-year experience at the Mayo Clinic. *Mayo Clin Proc* 2001; 76: 161.

WDHA syndrome See

- Diarrhoea.

Wegener's granulomatosis

Wegener's (Wegener) granulomatosis is the most common form of pulmonary vasculitis. It consists of a necrotizing granulomatous vasculitis of the upper respiratory tract (nose, sinuses), lungs and kidneys. A limited form may affect the lungs only. See Vasculitis.

Consideration has recently been given to renaming this condition without any eponymous recognition because of Dr Wegener's strong Nazi affiliations before and during World War II. Revised names such as 'granulomatous vasculitis', 'ANCA-positive vasculitis' and 'granulomatosis with polyangiitis (GPA)' have been suggested, and '**necrotizing granulomatous vasculitis**' (NGV) has become extensively adopted.

The aetiology is unknown, but the pathogenesis appears immunological since it is associated with the presence of a specific antibody. Epidemiologically, there appears to be an increased predisposition at higher latitudes.

The patient may be of either sex and any age but is most typically a middle-aged man. Clinical features are very variable, but they commonly comprise cough, pleuritic pain and haemoptysis (q.v.). Upper respiratory tract involvement is manifest by rhinorrhoea, ulcers, pain and purulent drainage.

There may be symptoms of multiorgan involvement, especially affecting the kidneys, but also the skin, joints and eyes.

Blood examination typically shows anaemia (q.v.), leukocytosis, thrombocytosis (q.v.) and raised ESR.

Serology is positive for rheumatoid factor but not antinuclear antibodies (q.v.). The presence of antineutrophil cytoplasmic autoantibodies (ANCAs) is nearly 100% specific and about 70% sensitive for the condition. The particular ANCA in Wegener's granulomatosis is directed against cytoplasmic proteinase-3, which is present in the lysosomes of neutrophils and monocytes. This autoantibody is therefore called c-ANCA or anti-PR3. BAL is also positive for ANCA and generally has about 50% neutrophils and a few eosinophils.

Some other vasculitides are also ANCA-associated, e.g. Churg–Strauss syndrome (q.v.), microscopic polyangiitis (see Vasculitis) and renal limited vasculitis. However, these conditions are generally positive for p-ANCA, i.e. the antigenic target is myeloperoxidase, MPO, which is perinuclear.

If the serological diagnosis is uncertain, histological confirmation should be sought.

The chest X-ray shows single or multiple densities of varying size, often with cavitation (q.v.), but sometimes there is a more general infiltration (see Pulmonary infiltrates).

The condition is often initially misdiagnosed as pulmonary malignancy, but histological examination establishes the diagnosis.

Treatment has traditionally been with the dual immunosuppressive agents **corticosteroids** and **cytotoxics** (formerly cyclophosphamide, currently azathioprine or methotrexate). The new immunosuppressive agent, **rituximab** (q.v.), appears to offer additional benefit, both for induction and for relapse (and possibly for maintenance). However, the use of **TNF-α blockers** (e.g. etanercept), while effective in some refractory cases, may be followed by an increased risk of malignancy.

The illness is fatal within 1 year if untreated, but long-term remission is now usual with treatment.

Variants of Wegener's granulomatosis probably include the following:

1. **Lymphomatoid granulomatosis** is an uncommon condition with histological features resembling both Wegener's granulomatosis and lymphoma. There is a pulmonary infiltrate which is angiocentric, destructive and lymphoreticular, with atypical cells showing mitoses. Similar lesions may be found in other organs, especially the skin and sometimes the mouth.

   Respiratory symptoms include cough, sputum and dyspnoea.

   The chest X-ray shows bilateral infiltrates, rounded lesions similar to metastases and cavitation (q.v.).

   *No consistently effective treatment is available, although combined **corticosteroid** and **cytotoxic** therapy is usually given.*

   There is a high mortality, often with progression to malignant lymphoma.

2. **Bronchocentric granulomatosis** is a destructive condition similar to Wegener's granulomatosis, except that the lesions are centred on bronchi and not on blood vessels. The distinction is important because its prognosis is much better.

   Many patients have asthma (q.v.), eosinophilia (q.v.), mucus plugs and hypersensitivity to *Aspergillus fumigatus* (see Aspergillosis). In these patients, the condition may represent a variant of 'mucoid impaction'. See Eosinophilia and lung infiltration.

   See
   - Interstitial lung diseases.

Bibliography

Aries PM, Lamprecht P, Gross WL. Biological therapies: new treatment options for ANCA-associated vasculitis? *Expert Opin Biol Ther* 2007; 7: 521.

Beaty MW, Toro J, Sorbara L, et al. Cutaneous lymphomatoid granulomatosis: correlation of clinical and biological features. *Am J Surg Pathol* 2001; 25: 1111.

Cordier JF, Valeyre D, Gullevin L, et al. Pulmonary Wegener's granulomatosis. *Chest* 1990; 97: 906.

European Vasculitis Study Group. A mulicenter randomized trial of cyclophosphamide versus azathioprine during remission in ANCA-associated systemic vasculitis. *Arthritis Rheum* 1999; 42 (suppl.): 225.

Falk RJ, Jennett JC. Wegener's granulomatosis, systemic vasculitis, and antineutrophil cytoplasmic autoantibodies. *Annu Rev Med* 1991; 42: 459.

Fauci AS, Haynes BF, Costa J, et al. Lymphomatoid granulomatosis. *N Engl J Med* 1982; 306: 68.

Frankel SK, Cosgrove GP, Fischer A, et al. Update in the diagnosis and management of pulmonary vasculitis. *Chest* 2006; 129: 452.

Gatenby PA. Anti-neutrophil cytoplasmic antibody-associated systemic vasculitis: nature or nurture? *Intern Med J* 2012; 42: 351.

Gomez-Puerta JA, Hernandez-Rodriguez J, Lopez-Soto A, et al. Antineutrophil cytoplasmic antibody-associated vasculitides and respiratory disease. *Chest* 2009; 136: 1101.

Hagen EC, Ballieux BEPB, van Es LA, et al. Antineutrophil cytoplasmic autoantibodies: a review of the antigens involved, the assays, and the clinical and possible pathogenetic consequences. *Blood* 1993; 81: 1996.

Hoffman G. Treatment of Wegener's granulomatosis: time to change the standard of care? *Arthritis Rheum* 1997; 40: 2099.

Hoffman GS, Specks U. Antineutrophil cytoplasmic antibodies. *Arthritis Rheum* 1998; 41: 1521.

Kallenberg C, Brouwer E, Weening J, et al. Anti-neutrophil cytoplasmic antibodies: current diagnostic and pathophysiological potential. *Kidney Int* 1994; 46: 1.

Ricketti AJ, Greenberger PA, Mintzer RA, et al. Allergic bronchopulmonary aspergillosis. *Arch Intern Med* 1983; 143: 1553.

Rosen MJ. Dr Friedrich Wegener and the ACCP, revisited. *Chest* 2007; 132: 1723.

Salama AD. Pathogenesis and treatment of ANCA-associated systemic vasculitis. *J R Soc Med* 1999; 92: 456.

Schuyler MR. Allergic bronchopulmonary aspergillosis. *Clin Chest Med* 1983; 4: 15.

Weil's disease *See*

- Leptospirosis.

Wernicke–Korsakoff syndrome

Wernicke–Korsakoff syndrome is the name given to the encephalopathy (q.v.) caused by thiamine deficiency (q.v.). It is seen in

- alcoholism,
- hyperemesis gravidarum,
- malnutrition,
- starvation,
- AIDS (q.v.).

The **Wernicke** component comprises
- acute delirium (q.v.),
- with associated ophthalmoplegia (q.v.), nystagmus and ataxia.

> The typical pathological changes in the brainstem, especially in the mamillary bodies, are best demonstrated by MRI. There may also be hypothalamic involvement, and associated polyneuropathy (q.v.) is common.
>
> *Although early treatment with **thiamine** 100 mg IV per day results in rapid improvement of the ophthalmoplegia (within 2 days) and subsequent improvement in the encephalopathy (within 2 weeks), some neurological deficits commonly remain.*
>
> *Glucose should not be administered without concomitant thiamine.*
>
> The **Korsakoff** component of the syndrome refers to a state of chronic and usually permanent dementia (q.v.).

Bibliography

Doherty MJ, Watson NF, Uchino K, et al. Diffusion abnormalities in patients with Wernicke encephalopathy. *Neurology* 2002; 58: 655.

Harper CG, Giles M, Finlay-Jones R. Clinical signs in the Wernicke-Korsakoff complex. *J Neurol Neurosurg Psychiatry* 1986; 49: 341.

Kopelman MD. The Korsakoff syndrome. *Br J Psychiatry* 1995; 166: 154.

Latt N, Dore G. Thiamine in the treatment of Wernicke encephalopathy in patients with alcohol use disorders. *Intern Med J* 2014; 44: 911.

Reuler JB, Girard DE, Cooney TG. Wernicke's encephalopathy. *N Engl J Med* 1985; 312: 1035.

West Nile virus encephalitis

West Nile virus (WNV) **encephalitis** was originally reported in 1937 in Uganda, and it has since spread throughout Africa, the Middle East, Europe and North America. In other countries, it may be seen in travellers. The responsible arbovirus is mosquito-borne, and its natural reservoir is wild birds. It is thus a zoonosis (q.v.). A closely related virus, Kunjin virus, is endemic in Northern Australia.

Its incubation period varies from 2 to 14 days. It has been estimated that 80% of infections with WNV are asymptomatic.

Clinical features in most patients comprise a nonspecific and self-limited febrile illness, with headache, myalgia and sometimes diarrhoea (q.v.). In 1% of patients, there are neurological complications, which may include encephalitis (q.v.), personality change, flaccid paralysis resembling Guillain–Barré disease (q.v.), seizures and focal deficits.

Diagnosis is made serologically.

Treatment is supportive, though a number of new therapies (such as new antiviral agents and monoclonal antibodies) are being studied. Mosquito control is the most important preventative measure.

In severe disease, the mortality is about 5%.

See
- Encephalitis,
- Mosquitoes,
- Zoonoses.

Bibliography

Campbell GL, Marfin AA, Lanciotti RS, et al. West Nile virus. *Lancet Infect Dis* 2002; 2: 519.

Hayes EB, Sejvar JJ, Zaki SR, et al. Virology, pathology and clinical manifestations of West Nile virus disease. *Emerg Infect Dis* 2005; 11: 1174

Solomon T, Ooi MH, Beasley DW, et al. West Nile encephalitis. *BMJ* 2003; 326: 865.

Whipple's disease

Whipple's disease is a rare systemic disorder due to infection with a Gram-positive actinomycete-like bacillus, *Tropheryma whippelii*. While it chiefly affects the small bowel, arthritis (q.v.) is also common, as in inflammatory bowel disease (q.v.). Although the organism is common in the environment, clinical infection has a prevalence of only about 1 per million of the population.

Clinical features are seen mainly in men and comprise fever (q.v.), weakness, weight loss, malabsorption (q.v.) and increased pigmentation (q.v.). Seronegative spondyloarthropathy (q.v.) and lymphadenopathy (q.v.) resembling sarcoidosis (q.v.) are common. There may also be digital clubbing, aortic and mitral valve disease and a slow dementia (q.v.), manifest by confusion and loss of memory. The patient is typically anergic.

PCR identification of the specific organism provides definitive diagnosis. The diagnosis may have been suggested by the finding of lymphadenopathy (q.v.) on abdominal CT scan.

*Treatment is with a prolonged course of **antibiotics**, initially ceftriaxone for 2–4 weeks, followed by cotrimoxazole for 12 months. The organism is also sensitive to penicillin, amoxicillin and tetracycline. For neurological involvement, **corticosteroids** are added to the antibiotic regimen.*

Whipple's disease can be fatal if untreated, but antibiotic treatment now produces long remissions, though about a quarter of the cases may later relapse.

See also other actinomycete infections
- Actinomycosis,
- Nocardiosis.

Bibliography
Relman DA, Schmidt TM, MacDermott RP, et al. Identification of the uncultured bacillus of Whipple's disease. *N Engl J Med* 1992; 327: 293.
Swartz MN. Whipple's disease: past, present and future. *N Engl J Med* 2000; 342: 648.

Whipple's triad *See*
- Islet cell tumour.

Wilson's disease *See*
- Copper.

Women's health *See*
- Obstetrics and gynaecology.

Woolsorter's disease *See*
- Anthrax.

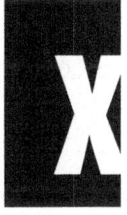

X-linked disorders

X-linked disorders are uncommon genetic conditions where the affected gene in on the X chromosome. They are therefore recessive disorders which affect predominantly hemizygotic men, whereas heterozygous women are carriers. However, women can sometimes have significant clinical disease due either to random X inactivation in different cells called lyonization (i.e. explained by the Lyon–Beutler hypothesis) or to rare inheritance of an affected X chromosome from both parents.

X-linked disorders of relevance to Intensive Care include
- Fabry's disease (q.v.),
- glucose-6-phosphate dehydrogenase deficiency (q.v.),
- haemophilia (q.v.), both A and B,
- some immunodeficiencies (see Agammaglobulinaemia, see Immunodeficiency),
- some muscular dystrophies (q.v.), specifically Duchenne's muscular dystrophy,
- some sideroblastic anaemias (q.v.), specifically hereditary benign sideroblastic anaemia.

Bibliography
Callego C, Korf BR. Practice of genetics in clinical medicine. In: *Scientific American Medicine. Human Genetics*. Hamilton: Decker Medicine. 2021.

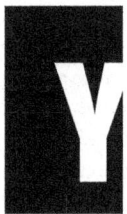

Yellow fever

Yellow fever is one of the viral zoonoses (q.v.). It is caused by a group B arbovirus or flavivirus, which is morphologically indistinguishable from other members of the togavirus family which cause encephalitis (q.v.) in the Americas. The disease occurs mainly in Central and South America and in sub-Saharan Africa. Typically, there is a tropical reservoir in monkeys and a mosquito vector (*Aedes aegypti*), though in urban areas the reservoir is in humans.

Epidemics of yellow fever were a recurrent scourge of armies and cities in the Americas in the eighteenth and nineteenth centuries, when tens of thousands of infected people could die on each occasion. At the time, the cause was attributed to miasmas or air-borne emanation from rotting or decayed matter. Eventually, in 1881, the responsible vector was identified, following which preventative measures became possible with quarantine, vector control and finally immunization.

After an average incubation period of 3–6 days (and possibly up to 16 days), there are non-specific symptoms of fever (q.v.), malaise, weakness, nausea, vomiting and back pain. The patient is highly infectious during this time.

These clinical features subside after 1–7 days. The patient then appears well for up to a day or so, only to relapse with
- jaundice, due to acute fulminant hepatitis (q.v.),
- shock,

- renal failure,
- coma,
- generalized bleeding tendency, due to disseminated intravascular coagulation (q.v.).

Diagnosis is made by viral isolation or serologically. A PCR method is available. Characteristic inclusion (Councilman) bodies and midzonal necrosis are seen on liver histology, usually, however, examined only postmortem.

Treatment is **supportive**, though early **ribavirin** administration has appeared promising in experimental studies.

The disease is best controlled by vector elimination. **Immunization** is available and is highly effective. In 2016, the WHO sponsored a major vaccination campaign to improve yellow fever control in Africa. However, the vaccine is in generally short supply, so that it is mainly reserved for travellers. Rarely, the live attenuated vaccine may lead to severe infection, particularly in the elderly.

The average mortality is 5% in endemic cases but about 40% in epidemics and 50% in severe cases. In those who survive, there is a prolonged convalescence (see Chronic fatigue syndrome).

Bibliography
Monath TP. Yellow fever: a medically neglected disease. *Rev Infect Dis* 1987; 9: 165.
Robertson SE, Hull BP, Tomori O, et al. Yellow fever: a decade of reemergence. *JAMA* 1996; 276: 1157.

Yellow nail syndrome See
- Nails.

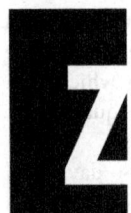

Zika virus infection

Zika virus infection was originally identified in Africa (in the Zika forest area of Uganda in 1947). It later spread progressively eastwards to South-East Asia, the Pacific and eventually to South and Central America, finally involving a complete worldwide equatorial belt. The Zika virus is mosquito-borne and is similar to the dengue virus (q.v.). It may also be transmitted by sexual contact.

It causes a flu-like illness, with fever (q.v.), headache, rash and arthralgia (q.v.), although asymptomatic infection is more common. Importantly, it has been associated with an increasing spectrum of birth defects, particularly microcephaly, hence the attention directed to it by the WHO. It has also been implicated in cases of Guillain–Barré syndrome (q.v.).

Specific diagnosis is made by serology. PCR in blood and urine should be added if exposure has been within the past month. Specific diagnosis is particularly recommended after exposure during pregnancy.

Treatment is symptomatic, and hospitalization is rarely required.

The outcome is almost always favourable. No vaccine is as yet available, and the enthusiasm for the development of a vaccine has been tempered by the theoretical possibility that, like the virus itself, it could cause an autoimmune complication (such as Guillain–Barré syndrome).

Bibliography
Haug CJ, Kieny MP, Murgue B. The Zika challenge. *N Engl J Med* 2016; 374: 1801.
Ong CW. Zika virus: an emerging infectious threat. *Intern Med J* 2016; 46: 525.
Petersen LR, Jamieson DJ, Powers AM, et al. Zika virus. *N Engl J Med* 2016; 374: 1552.

Zinc

Zinc (Zn, atomic number 30, atomic weight 65) is a metal with a low melting point and related to cadmium (q.v.) and mercury (q.v.). It has been a widely used metal since antiquity, primarily as an alloy, and it was first isolated as a separate substance in India in the thirteenth century.

Zinc is essential for many forms of life. It is present in carbonic anhydrase (and thus in high concentration in red blood cells) and in a number of gastrointestinal enzymes. It takes the place of iron in snails' blood. In addition to its presence in many enzymes, it is also needed for growth and tissue repair. It is thus an essential trace element (q.v.).

Zinc is also a cofactor in the toxic metalloproteinases present in the venom of some snakes, such as vipers. Thus, a chelate such as DMPS may bind to the zinc component and neutralize the venom, providing simple oral treatment in the field (see Bites and stings, see Chelating agents).

The usual dietary sources are meat and seafood, and deficient zinc intake is therefore common in situations of protein malnutrition. The normal daily requirement is

2.5–4 mg orally, and the recommended IV dose is 50–100 μmol per day. These doses should be increased if there are excessive gastrointestinal losses.

> Marked losses can occur in serious illness, especially from gastrointestinal fistulae. Significant and prolonged negative zinc balance occurs in the first week after major injury.
>
> The most obvious clinical feature of zinc deficiency is an eczematous rash, especially of the nasolabial folds on the face, but also in the perineum and on the extensor surfaces.
>
> Alopecia (q.v.), diarrhoea (q.v.), ileus, tremor, apathy and depression can also be produced.

Zinc overdose has been reported to cause nausea, vomiting, hypothermia (q.v.), hypotension, pulmonary oedema, oliguria, jaundice, coma and raised serum amylase.

Zinc chloride inhalation following exposure to a military smoke bomb may give rise to parenchymal lung damage.

Bibliography
Barceloux DG. Zinc. *J Toxicol Clin Toxicol* 1999; 37: 279.
Berger MM, Cavadini C, Chiolero R, et al. Copper, selenium and zinc status and balances after major trauma. *J Trauma* 1996; 40: 103.
McClain C, Soutor C, Zieve L. Zinc deficiency: a complication of Crohn's disease. *Gastroenterology* 1980; 78: 272.
Prasad AS. Clinical spectrum and diagnostic aspects of human zinc deficiency. In: Prasad AS, ed. *Essential and Toxic Trace Elements in Human Health and Disease*. New York: Liss. 1988, p 3.

Zollinger–Ellison syndrome

The **Zollinger–Ellison syndrome** refers to the condition of refractory, painful and often multiple peptic ulceration and diarrhoea (q.v.) associated with a gastrinoma or gastrin-secreting tumour.

The tumour arises either in the duodenal wall or more particularly in the pancreas, with about 25% of cases having other additional endocrine tumours. These include especially pancreatic insulinoma, but also adrenal, parathyroid and thyroid adenomas and pituitary chromophobe adenoma (see Multiple endocrine neoplasia). Two thirds of cases are malignant.

The diagnosis is based on increased basal gastric acid secretion (>15 mmol/hr) and increased fasting serum gastrin, which is always >200 ng/L and often up to 1000 ng/L, though similar levels can also be seen in renal failure or after omeprazole.

> The serum bicarbonate is typically high, often >40 mmol/L.

Since the tumour is often small, it can be difficult to locate even with sophisticated imaging.

Treatment is with **resection** *if possible, though the tumour cannot be located in 25% of cases or has metastasized in 50% of cases.*

Medical treatment is either with a high dose of H_2 ***antagonist*** *or preferably with a* **protein pump inhibitor** *if the tumour cannot be resected.*

See
- Diarrhoea – 2. Secretory diarrhoea.

Bibliography
Wolfe MM, Jensen RT. Zollinger-Ellison syndrome: current concepts in diagnosis and management. *N Engl J Med* 1987; 317: 1200.

Zoonoses

Zoonoses are animal infections which are incidentally transmitted to humans, either directly or via a vector (usually a blood-sucking arthropod – q.v.). It has been calculated that over 60% of the infectious pathogens involved in human disease originated previously in animals, although only those infections that currently involve animal reservoirs are currently considered zoonotic. The frequency of zoonoses probably escalated with the beginning of animal husbandry some 15,000 years ago, and it may now be increasing further because of climate change, deforestation and human encroachment on traditional wild animal habitat. However, potential animal sources of human disease may include domesticated, zoo and livestock animals as well as wildlife.

The quantification of the propensity of animal viruses to jump to humans has been the subject of the SpillOver project, in which a variety of risk factors pertaining to the virus, the host and the environment are calculated to obtain a total score. Interestingly, viruses which are insect-borne or derived from domesticated animals are not included in this platform. The highest scores are seen with the Influenza virus, Lassa virus, SARS-CoV-2 and Ebola virus, in that order (see these separate conditions).

Zoonoses can be caused by the transmission of viral, bacterial, fungal, parasitic or unclassified pathogens.

Viral zoonoses are generally the most troublesome of the zoonoses, as they can be severe and effectively untreatable. Fortunately, most animal viruses rarely spread to humans, but those that do so typically produce an entirely different disease in humans from that seen in the original animal reservoir. While the human disease may be asymptomatic or perhaps non-specific, the most serious presentations are encephalitis (q.v.), haemorrhagic fever (q.v.), or rash and arthralgia (q.v.). Most infected humans are dead-end hosts, as they do not then contribute to ongoing transmission (except for dengue, yellow fever and coronavirus infections).

The best-known examples of viral zoonoses are
- chikungunya (q.v.),
- coronavirus infections
    - COVID-19 (q.v.), in its initial transmission,
    - Middle East respiratory syndrome (MERS) (q.v.),
    - severe acute respiratory syndrome (SARS) (q.v.), in its initial transmission,
- dengue (q.v.),
- Hantavirus (q.v.),
- Hendra virus (q.v.),
- influenza (q.v.), namely, avian and swine variants,
- Japanese encephalitis,
- Lassa fever (q.v.),
- lyssavirus (q.v.),
- Murray Valley encephalitis (q.v.),
- rabies (q.v.),
- Ross River virus disease (q.v.),
- viral haemorrhagic fevers (including possibly Ebola fever) (q.v.),
- West Nile viral encephalitis (q.v.),
- yellow fever (q.v.).

Bacterial zoonoses include
- anthrax (q.v.),
- brucellosis (q.v.),
- *C. difficile* infection (see Colitis – 3. Antibiotic-associated colitis),
- food poisoning (q.v.) of some types,
- leptospirosis (q.v.),
- Lyme disease (q.v.),
- melioidosis (q.v.),
- psittacosis (q.v.),
- plague (q.v.),
- rickettsial diseases (q.v.).

Fungal zoonoses include
- cryptococcosis (q.v.),
- histoplasmosis (q.v.).

Parasitic zoonoses include
- echinococcosis (q.v.),
- giardiasis possibly (see Diarrhoea – 3. Exudative diarrhoea),
- infections with helminths (q.v.) (and see Parasitic infections),
- toxoplasmosis (q.v.).

Unclassified zoonoses include
- Creutzfeldt–Jacob disease (q.v.), which is due to a transmissible particle called a prion.

On the other hand, some human infections may be transmitted to animals (particularly primates), and this reverse zoonosis is referred to as **anthroponosis**. Such infections include
- hepatitis (q.v.),
- influenza (q.v.),
- leishmaniasis,
- measles,
- poliomyelitis (q.v.),
- tuberculosis (q.v.).

Bibliography

Meslin F-X. Global aspects of emerging and potential zoonoses: a WHO perspective. *Emerg Infect Dis* 1997; 3: 2.

Morse S, Mazet J, Woolhouse M, et al. Prediction and prevention of the next pandemic zoonosis. *Lancet* 2012; 380: 1956.

Petersen LR, Gubler DJ, Kuritzkes DR. Viral zoonoses. In: *Scientific American Medicine. Infectious Diseases*. Hamilton: Dekker Medicine. 2020.

Quammen D. *Spillover: Animal Infections and the Next Human Pandemic*. New York: Norton. 2012.

Zoster *See*
- Varicella-zoster.

Made in the USA
Monee, IL
03 May 2026

49437536R00289